Hale's
Medications & Mothers' Milk™

2021

A Manual of Lactational Pharmacology

Hale's
Medications & Mothers' Milk™
2021
A Manual of Lactational Pharmacology

19th Edition

Thomas W. Hale, R.Ph., Ph.D.

University Distinguished Professor

InfantRisk Center

Department of Pediatrics

Texas Tech University

School of Medicine

Amarillo, Texas

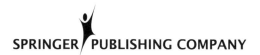

SPRINGER PUBLISHING COMPANY

Springer Publishing Company, LLC
11 West 42nd Street, New York, NY 10036
www.springerpub.com
connect.springerpub.com

Acquisitions Editor: Elizabeth Nieginski
Compositor: diacriTech

ISBN: 978-0-8261-8925-7
ebook ISBN: 978-0-8261-8926-4
DOI: 10.1891/9780826189264

21 22 23 / 5 4 3

The information contained in this publication is intended to supplement the knowledge of healthcare professionals regarding drug use during lactation. This information is advisory only and is not intended to replace sound clinical judgment or individualized patient care. The author disclaims all warranties, whether expressed or implied, of this information for any particular purpose.

The author and the publisher of this Work have made every effort to use sources believed to be reliable to provide information that is accurate and compatible with the standards generally accepted at the time of publication. Because medical science is continually advancing, our knowledge base continues to expand. Therefore, as new information becomes available, changes in procedures become necessary. We recommend that the reader always consult current research and specific institutional policies before performing any clinical procedure or delivering any medication. The author and publisher shall not be liable for any special, consequential, or exemplary damages resulting, in whole or in part, from the readers' use of, or reliance on, the information contained in this book. The publisher has no responsibility for the persistence or accuracy of URLs for external or third-party Internet websites referred to in this publication and does not guarantee that any content on such websites is, or will remain, accurate or appropriate.

Library of Congress Control Number: 2020913241

Publisher's Note: New and used products purchased from third-party sellers are not guaranteed for quality, authenticity, or access to any included digital components.

50356
Printed in the United States of America.

CONTENTS

CHANGES TO THIS EDITION

It seems the release of new drugs continues to increase each year, although the data published on breastfeeding mothers are still minimal. This new 2021 edition has many significant updates including the following:

New Drugs Added: 50

Drugs Updated With New Data: 356

Drugs With Updated LRC: 9

Drugs Updated Due to New Study/Research/Reference: 92

Drugs Updated Due to FDA Updates: 5

Drug References Updated: 817

Each year there are so many new FDA-approved medications that it is difficult to choose which to add. As usual, I chose those that a breastfeeding mother would most likely use. My laboratories have been publishing many new breastfeeding drug studies, and I have also added all of these new studies. I have added a number of infectious diseases and updated the old ones with current information.

I've added 50 new drugs, even though we don't know if and to what degree they transfer into human milk. As usual, I try to evaluate the relative risk of each drug and provided a lactation risk category.

Each year more than 3 million mothers visit the InfantRisk Center website seeking information about drugs and pregnancy and breastfeeding. So many breastfeeding mothers have volunteered for our drug studies that we simply cannot collect from all of them. But from these wonderful volunteers come the many new studies from my laboratories.

Thanks to all the lactation consultants and healthcare professionals that have helped us recruit patients for our studies. We will continue to pour out new studies that help moms continue breastfeeding their wonderful infants.

Thomas W. Hale

PREFACE

It is now well known that human milk is the best nutrition for infants. The benefits are simply enormous and supported by a world of excellent literature. However, the use of medications in breastfeeding mothers is often controversial and is steeped with misinformation in the healthcare field. This book has, for many years, been the primary source for drug information for breastfeeding mothers. The truth is, most drugs simply don't enter milk in levels that are hazardous to a breastfed infant. The problem, however, is determining which drugs are safe and which are hazardous.

Because so few clinicians understand lactational pharmacology, the number of women who are advised to discontinue breastfeeding in order to take a medication is still far too high. Fortunately, many mothers are now becoming aware of the enormous benefits of breastfeeding and simply refuse to follow some of the advice given by their healthcare professionals. They seek out the information on their own and invariably find this book or my websites.

Because almost all mothers ingest medications during the early neonatal period, it is not surprising that one of the most common questions encountered in pediatrics concerns the use of various drugs in the breastfeeding mother. Unfortunately, most healthcare professionals simply review the package insert or advise the mother not to breastfeed without having done a thorough study of the literature to find the true answer. Discontinuing breastfeeding is often the wrong decision, and most mothers could easily continue to breastfeed and take the medication without risk to the infant. Even the FDA has recognized this and now recommends that drug manufacturers carry out studies to determine milk levels of their drug.

It is generally accepted that all medications transfer into human milk to some degree, although it is almost always quite low. Only rarely does the amount transferred into milk produce clinically relevant doses in the infant. Ultimately, it is the clinician's responsibility to review the research I have on the drugs in this book and make a clear decision as to whether the mother should continue to breastfeed.

Drugs may transfer into human milk if they:

- Attain high concentrations in maternal plasma
- Are low in molecular weight (<800)
- Are low in protein binding
- Pass into the brain easily

However, once medications transfer into human milk, other kinetic factors are involved. One of the most important is the oral bioavailability of the medication to the infant. Numerous medications are either destroyed in the infant's gut, fail to be absorbed through the gut wall, or are rapidly picked up by the liver. Once in the liver, they are either metabolized or stored, but often never reach the mother's plasma.

Drugs normally enter milk by passive diffusion, driven by equilibrium forces between the maternal plasma compartment and the maternal milk compartment. They pass from the maternal plasma through capillaries into the lactocytes lining the alveolus. Medications must generally pass through both bilayer lipid membranes of the alveolar cell to penetrate milk; although early on, they may pass between the alveolar cells (first 72 hours postpartum). During the first 3 days postpartum, large gaps between the alveolar cells exist. These gaps permit enhanced access into the milk for most drugs, many immunoglobulins, maternal living cells (lymphocytes, leukocytes, macrophages), and other maternal proteins. By the end of the first week, the alveolar cells swell under the influence of prolactin and subsequently close the intracellular gaps, thus reducing the transcellular entry of most maternal drugs, proteins, and other substances into the milk compartment. While it is generally agreed that medications penetrate into milk at higher levels during the colostral period, nevertheless, the absolute dose transferred during the colostrum period is still low due to the minimal volume of colostrum (30-100 mL/day) for the first few days postpartum.

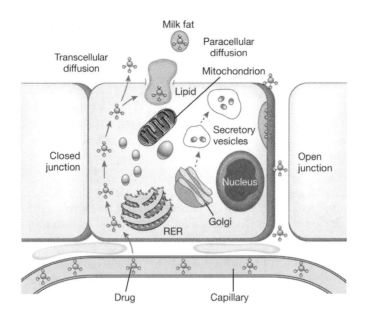

In most instances, the most important determinant of drug penetration into milk is the mother's plasma level. Almost without exception, as the level of the medication in the mother's plasma rises, the concentration in milk increases as well. Drugs enter and exit milk as a function of the mother's plasma level. As soon as the maternal plasma level of a medication begins to fall, equilibrium forces drive the medication out of the milk compartment back into the maternal plasma for elimination. In some instances, drugs may be trapped in milk (ion trapping) due to the lower pH of human milk (7.2). Drugs with a high pKa may become trapped in the milk compartment due to ion trapping. This is important in weakly basic drugs, such as the barbiturates (drugs with high pKa). There are some known cellular pumping systems that actively pump drugs into milk. The most important is iodine. The iodine pump is the same as found in everyone's thyroid gland. Its purpose is to make sure the infant receives iodine to maintain thyroxine production.

The iodides, such as ^{131}I or any "ionic" form of iodine, concentrate in milk due to this pump. Thus iodides, particularly radioactive ones, should be avoided as their milk concentrations are exceedingly high. Two other physicochemical factors are important in evaluating drugs in breastfeeding mothers—the degree of protein binding and lipid solubility. Drugs that are very lipid soluble penetrate into milk in higher concentrations almost without exception. Of particular interest are the drugs that are active in the central nervous system (CNS). CNS-active drugs invariably have the unique characteristics required to enter milk. Therefore, if a drug is active in the CNS, significant levels in milk can be expected; although the amounts still are often subclinical. Many of the neuroactive drugs produce Relative Infant Doses (RIDs) of >5%. Protein binding also plays an important role. Drugs circulate in the maternal plasma, either bound to albumin or freely soluble in the plasma. It is the free component (unbound fraction) that transfers into milk, while the bound fraction stays in the maternal circulation. Therefore, drugs that have high maternal protein binding (warfarin, most NSAIDs) have low milk levels simply because they are bound in the plasma compartment and cannot get out.

Once a drug has entered the mother's milk and has been ingested by the infant, it must traverse through the infant's GI tract prior to absorption. Some drugs are poorly stable in this environment due to the proteolytic enzymes and acids present in the infant's stomach. This includes the aminoglycoside family, omeprazole, and large peptide drugs, such as heparin, and most of the new monoclonal antibodies. Other drugs are poorly absorbed by the infant's GI tract and do not enter the infant's bloodstream. Thus, oral bioavailability is a useful tool to estimate just how much of the drug will be absorbed by the infant. Many drugs are sequestered in the liver (first pass) and may never actually reach the plasma compartment. Absorption characteristics such as these ultimately tend to reduce the overall effect of many drugs in breastfed infants. There are certainly exceptions to this rule, and one must always be aware that the action of a drug in the GI tract can be profound, producing diarrhea, constipation, and occasionally syndromes such as pseudomembranous colitis. One of the more popular methods for estimating risk to the infant is the RID. The RID is calculated by dividing the infant's dose via milk (mg/kg/day) by the mother's dose in mg/kg/day. The RID gives the clinician a feeling for just how much medication the infant is exposed to on a weight-normalized basis. However, many authors calculate the infant dose without normalizing for maternal and infant weight, so be cautious.

$$\text{Relative Infant Dose} \qquad \text{RID} = \frac{\text{Dose in infant } \frac{mg/kg}{d}}{\text{Dose in mother } \frac{mg/kg}{d}}$$

Dose.infant = dose in infant

Dose.mother = dose in mother

Key Points About Breastfeeding and Medications

- Avoid using medications that are not necessary. Herbal drugs, high dose vitamins, unusual supplements, iodine supplements, zinc supplements, and so on that are simply not necessary should be avoided.

- If the Relative Infant Dose is less than 10%, most medications are considered relatively safe to use, but again this is dependent on the type of drug taken.

- Choose drugs for which we have published data, rather than those recently introduced.

- Evaluate the infant for risks. Be more cautious with premature infants or neonates.

- Medications used in the first 3 to 4 days generally produce subclinical levels in the infant due to the limited volume of milk.

- Recommend that mothers with symptoms of depression or other mental disorders seek treatment. Most of the medications used to treat these syndromes are safe. **Remember, healthy moms make healthy babies.**

- Most drugs are quite safe in breastfeeding mothers, while the hazards of using formula are well known and documented. Use donor human milk when the drug is potentially dangerous.

- With some medications, discontinuing breastfeeding for some hours/days may be required, particularly with radioactive compounds and anticancer drugs. If the drug is hazardous to you, it is probably hazardous to your infant.

- Choose drugs with short half-lives, high protein binding, low oral bioavailability, or high molecular weight.

Lastly, it is very important to always evaluate the infant's ability to handle small amounts of medications. Some infants, such as premature or unstable infants, may not be suitable candidates for certain medications. But remember that in early postpartum (and in late stage lactation), the amount of milk produced (30-100 mL/day) is so low that the clinical dose of drug transferred is often low, so even premature neonates would receive only a limited amount from the milk.

Evaluation of the Infant

- Inquire about the infant—always inquire as to the infant's age, size, and stability. This is perhaps the most important criteria to be evaluated prior to using the medication.

- Infant age—premature and newborn infants are at somewhat greater risk. Older infants are at somewhat lower risk due to high metabolic capacity. Infants breastfeeding once or twice a day are at very low risk.

- Infant stability—unstable infants with poor GI stability may be at increased risk from certain medications.

- Pediatric Approved Drugs—generally are less hazardous if long-term history of safety is recognized.

- Dose vs. Age—the age of an infant is critical. Use medications cautiously in premature infants. Older, mature infants can metabolize and clear medications much easier. Remember the dose of the drug the infant receives is dependent on the milk supply. In mothers in late-stage lactation (>1 year), milk production is often low, so the dose of drug delivered is low as well.

- Drugs that alter milk production may profoundly affect infant growth and development—avoid medications that may alter the mother's milk production. These include estrogens, ergot alkaloids, and other drugs.

General Suggestions for the Clinician

Determine if the drug is absorbed from the GI tract. Many drugs, such as the aminoglycosides, vancomycin, cephalosporin antibiotics (third generation), magnesium salts, monoclonal antibodies, and large protein drugs (heparin), are so poorly absorbed that it is unlikely the infant will absorb significant quantities. At the same time, observe for GI side effects from the medication trapped in the GI compartment of the infant (e.g., diarrhea).

Review the Relative Infant Dose (RID) and compare that to the pediatric dose if known. Most older RIDs were derived using the C_{max} (highest milk concentration of the drug) that were published. In current research projects, I always calculate the average (C_{ave}) milk level throughout the dosing schedule. This estimate provided an average exposure rather than just the highest. I no longer use the milk/plasma ratio as it is virtually worthless unless you know the maternal plasma level. It does not provide the clinician with information as to the average amount of drug transferred to the infant via milk. Even if the drug has a high milk/plasma ratio, if the maternal plasma level of the medication is very small (such as with ranitidine), then the absolute amount (dose) of a drug delivered to the infant will still be quite small and often subclinical.

Be cautious of drugs (or their active metabolites) that have long pediatric half-lives as they can continually build up in the infant's plasma over time. The barbiturates, benzodiazepines, and meperidine are classic examples where higher levels in the infant can and do occasionally occur. Interestingly, the SSRI family have long half-lives, but are not retained in the infant's plasma.

If you are provided a choice, choose drugs that have higher protein binding because they are generally sequestered in the maternal circulation and do not transfer readily into the milk compartment or the infant. Remember, it is the free drug that transfers into the milk compartment. Without doubt, the most important parameter that determines drug penetration into milk is plasma protein binding. Choose drugs with high protein binding.

Although not always true, I have generally found centrally active drugs (anticonvulsants, antidepressants, antipsychotics) frequently penetrate milk in higher (not necessarily "high") levels simply due to their physicochemistry. If the drug in question produces sedation, depression, or other neuroleptic effects in the mother, it may produce similar effects in the infant. Thus, with CNS-active drugs, one should always check the data in this book closely and monitor the infant routinely.

For radioactive compounds, I have gathered much of the published data in this field into several tables. The Nuclear Regulatory Commission recommendations are quite good, but they differ from some published data. They can be copied and provided to your radiologist. They are available from the Nuclear Regulatory Commission's web page address in the appendix. With radioisotopes, I recommend you routinely call the InfantRisk Center for advice. Some are quite dangerous.

Use the Relative Infant Dose. In general, a Relative Infant Dose of <10% is considered safe, and its use is becoming increasingly popular by numerous investigators. But this depends on the drug. With risky anticancer drugs, a much lower RID should be used in your evaluation of risk.

Most importantly, it is rare that a breastfeeding mother needs to discontinue breastfeeding just to take a medication. It is simply not acceptable for the clinician to stop lactation merely because of heightened anxiety or ignorance on their part. The risks of formula feeding are significant and should not be trivialized. Few drugs have documented side effects in breastfed infants, and we know most of these.

The following review of drugs is a thorough review of what has been published and what I presently know about the use of medications in breastfeeding mothers.

The author makes no recommendations as to the safety of these medications during lactation, but only reviews what is currently published in the scientific literature. Individual use of medications must be left up to the judgment of the physician, the patient, and other healthcare consultants.

Thomas W. Hale

How to Use This Resource

This section of the book is designed to aid the reader in determining risk to an infant from maternal medications and in using the pharmacokinetic parameters throughout this reference.

Generic Name and Trade Name:

Each monograph begins with the generic name of the drug. The most common trade names are provided under the Trade section. With some pharmaceuticals, there may be more than one drug added to the product. In this case, I have added a table called "Combination Drugs" in the appendix where all the drugs present in that specific pharmaceutical are listed and you can then look up the individual products.

Other Trades:

This book is used all over the world. Thus many other trade names from other countries are now included in this section.

Category:

This lists the class or "family of drugs" that the medication belongs to and gives a general idea of the pharmacology, mechanism of action, and probable use of the drug.

Drug Monograph:

The drug monograph lists what we currently understand about the drug, its ability to enter milk, the concentration in milk at set time intervals, and other parameters that are important to a clinical consultant. I have attempted at great length to report only what the references have documented.

DR. HALE'S LACTATION RISK CATEGORIES:

L1 Compatible:

Drug which has been taken by a large number of breastfeeding mothers without any observed increase in adverse effects in the infant. Controlled studies in breastfeeding women fail to demonstrate a risk to the infant and the possibility of harm to the breastfeeding infant is remote; or the product is not orally bioavailable in an infant.

L2 Probably Compatible:

Drug which has been studied in a limited number of breastfeeding women without an increase in adverse effects in the infant. And/or the evidence of a demonstrated risk which is likely to follow use of this medication in a breastfeeding woman is remote.

L3 Probably Compatible:

There are no controlled studies in breastfeeding women; however, the risk of untoward effects to a breastfed infant is possible, or controlled studies show only minimal non-threatening adverse effects. Drugs should be given only if the potential benefit justifies the potential risk to the infant. (New medications that have absolutely no published data are automatically categorized in this category, regardless of how safe they may be.)

L4 Potentially Hazardous:

There is positive evidence of risk to a breastfed infant or to breastmilk production, but the benefits from use in breastfeeding mothers may be acceptable despite the risk to the infant (e.g., if the drug is needed in a life-threatening situation or for a serious disease for which safer drugs cannot be used or are ineffective).

L5 Hazardous:

Studies in breastfeeding mothers have demonstrated that there is significant and documented risk to the infant based on human experience, or it is a medication that has a high risk of causing significant damage to an infant. The risk of using the drug in breastfeeding women clearly outweighs any possible benefit from breastfeeding. The drug is contraindicated in women who are breastfeeding an infant.

Adult Concerns:

This section lists the most prevalent undesired or bothersome side effects listed for adults. As with most medications, the occurrence of these is often quite rare, generally less than 1% to 10%. Side effects vary from one patient to another, with most patients not experiencing untoward effects.

Pediatric Concerns:

This section lists the side effects noted in the published literature as associated with medications transferred via human milk. Pediatric concerns are those effects that were noted by investigators as being associated with drug transfer via milk. In some sections, I have added comments that may not have been reported in the literature, but are well-known attributes of this medication.

Infant Monitoring:

This section provides advice to the clinician regarding potential side effects that may occur in the infant from exposure to a medication in breastmilk. The infant monitoring parameters can be used by the clinician to educate the mother about potential side effects that could occur in the infant.

Relative Infant Dose:

The Relative Infant Dose (RID) is calculated by dividing the infant's dose via milk in "mg/kg/day" by the maternal dose in "mg/kg/day" (see page xi). This weight-normalizing method indicates approximately how much of the "maternal dose" the infant is receiving. Many authors now use this calculation because it gives a better indication of the relative dose transferred to the infant. I report RID ranges, as this gives the reader an estimate of all the RIDs published by the various authors.

Please understand, however, that many authors use different methods for calculating RID. Some are not weight-normalized. In these cases, their estimates may differ slightly from this book. While I often place these authors' estimates of RID in the text, the RID range that I calculate is weight-normalized in all instances when the maternal weight is provided. So RID may be slightly different according to how it is calculated.

Many researchers now suggest that anything less than 10% of the maternal dose is probably safe. This is usually correct. However, some drugs (metronidazole, acetaminophen) actually have much higher RIDs, but because they are quite non-toxic, they do not often bother an infant. To calculate this dose, I chose the data I felt were best, and these often included larger studies with AUC calculations of mean concentrations in milk. When maternal weights are not published, I choose an average body weight of 70 kg for an adult. Thus, most of the RIDs herein are calculated assuming a maternal average weight of 70 kg and a daily milk intake of 150 mL/kg/day in the infant.

Adult Dosage:

This is the usual adult oral dose provided in the package insert. While these are highly variable, I chose the dose for the most common use of the medication.

Alternatives:

Drugs listed in this section may be suitable alternate choices for the medication listed. In many instances, if the patient cannot take the medication or it is a poor choice due to high milk concentrations, these alternatives may be suitable candidates. WARNING: The alternatives listed are only suggestions and may not be at all appropriate for the syndrome in question. Only the clinician can make this judgment. For instance, nifedipine is a calcium channel blocker with good antihypertensive qualities, but poor antiarrhythmic qualities. In this case, verapamil would be a better choice.

T½ =

This lists the most commonly recorded adult half-life of the medication. It is very important to remember that short half-life drugs are preferred. Use this parameter to determine if the mother can successfully breastfeed around the medication by nursing the infant, then taking the medication. If the half-life is short enough (1-3 hours), then the drug level in the maternal plasma will be declining when the infant feeds again. This is ideal. If the half-life is significantly long (12-24 hours) and if your physician is open to suggestions, then find a similar medication with a shorter half-life (compare ibuprofen with naproxen). However, in today's world, longer half-life drugs are preferred and we simply have to accommodate these and rely on published data.

Vd=

The volume of distribution is a useful kinetic term that describes how widely the medication is distributed in the body. Drugs with high volumes of distribution (Vd) are distributed in higher concentrations in remote compartments of the body and may not stay in the blood. Marijuana is a classic example.

Another such drug, digoxin enters the blood compartment and then rapidly leaves to enter the heart and skeletal muscles. Most of the drug is sequestered in these remote compartments (100 fold). Therefore, drugs with high volumes of distribution (1-20 L/kg) generally require much longer to clear from the body than drugs with smaller volumes (<1 L/kg). For instance, whereas it may only require a few hours to totally clear gentamycin (Vd=0.28 L/kg), it may require weeks to clear amitriptyline (Vd=10 L/kg). Further, some drugs may have one half-life for the plasma compartment, but may have a totally different half-life for the peripheral compartment, as half-life is a function of volume of distribution. I have found that drugs with high Vd generally produce lower milk levels. For a complete description of Vd, please consult a good pharmacology reference. In this text, the units of measure for Vd are L/kg.

T_{max} =

This lists the time interval from administration of the drug until it reaches the highest level in the mother's plasma (C_{max}), which I call the peak or "time to max," hence T_{max}. Occasionally, you may be able to avoid nursing the baby when the medication is at the peak. Rather, wait until the peak is subsiding or has at least dropped significantly. Remember, drugs enter breastmilk as a function of the maternal plasma concentration. In general, the higher the mother's plasma level, the greater the entry of the drug into her milk. If possible, choose drugs that have short peak intervals, and suggest mom not breastfeed when the drug is at C_{max}.

MW=

The molecular weight of a medication is a significant determinant as to the entry of that medication into human milk. Medications with small molecular weights (<200) can easily pass into milk by traversing small pores in the cell walls of the mammary epithelium (see ethanol). Drugs with higher molecular weights must traverse the membrane by dissolving in the cells' lipid membranes, which may significantly reduce milk levels. As such, the smaller the molecular weight, the higher the relative transfer of that drug into milk. Protein medications (e.g., heparin), which have enormous molecular weights, transfer at much lower concentrations and are virtually excluded from human breastmilk. Therefore, when possible, choose drugs with higher molecular weights to reduce their entry into milk. A new class of drugs has risen in popularity in the last decade. These are the monoclonal antibodies. These very selective antibodies mostly derived from human IgG1-4, are used to treat a number of severe diseases, such as Crohn's disease, multiple sclerosis, rheumatoid conditions, migraine headache, and so on. Interestingly, IgG molecules are enormous in molecular weight (around 160,000 Da) and thus enter the milk compartment poorly. Further, they are largely destroyed by proteases in the GI tract of the infant if presented in milk. At this point, we do not think much, if any, of these monoclonals enter milk, or survive the GI tract of the infant. Thus far, all studies of these antibodies in human milk suggest levels in milk are far less than 1.0%, and virtually none of this would survive the GI tract of the infant. However, the use of these drugs in pregnant women in the last trimester may produce significant plasma levels in the fetus, and thus in the newborn infant. Thus some infants could be susceptible to problems associated with the fetal exposure to these drugs (immunosuppressed). Current data thus far do not suggest significant transfer of these products into human milk.

M/P=

This lists the milk/plasma ratio. This is the ratio of the concentration of drug in the mother's milk divided by the concentration in the mother's plasma. If high (>1-5), it is useful as an indicator of drugs that may sequester in milk in high levels. If low (<1), it is a good indicator that only minimal levels of the drug are transferred into milk (this is preferred). While it is best to try to choose drugs with LOW milk/plasma ratios, the amount of drug which transfers into human milk is largely determined by the level of drug in the mother's plasma compartment. Even with high M/P ratios and LOW maternal plasma levels, the amount of drug that transfers is still low. Therefore, the higher M/P ratios often provide an erroneous impression that large amounts of drug are going to transfer into milk. This simply may not be true.

PB=

This lists the percentage of maternal protein binding. Most drugs circulate in the blood bound to plasma albumin and other proteins. If a drug is highly protein bound, it cannot enter the milk compartment as easily. The higher the percentage of binding, the less likely the drug is to enter the maternal milk. Try to choose drugs that have high protein binding in order to reduce the infant's exposure to the medication. Good protein binding is typically greater than 90%.

Oral=

Oral bioavailability refers to the ability of a drug to reach the systemic circulation after oral administration. It is generally a good indication of the amount of medication that is absorbed into the bloodstream of the patient. Drugs with low oral bioavailability are generally either poorly absorbed in the gastrointestinal tract, are destroyed in the gut, or are sequestered by the liver prior to entering the plasma compartment. The oral bioavailability listed in this text is the adult value; almost none have been published for children or neonates. Recognizing this, these values are still useful in estimating if a mother or perhaps an infant will actually absorb enough drug to provide clinically significant levels in the plasma compartment of the individual. The value listed estimates the percent of an oral dose that would be found in the plasma compartment of the individual after oral administration. In many cases, the oral bioavailability of some medications is not listed by manufacturers, but instead terms such as "Complete," "Nil," or "Poor" are used. For lack of better data, I have included these terms when no data are available on the exact amount (percentage) absorbed.

pKa=

The pKa of a drug is the pH at which the drug is equally ionic and nonionic. The more ionic a drug is, the less capable it is of transferring from the milk compartment to the maternal plasma compartment. Hence, the drug becomes trapped in milk (ion-trapping). This term is useful because drugs that have a pKa higher than 7.2 may be sequestered to a slightly higher degree than those with a lower pKa. Drugs with higher pKa generally have higher milk/plasma ratios. Hence, choose drugs with a lower pKa.

With many drugs, the pharmacokinetics have not been described or published. In this case I leave this entry blank.

Common Abbreviations

ACEI	Angiotensin converting enzyme inhibitor
AUC	Area under the curve
BID	Twice daily
C_{max}	Plasma or milk concentration at peak
d	Day
et al	"and others"
g	Gram
GI	Gastrointestinal
h	Hour
LRC	Lactation risk category
M/P	Milk/plasma ratio
MAOI	Monoamine oxidase inhibitors
mg/L	Milligram per liter
mL	Milliliter. One cc
mmol	Millimole of weight
MW	Molecular weight
ng/L	Nanogram per liter
NR	Not rated
NSAID	Nonsteroidal anti-inflammatory drug
Oral	Oral bioavailability (adult)
PB	Percent of protein binding in maternal circulation
pg	Picogram
PHL	Pediatric elimination half-life
PRN	As needed
QD	Daily
QID	Four times daily
RID	Relative Infant Dose
SNRIs	Serotonin norepinephrine reuptake inhibitors
SSRIs	Selective serotonin reuptake inhibitors
T 1/2	Adult elimination half-life
TCAs	Tricyclic antidepressants
TID	Three times daily
T_{max}	Time to peak plasma level (PK)
Vd	Volume of distribution
X	Times
mCi	Millicurie of radioactivity
μCi	Microcurie of radioactivity
μg/L	Microgram per liter
μmol	Micromole of weight

Hale's

Medications & Mothers' Milk™

2021

A Manual of Lactational Pharmacology

ABACAVIR

Trade: Ziagen

Category: Antiviral

LRC: L5 - Limited Data-Hazardous if Maternal HIV Infection

Abacavir (ABC) is a nucleoside reverse transcriptase inhibitor (NRTI) that is used in combination with other agents for the treatment of HIV.[1]

In a study published in 2013, nine women receiving Trizivir (abacavir 300 mg + zidovudine 300 mg + lamivudine 150 mg) twice daily provided breast milk samples for analysis on day 30 postpartum.[2] The median abacavir level was 0.057 μg/mL and the highest level was about 0.5 μg/mL. The milk/plasma ratio was found to be 0.85. A typical infant would receive 0.0086 mg/kg/day when using the median milk sample and about 0.075 mg/kg/day when using the highest concentration. This corresponds to a relative infant dose of 0.1% and 0.9%, respectively. Of the nine infants in the study who were exposed to abacavir, only one had a detectable concentration of abacavir in plasma. No side effects were reported in these infants. However, the authors of this study raised the possibility of subinhibitory levels of abacavir promoting viral resistance to the drug, which could then affect the baby.

Note: This medication is an L5 to highlight the contraindication of breastfeeding when the mother is known to be infected with HIV; this medication is not an L5 based on its risk to the infant in breast milk. The Centers for Disease Control and Prevention recommend that HIV infected mothers do not breastfeed their infants to avoid postnatal transmission of HIV.

T 1/2	1.54 h	MW	670.74 Da	PB	50%
Tmax	0.7-1.7 h	RID	0.1%-0.88%	Vd	0.86 L/kg
Oral	83%	M/P		pKa	5.01

Adult Concerns: Headache, fatigue, depression, changes in sleep, abnormal dreams, nausea, vomiting, diarrhea, changes in liver function, elevated triglycerides, thrombocytopenia, severe rash.

Adult Dose: 300 mg twice a day or 600 mg daily.

Pediatric Concerns: In pediatric HIV clinical studies the most common side effects that occurred when this medication was administered directly to the infant (not via milk) included: fever and/or chills, nausea, vomiting, diarrhea, skin rashes, and ear/nose/throat infections.

Infant Monitoring: Breastfeeding is not recommended in mothers who have HIV.

Alternatives:

References:
1. Pharmaceutical manufacturers prescribing information.
2. Shapiro RL, Rossi S, Ogwu A, et al. Therapeutic levels of lopinavir in late pregnancy and abacavir passage into breast milk in the Mma Bana Study, Botswana. Antivir Ther. 2013;18(4):585-590.

ABATACEPT

Trade: Orencia

Category: Antirheumatic

LRC: L3 - No Data-Probably Compatible

Abatacept is a soluble fusion protein that is linked to a modified portion of human immunoglobulin G1 (IgG1).[1] The apparent molecular weight of abatacept is 92,000 Da. Abatacept inhibits T cell activation by binding to CD80 and CD86 receptors which down regulates the T cells implicated in inflammation of rheumatic disorders. In vitro, abatacept decreases T cell proliferation and inhibits the production of the cytokines TNF alpha, interferon-gamma, and interleukin-2. There are no data on the transfer of this antibody into human milk. Due to its large molecular weight and poor oral absorption, it is not likely to enter breast milk or the infant's systemic circulation in clinically relevant amounts; however, there are no data to confirm this at this time.

T 1/2	13.1 days	MW	92,000 Da	PB	
Tmax		RID		Vd	0.02-0.13 L/kg
Oral	Nil	M/P		pKa	

Adult Concerns: Headache, fever, dizziness, cough, nausea, abdominal pain, back pain or limb pain, rash, antibody formation, increased risk of infection.

Adult Dose: 500-1000 mg IV at 0, 2, and 4 weeks, then repeat every 4 weeks.

Pediatric Concerns: No adverse effects have been reported via milk at this time.

Infant Monitoring:

Alternatives: Infliximab(L3), Etanercept(L2)

References:
1. Pharmaceutical manufacturers prescribing information.

ACARBOSE

Trade: Glucobay, Prandase, Precose

Category: Antidiabetic, other

LRC: L3 - No Data-Probably Compatible

Acarbose is an oral alpha-glucosidase inhibitor used to delay the absorption of carbohydrates in the management of Type II diabetes.[1,2] The local action of this medication in the gastrointestinal tract reduces carbohydrate absorption and the rapid rise in glucose and insulin following a meal; hence, glycosylated hemoglobin (HbA1c) levels are reduced over time. No data are available on the transfer of acarbose into human milk. The oral bioavailability of this medication is less than 2%, thus little medication would be expected to enter maternal milk.

T 1/2	~2 h	MW	645 Da	PB	
Tmax	~1 h	RID		Vd	0.32 L/kg
Oral	0.7%-2%	M/P		pKa	11.23

Adult Concerns: Abdominal pain, flatulence, diarrhea, increases in liver enzymes.

Adult Dose: 50-100 mg TID.

Pediatric Concerns: None reported via milk.

Infant Monitoring: Flatulence, persistent diarrhea, weight gain.

Alternatives: Insulin(L2), Metformin(L1), Glyburide(L2)

References:
1. Pharmaceutical manufacturers prescribing information.
2. Balfour JA, McTavish D. Acarbose. An update of its pharmacology and therapeutic use in diabetes mellitus. Drugs. 1993;46(6):1025-1054.

ACEBUTOLOL

Trade: Monitan, Sectral

Category: Beta Adrenergic Blocker

LRC: L3 - Limited Data-Probably Compatible

Acebutolol predominately inhibits beta-1 receptors, but can block beta-2 receptors at high doses.[1] It is low in lipid solubility, and contains intrinsic sympathetic activity (partial beta agonist activity). Studies indicate that on a weight basis, acebutolol is approximately 10%-30% as effective as propranolol.

In a study of seven women receiving 200-1200 mg/day acebutolol, the highest milk concentration occurred in the women receiving 1200 mg/day and was 4123 µg/L.[2] In women receiving 200, 400, or 600 mg/day of acebutolol, milk levels were 286 µg/L, 666 µg/L, and 539 µg/L, respectively. Adverse effects of beta-blockade were reported.

Acebutolol and its major active metabolite, diacetolol, appear in breastmilk with a milk/plasma ratio of 1.9 to 9.2 (acebutolol) and 2.3 to 24.7 (diacetolol). These levels are considered relatively high and occurred following maternal doses of 400-1200 mg/day. When the metabolite is added, the infant dose may approach 10% of the maternal dose.

T 1/2	3-4 h	MW	336 Da	PB	26%
Tmax	2-4 h	RID	0.94%-3.61%	Vd	1.2 L/kg
Oral	35%-50%	M/P	7.1-12.2	pKa	13.91

Adult Concerns: Headache, dizziness, insomnia, depression, fatigue, chest pain, bradycardia, hypotension, heart failure, wheezing, vomiting, constipation, diarrhea, myalgia.

Adult Dose: 200-400 mg BID.

Pediatric Concerns: Hypotension, bradycardia, hypoxemia, and transient tachypnea have been reported.[2]

Infant Monitoring: Drowsiness, lethargy, pallor, poor feeding, and weight gain.

Alternatives: Labetalol(L2), Metoprolol(L2)

References:
1. Drug Facts and Comparisons 2017.
2. Boutroy MJ, Bianchetti G, Dubruc C, Vert P, Morselli PL. To nurse when receiving acebutolol: is it dangerous for the neonate? Eur J Clin Pharmacol. 1986;30(6):737-739.

ACETAMINOPHEN (PARACETAMOL)

Trade: 222 AF Extra Strength, Abenol, Feverall, Actamin Maximum Strength, Panadol, Aminofen, Tylenol, Genapap

Category: Analgesic

LRC: L1 - Extensive Data-Compatible

Acetaminophen is an analgesic/antipyretic used in the treatment of fever and pain. When taken orally, only minimal amounts are secreted into breast milk and are considered too small to be hazardous. In a study of 11 mothers who received 650 mg of acetaminophen orally, the highest milk levels reported were from 10-15 mg/L.[1] The milk/plasma ratio was 1.08. In another study of three patients who received a single 500 mg oral dose, the reported milk and plasma concentrations of acetaminophen were 4.2 mg/L and 5.6 mg/L respectively.[2] The milk/plasma ratio was 0.76. The maximum observed concentration in milk was 4.4 mg/L. In another study of women who ingested 1000 mg acetaminophen, milk levels averaged 6.1 mg/L and provided an average dose of 0.92 mg/kg/day according to the authors.[3] Although there seems to be wide variation in the milk concentrations in these studies, the amount of acetaminophen an infant could ingest via breast milk is most likely significantly less than the pediatric therapeutic dose.

Acetaminophen is increasingly being used intravenously for the relief of moderate to severe pain conditions. Some reports have suggested that the analgesic efficacy of intravenous acetaminophen is equivalent to that of intravenous morphine, and is probably preferred due to its minimal side effects.[4,5] Following a 1 g IV dose of acetaminophen, the peak plasma concentrations attained are in the order of 28 mg/L at the end of 15 minutes. According to one report, following a 2 g IV dose of acetaminophen in postpartum mothers, the plasma levels decreased from 22.5 mg/L to 3.9 mg/L within 6 hours postdose.[6] Following a single IV dose, a maternal peak plasma concentration of 28 mg/L suggests that a breastfed infant would receive a dose of 19.6-28 mg/day (M/P ratio = 1) or about 4-6 mg/kg/day. This is far lower than the clinical doses for infants (10-15 mg/kg/dose).

The dose ingested could be higher in premature or younger infants, but would probably still be lower than the clinically used pediatric doses. Nevertheless, some caution is advised. IV acetaminophen has been successfully used in premature infants born at 25-32 weeks of gestation, without any reported side effects.[7] The serum concentrations at the end of 8-12 doses ranged between 8-64 mg/L. The authors reported that the infants tolerated the drug well. Based on these studies it may be said that infants seem to tolerate IV acetaminophen well. The dose ingested by an infant following IV acetaminophen in a lactating mother would most probably not be clinically relevant.

There is growing evidence that acetaminophen use may be linked to an increased prevalence of asthma among children and adults. In one published paper, it has been recommended that any child with asthma or a family history of asthma avoid using acetaminophen.[8] Prenatal exposure and exposure to acetaminophen in the first year of life has also been linked to development of asthma later in life.[9-13] Subsequently, the issue of lactational exposure to acetaminophen and its association with development of asthma has also been addressed.

In one such short-term study, out of 11 wheezing, exclusively breastfed infants, mothers of seven of the infants had admitted intake of acetaminophen at the time of onset of wheezing symptoms in the infants.[14] However, these claims have been refuted by a few other authorities, based on various grounds. Nevertheless, due to the immaturity of metabolic pathways in the infant, a customary recommendation of judicious use of medications (including acetaminophen), during lactation has been advocated.

T 1/2	2 h	MW	151 Da	PB	10%-25%
Tmax	10-60 min	RID	6.41%-8.82%	Vd	0.8-1 L/kg
Oral	>85%	M/P	0.91-1.42	pKa	9.5

Adult Concerns: Few when taken in normal doses. Diarrhea, gastric upset. Note: numerous cases of liver toxicity have been reported following "chronic" use of acetaminophen at >200 mg/kg/day. Do not exceed 3000 mg in a 24-hour period or 1000 mg/dose. Exceedingly high doses can cause severe hepatic toxicity and death.

Adult Dose: 650 mg every 4-6 hours PRN.

Pediatric Concerns: None reported via milk at this time.

Infant Monitoring: Diarrhea, gastric upset; potential for liver toxicity if maternal overdose.

Alternatives: Ibuprofen(L1)

References:

1. Berlin CM Jr, Yaffe SJ, Ragni M. Disposition of acetaminophen in milk, saliva, and plasma of lactating women. Pediatr Pharmacol. 1980;1(2):135-141.
2. Bitzen PO, Gustafsson B, Jostell KG, Melander A, Wahlin-Boll E. Excretion of paracetamol in human breast milk. Eur J Clin Pharmacol. 1981;20(2):123-125.
3. Notarianni LJ, Oldham HG, Bennett PN. Passage of paracetamol into breast milk and its subsequent metabolism by the neonate. Br J Clin Pharmacol. July 1987;24(1):63-67.
4. Serinken M, Eken C, Turkcuer I, Elicabuk H, Uyanik E, Schultz CH. Intravenous paracetamol versus morphine for renal colic in the emergency department: a randomised double-blind controlled trial. Emerg Med J: EMJ. November 2012;29(11):902-905.
5. Craig M, Jeavons R, Probert J, Benger J. Randomised comparison of intravenous paracetamol and intravenous morphine for acute traumatic limb pain in the emergency department. Emerg Med J: EMJ. January 2012;29(1):37-39.
6. Kulo A, van de Velde M, de Hoon J, et al. Pharmacokinetics of a loading dose of intravenous paracetamol post caesarean delivery. Int J Obstet Anesth. April 2012;21(2):125-128.
7. van Ganzewinkel CJ, Mohns T, van Lingen RA, Derijks LJ, Andriessen P. Paracetamol serum concentrations in preterm infants treated with paracetamol intravenously: a case series. J Med Case Rep. 2012;6:1.
8. McBride JT. The association of acetaminophen and asthma prevalence and severity. Pediatrics. December 2011;128(6):1181-1185.
9. Eyers S, Weatherall M, Jefferies S, Beasley R. Paracetamol in pregnancy and the risk of wheezing in offspring: a systematic review and meta-analysis. Clin Exp Allergy: J Br Soc Allergy Clin Immunol. April 2011;41(4):482-489.
10. Etminan M, Sadatsafavi M, Jafari S, Doyle-Waters M, Aminzadeh K, Fitzgerald JM. Acetaminophen use and the risk of asthma in children and adults: a systematic review and metaanalysis. Chest. November 2009;136(5):1316-1323.
11. Rebordosa C, Kogevinas M, Sorensen HT, Olsen J. Pre-natal exposure to paracetamol and risk of wheezing and asthma in children: a birth cohort study. Int J Epidemiol. June 2008;37(3):583-590.
12. Shaheen SO, Newson RB, Henderson AJ, et al. Prenatal paracetamol exposure and risk of asthma and elevated immunoglobulin E in childhood. Clin Exp Allergy: J Br Soc Allergy Clin Immunol. January 2005;35(1):18-25.
13. Shaheen SO, Newson RB, Sherriff A, et al. Paracetamol use in pregnancy and wheezing in early childhood. Thorax. November 2002;57(11):958-963.
14. Verd S, Nadal-Amat J. Paracetamol and asthma and lactation. Acta paediatr. July 2011;100(7):e2-e3; author reply e3.

ACETAZOLAMIDE

Trade: Acetazolam, Dazamide, Diamox, Sequels

Category: Diuretic

LRC: L2 - Limited Data-Probably Compatible

Acetazolamide is a carbonic anhydrase inhibitor dissimilar to other thiazide diuretics. There are documented suggestions that diuretics in general decrease the volume of breast milk. In a patient who received 500 mg of acetazolamide twice daily, acetazolamide concentrations in milk were 1.3 to 2.1 mg/L while the maternal plasma levels ranged from 5.2-6.4 mg/L.[1] Plasma concentrations in the exposed infant were 0.2 to 0.6 µg/mL 2 to 12 hours after breastfeeding. These amounts are unlikely to cause adverse effects in the infant.

T 1/2	2.4-5.8 h	MW	222 Da	PB	70%-95%
Tmax	1-3 h	RID	1.37%-2.2%	Vd	0.2 L/kg
Oral	Complete	M/P	0.25	pKa	7.2

Adult Concerns: Anorexia, diarrhea, metallic taste, polyuria, muscular weakness, potassium loss. Malaise, fatigue, depression, renal failure have been reported.

Adult Dose: 500 mg BID.

Pediatric Concerns: None reported via milk.

Infant Monitoring: Observe for fluid loss, dehydration, lethargy.

Alternatives:

References:

1. Soderman P, Hartvig P, Fagerlund C. Acetazolamide excretion into human breast milk. Br J Clin Pharmacol. 1984;17(5):599-600.

ACETYLSALICYLIC ACID

Trade: Aspirin, ASA, Aspirtab, Ascriptin, Easprin, Ecotrin, Ecpirin, Entercote

Category: Analgesic

LRC: L2 - Limited Data-Probably Compatible

Acetylsalicylic acid (ASA) is an irreversible inhibitor of cyclooxygenase-1 and 2 (COX-1 and COX-2).[1] At low doses, COX-1 inhibition indirectly leads to decreased platelet aggregation. Anti-inflammatory, analgesic, and antipyretic effects also emerge at higher doses. ASA is rapidly metabolized to salicylic acid, which is a lower-potency, reversible inhibitor of a variety of processes. Few harmful effects have been reported with use in lactation.

In one study, salicylic acid (active metabolite) penetrated poorly into milk (454 mg dose ASA), with peak levels of only 1.12 to 1.60 µg/mL, whereas maternal peak plasma levels were 33 to 43.4 µg/mL.[2] In another study of a rheumatoid arthritis patient who received 4 g/day ASA, none was detectable in her milk (<5 mg/100 mL).[3] Extremely high doses in the mother could potentially produce slight bleeding in the infant. Because ASA is implicated in Reye syndrome, it is a poor choice of analgesic to use in breastfeeding mothers. However, in rheumatic fever patients, it is still one of the anti-inflammatory drugs of choice and a risk-versus-benefit assessment must be done in this case.

In a study of a patient consuming ASA chronically, salicylate concentrations in milk peaked at 3 hours at a concentration of 10 mg/L following a maternal dose of 975 mg.[4] Maternal plasma levels peaked at 2.25 hours at 108 mg/L. The milk/plasma ratio was reported to be 0.08. In a study of eight women following the use of 1 g (about three 325 mg tablets) oral doses of ASA, average milk levels of salicylic acid (active metabolite) were 2.4 mg/L at 3 hours.[5] The metabolite salicyluric acid, reached a peak of 10.2 mg/L at 9 hours. Averaging total salicylates and salicyluric acid metabolites, the author suggests the relative infant dose would be 9.4% of the maternal dose.

In a new study in seven breastfeeding mothers consuming 81 mg/day, milk samples were collected at 0, 1, 2, 4, 8, 12, and 24 hours.[6] Acetylsalicylic acid levels were below the limit of quantification (0.61 ng/ml) in all the milk samples, whereas salicylic acid was detected at very low concentrations. The average concentration of salicylic acid observed was 24 ng/ml and the estimated relative infant dose was 0.4%. Acetylsalicylic acid transfer to milk is so low that it is undetectable even by highly sophisticated methodology. Salicylic acid does appear in the human milk in comparatively low amounts, which are probably subclinical in infants. In one patient consuming 325 mg/day of aspirin, human milk levels of ASA were comparable with those taking 81 mg, or were undetectable (< 0.61 ng/ml). In this patient, the maximum concentration of SA was observed as 744.6 ng/ml, which peaked at 1 hour. The area under the curve was 2579 ng.hr/ml and the average concentration estimated was 107.4 ng/ml. The relative infant dose calculated was 0.45% at this dose. Thus, the daily use of an 81-mg dose or 325 mg/day of aspirin should be considered safe during lactation.

While the direct use of ASA in infants and children has been associated with Reye syndrome, the use of the 81 mg/day dose, or even a single 325 mg dose, in breastfeeding mothers has not been linked to an increased risk of this syndrome in the infant. Unfortunately, we do not presently know of any specific dose-response relationship between aspirin and Reye syndrome other than in older children where even low plasma levels of ASA were implicated in Reye syndrome during viral infections such as flu or chickenpox. Lastly, acetylsalicylic acid is rapidly metabolized to salicylic acid by the liver and no ASA apparently reaches the plasma compartment, hence from the latter study, none is present in milk. Unusually large oral doses could change the outcome of the latter study and produce higher levels in plasma. This is unknown at this time.

Consider ibuprofen or acetaminophen as better choices for pain relief in lactating women. Avoid this medication at higher doses in lactation when the infant has a viral syndrome.

T 1/2	3-10 h	MW	180 Da	PB	88-93%
Tmax	1-2 h	RID	2.5%-10.8%	Vd	0.15 L/kg
Oral	50%-75%	M/P	0.03-0.08	pKa	

Adult Concerns: Dizziness, confusion, tinnitus, Reye's syndrome, arrhythmias, dyspepsia, vomiting, stomach pain, gastrointestinal ulcers, changes in liver and kidney function, anemia, platelet dysfunction, increased risk of bleeding.

Adult Dose: 81 mg once daily; 325-650 mg q 4-6 hours (max 4 g/day).

Pediatric Concerns: One 16 day-old infant developed metabolic acidosis. Mother was consuming 3.9 g/day of ASA. Thrombocytopenia, petechiae, and anorexia were reported in an infant of 5 months following exposure to maternal milk containing aspirin. ASA has been associated with Reye syndrome in infants with viral fevers.

Infant Monitoring: Rare bruising on the skin, blood in urine or stool.

Alternatives: Ibuprofen(L1), Acetaminophen(L1)

References:
1. Pharmaceutical manufacturers prescribing information.
2. Findlay JW, DeAngelis RL, Kearney MF, Welch RM, Findlay JM. Analgesic drugs in breast milk and plasma. Clin Pharmacol Ther. 1981;29(5):625-633.
3. Erickson SH, Oppenheim GL. Aspirin in breast milk. J Fam Pract. 1979;8(1):189-190.
4. Bailey DN, Welbert RT, Naylor A. A study of salicylate and caffeine excretion in the breast milk of two nursing mothers. J Anal Toxicol. 1982;6:64-68.
5. Putter J, Satravaha P, Stockhausen H. Quantitative analysis of the main metabolites of acetylsalicylic acid. Comparative analysis in the blood and milk of lactating women. Z Geburtshilfe Perinatol. 1974;178:135-138.
6. Datta P, Rewers-Felkins K, Kallem RR, Baker T, Hale TW. Transfer of low dose aspirin into human milk. J Hum Lact. May 2017;33(2):296-299. doi:10.1177/0890334417695207. Epub March 20, 2017. PMID: 28418802.

ACITRETIN

Trade: Soriatane

Category: Antipsoriatic

LRC: L5 - Limited Data-Hazardous

Acitretin is used in the treatment of severe psoriasis. Its exact mechanism of action is unknown, but it helps to normalize cell differentiation and thin the cornified layer of the skin by reducing the rate of proliferation.[1] This product produces major human fetal anomalies, and is retained in the body for long periods of time. Chronic use in breastfeeding mothers is probably not recommended. In the only study conducted on the transfer of acitretin into human milk, a 31-year-old mother was taking 40 mg once daily and had milk concentrations of 30-40 µg/L. This indicated that an infant would receive only 0.8 to 1.8% of the maternal dose; however, due to the toxic potential of this medication, the authors concluded that acitretin should be avoided during breastfeeding.[2]

T 1/2	49 h	MW	326 Da	PB	>99.9%
Tmax	2-5 h	RID	0.79%-1.8%	Vd	
Oral	72%	M/P		pKa	

Adult Concerns: Alopecia, headache, hyperesthesia, fatigue, xerophthalmia, xerostomia, cheilitis, hypercholesterolemia, hypertriglyceridemia, changes in liver function, increased WBC, arthralgias, skin peeling.

Adult Dose: 25-50 mg/day.

Pediatric Concerns: No data are available.

Infant Monitoring: Signs of jaundice-yellowing of the eyes and skin: skin rash.

Alternatives:

References:
1. Pharmaceutical manufacturers prescribing information.
2. Rollman O, Pihl-Lundin I. Acitretin excretion into human breast milk. Acta Derm Venereol. 1990;70:487-490.

ACYCLOVIR

Trade: Aciclovir, Acyclo-V, Aviraz, Zovirax, Zyclir

Category: Antiviral

LRC: L2 - Limited Data-Probably Compatible

Acyclovir is converted by herpes simplex and varicella zoster virus to acyclovir triphosphate which interferes with viral HSV DNA polymerase. It is currently cleared for use in HSV infections, Varicella-Zoster, and under certain instances such as Cytomegalovirus and Epstein-Barr infections. There is virtually no percutaneous absorption following topical application and plasma levels are undetectable. The pharmacokinetics in children is similar to adults. In neonates, the half-life is 3.8-4.1 hours, and in children one year and older it is 1.9-3.6 hours.

Acyclovir levels in breastmilk are reported to be 0.6 to 4.1 times the maternal plasma levels.[1] Maximum ingested dose was calculated to be 1500 µg/day assuming 750 mL milk intake. This level produced no overt side effects in one infant. In a study by Meyer[2], a patient receiving 200 mg five times daily produced breastmilk concentrations averaging 1.06 mg/L. Using these values, an infant would ingest less than 1 mg acyclovir daily. In another study, doses of 800 mg five times daily produced milk levels that ranged from 4.16 to 5.81 mg/L (total estimated infant ingestion per day = 0.73 mg/kg/day).[3] Topical therapy on lesions other than nipple is probably safe. But mothers with lesions on or close to the nipple should not breastfeed on that side. Toxicities associated with acyclovir are few and usually minor. Acyclovir therapy in neonates is common and produces few toxicities. Calculated intake by infant would be less than 0.87 mg/kg/day.

T 1/2	2.4 h	MW	225 Da	PB	9%-33%
Tmax	1.5-2 h	RID	1.09%-1.53%	Vd	0.8 L/kg
Oral	15%-30%	M/P	0.6-4.1	pKa	7.99

Adult Concerns: Nausea, vomiting, diarrhea, sore throat, edema, and skin rashes.

Adult Dose: 200-800 mg every 4-6 hours.

Pediatric Concerns: None reported via milk in several studies.

Infant Monitoring: Vomiting, diarrhea.

Alternatives: Valacyclovir(L2)

References:
1. Lau RJ, Emery MG, Galinsky RE. Unexpected accumulation of acyclovir in breast milk with estimation of infant exposure. Obstet Gynecol. 1987;69(3 pt 2):468-471.
2. Meyer LJ, de Miranda P, Sheth N, Spruance S. Acyclovir in human breast milk. Am J Obstet Gynecol. 1988;158(3 pt 1):586-588.
3. Taddio A, Klein J, Koren G. Acyclovir excretion in human breast milk. Ann Pharmacother. 1994;28(5):585-587.

ADALIMUMAB

Trade: Humira

Category: Antirheumatic

LRC: L3 - Limited Data-Probably Compatible

Adalimumab is a recombinant humanized IgG1 monoclonal antibody specific for human tumor necrosis factor (TNF).[1] TNF is implicated in the pain and destructive component of arthritis and other autoimmune syndromes. This product would be similar to others such as etanercept (Enbrel) and infliximab (Remicade).

Two infants of women who took adalimumab 40 mg subcutaneously during lactation were followed until 14.5 and 15 months of age.[2] The first infant was exposed to adalimumab in pregnancy and lactation; the last dose was given 3.5 weeks before delivery. The maternal and infant serum levels on postpartum day 1 were 4900 ng/mL and 8400 ng/mL. Maternal serum and breast milk levels were taken again, this time they were drawn 7 days after an injection (about 21 weeks postpartum) and were found to be 6700 ng/mL and 4.83 ng/mL. In the second case maternal serum and breast milk levels were drawn 9 days after the last injection (at about 8 weeks postpartum) and were found to be 5500 ng/mL and 4.88 ng/mL; in this case the infant's serum level was undetectable. No adverse reactions were found in the infant to be attributed to exposure of the drug in breast milk. Both infants were reported to have met all developmental milestones. One infant did develop acute spasmodic laryngitis at 10 months of age; however, this is a common disease among infants and was not deemed to be drug related by the authors of these case reports. The authors of this study postulated that immunoglobulins such as adalimumab might be absorbed via the immunoglobulin G-transporting neonatal Fc receptor (FcRn) that is expressed in intestinal cells of adults and fetuses.

Although the molecular weight of this medication is very large and the amount in breast milk is very low, there are no long-term data concerning the safety of using immune modulating medications in breastfeeding mothers. Further there are current data that suggest that some IgG drugs do transfer into milk, and perhaps the breastfed infant. Therefore, some caution is recommended and each woman should understand the benefits and risk of using this type of medication in lactation.

T 1/2	2 weeks	MW	148,000 Da	PB	Nil
Tmax	131 h	RID	0.12%	Vd	4.7-6 L/kg
Oral	Low	M/P		pKa	

Adult Concerns: Headache, hypertension, nausea, changes in liver function, hematuria, hyperlipidemia, hypercholesterolemia, development of antibodies, infection, injection site reactions, and malignancies have been reported.

Adult Dose: 40 mg every other week subcutaneously.

Pediatric Concerns: None reported via milk.

Infant Monitoring: Vomiting, weight gain, frequent infections.

Alternatives: Infliximab(L3)

References:
1. Pharmaceutical manufacturers prescribing information.
2. Fritzsche J, Pilch A, Mury D, Schaefer C, Weber-Schoendorfer C. Infliximab and adalimumab use during breastfeeding. J Clin Gastroenterol. 2012;46(8):718-719.

ADAPALENE

Trade: Differin

Category: Antiacne

LRC: L3 - No Data-Probably Compatible

Adapalene is a retinoid-like compound (similar to Tretinoin) used topically for treatment of acne. No data are available on its transfer to human milk. However, adapalene is virtually unabsorbed when applied topically to the skin.[1] Plasma levels are almost undetectable (<0.25 mg/mL plasma), so milk levels would be infinitesimally low and probably undetectable.[2]

T 1/2	17 h	MW	412.52 Da	PB	
Tmax		RID		Vd	
Oral	Very low	M/P		pKa	

Adult Concerns: Exacerbation of sunburn, irritation of skin, erythema, dryness, scaling, burning, itching.

Adult Dose: Apply topical daily.

Pediatric Concerns: None reported via milk. Very unlikely due to minimal maternal absorption.

Infant Monitoring:

Alternatives: Tretinoin(L3)

References:
1. Pharmaceutical manufacturers prescribing information.
2. Drug Facts and Comparisons 2017.

ADEFOVIR

Trade: Hepsera

Category: Antiviral

LRC: L4 - No Data-Possibly Hazardous

Adefovir inhibits hepatitis B virus replication.[1] No data are available on the transfer of adefovir into human milk, yet based on the kinetic profile (low protein binding and moderate oral bioavailability, it is possible that the drug would cross into the milk compartment to some degree. Because this drug is potentially toxic to a rapidly growing infant, and because it is used over long periods of time, it is not recommended for use in lactating mothers at this time.

T 1/2	7.5 h	MW	501 Da	PB	<4%
Tmax	1.75 h	RID		Vd	0.4 L/kg
Oral	59%	M/P		pKa	

Adult Concerns: Headache, abdominal pain, vomiting, changes in renal function, hematuria, weakness, rash.

Adult Dose: 10 mg daily.

Pediatric Concerns: No data are available at this time.

Infant Monitoring: Breastfeeding is not recommended in mothers who have HIV.

Alternatives: Lamivudine(L5), if not resistant.

References:
1. Pharmaceutical manufacturers prescribing information.

ADENOSINE

Trade: Adenocard, Adenoscan

Category: Antiarrhythmic

LRC: L2 - No Data-Probably Compatible

Adenosine produces a direct negative chronotropic, dromotropic, and inotropic effect on the heart, presumably due to A1-receptor stimulation, and produces peripheral vasodilation, presumably due to A2-receptor stimulation. The net effect of adenosine in humans is typically a mild to moderate reduction in systolic, diastolic, and mean arterial blood pressure associated with a reflex increase in heart rate. Rarely, significant hypotension and tachycardia have been observed. There are no adequate well controlled studies in breastfeeding.[1] However, adenosine has a half-life <10 seconds and is not likely in the systemic circulation long enough to enter milk. Based on this information, it is probably safe to use in breastfeeding.

T 1/2	<10 secs	MW	267.2 Da	PB	
Tmax		RID		Vd	
Oral	Nil	M/P		pKa	

Adult Concerns: Flushing, chest discomfort, dyspnea or urge to breathe deeply, headache, throat, neck or jaw discomfort, gastrointestinal discomfort, lightheadedness/dizziness.

Adult Dose: 6-12 mg.

Pediatric Concerns:

Infant Monitoring: Drowsiness, lethargy, pallor, arrhythmias, poor feeding, weight gain.

Alternatives:

References:
1. Pharmaceutical manufacturing information. 2011.

AFLIBERCEPT

Trade: Eylea, Zaltrap

Category: vascular endothelial growth factor (VEGF) inhibitor

LRC: L3 - No Data-Probably Compatible

Aflibercept is a recombinant fusion protein (115,000 Da) that acts as a vascular endothelial growth factor inhibitor used in the treatment of various retinal degenerations. Aflibercept binds to the VEGF-A and PlGF receptors and acts as a decoy. Injected intravitreally, it is unlikely to attain significant plasma levels, and that present in the plasma it is inactive and is undetectable two weeks postdosing. This product is unlikely to enter the milk compartment, and would not be orally bioavailable in a human.

T 1/2	5-6 days	MW	115,000 Da	PB	N/A
Tmax	1-3 days	RID		Vd	0.086 L/kg
Oral	N/A	M/P		pKa	N/A

Adult Concerns: Conjunctival hemorrhage, eye pain, cataract, vitreous detachment, vitreous floaters, increased intraocular pressure, ocular hyperemia, corneal epithelium defect, detachment of the retina.

Adult Dose: Variable

Pediatric Concerns:

Infant Monitoring:

Alternatives:

References:
1. Pharmaceutical manufacturers prescribing information.

ALBENDAZOLE

Trade: Albenza, Eskazole, Zentel

Category: Anthelmintic

LRC: L2 - Limited Data-Probably Compatible

Albendazole is a broad-spectrum anthelmintic used to treat intestinal parasite infections.[1] It is a pro-drug that is rapidly metabolized by the liver to an active metabolite, albendazole sulfoxide; albendazole sulfoxide is then metabolized to its inactive form albendazole sulfone. In a study of 33 breastfeeding women given a single 400 mg dose of albendazole, the maternal serum samples at 6 hours of albendazole (ABZ), albendazole sulfoxide (ABSX) and albendazole sulfone (ABSO) were 63.7, 608 and 100.7 ng/mL, respectively.[2]

The levels of ABZ in milk were 31.9, 18.8, 7.5 ng/mL and undetectable at 6, 12, 24, and 36 hours. The levels of ABSX in milk were 312.8, 225.2, 94.1 and 57.1 ng/mL at 6, 12, 24, and 36 hours. The levels of ABSO were 52, 56, 19.9 ng/mL and undetectable at 6, 12, 24, and 36 hours. The milk/serum ratios for ABZ, ABSX and ABSO were 0.9, 0.6, and 0.7. Breast milk was withheld from the participants' infants (aged 2 weeks to 6 months) in this study. The authors suggest exposure to an infant via milk would be minimal. We calculated the RIDs (using the peak concentration for each component) to be: ABZ 0.08%, ABSX 0.82%, ABSO 0.15%.

T 1/2	8-12 h	MW	265 Da	PB	70%
Tmax	2-5 h	RID	0.08%-0.82%	Vd	
Oral	Poor	M/P	0.6	pKa	

Adult Concerns: Headache, dizziness, fever, nausea, vomiting, abdominal pain, changes in liver function, pancytopenia, rash.

Adult Dose: 400 mg once to twice daily for 1-3 days (dosing varies by parasite).

Pediatric Concerns: No data are available for infant exposure via breast milk. Milk levels are unlikely to be clinically relevant. Commonly used in infants and children.

Infant Monitoring:

Alternatives: Mebendazole(L3)

References:
1. Pharmaceutical manufacturers prescribing information.
2. Abdel-tawab AM, Bradley M, Ghazaly EA, Horton J, el-Setouhy M. Albendazole and its metabolites in the breast milk of lactating women following a single oral dose of albendazole. Br J Clin Pharmacol. 2009;68(5):737-742.

ALBUTEROL

Trade: Asmavent, Asmol, Proventil, Respax, Respolin, Salamol, Salbulin, Salbuvent, Ventolin

Category: Antiasthma

LRC: L1 - No Data-Compatible

Albuterol is a very popular beta-2 adrenergic agonist that is typically used to dilate constricted bronchi in asthmatics.[1] It is active orally but is most commonly used via inhalation. When used orally, significant plasma levels are attained, and transfer to breast milk is possible. When used via inhalation, less than 10% is absorbed into maternal plasma. Small amounts are probably secreted into milk, although no reports exist. It is very unlikely that pharmacologic doses will be transferred to the infant via milk following inhaler use. However, when used orally, breast milk levels could be sufficient to produce tremors and agitation in infants. Commonly used via inhalation in treating pediatric asthma. This product is safe to use in breastfeeding mothers.

T 1/2	3.8 h	MW	239 Da	PB	36%-93%
Tmax	5-30 min	RID		Vd	2.2 L/kg
Oral	100%	M/P		pKa	10.3

Adult Concerns: Headache, dizziness, insomnia, hypertension, tachycardia, angina, dry mouth, hyperglycemia, hypokalemia, tremor.

Adult Dose: 2-4 mg TID or QID.

Pediatric Concerns: None reported via milk. Observe infant for tremors and excitement.

Infant Monitoring: Irritability, insomnia, arrhythmias, weight loss, tremor.

Alternatives:

References:
1. Pharmaceutical manufacturers prescribing information.

ALCAFTADINE OPHTHALMIC SOLUTION

Trade: Lastacaft

Category: Antihistamine

LRC: L3 - No Data-Probably Compatible

Alcaftadine is an H1 histamine receptor antagonist used for allergic conjunctivitis. Following bilateral topical ocular administration of alcaftadine ophthalmic solution, 0.25%, the mean plasma C_{max} of alcaftadine was approximately 60 pg/mL and the median T_{max} occurred at 15 minutes. Plasma concentrations of alcaftadine were below the lower limit of quantification (10 pg/mL) by 3 hours after dosing. The mean C_{max} of the active carboxylic acid metabolite was approximately 3 ng/mL and occurred at 1 hour after dosing. Plasma concentrations of the carboxylic acid metabolite were below the lower limit of quantification (100 pg/mL) by 12 hours after dosing. There was no indication of systemic accumulation or changes in plasma exposure of alcaftadine or the active metabolite following daily topical ocular administration.

While no breastfeeding studies are available, the levels in plasma are so low that milk levels would be far subclinical.

T 1/2	2 h (metabolite)	MW	307 Da	PB	40%-60%
Tmax	15 min	RID		Vd	
Oral		M/P		pKa	

Adult Concerns: Eye irritation, burning and/or stinging upon instillation, eye redness, and eye pruritus.

Adult Dose: One drop twice daily.

Pediatric Concerns: Levels in maternal plasma too low to produce clinical effects in breastfed infant.

Infant Monitoring:

Alternatives:

References:
1. Pharmaceutical manufacturers prescribing information.

ALDESLEUKIN

Trade: Proleukin

Category: Anticancer

LRC: L4 - No Data-Possibly Hazardous

Aldesleukin is a human recombinant interleukin-2 product that is administered intravenously. It is a large peptide with a molecular weight of 15,300 Da, which is unlikely to enter milk, although low levels are known to be present. It is indicated for the treatment of metastatic renal cell carcinoma and patients with malignant melanoma. Aldesleukin is known to produce multiple immunological effects, but the exact mechanism by which it mediates its antitumor activity is unknown.[1] The transfer of Aldesleukin to human milk is still not known, but IL-2 is known to transfer into human milk. Following exposure to high levels of aldesleukin, it is not known if milk levels will increase. Caution is advised when using this medication, as it is accompanied with severe adverse events. Withholding breastfeeding for 24 hours is recommended to reduce risk.

T 1/2	85 min	MW	15,300 Da	PB	
Tmax		RID		Vd	
Oral		M/P		pKa	

Adult Concerns: Confusion, somnolence, fever, hypotension, arrhythmias, shortness of breath, diarrhea, vomiting, anorexia or weight gain, changes in renal function, thrombocytopenia, anemia, hyperbilirubinemia, and rash.

Adult Dose: 0.037 mg/kg every 8 hours.

Pediatric Concerns: None reported in the literature at this time.

Infant Monitoring: Drowsiness, lethargy, pallor, vomiting, diarrhea, weight gain. Recommend to avoid breastfeeding for 24 hours following use.

Alternatives:

References:
1. Pharmaceutical manufacturers prescribing information.

ALEFACEPT

Trade: Amevive

Category: Antipsoriatic

LRC: L3 - No Data-Probably Compatible

Alefacept is an immunosuppressant used in the treatment of chronic plaque psoriasis. It binds to the lymphocyte antigen CD2, thus inhibiting the LFA-3/CD2 interaction.[1] Although levels in milk have not been determined, its transfer to the milk compartment is highly unlikely due to its enormous molecular size (94,000 Da). Furthermore, due to low oral bioavailability, even if present in milk, it would be unabsorbed in an infant.

T 1/2	270 h	MW	91,400 Da	PB	
Tmax		RID		Vd	0.094 L/kg
Oral	63%	M/P		pKa	

Adult Concerns: Lymphopenia, malignancies, infections, and hypersensitivity.

Adult Dose: 7.5 mg IV weekly.

Pediatric Concerns: No data are available, but it is unlikely to transfer to milk.

Infant Monitoring:

Alternatives:

References:

1. Pharmaceutical manufacturers prescribing information.

ALEMTUZUMAB

Trade: Campath, MabCampath, Lemtrada

Category: Antineoplastic

LRC: L4 - No Data-Possibly Hazardous

Alemtuzumab is a recombinant DNA-derived humanized monoclonal antibody that is directed against specific cell receptors on leukemic cells.[1] It is indicated for treatment of chronic B-cell lymphocytic leukemia and is being investigated for possible use in multiple sclerosis. It is a large IgG1 antibody with a molecular weight of 150,000 Da. No data are available on its transfer to human milk, but it is very unlikely to enter milk, due to its large size.

Although the molecular weight of this medication is very large and the amount in breast milk is expected to be exceptionally low, there are no long-term data concerning the safety of using immune modulating medications in breastfeeding mothers. Further there are current data that suggest that some monoclonal antibody drugs do transfer to milk, and perhaps the breastfed infant. Therefore, some caution is recommended, and each woman should understand the benefits and risk of using this type of medication in lactation.

T 1/2	6 days	MW	150,000 Da	PB	
Tmax		RID		Vd	0.18 L/kg
Oral	Nil	M/P		pKa	

Adult Concerns: Headache, fever, fatigue, anxiety, insomnia, tachycardia, hyper or hypotension, dyspnea, vomiting, diarrhea, pruritus, rash, rigors, infusion reactions, cytopenias, and an elevated risk of infections. The FDA just issued a warning concerning a higher rate of ischemic and hemorrhagic stroke and cervicocephalic arterial dissection associated with alemtuzumab. In the nearly 5 years since the agency approved alemtuzumab for relapsing forms of multiple sclerosis (MS), such cases have been reported to the FDA.

Adult Dose: 30 mg IV infusion three times a week on alternate days (max 12 weeks).

Pediatric Concerns: None reported via milk at this time. Safety data are not available in the pediatric population at this time.

Infant Monitoring: Drowsiness, or insomnia, vomiting, poor feeding, weight gain, frequent infections.

Alternatives:

References:

1. Pharmaceutical manufacturers prescribing information.

ALENDRONATE SODIUM

Trade: Fosamax

Category: Calcium Regulator

LRC: L3 - No Data-Probably Compatible

Alendronate is a specific inhibitor of osteoclast-mediated bone resorption, thus reducing bone loss and bone turnover.[1] It is indicated for use in osteoporosis and Paget's disease of the bone. While incorporated in bone matrix, it is not pharmacologically active. Because concentrations in plasma are too low to be detected (<5 ng/mL), it is very unlikely that it would be secreted into human milk in clinically relevant concentrations. Concentrations in human milk have not been reported. Because this product has exceedingly poor oral bioavailability, particularly when ingested with milk, it is very unlikely that alendronate would be orally absorbed by a breastfeeding infant.

T 1/2	<3 h (plasma)	MW	325 Da	PB	78%
Tmax		RID		Vd	0.4 L/kg
Oral	<0.7%	M/P		pKa	1.45

Adult Concerns: Headache, abdominal pain, nausea, dyspepsia, acid regurgitation, constipation, hypophosphatemia, hypocalcemia, muscle cramps. There are a number of case reports of osteonecrosis of the jaw, esophagitis and esophageal ulceration in patients taking alendronate.

Adult Dose: 10 mg daily.

Pediatric Concerns: None reported via milk.

Infant Monitoring: Vomiting, reflux, constipation.

Alternatives:

References:
1. Pharmaceutical manufacturers prescribing information.

ALFENTANIL

Trade: Alfenta, Rapifen

Category: Analgesic

LRC: L2 - Limited Data-Probably Compatible

Alfentanil is an opiate used for pain relief during delivery and induction, and maintenance of analgesia during surgery. Alfentanil is secreted into human milk. Following a dose of 50 µg/kg IV (plus several additional 10 µg/kg doses during the procedure), the mean level of alfentanil in colostrum at 4 hours was 0.88 µg/L (range 0.21 to 1.56 µg/L), a level probably too small to produce overt toxicity in a breastfeeding infant.[1] The mean level 28 hours post alfentanil administration was 0.05 µg/L (range 0 to 0.26 µg/L).

T 1/2	1-2 h	MW	417 Da	PB	92%
Tmax	Immediate	RID	0.26%-0.4%	Vd	0.3-1 L/kg
Oral	43%	M/P		pKa	6.5

Adult Concerns: Observe for bradycardia, shivering, constipation, and sedation. In neonates observe for severe hypotension.

Adult Dose: 8-40 µg/kg IV (total dose).

Pediatric Concerns: None reported via milk.

Infant Monitoring: Sedation, slowed breathing rate, pallor, constipation, and appropriate weight gain.

Alternatives: Remifentanil(L3), Fentanyl(L2)

References:
1. Giesecke A, Rice L, Lipton J. Alfentanil in colostrum. Anesthesiology. 1985;63:A284.
2. Spigset O. Anaesthetic agents and excretion in breast milk. Acta Anaesthesiol Scand. 1994;38(2):94-103.

ALFUZOSIN

Trade: Uroxatral

Category: Alpha-Adrenergic Blocker

LRC: L4 - No Data-Possibly Hazardous

Alfuzosin is not approved for use in women, but is used in men for benign prostatic hyperplasia. It is occasionally used in women to assist in the passage of a kidney stone or for bladder motility problems. It works by antagonizing the alpha-1 adrenoreceptors, thus reducing ureter contractility. There are no data regarding alfuzosin transfer to breast milk. However, due to possibility of hypotension in the infant, breastfeeding while taking alfuzosin is not recommended.

T 1/2	10 h	MW	389 Da	PB	82%-90%
Tmax	8 h	RID		Vd	3.2 L/kg
Oral	49%	M/P		pKa	

Adult Concerns: Postural hypotension, syncope, dizziness, fatigue, constipation, abdominal pain, nausea, bronchitis, upper respiratory track infection.

Adult Dose: 10 mg once daily.

Pediatric Concerns:

Infant Monitoring: Drowsiness, low blood pressure, lethargy, pallor, poor feeding, and weight gain.

Alternatives:

References:
1. Pharmaceutical manufacturer prescribing information.

ALIROCUMAB

Trade: Praluent

Category: Monoclonal Antibody

LRC: L3 - No Data-Probably Compatible

Alirocumab is a monoclonal antibody used in combination with a statin medication to treat specific types of hyperlipidemia.[1] At this time there are no data regarding the transfer of this medication into human milk. Based on this medications large molecular weight, it is unlikely to enter milk in clinically relevant concentrations. The low oral bioavailability of this protein also suggests little absorption in the infant's gut. In addition, the manufacturer reports that although human IgG is present in milk, IgG antibodies do not appear to enter the infants circulation in clinically relevant amounts.

Despite the fact that the molecular weight of this medication is very large and the amount in breast milk is expected to be exceptionally low, there are no long-term data concerning the safety of using immune modulating medications in breastfeeding mothers. Further there are current data that suggest that other IgG drugs do transfer to milk, and perhaps the breastfed infant. Therefore, some caution is recommended, especially in the colostral phase. Each woman should understand the benefits and risk of using this type of medication in lactation.

T 1/2	17-20 days	MW	146,000 Da	PB	
Tmax	3-7 days	RID		Vd	0.04-0.05 L/kg
Oral	Nil	M/P		pKa	

Adult Concerns: Confusion, changes in memory, diarrhea, liver changes, myalgia, muscle spasms, influenza, infusion reactions, immunogenicity, hypersensitivity reactions.

Adult Dose: 75 mg subcutaneously once every 2 weeks.

Pediatric Concerns: At this time there are no lactation or pediatric safety data available.

Infant Monitoring: Diarrhea, poor feeding/poor weight gain. Based on clinical symptoms some infants may require monitoring of their liver enzymes.

Alternatives:

References:
1. Pharmaceutical manufacturer product monograph.

ALISKIREN

Trade: Tekturna, Tekturna HCT, Valturna

Category: Antihypertensive

LRC: L3 - No Data-Probably Compatible

Aliskiren is a direct renin inhibitor, blocking the formation of angiotensin II and thus decreasing blood pressure.[1] No data are available on its transfer into human milk. However, due to its high molecular weight and low oral absorption (3%), it is unlikely that an infant would absorb enough to receive a therapeutic dose from breast milk. Aliskiren should be avoided while breastfeeding premature infants, as the nephrons of the kidney are undeveloped. A risk versus benefit analysis should be conducted in each individual until lactation data are available. Other blood pressure medications with lactation data would be preferred (e.g., ramipril, captopril, nifedipine).

T 1/2	24 h	MW	609.8 Da	PB	47%-51%
Tmax	1-3 h	RID		Vd	
Oral	3%	M/P		pKa	14.56

Adult Concerns: Dizziness, hypotension, diarrhea, increased serum creatinine and BUN and creatine kinase, hyperkalemia, rash.

Adult Dose: 150-300 mg/day.

Pediatric Concerns: No data are available in lactation or pediatrics at this time.

Infant Monitoring: Drowsiness, lethargy, pallor, poor feeding, and weight gain.

Alternatives: Ramipril(L3), Captopril(L2), Enalapril(L2), Labetalol(L2), Nifedipine(L2)

References:
1. Pharmaceutical manufacturers prescribing information.

ALLERGY INJECTIONS

Trade:

Category: Other

LRC: L3 - No Data-Probably Compatible

Allergy injections consist of protein and carbohydrate substances from plants, animals, and other species. There are no reported untoward effects. They are unlikely to enter milk. Observe for allergic reactions, although adverse effects are unlikely in the breastfed infant.

Adult Concerns: Allergic pruritus, anaphylaxis, other immune reactions.

Adult Dose:

Pediatric Concerns: None reported in breastfeeding mothers.

Infant Monitoring:

Alternatives:

References:

ALLOPURINOL

Trade: Alloprin, Allorin, Aluline, Lopurin, Caplenal, Capurate, Cosuric, Zygout, Zyloprim, Zyloric

Category: Antigout

LRC: L2 - Limited Data-Probably Compatible

Allopurinol is a potent antagonist of xanthine oxidase, an enzyme involved in the production of uric acid. It is used in the treatment of gout to reduce uric acid levels. In a nursing mother receiving 300 mg/day allopurinol, the breast milk concentration at 2 and 4 hours was 0.9 and 1.4 µg/mL respectively.[1] The concentration of the metabolite, oxypurinol, was 53.7 and 48.0 µg/mL at 2 and 4 hours respectively. The milk/plasma ratio ranged from 0.9 to 1.4 for allopurinol and 3.9 for its metabolite, oxypurinol. The average daily dose that an infant would receive from milk would be approximately 0.14-0.2 mg/kg of allopurinol and 7.2-8 mg/kg of oxypurinol. No adverse effects were noted in the infant after 6 weeks of therapy.

T 1/2	1-3 h (allopurinol)	MW	136 Da	PB	0%
Tmax	2-6 h	RID	4.9%	Vd	1.6 L/kg
Oral	90%	M/P	0.9-1.4	pKa	9.4

Adult Concerns: Diarrhea, nausea, changes in liver function, skin rash.

Adult Dose: 100-400 mg BID.

Pediatric Concerns: No adverse effects were noted in one infant after 6 weeks of therapy.

Infant Monitoring: Vomiting, diarrhea.

Alternatives:

References:
1. Kamilli I, Gresser U. Allopurinol and oxypurinol in human breast milk. Clin Investig. February 1993;71(2):161-164.

ALMOTRIPTAN

Trade: Axert

Category: Antimigraine

LRC: L3 - No Data-Probably Compatible

Almotriptan is a 5-HT1B/1D/1F (serotonin) receptor agonist used to treat migraine headaches.[1] Activating these receptors is believed to constrict cranial blood vessels and block the release of pro-inflammatory neuropeptides from the trigeminal nerve. The oral bioavailability of almotriptan (70%) has not been found to be affected by the presence of a migraine and is about five times greater than sumatriptan (14%).

No studies examining almotriptan secretion into human milk or adverse effects in infants have been published. Some transfer is likely based on this medications size and low protein binding; however, the clinical significance of this is unknown. Consider sumatriptan as the preferred alternative.

T 1/2	3-4 h	MW	469.56 Da	PB	35%
Tmax	1-3 h	RID		Vd	2.85 L/kg
Oral	70%	M/P		pKa	8.77

Adult Concerns: Dizziness, drowsiness, flushing, hot tingling sensations, dry mouth, chest pain, arrhythmias, hypertension, nausea, vomiting, weakness, paresthesia.

Adult Dose: 6.25-12.5 mg orally, may repeat in 2 hours if needed.

Pediatric Concerns: None reported via milk at this time.

Infant Monitoring: Drowsiness, vomiting, poor feeding.

Alternatives: Sumatriptan(L3), NSAIDs, Acetaminophen(L1)

References:
1. Pharmaceutical manufacturers prescribing information.

ALOE VERA

Trade:

Category: Wound Care Agent

LRC: L3 - No Data-Probably Compatible

There are over 500 species of aloe.[1,2] The aloe plant yields two important products: aloe latex derived from the outer skin and aloe gel, a clear, gelatinous material derived from the inner leaf tissue. Aloe gel is commonly used in cosmetics, health food products and topically for minor burns and skin irritation. The gel contains minerals, vitamins, polysaccharides, organic acids, enzymes, and other products that are thought to relieve pain, decrease inflammation and itch. Thus far, the evidence regarding the efficacy of aloe vera is controversial.[3,4] Aloe latex, a bitter yellow product from the outer skin produces a strong laxative effect and may cause severe gastric cramping; aloe latex is not recommended for oral use in pregnant or breastfeeding women and children.[2]

Maternal use of aloe vera topically is probably suitable during lactation if used for a short period of time.

Adult Concerns: Severe gastric irritation, strong purgative effect and diarrhea when used orally.

Adult Dose:

Pediatric Concerns: No reports of untoward effects following exposure in milk at this time.

Infant Monitoring: Vomiting, diarrhea.

Alternatives:

References:
1. Review of Natural Products. St. Louis, MO: Facts and Comparisons; 1997.
2. Leung AY. Encyclopedia of Common Natural Ingredients Used in Food, Drugs and Cosmetics. Hoboken, NJ: John Wiley and Sons; 1980.
3. Fulton JE Jr. The stimulation of postdermabrasion wound healing with stabilized aloe vera gel-polyethylene oxide dressing. J Dermatol Surg Oncol. 1990;16(5):460-467.
4. Schmidt JM, Greenspoon JS. Aloe vera dermal wound gel is associated with a delay in wound healing. Obstet Gynecol. 1991;78(1):115-117.

ALOSETRON

Trade: Lotronex

Category: Antidiarrheal

LRC: L3 - No Data-Probably Compatible

Alosetron is a new 5-HT3 receptor antagonist that is used to control the symptoms of irritable bowel syndrome. No data are available on the transfer of this medication into human milk. While the manufacturer suggests it is present in animal milk, no data are provided.[1] The peak plasma levels (in young women) of this product are quite small, only averaging 9 ng/mL following a 1 mg dose. While the half-life of the parent alosetron is short (1.5 hours), its metabolites have much longer half-lives, although their importance is unknown. Bioavailability is lessened (<25%) when mixed with food. With this data, it is unlikely milk levels will be extraordinarily high, or that the infant will be exposed to clinically relevant drug levels. However, use of alosetron in breastfeeding patients should be approached with caution until we have more clinical experience with this new product.

T 1/2	1.5 h	MW	294 Da	PB	82%
Tmax	1 hour	RID		Vd	1.36 L/kg
Oral	50%-60%	M/P		pKa	

Adult Concerns: Headache, fatigue, vomiting, constipation.

Adult Dose: 1 mg twice daily.

Pediatric Concerns: None reported via milk, but no studies exist.

Infant Monitoring: Drowsiness, vomiting, and constipation.

Alternatives:

References:
1. Pharmaceutical manufacturers prescribing information.

ALPRAZOLAM

Trade: Kalma, Ralozam, Xanax

Category: Antianxiety

LRC: L3 - Limited Data-Probably Compatible

Alprazolam is a prototypic benzodiazepine drug similar to valium but is now preferred in many instances because of its shorter half-life. In a study of eight women who received a single oral dose of 0.5 mg, the peak alprazolam level in milk was 3.7 µg/L, which occurred at 1.1 hours; the observed milk/serum ratio (using AUC method) was 0.36.[1] The neonatal dose of alprazolam in breast milk is low. The author estimates the average between 0.3 to 5 µg/kg per day. While the infants in this study did not breastfeed, these doses would probably be too low to induce a clinical effect. In a brief letter, Anderson reports that the manufacturer is aware of withdrawal symptoms in infants following exposure in utero and via breast milk.[2] In a mother who received 0.5 mg 2-3 times daily orally during pregnancy, neonatal withdrawal syndrome was evident in the breastfed infant the first week postpartum. These data suggest that the amount of alprazolam in breast milk is insufficient to prevent a withdrawal syndrome following prenatal exposure. In another case of infant exposure solely via breast milk, the mother took alprazolam (dosage unspecified) for 9 months while breastfeeding and withdrew herself from the medication over a 3 week period. The mother reported withdrawal symptoms in the infant including irritability, crying, and sleep disturbances. The benzodiazepine family, as a rule, is not ideal for breastfeeding mothers due to relatively long half-lives and the development of dependence. However, it is apparent that the shorter-acting benzodiazepines are safest during lactation provided their use is short-term or intermittent, and at a low dose.[3]

T 1/2	12-15 h	MW	309 Da	PB	80%
Tmax	1-2 h	RID	8.5%	Vd	0.9-1.2 L/kg
Oral	90%	M/P	0.36	pKa	2.8

Adult Concerns: Drowsiness, fatigue, sedation, confusion, dry mouth, constipation, abnormal coordination.

Adult Dose: 0.5-1 mg three times a day.

Pediatric Concerns: Rarely, withdrawal syndrome reported in one breastfed infant.

Infant Monitoring: Sedation, slowed breathing rate, not waking to feed/poor feeding, and weight gain.

Alternatives: Lorazepam(L3), Midazolam(L2), Oxazepam(L2)

References:

1. Oo CY, Kuhn RJ, Desai N, Wright CE, McNamara PJ. Pharmacokinetics in lactating women: prediction of alprazolam transfer into milk. Br J Clin Pharmacol. 1995;40(3):231-236.
2. Anderson PO, McGuire GG. Neonatal alprazolam withdrawal—possible effects of breast feeding. DICP. 1989;23(7-8):614.
3. Maitra R, Menkes DB. Psychotropic drugs and lactation. N Z Med J. 1996;109(1024):217-218.

ALTEPLASE

Trade: Actilyse, Activase

Category: Thrombolytic

LRC: L3 - No Data-Probably Compatible

Alteplase is a thrombolytic agent commonly known as tissue-type plasminogen activator (tPA).[1,2] Alteplase is a large protein with 527 amino acids and with a large molecular weight. It binds to fibrin in a thrombus and converts the plasminogen to plasmin, which subsequently leads to a breakdown of the clot. Alteplase is rapidly cleared from the plasma, with an initial half-life of 5 minutes following rapid IV therapy and a somewhat longer half-life of 26-46 minutes following prolonged infusion. Its transfer into mature milk it expected to be negligible, but it could potentially pass in small amounts into colostrum. Significant amounts of endogenous tPA are naturally secreted into the milk compartment where it helps to maintain patency of the ducts.[3] Whether it would be bioavailable in the gut of a newborn infant is questionable, but it would almost certainly not be bioavailable in an older infant. It is very unlikely it would produce adverse effects in breastfed infants.

T 1/2	5 min	MW	59,000 Da	PB	
Tmax	20-40 min	RID		Vd	Approximates plasma volume L/kg
Oral	Nil	M/P		pKa	

Adult Concerns: Fever, hypotension, arrhythmias, nausea, vomiting, bruising, hemorrhage.

Adult Dose: 100 mg IV (dose depends on indication).

Pediatric Concerns: None reported.

Infant Monitoring: Bruising on the skin, blood in urine, vomit, or stool.

Alternatives:

References:

1. Pharmaceutical manufacturers prescribing information.
2. Verstraete M, Su CA, Tanswell P, Feuerer W, Collen D. Pharmacokinetics and effects on fibrinolytic and coagulation parameters of two doses of recombinant tissue-type plasminogen activator in healthy volunteers. Thromb Haemost. 1986;56(1):1-5.
3. Heegaard CW, Larsen LB, Rasmussen LK, Højberg KE, Petersen TE, Andreasen PA. Plasminogen activation system in human milk. J Pediatr Gastroenterol Nutr. 1997;25(2):159-166.

ALTRETAMINE

Trade: Hexalen

Category: Antineoplastic

LRC: L4 - No Data-Possibly Hazardous

Used to treat ovarian, breast, cervix, pancreatic, and other cancers, altretamine requires metabolism to the cytotoxic derivative. While it is well absorbed orally, its oral bioavailability is low, due to first pass metabolism and uptake by the liver. Its usefulness is limited by its toxicity. Following oral administration of radiolabeled altretamine, urinary recovery of radioactivity was 61% at 24 hours and 90% at 72 hours.[1] Human urinary metabolites were N-demethylated homologues of altretamine with <1% unmetabolized altretamine excreted at 24 hours. No data on entry into human milk are available. Withhold breastfeeding for at least 72 hours.

T 1/2	4.7-10.5 h	MW	210.3 Da	PB	94%
Tmax	0.5-3 h	RID		Vd	
Oral		M/P		pKa	

Adult Concerns: Anxiety, clumsiness, confusion, seizures, dizziness, mental depression, numbness in arms or legs, weakness, nausea, vomiting.

Adult Dose: 260 mg/m^2/day in four divided doses.

Pediatric Concerns:

Infant Monitoring: Withhold breastfeeding for 72 hours.

Alternatives:

References:
1. Pharmaceutical manufacturers prescribing information.

ALVIMOPAN

Trade: Entereg

Category: Opioid Antagonist

LRC: L3 - No Data-Probably Compatible

Alvimopan is a peripherally acting μ-opioid receptor antagonist indicated to accelerate the time to upper and lower gastrointestinal recovery following partial large or small bowel resection surgery with primary anastomosis.[1] No data are available on its transfer into human milk. However, adult plasma levels are incredibly low, the oral bioavailability is low, and the molecular weight is slightly high, so milk levels are anticipated to be quite low.

T 1/2	10-17 h	MW	460 Da	PB	80%-94%
Tmax	2 h	RID		Vd	0.42 L/kg
Oral	6%	M/P		pKa	9.75

Adult Concerns: Anemia, constipation, dyspepsia, flatulence, hypokalemia, back pain, and urinary retention.

Adult Dose: 12 mg BID.

Pediatric Concerns: None yet reported via milk.

Infant Monitoring: Constipation, flatulence, urinary retention.

Alternatives:

References:
1. Pharmaceutical manufacturers prescribing information.

AMANTADINE

Trade: Endantanine, Mantadine, Symadine, Symmetrel

Category: Antiviral

LRC: L3 - No Data-Probably Compatible

Amantadine is a unique compound that is effective in treating Parkinsonian symptoms and has antiviral activity against influenza A.[1] This medication has FDA approval for prevention and treatment of influenza in adults and pediatrics (ages 1-10); however, due to the increasing resistance of the influenza A virus to amantadine, its use is no longer recommended by the CDC.[2] Only trace amounts are believed to be secreted in milk although no reports are found. Adult plasma levels following doses of 200 mg daily are 400-900 ng/mL.[3] Even assuming a theoretical milk/plasma ratio of 1, the average daily dose to a breastfeeding infant would be far less than 0.9 mg, a dose that would be clinically irrelevant compared to the 5 mg/kg dose previously used in 1-year-old infants. However, amantadine is known to suppress prolactin production and should not be used in breastfeeding mothers or at least should be used with caution while observing for milk suppression.[4,5]

T 1/2	1-28 h	MW	151 Da	PB	67%
Tmax	1-4 h	RID		Vd	4.4 L/kg
Oral	86%-94%	M/P		pKa	10.71

Adult Concerns: Agitation, insomnia, confusion, depression, nausea, vomiting, constipation, urinary retention, anorexia, skin rash.

Adult Dose: 100 mg BID.

Pediatric Concerns: None reported via milk at this time.

Infant Monitoring: Can reduce breast milk production-not recommended in lactation.

Alternatives: Oseltamivir(L2), Zanamivir(L2)

References:
1. Pharmaceutical manufacturers prescribing information.
2. Centers for Disease Control. Influenza antiviral medications: summary for clinicians. https://www.cdc.gov/flu/professionals/antivirals/summary-clinicians.htm.
3. Cedarbaum JM. Clinical pharmacokinetics of anti-parkinsonian drugs. Clin Pharmacokinet. 1987;13(3):141-178.
4. Correa N, Opler LA, Kay SR, Birmaher B. Amantadine in the treatment of neuroendocrine side effects of neuroleptics. J Clin Psychopharmacol. 1987;7(2):91-95.
5. Siever LJ. The effect of amantadine on prolactin levels and galactorrhea on neuroleptic-treated patients. J Clin Psychopharmacol. 1981;1(1):2-7.

AMBRISENTAN

Trade: Letairis

Category: Antihypertensive

LRC: L4 - No Data-Possibly Hazardous

Ambrisentan is an antihypertensive indicated in the treatment of pulmonary hypertension.[1] It is an endothelin receptor antagonist that blocks vasoconstriction and cell proliferation. It works on vascular smooth muscles and endothelium of blood vessels, and hence decreases right atrial pressure in patients with pulmonary arterial hypertension.

It is not known if ambrisentan is excreted into human milk. Ambrisentan's low pKa (4) and high protein binding (99%) suggest that milk levels will probably be low. However, caution is advised until data are available regarding transfer to human milk, due to the potential for serious adverse effects in nursing infants.

T 1/2	9 h	MW	378.4 Da	PB	99%
Tmax	2 h	RID		Vd	
Oral	Unknown	M/P		pKa	4

Adult Concerns: Headache, dizziness, flushing, heart failure, palpitations, dyspepsia, constipation, anemia, peripheral edema.

Adult Dose: 5-10 mg daily.

Pediatric Concerns: None have been published.

Infant Monitoring: Drowsiness, lethargy, pallor, poor feeding, and weight gain.

Alternatives:

References:
1. Pharmaceutical manufacturers prescribing information.

AMIKACIN

Trade: Amikin

Category: Antibiotic, Aminoglycoside

LRC: L2 - Limited Data-Probably Compatible

Amikacin is a typical aminoglycoside antibiotic used for gram-negative infections. Other aminoglycoside antibiotics are poorly absorbed from the gastrointestinal tract in infants, although they could produce changes in the gastrointestinal flora. Only very small amounts are secreted into breast milk. Following 100 and 200 mg IM doses, only trace amounts have been found in breast milk in only two of four patients studied.[1] In another study of two to three patients who received 100 mg IM, undetectable to trace amounts were found in milk.[2]

T 1/2	2.3 h	MW	586 Da	PB	4%
Tmax	0.75-2 h	RID		Vd	0.28 L/kg
Oral	Poor	M/P		pKa	12.1

Adult Concerns: Ototoxicity, nausea, vomiting, diarrhea, changes in renal function.

Adult Dose: 5-7.5 mg/kg/dose TID.

Pediatric Concerns: None reported via milk. Commonly used in neonates.

Infant Monitoring: Vomiting, diarrhea, changes in gastrointestinal flora, and rash.

Alternatives: Gentamicin(L2)

References:
1. Matsuda S, Mori S, Tanno M, Kashiwagura T. [Evaluation of amikacin in obstetric and gynecological fields (author's transl)]. Jpn J Antibiot. October 1974;27(5):633-636.
2. Matsuda S. Transfer of antibiotics into maternal milk. Biol Res Pregnancy Perinatol. 1984;5(2):57-60.

AMILORIDE

Trade: Midamor

Category: Diuretic

LRC: L3 - No Data-Probably Compatible

Amiloride is a potassium-sparing diuretic agent used in the management of hypertension and congestive heart failure.[1] It is usually administered along with thiazide diuretics. Studies in rats have shown that the concentrations of amiloride in milk are higher than those in plasma. It is not known if amiloride is transferred to human milk, but a review of the drug's pharmacokinetic profile suggests that transfer to milk is likely. Due to the potential of untoward effects in the breastfed infant with its use, this drug is best avoided in breastfeeding mothers. Use in lactating mothers only if the potential benefit to the mother outweighs the potential risks to the infant.

T 1/2	6-9 h	MW	302.12 Da	PB	Not significant
Tmax	3-4 h	RID		Vd	5-5.4 L/kg
Oral	30%-90%	M/P		pKa	8.7

Adult Concerns: Headache, dizziness, nausea, vomiting, diarrhea, hyponatremia, hyperkalemia.

Adult Dose: 5-20 mg once daily.

Pediatric Concerns: None reported via milk at this time.

Infant Monitoring: Observe for changes in feeding, dehydration, lethargy, weight gain.

Alternatives: Spironolactone(L2)

References:
1. Pharmaceutical manufacturers prescribing information.

AMINOCAPROIC ACID

Trade: Amicar

Category: Hemostatic

LRC: L4 - No Data-Possibly Hazardous

Aminocaproic acid is an antifibrinolytic agent used in prevention of bleeding with cardiac surgery, bleeding disorders, or in patients who are currently on anticoagulant therapies.[1,2] It also prevents spontaneous fibrinolysis. There are no data on its transfer into human milk. If we were to assume a 1 to 1 milk/plasma ratio (which is probably high), and a normal maternal therapeutic plasma range of 130 µg/mL, then milk levels would be 130 µg/mL, with a relative infant dose of 19%. While high, this is very unlikely. Use caution. Observe the infant closely during therapy.

T 1/2	2 h	MW	131 Da	PB	
Tmax	2 h	RID		Vd	Oral: 0.32 L/kg
Oral	Complete	M/P		pKa	4.4

Adult Concerns: Headache, confusion, dizziness, fatigue, tinnitus, changes in vision, arrhythmias, hypotension, vomiting, diarrhea, anorexia, changes in renal function, agranulocytosis, increased bleeding time, myalgia.

Adult Dose: 50-100 mg/kg but variable.

Pediatric Concerns: None reported via milk at this time.

Infant Monitoring: Drowsiness, lethargy, vomiting, diarrhea, changes in feeding.

Alternatives:

References:
1. Lexi-Comp Online, Lexi-Drugs Online, Hudson, OH: Lexi-Comp, Inc.; July 11, 2011.
2. McAuley DF. The clinician's ultimate reference. http://www.globalrph.com/aminocaproic_acid_dilution.htm. Updated July 25, 2010. Accessed July 12, 2009.

AMINOLEVULINIC ACID

Trade: Levulan Kerastick

Category: Photosensitizing Agent

LRC: L3 - No Data-Probably Compatible

Aminolevulinic acid is used to treat minimally to moderately thick keratoses. It is a metabolic precursor of the pro-toporphyrin IX, which is a photosensitizer. Upon stimulation with light, accumulated protoporphyrin forms free radicals that work to break down thick keratoses.[1] However, when applied topically the transcutaneous absorption of this product is minimal to nil. Milk levels, although unreported, are likely to be nil.

T 1/2	0.7 h	MW	168 Da	PB	
Tmax		RID		Vd	
Oral	50%-60% (oral)	M/P		pKa	4.05

Adult Concerns: Burning, itching, redness, and swelling.

Adult Dose: Apply topically followed 14-18 hours later by blue light illumination.

Pediatric Concerns: No data are available, but milk levels are likely to be minimal to nil.

Infant Monitoring:

Alternatives:

References:
1. Pharmaceutical manufacturers prescribing information.

AMIODARONE

Trade: Aratac, Cordarone

Category: Antiarrhythmic

LRC: L5 - Limited Data-Hazardous

Amiodarone is a potent antiarrhythmic drug that requires close supervision by clinicians as it has numerous serious adverse effects.[1] Although poorly absorbed by the mother (35%-65%), maximum serum levels are attained after 3-7 hours. This drug has a very large volume of distribution, resulting in accumulation in the liver, spleen, lungs, and the adipose tissue.

A woman taking amiodarone 400 mg daily throughout pregnancy and lactation was followed for 2 months post-partum.[2] Milk samples were drawn on day 1, 4, 7, 14, and 31 postpartum. The concentrations of amiodarone and desethylamiodarone (active metabolite) in milk ranged from 1.06-3.65 mg/L and 0.5 to 1.24 mg/L, respectively. The highest levels correspond with a relative infant dose of about 9.6%. In this case the child was euthyroid and no concerns with goiter, growth, or corneal deposits were found.

Pitcher et al. reported amiodarone concentrations in milk from a woman receiving amiodarone 600 mg daily at 37 weeks, 400 mg daily at 36 weeks and 200 mg daily at 39 weeks.[3] In samples taken on the second and third day postpartum the concentrations of amiodarone and desethylamiodarone in milk ranged from 0.5 to 1.8 mg/L and 0.4 to 0.8 mg/L, respectively. In this case, the patient chose not to breastfeed her infant.

In one publication, the amount of drug secreted into breast milk was higher than the maternal plasma levels.[4] Breast milk samples obtained from birth to 3 weeks postpartum in two patients, receiving amiodarone 200 mg daily, contained levels of amiodarone and desethylamiodarone ranging 1.7 to 3.04 mg/L and 0.75 to 1.81 mg/L, respectively. In a third patient receiving amiodarone 200 mg/day in pregnancy and for one week postpartum, milk samples were checked at week 4 and 6 after delivery. The concentrations of amiodarone and desethylamiodarone in milk declined from 0.55 to 0.03 mg/L and 0.44 to 0.002 mg/L, respectively. Despite the concentrations of amiodarone in milk, the amounts were apparently not high enough to produce infant plasma levels higher than about 0.03 mg/L of amiodarone, which were minimal compared to the maternal plasma levels of 0.13 to 0.66 mg/L of amiodarone. In one case where an infant was exposed to the medication in pregnancy and lactation, the infant was hypothyroid at day 9 of life. Because this persisted at day 24 of life, the infant was initiated on treatment and breastfeeding was stopped at 5 weeks.

McKenna et al. reported amiodarone milk levels in a mother treated with 400 mg daily.[5] In this study, at 6 weeks postpartum, breast milk levels of amiodarone and desethylamiodarone varied during the day from 2.8-16.4 mg/L and 1.1-6.5 mg/L respectively. Reported infant plasma levels of amiodarone and desethylamiodarone were 0.4 mg/L and 0.25 mg/L respectively. The dose ingested by the infant was approximately 1.5 mg/kg/day. The authors suggest that the amount of amiodarone ingested was moderate and could expose the developing infant to a significant dose of the drug and should be avoided.

In another case, a woman took 200 mg of amiodarone twice daily to treat fetal ascites and tachycardia.[6] Upon delivery, the mother stopped taking amiodarone. Her breast milk was tested and the amiodarone levels in milk were 0.6 mg/L, 2.1 mg/L, and undetectable on days 5, 11, and 25, respectively. The baby was monitored closely during this lactation period and thyroid function was reported as normal.

Khurana et al. published a case report of a woman started on an IV amiodarone infusion a few hours after delivery until 6 days postpartum (total 7.6 g given IV) for a cardiac condition diagnosed around the time of delivery.[7] The patient was also given two oral doses of amiodarone 200 mg on day 6 and 7 postpartum. The patient manually expressed and discarded her milk until her care providers were able to assess her new medication in milk. Samples were initially taken on day 18 postpartum (11 days after the last dose); the estimated infant dose was 1.81 mg or 0.72 mg/kg/day. A subsequent sample was drawn 5 days later and the estimated infant dose was 0.32 mg/kg/day. In this case report the infant was never given any maternal milk.

In a more recent case report of a breastfeeding mother who received a single intravenous dose of 450 mg, milk levels peaked at day 4 at 233 µg/L.[8] Milk to plasma ratio was reported at 3.5 at this time. Levels in milk were still detectable on day 10 at 132 µg/L. The authors calculated the maximum relative infant dose at 0.6%. This dose is far less than used clinically in an infant.

Although not demonstrated in the data above, amiodarone concentrations could theoretically accumulate in the infant with ongoing maternal use because of its long half-life and distribution in various organs.[2-8] This product should only be used under rare conditions when other alternative therapies are not appropriate. If used briefly (3-7 days) a 24-48 hour interruption is recommended before re-instating breastfeeding; the infant should be closely monitored for cardiovascular and thyroid function. Breastfeeding is not recommended if this product is used chronically.

T 1/2	26-107 days	MW	645 Da	PB	96%
Tmax	3-7 h	RID	0.54%-43.1%	Vd	18-148 L/kg
Oral	35%-65%	M/P	4.6-13	pKa	6.6

Adult Concerns: Headache, insomnia, malaise, altered sense of smell, hypothyroidism and hyperthyroidism, hypotension, arrhythmias, heart failure, pulmonary toxicity, anorexia, nausea, vomiting, serious liver injury, tremor, abnormal gait, blue-gray skin pigmentation.

Adult Dose: 200-800 mg once to twice daily (variable based on indication).

Pediatric Concerns: Hypothyroidism has been reported in one case with exposure in utero and breast milk.[4]

Infant Monitoring: Drowsiness, lethargy, pallor, changes in feeding, or weight gain. Based on clinical symptoms some infants may require monitoring of thyroid or liver function.

Alternatives: Disopyramide(L2), Mexiletine(L2)

References:

1. Pharmaceutical manufacturers prescribing information.
2. Strunge P, Frandsen J, Andreasen F, et al. Amiodarone during pregnancy. Eur Heart J. 1988;9:106-109.
3. Pitcher D, Leather HM, Storey GCA, et al. Amiodarone in pregnancy. Lancet. 1983;321(8324):597-598.
4. Plomp TA, Vulsma T, de Vijlder JJ. Use of amiodarone during pregnancy. Eur J Obstet Gynecol Reprod Biol. 1992;43(3):201-207.

5. McKenna WJ, Harris L, Rowland E, Whitelaw A, Storey G, Holt D. Amiodarone therapy during pregnancy. Am J Cardiol. 1983;51(7):1231-1233.
6. Hall CM, McCormick KPB. Amiodarone and breast feeding. Arch Dis Child Fetal Neonatal Ed. May 2003;88(3):F255-F254.
7. Khurana R, Bin Jardan YA, Wilkie J, et al. Breast milk concentrations of amiodarone, desethylamiodarone, and bisoprolol following short-term drug exposure: two case reports. J Clin Pharmacol. 2014;54(7):828-831.
8. Javot L, Pape E, Yelehe-Okouma M, et al. Intravenous single administration of amiodarone and breastfeeding. Fundam Clin Pharmacol. June 2019;33(3):367-372.

AMITRIPTYLINE

Trade: Domical, Elavil, Endep, Lentizol, Mutabon D, Tryptanol

Category: Antidepressant, Tricyclic

LRC: L2 - Limited Data-Probably Compatible

Amitriptyline and its active metabolite, nortriptyline, are secreted into breastmilk in small amounts. In one report of a mother taking 100 mg/day of amitriptyline, milk levels of amitriptyline and nortriptyline (active metabolite) averaged 143 µg/L and 55.5 µg/L respectively; maternal serum levels averaged 112 µg/L and 72.5 µg/L respectively.[1] No drug was detected in the infants serum. From this data, an infant would consume approximately 21.5 µg/kg/day, a dose that is unlikely to be clinically relevant.

In another study following a maternal dose of 25 mg/day, the amitriptyline and nortriptyline (active metabolite) levels in milk were 30 µg/L and <30 µg/L respectively.[2,3] In the same study when the dosage was 75 mg/day, milk levels of amitriptyline and nortriptyline averaged 88 µg/L and 69 µg/L respectively. Both drugs were essentially undetectable in the infant's serum. Therefore, the authors estimated that a nursing infant would receive less than 0.1 mg/day.

Amitriptyline 100 mg daily was initiated 16 days postpartum in a women who had a c-section at 34 weeks for severe preeclampsia.[4] Milk samples were collected after 4 days of treatment 30 min before the woman's dose, then 1.5, 6, 12, 18, and 24 hours postdose. The peak amitriptyline and nortriptyline milk concentration occurred at 1.5 hours (103 ng/mL) and 18 hours (58 ng/mL), respectively. The authors provided no specific comments regarding any adverse effects in this premature infant with exposure in lactation.

One small study which followed four groups of women prescribed TCAs throughout different stages of reproduction found no adverse events in the group of infants whose mothers were prescribed these medications in lactation.[5] This study included 21 women (1 on amitriptyline) that initiated tricyclic antidepressant therapy at a mean of 10.3 weeks postpartum and breastfed on treatment for a mean of 12 weeks.

In another mother taking 175 mg/day, amitriptyline levels in the mother's milk were the same as in her serum on day one (24-27 µg/mL), but milk levels decreased to 54% of the serum concentration on days 2 to 26. Milk concentrations of nortriptyline were 74 percent of that in the mother's serum (87 ng/mL). Thus, the authors reported the absolute infant dose as 35 µg/kg, 80 times lower than the mother's dose. Neither compound could be detected in the infant's serum on day 26, nor were there any signs of sedation or other adverse effects.[6]

Ten breastfeeding women taking tricyclic antidepressants were followed throughout lactation to determine medication transfer into breast milk and infant safety after exposure to medication in milk.[7] In this study two women were taking amitriptyline, the first woman started medication 11 weeks postpartum and breastfed while on medication for 4 weeks. The second woman started medication 6 weeks postpartum and breastfed while on medication for 28 weeks. Fore and hind-milk samples were collected about 12-15 hours postdose and were reported as combined concentrations of both parent drug and active metabolite. In the fist case the woman was taking 100 mg/day and her fore and hind-milk concentrations were 30 ng/mL and 113 ng/mL, respectively. In the second case the woman was taking 175 mg/day and her fore and hind-milk concentrations were undetectable and 197 ng/mL, respectively. Among the ten infants exposed to tricyclic antidepressants no significant differences were noted in psychomotor and mental scores when compared to 15 bottle-fed infants (compared up to 12 months of age).

Although the data thus far have reported low levels of amitriptyline in breast milk, there is one case report of an infant with poor feeding and severe sedation after amitriptyline exposure in milk.[8] In this case report, the mother was initiated on amitriptyline 10 mg/day for severe insomnia and anxiety starting 15 days postpartum. About 72 hours after maternal treatment was started the woman reported her infant had a 48-hour history of sedation and poor feeding (number and duration of feeds decreased by 80%). Once maternal therapy was stopped the infant's symptoms fully resolved within 48 hours. The medication was rechallenged and the same concerns recurred. The pediatrician caring for the infant could not attribute these symptoms to any other causes.

T 1/2	31-46 h	MW	277 Da	PB	94.8%
Tmax	2-4 h	RID	1.08%-2.8%	Vd	6-10 L/kg
Oral	Complete	M/P	1	pKa	9.4

Adult Concerns: Sedation, dizziness, confusion, dilated pupils, drying of secretions, arrhythmias, anorexia, constipation.

Adult Dose: 10-300 mg daily (varies by indication).

Pediatric Concerns: At this time, there is one case report of severe sedation and poor feeding in a 15-day-old infant.[8]

Infant Monitoring: Sedation or irritability, dry mouth, not waking to feed/poor feeding, constipation, urinary retention, weight gain.

Alternatives: Nortriptyline(L2), SSRIs, SNRIs.

References:
1. Bader TF, Newman K. Amitriptyline in human breastmilk and the nursing infant's serum. Am J Psychiatry. 1980;137(7):855-856.
2. Brixen-Rasmussen L, Halgrener J, Jorgensen A. Amitriptyline and nortriptyline excretion in human breastmilk. Psychopharmacology (Berl). 1982;76(1):94-95.
3. Matheson I, Skjaeraasen J. Milk concentrations of flupenthixol, nortriptyline and zuclopenthixol and between-breast differences in two patients. Eur J Clin Pharmacol. 1988;35(2):217-220.
4. Pittard WB, O'Neal W. Amitriptyline excretion in human milk. J Clin Psychopharmacol. 1985;6(6):383-384.
5. Misri S, Sivertz K. Tricyclic drugs in pregnancy and lactation: a preliminary report. Int J Psychiatry Med. 1991;21:157-171.
6. Breyer-Pfaff U, Nill K, Entenmann A, Gaertner HJ. Secretion of amitriptyline and metabolites into breast milk. Am J Psychiatry. 1995;152(5):812-813.
7. Yoshida K, Smith B, Craggs M, et al. Investigation of pharmacokinetics and of possible adverse effects in infants exposed to tricyclic antidepressants in breast-milk. J Affect Disord. 1997;43:225-237.
8. Uguz F. Poor feeding and severe sedation in a newborn nursed by a mother on a low dose of amitriptyline. Breastfeeding Medicine 2017;12(1):67-68.

AMLODIPINE BESYLATE

Trade: Istin, Norvasc

Category: Calcium Channel Blocker

LRC: L3 - Limited Data-Probably Compatible

Amlodipine is a calcium channel blocker used to treat hypertension.[1] Historically, amlodipine was not recommended for use in lactation because of its long elimination half-life. Up until recently, only three case reports existed about the use of amlodipine in breastmilk. The first case report was of a woman who took amlodipine 5 mg daily starting two weeks postpartum.[2] Her term baby girl was exclusively breastfed; at 3 months of age no adverse events were noted during a follow-up appointment with the pediatrician. The infant continued to breastfeed but no further follow-up occurred. The second case was of a woman who took amlodipine 5 mg twice a day. She breastfed her full term infant exclusively and her infant was reported to have normal growth and development at each pediatrician visit.[3] The third case was of a 32 week preterm infant who exclusively breastfed from day 7 to 20 of life; the infants blood level was undetectable on day 4 of exposure in milk and no adverse events were observed.[4]

In 2015, a study was published which determined the amount of drug transfer into human milk.[5] This study included 31 women who took a mean dose of 6 mg of amlodipine once daily. When maternal blood and milk samples were taken between day 6-21 postpartum (24 hours postdose), the median milk concentration was 11.5 μg/L. The median milk/plasma ratio was 0.85. The median infant dose and RID estimated by the authors were 4.17 μg/kg/day and 4.18%, respectively. The authors did report that the highest RID was 15.2%. In addition, no circulatory adverse effects were reported in these breastfed infants.

In a study of 8 nursing mothers consuming amlodipine at 2.5 to 5 mg/day while nursing newborn infants (range 5-7 days), amlodipine reached a peak at 4-8 hours in infant plasma and 8 hours in milk.[6] The average RID of amlodipine observed in this study was 3.4% and ranged from 1.56% to 4.32%). Plasma level in infants were all less than 0.4 ng/mL, which was their limit of quantification.

At this time, the pharmacokinetics, estimated RID, and clinical experience with nifedipine make it the preferred calcium channel blocker in lactation; however, the use of this product should not deter a woman from breastfeeding if this medication is required.

T 1/2	30-50 h	MW	567 Da	PB	93%
Tmax	6-12 h	RID	1.72%-4.32%	Vd	21 L/kg
Oral	64%-90%	M/P		pKa	8.7

Adult Concerns: Headache, fatigue, dizziness, hypotension, palpitations, flushing, edema, constipation.

Adult Dose: 5-10 mg daily.

Pediatric Concerns: None reported via milk at this time.

Infant Monitoring: Drowsiness, lethargy, pallor, poor feeding, and weight gain.

Alternatives: Nifedipine(L2), Labetalol(L2)

References:

1. Pharmaceutical manufacturers prescribing information.
2. Ahn HK, Nava-Ocampo AA, Han JY, et al. Exposure to amlodipine in the first trimester of pregnancy and breastfeeding. Hypertens Pregnancy. 2007;26(2):179-187.
3. Szucs KA, Axline SE, Rosenman MC. Maternal membranous glomerulonephritis and successful exclusive breastfeeding. Breastfeed Med. 2010;5(3):123-126.
4. Vasa R, Ramirez M. Amlodipine exposure through breastfeeding in a 32 week preterm newborn. Breastfeed Med. 2013;8(suppl 1):S15.
5. Naito T, Kubono N, Deguchi S, et al. Amlodipine passage into breast milk in lactating women with pregnancy-induced hypertension and its estimation of infant risk for breastfeeding. J Hum Lact. 2015;31(2):301-306.
6. Aoki H, Ito N, Kaniwa N, et al. Low levels of amlodipine in breast milk and plasma. Breastfeed Med. November 2018;13(9):622-626. PMID: 30265578.

AMOXAPINE

Trade: Asendin, Asendis

Category: Antidepressant, Tricyclic

LRC: L2 - Limited Data-Probably Compatible

Amoxapine and its metabolite are both secreted into breast milk at relatively low levels. Following a dose of 250 mg/day, milk levels of amoxapine were less than 20 µg/L and 113 µg/L of the active metabolite.[1] Milk levels of the active metabolite varied from 113 to 168 µg/L in two other milk samples. Maternal serum levels of amoxapine and metabolite at steady state were 97 µg/L and 375 µg/L, respectively.

T 1/2	8 h	MW	314 Da	PB	15%-25%
Tmax	2 h	RID	0.6%	Vd	65.7 L/kg
Oral	18%-54%	M/P	0.21	pKa	

Adult Concerns: Dry mouth, constipation, urine retention, drowsiness or sedation, anxiety, emotional disturbances, parkinsonism, tardive dyskinesia, seizures.

Adult Dose: 25 mg BID or TID.

Pediatric Concerns: None reported via milk.

Infant Monitoring: Sedation or irritability, dry mouth, not waking to feed/poor feeding, constipation, urinary retention, weight gain.

Alternatives:

References:

1. Gelenberg AJ. Single case study. Amoxapine, a new antidepressant, appears in human milk. J Nerv Ment Dis. 1979;167(10):635-636.

AMOXICILLIN

Trade: Alphamox, Amoxil, Betamox, Cilamox, Larotid, Moxacin

Category: Antibiotic, Penicillin

LRC: L1 - Limited Data-Compatible

Amoxicillin is a popular oral penicillin used for the treatment of many types of infections in both children and adults (e.g., respiratory, urinary tract, skin infections).[1] In one group of six mothers who received a single 1 gram oral dose of amoxicillin, the peak concentrations of amoxicillin occurred in serum at about 2 hours and in breast milk at about 4-5 hours postdose. The breast milk concentrations ranged from 0.68 µg/mL to 1.3 µg/mL (mean 0.9 µg/mL). The milk/plasma ratios at 1, 2, and 3 hours were 0.014, 0.013, and 0.043. The relative infant dose was 0.95%, this correlates to an absolute infant dose of 0.14 mg/kg/day. This amounts to less than 0.5% of the typical therapeutic dose of amoxicillin given to infants.

T 1/2	1.7 h	MW	365 Da	PB	18%
Tmax	1.5 h	RID	0.95%	Vd	0.3 L/kg
Oral	89%	M/P	0.014-0.043	pKa	3.23

Adult Concerns: Diarrhea, rashes, and changes in GI flora. Pancytopenia, rarely pseudomembranous colitis.

Adult Dose: 500 mg TID or 875 mg BID.

Pediatric Concerns: None reported via milk at this time, medication is commonly used in infants and children.

Infant Monitoring: Vomiting, diarrhea, changes in gastrointestinal flora, and rash.

Alternatives: Ampicillin(L1), Cephalexin(L1)

References:

1. Kafetzis DA, Siafas CA, Georgakopoulos PA, Papadatos CJ. Passage of cephalosporins and amoxicillin into the breast milk. Acta Paediatr Scand. 1981;70(3):285-288.

AMOXICILLIN + CLARITHROMYCIN + LANSOPRAZOLE

Trade: Prevpac

Category: Antiulcer

LRC: L3 - No Data-Probably Compatible

Amoxicillin + clarithromycin + lansoprazole is a combined drug product indicated for treatment of Helicobacter pylori infections that cause stomach ulcers.[1]

Amoxicillin is a popular oral penicillin used for the treatment of many types of infections in both children and adults.[2] In one group of six mothers who received a single 1 gram oral dose of amoxicillin, the peak concentrations of amoxicillin occurred in serum at about 2 hours and in breast milk at about 4-5 hours postdose. The breast milk concentrations ranged from 0.68 µg/mL to 1.3 µg/mL (mean 0.9 µg/mL). The milk/plasma ratios at 1, 2, and 3 hours were 0.014, 0.013, and 0.043. The relative infant dose was 0.95%, this correlates to an absolute infant dose of 0.14 mg/kg/day. This amounts to less than 0.5% of the typical therapeutic dose of amoxicillin given to infants.

Clarithromycin is an antibiotic that belongs to the macrolide family. In a study of 12 mothers receiving 250 mg twice daily, the maximum concentration occurred at 2.2 hours and was reported to be 0.85 mg/L.[3] The estimated average dose of clarithromycin via milk was reported to be 150 µg/kg/day, or 2% of the maternal dose.

Lansoprazole is a new proton pump inhibitor that suppresses the release of acid protons from the parietal cells in the stomach, effectively raising the pH of the stomach.[4] Lansoprazole is secreted in animal milk; however, there are no human data at this time. Lansoprazole is structurally similar to omeprazole and it is very unstable in stomach acid and to a large degree, is denatured by acidity of the infant's stomach. A new study shows milk levels of omeprazole are minimal, it is likely milk levels of lansoprazole would be similar.

T 1/2	Amox/clar/lan: 1.7 h/5-7 h/1.5 h	MW	Amox/clar/lan: 365/748/369 Da	PB	Amox/clar/lan: 18%/40%-70%/97%
Tmax	Amox/clar/lan: 1.5 h/1.7 h/1.7 h	RID		Vd	Amox/clar/lan: 0.3/3-4/0.5 L/kg
Oral	Amox/clar/lan: 89%/50%/80%	M/P	Amox/clar/lan: 0.014-0.043/>1 /	pKa	Amox/clar/lan: 9.48/12.94/8.85

Adult Concerns: Headache, alterations of taste, abdominal pain, diarrhea, oral candidiasis, rash.

Adult Dose: Amox/clar/lan: 1 g/500 mg/30 mg once daily for 10-14 days.

Pediatric Concerns:

Infant Monitoring: Vomiting, diarrhea, changes in gastrointestinal flora, and rash.

Alternatives:

References:

1. Pharmaceutical manufacturers prescribing information.
2. Kafetzis DA, Siafas CA, Georgakopoulos PA, Papadatos CJ. Passage of cephalosporins and amoxicillin into the breast milk. Acta Paediatr Scand. 1981;70(3):285-288.
3. Sedlmayr T, Peters F, Raasch W, Kees F. Clarithromycin, a new macrolide antibiotic. Effectiveness in puerperal infections and pharmacokinetics in breast milk. Geburtshilfe Frauenheilkd. July 1993;53(7):488-491.
4. Pharmaceutical manufacturers prescribing information.

AMOXICILLIN + CLAVULANATE

Trade: Amoclan, Augmentin, Augmentin ES-600, Augmentin XR, Clavulin

Category: Antibiotic, Penicillin

LRC:

Amoxicillin and clavulanate potassium is a combination oral antibiotic that is used for the treatment of many types of infections in both children and adults (e.g., pneumonia, otitis media, sinusitis, urinary tract, skin infections).[1] The addition of clavulanate extends the spectrum of amoxicillin by inhibiting beta-lactamases which are enzymes that can inactivate amoxicillin.

Amoxicillin is a popular oral penicillin used for the treatment of many types of infections in both children and adults.[2] In one group of six mothers who received a single 1 gram oral dose of amoxicillin, the peak concentrations of amoxicillin occurred in serum at about 2 hours and in breast milk at about 4-5 hours postdose. The breast milk concentrations ranged from 0.68 μg/mL to 1.3 μg/mL (mean 0.9 μg/mL). The milk/plasma ratios at 1, 2, and 3 hours were 0.014, 0.013, and 0.043. The relative infant dose was 0.95%, this correlates to an absolute infant dose of 0.14 mg/kg/day. This amounts to less than 0.5% of the typical therapeutic dose of amoxicillin given to infants.

In another study of 67 breastfeeding mothers, 27 mothers were treated with amoxicillin + clavulanic acid and 40 mothers were treated with only amoxicillin. In the amoxicillin + clavulanic acid group, 22.3% of the infants had mild adverse effects.[3] Only 7.5% of the control group (amoxicillin-only) infants had adverse effects. However, the authors suggest that this difference in untoward effects is not clinically significant. The reported side effects included constipation (1), rash (4), diarrhea (4), and irritability (6). This amounts to less than 0.5% of a typical infant dose of amoxicillin.

One published abstract in 2009 reported the case of a 2-month-old infant whose mother was breastfeeding while taking amoxicillin + clavulanate 1 gram orally every 12 hours and gentamicin 160 mg IM every other day.[1,4] The mother noted that she breastfed her infant 15 minutes after her first dose of therapy for 10 minutes. About 20 minutes after this, the child developed a general urticaria, which resolved within 30 minutes. This repeated itself a few hours later, urticaria started 15 minutes after starting to feed and resolved within 1 hour. The mother stopped breastfeeding and no further episodes occurred. The authors of this report query if the infant could be allergic to penicillin.

T 1/2	Amox/Clav: 1.7 h/1h	MW	Amox/Clav: 365/199 Da	PB	Amox/Clav: 18%/22%-30%
Tmax	Amox/Clav: 1.5 h/1 h	RID	0.9%	Vd	Amox/Clav: 0.3/ L/kg
Oral	Amox/Clav: 89%/75%	M/P	Amox/Clav: 0.014-0.043	pKa	Amox/Clav: 3.23/3.32

Adult Concerns: Diarrhea, rashes, and changes in GI flora. Pancytopenia, rarely pseudomembranous colitis.

Adult Dose: 875 mg BID.

Pediatric Concerns: One case report of urticaria.[3]

Infant Monitoring: Vomiting, diarrhea, changes in gastrointestinal flora, and rash.

Alternatives:

References:
1. Pharmaceutical manufacturer prescribing information.
2. Kafetzis DA, Siafas CA, Georgakopoulos PA, Papadatos CJ. Passage of cephalosporins and amoxicillin into the breast milk. Acta Paediatr Scand. 1981;70(3):285-288.
3. Benyamini L, Merlob P, Stahl B, et al. The safety of amoxicillin/clavulanic acid and cefuroxime during lactation. Ther Drug Monit. August 2005;27(4):499-502.
4. Cherif F, El Aidli S, Kastalli S, et al. Drug induced urticaria via breastfeeding. Fundam Clin Pharmacol. 2009;23(suppl 1):37. (Abstract 203).

AMPHOTERICIN B

Trade: Abelcet, Ambisome, Amphocel, Amphotec, Fungilin, Fungizone

Category: Antifungal

LRC: L3 - No Data-Probably Compatible

Amphotericin B is an intravenous antifungal effective for the treatment of a range of different organisms, including Candida albicans. Amphotericin is significantly toxic when given intravenously, and is reserved for life-threatening infections. No data are available on its transfer to human milk; however, it is virtually unabsorbed orally (<9%), has high protein binding, and a large molecular weight.[1,2] It is unlikely the amount in milk would be clinically relevant to a breastfeeding infant.

T 1/2	15 days	MW	924 Da	PB	>90%
Tmax	<1 h	RID		Vd	4 L/kg
Oral	<9%	M/P		pKa	3.58

Adult Concerns: Headache, malaise, fever, chills, hypotension, tachypnea vomiting, diarrhea, anorexia, changes in electrolytes, changes in liver and renal function, anemia.

Adult Dose: 0.25 to 1 mg/kg daily IV.

Pediatric Concerns: None reported via milk at this time.

Infant Monitoring: Vomiting, diarrhea, weight gain.

Alternatives:

References:
1. Pharmaceutical manufacturers prescribing information.
2. Mactal-Haaf C, Hoffman M, Kuchta A. Use of anti-infective agents during lactation, Part 3: antivirals, antifungals, and urinary anti-septics. J Hum Lact. May 2001;17(2):160-166.

AMPICILLIN

Trade: Amfipen, Ampicyn, Austrapen, Britcin, Omnipen, Polycillin, Vidopen

Category: Antibiotic, Penicillin

LRC: L1 - Limited Data-Compatible

Ampicillin is an antibiotic in the penicillin family.[1] In a study by Matsuda of three breastfeeding patients who received 500 mg of ampicillin orally, levels in milk peaked at 6 hours and averaged only 0.14 mg/L of milk.[2] The milk/plasma ratio was reported to be 0.03 at 2 hours. In a group of nine9 breastfeeding women sampled at various times and who received doses of 350 mg TID orally, milk concentrations ranged from 0.06 to 0.17 mg/L with peak milk levels at 3-4 hours after the dose.[3] Milk/plasma ratios varied between 0.01 and 0.58. The highest reported milk level (1.02 mg/L) was in a patient receiving 700 mg TID. Ampicillin was not detected in the plasma of any infant. Ampicillin is one of the most commonly used prophylactic antibiotics in pediatric neonatal nurseries. Neonatal half-life is 2.8 to 4 hours.

T 1/2	1.3 h	MW	349 Da	PB	8-20
Tmax	1-2 h	RID	0.17%-0.51%	Vd	0.38 L/kg
Oral	50%	M/P	0.58	pKa	3.24

Adult Concerns: Diarrhea, rash, fungal overgrowth, agranulocytosis, pseudomembranous colitis.

Adult Dose: 250-500 mg orally four times a day; 1-2 g IV every 4-6 hours.

Pediatric Concerns: None reported via milk at this time.

Infant Monitoring: Vomiting, diarrhea, changes in gastrointestinal flora, and rash.

Alternatives: Amoxicillin(L1), Cefazolin(L1), Cephalexin(L1)

References:
1. Kafetzis DA, Siafas CA, Georgakopoulos PA, Papadatos CJ. Passage of cephalosporins and amoxicillin into the breast milk. Acta Paediatr Scand. 1981;70(3):285-288.
2. Matsuda S. Transfer of antibiotics into maternal milk. Biol Res Pregnancy Perinatol. 1984;5(2):57-60.
3. Branebjerg PE, Heisterberg L. Blood and milk concentrations of ampicillin in mothers treated with pivampicillin and in their infants. J Perinat Med. 1987;15(6):555-558.

AMPICILLIN + SULBACTAM

Trade: Dicapen, Unasyn

Category: Antibiotic, Penicillin

LRC: L1 - Limited Data-Compatible

Ampicillin sodium and Sulbactam sodium is a drug combination product indicated for use in pelvic inflammatory disease and in infections of the skin and subcutaneous tissues.

Small amounts of ampicillin may transfer (1 mg/L).[1] Possible rash, sensitization, diarrhea, or candidiasis could occur, but unlikely. This drug may alter gastrointestinal flora. Ampicillin is considered compatible with breastfeeding.

The absorption of sulbactam from GI tract is poor.[2] After a dose of 0.5 to 1 gram, sulbactam is secreted into milk at an average concentration of 0.52 μg/mL. This would lead to a maximal dose of 0.7 mg/kg/day in a breastfeeding infant, which equates to less than 1% of the maternal dose. Therefore, untoward effects are unlikely in a breastfeeding infant.[3]

T 1/2	Amp/sulb: 1.3 h/	MW	Amp/sulb: 349/233 Da	PB	Amp/sulb: 8%-20%/
Tmax	Amp/sulb: 1-2 h/	RID	0.5%-1.5%	Vd	Amp/sulb: 0.38/ L/kg
Oral	Amp/sulb: 50%/	M/P	Amp/sulb: 0.58/	pKa	Amp/sulb: 3.24/12.48

Adult Concerns: Diarrhea, rash, fungal overgrowth, agranulocytosis, pseudomembranous colitis.

Adult Dose: 1.5-3 g IV every 6 hours.

Pediatric Concerns: None reported via milk.

Infant Monitoring: Vomiting, diarrhea, changes in gastrointestinal flora, and rash.

Alternatives:

References:
1. Kafetzis DA, Siafas CA, Georgakopoulos PA, Papadatos CJ. Passage of cephalosporins and amoxicillin into the breast milk. Acta Paediatr Scand. 1981;70(3):285-288.
2. Sweetman S, ed. Martindale: the Complete Drug Reference. London, England: Pharmaceutical Press; 2010. Electronic version.
3. Foulds G, Miller RD, Knirsch AK, Thrupp LD. Sulbactam kinetics and excretion into breast milk in postpartum women. Clin Pharmacol Ther. 1985;38(6):692-696.

ANAGRELIDE

Trade: Agrylin

Category: Platelet Reducing Agent

LRC: L4 - No Data-Possibly Hazardous

Anagrelide hydrochloride is used in the treatment of essential thrombocythemia and thrombocythemia associated with chronic myelogenous leukemia, polycythemia vera, and other myeloproliferative disorders. It inhibits the release of arachidonic acid from phospholipase, possibly by inhibiting phospholipase A2.[1] We do not have any data on its use in breastfeeding mothers, but some probably enters milk and would be orally absorbed by the infant. Since this drug is used for prolonged periods, untoward effects such as reduction of blood platelets (thrombocytopenia) and cardiovascular disorders in the infant are a possibility. While the risks of this drug are rather remote, chronic use in breastfeeding mothers should be discouraged or the infant closely monitored.

T 1/2	1.3 h	MW	310 Da	PB	
Tmax	1 h	RID		Vd	
Oral	70%	M/P		pKa	

Adult Concerns: Headache, palpitations, edema, dyspnea, diarrhea, weakness.

Adult Dose: 0.5 mg 4 times a day or 1 mg twice a day.

Pediatric Concerns: No data are available, but chronic use is discouraged.

Infant Monitoring:

Alternatives:

References:
1. Pharmaceutical manufacturers prescribing information.

ANAKINRA

Trade: Kineret

Category: Antirheumatic

LRC: L3 - No Data-Probably Compatible

Anakinra is a recombinant form of the human interleukin-1 receptor antagonist (IL-1RA) and is used to reduce the inflammatory stimuli that mediate various inflammatory and immunological responses common in rheumatoid arthritis.[1] It is a large molecular weight protein (17,300 Da) administered subcutaneously. Due to its size, it is very unlikely to enter milk after the first week postpartum. In addition, it is not likely to be orally bioavailable in an infant. However, we do not have data on its transfer to human milk and if used the infant should be observed for increased risk of gastrointestinal infections.

T 1/2	4-6 h	MW	17,300 Da	PB	Nil
Tmax	3-7 h	RID		Vd	
Oral	Nil	M/P		pKa	

Adult Concerns: Adverse events include a high risk of serious infections (2%), URI, headache, nausea, and diarrhea.

Adult Dose: 100 mg SC daily.

Pediatric Concerns: None reported via milk. This agent is too large to enter milk effectively after the first week postpartum.

Infant Monitoring: Observe for serious infections, URI, headache, nausea, and diarrhea.

Alternatives:

References:
1. Pharmaceutical manufacturers prescribing information.

ANASTROZOLE

Trade: Arimidex

Category: Antineoplastic

LRC: L5 - No Data-Hazardous

Anastrozole is a potent and selective non-steroidal aromatase inhibitor indicated for the treatment of postmenopausal women with hormone receptor-positive breast cancer. It significantly lowers serum estradiol concentrations and has no detectable effect on formation of adrenal corticosteroids or aldosterone. Orally administered anastrozole is well absorbed into the systemic circulation with 83% to 85% of the drug recovered in urine and feces. Anastrozole has a mean terminal elimination half-life of approximately 50 hours in postmenopausal women.[1] The major circulating metabolite of anastrozole, triazole, lacks pharmacologic activity. As with other aromatase inhibitors, this product, even in low concentrations in milk, could permanently bind to specific receptors, and potentially suppress estrogen formation completely in a breastfed infant.

Mothers should discontinue breastfeeding for at least 15 days after consuming this medication.

T 1/2	50 h	MW	293.4 Da	PB	40%
Tmax	2 h	RID		Vd	
Oral	Complete	M/P		pKa	

Adult Concerns: Blurred vision, chest pain or discomfort, dizziness, headache, nervousness, pounding in the ears, shortness of breath, slow or fast heartbeat, swelling of the feet or lower legs.

Adult Dose: 1 mg daily.

Pediatric Concerns: None yet reported, but this drug should not be used in breastfeeding mothers.

Infant Monitoring: Discontinue breastfeeding for at least 15 days after use.

Alternatives:

References:
1. Pharmaceutical manufacturers prescribing information.

ANIDULAFUNGIN

Trade: Eraxis

Category: Antifungal

LRC: L3 - No Data-Probably Compatible

Anidulafungin is an injectable antifungal used in the treatment of Candida infections. It inhibits the formation of 1,3-beta-D-glucan, an essential polysaccharide in the cell wall of Candida albicans. This leads to cell lysis.[1] No data are available on levels in human milk, but due to the large molecular weight, its high protein binding, and its large volume of distribution, it is highly unlikely that it will transfer to breast milk. Lastly, it would not be orally bioavailable in the infant.

T 1/2	27 h	MW	1140.2 Da	PB	>99%
Tmax		RID		Vd	0.43-0.71 L/kg
Oral	Nil	M/P		pKa	9.5

Adult Concerns: Fever, insomnia, shortness of breath, hyper or hypotension, nausea, vomiting, diarrhea, constipation, changes in liver and renal function, changes in electrolytes, anemia, thrombocytopenia.

Adult Dose: 100 mg IV daily for 14 days.

Pediatric Concerns: No data are available.

Infant Monitoring: Lethargy, pallor, vomiting, diarrhea, constipation, weight gain.

Alternatives: Fluconazole(L2)

References:
1. Pharmaceutical manufacturers prescribing information.

ANTHRALIN

Trade: Alphodith, Anthra-Derm, Anthraforte, Anthranol, Anthrascalp, Dithranol, Dritho-Scalp, Drithocreme, Micanol

Category: Antipsoriatic

LRC: L3 - No Data-Probably Compatible

Anthralin is a synthetic tar derivative used topically for suppression of psoriasis. Anthralin, when applied topically, induces burning and inflammation of the skin but is one of the most effective treatments for psoriasis. Absorbed medication is rapidly excreted via the kidneys almost instantly; plasma levels are very low to undetectable.[1] No data are available on its transfer into human milk. Most anthralin is eliminated by washing off and desquamation of dead surface cells.[2] For this reason, when placed directly on lesions on the areola or nipple, breastfeeding should be discouraged. Another similar anthraquinone is Senna (laxative), which even in high doses does not enter milk. While undergoing initial intense treatment, it would perhaps be advisable to interrupt breastfeeding temporarily, but this may be overly conservative. It has been used in children over 2 years of age for psoriasis.

T 1/2	Brief	MW	226 Da	PB	
Tmax		RID		Vd	
Oral	Complete	M/P		pKa	

Adult Concerns: Pruritus, skin irritation, and inflammation. Purple-brown staining of skin and permanent staining of clothing and porcelain bathroom fixtures is frequent. Anthralin may have carcinogenic properties following high doses in mice; relevance to humans is unknown.

Adult Dose: Apply topical BID.

Pediatric Concerns: None reported via milk at this time.

Infant Monitoring: Vomiting, diarrhea.

Alternatives:

References:
1. Goodfield MJ, Hull SM, Cunliffe WJ. The systemic effect of dithranol treatment in psoriasis. Acta Derm Venereol. 1994;74(4):295-297.
2. Shroot B. Mode of action of dithranol, pharmacokinetics/dynamics. Acta Derm Venereol Suppl (Stockh). 1992;172:10-12.

ANTHRAX (BACILLUS ANTHRACIS)

Trade: Anthrax Infection, Bacillus Anthracis

Category: Infectious Disease

LRC: L5 - No Data-Hazardous

Anthrax is an acute infection usually involving skin, lungs, and gastrointestinal tract. Anthrax is caused by the gram-positive, spore-forming bacterium bacillus anthracis. The spore may persist in nature for many years and infect grazing animals such as sheep, goats, and cattle. The most common forms of the disease are inhaled, oral, and cutaneous.

The Center for Disease Control has recently published guidelines for treating or prophylaxing exposed breastfeeding mothers.[1] Thus far, all of the anthrax strains released by bioterrorists have been sensitive to ciprofloxacin, doxycycline, and the penicillin family. In breastfeeding women, amoxicillin (80 mg/kg/day in 3 divided doses) is an option for antimicrobial prophylaxis when B. anthracis is known to be penicillin-susceptible and no contraindication to maternal amoxicillin use is indicated. The American Academy of Pediatrics also considers ciprofloxacin and tetracyclines (which include doxycycline) to be usually compatible with breastfeeding because the amount of either drug absorbed by infants is small, but little is known about the safety of long-term use. Until culture sensitivity tests have been completed, the breastfeeding mother should be treated with ciprofloxacin (see ofloxacin or levofloxacin as alternates) or doxycycline (< 3 weeks). Once cultures show that the anthrax strain is sensitive to penicillins, then the mother can switch to amoxicillin for long-term use up to 60 days or more. Due to possible dental staining following prolonged exposure, we would not suggest long-term use (60 days) of doxycycline in a breastfeeding mother. The CDC offers several alternative antibiotics such as rifampin, vancomycin, imipenem, clindamycin, and clarithromycin in those patients with allergic conditions.[2] Check the CDC web sites for the most current recommendations.[1] Due to the risks posed by infection with anthrax, mothers who test positive for this infection should probably not breastfeed their infants until after treatment has been started and testing negative for this species.

Adult Concerns: Inhalation anthrax: Flu like symptoms progressing to respiratory distress. Usually fatal. GI anthrax: Fever, nausea, vomiting blood, severe diarrhea. Cases are fatal 25%-60% of the time.

Adult Dose:

Pediatric Concerns:

Infant Monitoring: Potentially hazardous. Do not breastfeed.

Alternatives:

References:

1. Centers for Disease Control and Prevention. https://www.cdc.gov/anthrax/basics/index.html
2. Centers for Disease Control and Prevention. Update: investigation of bioterrorism-related anthrax and interim guidelines for exposure management and antimicrobial therapy. MMWR Morb Mortal Wkly Rep. October 2001;50(42):909-919.

ANTHRAX VACCINE

Trade: Anthrax Vaccine, BioThrax

Category: Vaccine

LRC: L3 - No Data-Probably Compatible

The anthrax vaccine for humans licensed for use in the United States is a cell-free filtrate vaccine, which means it uses dead bacteria as opposed to live bacteria. The vaccine is reported to be 93% effective in protecting against cutaneous anthrax.[1] The vaccine should only be administered to healthy men and women from 18 to 65 years of age since investigations to date have been conducted exclusively in that population. Because it is not known whether the anthrax vaccine can cause fetal harm, pregnant women should not be vaccinated. There are no data or indications relative to its use in breastfeeding mothers. While it consists primarily of protein fragments of anthrax bacteria, it is very unlikely any would transfer into milk or even be bioavailable in the infant.

The CDC states that, "No data suggest increased risk for side effects or temporally related adverse events associated with receipt of anthrax vaccine by breastfeeding women or breastfed children. Administration of nonliving vaccines (e.g., anthrax vaccine) during breast-feeding is not medically contraindicated." According to the Advisory Committee on Immunization Practices (ACIP), while vaccination of breastfeeding women with the anthrax vaccine is generally not recommended, it may be administered as postexposure prophylaxis along with antibiotics after an incident of high risk exposure to Bacillus anthracis, or it may also be given when the mother faces an occupational risk of exposure to anthrax.[2]

Adult Concerns: Mild local reactions occur in 30% of recipients and consist of slight tenderness and redness at the injection site. A moderate local reaction can occur if the vaccine is given to anyone with a past history of anthrax infection. Severe local reactions are very infrequent and consist of extensive swelling of the forearm in addition to the local reaction. Systemic reactions occur in fewer than 0.2% of recipients and are characterized by flu-like symptoms.

Adult Dose: 0.5 mL injection (IM).

Pediatric Concerns: None reported via milk.

Infant Monitoring:

Alternatives:

References:

1. Centers for Disease Control and Prevention. https://www.cdc.gov/anthrax/index.html
2. Bower WA, Schiffer J, Atmar RL, et al. Advisory Committee on Immunization Practices (ACIP): use of anthrax vaccine in the United States. MMWR Recomm Rep. 2010;59(RR-6):1-30.

ANTIHEMOPHILIC FACTOR (RECOMBINANT FACTOR VIII)

Trade: Kogenate FS, Helixate FS, Advate, Kovaltry

Category: Other

LRC: L3 - No Data-Probably Compatible

Recombinant factor VIII is a large molecular weight protein use intravenously to treat hemophilia A by replacing the missing clotting factor VIII that is needed for hemostasis.[1] This product can be used for the acute treatment of bleeding, during surgery or as routine prophylaxis to reduce the number of bleeding episodes in those with hemophilia A. No data are available on its transfer to human milk, but due to its extraordinary size, it is unlikely to enter the milk compartment, or be bioavailable orally.

T 1/2	14 h	MW	>80,000 Da	PB	
Tmax		RID		Vd	
Oral	Nil	M/P		pKa	

Adult Concerns: Hypersensitivity reactions (bronchospasm, hypotension, anaphylaxis), skin rash, pruritus, urticaria, infusion related reactions (inflammation, pain).

Adult Dose: Variable

Pediatric Concerns:

Infant Monitoring: Observe for unusual blood clots in feces.

Alternatives:

References:
1. Pharmaceutical manufacturer prescribing information.

ANTIHEMOPHILIC FACTOR-VON WILLEBRAND FACTOR COMPLEX

Trade: Alphanate, Humate-P, Wilate

Category: Antihemophilic Agent

LRC: L3 - No Data-Probably Compatible

This antihemophilic agent is used in hemophilia A and factor VIII deficiency to prevent and treat hemorrhagic episodes. It is also used to treat bleeding and as prophylaxis during procedures in patients with von Willebrand disease.[1] No data are available on the excretion of this antihemophilic agent into breast milk, however, it is highly unlikely due to the large molecular weight. Further, it is minimally bioavailable when ingested orally.

T 1/2	10-12 h	MW	264,726 Da	PB	
Tmax		RID		Vd	0.36-0.57 L/kg
Oral	Nil	M/P		pKa	

Adult Concerns: Adverse reactions include epistaxis, body pain, nausea, dyspnea, cardiorespiratory arrest, and chills.

Adult Dose: 15-80 IU/kg (individualize).

Pediatric Concerns: No data available in infants.

Infant Monitoring:

Alternatives:

References:
1. Pharmaceutical manufacturers prescribing information.

APIXABAN

Trade: Eliquis

Category: Anticoagulant

LRC: L4 - No Data-Possibly Hazardous

Apixaban is an anticoagulant (Factor Xa inhibitor) used to reduce the risk of stroke in atrial fibrillation, reduce the risk and treat deep vein thrombosis and pulmonary embolism.[1] At this time there are no data regarding the transfer of apixaban into human milk. The manufacturer reports that apixaban is excreted into rodent milk (about 12% of the maternal dose). Based on this medication's small volume of distribution and high pKa it will likely enter human milk. At this time we recommend the use of alternatives with more data in lactation (e.g. LMWH, Rivaroxaban warfarin) when suitable to treat the maternal condition.

T 1/2	12 h	MW	459.5 Da	PB	87%
Tmax	3-4 h	RID		Vd	0.3 L/kg
Oral	50%	M/P		pKa	13.12

Adult Concerns: Nausea, changes in liver function, anemia, bruising on the skin, hemorrhage (blood in vomit, stool, urine, etc.).

Adult Dose: 5 mg twice daily.

Pediatric Concerns: No known adverse events at this time.

Infant Monitoring: Rare-bruising on the skin, blood in vomit, stool, or urine.

Alternatives: Low molecular weight heparins, Warfarin(L2)

References:
1. Pharmaceutical manufacturers prescribing information.

APREMILAST

Trade: Otezla

Category: Antiarthritic

LRC: L4 - No Data-Possibly Hazardous

Apremilast is a phosphodiesterase-4 inhibitor used in the treatment of adults with active psoriatic arthritis. It is currently unknown if it is secreted in human milk. Due to its high pKa, low molecular weight, and good oral absorption, care should be exercised when apremilast is given to a nursing woman.[1]

T 1/2	6-9 h	MW	460.5 Da	PB	68%
Tmax	2.5 h	RID		Vd	1.24 L/kg
Oral	73%	M/P		pKa	12.58

Adult Concerns: Observe for weight decrease (5%-10%), nausea, diarrhea, headache, upper respiratory tract infection, vomiting, nasopharyngitis, upper abdominal pain, depression.

Adult Dose: 30 mg once to twice daily.

Pediatric Concerns:

Infant Monitoring: Observe for weight decrease (5%-10%), nausea, diarrhea, upper respiratory tract infection, vomiting, nasopharyngitis, upper abdominal pain.

Alternatives:

References:
1. Pharmaceutical manufacturers prescribing information.

APREPITANT

Trade: Emend, Ivemend

Category: Antiemetic

LRC: L3 - No Data-Probably Compatible

Aprepitant is a neurokinin-1 receptor antagonist. It is used as an antiemetic agent for the prevention of nausea and vomiting following chemotherapy or surgeries.[1] Side effect profiles appear minimal. Levels in milk will likely be minimal due to moderately large molecular weight. Currently there are no data available on the transfer of aprepitant in to human milk although it will likely be minimal.

T 1/2	9-13 h	MW	534.43 Da	PB	>95%
Tmax	3 h	RID		Vd	1 L/kg
Oral	60%-65%	M/P		pKa	

Adult Concerns: Dizziness, fatigue, hiccups, hypotension, bradycardia, constipation, changes in liver and renal function, weakness.

Adult Dose: Chemotherapy-induced N/V: 125 mg 1 hour prior, 80 mg on days 2 and 3. Postoperative N/V: 40 mg 3 hours before surgery.

Pediatric Concerns:

Infant Monitoring: Drowsiness, constipation, diarrhea, and weight gain.

Alternatives:

References:
1. Pharmaceutical manufacturers prescribing information.

ARFORMOTEROL

Trade: Brovana

Category: Antiasthma

LRC: L3 - No Data-Probably Compatible

Arformoterol tartrate is used for long-term treatment of bronchoconstriction in COPD. It is the (R,R)-enantiomer of the racemic formoterol, which relaxes bronchial smooth muscle by selective action on beta 2-receptors.[1] The average steady-state peak plasma concentration is 4.3 pg/mL, which means levels in milk would be incredibly low if even present. There have been no studies on the transfer of arformoterol tartrate into human breast milk. However, due to the extremely low plasma levels, any transfer to milk would be minimal to nil. Just like all the other beta agonists used in asthma, it is unlikely that this product would pose a problem to a breastfeeding infant.

T 1/2	26 h	MW	494.5 Da	PB	52-65%
Tmax	0.5-3 h	RID		Vd	
Oral		M/P		pKa	8.61

Adult Concerns: Chest pain, edema, rash, diarrhea, back pain, sinusitis, and dyspnea.

Adult Dose: 15 µg twice daily.

Pediatric Concerns: No data are available.

Infant Monitoring: Irritability, insomnia, arrhythmias, weight loss, tremor.

Alternatives: Formoterol(L3), Albuterol(L1)

References:
1. Pharmaceutical manufacturers prescribing information.

ARGATROBAN

Trade: Arganova, Argata

Category: Anticoagulant

LRC: L4 - No Data-Possibly Hazardous

Argatroban is a synthetic inhibitor of thrombin and is derived from L-arginine.[1] It reversibly binds to the thrombin active site and exerts an anticoagulant effect by inhibiting thrombin-catalyzed reactions. It is primarily indicated as an anticoagulant for treatment of thrombosis in patients with heparin-induced thrombocytopenia. It is primarily in the extracellular fluid as evidenced by its low volume of distribution. No data are available on its transfer to human milk but it is reported to be present in rodent milk. The oral bioavailability of this product is unknown but expected to be poor. Extreme caution is recommended until we know levels present in milk and more about its gastrointestinal stability and absorption.

T 1/2	39-51 min	MW	526 Da	PB	55%
Tmax	1-3 h	RID		Vd	0.174 L/kg
Oral	Unknown	M/P		pKa	10.28

Adult Concerns: Headache, cough, dyspnea, chest pain, hypotension, arrhythmias, nausea, vomiting, abdominal pain, hemorrhage.

Adult Dose: 2-25 µg/kg/min (highly variable based on indication).

Pediatric Concerns: None reported via milk.

Infant Monitoring: Rare-bruising on the skin, blood in urine, vomit or stool.

Alternatives:

References:
1. Pharmaceutical manufacturers prescribing information.

ARIPIPRAZOLE

Trade: Abilify, Abilitat, Aristada

Category: Antipsychotic, Atypical

LRC: L3 - Limited Data-Probably Compatible

Aripiprazole is a second-generation antipsychotic, used for the treatment for schizophrenia. In a case report of a patient who started therapy on 10 mg daily and then had a subsequent dose increase to 15 mg daily, milk levels were drawn prior to dose administration on day 15 and 16 after therapy initiation.[1] Levels of aripiprazole in milk were reported to be 13 and 14 µg/L on the two consecutive days and maternal plasma levels drawn at the same time as the milk samples were both 71 µg/L.

In a second case report published in 2010, a woman took aripiprazole 15 mg daily throughout pregnancy and lactation.[2] In this case two breast milk (colostrum) samples were taken on day 3 after birth, in both specimens aripiprazole was undetectable (limit of detection 10 ng/mL). Due to concerns with difficulty of measuring the drug in the colostral phase and potential interactions of colostrum with the measuring device (HPLC), three samples were re-taken on day 27 after birth. These samples were taken 24 hours after the last dose, 4 hours after dose administration and 10 hours after dose administration. The maternal serum concentration was 207 ng/mL of aripiprazole and 42 ng/mL for the metabolite dehydroaripiprazole. Again, neither the drug nor its metabolite were detected in the three milk samples. The authors reported the milk plasma ratio was less than 0.04 and the RID was 0.7% (using the limit of detection milk concentration of 10 ng/mL). Following a 3 month follow up period the infant was reported to be growing normally.

In a third case report of a mother who took aripiprazole 18 mg daily in pregnancy (starting at 22 weeks gestation) and while breastfeeding, the maternal breast milk and infant plasma levels were found to be 38.7 µg/L and 7.6 µg/L.[3] The milk and blood levels were drawn on postpartum day 6 as the mother discontinued breastfeeding at this time due to concerns of maternal fatigue. There was some speculation that the infants blood levels were more reflective of in utero exposure to the medication, rather than breast milk exposure because of the timing of the level being so close to birth and the long half life of the medication (75 hours).

In 2014, a fourth case report of a mother who took 10 mg of aripiprazole daily in pregnancy (up to 5 weeks and re-started at 9 weeks gestation) and throughout breastfeeding.[4] After 6 weeks of breastfeeding a milk substitute was introduced because of poor maternal milk supply. By week 7 the infant was feeding 8 x per day with 40 mL of breast milk per feed. Breast milk samples were taken during week 8 and 10 postpartum prior to the morning dose (time 0), and then at 2, 3, 6, 9, 12, and 24 hours after drug administration. Mid-feed samples were hand expressed by this patient. The average milk concentrations of aripiprazole and its metabolite, dehydroaripiprazole, were 52.6 ng/mL and 8.8 ng/mL during week 8 and 53.6 ng/mL and 6.3 ng/mL during week 10. The average infant dose of an exclusively breastfed infant weighing 5 kg was estimated to be 47 µg/day and the relative infant dose was 8.3% (authors used maternal weight of 87 kg). The infant was still breastfeeding at 4 months of age and was found to have normal psychomotor and behavioral development and had reached all milestones for her age. We calculated the relative infant dose using the standard maternal weight of 70 kg and found the RID to be 6.4%. In addition, the authors reported that this mother's poor milk supply was most likely due to her low prolactin levels, 35-40 ng/mL. The authors attribute aripiprazole use to these low prolactin levels as there has been another case report where a woman who took aripiprazole during pregnancy had lactation failure (other confounders were present in this particular pregnancy/delivery).[5] The potential mechanism for aripiprazole use and lactation failure is thought to be the partial agonist effect of the medication in the tuberoinfundibulnar dopaminergic system, as this could interfere with prolactin release and inhibit lactation.[5]

Several reports (personal communication) of somnolence have been reported to this author. The infant should be monitored for somnolence. Aripiprazole may suppress prolactin levels, use caution.

T 1/2	75 h	MW	448 Da	PB	99%
Tmax	3-5 h	RID	0.7%-6.44%	Vd	4.9 L/kg
Oral	87%	M/P	0.2	pKa	

Adult Concerns: Headache, dizziness, sedation, insomnia, anxiety, agitation, chest pain, tachycardia, QTc prolongation, hypertension, orthostatic hypotension, dry mouth, dyspepsia, nausea, vomiting, constipation, changes in liver function, extrapyramidal symptoms (e.g., dystonia, akathisia, tremor). May increase urge to gamble.

Adult Dose: 10-15 mg/day.

Pediatric Concerns: Several cases of somnolence in breastfed infants have been unofficially reported, no adverse effects in published case reports.

Infant Monitoring: Sedation or irritability, apnea, not waking to feed, poor feeding, extrapyramidal symptoms and weight gain.

Alternatives: Risperidone(L2), Olanzapine(L2), Quetiapine(L2)

References:

1. Schlotterbeck P, Leube D, Kircher T, Hiemke C, Grunder G. Aripiprazole in human milk. Int J Neuropsychopharmacol. 2007;10:433.
2. Lutz UC, Hiemke C, Wiatr G. Aripiprazole in pregnancy and lactation: a case report. J Clin Psychopharmacol. 2010;30:204-205.
3. Watanabe N, Kasahara M, Sugibayashi R, et al. Perinatal use of aripiprazole: a case report. J Clin Psychpharmacol. 2011;31(3):377-379.
4. Nordeng H, Gjerdalen G, Brede WR, Michelsen LS, Spigset O. Transfer of aripiprazole to breast milk: a case report. J Clin Psychopharamcology. 2014;34(2):272-275.
5. Mendhekar DN, Sunder KR, Andrade C. Aripiprazole use in pregnant schizoaffective woman. Bipolar Disord. 2006;8:229-300.

ARMODAFINIL

Trade: Nuvigil

Category: CNS Stimulant

LRC: L4 - No Data-Possibly Hazardous

Armodafinil is the R-enantiomer of modafinil which is a 1:1 mixture of the R- and S-enantiomers. Armodafinil is a wakefulness-promoting agent used for the treatment of narcolepsy.[1] Although its pharmacologic results are similar to amphetamines and methylphenidate, its method of action is unknown.

In a recent study of armodafinil, a 27-year-old mother who was receiving 250 mg/day armodafinil, delivered an infant at 37 weeks gestational age.[2] Following a dose of 250 mg, the maximum concentration of armodafinil in milk was 2.3 µg/mL and was observed at 2 hours. This level decreased gradually over 24 hours. As the patient was at steady-state, the authors observed a milk level of 0.43 µg/mL at zero hour. The calculated area under the curve was 28.96 mg.hr/L. The average infant dose was 0.181 mg/kg/day based on the assumption of the infant's daily intake of 150 mL/kg/ day. The relative infant dose (RID) was estimated to be 5.3%.

T 1/2	15 h	MW	273 Da	PB	60
Tmax	2 h	RID	5.29%	Vd	0.6 L/kg
Oral		M/P		pKa	

Adult Concerns: Headache, insomnia, dizziness, anxiety, dry mouth, nausea, diarrhea, serious rash, tremor.

Adult Dose: 150-250 mg daily.

Pediatric Concerns: None reported via milk at this time.

Infant Monitoring: Agitation, irritability, poor sleeping patterns, poor weight gain, tremor.

Alternatives:

References:

1. Pharmaceutical manufacturers prescribing information.

ARTICAINE

Trade: Orabloc, Septocaine

Category: Anesthetic, Local

LRC: L3 - No Data-Probably Compatible

Articaine is a local anesthetic with an intermediate-duration. It has a structure similar to lidocaine, etidocaine, and prilocaine. It has an ester bond mid-structure that permits it to be rapidly hydrolyzed by blood and tissue esterases.[1] Although its potency is approximately equal to or slightly more than that of lidocaine, it may be less toxic due to its more rapid metabolism. No data are available on its use in breastfeeding mothers. As with lidocaine, however, its transfer into human milk is probably minimal. If ingested, it would be rapidly hydrolyzed by gastric esterases.

T 1/2	1.8	MW	284 Da	PB	60%-80%
Tmax		RID		Vd	
Oral		M/P		pKa	7.8

Adult Concerns: Headache, pain, facial edema, gingivitis.

Adult Dose: 20-204 mg (varies).

Pediatric Concerns: None reported.

Infant Monitoring:

Alternatives:

References:
1. Pharmaceutical manufacturers prescribing information.

ASCORBIC ACID

Trade: Ascorbicap, Ce-Vi-Sol, Cecon, Cevi-Bid, Vitamin C

Category: Vitamin

LRC: L1 - No Data-Compatible

Ascorbic acid is an essential vitamin, commonly referred to as vitamin C. Vitamin C is popularly used for various reasons, the most common being prevention and treatment of infections, fatigue, and cancer. Without supplementation, 75 mg/day is excreted in the urine of the average individual due to overabundance. Renal control of vitamin C is significant and maintains plasma levels at 0.4 to 1.5 mg/dL regardless of dose.

Ascorbic acid is secreted into human milk in well-controlled sequence and mature milk. In a large number of studies, ascorbic acid levels in milk ranged from 35 to 200 mg/L depending on the oral intake of the mother.[1] Excessive vitamin C intake in the mother only modestly changes the controlled secretion into breast milk. The recommended daily allowance for the mother is 100 mg/day. Maternal supplementation is only required in undernourished mothers. In a study of 25 lactating women given 90 mg of ascorbic acid for 1 day, followed by 250, 500, or 1000 mg/day for 2 days, the levels of vitamin C in maternal milk were not significantly influenced.[2] Mean vitamin C intakes of infants ranged between 49 ± 9 and 86 ± 11 mg/day and were not statistically different among the five levels of maternal vitamin C intake. This lack of change in vitamin C content in milk suggests a regulatory mechanism for vitamin C levels. In cases where supplementation has reached 1000 to 1500 mg/day, reported milk levels were only slightly increased to 100 and 105 mg/L.[2,3] Whereas the half-life in normal non-supplemented patients is 16 days, high oral doses can induce the metabolism of ascorbic thereby reducing the half-life of ascorbic acid to as little as 3.4 hours. Pregnant women should not use excessive ascorbic acid due to metabolic induction in the maternal or fetal liver, followed by a metabolic rebound scurvy early postpartum in the neonate.

Intravenous vitamin C is used extensively by complementary and alternative medicine (CAM) practitioners. From surveys conducted at annual CAM conferences in 2006 and 2008, it was found that average doses administered were in the order of 28 grams intravenously, but doses ranged from as low as 1 gram to as high as 200 grams.[4] While plasma concentrations following oral administration are strictly controlled by the kidneys between the ranges of 70-85 µmol/L, plasma concentrations are 30-70 times higher with intravenous vitamin C use.[5] Intravenous vitamin C may produce concentrations as high as 15,000 µmol/L. Recent trials in animals and in vitro studies have indicated that high plasma concentrations of vitamin C in the order of 1000 µmol/L has anticancer properties.[6-10] Although similarly high plasma concentrations were achieved with IV vitamin C use in humans, the antitumor role of high vitamin C doses in humans is still in question.[11] Adverse effects with IV vitamin C have been rarely reported and include minor side-effects such as lethargy, fatigue, vein irritation, nausea and vomiting. Three cases of renal failure in those with preexisting renal disease and two cases of hemolysis in those with G6PD deficiency have been reported.[12-16] Intravenous vitamin C appears to have a moderately safe profile, but avoid use in mothers with preexisting renal impairment, history of kidney stones, G6PD deficiency or paroxysmal nocturnal hematuria. The use of intravenous vitamin C in breastfeeding women has not been studied. The very high plasma concentrations achieved with IV vitamin C use would probably result in high concentrations in milk as well. This might predispose infants to a higher risk of kidney stones with excessive vitamin C exposure. Mothers of infants with compromised renal function and G6PD deficiency should avoid excessively high doses of vitamin C.

Ascorbic acid should not routinely be administered to breastfed infants unless to treat clinical scurvy. Even following high maternal oral doses, ascorbic acid levels only rise moderately in milk. Recommend normal RDA (100 mg/day) in mothers, and avoid excessively high oral doses. Avoid intravenous vitamin C during breastfeeding, or in those cases where it is used, mothers should avoid breastfeeding, pump and discard milk, for a minimum of 12-24 hours after therapy.

T 1/2	16 days (3.4 h in heavy users)	MW	176 Da	PB	25%
Tmax	2-3 h	RID		Vd	
Oral	Complete	M/P		pKa	9.07

Adult Concerns: Faintness, flushing, dizziness, nausea, vomiting, gastritis, renal stones with large doses. IV Vitamin C: dizziness, lethargy, fatigue, heartburn, nausea, vomiting, hypersensitivity reactions, local vein irritation, renal stones, renal failure.

Adult Dose: 75 mg orally per day.

Pediatric Concerns: None reported via breastmilk at this time.

Infant Monitoring: Vomiting.

Alternatives:

References:
1. Picciano MF. Vitamins in milk. Water-soluble vitamins in human milk. In: Jensen RG, ed. Handbook of Milk Composition. San Diego, CA: Academic Press; 1995.
2. Byerley LO, Kirksey A. Effects of different levels of vitamin C intake on the vitamin C concentration in human milk and the vitamin C intakes of breast-fed infants. Am J Clin Nutr. April 1985;41(4):665-671.
3. Kirksey A, Rahmanifar A. Vitamin and mineral composition of preterm human milk: Implications for the nutritional management of the preterm infant. In: H. Berger, ed. Vitamins and Minerals in Pregnancy and Lactation. Raven Press; 1988:301-329.
4. Padayatty SJ, Sun AY, Chen Q, Espey MG, Drisko J, Levine M. Vitamin C: intravenous use by complementary and alternative medicine practitioners andadverse effects. PLoS One. July 7, 2010;5(7):e11414.
5. Padayatty SJ, Sun H, Wang Y, et al. Vitamin C pharmacokinetics: implications for oral and intravenous use. Ann Intern Med. April 6, 2004;140(7):533-537.
6. Chen Q, Espey MG, Sun AY, et al. Ascorbate in pharmacologic concentrations selectively generates ascorbate radical and hydrogen peroxide in extracellular fluid in vivo. Proc Natl Acad Sci U S A. 2007;104:8749-8754.
7. Chen Q, Espey MG, Sun AY, et al. Pharmacologic doses of ascorbate act as a prooxidant and decrease growth of aggressive tumor xenografts in mice. Proc Natl Acad Sci USA. 2008;105:11105-11109.
8. Verrax J, Calderon PB. Pharmacologic concentrations of ascorbate are achieved by parenteral administration and exhibit antitumoral effects. Free Radic Biol Med. 2009;47:27-29.
9. Leung PY, Miyashita K, Young M, Tsao CS. Cytotoxic effect of ascorbate and its derivatives on cultured malignant and nonmalignant cell lines. Anticancer Res. 1993;13:475-480.
10. Sakagami H, Satoh K, Hakeda Y, Kumegawa M. Apoptosis-inducing activity of vitamin C and vitamin K. Cell Mol Biol (Noisy-le-grand). 2000;46:129-143.
11. Hoffer LJ, Levine M, Assouline S, et al. Phase I clinical trial of i.v. ascorbicacid in advanced malignancy. Ann Oncol. November 2008;19(11):1969-1974. Epub June 9, 2008. Erratum in: Ann Oncol. December 2008;19(12):2095.
12. Lawton JM, Conway LT, Crosson JT, Smith CL, Abraham PA. Acute oxalate nephropathy after massive ascorbic acid administration. Arch Intern Med. 1985;145:950-951.
13. Wong K, Thomson C, Bailey RR, McDiarmid S, Gardner J. Acute oxalate nephropathy after a massive intravenous dose of vitamin C. Aust N Z J Med. 1994;24:410-411.
14. McAllister CJ, Scowden EB, Dewberry FL, Richman A. Renal failure secondary to massive infusion of vitamin C. JAMA. 1984;252:1684.
15. Campbell GD Jr, Steinberg MH, Bower JD. Ascorbic acid-induced hemolysis in G-6-PD deficiency. Ann Intern Med. 1975;82:810.
16. Rees DC, Kelsey H, Richards JD. Acute haemolysis induced by high dose ascorbic acid in glucose-6- phosphate dehydrogenase deficiency. BMJ. 1993;306:841-842.

ASENAPINE

Trade: Saphris

Category: Antipsychotic, Atypical

LRC: L3 - No Data-Probably Compatible

Asenapine is an atypical antipsychotic used to treat schizophrenia and bipolar disorder.[1] According to the manufacturer, asenapine appears in rat milk. At this time there are no data regarding asenapine in human milk; however, levels will probably be low-moderate as with other members of this family because of its high protein binding and large volume of distribution. Galactorrhea may occur due to hyperprolactinemia.

T 1/2	24 h	MW	285.8 Da	PB	95%
Tmax	0.5-1.5 h	RID		Vd	20 to 25 L/kg
Oral	Sublingual 35%; <2% if swallowed	M/P		pKa	

Adult Concerns: Headache, somnolence, insomnia, anxiety, irritability, hypertension, dyspepsia, elevated prolactin and triglyceride levels, increased appetite, weight gain, changes in liver function, extrapyramidal symptoms.

Adult Dose: 5-10 mg twice daily.

Pediatric Concerns: None reported via milk at this time.

Infant Monitoring: Sedation or irritability, apnea, not waking to feed, poor feeding, extrapyramidal symptoms, and weight gain.

Alternatives: Risperidone(L2), Quetiapine(L2), Aripiprazole(L3)

References:
1. Pharmaceutical manufacturers prescribing information.

ASPARAGINASE

Trade: Colaspase, Crasnitin, Elspar, Kidrolase, L-ASP, L-asparaginase, Erwinaze

Category: Antineoplastic

LRC: L4 - No Data-Possibly Hazardous

Asparaginase is used for a number of different cancers.[1] Asparaginase contains the enzyme L-asparagine amidohydrolase derived from E. coli. Asparaginase removes asparagine from leukemic cells, thus requiring that these cells obtain it from an exogenous source for survival, which cancer cells are unable to do. Fortunately, normal cells are able to synthesize asparagine. It does not have active metabolites and does not pass the blood brain barrier (<1%). No data are available on its transfer to human milk. But due to its long half-life some asparaginase may be present in milk.

Withhold breastfeeding for a minimum of 7 days.

T 1/2	8-49 h	MW	35,000 Da	PB	
Tmax	14-24 h (IM)	RID		Vd	70%-80% of plasma volume L/kg
Oral	Nil	M/P		pKa	

Adult Concerns: Disorientation, fever, dyspnea, nausea, vomiting, changes in liver function, pancreatitis, thrombosis, bone marrow depression, coagulation disorders, weight loss.

Adult Dose: Varies by indication.

Pediatric Concerns:

Infant Monitoring: Avoid breastfeeding for a minimum of 7 days.

Alternatives:

References:
1. Pharmaceutical manufacturers prescribing information.

ATENOLOL

Trade: Anselol, Antipress, Noten, Tenlol, Tenoretic, Tenormin, Tensig

Category: Beta Adrenergic Blocker

LRC: L3 - Limited Data-Probably Compatible

Atenolol is a potent cardio-selective beta-blocker. Data conflict on the secretion of atenolol into breastmilk.

One author reports an incident of significant bradycardia, cyanosis, low body temperature, and low blood pressure in breastfeeding infant of mother consuming 100 mg atenolol daily while a number of others have failed to detect plasma levels in the neonate or untoward side effects.[1] Data seem to indicate that atenolol secretion into breast milk is highly variable but may be as high as 10 times greater than for propranolol.

In one study, women taking 50-100 mg/day were found to have milk/plasma ratios of 1.5-6.8. However, even with high M/P ratios, the calculated intake per day (at peak levels) for a breastfeeding infant would only be 0.13 mg.[2] In a study by White et al, breast milk levels in one patient were 0.7, 1.2, and 1.8 mg/L of milk at doses of 25, 50, and 100 mg daily respectively.[3] In another study, the estimated daily intake for an infant receiving 500 mL milk per day, would be 0.3 mg.[4] In these five patients who received 100 mg daily, the mean milk concentration of atenolol was 630 μg/L. In a study by Kulas et al , the amount of atenolol transferred into milk varied from 0.66 mg/L with a maternal dose of 25 mg, 1.2 mg/L with a maternal dose of 50 mg, and 1.7 mg/L with a maternal dose of 100 mg per day.[5] Although atenolol is approved by the AAP, some caution is recommended due to the milk/plasma ratios and the reported problem with one infant.

T 1/2	6-7 h	MW	266 Da	PB	6%-16%
Tmax	2-4 h	RID	6.6%	Vd	1.3 L/kg
Oral	50%-60%	M/P	1.5-6.8	pKa	9.6

Adult Concerns: Headache, dizziness, insomnia, depression, fatigue, chest pain, bradycardia, hypotension, heart failure, wheezing, vomiting, constipation, diarrhea, myalgia.

Adult Dose: 50-100 mg daily.

Pediatric Concerns: One report of bradycardia, cyanosis, low body temperature, and hypotension in a breastfeeding infant of mother consuming 100 mg atenolol daily, but other reports do not suggest clinical effects on breastfed infants.

Infant Monitoring: Drowsiness, lethargy, pallor, poor feeding, and weight gain.

Alternatives: Propranolol(L2), Metoprolol(L2)

References:
1. Schimmel MS, Eidelman AI, Wilschanski MA, et al. Toxic effects of atenolol consumed during breast feeding. J Pediatr. 1989;114(3):476-478.
2. Liedholm H, Melander A, Bitzen PO, et al. Accumulation of atenolol and metoprolol in human breast milk. Eur J Clin Pharmacol. 1981;20(3):229-231.
3. White WB, Andreoli JW, Wong SH, Cohn RD. Atenolol in human plasma and breast milk. Obstet Gynecol. 1984;63(3 suppl):42S-44S.
4. Thorley KJ, McAinsh J. Levels of the beta-blockers atenolol and propranolol in the breast milk of women treated for hypertension in pregnancy. Biopharm Drug Dispos. 1983;4(3):299-301.
5. Kulas J, Lunell NO, Rosing U, Steen B, Rane A. Atenolol and metoprolol. A comparison of their excretion into human breast milk. Acta Obstet Gynecol Scand Suppl. 1984;118:65-69.

ATOMOXETINE

Trade: Strattera

Category: Adrenergic

LRC: L4 - No Data-Possibly Hazardous

Atomoxetine is a selective norepinephrine reuptake inhibitor that is presently indicated for the treatment of Attention Deficit Hyperactivity Disorder (ADHD).[1] Atomoxetine metabolism is highly variable. One group of poor metabolizers (7%) may have extended half-lives (22 h) and higher plasma levels, while another group of normal metabolizers has a half-life of about 5 hours. No data are available on the transfer of Atomoxetine into human milk. Because this is a lipophilic, neuroactive drug, there is some potential risk with its use in a breastfeeding mother, and mothers should probably be cautioned about its use while breastfeeding.

T 1/2	5.2 h	MW	291 Da	PB	98%
Tmax	1-2 h	RID		Vd	0.85 L/kg
Oral	63%-94%	M/P		pKa	

Adult Concerns: Headache, dizziness, abdominal pain, dyspepsia, vomiting, decreased appetite.

Adult Dose: 80 mg/day.

Pediatric Concerns: None reported via milk at this time.

Infant Monitoring: Observe for irritability, poor sleep, tremors, and weight gain.

Alternatives: Methylphenidate(L2)

References:
1. Pharmaceutical manufacturers prescribing information.

ATORVASTATIN

Trade: Caduet, Lipitor

Category: Antihyperlipidemic

LRC: L3 - No Data-Probably Compatible

Atorvastatin is an HMG Co-A reductase inhibitor for lowering plasma cholesterol levels. It is known to transfer into animal milk, but human studies are not available.[1] Due to its poor oral absorption and high protein binding, it is unlikely that clinically relevant amounts would transfer into human milk. However, the effect on the infant is unknown and statins could reduce cholesterol synthesis. Cholesterol and other products of cholesterol biosynthesis are essential components for neonatal development; therefore, it is not clear if it would be safe for use in a breastfed infant who needs high levels of cholesterol. Caution is recommended until more data are available.

T 1/2	14 h	MW	1209 Da	PB	>98%
Tmax	1-2 h	RID		Vd	5.44 L/kg
Oral	14%	M/P		pKa	4.33

Adult Concerns: Headache, dizziness, nausea, abdominal pain, diarrhea, changes in liver function, weakness, myalgia.

Adult Dose: 10-80 mg daily.

Pediatric Concerns: None reported, but the use of these products in lactating women is not recommended.

Infant Monitoring: Weight gain, growth.

Alternatives:

References:
1. Pharmaceutical manufacturers prescribing information.

ATOVAQUONE

Trade: Mepron, Meprone, Malarone

Category: Antiprotozoal agent

LRC: L3 - No Data-Probably Compatible

Atovaquone is an antiprotozoal used to treat and prevent infections such as Pneumocystis jiroveci pneumonia (formerly P. carinii pneumonia or PCP) and malaria.[1] Due to increasing resistance atovaquone is given with proguanil when used for malaria (combination tablet commercially available). At this time there are no data regarding the transfer of atovaquone into human milk; however, the manufacturer reports that atovaquone enters rodent milk at 30% of maternal concentrations. At this time, this medication is not recommended by the WHO for malaria in lactation[2], however, the risk to the infant is probably minimal.

Please note that regardless of maternal malaria therapy, concentrations achieved in human milk are too low to be therapeutic in the infant.[2] Therefore, a nursing infant should be assessed and given appropriate prophylaxis or treatment for malaria based on their individual needs.

T 1/2	2.9 days	MW	366.84 Da	PB	>99%
Tmax		RID		Vd	8.8 L/kg
Oral	21%	M/P		pKa	

Adult Concerns: Fever, headache, insomnia, depression, hypotension, anorexia, nausea, vomiting, diarrhea, abdominal pain, changes in liver and renal function, weakness, anemia, neutropenia, infection, pruritus, rash.

Adult Dose: 750 mg twice a day (varies by indication).

Pediatric Concerns: None reported via milk at this time.

Infant Monitoring: Insomnia, weakness, vomiting, diarrhea, decreased feeding/poor weight gain. If clinical signs of jaundice, check liver enzymes or if ongoing infection check CBC. Breastfeeding is not recommended in mothers who have HIV.

Alternatives:

References:
1. Pharmaceutical manufacturers prescribing information.
2. World Health Organization (WHO). Malaria. In: International Travel and Health. 2010:chap 7. Geneva, Switzerland: WHO. http://www.who.int/ith/ITH_chapter_7.pdf.

ATROPINE

Trade: Atropine, Atropine Minims, Atropisol, Atropt, Belladonna, Eyesule, Isopto-Atropine

Category: Anticholinergic

LRC: L3 - No Data-Probably Compatible

Atropine is a powerful anticholinergic that is well distributed throughout the body.[1] Only small amounts are believed to be secreted in milk. Effects may be highly variable. Slight absorption together with enhanced neonatal sensitivity creates hazardous potential. Use caution. Avoid if possible but not definitely contraindicated. Note that anticholinergics have been found in sheep to reduce prolactin production.

T 1/2	4.3 h	MW	289 Da	PB	14%-22%
Tmax	1 h	RID		Vd	2.3-3.6 L/kg
Oral	90%	M/P		pKa	9.8

Adult Concerns: Drowsiness, insomnia, dizziness, dilated pupils, xerostomia, increased heart rate, hypotension, arrhythmias, constipation, urinary retention, dry hot skin.

Adult Dose: 0.6 mg every 6 hours.

Pediatric Concerns: No reports are available, although caution is urged.

Infant Monitoring: Drowsiness or insomnia, dry hot skin, dry mouth, increased heart rate, constipation, urinary retention.

Alternatives:

References:
1. Pharmaceutical manufacturers prescribing information.

ATROPINE + DIPHENOXYLATE

Trade: Lofene, Lofenoxal, Lomocot, Lomotil, Lonox, Vi-Atro

Category: Antidiarrheal

LRC: L3 - No Data-Probably Compatible

Atropine sulfate and diphenoxylate hydrochloride is a drug combination product used for the treatment of diarrhea. There are no reports on the transfer of this drug product in breast milk. Atropine is a powerful anticholinergic that is well distributed throughout the body.[1] Only small amounts are believed to be secreted in milk. Effects may be highly variable. Slight absorption together with enhanced neonatal sensitivity creates hazardous potential. Use caution. Avoid if possible but not definitely contraindicated.

Diphenoxylate belongs to the opiate family (meperidine) and acts on the intestinal tract inhibiting gastrointestinal motility and excessive gastrointestinal propulsion.[2] The drug has no analgesic activity. Although no reports on its transfer to human milk are available, it is probably secreted in breast milk in very small quantities.[4] Some authors consider diphenoxylate to be contraindicated, but this is questionable.

T 1/2	Atro/diph: 4.3 h/2.5 h	MW	Atro/diph: 289/453 Da	PB	Atro/diph: 14%-22%/
Tmax	Atro/diph: 1 h/2 h	RID		Vd	Atro/diph: 2.3-3.6/3.8 L/kg
Oral	Atro/diph: 90%/90%	M/P		pKa	Atro/diph: 9.8/7.1

Adult Concerns: Headache, drowsiness, irritability, confusion, dry skin, dry mouth, nausea, pancreatitis, constipation, toxic megacolon, anorexia, urinary retention.

Adult Dose: Atropine/diphenoxylate: 0.025/2.5 mg, two tablets 4 times daily. Do not exceed 20 mg/day diphenoxylate.

Pediatric Concerns: No known adverse reactions in breast milk at this time.

Infant Monitoring: Drowsiness or insomnia, dry hot skin, dry mouth, increased heart rate, constipation, urinary retention, weight gain.

Alternatives: Loperamide(L2)

References:

1. Pharmaceutical manufacturers prescribing information.
2. Stewart JJ. Gastrointestinal drugs. In: Wilson JT, ed. Drugs in Breast Milk. Balgowlah, Australia: ADIS Press; 1981;71.

AZATHIOPRINE

Trade: Imuran, Thioprine, Azapress

Category: Immune Suppressant

LRC: L3 - Limited Data-Probably Compatible

Azathioprine is a powerful immunosuppressive agent that is metabolized to 6-Mercaptopurine (6-MP).

In two mothers receiving 75 mg azathioprine, the concentration of 6-MP in milk varied from 3.5-4.5 µg/L in one mother and 18 µg/L in the second mother.[1] Both levels were peak milk concentrations at 2 hours following the dose. The authors conclude that these levels would be too low to produce clinical effects in a breastfed infant. Using these data for 6-MP, an infant would absorb only 0.1 % of the weight-adjusted maternal dose, which is probably too low to produce adverse effects in a breastfeeding infant. Plasma levels in treated patients is maintained at 50 ng/mL or higher. One infant continued to breastfeed during therapy and displayed no immunosuppressive effects. In another study of two infants who were breastfed by mothers receiving 75-100 mg/day azathioprine, milk levels of 6-MP were not measured. But both infants had normal blood counts, no increase in infections, and above-average growth rate.[2] However, caution is recommended.

Four mothers who were receiving 1.2-2.1 mg/kg/day of azathioprine throughout pregnancy and continued post-partum were studied while breastfeeding. The mothers' blood concentrations of 6-TGN (active metabolite) and 6-MMPN (most hepatotoxic metabolite) ranged from 234-291 and 284 to 1178 pmol/100 million RBC, respectively. Neither 6-TGN nor 6-MMPN could be detected in the exposed infants. The authors suggest that breastfeeding while taking azathioprine may be safe in mothers with "normal" TPMT enzyme activity (the enzyme responsible for metabolizing 6-TGN).[3] The authors of this study also published an updated report, which then included six mother-infant pairs in 2007; the conclusions of this report were the same, both metabolites were undetectable in the infants and no adverse effects were reported.[4]

Four case reports were performed with mothers taking between 50 to 100 mg/day of azathioprine. No adverse events were reported in any of the infants, and milk concentrations in two mothers proved to be undetectable.[5] Ten women at steady state on 75 to 150 mg/day azathioprine provided milk samples on days 3-4, days 7-10, and day 28 after delivery, between 3 and 18 hours after azathioprine administration. 6-MP was detected in only one case, at 1.2 and 7.6 ng/mL at 3 and 6 hours after azathioprine intake on day 28. However, 6-MP and 6-TGN were undetectable in the infants blood. There were no signs of immunosuppression, even in three preterm neonates. The authors suggest that azathioprine therapy should not deter mothers from breastfeeding.[6]

Another study of three mothers taking azathioprine while breastfeeding (doses of 100-175 mg) reported normal blood cell counts in all three infants, and only a low amount of 6-TGN in one infant on day 3. At age 3 weeks, this level decreased below the detectable range.[7] In a group of eight lactating women who received azathioprine (75-200 mg/day), levels in milk ranged from 2-50 µg/L.[8] After 6 hours an average of 10% of the peak values were measured. The authors estimate the infants dose to be <0.008 mg/kg body weight per 24 hours. They suggest that breastfeeding during treatment with azathioprine seems safe and should be recommended. In a 31-year-old mother with Crohn's disease being treated with 100 mg/day azathioprine, peripheral blood levels of 6-MP and 6-TGN in the infant were undetectable at day 8 or after 3 months of therapy.[9] The infant was reported to be normal after 6 months. In a recent study of the long-term follow-up (median 3.3 years) of fetal and breastfeeding exposure to azathioprine (n = 11 infants), there were no differences in rates of infectious disease in azathioprine-treated groups compared to non-treated controls. The authors suggest that breastfeeding following exposure to azathioprine does not increase the risk of infections.[10]

One published abstract in 2003 found that five of six infants breastfeeding on azathioprine had normal monthly blood counts, and no signs of infection.[11] One infant required cessation of breastfeeding due to low blood counts; however, details of this scenario were not reported.

In summary, the transport of 6-mercaptopurine into human milk is apparently quite low. However, this is a strong immunosuppressant and some caution is still recommended if it is used in a breastfeeding mother. Monitor the infant closely for signs of immunosuppression, leukopenia, thrombocytopenia, hepatotoxicity, pancreatitis, and other symptoms of 6-mercaptopurine exposure. The risks to the infant are probably low. Recent long-term data suggest that the rate of infections in treated groups is no different from non-treated controls.

T 1/2	2 h	MW	277 Da	PB	30%
Tmax	1-2 h	RID	0.07%-0.3%	Vd	0.9 L/kg
Oral	41%-44%	M/P		pKa	8.2

Adult Concerns: Fever, malaise, vomiting, diarrhea, changes in liver function, leukopenia, thrombocytopenia, myalgia. Recent long-term data suggest that the rate of infections in treated groups is no different from non-treated controls.

Adult Dose: 1-3 mg/kg/day.

Pediatric Concerns: One infant required cessation of breastfeeding due to low blood counts, details of this scenario were not reported.[11]

Infant Monitoring: If signs of immunosuppression or anemia check CBC; if signs of liver dysfunction (yellowing of skin or whites of eyes) check liver enzymes and bilirubin.

Alternatives:

References:

1. Coulam CB, Moyer TP, Jiang NS, Zincke H. Breast-feeding after renal transplantation. Transplant Proc. 1982;14(3):605-609.
2. Grekas DM, Vasiliou SS, Lazarides AN. Immunosuppressive therapy and breast-feeding after renal transplantation. Nephron. 1984;37(1):68.
3. Gardiner SJ, Gearry RB, Roberts RL, Zhang M, Barclay ML, Begg EJ. Exposure to thiopurine drugs through breast milk is low based on metabolite concentrations in mother-infant pairs. Br J Clin Pharmacol. 2006;62(4):453-456.
4. Gardiner SJ, Gearry RB, Roberts RL, Zhang M, Barclay ML, Begg EJ. Comment: breast-feeding during maternal use of azathioprine. Ann Pharmacother. 2007;41:719-720.
5. Moretti ME, Verjee Z, Ito S, Koren G. Breast-feeding during maternal use of azathioprine. Ann Pharmacother. 2006;40:2269-2272.
6. Sau A, Clarke S, Bass J, Kaiser A, Marinaki A, Nelson-Piercy C. Azathioprine and breastfeeding- is it safe? BJOG. 2007;114:498-501.
7. Bernard N, Garayt C, Chol F, Vial T, Descotes J. Prospective clinical and biological follow-up of three breastfed babies from azathioprine-treated mothers. Fundam Clin Pharmacol. 2007;21(suppl 1):62-63. Abstract.
8. Christensen LA, Dahlerup JF, Nielsen MJ, Fallingborg JF, Schmiegelow K. Azathioprine treatment during lactation. Aliment Pharmacol Ther. November 15, 2008;28(10):1209-1213. Epub August 30, 2008.
9. Zelinkova Z, De Boer IP, Van Dijke MJ, Kuipers EJ, Van Der Woude CJ. Azathioprine treatment during lactation. Aliment Pharmacol Ther. July 2009;30(1):90-91.
10. Angelberger S, Reinisch W, Messerschmidt A, et al. Long-term follow-up of babies exposed to azathioprine in utero and via breast-feeding. J Crohns Colitis. April 2011;5(2):95-100. Epub December 9, 2010.
11. Khare MM, Lott J, Currie A, et al. Is it safe to continue azathioprine in breast feeding mothers? J Obstet Gynaecol. 2003;23(suppl 1):S48. (Abstract 53).

AZELAIC ACID

Trade: Azelex, Finacea, Finevin, Skinoren

Category: Antiacne

LRC: L3 - No Data-Probably Compatible

Azelaic acid is a dicarboxylic acid derivative normally found in whole grains and animal products. Azelaic acid, when applied as a cream, produces a significant reduction of Propionibacterium acnes (implicated in the causation of acne) and has an anti-keratinizing effect as well. Small amounts of azelaic acid are normally present in human milk.[1] Azelaic acid is only modestly absorbed via skin (<4%), and it is rapidly metabolized. The amount absorbed does not change the levels normally found in plasma nor milk. Due to its poor penetration into plasma and rapid half-life (45 min), it is not likely to penetrate milk or produce untoward effects in a breastfed infant.

T 1/2	45 min	MW	188 Da	PB	
Tmax		RID		Vd	
Oral		M/P		pKa	4.98

Adult Concerns: Pruritus, burning, stinging, erythema, dryness, peeling, and skin irritation.

Adult Dose: Apply topically twice a day.

Pediatric Concerns: None reported via milk. Normal constituent of milk.

Infant Monitoring:

Alternatives:

References:

1. Pharmaceutical manufacturers prescribing information.

AZELASTINE

Trade: Astelin, Astepro, Azep, Dymista, Optilast, Optivar, Rhinolast

Category: Antihistamine

LRC: L3 - No Data-Probably Compatible

Azelastine (Astelin) is an antihistamine for oral, intranasal, and ophthalmic administration.[1] It is effective in treating seasonal and perennial rhinitis and nonallergic vasomotor rhinitis. Ophthalmically, it is effective for allergic conjunctivitis (itchy eyes). Oral bioavailability is 80%, and intranasal bioavailability is only 40%. No data are available on the transfer of azelastine into human milk. The doses used intranasally and ophthalmically are so low that it is extremely unlikely to produce clinically relevant levels in human milk. Oral administration could potentially lead to slightly higher levels but azelastine is relatively devoid of serious side effects and it is doubtful that any would occur in a breastfed infant. However, this is an extremely bitter product. It is possible that even minuscule amounts in milk could alter the taste of milk leading to rejection by the infant.

Dymista is an intranasal spray that contains both azelastine and fluticasone.

T 1/2	22 h	MW	418 Da	PB	88%
Tmax	2-3 h	RID		Vd	14.5 L/kg
Oral	80%	M/P		pKa	9.5

Adult Concerns: Intranasal: nasal burning and bitter taste, headache, somnolence. Orally: drowsiness and bitter taste. Ophthalmic: transient eye burning/stinging, headache, and bitter taste.

Adult Dose: Variable: 1-2 sprays (137 µg/spray) per nostril BID.

Pediatric Concerns: None reported via milk. Levels in milk are unlikely to pose a problem. May impart bitter taste to milk, infant may reject milk.

Infant Monitoring:

Alternatives: Loratadine(L1), Cetirizine(L2)

References:
1. Pharmaceutical manufacturers prescribing information.

AZITHROMYCIN

Trade: Zithromax

Category: Antibiotic, Macrolide

LRC: L2 - Limited Data-Probably Compatible

Azithromycin is a macrolide antibiotic that is excreted minimally into breast milk; the level of exposure to the infant is unlikely to be clinically relevant. However, rare but serious toxicities have been associated with direct administration of azithromycin to neonates. At therapeutic levels, this drug has caused anaphylactic reactions, pseudomembranous colitis, and hypertrophic pyloric stenosis.[1,2] The incidence of these effects caused by incidental exposure to azithromycin via breast milk has not been documented.

In one study of a patient who received 1 g initially followed by 500 mg per day, the concentration of azithromycin in breast milk varied from 0.64 mg/L initially to 2.8 mg/L on the third day.[3] The predicted dose of azithromycin received by the infant would be approximately 0.4 mg/kg/day. In contrast, a typical direct dose for a neonate is 10 mg/kg initially followed by 5 mg/kg/day.[4]

T 1/2	48-68 h	MW	749 Da	PB	7%-51%
Tmax	3-4 h	RID	5.9%	Vd	23-31 L/kg
Oral	37%	M/P		pKa	12.43

Adult Concerns: QTc prolongation, arrhythmias, nausea, vomiting, abdominal cramping diarrhea, cholestatic jaundice, and severe rashes.

Adult Dose: 250-500 mg daily.

Pediatric Concerns: None reported via breastmilk. Pediatric formulations are available.

Infant Monitoring: Vomiting, diarrhea, changes in gastrointestinal flora, and rash.

Alternatives: Clarithromycin(L1), Erythromycin(L3)

References:
1. Eberly MD, Eide MB, Thompson JL, Nylund CM. Azithromycin in early infancy and pyloric stenosis. Pediatrics. March 2015;135(3):483-488.
2. Pharmaceutical manufacturer prescribing information.
3. Kelsey JJ, Moser LR, Jennings JC, Munger MA. Presence of azithromycin breast milk concentrations: a case report. Am J Obstet Gynecol. May 1994;170(5 pt 1):1375-1376.
4. Engorn B, Flerlage J, eds. The Harriet Lane Handbook: Mobile Medicine Series. 20th ed. Philadelphia, PA: Saunders; 2014.

AZTREONAM

Trade: Azactam

Category: Antibiotic, Other

LRC: L2 - Limited Data-Probably Compatible

Aztreonam is a monobactam antibiotic whose structure is similar but different from the penicillins and is used for documented gram-negative sepsis. Following a single 1 gm IV dose, breast milk level was 0.18 mg/L at 2 hours and 0.22 mg/L at 4 hours.[1] An infant would ingest approximately 33 µg/kg/day or <0.03% of the maternal dose per day (not weight adjusted). The manufacturer reports that less than 1% of a maternal dose is transferred into milk.[2] Due to poor oral absorption (<1%), no untoward effects would be expected in nursing infants, aside from changes in gastrointestinal flora. Aztreonam is commonly used in pediatric units. In another study of a patient early postpartum receiving a 1 gm intravenous injection, aztreonam levels in milk at 6 hours were 0.4 µg/mL to 1 µg/mL.[3]

T 1/2	1.7 h	MW	435 Da	PB	60%
Tmax	0.6-1.3 h	RID	0.2%-1%	Vd	0.26-0.36 L/kg
Oral	<1%	M/P	0.005	pKa	2.87

Adult Concerns: Changes in gastrointestinal flora, diarrhea, rash, elevations of hepatic function tests.

Adult Dose: 1-2 g every 8-12 hours.

Pediatric Concerns: None reported via milk in two cases.

Infant Monitoring: Vomiting, diarrhea, changes in gastrointestinal flora, and rash.

Alternatives:

References:
1. Fleiss PM, Richwald GA, Gordon J, Stern M, Frantz M, Devlin RG. Aztreonam in human serum and breast milk. Br J Clin Pharmacol. 1985;19(4):509-511.
2. Pharmaceutical manufacturers prescribing information.
3. Ito K, Hirose R, Tamaya T, Yamada Y, Izumi K. Pharmacokinetic and clinical studies on aztreonam in the perinatal period. Jpn J Antibiot. April 1990;43(4):719-726.

BACILLUS CALMETTE-GUERIN

Trade: BCG Vaccine, Bacillus of Calmette

Category: Vaccine

LRC: L3 - No Data-Probably Compatible

Bacillus Calmette-Guerin is a live attenuated bacterial preparation of *mycobacterium bovis* primarily used to prevent tuberculosis in countries with high prevalence of tuberculosis. It is commonly used in infants, children, and adults.[1] More recently, it is used as infusions in the bladder in the treatment of the bladder cancer.

While there are no literature reports of BCG vaccine in breastfeeding women, both the World Health Organization and American Advisory Committee on Immunization Practices suggest that the use of vaccines (live or inactivated) are considered safe. It is possible that the vaccine or antibodies may enter the breast milk but a preclinical study by the Swiss Serum and Vaccine Institute Berne suggested that breastfed infants of mothers inoculated with the BCG vaccine experienced no effects. It should be considered reasonably safe to administer this vaccine to nursing mothers when necessary.

Adult Concerns: BCG vaccine should not be used in infants, children, or adults with severe immune deficiency syndromes.

Adult Dose: Variable by indication.

Pediatric Concerns: BCG vaccine should not be used in infants or children, with severe immune deficiency syndromes.

Infant Monitoring: Disseminated infection in immunocompromised infants. Local tissue reactions. None reported via milk.

Alternatives:

References:

1. Centers for Disease Control and Prevention. The role of BCG VACCINE in the prevention and control of tuberculosis in the United States. MMWR. 1996;45(RR-4):1-18.

BACITRACIN

Trade: Bacitin, BACiiM, Baciject

Category: Antibiotic, Other

LRC: L2 - No Data-Probably Compatible

Bacitracin is a polypeptide antibiotic with bactericidal activity primarily against gram-positive organisms.[1] There are no adequate and well-controlled studies or case reports in breastfeeding women. It is unknown if bacitracin is distributed in human milk; however, it is unlikely as the minimal transcutaneous absorption after topical use should limit the amount of medication available for transfer into milk.

T 1/2	1.5 h	MW	1422 Da	PB	Minimal
Tmax	1-2 h (IM)	RID		Vd	Nil L/kg
Oral	Nil	M/P		pKa	3.95

Adult Concerns: Skin rashes or allergic reaction when used topically.

Adult Dose: Apply topically to affected area one to three times per day.

Pediatric Concerns: None reported via milk. Intramuscular use of this medications is restricted for the treatment of infants with pneumonia and empyema from staphylococci. When given IM can cause nausea, vomiting, albuminuria, renal failure, azotemia, pain at injection site, and skin rashes.

Infant Monitoring: Not required with topical maternal use.

Alternatives:

References:

1. Pharmaceutical manufacturers prescribing information.

BACLOFEN

Trade: Gablofen, Lioresal, Clofen

Category: Skeletal Muscle Relaxant

LRC: L2 - Limited Data-Probably Compatible

Baclofen inhibits spinal reflexes and is used to reverse spasticity associated with multiple sclerosis or spinal cord lesions.[1] Animal studies indicate baclofen inhibits prolactin release and may inhibit lactation. Small amounts of baclofen are secreted into milk. In one mother given a 20 mg oral dose, total consumption by the infant over a 26-hour period was estimated to be 22 µg, about 0.1% of the maternal dose (authors estimate). Milk levels ranged from 0.6 µmol/L (138 µg/L C_{max}) to 0.052 µmol/L at 26 hours. The maternal plasma and milk half-lives were 3.9 hours and 5.6 hours, respectively. It is quite unlikely that baclofen administered intrathecally would be secreted into milk in clinically relevant quantities.

T 1/2	3-4 h	MW	214 Da	PB	30%
Tmax	2-3 h	RID	6.9%	Vd	0.84 L/kg
Oral	Complete	M/P		pKa	

Adult Concerns: Headache, ataxia, drowsiness, dizziness, insomnia, dilated pupils, dry mouth, hypotension, palpitations, nausea, constipation, urinary retention or polyuria, weakness, tremor, rigidity and skin rashes. Withdrawal symptoms can occur; avoid abrupt discontinuation of intrathecal use as this can result in fever, muscle rigidity or spasticity, multiple organ failure, and death.

Adult Dose: 5-10 mg TID to QID.

Pediatric Concerns: None reported via milk. When an infant is exposed in utero, there is a risk of discontinuation syndrome after birth.

Infant Monitoring: Drowsiness, dry mouth, tremor, rigidity, wide pupils.

Alternatives:

References:
1. Eriksson G, Swahn CG. Concentrations of baclofen in serum and breast milk from a lactating woman. Scand J Clin Lab Invest. 1981;41(2):185-187.

BALOXAVIR

Trade: Xofluza

Category: Antiviral

LRC: L3 - No Data-Probably Compatible

Baloxavir is a polymerase acidic endonuclease inhibitor indicated for the treatment of acute uncomplicated influenza in patients 12 years of age and older who have been symptomatic for no more than 48 hours.[1] It is rather large in molecular weight (571 Da), which would limit high levels in milk. While it is known that it enters milk of rodents, drug levels in rodent milk are always higher and in no way correlates with human levels. Without any data, this product is probably relatively safe to use in breastfeeding mothers.

T 1/2	79.1 h	MW	571.55 Da	PB	93.9%
Tmax	4 h	RID		Vd	16.85 L/kg
Oral		M/P		pKa	

Adult Concerns: Diarrhea, bronchitis, nausea, nasopharyngitis, headache.

Adult Dose: 40-80 mg depending on weight, single dose.

Pediatric Concerns:

Infant Monitoring: Baloxavir is a polymerase acidic endonuclease inhibitor indicated for the treatment of acute uncomplicated influenza in patients 12 years of age and older who have been symptomatic for no more than 48 hours. It is rather large in molecular weight (571 Da), which would limit high levels in milk. While it is known that it enters milk of rodents, drug levels in rodent milk are always higher and in no way correlates with human levels.

Without any data, this product is probably relatively safe to use in breastfeeding mothers.

Alternatives:

References:
1. Pharmaceutical manufacturers prescribing information.

BALSALAZIDE

Trade: Colazal

Category: Salicylate, Non-Aspirin

LRC: L3 - Limited Data-Probably Compatible

Balsalazide disodium is a prodrug that is metabolized to mesalamine (5-aminosalicylic acid).[1] Balsalazide is delivered intact to the colon where it is cleaved by bacterial enzymes to release the active drug. The oral absorption of balsalazide is very low; less than 1% of the parent drug is recovered in the urine. Safety and side-effect profiles of balsalazide are expected to be similar to enteric-coated mesalamine. See the mesalamine monograph for more information.

T 1/2		MW	437 Da	PB	99%
Tmax	1-2 h	RID		Vd	
Oral	<1%	M/P		pKa	

Adult Concerns: Headache, abdominal pain, nausea, diarrhea, vomiting, respiratory infection, arthralgia have been reported.

Adult Dose: 2.25 g TID.

Pediatric Concerns: Watery diarrhea with mesalamine in one breastfeeding infant. Close observation recommended but it can probably be used relatively safely in breastfeeding mothers.

Infant Monitoring: Vomiting, diarrhea.

Alternatives: Mesalamine(L3), Olsalazine(L3)

References:
1. Pharmaceutical manufacturers prescribing information.

BARIUM SULFATE

Trade: Volumen, Entero VU, E-Z-CAT DRY, E-Z-PAQUE, E-Z-HD, Tagitol V

Category: Diagnostic Agent, Radiological Contrast Media

LRC: L1 - No Data-Compatible

Barium sulfate is used as a radiocontrast agent for X-ray imaging. Barium sulfate is available in a wide variety of concentrations, from 1.5% to 210%, under many trade names. It is not absorbed orally; therefore, none will enter the maternal milk compartment and reach the breastfeeding infant. No interruption in breastfeeding is required.[1]

T 1/2		MW	233.4 Da	PB	
Tmax		RID		Vd	
Oral	none	M/P		pKa	

Adult Concerns: Hypersensitivity, constipation, cramping. Serious side effects: emboli formation (venous intravasation), peritonitis (bowel perforation), pneumonitis (lung aspiration).

Adult Dose:

Pediatric Concerns: None reported via breast milk.

Infant Monitoring:

Alternatives:

References:
1. Pharmaceutical manufacturers prescribing information.

BECLOMETHASONE

Trade: AeroBec, Becloforte, Beclovent, Beconase, Qnasl, Qvar

Category: Anti-Inflammatory

LRC: L2 - No Data-Probably Compatible

Beclomethasone is a potent steroid that is generally used via oral inhalation in asthma or via intranasal administration for allergic rhinitis.[1] Plasma levels of both beclomethasone dipropionate (BDP) and its active metabolite beclomethasone-17-monopropionate (17-BMP) have been measured after both intranasal and oral inhalation. Systemic concentrations have been reported to be very low; therefore, it is unlikely that maternal use would produce significant levels in milk. See corticosteroids.

T 1/2	0.3 h (BDP); 3-4.5 h (17-BMP)	MW	521 Da	PB	87%-96%
Tmax	0.5-0.7 h	RID		Vd	0.28 (BDP); 6.05 (17-BMP) L/kg
Oral	43% (17-BMP)	M/P		pKa	13.85

Adult Concerns: Headache, oral candidiasis, hoarseness, bronchial irritation, cough.

Adult Dose: 40-400 µg twice daily.

Pediatric Concerns: None reported via milk.

Infant Monitoring: Feeding, growth and weight gain.

Alternatives:

References:
1. Pharmaceutical manufacturers prescribing information.

BELIMUMAB

Trade: Benlysta

Category: Immune Modulator

LRC: L3 - No Data-Probably Compatible

It is a B-lymphocyte stimulator (BLyS) inhibitor which is indicated for the treatment of patients with active, autoantibody-positive, systemic lupus erythematosus (SLE).[1] It blocks the binding of soluble BLyS, a B-cell survival factor, to its receptors on B cells and cause reduction in IgG and anti-dsDNA and increases complement (C3 and C4).

It is not known whether it is transferred into human milk or absorbed systemically after ingestion. Belimumab was excreted into the milk of cynomolgus monkeys, although levels were not reported. However, due to its size and structure, its transfer into human milk will probably be exceedingly low.

Although the molecular weight of this medication is very large and the amount in breast milk is expected to be exceptionally low, there are no long-term data concerning the safety of using immune modulating medications in breastfeeding mothers. Further there are current data that suggest that some IgG drugs do transfer to milk, and perhaps the breastfed infant. Therefore, some caution is recommended, and each woman should understand the benefits and risk of using this type of medication in lactation.

T 1/2	19.4 days	MW	151,800 Da	PB	
Tmax		RID		Vd	0.08 L/kg
Oral	Minimal	M/P		pKa	

Adult Concerns: Nausea, diarrhea, fever, hypersensitivity, infusion-site reactions, infections.

Adult Dose: 10 mg/kg at 2 week intervals for the first three doses, then every 4 weeks.

Pediatric Concerns: Safety and effectiveness have not been established in infants.

Infant Monitoring: Vomiting, diarrhea, fever, frequent infections.

Alternatives:

References:
1. Pharmaceutical manufacturers prescribing information.

BENAZEPRIL

Trade: Lotensin

Category: ACE Inhibitor

LRC: L2 - Limited Data-Probably Compatible

Benazepril hydrochloride belongs to the ACE inhibitor family. Oral absorption is rather poor (37%). The active component (benazeprilat) reaches its peak at approximately 2 hours after ingestion.[1] In a group of nine women taking benazepril 20 mg/day for 3 days, C_{max} levels of benazepril and benazeprilate were 0.89 µg/L and 2.048 µg/L respectively. This is 0.046% of the maternal dose of Benazepril, and 0.1% of the dose of the metabolite benazeprilate. Thus, the levels in milk are almost unmeasurable.

T 1/2	10-11 h	MW	424 Da	PB	96.7%
Tmax	0.5-1 h	RID	0.05%-0.11%	Vd	0.124 L/kg
Oral	37%	M/P	0.003	pKa	3.53

Adult Concerns: Headache, dizziness, fatigue, hypotension, abnormal taste, cough, nausea, diarrhea, constipation, changes in renal function/urine output, hyperkalemia, rash.

Adult Dose: 20-40 mg daily.

Pediatric Concerns: None reported via milk at this time.

Infant Monitoring: Drowsiness, lethargy, pallor, poor feeding, and weight gain.

Alternatives: Ramipril(L3), Enalapril(L2), Captopril(L2)

References:
1. Kaiser G, Ackerman R, Dieterle W, et al. Benazepril and benazeprilat in human plasma and breast milk. Eur J Clin Pharmacol. 1989;36(suppl):A303. Abstract.

BENDROFLUMETHIAZIDE

Trade: Aprinox, Berkozide, Centyl, Naturetin, Urizid

Category: Diuretic

LRC: L4 - Limited Data-Possibly Hazardous

Bendroflumethiazide is a thiazide diuretic sometimes used to suppress lactation. In one study, the clinician found this thiazide to effectively inhibit lactation.[1] Use with caution. Not generally recommended in breastfeeding mothers.

T 1/2	3-3.9 h	MW	421 Da	PB	94%
Tmax	2-4 h	RID		Vd	1.48 L/kg
Oral	Complete	M/P		pKa	9.04

Adult Concerns: Headache, dizziness, vertigo, hypotension, changes in electrolytes, leukopenia, reduced milk production.

Adult Dose: 2.5-10 mg daily.

Pediatric Concerns: None reported, but may inhibit lactation.

Infant Monitoring: Observe for fluid loss, dehydration, lethargy; monitor maternal milk supply.

Alternatives: Hydrochlorothiazide(L2)

References:
1. Healy M. Suppressing lactation with oral diuretics. Lancet. 1961;1:1353-1354.

BENOXINATE

Trade:

Category: Anesthetic, Local

LRC: L3 - No Data-Probably Compatible

Benoxinate hydrochloride is a derivative of para-aminobenzoic acid and is structurally similar to procaine. The anesthetic activity of benoxinate is ten times that of cocaine and twice that of tetracaine (amethocaine).[1] Its transfer to milk is probably minimal. Further, the ophthalmic dose would be minuscule and unlikely to produce significant plasma levels.

T 1/2		MW	344 Da	PB	
Tmax	1-15 min	RID		Vd	
Oral		M/P		pKa	

Adult Concerns: Conjunctivitis, keratitis, corneal damage due to prolonged, chronic use.

Adult Dose:

Pediatric Concerns:

Infant Monitoring:

Alternatives:

References:
1. Pharmaceutical manufacturers prescribing information.

BENRALIZUMAB

Trade: Fasenra

Category: Antiasthma

LRC: L3 - No Data-Probably Compatible

Benralizumab is a humanized monoclonal antibody (IgG1/κ-class) selective for interleukin-5 receptor alpha subunit (IL-5Rα). It is a monoclonal antibody that has a molecular weight of 150,000 Da. It is used to reduce eosinophil levels in the blood and tissues of asthmatics, and to reduce asthmatic allergic symptoms. Benralizumab, by binding to IL-5, reduces eosinophils through antibody-dependent cellular cytotoxicity. Not absorbed orally, benralizumab requires injection and has a biological half-life of about 15 days. This large monoclonal antibody is not likely to enter milk in clinically relevant amounts, nor to be orally absorbed by the infant.

T 1/2	15 days	MW	146,000 Da	PB	
Tmax		RID		Vd	
Oral	Nil	M/P		pKa	

Adult Concerns: Headache, fever, pharyngitis, hypersensitivity reactions, treatment emergent anti-drug antibody formation.

Adult Dose: 30 mg once every 4 weeks for the first three doses, and then once every 8 weeks.

Pediatric Concerns:

Infant Monitoring: No data on human milk. Probably compatible due to large molecular weight and poor oral absorption.

Alternatives:

References:
1. Pharmaceutical manufacturers prescribing information.

BENZALKONIUM CHLORIDE

Trade:

Category: Antibiotic, Other

LRC: L3 - No Data-Probably Compatible

Benzalkonium chloride is cationic detergent for topical use with bactericidal activity against bacteria, fungi, and viruses.[1] There are no adequate and well-controlled studies in lactating women. However, benzalkonium chloride is used in topical preparations (weak < 0.001%) and not absorbed systemically. Benzalkonium chloride is very soluble in water and is not likely to cause any problems in breastfeeding mothers.

T 1/2		MW	Variable Da	PB	
Tmax		RID		Vd	
Oral	Good	M/P		pKa	

Adult Concerns: Hypersensitivity reaction, bronchoconstriction, nausea, vomiting, contact dermatitis.

Adult Dose:

Pediatric Concerns:

Infant Monitoring:

Alternatives:

References:
1. Pharmaceutical manufacturer prescribing information.

BENZOCAINE

Trade: Americaine, Anacaine, Anusol, Benzodent, Ciggerex, Dent's, Orajel

Category: Anesthetic, Local

LRC: L2 - No Data-Probably Compatible

Benzocaine is a local anaesthetic.[1] It temporarily relieves pain associated with minor cuts, minor burns, scrapes itching. There are no adequate and well-controlled studies or case reports in breastfeeding women. Due to its poor bioavailability after topical application, concentrations achieved in maternal plasma are probably too low to produce any significant clinical effects in the breastfed infant. Dental procedure benzocaine usage is minimal and should pose no harm to the breastfed infant. Maternal plasma and milk levels do not seem to approach high concentrations and the oral bioavailability in the infant would be quite low (<35%). Probably safe during breastfeeding when used topically or orally.

T 1/2		MW		PB	
Tmax		RID		Vd	
Oral	Poor	M/P		pKa	2.51

Adult Concerns: Burning, contact dermatitis, edema, erythema, pruritis, rash, stinging, tenderness, uticaria.

Adult Dose: Apply topical 3-4 times a day.

Pediatric Concerns:

Infant Monitoring:

Alternatives:

References:
1. Pharmaceutical manufacturers prescribing information.

BENZONATATE

Trade: Tessalon Perles

Category: Antitussive

LRC: L4 - No Data-Possibly Hazardous

Benzonatate is a non-narcotic cough suppressant similar to the local anesthetic tetracaine. It anesthetizes stretch receptors in respiratory passages, dampening their activity and reducing the cough reflex.[1] There are minimal pharmacokinetic data on this product and no data on transfer to human milk. Milk transfer is expected to be low-moderate based on the medication's size (molecular weight 603 Da).

Benzonatate is a very dangerous product when taken directly by a child, with as little as 200 mg (typical dose 200 mg three times a day) serious toxicity can occur. There have been at least four deaths with this product (two infants, one toddler and one adult), and numerous serious adverse events such as agitation, seizure, coma, hypotension, cardiac arrhythmias, and cardiac arrest.[2,3] Due to this potential for severe toxicity at doses less than the typical recommended dose for cough suppressant effects this medication should be avoided in lactation.

Note: Although non-drug measures are preferred, an alternative cough suppressant that could be considered is dextromethorphan. Please see dextromethorphan monograph for specific details regarding suitability in lactation. Codeine is no longer recommended as a cough suppressant in lactation.

T 1/2	3-8 h	MW	603 Da	PB	
Tmax	20 min	RID		Vd	
Oral	Good	M/P		pKa	

Adult Concerns: Headache, dizziness, sedation, confusion, hallucinations, seizures, chest numbness, nausea, constipation, skin rash, pruritus have been reported. Para-aminobenzoic acid (PABA) is a metabolite of benzonatate, severe allergic reactions have been reported in patients who are allergic to PABA.

Adult Dose: 100 mg to 200 mg three times a day as needed.

Pediatric Concerns: Not approved for use in young children. No adverse effects reported via milk at this time. Significant risk of toxicity, even with typical dose recommendations; avoid use.

Infant Monitoring: AVOID in lactation.

Alternatives: Dextromethorphan(L3)

References:
1. Pharmaceutical manufacturers prescribing information.
2. Crouch BI, Knick KA, Crouch DJ, et al. Benzonatate overdose associated with seizures and arrhythmias. J Toxicol: Clin Toxicol. 1998;36(7):713-718.
3. Winter ML, Spiller HA, Griffith JRK. Benzonatate ingestion reported to the National Poison Centre Database System (NPDS). J Med Toxicol. 2010;6:398-.402.

BENZOYL PEROXIDE

Trade: Acne derm, Acne Gel, Banzagel, Benziq

Category: Antiacne

LRC: L2 - No Data-Probably Compatible

Benzoyl peroxide is an organic peroxide commonly used in many products for the treatment of acne, for bleaching hair and teeth, and many other uses.[1] Thus far, there are no data on its transfer into human milk. Benzoyl peroxide if ingested would be largely destroyed almost instantly by tissue and stomach esterases. It is unlikely that any would be absorbed systemically. Because only about 5% of topically applied benzoyl peroxide is absorbed (and rapidly converted to benzoic acid in the skin), it is thought to be of low risk to a nursing infant.

T 1/2		MW	242.23 Da	PB	
Tmax		RID		Vd	
Oral	Nil	M/P		pKa	

Adult Concerns: Erythema, irritation, allergy contact sensitization.

Adult Dose: Apply to affected area sparingly 1-3 times a day.

Pediatric Concerns:

Infant Monitoring:

Alternatives:

References:
1. Leachman SA, Reed BR. The use of dermatologic drugs in pregnancy and lactation. Dermatol Clin. 2006;24(2):167-197.

BENZTROPINE

Trade: Cogentin

Category: Cholinergic Antagonist

LRC: L3 - No Data-Probably Compatible

Benztropine mesylate is commonly used for the relief of parkinsonian signs (extrapyramidal reactions) commonly seen following the use of antipsychotic agents.[1] Benztropine has about one-half the anticholinergic effects of atropine, and has antihistamine effects. Its transfer into human milk has not been studied. Some caution is recommended if this product is used in breastfeeding mothers as some animal studies suggest anticholinergics reduce prolactin levels.

T 1/2		MW	403.55 Da	PB	95%
Tmax	7 h	RID		Vd	
Oral	29%	M/P		pKa	9.54

Adult Concerns: Confusion, hallucinations, blurred vision, mydriasis, hyperthermia, fever, tachycardia, urinary retention, constipation.

Adult Dose: 1-2 mg daily.

Pediatric Concerns: None reported via milk at this time.

Infant Monitoring: Sedation or irritability, hyperthermia, drying of oral and ophthalmic secretions, urinary retention, constipation.

Alternatives:

References:
1. Pharmaceutical manufacturers prescribing information.

BESIFLOXACIN

Trade: Besivance

Category: Antibiotic, Quinolone

LRC: L3 - No Data-Probably Compatible

Besifloxacin hydrochloride ophthalmic suspension, is a quinolone antimicrobial indicated for the treatment of bacterial conjunctivitis. No data are available on the transfer of this fluoroquinolone antibiotic into human milk. Plasma concentrations of besifloxacin following ophthalmic use indicated the maximum plasma besifloxacin concentration in each patient was less than 1.3 ng/mL.[1] The mean besifloxacin C_{max} was 0.37 ng/mL on day 1 and 0.43 ng/mL on day 6. The average elimination half-life of besifloxacin in plasma following multiple dosing was estimated to be

7 hours. While there are no milk studies available, plasma levels are so low that the amount likely present in milk is probably miniscule.

Because fluoroquinolones have limited safety data in pediatric and breastfeeding patients, use in lactation is not recommended if alternative therapies exist.1

T 1/2	7 h	MW		PB	
Tmax		RID		Vd	
Oral		M/P		pKa	

Adult Concerns: Headache, conjunctival redness, blurred vision, eye pain, eye irritation, eye pruritus.

Adult Dose: Instill one drop TID for 7 days.

Pediatric Concerns:

Infant Monitoring:

Alternatives:

References:
1. Pharmaceutical manufacturers prescribing information

BETA-CAROTENE

Trade: A-Caro-25, B-Caro-T, Lumitene

Category: Vitamin

LRC: L3 - No Data-Probably Compatible

Beta-carotene is a provitamin A that requires conversion to the active form of vitamin A (retinol) in the liver and intestinal mucosa.[1] Beta-carotene conversion in the liver is regulated by the concentration of retinol in the body. Recommended daily vitamin A intake is equivalent to 8000 IU or 4.8 mg of beta-carotene. Large doses of beta-carotene are used in the treatment of vitamin A deficiency (up to 162,000 IU) and cutaneous lesions of porphyria (up to 540,000 IU).[2]

In a study of 21 lactating women, ingestion of 31-35 mg/day (51,667-58,333 IU) of beta-carotene did not significantly increase beta-carotene concentrations in breast milk, suggesting that beta-carotene supplementation does increase levels in milk at least during the first 27 days postpartum.[3] Another study of lactating women approximately 279 days postpartum, beta-carotene supplementation (30 mg or 50,000 IU for 28 days) increased milk beta-carotene concentration 6.4 times (max around 190 μg/L); however, milk retinoid concentration did not increase significantly.[4]

There are no reports of adverse effects in breastfed infants from maternal beta-carotene supplementation.

T 1/2		MW	537 Da	PB	
Tmax		RID		Vd	
Oral	30%	M/P		pKa	

Adult Concerns: Carotenodermia, diarrhea, bruising, dizziness.

Adult Dose: 6-15 mg/day.

Pediatric Concerns:

Infant Monitoring: Diarrhea, bruising.

Alternatives:

References:
1. Polifka JE, Dolan CR, Donlan MA, Friedman JM. Clinical teratology counseling and consultation report: high dose beta-carotene use during early pregnancy. Teratology. August 1996;54(2):103-107.
2. Lewis JM, Bodansky O, Lillienfeld MCC, Schneider H. Supplements of vitamin A and of carotene during pregnancy. Their effect on the levels of vitamin A and carotene in the blood of mother and of newborn infant. Am J Dis Child. 1947;73:143-150.
3. Gossage CP, Deyhim M, Yamini S, Douglass LW, Moser-Veillon PB. Carotenoid composition of human milk during the first month postpartum and the response to beta-carotene supplementation. Am J Clin Nutr. July 2002;76(1):193-197.
4. Canfield LM, Giuliano AR, Neilson EM, Blashil BM, Graver EJ, Yap HH. Kinetics of the response of milk and serum beta-carotene to daily beta-carotene supplementation in healthy, lactating women. Am J Clin Nutr. February 1998;67(2):276-283. Erratum in: Am J Clin Nutr. June 1998;67(6):1286.

BETAHISTINE

Trade: Betaserc, Hiserc, Serc

Category: Other

LRC: L4 - No Data-Possibly Hazardous

Betahistine hydrochloride is an anti-vertigo drug used for the treatment of Meniere's disease. It is a histamine analog and has agonistic action on the histamine-1 receptors. It also causes the release of histamine from nerve terminals. Therefore, its pharmacological effects are similar to that of histamine. At this time there are no data regarding the transfer of this medication into human milk. Betahistine is completely absorbed orally and has very low protein binding (<5%) that would encourage transfer into milk; however, this medication is primarily metabolized to an inactive metabolite (peaks 1 hour) and thus we do not anticipate a significant amount of active drug in milk.

Due to the possibility of major side effects in the breastfed infant, and poorly characterized active component, it is advisable to avoid the use of this drug in lactating women until data that quantify drug transfer to milk and report on infant safety are available. Consider alternatives such as dimenhydrinate or meclizine if appropriate.

T 1/2	3-4 h	MW	209 Da	PB	<5%
Tmax	1 h	RID		Vd	
Oral	Complete	M/P		pKa	

Adult Concerns: Headache, dizziness, confusion, flushing, hypotension, nausea, vomiting, diarrhea, skin rash, pruritus. Exacerbation of asthma and peptic ulcers.

Adult Dose: 8-16 mg three times a day.

Pediatric Concerns: No data in lactation at this time.

Infant Monitoring: Lethargy, vomiting, diarrhea, skin rash.

Alternatives: Dimenhydrinate(L2), Diphenhydramine(L2), Meclizine(L3)

References:
1. Pharmaceutical manufacturer prescribing information.

BETAMETHASONE

Trade: Betaject, Betaderm, Betnovate, Betnelan, Celestone Soluspan, Diprosone

Category: Corticosteroid

LRC: L3 - No Data-Probably Compatible

Betamethasone is a potent long-acting steroid and is about 25 times as potent as hydrocortisone. It generally produces less sodium and fluid retention than other steroids.[1] In small doses, most steroids are certainly not contraindicated in nursing mothers. Whenever possible use low-dose alternatives such as aerosols or inhalers. Following administration, wait at least 4 hours if possible prior to feeding infant to reduce exposure. With high doses (>40 mg/day), particularly for long periods, steroids could potentially produce problems in infant growth and development, although we have absolutely no data in this area, or which doses would pose problems. Brief applications of high dose steroids are probably not contraindicated as the overall exposure is low. With prolonged high dose therapy, the infant should be closely monitored for growth and development.

T 1/2	5.6 h	MW	392 Da	PB	64%
Tmax	10-36 min	RID		Vd	
Oral	Complete	M/P		pKa	12.42

Adult Concerns: Gastric distress, gastric ulceration, glaucoma, thinning of skin.

Adult Dose: 0.25-12 mg IM per dose (variable based on indication).

Pediatric Concerns: None reported, used in pediatric patients.

Infant Monitoring: Feeding, growth, and weight gain.

Alternatives:

References:

maceutical manufacturers prescribing information.

BETAXOLOL

Trade: Betoptic, Kerlone

Category: Beta Adrenergic Blocker

LRC: L3 - Limited Data-Probably Compatible

Betaxolol is a long-acting, cardioselective beta blocker primarily used for glaucoma but can be used orally for hypertension. One report by the manufacturer reports side effects that occurred in one nursing infant.[1] Many in this family of drugs readily transfer to human milk (see atenolol, acebutolol), others do so poorly (propranolol, metoprolol).[2] Betaxolol when used ophthalmically, is apparently poorly absorbed systemically as no evidence of beta-blockade can be found in patients following its use ophthalmically. Since maternal plasma levels with ophthalmic are low, levels in mature milk should be low as well, although there are currently no studies to confirm this. In a study of 28 women consuming 10 mg betaxolol during the perinatal period, the milk/plasma ratio in three patients was 3.[3] Note this was done early postnatally in colostrum and may not at all reflect postnatal levels in mature milk. In one case where the drug was administered 3 hours prior to delivery, colostrum levels were 48 µg/L at 24 hours postpartum and 3 µg/L at 72 hours postpartum. Nothing in this study should reflect levels in mature milk.

T 1/2	14-22 h	MW	307 Da	PB	50%
Tmax	3 h	RID		Vd	4.9 L/kg
Oral	89%	M/P	2.5-3	pKa	9.4

Adult Concerns: Headache, dizziness, insomnia, depression, fatigue, chest pain, bradycardia, hypotension, heart failure, wheezing, vomiting, heartburn, diarrhea, myalgia.

Adult Dose: 10 mg daily.

Pediatric Concerns: No data is available on its transfer to milk. However, when used ophthalmically, no systemic beta-blockade was noted, suggesting plasma levels are low to nil. Milk levels are likely low as well.

Infant Monitoring: Drowsiness, lethargy, pallor, poor feeding, and weight gain.

Alternatives: Propranolol(L2), Metoprolol(L2)

References:
1. Pharmaceutical manufacturers prescribing information.
2. Beresford R, Heel RC. Betaxolol: a review of its pharmacodynamic and pharmacokinetic properties, and therapeutic efficacy in hypertension. Drugs. 1986;31:6-28.
3. Morselli PL, Boutroy MJ, Thenot JP. Pharmacokinetics of antihypertensive drugs in the neonatal period. Dev Pharmacol Ther. 1989;13:190-198.

BETHANECHOL

Trade: Duvoid, Myotonine, Urabeth, Urecholine, Urocarb

Category: Renal-Urologic Agent

LRC: L4 - No Data-Possibly Hazardous

Bethanechol chloride is a cholinergic stimulant useful for urinary retention. Although poorly absorbed from gastrointestinal tract, no reports on entry into breast milk are available. However, it could conceivably cause abdominal cramps, colicky pain, nausea, salivation, bronchial constriction, or diarrhea in infants. There are several reports of discomfort in nursing infants.[1] Use with great caution.

T 1/2	1-2 h	MW	197 Da	PB	
Tmax	60-90 min (oral)	RID		Vd	
Oral	Poor	M/P		pKa	

Adult Concerns: Headache, salivation, hypotension, heart block, breathing difficulties, nausea, cramping, diarrhea, urinary urgency. Contraindicated in patients with asthma, bradycardia, hypotension, epilepsy, etc.

Adult Dose: 10-50 mg BID-QID.

Pediatric Concerns: Gastrointestinal distress, discomfort, diarrhea.

Infant Monitoring: Colic, diarrhea.

Alternatives:

References:
1. Shore MF. Drugs can be dangerous during pregnancy and lactation. Can Pharmaceut J. 1970;103:358.

BEVACIZUMAB

Trade: Avastin

Category: Immune Modulator

LRC: L3 - No Data-Probably Compatible

Bevacizumab is a monoclonal IgG antibody that binds to vascular endothelial growth factor, preventing it from binding to endothelial receptors, thus blocking angiogenesis. This slows the growth of all tissues, including metastatic tissues. It is used in colorectal, lung, breast, prostate, and ovarian cancers, as well as for age-related macular degeneration.[1]

Following intravitreal injections in two breastfeeding mothers over the course of 16 months, enzyme-linked immunosorbent assay and Western blot analysis was used to determine the levels of bevacizumab in the milk samples.[2] All breast milk samples assayed from the two patients actively undergoing treatment did not have detectable levels of bevacizumab. Samples collected 1.5 hours and 7 hours after an injection and two randomly chosen samples were negative by Western blot analysis.

When used intravitreally, the dose (1.25 mg) is much lower than via systemic administration (5-10 mg/kg), and it is largely sequestered in the eye[3], thus plasma levels (and milk) would be exceedingly low. The intravitreal use of this drug is probably compatible with breastfeeding. The systemic use of this drug may not be compatible with breastfeeding.

T 1/2	20 days	MW	149,000 Da	PB	
Tmax		RID		Vd	0.046 L/kg
Oral	Nil	M/P		pKa	

Adult Concerns: Gastrointestinal perforations, surgery and wound healing complications, hemorrhage, venous thromboembolic events, neutropenia and infection, slight proteinuria, congestive heart failure, hypertension, diarrhea, leukopenia.

Adult Dose: 5-15 mg/kg every 2-3 weeks.

Pediatric Concerns: None reported via milk. Reduced growth in epiphyseal growth plates in monkey studies.

Infant Monitoring: Vomiting, diarrhea, fever, frequent infections.

Alternatives:

References:
1. Pharmaceutical manufacturers prescribing information.
2. McFarland TJ, Rhoads AD, Hartzell M, Emerson GG, Bhavsar AR, Stout JT. Bevacizumab levels in breast milk after long-term intravitreal injections. Retina. August 2015;35(8):1670-1673.
3. Julien S, Heiduschka P, Hofmeister S, Schraermeyer U. Immunohistochemical localisation of intravitreally injected bevacizumab at the posterior pole of the primate eye: implication for the treatment of retinal vein occlusion. Br J Ophthalmol. October 2008;92(10):1424-1428.

BIFIDOBACTERIUM INFANTIS

Trade: Align

Category: Probiotic

LRC: L3 - No Data-Probably Compatible

Bifidobacteria infantis is a probiotic strain that may help in relieving common digestive problems, including: constipation, diarrhea, abdominal discomfort, urgency, gas, and bloating. According to the WHO, probiotics are live microorganisms, which when administered in adequate amounts, confer a health benefit to the host.[1]

In a study that explored the immunomodulatory potential of Bifidobacteria compared with three other commercial strains, the researchers suggested that it enhances Natural Killer activity and production of interferons.[2]

Due to the fact that probiotics are not often absorbed systemically, it is unlikely that they will transfer into breast milk. There are currently no published data regarding adverse effects in breastfed infants whose mothers were actively taking probiotics.[3] However, these should probably not be used in a mother with a premature infant with a poorly developed GI tract.

Adult Concerns: Gastric side effects include temporary increase in gas and bloating.

Adult Dose: One capsule daily.

Pediatric Concerns: None reported.

Infant Monitoring:

Alternatives:

References:
1. Ciorba MA. A gastroenterologist's guide to probiotics. Clin Gastroenterol Hepatol. September 2012;10(9):960-968.
2. You J, Yaqoob P. Evidence of immunomodulatory effects of a novel probiotic, Bifidobacterium longum bv. infantis CCUG 52486. FEMS Immunol Med Microbiol. December 2012;66(3):353-362. doi:10.1111/j.1574-695X.2012.01014.x. Epub August 31, 2012.
3. Bozzo P, Einarson A, Elias J. Are probiotics safe for use during pregnancy and lactation? Can Fam Physician. March 2011;57:299-301.

BIMATOPROST

Trade: Latisse, Lumigan

Category: Antiglaucoma

LRC: L3 - No Data-Probably Compatible

Bimatoprost is used in open-angle glaucoma or ocular hypertension to reduce intraocular pressure. It is a synthetic structural analog of prostaglandin, and it mimics the effects of naturally occurring prostaglandins. Bimatoprost increases the outflow of aqueous humor through the trabecular meshwork and uveoscleral routes.[1] No breastfeeding data are available. However, after intraocular administration, plasma levels peak at 10 minutes, then fall rapidly to undetectable levels within 1.5 hours. Combined with low plasma levels and high protein binding, it is unlikely this product would produce measurable levels in human milk.

T 1/2	45 min	MW	415 Da	PB	88%
Tmax	10 min	RID		Vd	0.67 L/kg
Oral		M/P		pKa	14.35

Adult Concerns: Adverse effects include conjunctival hyperemia, growth of eyelashes, and ocular pruritus.

Adult Dose: One drop every evening.

Pediatric Concerns: No data are available.

Infant Monitoring:

Alternatives:

References:
1. Pharmaceutical manufacturers prescribing information.

BIOTIN

Trade: Coenzyme R, Vitamin B7, Vitamin H

Category: Vitamin

LRC:

Biotin, also known as vitamin H or B7, is a coenzyme that participates in many metabolic processes. It is part of gluconeogenesis as well as the metabolism of fatty acids and leucine. It is also required for normal neuronal and hematopoietic function. Symptoms of biotin deficiency include thinning hair, skin rash, and depression. The recommended daily dose of biotin for a pregnant woman is 30 µg/day, and for a lactating woman is 35 µg/day. An infant less than 6 months old needs 0.9 µg/kg/day, while an infant over 6 months should get 6 µg/day.[1] Levels of biotin in human milk range from 5 to 9 µg/L, indicating that there is active transport of biotin into milk.[2] No adverse effects have been found, nor has a toxic upper intake been established.

T 1/2		MW	244 Da	PB	
Tmax		RID		Vd	
Oral	Complete	M/P		pKa	

Adult Concerns: None. Supplements that contain biotin above recommended amounts may cause false results in some lab tests, including those that measure levels of certain hormones, like thyroid hormone. One patient consuming 2400 micrograms of biotin daily reported gastrointestinal upset.

Adult Dose: 35 micrograms per day.

Pediatric Concerns: None reported via milk at this time.

Infant Monitoring:

Alternatives:

References:

1. Food and Nutrition Board. Institute of Medicine. Dietary Reference Intakes for Thiamin, Riboflavin, Niacin, Vitamin B6, Folate, Vitamin B12, Pantothenic Acid, Biotin, and Choline. Washington, DC: National Academy Press; 1998.
2. Picciano MF. Vitamins in milk. Water-soluble vitamins in human milk. In: Jensen RG, ed. Handbook of Milk Composition. San Diego, CA: Academic Press; 1995.

BISACODYL

Trade: Bisacolax, Dulcolax

Category: Laxative

LRC: L2 - Limited Data-Probably Compatible

Bisacodyl is a stimulant laxative that selectively stimulates colon contractions and defecation. It has only limited secretion into breast milk due to poor gastric absorption and subsequently minimal systemic levels.[1] Little or no known harmful effects on infants.

T 1/2	16 h	MW	361 Da	PB	
Tmax		RID		Vd	
Oral	<5%	M/P		pKa	

Adult Concerns: Diarrhea, gastrointestinal cramping, rectal irritation.

Adult Dose: 5-15 mg as a single dose.

Pediatric Concerns: None reported via milk.

Infant Monitoring: Diarrhea.

Alternatives:

References:

1. Vorherr H. Drug excretion in breast milk. Postgrad Med. 1974;56(4):97-104.

BISMUTH SUBGALLATE

Trade: Devrom

Category: Dietary Supplement

LRC: L3 - No Data-Probably Compatible

Bismuth subgallate is used as an internal deodorant commonly used by people who have fecal incontinence and those who have had an ileostomy, colostomy and bariatric surgery (duodenal switch, gastric bypass, biliopancreatic diversion). It is used to deodorize embarrassing flatulence odor. Bismuth subgallate has poor oral bioavailability of less than 1%.[1] Since it is poorly absorbed, bismuth subgallate is unlikely to be present in breastmilk.

T 1/2		MW	394 Da	PB	
Tmax		RID		Vd	
Oral	<1%	M/P		pKa	

Adult Concerns: Reversible darkening of stool and tongue, constipation.

Adult Dose: 200-400 mg four times daily. Not to exceed 8 capsules per day.

Pediatric Concerns:

Infant Monitoring:

Alternatives:

References:
1. Dresow B, Fischer R, Gabbe EE, Wendel J, Heinrich HC. Bismuth absorption from 205Bi-labelled pharmaceutical bismuth compounds used in the treatment of peptic ulcer disease. Scand J Gastroenterol. April 1992;27(4):333-336. Abstract.

BISMUTH SUBSALICYLATE

Trade: Pepto-Bismol

Category: Antidiarrheal

LRC: L3 - No Data-Probably Compatible

Bismuth subsalicylate is present in many diarrhea mixtures. Although bismuth salts are poorly absorbed from the maternal GI tract, significant levels of salicylate could be absorbed from these products.[1] While to date, bismuth subsalicylate and other nonacetylated salicylates have not been associated with Reye syndrome, this drug should not be routinely used in breastfeeding women.

T 1/2	Highly variable	MW	362 Da	PB	
Tmax		RID		Vd	
Oral	Poor	M/P		pKa	

Adult Concerns: Constipation, black tongue, black stool, salicylate poisoning (tinnitus, weakness).

Adult Dose: 524 mg every 30 minutes to 1 hour as needed up to eight doses per 24 hour.

Pediatric Concerns: Risk of Reye syndrome in neonates, but has not been reported with this product in a breastfed infant.

Infant Monitoring:

Alternatives:

References:
1. Findlay JW, DeAngelis RL, Kearney MF, Welch RM, Findlay JM. Analgesic drugs in breast milk and plasma. Clin Pharmacol Ther. 1981;29(5):625-633.

BISOPROLOL

Trade: Emcor, Monocor, Zebeta

Category: Beta Adrenergic Blocker

LRC: L3 - Limited Data-Probably Compatible

Bisoprolol fumarate is a beta-blocker used to treat hypertension.[1] The manufacturer states that small amounts (<2%) are secreted into milk of animals.

In one case report a woman was started on bisoprolol 5 mg once daily 6 days postpartum for a cardiac condition diagnosed around the time of delivery.[2] The patient manually expressed and discarded her milk until her care providers were able to assess her new medication in milk. She provided milk samples taken between 11 and 18 days after bisoprolol was initiated and they were undetectable. In this case the infant was not given any of the maternal breast milk, thus no infant safety data is available at this time.

T 1/2	9-12 h	MW	325 Da	PB	30%
Tmax	2-4 h	RID		Vd	3.5 L/kg
Oral	80%	M/P		pKa	9.5

Adult Concerns: Headache, dizziness, insomnia, depression, fatigue, chest pain, bradycardia, hypotension, heart failure, wheezing, vomiting, diarrhea, myalgia.

Adult Dose: 5-10 mg daily.

Pediatric Concerns: None reported via milk at this time.

Infant Monitoring: Drowsiness, lethargy, pallor, poor feeding, and weight gain.

Alternatives: Labetalol(L2), Metoprolol(L2), Nifedipine(L2)

References:
1. Pharmaceutical manufacturers prescribing information.
2. Khurana R, Bin Jardan YA, Wilkie J, et al. Breast milk concentrations of amiodarone, desethylamiodarone, and bisoprolol following short-term drug exposure: two case reports. J Clin Pharmacol. 2014;54(7):828-831.

BIVALIRUDIN

Trade: Angiomax, Angiox

Category: Anticoagulant

LRC:

Bivalirudin Injection is a direct thrombin inhibitor indicated for use as an anticoagulant in patients undergoing percutaneous coronary intervention.[1] It is a specific and reversible direct thrombin inhibitor. Bivalirudin is a synthetic, 20 amino acid peptide, with a molecular weight of 2180 Da. It has a brief 25 minute half-life and is large in molecular weight. It is unlikely to enter milk or be orally bioavailable as it is metabolized by various proteases. It is only presently used during cardiac surgery.

T 1/2	25 min	MW	2180.29 Da	PB	None
Tmax		RID		Vd	
Oral	Nil	M/P		pKa	

Adult Concerns: Hemorrhage.

Adult Dose: 0.75 mg/kg IV followed by a 1.75 mg/kg/h intravenous infusion for the duration of the procedure.

Pediatric Concerns:

Infant Monitoring: None required.

Alternatives:

References:
1. Pharmaceutical manufacturers prescribing information.

BLACK COHOSH

Trade: Actaea racemosa

Category: Herb

LRC: L4 - No Data-Possibly Hazardous

The roots and rhizomes of this herb are used medicinally. Traditional uses include the treatment of dysmenorrhea, dyspepsia, rheumatism, and as an antitussive. It has also been used as an insect repellent. The standardized extract, called Remifemin, has been used in Germany for menopausal management.[1]

Black cohosh contains a number of alkaloids including N-methylcytosine, other tannins, and terpenoids. It is believed that the isoflavones or formononetin components may bind to estrogenic receptors.[2] Intraperitoneal injection of the extract selectively inhibits release of luteinizing hormone with no effect on the follicle-stimulating hormone (FSH) or prolactin.[3] The data seem to suggest that this product interacts strongly at certain specific estrogen receptors and might be useful as estrogen replacement therapy in postmenopausal women although this has not been well studied. More studies are needed to address its usefulness in postmenopausal women and osteoporotic states.[1]

No data are available on the transfer of black cohosh to human milk, but due to its estrogenic activity, it could lower milk production although this is not known at this time. Caution is recommended in breastfeeding mothers.[5]

Adult Concerns: Hypotension, hypocholesterolemic activity, and peripheral vasodilation in vasospastic conditions. Overdose may cause nausea, vomiting, dizziness, visual disturbances, bradycardia, and perspiration. Large doses may induce miscarriage. This product should not be used in pregnant women.

Adult Dose: 20-40 mg twice daily (varies by indication).

Pediatric Concerns: None reported via milk.

Infant Monitoring:

Alternatives:

References:
1. Murray M. Remifemin: answers to some common questions. Am J Nat Med. 1997;4(3):3-5.
2. Jarry H, et al. Planta Medica. 1885;4:316-319.

3. Jarry H, et al. Planta Medica. 1885;1:46-49.
4. Newall C. Black Cohosh Herbal Medicines. London, UK: Pharmaceutical Press; 1996:80-81.
5. The Complete German Commission E Monographs. Ed. M. Blumenthal. Austin, TX/Boston, MA: American Botanical Council 1998.

BLEOMYCIN

Trade: Blenoxane, Bleo-S, Bleo-cell, Bleocin

Category: Antineoplastic

LRC: L4 - No Data-Possibly Hazardous

Bleomycin sulfate is used for a number of different cancers including: testicular, head and neck cancer, Hodgkin's and non-Hodgkin's lymphomas, and cervical cancer. Seventy percent of the dose is recovered in urine 24 hours after dosing.[1] The elimination of bleomycin is described by two bioexponential curves with a terminal T(beta) of 134-238 minutes. In patients with severely reduced kidney function, the T(beta) increases to 13.5 hours. No data are available on its transfer to milk, but its transfer to milk in clinically relevant levels is remote as its molecular weight is 1415 Da. Secondly, its oral bioavailability is probably low to nil.

Withhold breastfeeding for at least 24 hours. Extend this recommendation in mothers with poor renal function.

T 1/2	134-238 min	MW	1415.56 Da	PB	1%
Tmax	<30 min	RID		Vd	0.35-0.45 L/kg
Oral		M/P		pKa	11.34

Adult Concerns: Nausea, vomiting, weight loss, stomatitis, dermatitis, mucositis, alopecia, fever.

Adult Dose: Varies depending on indication.

Pediatric Concerns:

Infant Monitoring: Avoid breastfeeding for at least 24 hours or longer in mothers with poor renal function.

Alternatives:

References:
1. Grochow LB, Ames MM. A Clinician's Guide to Chemotherapy Pharmacokinetics and Pharmacodynamics. 1st ed. Baltimore, MD: Williams & Wilkins; 1998.

BLESSED THISTLE

Trade: Blessed Thistle

Category: Herb

LRC: L3 - No Data-Probably Compatible

Blessed thistle contains an enormous array of chemicals, polyenes, steroids, terpenoids, and volatile oils. It is thought to be useful for diarrhea, hemorrhage, fevers, as an expectorant, as a bacteriostatic, for loss of appetite, indigestion, for promoting lactation, and other antiseptic properties. Traditionally it has been used for loss of appetite, flatulence, cough and congestion, gangrenous ulcers, and dyspepsia. It has been documented to be antibacterial against: *Bacillus subtilis*, *Brucella abortus*, *Bordatella bronchiseptica*, *E. coli*, Proteus species, *P. aeruginosa*, *Staphylococcus aureus*, and *Streptococcus faecalis*.

The antibacterial and anti-inflammatory properties are due to its cnicin component.[1] While it is commonly use as a galactagogue, no data could be found supporting its use in this application in the German E commission, nor a number of other herbal references. Although this herb lacks good safety data in adult and pediatric patients, there are only occasional suggestions that high doses may induce gastrointestinal symptoms.[2] Some sources mention that it is an abortifacient, do not use in pregnant patients.

Adult Concerns: Virtually non-toxic, but may be an abortifacient. In doses > 5 grams per cup, it has been associated with stomach irritation, nausea, and vomiting. It also may induce allergies in individuals sensitive to ragweed, daisies, marigolds, and chrysanthemums.

Adult Dose: 1.5-3 g as a tea up to three times daily.

Pediatric Concerns: None reported via milk but it lacks justification as a galactagogue.

Infant Monitoring:

Alternatives:

References:
1. Vanhaelen-Fastre R. Cnicus benedictus: seperation of antimicrobial constituents. Plant Med Phytother. 1968;2:294-299.
2. Newall C. Black Cohosh Herbal Medicines. London, UK: Pharmaceutical Press; 1996:80-81.

BLUE COHOSH

Trade: Blue ginseng, Papoose root, Squaw root, Yellow ginseng

Category: Herb

LRC: L5 - Limited Data-Hazardous

Blue cohosh is also known as blue ginseng, squaw root, papoose root, or yellow ginseng. It is primarily used as a uterotonic drug to stimulate uterine contractions. In one recent paper, an infant born of a mother who ingested blue cohosh root for 3 weeks prior to delivery, suffered from severe cardiogenic shock and congestive heart failure.[1] Subsequent studies have found it cardiotoxic in animals. Blue cohosh root contains a number of chemicals, including the alkaloid methylcytosine and the glycosides caulosaponin and caulophyllosaponin. Methylcytosine is pharmacologically similar to nicotine and may result in elevated blood pressure, gastric stimulation, and hyperglycemia. Caulosaponin and caulophyllosaponin are uterine stimulants. They also, apparently, produce severe ischemia of the myocardium due to intense coronary vasoconstriction. This product should not be used in pregnant women. No data are available concerning its transfer into human milk. Do not use in breastfeeding mothers at any time.

Adult Concerns: The leaves and seeds contain alkaloids and glycosides that can cause severe stomach pain when ingested. Poisonings have been reported. Symptoms include irritation of mucous membranes, diarrhea, cramping, chest pain, and hyperglycemia.

Adult Dose:

Pediatric Concerns: No adverse events reported in lactation at this time.

Infant Monitoring: Severe cardiac toxin. Avoid.

Alternatives:

References:
1. Jones TK, Lawson BM. Profound neonatal congestive heart failure caused by maternal consumption of blue cohosh herbal medication. J Pediatr. 1998;132(3 pt 1):550-552.

BOCEPREVIR

Trade: Victrelis

Category: Antiviral

LRC: L4 - Limited Data-Possibly Hazardous

Boceprevir is an antiviral drug for treatment of chronic hepatitis C virus (HCV). It functions by inhibiting hepatitis C virus replication in infected cells. It is usually used in combination with ribavirin and interferon alfa. There are no studies of its use in breastfeeding women. In one animal study peak serum concentration of boceprevir and its metabolite in nursing pups was about 1% of maternal serum concentration.[1] Although data show limited entry in rodent milk, its use for the treatment of hepatitis C in lactation may be problematic as it is used in combination with ribavirin. High concentrations of ribavirin could accumulate in the breastfed infant (see ribavirin monograph).

T 1/2	3.4 h	MW	520 Da	PB	75%
Tmax	2 h	RID		Vd	11 L/kg
Oral	65%	M/P		pKa	

Adult Concerns: Fatigue, insomnia, chills, anemia, neutropenia, thrombocytopenia, nausea, vomiting, headache, abnormal taste, xerostomia, arthralgia, thromboembolic events.

Adult Dose: 800 mg TID.

Pediatric Concerns:

Infant Monitoring: Not recommended for chronic exposure via breast milk.

Alternatives:

References:
1. Pharmaceutical manufacturers prescribing information.

BORAGE

Trade: Bee plant, Beebread, Borage, Borage oil, Burrage, Ox, Starflower

Category: Herb

LRC: L5 - No Data-Hazardous

Borage is also called Beebread, Bee Plant, Burrage, Starflower. Borage oil or other products may contain the powerful and dangerous pyrrolizidine-type alkaloids. Native borage oil contains, amabiline, which is hepatotoxic pyrrolizidine alkaloid. The use of this product in breastfeeding women is contraindicated unless it is certified to be free of amabiline. Ingestion of 1-2 grams of borage oil per day could provide doses of unsaturated pyrrolizidine alkaloids equal to 10 µg, which is in excess of the 1 µg/day limit recommended by the German Federal Health Agency.

Adult Concerns: May contain amabiline, which is hepatotoxic pyrrolizidine alkaloid.

Adult Dose: 1-4 grams.

Pediatric Concerns:

Infant Monitoring: Liver toxicity.

Alternatives:

References:
1. Newell C, Anderson LA, Phillipson JD. Borage. In: Herbal Medicine: a guide for the healthcare professionals. London, UK: The Pharmaceutical Press; 1996.

BOSENTAN

Trade: Tracleer

Category: Antihypertensive

LRC: L4 - No Data-Possibly Hazardous

Bosentan is used in the treatment of pulmonary artery hypertension. It blocks endothelin receptors on vascular endothelium and smooth muscle, thus blocking vasoconstriction.[1] No data are available on the transfer into human milk, but bosentan is highly protein bound (98%), with a large molecular weight; therefore, only small amounts are likely to be found unbound in the plasma. As a result, the amount in the milk compartment would probably be very low. However, this product is 50% orally bioavailable, and is known to have a high incidence of liver toxicity. Great caution is recommended with this product in breastfeeding mothers until we have published milk levels.

T 1/2	5 h	MW	569 Da	PB	98%
Tmax	3-5 h	RID		Vd	0.26 L/kg
Oral	50%	M/P		pKa	5.8

Adult Concerns: Headache, hypotension, palpitations, flushing, changes in liver function, anemia, lower extremity edema.

Adult Dose: 125 mg BID.

Pediatric Concerns: No data are available in lactation. Used in pediatrics (children > 10 kg) to treat pulmonary artery hypertension.

Infant Monitoring: Drowsiness, lethargy, pallor, poor feeding, and weight gain.

Alternatives:

References:
1. Pharmaceutical manufacturers prescribing information.

BOTULINUM TOXIN

Trade: Botox, Botulism, Clostridium botulinum, Onabotulinumtoxin A, Dysport, Xeomin, Azzalure

Category: Neuromuscular Blocker

LRC: L3 - No Data-Probably Compatible

Botulism is a syndrome produced by the deadly toxin secreted by the bacteria *Clostridium botulinum*. Botulinum toxins are neuromuscular blocking agents that produce muscular paralysis. Although the bacteria are widespread, their colonization in food or the intestine of infants produces a deadly toxin. The syndrome is characterized by GI distress, weakness, malaise, lightheadedness, sore throat, and nausea. Dry mouth is almost universal. In most adult poisoning, the bacteria are absent; only the toxin is present. In most pediatric poisoning, the stomach is colonized by the bacteria, often from contaminated honey.

In one published report, a breastfeeding woman severely poisoned by botulism toxin continued to breastfeed her infant throughout the illness.[1] Four hours after admission, her milk was tested and was free of botulinum toxin or C. botulinum bacteria, although she was still severely ill. The infant showed no symptoms of poisoning. It is apparent from this case that neither botulinum bacteria, nor the toxin is secreted in breast milk.

Onabotulinumtoxin A (Botox): The pharmaceutical product Botox contains a purified Botulinum A toxin.[2] It is commonly used for numerous cosmetic, as well as other procedures, such as for treatment of rectal tears, spasticity, cerebral palsy, strabismus, etc. When injected into the muscle, it produces a partial chemical denervation resulting in paralysis of the muscle. When injected properly, and directly into the muscle, the toxin does not enter the systemic circulation. Thus, levels in maternal plasma and milk are very unlikely. Waiting a few hours for dissipation of any toxin would all but eliminate any risk to the infant. Also, avoid use of generic or unknown sources of botulinum toxin, as some are known to produce significant plasma levels in humans.

Abobotulinumtoxin A (Dysport): The pharmaceutical product Dysport contains a purified Botulinum A toxin that is essentially the same at Botox.

Xeomin is another manufacturer's product similar to Botox.

T 1/2	High	MW		PB	
Tmax		RID		Vd	
Oral		M/P		pKa	

Adult Concerns: Gastrointestinal distress, weakness, malaise, lightheadedness, sore throat, nausea, dry mouth, hypersensitvity reactions. The effects of botulinum toxin may sometimes spread from the site of injection and involve other organs of the body, sometimes to cause life-threatening respiratory difficulties. These side-effects may occur hours to weeks after the injection. More pronounced in children, rather than adults.

Adult Dose: 1.25-5 units IM injection. Do not exceed 360 units in a 3 month period.

Pediatric Concerns: No data on its use in breastfeeding mothers.

Infant Monitoring: Weakness, difficulty breathing, GI distress.

Alternatives:

References:
1. Middaugh J. Botulism and breast milk. N Engl J Med. 1978;298(6):343.
2. Pharmaceutical manufacturers prescribing information.

BREMELANOTIDE

Trade: Vyleesi

Category: Melanocortin receptor agonist

LRC: L3 - No Data-Probably Compatible

Bremelanotide is a receptor agonist indicated for the treatment of premenopausal women with acquired, generalized hypoactive sexual desire disorder as characterized by low sexual desire that causes marked distress or interpersonal difficulty. It consists of seven amino acids. As such it would not be orally bioavailable. It is administered as a subcutaneous injection about 45 minutes before an anticipated sexual activity. Observe for nausea, flushing, injection site reactions, headache, and vomiting. There are no data available on the transfer of bremelanotide to human milk.

T 1/2	1.9–4 h	MW	1025.2 Da	PB	21%
Tmax	1	RID		Vd	0.358 L/kg
Oral	Nil	M/P		pKa	

Adult Concerns: Transient increase in blood pressure and decrease in heart rate. Focal hyperpigmentation reported by 1% of patients who received up to 8 doses per month, including involvement of the face, gingiva, and breasts. Nausea reported by 40% of patients who received up to 8 doses per month. Most common adverse reactions (incidence > 4%) are nausea, flushing, injection site reactions, headache, and vomiting.

Adult Dose: 1.75 mg SC

Pediatric Concerns:

Infant Monitoring: Nausea, vomiting, hypotension.

Alternatives:

References:
1. Pharmaceutical manufacturers prescribing information.

BREXANOLONE

Trade: Zulresso

Category: Antidepressant, other

LRC: L3 - Limited Data-Probably Compatible

Brexanolone is a neuroactive steroid modulator similar in structure to allopregnanolone. It is active at the steroid gamma-aminobutyric acid (GABA) receptor. The manufacturer reports that data from a lactation study in 12 women who received intravenous doses of 90 mg/kg/hour for 60 hours, that levels of brexanolone transferred to breast milk was exceedingly low with an RID of 1%-2% of maternal dose.[1] In addition, because brexanolone has low oral bioavailability (<5%) in adults, infant exposure is expected to be low. Concentrations of brexanolone in breast milk were at low levels (<10 ng/mL) in >95% of women by 36 hours after the end of the infusion. Adverse events in breastfeeding infants are not expected.

T 1/2	9 h	MW	318.5 Da	PB	99%
Tmax		RID	1%-2%	Vd	3 L/kg
Oral	<5%	M/P		pKa	

Adult Concerns: Excessive Sedation and Sudden Loss of Consciousness. Brexanolone is a neuroactive steroid modulator similar in structure to allopregnanolone. It is active at the steroid gamma-aminobutyric acid (GABA) receptor. The manufacturer reports that data from a lactation study in 12 women who received intravenous doses of 90 mg/kg/hour for 60 hours, that levels of brexanolone transferred to breast milk was exceedingly low with an RID of 1%-2% of maternal dose. In addition, because brexanolone has low oral bioavailability (<5%) in adults, infant exposure is expected to be low. Concentrations of brexanolone in breast milk were at low levels (<10 ng/mL) in >95% of women by 36 hours after the end of the infusion. Adverse events in breastfeeding infants are not expected.

Adult Dose: Administered IV over 60 hours. See prescribing inform.

Pediatric Concerns:

Infant Monitoring: Side effects in mothers were sedation and loss of consciousness.

Alternatives:

References:
1. Pharmaceutical manufacturers prescribing information.

BREXPIPRAZOLE

Trade: Rexulti

Category: Antipsychotic, Atypical

LRC: L3 - No Data-Probably Compatible

Brexpiprazole is an atypical antipsychotic used as an adjunct therapy in major depressive disorder and for treatment of schizophrenia. At this time there are no human data regarding this medication in lactation. Based on this medication's molecular weight (434 Da) and high protein binding (99%) we do not anticipate significant entry into human milk; however, caution is recommended until human data are available as this medication has a very long half-life (91 hours). Depending on the maternal indication for treatment other options with lactation data are recommended (e.g., quetiapine, aripiprazole, risperidone).

T 1/2	91 h	MW	434 Da	PB	99%
Tmax	4 h	RID		Vd	1.56 L/kg
Oral	95%	M/P		pKa	

Adult Concerns: Headache, drowsiness, anxiety, insomnia, abnormal dreams, orthostatic hypotension, dry mouth, dyspepsia, abdominal pain, diarrhea, increased appetite, changes in liver function, extrapyramidal symptoms (e.g., dystonia, akathisia, tremor).

Adult Dose: 2 mg once daily (varies by indication).

Pediatric Concerns: No data in lactation at this time. Safety has not been established in pediatric patients at this time.[1]

Infant Monitoring: Sedation or irritability, apnea, not waking to feed, poor feeding, extrapyramidal symptoms and weight gain.

Alternatives: Quetiapine(L2), Risperidone(L2), Aripiprazole(L3)

References:
1. Pharmaceutical manufacturers prescribing information.

BRIMONIDINE

Trade: Alphagan, Combigan, Enidin, Mirvaso

Category: Alpha agonist

LRC: L3 - No Data-Probably Compatible

Brimonidine is a selective alpha-2 adrenergic receptor agonist used to reduce intraocular pressure in open-angle glaucoma by reducing aqueous humor production and increasing uveoscleral outflow.[1] It may also be used topically to treat rosacea. The absorption of topical brimonidine gel was evaluated in a clinical trial in 24 adult subjects with facial erythema. All subjects applied Mirvaso topical gel (1 gram) to the entire face for 29 days. Pharmacokinetic assessments were performed on day 1, day 15, and day 29. The mean plasma maximum concentration was highest on day 15, with a C_{max} of 46 ± 62 pg/mL.[1]

No data are available on its transfer into human milk. Pharmacokinetic properties suggest the potential for significant transfer to breast milk. However, the degree of systemic absorption is not well established and may be variable from patient to patient. There are no data on oral bioavailability in adults or babies.

T 1/2	2 h	MW	442 Da	PB	Not studied
Tmax	0.5-2.5 h	RID		Vd	
Oral	Not studied	M/P		pKa	7.4

Adult Concerns: Allergic conjunctivitis, conjunctival hyperemia, pruritus or burning in the eye, blurry vision, abnormal taste, oral dryness, hypertension. Topical brimonidine may produce local erythema and worsen acne.

Adult Dose: One drop in each eye three times daily. Topical gel dosage varies.

Pediatric Concerns: No adverse effects have been reported in lactation at this time.

Infant Monitoring: Drowsiness, not waking to feed, dry mouth.

Alternatives:

References:
1. Pharmaceutical manufacturer prescribing information.

BRINZOLAMIDE

Trade: Azopt, Befardin

Category: Antiglaucoma

LRC: L3 - No Data-Probably Compatible

Brinzolamide is a carbonic anhydrase inhibitor used in the treatment of increased intraocular pressure in patients with ocular hypertension or open-angle glaucoma. It is currently unknown if brinzolamide is excreted in human milk. Due to a long half-life, some concern should be considered following prolonged use in breastfeeding mothers.[1]

T 1/2	111 days	MW	383.5 Da	PB	60%
Tmax	4 weeks	RID		Vd	
Oral		M/P		pKa	7.5

Adult Concerns: Observe for: blurred vision and bitter, sour or unusual taste, blepharitis, dermatitis, dry eye, foreign body sensation, headache, hyperemia, ocular discharge, ocular discomfort, ocular keratitis, ocular pain, ocular pruritus and rhinitis, allergic reactions, alopecia, chest pain, conjunctivitis, diarrhea, diplopia, dizziness, dry mouth, dyspnea, dyspepsia, eye fatigue, hypertonia, keratoconjunctivitis, keratopathy, kidney pain, lid margin crusting or sticky sensation, nausea, pharyngitis, tearing, and urticaria.

Adult Dose: One drop (10 mg/mL) TID

Pediatric Concerns:

Infant Monitoring: Sour, bitter taste, diarrhea, dyspnea, nausea.

Alternatives:

References:
1. Pharmaceutical manufacturers prescribing information, 1998.

BRIVARACETAM

Trade: Briviact

Category: Anticonvulsant

LRC: L3 - No Data-Probably Compatible

Brivaracetam is a new anticonvulsant that can be helpful as an adjunctive treatment for partial-onset seizures.[1] At this time there are no data regarding the transfer of brivaracetam into human milk. Based on this medication's low molecular weight, low protein binding, and small volume of distribution we anticipate brivaracetam will enter human milk to some degree. Caution is warranted until further information is available.

T 1/2	9 h	MW	212.29 Da	PB	< 20%
Tmax	1 h	RID		Vd	0.5 L/kg
Oral	Complete	M/P		pKa	

Adult Concerns: Somnolence, sedation, fatigue, weakness, dizziness, irritability, anxiety, changes in mood, changes in balance and coordination, nausea, vomiting, constipation, leukopenia, neutropenia. Increased thoughts concerning suicide.

Adult Dose: 50 to 100 mg twice a day.

Pediatric Concerns: No data in lactation or pediatric patients under 16 years of age at this time.

Infant Monitoring: Sedation, weakness, irritability, vomiting, constipation. If clinical symptoms or signs of ongoing infection, consider checking a CBC.

Alternatives: Levetiracetam, lamotrigine.

References:
1. Pharmaceutical manufacturer product monograph, 2016.

BROLUCIZUMAB

Trade: Beovu

Category: vascular endothelial growth factor (VEGF) inhibitor

LRC: L3 - No Data-Probably Compatible

Brolucizumab-dbll is a recombinant human vascular endothelial growth factor inhibitor and is a humanized monoclonal single-chain Fv (scFv) antibody fragment. It is indicated for the treatment of Neovascular (Wet) Age-Related Macular Degeneration. Brolucizumab is an approximate molecular weight of 26,000 Da. It is a human VEGF inhibitor. Brolucizumab binds to the three major isoforms of VEGF-A (e.g., VEGF110, VEGF121, and VEGF165), thereby preventing interaction with receptors VEGFR-1 and VEGFR-2. By inhibiting VEGF-A, brolucizumab suppresses endothelial cell proliferation, neovascularization, and vascular permeability. As it is administered by intravitreal injection, the amount present in plasma and subsequently milk would be infinitesimally low. If even present in human milk, it would be largely metabolized by proteases in the GI tract of the infant.

T 1/2	4.4 days	MW	26,000 Da	PB	
Tmax		RID		Vd	
Oral	Nil	M/P		pKa	

Adult Concerns: The most common adverse reactions (≥ 5%) reported in patients are vision blurred (10%), cataract (7%), conjunctival hemorrhage (6%), eye pain (5%), and vitreous floaters (5%).

Adult Dose: Intravitreal Injection: 6 mg/0.05 mL.

Pediatric Concerns: None likely.

Infant Monitoring: Minimal to no effect on infant via oral absorption in milk.

Alternatives:

References:
1. Pharmaceutical manufacturers prescribing information.

BROMOCRIPTINE

Trade: Parlodel, Bromolactin, Kripton

Category: Antiparkinsonian

LRC: L5 - Limited Data-Hazardous

Bromocriptine mesylate is an antiparkinsonian, synthetic ergot alkaloid which inhibits prolactin secretion and hence physiologic lactation. Maternal serum prolactin levels remain suppressed for up to 14 hours after a single dose. Most of the dose of bromocriptine is absorbed by first-pass by the liver, leaving less than 6% to remain in the plasma.

The FDA approved indication for lactation suppression has been withdrawn, and it is no longer approved for this purpose due to numerous maternal deaths. It is sometimes used in hyperprolactinemic patients who have continued to breastfeed although the incidence of maternal side-effects is significant and newer products are preferred.[1,2] Several studies have shown the possibility of breastfeeding during bromocriptine therapy for pituitary tumors with no untoward effects in infants.[3,4]

In 2015, the French pharmacovigilance program published a review of the adverse events associated with bromocriptine use to cease lactation.[5] This group reported 105 serious adverse reactions including cardiovascular (70.5%), neurological (14.4%) and psychiatric (8.6%) events. There were also two fatalities, one 32-year-old female had a myocardial infarction with an arrhythmia, and a 21-year-old female had an ischemic stroke.

Although medications to suppression lactation are no longer recommended for routine use, cabergoline would be preferred to bromocriptine if a medication is required.

T 1/2	5 h	MW	750 Da	PB	90%-96%
Tmax	0.5-4.5 h	RID		Vd	0.87 L/kg
Oral	<28%	M/P		pKa	

Adult Concerns: Dizziness, headache, hallucinations, psychosis, confusion, stroke, hypotension, hypertension, myocardial infarction, nausea, abdominal cramps, diarrhea. A number of deaths have been associated with this product and it is no longer approved for postpartum use to inhibit lactation[5].

Adult Dose: 1.25-2.5 mg BID-TID.

Pediatric Concerns: No reports of direct toxicity to infant via milk but use with caution.

Infant Monitoring: Can reduce breast milk production-not recommended in lactation.

Alternatives: Cabergoline(L3)

References:
1. Meese MG. Reassessment of bromocriptine use for lactation suppression. P & T. 1992;17:1003-1004.
2. Spalding G. Bromocriptine (Parlodel) for suppression of lactation. Aust N Z J Obstet Gynaecol. 1991;31(4):344-345.
3. Canales ES, Garcia IC, Ruiz JE, Zarate A. Bromocriptine as prophylactic therapy in prolactinoma during pregnancy. Fertil Steril. 1981;36(4):524-526.
4. Verma S, Shah D, Faridi MMA. Breastfeeding a baby with mother on bromocriptine. Indian J Pediatr. 2006;73(5):435-436.
5. Bernard N, Jantzem H, Pecriaux C, et al. Severe adverse effects of bromocriptine in lactation inhibition: a pharmacovigilance survey. BJOG. 2015;122:1244-1251.

BROMPHENIRAMINE

Trade: VaZol, Bromine, Dimetane Extentab, Dimetapp, Lodrane, J-Tan PD

Category: Antihistamine

LRC: L3 - Limited Data-Probably Compatible

Brompheniramine is a popular antihistamine typically sold in combination cough and cold products. Although only insignificant amounts of brompheniramine appear to be secreted into breast milk, there are a number of reported cases of irritability, excessive crying, and sleep disturbances that have been reported in breastfeeding infants.[1]

Note, many cough and cold combination products may contain pseudoephedrine, and should be avoided in breastfeeding mothers if possible.

T 1/2	24.9 h	MW	319 Da	PB	
Tmax	3.1 h	RID		Vd	11.7 L/kg
Oral	Complete	M/P		pKa	3.9

Adult Concerns: Drowsiness, dry mucosa, excessive crying, irritability, sleep disturbances.

Adult Dose: 4 mg every 4-6 hours.

Pediatric Concerns: Irritability, excessive crying, and sleep disturbances have been reported.

Infant Monitoring: Drowsiness or irritability, sleep disturbances, dry mouth.

Alternatives: Loratadine(L1), Cetirizine(L2)

References:
1. Paton DM, Webster DR. Clinical pharmacokinetics of H1-receptor antagonists (the antihistamines). Clin Pharmacokinet. 1985;10(6):477-497.

BUDESONIDE

Trade: Entocort, Entocort EC, Rhinocort, Rhinocort Turbuhaler, Pulmicort, Pulmicort Turbuhaler

Category: Corticosteroid

LRC: L1 - Extensive Data-Compatible

Budesonide is a potent corticosteroid available in intranasal, inhaled, and oral forms for treatment of a variety of inflammatory disease processes. This drug is typically used for its topical glucocorticoid effects on mucosa in the respiratory and gastrointestinal tracts.[1]

Budesonide is an excellent drug choice in terms of breastfeeding safety. Limited systemic absorption, relatively rapid clearance, and weak mineralocorticoid activity reduce the potential risk to the baby. In a study of eight asthmatic women using 400-800 μg of inhaled budesonide per day, the authors estimated relative infant dose at 0.3%.[2] This works out to an oral dose of 7-14 ng/kg/day to the infant. A study of children aged 2-7 receiving 200 μg of inhaled budesonide per day found no differences in growth or pituitary-adrenal function compared with unmedicated controls.[3]

Oral budesonide administration requires much larger doses than inhalation, but also exhibits reduced bioavailability. Maternal peak plasma levels following 9 mg oral dosing are roughly 10 times maternal average plasma levels following 800 μg inhalation daily.[1,2] Typical levels of budesonide in the milk are unlikely to be clinically relevant to the breastfeeding infant.

T 1/2	2.8 h	MW	430 Da	PB	85%-90%
Tmax	32-43 min (Inh)	RID	0.3%	Vd	4.3 L/kg
Oral	10.7% (oral)	M/P	0.50	pKa	13.74

Adult Concerns: Intranasal use: irritation, pharyngitis, cough, bleeding, candidiasis, dry mouth. Oral use: headache, acne, bruising, nausea.

Adult Dose: Intranasal: 200-400 μg BID; Oral: 9 mg daily.

Pediatric Concerns: None reported via milk.

Infant Monitoring: Feeding, growth and weight gain.

Alternatives:

References:
1. Pharmaceutical manufacturer prescribing information.
2. Falt A, Bengtsson T, Kennedy BM, et al. Exposure of infants to budesonide through breast milk of asthmatic mothers. J Allergy Clin Immunol. October 2007;120(4):798-802.
3. Volovitz B, Amir J, Malik H, Kauschansky A, Varsano I. Growth and pituitary-adrenal function in children with severe asthma treated with inhaled budesonide. N Engl J Med. December 2, 1993;329(23):1703-1708.

BUDESONIDE + FORMOTEROL

Trade: Symbicort

Category: Antiasthma

LRC: L3 - No Data-Probably Compatible

Budesonide and Formoterol fumarate is a drug combination product of an anti-inflammatory (budesonide) agent along with a bronchodilator (formoterol). It is FDA approved for treatment of asthma and chronic obstructive pulmonary disease (COPD).[1] The transfer of this combination product to breast milk has not been studied.

Budesonide is a potent corticosteroid used intranasally for allergic rhinitis, inhaled for asthma, and orally for Crohn's disease.[2] As such, the lung bioavailability is estimated to be 34% of the inhaled dose.[3] Once absorbed systemically, budesonide is a weak systemic steroid and should not be used to replace other steroids. In one 5 year study of children aged 2-7 years, no changes in linear growth, weight, and bone age were noted following inhalation.[4] Adrenal suppression at these doses is extremely remote. Using normal doses, it is unlikely that clinically relevant concentrations of inhaled budesonide would ever reach the milk nor be systemically bioavailable to a breastfed infant. One study tested breast milk samples from eight women before and after their first morning dose of 200 or 400 µg inhaled budesonide (Pulmicort Turbuhaler). Average milk level of budesonide (Cav) was 0.105-0.219 nmol/L with doses of 200 and 400 µg twice daily, respectively. Maternal plasma levels of budesonide reported (Cav) were 0.246-0.437 nmol/L at the doses above. Milk/plasma ratios were 0.428 and 0.502 at the doses above. Plasma samples from infants 1-1.5 hours after feeding showed levels below the limit of quantification. Therefore, the estimated daily infant dose is 0.3% of the mother's daily dose or approximately 0.0068-0.0142 µg/kg/day.[3] Relative Infant Dose for budesonide is 0.29%.

Formoterol is a long-acting selective beta-2 adrenoceptor agonist used for asthma and COPD. Following inhalation of a 120 µg dose, the maximum plasma concentration of 92 pg/mL occurred within 5 minutes.[5] No data are available on its transfer to human milk, but the extremely low plasma levels would suggest that milk levels would be incredibly low, if even measurable. Studies of oral absorption in adults suggests that while absorption is good, plasma levels are still below detectable levels and may require large oral doses prior to attaining measurable plasma levels.[6,7] It is not likely the amount present in human milk would be clinically relevant to a breastfed infant.

T 1/2	Budes/form: 2.8 h/10 h	MW	Budes/form: 430/840 Da	PB	Budes/form: 85%-90%(oral)/64%
Tmax	Budes/form: 32-43 min/ 5 min	RID		Vd	Budes/form: 4.3/ L/kg
Oral	Budes/form: 10.7%/good	M/P	Budes/form: 0.5/	pKa	Budes/form: 13.74/

Adult Concerns: Oral candidiasis, vomiting, headache, nasal congestion, nasopharyngitis, sinusitis are the commonly reported side-effects. Less common are hypokalemia, cataract, glaucoma.

Adult Dose: Budesonide/formoterol: 80-160 µg/4.5µg twice daily.

Pediatric Concerns:

Infant Monitoring: Irritability, insomnia, arrhythmias, feeding, growth, weight gain, tremor.

Alternatives:

References:
1. Pharmaceutical manufacturer prescribing information.
2. Pharmaceutical manufacturer prescribing information.
3. Falt A, Bengtsson T, Gyllenberg A, Lindberg B, Strandgarden K. Negligible exposure of infants to budesonide via breast milk. J Allergy Clin Immunol. 2007;120(4):798-802.
4. Volovitz B, Amir J, Malik H, Kauschansky A, Varsano I. Growth and pituitary-adrenal function in children with severe asthma treated with inhaled budesonide. N Engl J Med. 1993;329(23):1703-1708.
5. Pharmaceutical manufacturers prescribing information.
6. Tattersfield AE. Long-acting beta 2-agonists. Clin Exp Allergy. 1992;22(6):600-605.
7. Maesen FP, Smeets JJ, Gubbelmans HL, Zweers PG. Bronchodilator effect of inhaled formoterol vs salbutamol over 12 hours. Chest. 1990;97(3):590-594.

BUMETANIDE

Trade: Bumex, Burinex

Category: Diuretic

LRC: L3 - No Data-Probably Compatible

Bumetanide is a potent loop diuretic similar to furosemide.[1] As with all diuretics, some reduction in breast milk production may result but it is rare. It is not known if bumetanide transfers to human milk. If needed furosemide may be a better choice, as the oral bioavailability of furosemide in neonates is minimal.

T 1/2	1-1.5	MW	364 Da	PB	97%
Tmax	1 h (oral)	RID		Vd	0.129-0.357 L/kg
Oral	59%-89%	M/P		pKa	9.62

Adult Concerns: Dizziness, hypotension, ototoxicity, hyperglycemia, hyponatremia, hypokalemia, hyperuricemia, changes in renal function, muscle cramps.

Adult Dose: 0.5-2 mg one to two times a day.

Pediatric Concerns: None reported via milk at this time.

Infant Monitoring: Observe for fluid loss, dehydration, lethargy.

Alternatives: Furosemide(L3)

References:
1. Pharmaceutical manufacturers prescribing information.

BUPIVACAINE

Trade: Exparel, Marcain, Marcaine, Sensorcaine

Category: Anesthetic, Local

LRC: L2 - Limited Data-Probably Compatible

Bupivacaine is the most commonly employed regional anesthetic used in delivery because its concentrations in the fetus are the least of the local anesthetics. In one study of five patients, levels of bupivacaine in breastmilk were below the limits of detection (<0.02 mg/L) at 2 to 48 hours postpartum.[1] These authors concluded that bupivacaine is a safe drug for perinatal use in mothers who plan to breastfeed.

In a study of 27 patients who received an average of 183.3 mg lidocaine and 82.1 mg bupivacaine via an epidural catheter, lidocaine plasma levels at 2, 6, and 12 hours post administration were 0.86, 0.46, and 0.22 mg/L respectively.[2] Levels of bupivacaine in milk at 2, 6, and 12 hours were 0.09, 0.06, 0.04 mg/L respectively. The milk/serum ratio based upon area under the curve values (AUC) were 1.07 and 0.34 for lidocaine and bupivacaine respectively. Based on AUC data of lidocaine and bupivacaine milk levels, the average milk concentration of these agents over 12 hours was 0.5 and 0.07 mg/L. Most of the infants had a maximal APGAR score.

In a study of one patient with a 9.35 kg infant (10 months postpartum), who received a bolus intrapleural injection of 20 mL of 0.25% bupivacaine (50 mg), followed by a continuous infusion of bupivacaine (10 mL/hour 0.25% or 25 mg) for 5 days, breast milk samples were collected at 6, 24, 48, and 72 hours after beginning the infusion. Breast milk levels ranged from a high of approximately 0.4 µg/mL at 6 hours to 0.15 µg/mL at 70 hours. The maternal C_{max} was approximately 1.67 µg/mL at 47 hours. The authors using the highest dose in milk estimated the RID at 0.1%.[3]

In 2014, a prospective study was published which included 20 women undergoing elective cesarean section, half of the women were randomized to receive epidurals with 0.5% levobupivacaine and the other 0.5% racemic bupivacaine.[4] Both groups had their milk levels quantified for the first 24 hours after epidural drug administration. Although levobupivacaine was detectable 30 minutes after administration, the levels were three times lower than that of plasma and undetectable by 24 hours. The mean milk/plasma ratios for levobupivacaine and bupivacaine were 0.34 and 0.37 respectively. Although milk C_{max} were not reported, the mean peak milk concentrations were approximately 0.25 µg/mL and 0.2 µg/mL for levobupivacaine and bupivacaine.

Exparel (Microsomal Bupivacaine): Exparel is a slow-release formulation of bupivicaine that when injected into the margins of a surgical wound, continues to provide local anesthesia for several days. We believe that use of Exparel at typical dosages is probably compatible with breastfeeding without restriction. A typical dose used in Cesarean sections is 266 mg but this is variable. The available pharmacokinetic data on Exparel suggest that 266 mg produces an immediate peak (due to a small amount of "extraliposomal" bupivacaine in the formulation), which drops off at 2 hours to a plateau of around 360 ng/mL. The elimination half-life of liposomal bupivacaine varies by route of administration between 12 and 34 hours. During early postpartum (colostral phase), the lactocyte barrier is not fully formed and the milk/plasma ratio of most drugs is near 1:1. However, mothers only produce about 60 mL of colostrum per day, so not much drug actually reaches the baby. Circulating bupivacaine derived from Exparel is no different from regular bupivacaine. Assuming a sustained plasma level of 360 ng/mL in both milk and plasma, only 21 µg/day of bupivacaine would be delivered to the infant. The oral bioavailability of bupivacaine is not known, but using lidocaine as a model (~30%), then 7 µg per day may end up in the infant's plasma. In addition, the volume of distribution for bupivacaine is high (0.4-1.0 L/kg), implying that plasma levels in the baby will be very low with this level of exposure. In adults, toxic effects are first seen at around 2000 ng/mL. It is my opinion that plasma levels in the baby are highly unlikely to come anywhere close to this, however this conclusion requires confirmation by patient studies.

T 1/2	2.7 h (Exparel longer)	MW	288 Da	PB	95%
Tmax	30-45 min	RID	0.85%-2.92%	Vd	0.4-1 L/kg
Oral		M/P		pKa	8.1

Adult Concerns: Sedation, bradycardia, respiratory depression.

Adult Dose: 25-100 mg once.

Pediatric Concerns: None reported via milk.

Infant Monitoring:

Alternatives:

References:

1. Naulty JS. Bupivacaine in breast milk following epidural anesthesia for vaginal delivery. Regional Anesthesia. 1983;8(1):44-45.
2. Ortega D, Viviand X, Lorec AM, Gamerre M, Martin C, Bruguerolle B. Excretion of lidocaine and bupivacaine in breast milk following epidural anesthesia for cesarean delivery. Acta Anaesthesiol Scand. 1999;43(4):394-397.
3. Baker PA, Schroeder D. Interpleural bupivacaine for postoperative pain during lactation. Anesth Analg. September 1989;69(3):400-402.
4. Bolat E, Bestas A, Bayar MK, et al. Evaluation of levobupivacaine passage to breast milk following epidural anesthesia for cesarean delivery. Int J Obstet Anesth. 2014;23:217-221.

BUPRENORPHINE

Trade: Buprenex, Butrans, Subutex, Temgesic, Probuphine

Category: Analgesic

LRC: L2 - Limited Data-Probably Compatible

Buprenorphine is a potent, long-acting narcotic agonist and antagonist and may be useful as a replacement for methadone treatment in addiction.[1] It is also recently approved for the treatment of opiate dependence in the form of a transdermal patch. Its elimination half-life varies from paper to paper, but new recent sublingual studies suggest it ranges from 23-30 hours.

In one patient who received 4 mg/day to facilitate withdrawal from other opiates, the amount of buprenorphine transferred via milk was only 3.28 µg/day, an amount that was clinically insignificant.[2] No symptoms were noted in this breastfed infant. In another study of continuous epidural bupivacaine and buprenorphine in post cesarean women for 3 days, it was suggested that buprenorphine may suppress the production of milk (and infant weight gain), although this was not absolutely clear.[3] In another study of one patient on buprenorphine maintenance for 7 months, and who received 8 mg daily sublingually over 4 days, milk levels of buprenorphine and norbuprenorphine ranged from 1 to 14.7 ng/mL and 0.6 to 6.3 ng/mL, respectively.[4] Plasma concentrations of both analytes ranged from 0.2 to 20.1 ng/mL (buprenorphine) and 1.2 to 4.4 ng/mL (norbuprenorphine) over 4 days of study. Using peak levels only, the concentration of buprenorphine and norbuprenorphine were 1.47 and 0.63 µg/100 mL of breast milk, respectively. Assuming an intake of 150 mL/kg/day, the authors estimated the daily dose would be less than 10 µg for a 4 kg infant, a dose that is probably far subclinical.

In a recent study of 7 women who were taking a median of 0.32 mg/kg/day buprenorphine, the median area under the curve estimates of milk levels were 0.12 mg.h/L for buprenorphine and 0.10 mg.h/L for norbuprenorphine.[5] Levels of buprenorphine and norbuprenorphine in the infant plasma were approximately 4.5% and 11.7% of maternal levels.

In another study of 7 women who received a mean buprenorphine dose of 7 mg/day (2.4-24 mg sublingually), the mean milk concentrations of buprenorphine and norbuprenorphine were 3.65 µg/L and 1.94 µg/L respectively.[6] The authors calculated the relative infant dose to be 0.38% for buprenorphine, and 0.18% for norbuprenorphine. The authors concluded that the doses of buprenorphine and norbuprenorphine received by the infant through breast milk were clinically insignificant. The authors also published a second outcomes paper in 2014 where the seven infants were followed for the first 4 weeks of life to determine the effects of buprenorphine via breast milk.[7] Of the seven participating mother-infant pairs, four infants received breastmilk exclusively and three received breast milk plus 260 to 700 mL of formula per 24 hour period. The feeding, sleeping, bladder and bowel patterns, skin color, hydration status and weight gain were assessed for each infant at 3 and 4 weeks after birth; all neonatal outcomes were found to be within normal limits. The authors also looked at Neonatal Abstinence Scores and reported four infants had elevated scores, three of which were admitted to a level II nursery. Two infants had elevated scores greater than 15, one was attributed to sepsis and was given antibiotics and the other was attributed to withdrawal and was given morphine.

In another study of 10 breastfeeding mothers receiving 2-22 mg sublingually and their infants provided samples at day 2, 3, 4, 14, and 30 days postpartum at peak times.[8] Median milk levels of buprenorphine ranged from 1.4 to 4.8 µg/L. Infants provided blood samples on day 14 of life. Buprenorphine plasma levels in infants were exceedingly low at concentrations of 0.2, 0.7, 1.0, and 2.9 µg/L in four of nine infants. It was undetectable in the five remaining infants. Milk/plasma ratios ranged from 0.9 to 2.0.

Based on these studies, it may be concluded that although experience with the use of buprenorphine in breastfeeding women is limited, there is no evidence that the use of this drug will have major adverse effects in the breastfed infants.

Note: The buprenorphine patch produces significant plasma levels for up to 7 days, with steady-state achieved at day 3. Plasma levels drop to zero approximately 5-6 days after patch removal. At this time we have no data regarding the use of the transdermal form in lactation. Note: A new buprenorphine sustained release pellet (provides 74.2 mg of buprenorphine (equivalent to 80 mg of buprenorphine hydrochloride) is now available and provides a dose similar to 8 mg/day or less of Subutex or Suboxone. It provides low daily doses of buprenorphine over weeks of time depending on the number of pellets injected.

T 1/2	2-3 h IV; 37 h sl; 26 h transdermal	MW	504 Da	PB	96%
Tmax	1 h IM; 15-30 min sl; 3 days transdermal	RID	0.09%-2.52%	Vd	97-187 L/kg
Oral	70% IM; 29% sl; 15% transdermal	M/P	1.7	pKa	8.24, 9.92

Adult Concerns: Sedation, respiratory depression/apnea, nausea, vomiting, constipation, urinary retention, weakness, pruritus.

Adult Dose: 12-16 mg/day sl for withdrawal; 5 µg/hour transdermal patch applied once every 7 days.

Pediatric Concerns: Low weight gain and reduced breast milk levels in one study, and no effects in two other studies.

Infant Monitoring: Sedation, slowed breathing rate/apnea, pallor, constipation and not waking to feed/poor feeding.

Alternatives: Methadone(L2)

References:

1. McAleer SD, Mills RJ, Polack T, et al. Pharmacokinetics of high-dose buprenorphine following single administration of sublingual tablet formulations in opioid naive healthy male volunteers under a naltrexone block. Drug Alcohol Depend. 2003;72:75-83.
2. Marquet P, Chevrel J, Lavignasse P, Merle L, Lachatre G. Buprenorphine withdrawal syndrome in a newborn. Clin Pharmacol Ther. 1997;62(5):569-571.
3. Hirose M, Hosokawa T, Tanaka Y. Extradural buprenorphine suppresses breast feeding after caesarean section. Br J Anaesth. 1997;79(1):120-121.
4. Grimm D, Pauly E, Poschl J, et al. Buprenorphine and norbuprenorphine concentrations in human breast milk samples determined by liquid chromatography-tandem mass spectrometry. Ther Drug Monit. 2005;27:526-530.
5. Lindemalm S, Nydert P, Svensson JO, Stahle L, Sarman I. Transfer of buprenorphine into breast milk and calculation of infant drug dose. J Hum Lact. May 2009;25(2):199-205.
6. Ilett K, Hackett LP, Gower S, Doherty D, Hamilton D, Bartu AE. Estimated dose exposure of the neonate to buprenorphine and its metabolite norbuprenorphine via breast milk during maternal buprenorphine substitution treatment. Breastfeed Med. 2012;7:269-274.
7. Gower S, Bartu A, Ilett KF, et al. The wellbeing of infants exposed to buprenorphine via breast milk at 4 weeks of age. J Hum Lact. 2014;30(2):217-223.
8. Jansson LM, Spencer N, McConnell K, et al. Maternal buprenorphine maintenance and lactation. J Hum Lact. November 2016;32(4):675-681. PubMed PMID: 27563013.

BUPRENORPHINE + NALOXONE

Trade: Suboxone

Category: Opioid Dependency

LRC: L3 - No Data-Probably Compatible

Buprenorphine + naloxone is a combination drug product indicated for use in opioid dependence.[1] Buprenorphine and naloxone are combined in a sublingual tablet that contains a partial opioid agonist (buprenorphine) and an opioid antagonist (naloxone) in a 4:1 (buprenorphine: naloxone) ratio. Buprenorphine reduces the patients' craving for opioids, and naloxone discourages the use of other opioids by blocking the opiate receptor. Naloxone and buprenorphine are both poorly absorbed orally.[1,2]

In one patient who received 4 mg/day to facilitate withdrawal from other opiates, the amount of buprenorphine transferred via milk was only 3.28 µg/day, an amount that was clinically insignificant.[3] No symptoms were noted in this breastfed infant. In another study of continuous epidural bupivacaine and buprenorphine in post cesarean women for 3 days, it was suggested that buprenorphine may suppress the production of milk (and infant weight gain) although this was not absolutely clear.[4] In another study of one patient on buprenorphine maintenance for 7 months, and who received 8 mg daily sublingually over 4 days, milk levels of buprenorphine and norbuprenorphine ranged from 1 to 14.7 ng/mL and 0.6 to 6.3 ng/mL, respectively.[5] Plasma concentrations of both analytes ranged from 0.2 to 20.1 ng/mL (buprenorphine) and 1.2 to 4.4 ng/mL (norbuprenorphine) over 4 days of study. Using peak levels only, the concentration of buprenorphine and norbuprenorphine were 1.47 and 0.63 µg/100 mL of breast milk, respectively. Assuming an intake of 150 mL/kg/day, the authors estimated the daily dose would be less than 10 µg for a 4 kg infant, this dose is probably not clinically relevant.

In a recent study of 7 women who were taking a median of 0.32 mg/kg/day buprenorphine, the median area under the curve estimates of milk levels were 0.12 mg.h/L for buprenorphine and 0.10 mg.h/L for norbuprenorphine.[6] Levels of buprenorphine and norbuprenorphine in the infant plasma were approximately 4.5% and 11.7% of maternal levels.

In another study of seven women who received a mean buprenorphine dose of 7 mg/day (2.4-24 mg sublingually), the mean milk concentrations of buprenorphine and norbuprenorphine were 3.65 µg/L and 1.94 µg/L respectively.[7] The authors calculated the relative infant dose to be 0.38% for buprenorphine and 0.18% for norbuprenorphine. The authors concluded that the doses of buprenorphine and norbuprenorphine received by the infant through breastmilk were clinically insignificant. The authors also published a second outcomes paper in 2014 where the seven infants were followed for the first 4 weeks of life to determine the effects of buprenorphine via breast milk.[8] Of the seven participating mother-infant pairs, four infants received breast milk exclusively and three received breast milk plus 260 to 700 mL of formula per 24 hour period. The feeding, sleeping, bladder and bowel patterns, skin color, hydration status, and weight gain were assessed for each infant at 3 and 4 weeks after birth; all neonatal outcomes were found to be within normal limits. The authors also looked at Neonatal Abstinence Scores and reported four infants had elevated scores, three of which were admitted to a level II nursery. Two infants had elevated scores greater than 15, one was attributed to sepsis and was given antibiotics and the other was attributed to withdrawal and was given morphine.

In another study of 10 breastfeeding mothers receiving 2-22 mg sublingually and their infants provided samples at day 2, 3, 4, 14, and 30 days postpartum at peak times.[9] Median milk levels of buprenorphine ranged from 1.4 to 4.8 µg/L. Infants provided blood samples on day 14 of life. Buprenorphine plasma levels in infants were exceedingly low at concentrations of 0.2, 0.7, 1.0, and 2.9 µg/L in 4 of 9 infants. It was undetectable in the five remaining infants. Milk/plasma ratios ranged from 0.9 to 2.0.

Based on these studies and other studies it may be concluded that although experience with the use of buprenorphine in breastfeeding women is limited, there is no evidence that the use of this drug will have major adverse effects in the breastfed infants. The relative infant dose of buprenorphine ranges from 0.09%-2.5%.

Naloxone is commonly used for the treatment of opiate overdose, and now to prevent opiate abuse in patients undergoing withdrawal treatment. Naloxone is poorly absorbed orally and plasma levels in adults are undetectable (<0.05 ng/mL) 2 hours after oral doses. Following intravenous use (0.4 mg), plasma naloxone levels averaged <0.084 µg/mL. Side effects are minimal except in narcotic-addicted patients. Its use in breastfeeding mothers would be unlikely to cause problems as its milk levels would likely be low and its oral absorption is minimal to nil.

In summary, it is unlikely that the breast milk levels of the combination of buprenorphine + naloxone would be significant. Therefore the use of buprenorphine + naloxone is probably compatible with breastfeeding.

T 1/2	Bup/nalox: 26-37 h/64 min	MW	Bup/nalox: 504/399 Da	PB	Bup/nalox: 96%/45%
Tmax	Bup/nalox: day3/	RID	0.13%-2.52%	Vd	Bup/nalox: 97-187/2.6-2.8 L/kg
Oral	Bup/nalox: 15%/nil	M/P	1-2	pKa	Bup/nalox: 8.24,9.92/7.9

Adult Concerns: Headache, sedation, respiratory depression/apnea, hypotension, nausea, vomiting, constipation, weakness, pruritus. Withdrawal symptoms on discontinuation of drug.

Adult Dose: 16 mg buprenorphine/4 mg naloxone daily for maintenance therapy.

Pediatric Concerns: None reported via milk at this time, but data is limited at these doses.

Infant Monitoring: Sedation, slowed breathing rate/apnea, pallor, constipation and not waking to feed/poor feeding.

Alternatives: Methadone(L2)

References:

1. Pharmaceutical manufacturers prescribing information.
2. McAleer SD, Mills RJ, Polack T, et al. Pharmacokinetics of high-dose buprenorphine following single administration of sublingual tablet formulations in opioid naive healthy male volunteers under a naltrexone block. Drug Alcohol Depend. 2003;72:75-83.

3. Marquet P, Chevrel J, Lavignasse P, Merle L, Lachatre G. Buprenorphine withdrawal syndrome in a newborn. Clin Pharmacol Ther. 1997;62(5):569-571.

4. Hirose M, Hosokawa T, Tanaka Y. Extradural buprenorphine suppresses breast feeding after caesarean section. Br J Anaesth. 1997;79(1):120-121.

5. Grimm D, Pauly E, Poschl J, et al. Buprenorphine and norbuprenorphine concentrations in human breast milk samples determined by liquid chromatography-tandem mass spectrometry. Ther Drug Monit. 2005;27:526-530.

6. Lindemalm S, Nydert P, Svensson JO, Stahle L, Sarman I. Transfer of buprenorphine into breast milk and calculation of infant drug dose. J Hum Lact. May 2009;25(2):199-205.

7. Ilett K, Hackett LP, Gower S, Doherty D, Hamilton D, Bartu AE. Estimated dose exposure of the neonate to buprenorphine and its metabolite norbuprenorphine via breast milk during maternal buprenorphine substitution treatment. Breastfeed Med. 2012;7:269-274.

8. Gower S, Bartu A, Ilett KF, et al. The wellbeing of infants exposed to buprenorphine via breast milk at 4 weeks of age. J Hum Lact. 2014;30(2):217-223.

9. Jansson LM, Spencer N, McConnell K, et al. Maternal buprenorphine maintenance and lactation. J Hum Lact. November 2016;32(4):675-681. doi:10.1177/0890334416663198. Epub September 26, 2016. PubMed PMID: 27563013.

BUPROPION

Trade: Aplenzin, Wellbutrin, Zyban

Category: Antidepressant, other

LRC: L3 - Limited Data-Probably Compatible

Bupropion is an NDRI (norepinephrine, dopamine reuptake inhibitor) that is used for both depression and smoking cessation. Following one 100 mg dose in a mother, the milk/plasma ratio ranged from 2.51 to 8.58, clearly suggesting a concentrating mechanism for this drug in human milk.[1] However, plasma levels of bupropion (and its metabolites) in the infant were undetectable, indicating that the dose transferred to the infant was low, and accumulation in infant plasma apparently did not occur under these conditions (infant was fed 7.5 to 9.5 hours after dosing). The peak milk bupropion level (0.189 mg/L) occurred two hours after the 100 mg dose. This peak milk level would provide 0.66% of the maternal dose, a dose that is likely to be clinically insignificant to a breastfed infant.

In a recent study of two breastfeeding patients consuming 75 mg twice daily and 150 mg (sustained release) daily respectively, no bupropion and its metabolites were detected in either breastfed infant.[2] In the first patient at 17 weeks postpartum, plasma levels were drawn at 2 hours postdose and bupropion and hydroxybupropion levels were undetectable. In the second patient at 29 weeks postpartum, bupropion and hydroxybupropion were undetectable as well. The limit of detection for bupropion was 5-10 ng/mL and for hydroxybupropion was 100-200 ng/mL.

There are now two case reports of infants whom have had seizures while being exposed to bupropion in milk.[3,4] In the first case report the infant had a seizure at 6 months of age, this seizure occurred after the mother had taken two doses of 150 mg SR about 36 hours apart (she had been on the drug pre-pregnancy/then stopped during pregnancy).[3] At the time of the seizure the infant was not known to be febrile but did have a respiratory tract infection; therefore, a febrile seizure could not be ruled out. The seizure did not recur (although the mother switched to sertraline for a few days then stopped all drug therapy and continued breastfeeding).

In the second case report, the infant had severe emesis with tonic-clonic seizure like symptoms at 6.5 months of age.[4] This infant was exclusively breastfed until 6 months of age, during this time the mother was taking escitalopram 10 mg/day, three weeks prior to presentation bupropion 150 mg XL/day was added. The mother noted that one week after starting bupropion the infant had a change in sleep pattern, the following week the infant had an episode during a feed of grinning, staring with outstretched limbs, was unresponsive for 1-2 minutes and then drowsy for 20 minutes; this was not investigated. Then on the day of the seizure the infant was breastfed, 20 minutes later started to vomit six times, and then became somnolent for several hours. In ER, the infant was unresponsive, hypertonic, and cyanotic. The symptoms resolved by 48 hours with supportive care and discontinuation of breastfeeding. In this case four milk samples from 5-7 days pre-episode revealed, bupropion and hydroxybupropion concentrations of 15.8-24.4 µg/L and 46-87 µg/L, respectively. The infants serum levels on arrival and 14 hours later for bupropion and hydroxybupropion were detectable but not quantifiable (< 4.8 µg/L) and 11.2-17.1 µg/L (metabolite higher than expected), respectively.

In a study of 10 breastfeeding patients who received 150 mg bupropion SR daily for 3 days and then 300 mg bupropion SR daily thereafter for 4 more days, milk concentrations of bupropion averaged 45 µg/L.[5] The average infant dose via milk was 6.75 µg/kg/day. The reported relative infant dose was 0.14% of the weight-normalized maternal dose. When the active metabolites present in milk were added, the RID would be 2% of the maternal dose. No side effects were noted in any of the infants.

In a study of four mothers consuming 150 to 300 mg/day of bupropion SR, peak and trough blood levels were highly variable, but averaged 64 ng/mL at peak and 9.2 ng/mL at trough.[6] Bupropion was detected in urine in only one of four infants (infant was 6 week premature). The average milk/serum ratio was 1.3.

Due to persistent case reports to the author, bupropion may, in some women, suppress milk production; further data and evaluation is needed to assess this finding. Some caution is recommended concerning changes to milk supply.

T 1/2	8-24 h	MW	240 Da	PB	84%
Tmax	2 h	RID	0.11%-1.99%	Vd	20-47 L/kg
Oral	85%	M/P	2.51-8.58	pKa	8

Adult Concerns: Headache, restlessness, agitation, sleep disturbances, seizures, blurred vision, dry mouth, tachycardia, nausea, constipation or diarrhea. Use is contraindicated in patients with seizure disorders.

Adult Dose: 150 mg twice a day Sustained Release.

Pediatric Concerns: Two cases of seizure have been reported via breastmilk exposure; however, a febrile seizure could not be ruled out in one of the cases.[3,4]

Infant Monitoring: Sedation or irritability, seizures, not waking to feed/poor feeding and poor weight gain.

Alternatives: Sertraline(L2), Citalopram(L2)

References:
1. Briggs GG, Samson JH, Ambrose PJ, Schroeder DH. Excretion of bupropion in breast milk. Ann Pharmacother. 1993;27(4):431-433.
2. Baab SW, Peindl KS, Piontek CM, Wisner KL. Serum bupropion levels in 2 breastfeeding mother-infant pairs. J Clin Psychiatry. 2002;63:910-911.
3. Chaudron LH, Schoenecker CJ. Bupropion and breastfeeding: a case of possible infant seizure. J Clin Psychiatry. 2004:64(6):881-882.
4. Neuman G, Colantonio D, Delaney S, et al. Bupropion and escitalopram during lactation. Ann Pharmacotherapy. 2014;48(7):928-931.
5. Haas JS, Kaplan CP, Barenboim D, Jacob P III, Benowitz NL. Bupropion in breast milk: an exposure assessment for potential treatment to prevent post-partum tobacco use. Tob Control. March 2004;13(1):52-56.
6. Davis MF, Miller HS, Nolan PE Jr. Bupropion levels in breast milk for 4 mother-infant pairs: more answers to lingering questions. J Clin Psychiatry. February 2009;70(2):297-298.

BUSPIRONE

Trade: Bustab, Buspar, Buspon

Category: Antianxiety

LRC: L3 - No Data-Probably Compatible

Buspirone is an anxiolytic agent indicated for the treatment of generalized anxiety disorder.[1] This drug's mechanism of action is unknown; however, it has high affinity for 5-HT1A and 5-HT2 receptors, moderate affinity for D2 receptors, and no affinity for GABA receptors in the brain.

Currently there are no data regarding buspirone excretion into human milk.[1] Several properties of this medication suggest it has difficulty entering breastmilk: high protein binding, short half-life, large volume of distribution, low oral bioavailability, and minimally active metabolites. In addition, no data are available regarding the effect of buspirone on milk production.

T 1/2	2-3 h	MW	422 Da	PB	86%
Tmax	40-90 min	RID		Vd	5.3 L/kg
Oral	1%	M/P		pKa	7.32

Adult Concerns: Headache, dizziness, drowsiness, fatigue, excitement, confusion, chest pain, nausea, diarrhea, sweating, rash.

Adult Dose: 10-15 mg twice daily.

Pediatric Concerns: None reported via milk at this time.

Infant Monitoring: Behavioral changes, feeding problems, weight gain.

Alternatives: Lorazepam(L3)

References:
1. Pharmaceutical manufacturer prescribing information.

BUSULFAN

Trade: Busilvex, Myleran

Category: Alkylating Agent

LRC: L5 - No Data-Hazardous

Busulfan is an alkylating agent used in chronic myeloid leukemia and bone marrow transplant. Oral absorption varies enormously but is probably 100%. Its elimination is described by a monoexponential curve with a plasma elimination half-life of approximately 2.6 hours. Volume of distribution varies but is reported to be two- to three-fold higher in young children.[1] No data are available on the transfer of busulfan into human milk. However, approximately 20% enters the CNS, which suggests similar amounts could enter the milk compartment. Busulfan is a potent antineoplastic agent that can produce severe bone marrow suppression, anemia, loss of blood cells, and elevated risk of infection.[1] It is not known if busulfan is distributed to human milk. No data is available concerning breast milk concentrations, but this agent would be extremely toxic to growing infants and continued breastfeeding would not be justified. Use of this drug during breastfeeding is definitely not recommended.

Breastfeeding should be interrupted for a minimum of 24 hours following exposure to this agent.

T 1/2	2.6 h	MW	246 Da	PB	14%
Tmax	0.5-2 h	RID		Vd	0.94 L/kg
Oral	Complete	M/P		pKa	

Adult Concerns: Severe bone marrow suppression, anemia, leukopenia, pulmonary fibrosis, cholestatic jaundice.

Adult Dose: 1 mg/kg/dose every 6 hours (16 doses total).

Pediatric Concerns: Extremely cytotoxic, use is not recommended in nursing women. Withhold breastfeeding for at least 24 hours following its use.

Infant Monitoring: Hazardous, withhold breastfeeding.

Alternatives:

References:
1. Pharmaceutical manufacturers prescribing information.

BUTALBITAL

Trade:

Category: Analgesic

LRC: L3 - No Data-Probably Compatible

Butalbital is a short-acting barbiturate used as a mild analgesic in combination products with caffeine and may include acetaminophen, aspirin, or codeine as the analgesic.[1] Butalbital has a small molecular weight (224 Da), low protein binding (45%) and a long half-life (35 hours), thus it most likely will enter milk. While this product is probably compatible with breastfeeding, other analgesics are preferred (acetaminophen, NSAIDs, narcotics as needed).

T 1/2	35 h	MW	224 Da	PB	45%
Tmax	40-60 min	RID		Vd	0.8 L/kg
Oral	Complete	M/P		pKa	8.48

Adult Concerns: Headache, dizziness, sedation, confusion, dry mouth, heartburn, nausea, vomiting, constipation, skin rashes.

Adult Dose: 50-100 mg every 4 hours.

Pediatric Concerns: None reported via milk at this time.

Infant Monitoring: Sedation, slowed breathing rate/apnea, pallor, not waking to feed at regular intervals.

Alternatives: Acetaminophen(L1), Ibuprofen(L1), Hydromorphone(L3)

References:
1. Pharmaceutical manufacturers prescribing information.

BUTENAFINE

Trade: Lotrimin Ultra, Mentax

Category: Antifungal

LRC: L3 - No Data-Probably Compatible

Butenafine is a topical antifungal available in OTC medications.[1] It absorbs well into the skin, but does not appear to absorb greatly into the systemic circulation. It is unlikely that it would enter the milk compartment when applied through the topical route. There are currently no adequate and well-controlled studies or case reports in breastfeeding women.

T 1/2	35 h and >150 (biphasic)	MW	353.93 Da	PB	
Tmax	6-15 h	RID		Vd	
Oral		M/P		pKa	

Adult Concerns: Contact dermatitis, burning sensation, erythema, pruritus, local irritation.

Adult Dose: Apply topically once daily for 2 weeks.

Pediatric Concerns:

Infant Monitoring:

Alternatives:

References:
1. Pharmaceutical manufacturers prescribing information.

BUTOCONAZOLE

Trade: Femstat One, Gynazole-1, Mycelex-3

Category: Antifungal

LRC: L3 - No Data-Probably Compatible

Butoconazole nitrate is an imidazole derivative that has fungicidal activity in vitro against Candida species and has been demonstrated to be clinically effective against vaginal *Candida albicans*.[1] It is not known whether this drug is excreted in human milk. Absorption of the drug vaginally is about 1.7%. Peak plasma levels are 13.6-18.6 ng/mL. While it is not known whether this drug is excreted in human milk, vaginal absorption is low and plasma levels even lower. It is not likely this would produce untoward effects in a breastfed infant.

T 1/2	12-24 h	MW	474.8 Da	PB	
Tmax	12-24 h	RID		Vd	
Oral	5.5% (vaginal)	M/P		pKa	

Adult Concerns: Local irritation, burning, cramping, abdominal pain.

Adult Dose: Insert one applicator as a single dose.

Pediatric Concerns:

Infant Monitoring:

Alternatives: Ketoconazole(L2), Clotrimazole(L2), Miconazole(L2)

References:
1. Pharmaceutical manufacturers prescribing information.

BUTORPHANOL

Trade: Stadol

Category: Analgesic

LRC: L2 - Limited Data-Probably Compatible

Butorphanol is a potent narcotic agonist-antagonist analgesic that can be administered IV, IM, and intranasally.[1] In one study of 12 breastfeeding women, six of whom received a single 2 mg IM dose, and six of whom received a single 8 mg oral dose, the milk/serum ratios were constant over time, 0.7 (IM) and 1.9 (oral).[2] The average milk concentrations following a 2 mg IM dose, were 1.5, 0.7, and 0.3 µg/L at 2, 4, and 8 hours respectively. Following an oral dose of 8 mg, milk levels were 3.6, 1.8, and 1.1 µg/L at 3, 5, and 8 hours respectively. The elimination half-life in milk was approximately 2 hours. The estimated dose via milk is 0.1 µg/kg following an 8 mg oral dose, or 0.04 µg/kg following a 2 mg IM dose. The authors estimate that the infant would receive a maximum of 4 µg of butorphanol per day. Levels received by infants via milk are considered very low to insignificant. In addition, butorphanol undergoes first-pass metabolism by the liver, thus only 5%-17% of the oral dose reaches the plasma.

Butorphanol was used in labor and delivery in women who subsequently nursed their infants, although it has been noted to produce a sinusoidal fetal heart rate pattern and dysphoric or psychotomimetic responses in the fetus. Butorphanol use in breastfeeding is expected to be of minimal risk to the normal term infant; however, other pain medications are preferred in lactation.

T 1/2	4.56 h	MW	477.6 Da	PB	80%
Tmax	0.5-1 h IV/IM; 1-2 h nasal	RID	0.5%	Vd	4.36-12.87 L/kg
Oral	5%-17 %	M/P	0.7(IM)-1.9 (oral)	pKa	8.6

Adult Concerns: Sedation, respiratory depression/apnea, nausea, vomiting, constipation, urinary retention, weakness.

Adult Dose: 1-4 mg IM every 3-4 hours or 0.5-2 mg IV every 3-4 hours or 1 mg intranasally every 3-4 hours.

Pediatric Concerns: None reported via milk at this time. There have been rare reports of infant respiratory distress/apnea following the administration of butorphanol injection during labor.

Infant Monitoring: Sedation, slowed breathing rate/apnea, pallor, constipation, and not waking to feed/poor feeding.

Alternatives: Ibuprofen(L1), Acetaminophen(L1), Hydromorphone(L3)

References:
1. Pharmaceutical manufacturers prescribing information.
2. Pittman KA, Smyth RD, Losada M, Zighelboim I, Maduska AL, Sunshine A. Human perinatal distribution of butorphanol. Am J Obstet Gynecol. 1980;138(7 pt 1):797-800.

CABERGOLINE

Trade: Dostinex

Category: Prolactin Secretion Inhibitor

LRC: L3 - No Data-Probably Compatible

Cabergoline is a long-acting synthetic ergot alkaloid derivative that produces a dopamine agonist effect similar to bromocriptine. Cabergoline directly inhibits prolactin secretion by the pituitary.[1,2] It is primarily indicated for pathological hyperprolactinemia, but in several European studies, it has been used for inhibition of lactation.[3]

Although drug therapy is not required to cease lactation, a dose regimen used to inhibit lactation is cabergoline 1 mg administered as a single dose on the first day postpartum. For the suppression of established lactation, cabergoline 0.25 mg is taken every 12 hours for 2 days for a total of 1 mg. Single doses of 1 mg have been found to completely inhibit lactation.[4]

Transfer to human milk is not reported. In patients with hyperprolactinemia, it is possible to carefully administer doses to lower the prolactin to safe ranges, but high enough to retain lactation. In such cases, the infant should be observed for potential ergot side effects, if any.

In addition, mothers treated with cabergoline early postpartum, some cabergoline will pass into the milk supply. In some cases, the mothers may recover their milk supply following heavy pumping. Caution is recommended in feeding milk to infants following maternal exposure to cabergoline.

T 1/2	63-69 h	MW	451 Da	PB	40%-42%
Tmax	2-3 h	RID		Vd	
Oral	Complete	M/P		pKa	9.3, 6.4

Adult Concerns: Headache, dizziness, fatigue or insomnia, palpitations, orthostatic hypotension, edema, nose bleed, dry mouth, inhibition of lactation, nausea, constipation, anorexia, weakness.

Adult Dose: 0.25-1 mg twice a week.

Pediatric Concerns: Transfer via milk is unknown. Completely suppresses lactation and should not be used in mothers who are breastfeeding.

Infant Monitoring: Drowsiness or insomnia, dry mouth, constipation, weight gain, maternal decrease in milk supply.

Alternatives:

References:

1. Caballero-Gordo A, Lopez-Nazareno N, Calderay M, Caballero JL, Mancheno E, Sghedoni D. Oral cabergoline. Single-dose inhibition of puerperal lactation. J Reprod Med. 1991;36(10):717-721.
2. Rains CP, Bryson HM, Fitton A. Cabergoline. A review of its pharmacological properties and therapeutic potential in the treatment of hyperprolactinaemia and inhibition of lactation. Drugs. February 1995;49(2):255-279. Review.
3. Single dose cabergoline versus bromocriptine in inhibition of puerperal lactation: randomised, double blind, multicentre study. European Multicentre Study Group for Cabergoline in Lactation Inhibition. BMJ. 1991;302(6789):1367-1371.
3. Bravo-Topete EG, Mendoza-Hernandez F, Cejudo-Alvarez J, Briones-Garduno C. Cabergoline for inhibition of lactation. Cir Cir. 2004;72(1):5-9.

CAFFEINE

Trade:

Category: CNS Stimulant

LRC: L2 - Limited Data-Probably Compatible

Caffeine is a naturally occurring CNS stimulant present in many foods and drinks. While the half-life in adults is 4.9 hours, the half-life in neonates is as high as 97.5 hours. The half-life decreases with age to 14 hours at 3-5 months and 2.6 hours at 6 months and older. The average cup of coffee contains 100-150 mg of caffeine depending on preparation and country of origin.

Peak levels of caffeine are found in breastmilk 60-120 minutes after ingestion. In a study of five patients following an ingestion of 150 mg caffeine, peak concentrations of caffeine in serum ranged from 2.39 to 4.05 µg/mL and peak concentrations in milk ranged from 1.4 to 2.41 mg/L with a milk/serum ratio of 0.52.[1] The average milk concentration at 30, 60, and 120 minutes post dose was 1.58, 1.49, and 0.926 mg/L, respectively. In another study of seven breastfeeding mothers who consumed 750 mg caffeine/day for 5 days, and were 11-22 days postpartum, the average milk concentration was 4.3 mg/L.[2] Values ranged significantly from undetectable to 15.7 mg/L. The mean concentration of caffeine in sera of the infants on day 5 was 1.4 µg/mL (range undetectable to 2.8 µg/mL). In two patients whose milk levels were 13.4 and 28 mg/L, the respective infant serum levels were 0.25 and 3.2 µg/mL.

In a study of six breastfeeding mothers who received one dose of 100 mg orally, peak levels (C_{max}) in maternal serum ranged from 0.5 to 1 hour and 0.75 to 2 hours in milk.[3] The maternal plasma C_{max} ranged from 3.6 to 6.15 µg/mL, while the C_{max} for their milk ranged from 1.98 to 4.3 mg/L. The average concentration of caffeine in milk was 2.45 mg/L at 1 hour. The average milk/plasma ratio (AUC) was 0.812 for both breasts. This elegant study shows that caffeine rapidly enters milk and that the decay of caffeine in milk is similar to that of plasma. In infants from 4 to 7 kg body weight, the estimated dose to the infant would be 1.77 to 3.10 mg/d following a 100 mg maternal dose.

In a group of mothers who ingested from 35 to 336 mg of caffeine daily, the level of caffeine in milk ranged from 2.09 to 7.17 mg/L.[4] The author estimates the dose to infant is at 0.01 to 1.64 mg/d or 0.06% to 1.5% of the maternal dose. An interesting review of the nutritional effects of caffeine ingestion on infants is provided by Nehlig.[5] There is some evidence that chronic coffee drinking may reduce the iron content of milk. Irritability and insomnia may occur and have been reported.[6] Occasional use of caffeine is not contraindicated, but persistent, chronic use may lead to high plasma levels in the infant particularly during the neonatal period.

T 1/2	4.9 h	MW	194 Da	PB	36%
Tmax	60 min	RID	6%-25.9%	Vd	0.4-0.6 L/kg
Oral	100%	M/P	0.52 - 0.76	pKa	

Adult Concerns: Agitation, irritability, poor sleeping patterns.

Adult Dose:

Pediatric Concerns: Rarely, irritability and insomnia.

Infant Monitoring: Agitation, irritability, poor sleeping patterns, rapid heart rate, tremor.

Alternatives:

References:

1. Tyrala EE, Dodson WE. Caffeine secretion into breast milk. Arch Dis Child. 1979;54(10):787-800.
2. Ryu JE. Caffeine in human milk and in serum of breast-fed infants. Dev Pharmacol Ther. 1985;8(6):329-337.
3. Stavchansky S, Combs A, Sagraves R, Delgado M, Joshi A. Pharmacokinetics of caffeine in breast milk and plasma after single oral administration of caffeine to lactating mothers. Biopharm Drug Dispos. 1988;9(3):285-299.
4. Berlin CM Jr, Denson HM, Daniel CH, Ward RM. Disposition of dietary caffeine in milk, saliva, and plasma of lactating women. Pediatrics. 1984;73(1):59-63.

5. Nehlig A, Debry G. Consequences on the newborn of chronic maternal consumption of coffee during gestation and lactation: a review. J Am Coll Nutr. 1994;13(1):6-21.
6. Munoz LM, Lonnerdal B, Keen CL, Dewey KG. Coffee consumption as a factor in iron deficiency anemia among pregnant women and their infants in Costa Rica. Am J Clin Nutr. 1988;48:645-651.

CALCIPOTRIENE

Trade: Dovonex, Sorilux Foam, Taclonex Scalp

Category: Antipsoriatic

LRC: L3 - No Data-Probably Compatible

Calcipotriene is a synthetic vitamin D3 derivative used topically for the treatment of plaque psoriasis.[1] Only 5%-6% is transcutaneously absorbed into the systemic circulation (via ointment). It is rapidly bound to plasma proteins and excreted by the liver via bile. Less than 1% is absorbed from the scalp when the solution is used. It is unlikely plasma levels of calcipotriene would be elevated at all, and milk levels would be virtually nil because vitamin D transport to milk is normally quite low. Calcipotriene is active, however, and if used over wide areas of the body could (but unlikely) lead to some absorption. However, hypercalcemia in treated patients has been reported only rarely.

Taclonex Scalp Topical Suspension contains 52.18 µg of calcipotriene hydrate and 0.643 mg of betamethasone dipropionate.

Sorilux Foam is a vitamin D analog indicated for the topical treatment of plaque psoriasis in patients aged 18 years and older.

T 1/2		MW	430 Da	PB	
Tmax		RID		Vd	
Oral	Variable	M/P		pKa	

Adult Concerns: Skin irritation, rare but reversible hypercalcemia, rash, pruritus, worsening of psoriasis.

Adult Dose: Apply to skin lesions twice daily.

Pediatric Concerns: None reported via milk but no studies are available.

Infant Monitoring: Adverse effects in a breastfed infant are unlikely if the surface area treated is moderate to low.

Alternatives:

References:
1. Pharmaceutical manufacturers prescribing information.

CALCITRIOL

Trade: Rocaltrol

Category: Vitamin

LRC: L3 - Limited Data-Probably Compatible

Vitamin D typically undergoes a series of metabolic steps to become active. Calcitriol (1,25-dihydroxycholecalciferol) is believed to be the active metabolite of vitamin D metabolism. Calcitriol is the most potent of the synthetic vitamin D analogs. It is indicated for treatment of hypocalcemia in patients undergoing chronic renal dialysis and renal osteodystrophy. Because calcitriol works more quickly, it is useful in the treatment of patients with severe hypocalcemia. Calcitriol is well absorbed from the GI tract with a peak at 3-6 hours.[1] It is 99.9% protein bound to a specific alpha-globulin vitamin D binding protein. The elimination half-life is about 5-8 hours in adults and 27 hours in pediatric age patients. However, plasma levels are quite low, averaging approximately 40 pg/mL. Transfer of calcitriol to human milk is reported to be 2.2 pg/mL.[2] It is not likely that normal doses of this vitamin D analog would lead to clinically relevant levels in human milk, particularly since vitamin D transfers only minimally into human milk anyway. While plasma levels of vitamin D are normally quite low in human milk (<20 IU/L), at least one study now suggests that supplementing a mother with extraordinarily high levels of vitamin D2 can elevate milk levels, and subsequently lead to hypercalcemia in a breastfed infant.[3] See Vitamin D for new data.

T 1/2	5-8 h	MW	416 Da	PB	99.9%
Tmax	3-6 h	RID		Vd	
Oral	Complete	M/P		pKa	14.39

Adult Concerns: Overdosage of any form of vitamin D is dangerous and could lead to severe hypercalcemia, hypercalciuria, and hyperphosphatemia. Hypercalcemia may subsequently lead to vascular calcification, nephrocalcinosis, and other soft-tissue calcification.

Adult Dose: 0.25-2 µg daily (dose depends on indication).

Pediatric Concerns: None reported via milk, but caution recommended at higher doses.

Infant Monitoring: Weakness, dry mouth, constipation.

Alternatives: Vitamin d(L1)

References:
1. Pharmaceutical manufacturers prescribing information.
2. Teva Pharmaceuticals USA manufacturer prescribing information, 2008.
3. Greer FR, Hollis BW, Napoli JL. High concentrations of vitamin D2 in human milk associated with pharmacologic doses of vitamin D2. J Pediatr. 1984;105(1):61-64.

CALCIUM SALT

Trade:

Category: Calcium Supplement

LRC: L3 - No Data-Probably Compatible

Calcium salts come in different forms such as calcium carbonate, calcium lactate, calcium gluconate, calcium citrate, etc. Calcium salts can be used as an antacid and for treatment and prevention of calcium deficiency or hyperphosphatemia (such as osteoporosis or mild to moderate renal insufficiency). Recommended dietary allowance for calcium in breastfeeding women is 1000 mg/day. Milk-alkali syndrome during pregnancy has been associated with excessive intake of calcium carbonate antacids.[1] Calcium supplementation does not provide lactation benefits during late pregnancy or lactation.[2,3] Symptoms of milk-alkali syndrome (hypercalcemia) are nausea, vomiting, weight loss, thirst, muscle weakness, and confusion.

Adult Concerns: Headache, dry mouth, nausea, vomiting, constipation, flatulence, hypercalcemia, hypophosphatemia, milk-alkali syndrome.

Adult Dose: 1000 mg daily.

Pediatric Concerns:

Infant Monitoring:

Alternatives:

References:
1. Ullian ME, Linas SL. The milk-alkali syndrome in pregnancy. Case report. Miner Electrolyte Metab. 1988;14(4):208-210.
2. Karandish M, Djazayery A, Mahmoodi M, Behrooz A, Moremazi F. The effect of calcium supplementation during pregnancy on breast milk calcium concentration: a double blind placebo controlled clinical trial. J Pediatr Gastroenterol Nutr. 2004;39(suppl 1):S472.
3. Prentice A, Jarjou LM, Cole TJ, et al. Calcium requirements of lactating Gambian mothers: effects of a calcium supplement on breast-milk calcium concentration, maternal bone mineral content, and urinary calcium excretion. Am J Clin Nutr. 1995;62:58-67.

CALENDULA

Trade:

Category: Herb

LRC: L3 - No Data-Probably Compatible

Calendula, grown worldwide, has been used topically to promote wound healing and to alleviate conjunctivitis and other ocular inflammations. It consists of a number of flavonol glycosides and saponins, but the active ingredients are unknown.[1] Despite these claims, there are almost no studies regarding its efficacy in any of these disorders. Further, there are no suggestions of overt toxicity, with exception of allergies.[2] Although it may have some uses externally, its internal use as an antiphlogistic and spasmolytic is largely obsolete.

No data are available on its transfer into human milk.

T 1/2		MW		PB	
Tmax		RID		Vd	
Oral	Good	M/P		pKa	

Adult Concerns: Allergic reactions.

Adult Dose: One cup of the tea (1-2 grams of the dried flowers) three times daily.

Pediatric Concerns: None reported via milk.

Infant Monitoring:

Alternatives:

References:
1. Bissett NG. Herbal Drugs and Phytopharmaceuticals. Boca Raton, FL: Medpharm Scientific Publishers, CRC Press; 1994.
2. Natural Medicines Comprehensive Database, 2010.

CANAGLIFLOZIN

Trade: Invokana

Category: Antidiabetic, other

LRC: L4 - No Data-Possibly Hazardous

Canagliflozin is a medication used to treat type II diabetes. At this time there are no data regarding the transfer of canagliflozin to human milk. Based on this medications high protein binding, moderate molecular weight and volume of distribution milk levels are expected to be low. However, this medication has a number of adverse effects reported in the adult population, which would be concerning in a breastfed infant (e.g., dehydration, changes in electrolytes, renal dysfunction, changes in cholesterol and bone mineral density), thus caution is recommended. There are numerous other medications with breastfeeding data that would be preferred for use in lactation (e.g., insulin, metformin, glyburide).

T 1/2	10.6-13.1 h	MW	453.53 Da	PB	99%
Tmax	1-2 h	RID		Vd	1.19 L/kg
Oral	65%	M/P		pKa	

Adult Concerns: Dizziness, fatigue, orthostatic hypotension, abdominal pain, constipation, genitourinary infections, renal dysfunction, dehydration, hyperkalemia, hypermagnesemia, increased cholesterol, increased hemoglobin, decreased bone mineral density.

Adult Dose: 100-300 mg once daily.

Pediatric Concerns: No data in lactation at this time.

Infant Monitoring: Lethargy, changes in feeding, weight gain, constipation; should clinical signs of dehydration occur consider checking electrolytes.

Alternatives: Insulin(L2), Metformin(L1), Glyburide(L2)

References:
1. Pharmaceutical manufacturers prescribing information.

CANDESARTAN

Trade: Amias, Atacand

Category: Angiotensin II Receptor Antagonist

LRC: L3 - No Data-Probably Compatible

Candesartan is a specific blocker of the angiotensin II receptor. It is typically used as an antihypertensive similar to the ACE inhibitor family.[1]

Some of the ACE inhibitors can be used in breastfeeding mothers postpartum. However, no data are available on candesartan in human milk although the manufacturer states that it is present in rodent milk. Some caution is recommended in the neonatal period, particularly when used in mothers with premature infants as exposure to medications that act directly on the renin-angiotensin system (RAS) may have effects on the development of immature kidneys.

Both the ACE inhibitor family and the specific angiotensin II receptor blockers are contraindicated in pregnancy and thus should be used with caution in women who are planning a subsequent pregnancy in the near future.

T 1/2	9 h	MW	611 Da	PB	>99%
Tmax	3-4 h	RID		Vd	0.13 L/kg
Oral	15%	M/P		pKa	8.15

Adult Concerns: Headache, dizziness, fatigue, hypotension, nausea, diarrhea, constipation, changes in renal function/urine output, hyperkalemia.

Adult Dose: 4-32 mg daily.

Pediatric Concerns: None reported via milk at this time.

Infant Monitoring: Drowsiness, lethargy, pallor, poor feeding, and weight gain.

Alternatives: Captopril(L2), Enalapril(L2), Ramipril(L3)

References:
1. Pharmaceutical manufacturers prescribing information.

CANDIN

Trade: Candida albicans skin test antigen

Category: Dermatologic Agents

LRC: L3 - No Data-Probably Compatible

Candin is a *Candida albicans* skin test antigen used to evaluate for cellular immune response in those suspected to have reduced cellular immunity.[1] This product is prepared from the culture filtrate and strains of C. albicans. When administered intradermally in immuno-competent individuals, a delayed type hypersensitivity response is elicited within 48 hours. An induration of >=5 mm at the site of injection represents adequate cellular immununity. There are currently no studies done on its use in breastfeeding women. However, since only minimal amounts of the antigen is used for this test (0.1 mL), plasma concentrations attained after its injection are probably too low to cause significant transfer into breast milk.

Adult Concerns: Redness, swelling, itching, excoriation at the site of injection. Severe hypersensitivity reactions may occur.

Adult Dose: 0.1 mL intradermal.

Pediatric Concerns:

Infant Monitoring:

Alternatives:

References:
1. Pharmaceutical manufacturers prescribing information.

CANNABIS

Trade: Marijuana, Tetrahydrocannabinol, THC

Category: Sedative-Hypnotic

LRC: L4 - Limited Data-Possibly Hazardous

Cannabis, more commonly referred to as marijuana, contains the active component delta-9-THC (Tetrahydrocannabinol or THC).[1] THC can be measured in the blood within seconds after inhalation and peak within 3-10 minutes of smoking. The systemic bioavailability is dependent on numerous factors including the depth of inhalation, duration of use, breath holding, and frequency of use. Occasional users may have a bioavailability of 10%-14%, where chronic users tend to be higher, 23%-27%. With oral use, THC can be measured in blood 1-2 hours post ingestion and peak around 4 hours. Although oral absorption appears to be very good, an extensive first pass effect results in a low systemic bioavailability of 4%-12%.

THC is highly protein bound (95%-99%) and initially distributed in plasma (Vd=2.5-3.5 L); however, this lipophilic drug has a highly variable and large volume of distribution at steady state (3.4-10 L/kg).[1] THC is also known to enter well-vascularized areas such as the liver, heart, lung, and breast and then eventually accumulate in fat tissue.

Multiple articles examining the correlation between exposure to marijuana and prolactin levels have found decreased prolactin levels in chronic users as the binding of THC to cannabinoid receptors may regulate a variety of hormone secretions from the anterior pituitary.[2,3] Thus, major changes in the reproductive system, lactation, metabolism, and stress systems are possible.

Small to moderate secretion of THC in breast milk has been documented. In one report of a mother who smoked marijuana once daily for 7 months, up to 105 μg/L of THC was quantified in her milk.[4] Her infant had negative urine samples and was reported to have normal development by the pediatrician. Another mother who used the drug seven times per day for 8 months was found to have 340 μg/L of THC and 4.2 μg/L of 11-OH-THC (active metabolite) in her first milk sample. In her second milk sample, she had 60.3 μg/L of THC, 1.1 μg/L of 11-OH-THC, and 1.6 μg/L 9-carboxy-THC (inactive metabolite). In this case, the mother had eight times more THC in her milk than plasma. Her infant had negative urine samples but positive fecal samples for 347 ng of THC, 67 ng of 11-OH-THC, and 611 ng 9-carboxy-THC. This infant was also reported to have normal development by the pediatrician.

A 2011 study that verified a method to quantify illicit substances in human milk obtained one milk sample from a woman using cannabis in lactation. Her milk sample contained 86 μg/L of THC and 5 μg/L of 11-OH-THC.[5] No details were provided regarding maternal use, timing of milk sample or infant outcomes in this paper. In addition, numerous animal studies have also reported the transfer of THC to milk.[6,7]

At this time, safety data for maternal marijuana use in lactation is lacking for both short- and long-term infant outcomes. In addition, most of the data is limited by small sample sizes, shortcomings in study design, poor dose characterization, in-utero exposure, and other concomitant maternal medications.

In one study comparing 27 women who smoked marijuana routinely during breastfeeding to 35 non-marijuana smoking women, no differences were noted in their children's growth, mental, and motor development.[8] A 1990 prospective study evaluated the motor and mental abilities of infants exposed to marijuana via milk.[9] This study used participants from a previous study, which evaluated diet, alcohol use, and smoking in lactation and their influence on infant growth and development. Of these participants, 68 women used marijuana in lactation (largely first and third month). When matched to 68 women with similar exposures in pregnancy that did not use marijuana in lactation, it was found that those infants with higher marijuana exposure in first trimester or the first month of lactation had significantly lower psychomotor development index scores than infants with no exposure in these periods at 1 year of age. No differences in mental development were noted.

Of 109 breast milk samples randomly collected from a Poison Center along with a questionnaire that identified life-long drug use and use in pregnancy, 19 participants reported drug use and one had a detectable level.[10] In this one sample the concentration of THC was 20 ng/mL, both cannabidiol (CBD) and cannabinol (CBN) were undetectable. This woman's urine was also found to be positive for cannabinoids during her hospital stay. A second sample was also positive for THC at 31 ng/mL and CBD (concentration below limit of quantification); however, this woman did not report drug use on her questionnaire. The authors estimated that the infants of these two participants would receive 2-3.1 μg of THC per 100 mL feed. After accounting for poor oral absorption the authors reduced the dose that could be absorbed by the infants after a feed to 0.24-0.37 μg of THC. Please note that the maternal dose, timing of use, and milk samples were not available in this study, thus a relative infant dose cannot be calculated and the absolute infant dose could vary based on these parameters.

In a recent study, THC was detected at low concentrations at all the time points beyond time zero.[11] THC was transferred to mother's milk such that exclusively breastfeeding infants ingested an estimated mean of 2.5% of the maternal dose (the calculated relative infant dose was 2.5%, with a range of 0.4%–8.7%). The estimated daily infant dose was 8 micrograms per kilogram per day. Because the oral bioavailability of THC is low (< 1-6%), the dose absorbed by the infant is likely minimal.

In summary, there is increasing concern about the use of marijuana or other cannabis products, in breastfeeding mothers. Both human and animal studies suggest that early exposure to cannabis may not be benign, and that cannabis exposure in the perinatal period may produce long-term changes in mental and motor development.[1-13] While this data poses numerous limitations, and does not directly examine the benefits of breast milk versus risks of exposure to marijuana in milk, cannabis use in breastfeeding mothers should be discouraged at this time. Healthcare professionals should encourage alternative treatment options for maternal health conditions requiring the use of marijuana.

T 1/2	25-57 h	MW	314 Da	PB	95%-99%
Tmax		RID		Vd	3.4 L/kg; variable L/kg
Oral	4%-12%	M/P	8	pKa	

Adult Concerns: Sedation, fatigue, hallucinations, increased sensory perception, poor memory, seizures, tachycardia, dry mouth, constipation, changes in menstrual cycle, inhibition of platelet aggregation, weakness, changes in motor coordination.[1] Possible decreased milk production.

Adult Dose:

Pediatric Concerns: Limited information in lactation and pediatrics at this time. Infants may eliminate drug in urine for weeks after exposure.[10]

Infant Monitoring: Sedation, not waking to feed/poor feeding, weight gain, potential neurobehavioral or psychomotor delays.

Alternatives:

References:

1. Grotenhermen F. Pharmacokinetics and pharmacodynamics of cannabinoids. Clin Pharmacokinet. 2003;42(4):327-360.
2. Ranganathan M, Braley G, Pittman B, et al. The effects of cannabinoids on serum cortisol and prolactin in humans. Pyschopharmacology (Berl). 2009;203(4):737-744.
3. Mendelson JH, Mello NK, Ellingboe J. Acute effects of marihuana smoking on prolactin levels in human females. J Pharmacol Exp Ther. 1985;232(1):220-222.
4. Perez-Reyes M, Wall ME. Presence of delta9-tetrahydrocannabinol in human milk. N Engl J Med. 1982;307(13):819-820.
5. Marchei E, Escuder D, Pallas CR, et al. Simultaneous analysis of frequently used licit and illicit psychoactive drugs in breast milk by liquid chromatography tandem mass spectrometry. J Pharmaceut Biomed Anal. 2011;55:309-316.
6. Ahmad GR, Ahmad N. Passive consumption of marijuana through milk: a low level chronic exposure to delta-9-tetrahydrocannabinol (THC). J Toxicol Clin Toxicol. 1990;28(2):255-260.
7. Chao FC, Green DE, Forrest IS, Kaplan JN, Winship-Ball A, Braude M. The passage of 14C-delta-9-tetrahydrocannabinol into the milk of lactating squirrel monkeys. Res Commun Chem Pathol Pharmacol. 1976;15(2):303-317.
8. Tennes K, Avitable N, Blackard C, et al. Marijuana: prenatal and postnatal exposure in the human. NIDA Res Monogr. 1985;59:48-60.
9. Astley SJ, Little RE. Maternal marijuana use during lactation and infant development at one year. Neurotoxicol Teratol. 1990;12:161-168.
10. de Oliveira Silveira G, Loddi S, Dizioli Rodrigues de Oliveira C, et al. Headspace solid-phase microextraction and gas chromatography-mass spectrometry for determination of cannabinoids in human breast milk. Forensic Toxicol. 2017;35:125-132.
11. Baker T, Datta P, Rewers-Felkins K, Thompson H, Kallem RR, Hale TW. Transfer of inhaled cannabis into human breast milk. Obstet Gynecol. May 2018;131(5):783-788.
12. Jutras-Aswad D, DiNieri JA, Harkany T, Hurd YL. Neurobiological consequences of maternal cannabis on human fetal development and its neuropsychiatric outcome. Eur Arch Psychiatry Clin Neurosci. October 2009;259(7):395-341.
13. Liston J. Breastfeeding and the use of recreational drugs-alcohol, caffeine, nicotine and marijuana. Breastfeed Rev. 1998;6(2):27-30.

CAPECITABINE

Trade: Xeloda

Category: Antineoplastic

LRC: L5 - Limited Data-Hazardous

Capecitabine is an antineoplastic agent commonly used in the treatment of colon cancer. It is converted enzymatically to the active drug 5-Fluorouracil (5-FU).[1] Capecitabine is readily absorbed orally and rapidly metabolized in most tissues to 5-FU in about 2 hours following administration.

5-Fluorouracil is well absorbed orally, but poorly absorbed transcutaneously. Milk levels have not yet been published. Breastfeeding is probably fine if exposure is due to topical application over small to moderate areas (not large areas). If used orally, or intravenously in significant doses, a suitable waiting period should be used to avoid infant exposure. Because it has only a 12 minute half-life, a few hours, or better, 24 hours would probably reduce any risk from this agent. The injection into the intraocular space would prolong the release of 5FU into the plasma. But the dose is so low, it is unlikely to cause significant exposure to a breastfeeding infant via breast milk.

T 1/2	38-45 min	MW	359.4 Da	PB	<60%
Tmax	1.5 h	RID		Vd	
Oral		M/P		pKa	8.23

Adult Concerns: Diarrhea, pain, blistering, peeling, redness, or swelling of palms of hands and/or bottoms of feet; sores, or ulcers in mouth or on lips.

Adult Dose: 1000 mg/m² twice daily for two weeks every 21 days.

Pediatric Concerns:

Infant Monitoring: Wait 24 hours to resume breastfeeding to minimize risk.

Alternatives:

References:
1. Pharmaceutical manufacturers prescribing information.

CAPSAICIN

Trade: Pepper Spray

Category: Analgesic

LRC: L3 - No Data-Probably Compatible

Capsaicin is an alkaloid derived from peppers from the Solanaceae family. It is commonly found in pepper spray devices. Used topically, it increases, depletes, and then suppresses substance P release from sensory neurons, thus preventing pain sensation. Substance P is the principal chemomediator of pain from the periphery to the CNS.[1,2] After repeated application (days to weeks), it depletes substance P and prevents reaccumulation in the neuron. Very little or nothing is known about the kinetics of this product. It is approved for use in children >2 years of age. No data are available on transfer into human milk. However, topical application to the nipple or areola should be avoided unless it is thoroughly removed prior to breastfeeding.

T 1/2	1.64 h	MW	305 Da	PB	
Tmax		RID		Vd	
Oral	None	M/P		pKa	9.5

Adult Concerns: Local irritation, burning, stinging, erythema. Cough and infrequently neurotoxicity. Avoid use near eyes, or on the nipple.

Adult Dose: Apply to affected area 3-4 times a day.

Pediatric Concerns: None reported. Avoid transfer to eye and other sensitive surfaces via hand contact.

Infant Monitoring:

Alternatives:

References:
1. Bernstein JE. Capsaicin in dermatologic disease. Semin Dermatol. 1988;7(4):304-309.
2. Watson CP, Evans RJ, Watt VR. The post-mastectomy pain syndrome and the effect of topical capsaicin. Pain. 1989;38(2):177-186.

CAPTOPRIL

Trade: Acepril, Capoten

Category: ACE Inhibitor

LRC: L2 - Limited Data-Probably Compatible

Captopril is a typical angiotensin converting enzyme inhibitor (ACEI) used to reduce hypertension. In one report of 12 women treated with 100 mg three times daily, maternal serum levels averaged 713 µg/L while breast milk levels averaged 4.7 µg/L at 3.8 hours after administration.[1] Data from this study suggest that an infant would ingest approximately 0.016% of the free captopril consumed by its mother (300 mg) on a daily basis. No adverse effects have been reported in this study. Use with care in mothers with premature infants.

Both the ACE inhibitor family and the specific angiotensin II receptor blockers are contraindicated in the second and third trimester of pregnancy.

T 1/2	2.2 h	MW	217 Da	PB	30%
Tmax	1 h	RID	0.02%	Vd	0.7 L/kg
Oral	60%-75%	M/P	0.012	pKa	4.02

Adult Concerns: Headache, dizziness, fatigue, hypotension, abnormal taste, cough, nausea, diarrhea, constipation, changes in renal function/urine output, hyperkalemia, rash.

Adult Dose: 50 mg TID.

Pediatric Concerns: None reported via milk at this time.

Infant Monitoring: Drowsiness, lethargy, pallor, poor feeding, and weight gain.

Alternatives: Enalapril(L2), Benazepril(L2), Ramipril(L3)

References:
1. Devlin RG, Fleiss PM. Captopril in human blood and breast milk. J Clin Pharmacol. February-March 1981;21(2):110-113.

CARBAMAZEPINE

Trade: Carbatrol, Epitol, Mazepine, Tegretol, Teril

Category: Anticonvulsant

LRC: L2 - Limited Data-Probably Compatible

Carbamazepine (CBZ) is a unique anticonvulsant commonly used for grand mal, tonic-clonic, simple, and complex seizures. It is also used in manic depression and a number of other neurologic syndromes.

In a brief study by Kaneko, with maternal plasma levels averaging 4.3 µg/mL, milk levels were 1.9 mg/L.[1] In a study of 3 patients who received from 5.8 to 7.3 mg/kg/day carbamazepine, milk levels were reported to vary from 1.3 to 1.8 mg/L, while the epoxide metabolite varied from 0.5 to 1.1 mg/L.[2] No adverse effects were noted in any of the infants. In another study by Niebyl, breast milk levels were 1.4 mg/L in the lipid fraction and 2.3 mg/L in the skim fraction in a mother receiving 1000 mg daily of carbamazepine.[3] This author estimated a daily intake of 2 mg carbamazepine (0.5 mg/kg) in an infant ingesting 1 liter of milk per day. In a study of CBZ and its epoxide metabolite (ECBZ) in milk, 16 patients received an average dose of 13.8 mg/kg/day.[4] The average maternal serum levels of CBZ and ECBZ were 7.1 and 2.6 µg/mL, respectively. The average milk levels of CBZ and ECBZ were 2.5 and 1.5 mg/L respectively. The relative percent of CBZ and ECBZ in milk were 36.4% and 53% of the maternal serum levels. A total of 50 milk samples in 19 patients were analyzed. Of these, the lowest CBZ concentration in milk was 1 mg/L; the highest was 4.8 mg/L. The CBZ level was determined in seven infants 4-7 days postpartum. All infants have CBZ levels below 1.5 µg/mL. In a study of 7 women receiving 250-800 mg/d carbamazepine, the CBZ level ranged from 2.8-4.5 mg/L in milk to 3.2-15 mg/L in plasma.[5] The levels of ECBZ ranged from 0.5-1.7 mg/L in milk to 0.8-4.8 mg/L in plasma. We also have one report of a mother taking carbamazepine 200 mg in the morning and 300 mg at bedtime, at 3 months, the infants total serum levels were 0.7 µg/mL and free levels were 0.22 µg/mL (levels drawn 14 hours after the dose).[6] The amount of CBZ transferred to the infant is apparently quite low. Although the half-life of CBZ in infants appears shorter than in adults, infants should still be monitored for sedative effects.

In one case report of a mother consuming 600 mg/d during pregnancy and lactation, the infant was treated for physiologic jaundice from day 4-5.[7] On day 21, the infant was hospitalized for persistent jaundice (yellow skin color, slightly enlarged liver and spleen), with elevated direct bilirubin, GGT, and ALP (peaked at 6.5 weeks). The authors reported histological findings of intracellular cholestasis and subacute portal triad inflammation with eosinophils, which subsequently resolved with no long-term sequelae. In-utero exposure cannot be ruled out as fetal exposure is 50%-80% of maternal levels.

In a second case with a mother consuming 400 mg/day carbamazepine during pregnancy and lactation, the infant at term was noted to be jaundiced.[8] Levels of GGT and direct bilirubin peaked on day 5. In addition, the infant had ABO hemolytic disease with tachypnea, pallor, and a venous hematocrit of 0.3 on day 8 of life that required a packed-cell transfusion. On day 9 of life, the breastfeeding frequency was reduced and supplementation was started. Levels of carbamazepine on day 2 in maternal serum, milk, and infant serum were 5.5 µg/mL, 2.8 µg/mL, and 1.8 µg/mL, respectively. On day 63 carbamazepine levels were 6.5 µg/mL, 2.2 µg/mL, 1.1 µg/mL, respectively. Based on the information provided, we believe that this toxicity was most likely due to in-utero exposure.

A Norwegian study published in 2013 assessed the adverse effects of antiepileptic medications via breast milk in infants who were also exposed in utero.[9] The study evaluated mothers' reports of their child's behavior, motor, social, and language skills at 6, 18, and 36 months using validated screening tools. At age 6 months, infants of mothers using antiepileptic drugs in utero had a significantly higher risk of impaired fine motor skills when compared to control group infants. In addition, infants exposed to multiple antiepileptics also had a greater risk of fine motor and social impairment when compared to control group infants. However, it was noted that continuous breastfeeding in the first 6 months did demonstrate a trend toward improvement in all of the developmental domains. In addition, the study demonstrated that continuous breastfeeding (daily for more than 6 months) in children of women using antiepileptic drugs in utero reduced the impairment in development at 6 and 18 months when compared with those with no breastfeeding or breastfeeding for less than 6 months. At 18 months, children in the drug-exposed group had an increased risk of impaired development compared with the reference group; the risks were highest in children who stopped breastfeeding early. Within the drug-exposed group, this impairment was statistically significant for autistic traits, 22.4% with discontinued breastfeeding were affected compared with 8.7% with prolonged breastfeeding. By 36 months, prenatal antiepileptic drug exposure was associated with impaired development such as autistic traits, reduced sentence completeness and aggressive symptoms, regardless of breastfeeding during the first year of life. The authors concluded that women with epilepsy should be encouraged to breastfeed regardless of their antiepileptic medication.

In 2014, a prospective observational study looked at long-term neurodevelopment of infants exposed to antiepileptic drugs in utero and lactation.[10] This study included women taking carbamazepine, lamotrigine, phenytoin, or valproate as monotherapy for epilepsy. In this study, 42.9% of the infants were breastfed for a mean of 7.2 months. The IQ of these children at 6 years of age was statistically significantly lower in children who were exposed to valproate in utero (7-13 IQ points lower). It was also noted that higher doses of medication (primarily with valproate) were associated with lower IQ scores. The children's IQ scores were found to be higher if the maternal IQ was higher, the mother took folic acid near the time of conception and if the child was breastfed (4 points higher). In addition, verbal abilities were also found to be significantly higher in children that were breastfed. Although this study has many limitations (e.g., small sample size, difficulties with patient follow-up) it does provide data up to age 6 that suggest benefits of breastfeeding are not outweighed by risks of maternal drug therapy in milk.

Infants of epileptic mothers treated with carbamazepine throughout pregnancy and breastfeeding should be carefully monitored for possible adverse effects.

T 1/2	18-54 h	MW	236 Da	PB	74%
Tmax	4-5 h	RID	3.8%-5.9%	Vd	0.8-1.8 L/kg
Oral	100%	M/P	0.69	pKa	7

Adult Concerns: Sedation, dizziness, headache, confusion, hypertension, tachycardia, respiratory depression, nausea, vomiting, diarrhea, changes in thyroid function, hypocalcemia, hyponatremia, blood dyscrasias. The FDA warns that patients of Asian ancestry should be screened for the human leukocyte antigen (HLA) allele HLA-B*1502 before receiving carbamazepine. The risk for Stevens-Johnson syndrome (SJS) and toxic epidermal necrolysis (TEN) is higher among these patients.

Adult Dose: 800-1200 mg daily divided TID or QID.

Pediatric Concerns: Two case reports of liver toxicity; however, in both cases in-utero exposure was most likely the cause.[7,8]

Infant Monitoring: Sedation or irritability, not waking to feed/poor feeding, and weight gain. Based on clinical symptoms some infants may require monitoring of liver enzymes.

Alternatives:

References:

1. Kaneko S, Sato T, Suzuki K. The levels of anticonvulsants in breast milk. Br J Clin Pharmacol. 1979;7(6):624-627.
2. Pynnonen S, Kanto J, Sillanpaa M, Erkkola R. Carbamazepine: placental transport, tissue concentrations in foetus and newborn, and level in milk. Acta Pharmacol Toxicol (Copenh). 1977;41(3):244-253.
3. Niebyl JR, Blake DA, Freeman JM, Luff RD. Carbamazepine levels in pregnancy and lactation. Obstet Gynecol. 1979;53(1):139-140.
4. Froescher W, Eichelbaum M, Niesen M, Dietrich K, Rausch P. Carbamazepine levels in breast milk. Ther Drug Monit. 1984;6(3):266-271.
5. Shimoyama R, Ohkubo T, Sugawara K. Monitoring of carbamazepine and carbamazepine 10,11-epoxide in breast milk and plasma by high-performance liquid chromatography. Ann Clin Biochem. 2000;37(pt 2):210-215.
6. Wisner K, Perel J. Serum levels of valproate and carbamazepine in breastfeeding mother-infant pairs. J Clin Psychopharmacol. 1998;18:167-169.
7. Frey B, Schubiger G, Musy JP. Transient cholestatic hepatitis in a neonate associated with carbamazepine exposure during pregnancy and breast-feeding. Eur J Pediatr. 1990;150:136-138.
8. Merlob P, Mor N, Litwin A. Transient hepatic dysfunction in an infant of an epileptic mother treated with carbamazepine during pregnancy and breastfeeding. Ann Pharmacother. December 1992;26(12):1563-1565.
9. Veiby G, Engelsen BA, Gilhus NE. Early child development and exposure to antiepileptic drugs prenatally and through breastfeeding: a prospective cohort study on children of women with epilepsy. JAMA Neurol. 2013;70:1367-1374.
10. Meador KJ, Baker GA, Browning N, et al. Breastfeeding in children of women taking antiepileptic drugs cognitive outcomes at age 6. JAMA Pediatr. 2014;168(8):729-736.

CARBAMIDE PEROXIDE

Trade: Audiologist's choice, Auraphene-B, Auro ear drops, Cankaid, Debrox, Dewax

Category: Ceruminolytic

LRC: L1 - Limited Data-Compatible

Carbamide peroxide, also called urea peroxide, is stable while immersed in glycerin, but on contact with moisture, releases hydrogen peroxide and nascent oxygen, both strong oxidizing agents.[1] It is used to disinfect infected lesions, for the removal of earwax, and for whitening of teeth and dental appliances. Hydrogen peroxide is rapidly metabolized by hydroperoxidases, peroxidases, and catalase present in all tissues, plasma, and saliva. Its transfer to the plasma is minimal if at all. It would be all but impossible for any to reach breast milk unless under extreme overdose.

T 1/2		MW	94 Da	PB	
Tmax		RID		Vd	
Oral		M/P		pKa	

Adult Concerns: Dermal irritation, mucous membrane irritation, inflammation. Overgrowth of Candida and other opportunistic infections.

Adult Dose: Apply several drops on affected area for four times a day after meals and at bedtime.

Pediatric Concerns: Possibly toxic in major oral overdose. Exposure to small amounts may lead to inflamed membranes.

Infant Monitoring:

Alternatives:

References:
1. Pharmaceutical manufacturers prescribing information.

CARBETOCIN

Trade: Duratocin

Category: Pituitary Hormone

LRC: L3 - Limited Data-Probably Compatible

Carbetocin is a long acting version of oxytocin that is used for the prevention of hemorrhage following delivery by cesarean section.[1] Although this medication is a longer acting version of oxytocin, its half-life is still considerably short (29-53 minutes), thus it does not have much time to enter milk in significant quantities.

Silcox et al. reported that after five women were given a single 70 µg dose of carbetocin intramuscularly, 7 to 14 weeks postpartum, the mean peak milk concentration was 56 times lower than the mean peak maternal plasma concentration.[1,2] The mean peak milk concentrations from both left and right breast samples were 19.6 pg/mL and 17.8 pg/mL. Using this data, we calculated the relative infant dose to be less than 0.3%. In addition, very little of the medication found in milk is thought to be absorbed by the infant as most of the drug should be quickly broken down by peptidases in the infants stomach.

Although the shorter acting version of this medication, oxytocin, is known to cause contraction of the myoepithelial cells around the alveoli, it is not known if carbetocin has the same effect.[1,2] However, four of five women given the single dose of carbetocin reported an increased ease of obtaining milk samples. The authors suggested that carbetocin may enhance let down.[2]

T 1/2	29-53 min	MW	988.1 Da	PB	
Tmax	15-30 min	RID	0.27%-0.29%	Vd	
Oral		M/P		pKa	

Adult Concerns: Headache, dizziness, anxiety, hypotension, chest pain, tachycardia, flushing/feeling of warmth/chills, dyspnea, metallic taste, nausea, vomiting, abdominal pain, hyperstimulation of the uterus, sweating, tremor, pruritis.

Adult Dose: 100 µg IV x 1 dose.

Pediatric Concerns: None reported via breast milk at this time.

Infant Monitoring:

Alternatives: Oxytocin(L2)

References:
1. Pharmaceutical manufacturers prescribing information.
2. Silcox J, Schulz P, Horbay GLA, et al. Transfer of carbetocin into human breast milk. Obstet Gynecol. 1993;82:456-459.

CARBIDOPA + LEVODOPA

Trade: Brocadopa, Dopar, Kinson, Larodopa, Madopar, Prolopa, Sinemet

Category: Antiparkinsonian

LRC: L4 - Limited Data-Possibly Hazardous

Levodopa (l-dopa) is a prodrug of dopamine used primarily for treatment of parkinsonian symptoms. Carbidopa inhibits the metabolic activation of levodopa but does not cross the blood-brain barrier, thereby increasing the amount of levodopa that becomes active in the central nervous system.[1]

In a study of one mother with Parkinsonism, peak breast milk levodopa was measured to be 1.6 nmol/mL 3 hours after Sinemet CR 50/200 at steady state, and returned to baseline after 6 hours. This would constitute an RID of 1.65% of maternal dose. Following administration of immediate release Sinemet, milk concentrations peaked at 3.47 nmol/mL after 3 hours, and returned to baseline in 6 hours. Based on milk concentrations, the infant would have ingested a maximum of 0.1 mg/kg/day or an RID of 3.6%. No adverse reactions were noted in the breastfed infant.[2]

However, dopamine inhibits the release of prolactin from the anterior pituitary. Levodopa is known to decrease plasma prolactin levels by as much as 78%, which has been associated with diminished milk production.[3-7]

T 1/2	levo/carb: 1.5 h/1-2 h	MW	levo/carb: 197.2/244.3 Da	PB	both: <36%
Tmax	0.5-2 h (combination)	RID	1.66%-3.59%	Vd	levo: 0.9-1.6 L/kg
Oral	both: 40%-70%	M/P		pKa	levo/carb: 9.69/9.29

Adult Concerns: Headache, dizziness, confusion, agitation, insomnia, hypotension, chest pain, arrhythmias, nausea, vomiting, anorexia, changes in liver function.

Adult Dose: levo/carb: 100 mg/25 mg four to six times a day (max 1500 mg/200 mg).

Pediatric Concerns: None reported via milk, but reduced prolactin levels may reduce milk production.

Infant Monitoring: Can reduce breast milk production-not recommended in lactation.

Alternatives:

References:
1. Pharmaceutical manufacturers prescribing information. Merck Sharp & Dohme Corp., 2014.
2. Thulin PC, Woodward WR, Carter JH, Nutt JG. Levodopa in human breast milk: clinical implications. Neurology. 1998;50:1920-1921.
3. Ayalon D, Peyser MR, Toaff R, et al. Effect of L-dopa on galactopoiesis and gonadotropin levels in the inappropriate lactation syndrome. Obstet Gynecol. 1974;44:159-170.
4. Leblanc H, Yen SS. The effect of L-dopa and chlorpromazine on prolactin and growth hormone secretion in normal women. Am J Obstet Gynecol. 1976;126:162-164.
5. Board JA, Fierro RJ, Wasserman AJ, Bhatnagar AS. Effects of alpha- and beta-adrenergic blocking agents on serum prolactin levels in women with hyperprolactinemia and galactorrhea. Am J Obstet Gynecol. 1977;127:285-287.
6. Rao R, Scommegna A, Frohman LA. Integrity of central dopaminergic system in women with postpartum hyperprolactinemia. Am J Obstet Gynecol. 1982;143:883-887.
7. Barbieri C, Ferrari C, Caldara R, Curtarelli G. Growth hormone secretion in hypertensive patients: evidence for a derangement in central adrenergic function. Clin Sci (Lond). 1980;58(2):135-138.

CARBIMAZOLE

Trade: Neo-Mercazole, NeoMercazole

Category: Antithyroid Agent

LRC: L3 - Limited Data-Probably Compatible

Carbimazole, a prodrug of methimazole, is rapidly and completely converted to the active metabolite methimazole in the plasma. Only methimazole is detected in plasma, urine, and thyroid tissue. See breastfeeding specifics for methimazole.

In a study, Rylance et al. suggests that subclinical levels of methimazole enter milk subsequent to a maternal dose of 30 mg/day carbimazole.[1] Free methimazole measured in milk on 10 occasions averaged 43 µg/L. Plasma methimazole in twins was 45 to 52 ng/mL. Thyroid suppression is believed to occur only when plasma levels exceed 50-100 ng/mL. No thyroid suppression was noted in these two twins. Peak transfer into milk occurred at 2-4 hours, and the lowest at 6 hours after the dose. The authors suggest that breastfeeding is permissible if the maternal dose is less than 30 mg/day. In another study of 5 five lactating women receiving 40 mg/d, the mean concentration of methimazole in milk was 182 µg/L, with a mean milk/serum ratio of 0.98.[2] The mean total amount of methimazole excreted in milk over 8 h was 34 µg. The limited data above suggest that the transfer of carbimazole is too low to affect thyroid function in breastfeeding infants. However, close monitoring of infant thyroid function is probably advisable. See propylthiouracil as alternative.

T 1/2	6-13 h	MW	186 Da	PB	0%
Tmax	4 h	RID	2.3%-5.3%	Vd	
Oral	Complete	M/P	0.3-0.7	pKa	

Adult Concerns: Hypothyroidism, hepatic dysfunction, bleeding, drowsiness, skin rash, nausea, vomiting, fever.

Adult Dose: 15-60 mg daily taken in two to three divided doses.

Pediatric Concerns: None reported via milk, but propylthiouracil is generally preferred in breastfeeding women.

Infant Monitoring:

Alternatives: Propylthiouracil(L2)

References:
1. Rylance GW, Woods CG, Donnelly MC, Oliver JS, Alexander WD. Carbimazole and breastfeeding. Lancet. 1987;1(8538):928.
2. Johansen K, Andersen AN, Kampmann JP, Molholm Hansen JM, Mortensen HB. Excretion of methimazole in human milk. Eur J Clin Pharmacol. 1982;23(4):339-341.

CARBINOXAMINE

Trade: Arbinoxa, Palgic

Category: Antihistamine

LRC: L2 - No Data-Probably Compatible

Carbinoxamine is an antihistamine used over-the-counter.[1] The main adverse effect is sedation. The use of this sedating antihistamine in breastfeeding mothers is not ideal. Non-sedating antihistamines are generally preferred.

T 1/2	10-20 h	MW	407 Da	PB	
Tmax		RID		Vd	
Oral		M/P		pKa	8.1

Adult Concerns: Sedation, urticaria, hypotension, epigastric distress, thickening of bronchial secretions, dizziness, disturbed coordination.

Adult Dose: 4-8 mg three to four times a day.

Pediatric Concerns:

Infant Monitoring: Sedation, vomiting.

Alternatives:

References:
1. Pharmaceutical manufacturers prescribing information.

CARBON MONOXIDE

Trade:

Category: Other

LRC: L3 - No Data-Probably Compatible

Carbon monoxide (CO) is an odorless, colorless gas. It is a gaseous component of the atmospheric air. In fact, it is the most abundant air pollutant in the lower atmosphere, produced from the incomplete combustion of carbonaceous fuels such as gasoline, natural gas, oil, coal, and wood, and other materials such as tobacco.

Acute CO poisoning due to environmental exposure in mother or baby should be considered an emergency and treated immediately. It should be noted the effects of CO toxicity in an infant are more than those in an adult. An infant or child experiences an earlier onset of hypoxia as compared to an adult. Further, an infant up to the age of 6 months has fetal hemoglobin. Fetal hemoglobin has a 2.5-3 times higher affinity for carbon monoxide as compared to adult hemoglobin, causing the infant carboxyhemoglobin levels to be 10%-15% higher than maternal levels.[1-3] Therefore, the hypoxia that occurs in an infant is more severe than that which occurs in an adult for the same amount of exposure. Chronic CO poisoning generally occurs when incomplete combustion of fuels occurs in poorly ventilated, closed spaces. Some of the most common sources of exposure in infants is when heavy smoking occurs in poorly ventilated areas, or when gas ranges or vehicles are turned on in unvented garages. Some of the other common sources of chronic CO exposure are gas furnaces, water and space heaters, wood and coal stoves or fireplaces, regularly used in poorly ventilated spaces. Chronic CO exposure over prolonged periods has been known to cause neurological, neurodevelopmental, and cognitive effects. Symptoms may include personality changes, mental confusion, and movement disorders.

There are no studies of transfer of CO in human milk following maternal exposure. Following CO exposure, almost all of it is absorbed into the bloodstream via lungs, where it forms carboxyhemoglobin (COHb). The remaining 1% is oxidized by metabolic processes to produce carbon dioxide. The half-life of COHb is 4-5 hours, which is significantly decreased following exposure to oxygen. It is not known if COHb enters human milk, but it is highly unlikely that COHb would be capable of entry in to human milk as there is no binding protein. Therefore, it would be almost impossible for a breastfed infant to be exposed to CO strictly through breast milk. Further, even if it is assumed that some does enter breast milk, the absorption of CO following oral absorption would probably be negligible to nil. Although there are no data on the oral absorption of CO in humans, a study conducted in monkeys where the oral and nasal cavities were exposed to large amounts of smoke containing CO, the amount of CO absorbed through the nasal and oral mucosa was found to be nil.[4]

Therefore, a mother exposed to high levels of CO may safely continue to breastfeed once she is treated with oxygen or released from care. Although, the exposed mother may suffer some long-term effects of acute CO poisoning for up to 1-3 months, such clinical effects are not expected in the breastfed infant.

T 1/2	4-5 h	MW	28.01 Da	PB	
Tmax		RID		Vd	
Oral		M/P		pKa	

Adult Concerns: Acute CO poisoning: Headache, nausea, malaise, and fatigue. Increasing exposures causes increase in heart rate, hypotension, and cardiac arrhythmias. Central nervous system involvement is manifested with delirium, hallucinations, dizziness, ataxia, confusion, and seizures. Delayed neurological manifestation up to 1-3 months following CO exposure have been reported. Some of these manifestations include mood disturbances, amnesia, dementia, memory loss, ataxia, speech disturbances, and personality disorders. Chronic CO poisoning: Persistent headaches, lightheadedness, depression, confusion, memory loss, nausea, and vomiting. Chronic exposure to carbon monoxide causes accelerated development of atherosclerosis and increases the risk for heart disease and myocardial infarction.

Adult Dose:

Pediatric Concerns: Manifestations of CO exposures in children and infants are more subtle and difficult to recognize. Excessive sleepiness or somnolence, change in mental status or mental confusion should arouse suspicion of CO poisoning.

Infant Monitoring: Delirium, seizures, malaise, fatigue, vomiting.

Alternatives:

References:
1. Hill EP, Hill JR, Power GG, et al. Carbon monoxide exchanges between the human fetus and mother: a mathematical model. Am J Physiol. 1977;232:H311–H323.
2. Longo LD, Hill EP. Carbon monoxide uptake and elimination in fetal and maternal sheep. Am J Physiol. 1977;232:H324–H330.
3. Yildiz H, Aldemir E, Altuncu E, Celik M, Kavuncuoglu S. A rare cause of perinatal asphyxia: maternal carbon monoxide poisoning. Arch Gynecol Obstet. February 2010;281(2):251-254. Epub June 6, 2009.
4. Schoenfisch WH, Hoop KA, Struelens BS. Carbon monoxide absorption through the oral and nasal mucosae of cynomolgus monkeys. Arch Environ Health. May-June 1980;35(3):152-154.

CARBOPLATIN

Trade: Carboplat, Carbosin, Emorzim, Paraplatin

Category: Antineoplastic

LRC: L5 - Limited Data-Hazardous

Carboplatin is a platinum derivative anticancer agent similar to cisplatin. Although carboplatin is not bound to plasma proteins, platinum is irreversibly bound to plasma proteins.[1] Carboplatin is apparently more rapidly cleared as compared to cisplatin. About 65% of carboplatin is eliminated renally in the first 12 hours, and 71% by 24 hours. Only 3%-5% of the platinum is eliminated by 24-96 hours. In addition, the half-life of platinum is long, depending on the resource the half-life has been reported as greater than 5 days to more than 12 days.[1-3] In a study of one mother undergoing carboplatin chemotherapy (233 mg/week) for papillary thyroid cancer, milk levels were determined at 4, 28, 172, and 316 hours following infusion. The AUC0-316 h was 127.92 mg.h/L.[4] The C_{ave} was 0.404 mg/L with an RID of 1.82%. Levels were demonstrable in milk even 300 hours after the final infusion. See cisplatin for additional information regarding levels present in human milk.

Two options are suggested. One, the breast milk should be tested for platinum levels and not used as long as they are measurable. Or two, without measuring platinum levels, breastfeeding should be interrupted for at least 20 days for low doses as above, or much longer (permanently) for higher doses.

T 1/2	Carb: 2.6-5.9 h; plat: >5 days	MW	371.3 Da	PB	Carb: 0%; plat: irreversibly bound
Tmax		RID	1.8%	Vd	0.23 L/kg
Oral	None	M/P		pKa	

Adult Concerns: Alopecia, ototoxicity, unusual tiredness or weakness, nausea, vomiting, changes in liver enzymes and renal function, changes in electrolytes, myelosuppression, bleeding, increased risk of infection.

Adult Dose: Varies depending on indication.

Pediatric Concerns: No case reports of infant adverse effects in lactation at this time (in lactation data thus far infants were not breastfed).

Infant Monitoring: Interrupt breastfeeding for at least 20 days for low doses, or longer (permanently) for higher doses.

Alternatives:

References:

1. Pharmaceutical manufacturers prescribing information.
2. Grochow LB, Ames MM. A Clinician's Guide to Chemotherapy Pharmacokinetics and Pharmacodynamics. 1st ed. Baltimore, MD: Williams & Wilkins; 1998.
3. van der Vijgh WJF. Clinical pharmacokinetics of carboplatin. Clin Pharmacokinet. 1991;21(4):242-261.
4. Griffin SJ, Milla M, Baker TE, Liu T, Wang H, Hale TW. Transfer of carboplatin and paclitaxel into breast milk. J Hum Lact. November 2012;28(4):457-459.

CARBOPROST

Trade: Hemabate

Category: Prostaglandin

LRC: L3 - No Data-Probably Compatible

Carboprost tromethamine is a prostaglandin analog (15-methyl prostaglandin F2-alpha), which stimulates the myometrial contractions in a gravid uterus simulating labor.[1] It is used to treat postpartum hemorrhage. No data are available on its transfer to human milk. Prostaglandins have brief half-lives and little distribution out of the plasma compartment. Even then, rather large intramuscular doses only produce picogram concentrations in the plasma of recipients. It is not likely it will penetrate milk in clinically relevant amounts.

T 1/2	<1 h	MW	489 Da	PB	
Tmax	15-30 min	RID		Vd	
Oral	None	M/P		pKa	4.36

Adult Concerns: Headache, fever, hypertension, palpitations, chest pain, bronchoconstriction, vomiting, diarrhea, leukocytosis, dystonic reactions, uterine rupture, flushing of the skin.

Adult Dose: 250 µg initially, doses may be repeated if needed (max 8 doses).

Pediatric Concerns: None reported via milk. Commonly used in obstetrics without complications in breastfeeding infants.

Infant Monitoring: Vomiting, diarrhea, flushing.

Alternatives:

References:

1. Pharmaceutical manufacturers prescribing information.

CARISOPRODOL

Trade: Carisoma, Vanadom, Soma

Category: Skeletal Muscle Relaxant

LRC: L3 - Limited Data-Probably Compatible

Carisoprodol is a commonly used skeletal muscle relaxant that is a CNS depressant. It is metabolized to an active metabolite called meprobamate. At this time there are two case reports in lactation, in the first case a breastfeeding mother receiving 2100 mg/day had average milk concentrations of carisoprodol and meprobamate of 0.9 mg/L and 11.6 mg/L respectively.[1] The authors noted the infant would receive about 1.9 mg/kg/day of both carisoprodol and its metabolite which correlated to a RID of 4.1%. No adverse effects in the infant were noted.

In the second case, a breastfeeding mother receiving 2800 mg/day had peak and trough milk concentrations of carisoprodol and meprobamate taken 1 week postpartum, the highest concentrations of this medication and its metabolite were 1.4 µg/mL and 17.1 µg/mL, respectively.[2] Serum samples in the infant were below the limit of detection, the authors estimated the infant received 2.7 mg/kg/day of carisoprodol and its metabolite, which correlated to a RID of 6.9%. The authors noted the infant had slight sedation, but it was not thought to be harmful and the infants growth was considered normal at 14 months of age. In this case, the infant was only breastfed for one month due to a maternal milk supply issue.

T 1/2	8 h	MW	260 Da	PB	60%
Tmax		RID	0.5%-6.41%	Vd	
Oral	Complete	M/P	2-4	pKa	15.06

Adult Concerns: Nausea, vomiting, hiccups, sedation, weakness, mild withdrawal symptoms after chronic use.

Adult Dose: 250-350 mg TID-QID.

Pediatric Concerns: One case report of sedation.[2]

Infant Monitoring: Sedation, vomiting, hiccups, weakness.

Alternatives:

References:
1. Nordeng H, Zahlsen K, Spigset O. Transfer of carisoprodol to breast milk. Ther Drug Monit. 2001;23(3):298-300.
2. Briggs GG, Ambrose PJ, Nageotte MP, Padilla G. High-dose carisoprodol during pregnancy and lactation. Ann Pharmacother. 2008;42:898-901.

CARMUSTINE

Trade: BCNU, BiCNU, Carmubris, Gliadel, Nitrumon

Category: Antineoplastic

LRC: L5 - No Data-Hazardous

Carmustine is an alkylating agent of the nitrosourea type. Among its indications are brain tumors, gastric carcinoma, Hodgkin's lymphomas, and other syndromes. With a rather low molecular weight (214), it is best known for its ability to enter the CNS by crossing the blood-brain barrier.[1] This would suggest its ability to enter the milk compartment is significant. No data are available on its transfer to milk; however, initial transfer may be significant. The metabolism of this product is somewhat obscure and may account to some degree for its lasting side effects. Further, the half-life is highly varied among patients (15-20 fold). Because of the prolonged and delayed side effect profiles (pulmonary injury) associated with this drug, mothers should delay breastfeeding for a minimum of 24-48 hours.

T 1/2	12-45 min	MW	214.05 Da	PB	80%
Tmax		RID		Vd	3.3 L/kg
Oral	5%-28%	M/P		pKa	

Adult Concerns: Ataxia, dizziness, arrhythmia, chest pain, hypotension, flushing, vomiting, mucositis, changes in liver or renal function, leukopenia, anemia.

Adult Dose: IV: 150-200 mg/m² every 6 weeks or 75-100 mg/m² for 2 days every 6 weeks.

Pediatric Concerns:

Infant Monitoring: Withhold breastfeeding for a minimum of 24-48 hours.

Alternatives:

References:
1. Pharmaceutical manufacturers prescribing information.

CARNITINE

Trade: Carnitor, L-Carnitine

Category: Dietary Supplement

LRC: L2 - Limited Data-Probably Compatible

Carnitine is biosynthesized from lysine and methionine and its main function is to facilitate fatty acid metabolism. Carnitine supplementation comes in the form of L-carnitine, acetyl l-carnitine, and propionyl l-carnitine. Carnitine supplementation is used for primary carnitine deficiency in hemodialysis patients.[1] L-carnitine is present in some formulas and many foods. Carnitine is present in breast milk with a concentration of 45 μmol/L.[2] Carnitine levels in breast milk are not dependent on dietary carnitine supplementation, but rather is transported into milk by the mother.[2] Another study suggests that the levels of carnitine in breast milk are constant around 56-69.8 μmol/L for the first 21 days and reduces to 35.2 μmol/L around 40-50 days postpartum.[3] Because carnitine is naturally present in breast milk and its concentration is not affected by supplementation, the risk to the infant is probably remote from exogenous sources.

T 1/2	17.4 h	MW	161 Da	PB	
Tmax		RID		Vd	
Oral	15%	M/P		pKa	

Adult Concerns: Diarrhea, abdominal pain, hypertension, headache, hypercalcemia, weakness, cough, infection, rash.

Adult Dose: 990 mg 2-3 times/day (oral).

Pediatric Concerns: None reported. Natural component of breast milk.

Infant Monitoring:

Alternatives:

References:
1. Ulbricht C, Costa D, M Grimes Serrano J, et al. An evidence-based systematic review of L-carnitine by the natural standard research collaboration. www.naturalstandard.com. Accessed July 13, 2011.
2. Mitchell ME, Snyder EA. Dietary carnitine effects on carnitine concentrations in urine and milk in lactating women. Am J Clin Nutr. November 1991;54(5):814-820.
3. Sandor A, Pecsuvac K, Kerner J, Alkonyi I. On carnitine content of the human breast milk. Pediatr Res. February 1982;16(2):89-91. Abstract.

CARTEOLOL

Trade: Cartrol, Teoptic

Category: Beta Adrenergic Blocker

LRC: L3 - No Data-Probably Compatible

Carteolol is a nonselective beta-blocker used to lower intraocular pressure in patients with intraocular hypertension or open-angle glaucoma.[1] Carteolol is reported to be excreted in breastmilk of lactating animals; however, no data are available regarding carteolol concentrations in human milk.

T 1/2	6 h	MW	328.84 Da	PB	
Tmax		RID		Vd	
Oral		M/P		pKa	13.41

Adult Concerns: Ocular use: conjunctival hyperemia, eye pain, changes in vision, decreased corneal sensitivity, corneal staining.

Adult Dose: Instill one drop in affected eye twice daily.

Pediatric Concerns: None reported at this time.

Infant Monitoring:

Alternatives:

References:
1. Pharmaceutical manufacturers prescribing information.

CARVEDILOL

Trade: Coreg, Dilatrend, Eucardic, Proreg

Category: Beta Adrenergic Blocker

LRC: L3 - No Data-Probably Compatible

Carvedilol is a nonselective beta-adrenergic blocking agent (with partial alpha-1 blocking activity) with no intrinsic sympathomimetic activity.[1] There are no data available on the transfer of this drug to human milk. However, due to its high lipid solubility, some may transfer. As with any beta-blocker, some caution is recommended until milk levels are reported.

T 1/2	7-10 h	MW	406.47 Da	PB	>98%
Tmax	1-1.5 h; Extended release 5 h	RID		Vd	1.64 L/kg
Oral	25%-35%	M/P		pKa	14.03

Adult Concerns: Headache, dizziness, insomnia, depression, fatigue, chest pain, bradycardia, hypotension, heart failure, wheezing, vomiting, diarrhea, myalgia.

Adult Dose: 6.25-12.5 mg BID.

Pediatric Concerns: None reported via milk at this time.

Infant Monitoring: Drowsiness, lethargy, pallor, poor feeding, and weight gain.

Alternatives: Metoprolol(L2), Labetalol(L2)

References:
1. Pharmaceutical manufacturers prescribing information.

CASPOFUNGIN ACETATE

Trade: Cancidas

Category: Antifungal

LRC: L3 - No Data-Probably Compatible

Caspofungin is a unique semisynthetic lipopeptide that is active against Aspergillus fumigatus. It has a large polycyclic structure with a molecular weight of 1213 Da. The half-life of this product is unique with a polyphasic elimination curve with three distinct phases. The half-life varies from 11 hours in one phase to 40-50 hours in the last phase.[1] This is a new product; however, newer data provide dosing regimens for infants. The pharmaceutical manufacturer states that it was found in rodent milk; no data are available for human milk. Nevertheless, the oral bioavailability is reported as poor and it is unlikely an infant would absorb enough to be clinically relevant, but this is only speculative.

T 1/2	9-11 h	MW	1213 Da	PB	97%
Tmax		RID		Vd	0.138 L/kg
Oral	Poor	M/P		pKa	8.75

Adult Concerns: Fever, nausea, vomiting, flushing, phlebitis, anemia, headache, etc.

Adult Dose: 70 mg IV on day one, then 50 mg IV daily.

Pediatric Concerns: None reported via milk. Not cleared for pediatric patients.

Infant Monitoring:

Alternatives:

References:
1. Pharmaceutical manufacturers prescribing information.

CASTOR OIL

Trade: Purge

Category: Laxative

LRC: L3 - No Data-Probably Compatible

Castor oil is converted to ricinoleic acid in the gut.[1] It is indicated for use in constipation and for preoperative bowel preparation. Its transfer to milk is unknown. Caution should be used. Usage in excess amounts could produce diarrhea, insomnia, and tremors in exposed infants.

T 1/2		MW	932 Da	PB	
Tmax	2-3 h	RID		Vd	
Oral	Unknown	M/P		pKa	

Adult Concerns: Insomnia, tremors, diarrhea.

Adult Dose:

Pediatric Concerns: Observe for diarrhea, insomnia, tremors in infants.

Infant Monitoring: Diarrhea.

Alternatives:

References:
1. Pharmaceutical manufacturers prescribing information.

CEFACLOR

Trade: Ceclor, Distaclor, Keflor

Category: Antibiotic, Cephalosporin

LRC:

Cefaclor is a second generation cephalosporin antibiotic; small amounts are known to be secreted into human milk. Following a single dose of 250 mg orally in two mothers, the levels in milk were undetectable in one, and ranged from 0.15 to 0.19 mg/L 2 to 4 hours postdose. Following a 500 mg oral dose in five mothers, milk levels averaged 0.16 to 0.21 mg/L. Average levels were 0.18, 0.20, 0.21, and 0.16 µg/mL at 2, 3, 4, and 5 hours respectively.[1] Trace amounts were detected at 1 hour.

T 1/2	0.5-1 h	MW	386 Da	PB	23.5%
Tmax	0.5-1 h	RID	0.4%-0.8%	Vd	0.35 L/kg
Oral	100%	M/P		pKa	

Adult Concerns: Nausea, vomiting, diarrhea, changes in liver function, eosinophilia, rash, allergic reaction, serum sickness.

Adult Dose: 250-500 mg every 8 hours.

Pediatric Concerns: None reported via milk.

Infant Monitoring: Vomiting, diarrhea, changes in gastrointestinal flora, and rash.

Alternatives:

References:
1. Takase Z. Clinical and laboratory studies of cefaclor in the field of obstetrics and gynecology. Chemotherapy. 1979;27(suppl):668.

CEFADROXIL

Trade: Baxan, Duricef, Ultracef

Category: Antibiotic, Cephalosporin

LRC: L1 - Limited Data-Compatible

Cefadroxil is a first generation cephalosporin antibiotic. Small amounts are known to be secreted into milk. Milk concentrations following a 1000 mg oral dose were 0.10 mg/L at 1 hour and 1.24 mg/L at 5 hours.[1] Milk/serum ratios were 0.009 at 1 hour and 0.019 at 3 hours.

In a study of two to three patients who received an oral dose of 500 mg cefadroxil, milk levels peaked at 4 hours at an average of 0.4 mg/L, which is only about 0.8% of the maternal dose.[2] The milk/plasma ratio was 0.085.

T 1/2	1-2 h	MW	381 Da	PB	20%
Tmax	1-1.5 h	RID	0.8%-1.3%	Vd	0.31 L/kg
Oral	100%	M/P	0.009-0.085	pKa	3.45

Adult Concerns: Diarrhea, allergic rash.

Adult Dose: 0.5-1 g BID.

Pediatric Concerns: None reported via milk.

Infant Monitoring: Vomiting, diarrhea, changes in gastrointestinal flora, and rash.

Alternatives:

References:

1. Kafetzis DA, Siafas CA, Georgakopoulos PA, Papadatos CJ. Passage of cephalosporins and amoxicillin into the breast milk. Acta Paediatr Scand. 1981;70(3):285-288.
2. Matsuda S. Transfer of antibiotics into maternal milk. Biol Res Pregnancy Perinatol. 1984;5(2):57-60.

CEFAZOLIN

Trade: Ancef, Cefamezin, Kefzol

Category: Antibiotic, Cephalosporin

LRC: L1 - Limited Data-Compatible

Cefazolin is a first generation cephalosporin antibiotic that has adult and pediatric indications. In 20 patients who received a 2 g STAT dose over 10 minutes, the average concentration of cefazolin in milk 2, 3, and 4 hours after the dose was 1.25, 1.51, and 1.16 mg/L respectively.[1] A very small milk/plasma ratio (0.023) indicates insignificant transfer to milk. Cefazolin is poorly absorbed orally, therefore the infant would absorb a minimal amount. Plasma levels in breastfed infants are reported to be too small to be detected.

T 1/2	1.5-2.5 h	MW	476.5 Da	PB	74%-86%
Tmax	5 min (IV); 0.5-2 h (IM)	RID	0.8%	Vd	0.143 L/kg
Oral	Poor	M/P	0.023	pKa	3.03

Adult Concerns: Nausea, vomiting, diarrhea, abdominal pain, changes in liver function, neutropenia, skin rashes.

Adult Dose: 1-2 g IV every 8 hours.

Pediatric Concerns: None reported via milk at this time.

Infant Monitoring: Vomiting, diarrhea, changes in gastrointestinal flora, and rash.

Alternatives:

References:

1. Yoshioka H, Cho K, Takimoto M, Maruyama S, Shimizu T. Transfer of cefazolin into human milk. J Pediatr. 1979;94(1):151-152.

CEFDINIR

Trade: Omnicef

Category: Antibiotic, Cephalosporin

LRC: L1 - Limited Data-Compatible

Cefdinir is a broad-spectrum third generation cephalosporin antibiotic. The manufacturer reports that after administration of 600 mg single oral doses, no cefdinir was detected in human milk.[1]

T 1/2	1.7 h	MW	395 Da	PB	60%-70%
Tmax	2-4 h	RID		Vd	0.35 L/kg
Oral	16%-21%	M/P		pKa	1.74

Adult Concerns: Nausea, vomiting, diarrhea, skin rash.

Adult Dose: 300 mg twice daily.

Pediatric Concerns: None reported via milk.

Infant Monitoring: Vomiting, diarrhea, changes in gastrointestinal flora, and rash.

Alternatives:

References:

1. Pharmaceutical manufacturers prescribing information.

CEFDITOREN

Trade: Spectracef

Category: Antibiotic, Cephalosporin

LRC: L2 - No Data-Probably Compatible

Cefditoren is a third generation cephalosporin antibiotic that is indicated in the treatment of acute bacterial exacerbations of chronic bronchitis, community acquired pneumonia, pharyngitis, tonsillitis, and uncomplicated skin infections.[1] No data are available on its transfer to breast milk at this time.

T 1/2	1.6 h	MW	620 Da	PB	88%
Tmax	1-3 h	RID		Vd	0.13 L/kg
Oral	14%	M/P		pKa	3.4

Adult Concerns: Headache, dyspepsia, nausea, vomiting, diarrhea, skin rash.

Adult Dose: 200-400 mg BID.

Pediatric Concerns: No data reported in breastfed infants.

Infant Monitoring: Vomiting, diarrhea, changes in gastrointestinal flora, and rash.

Alternatives: Cefdinir(L1)

References:
1. Pharmaceutical manufacturers prescribing information.

CEFEPIME

Trade: Maxipime

Category: Antibiotic, Cephalosporin

LRC: L2 - Limited Data-Probably Compatible

Cefepime is a fourth generation parenteral cephalosporin. Cefepime is secreted in human milk in small amounts averaging 0.5 mg/L.[1,2] In a mother consuming 2 g/day, an infant would ingest approximately 75 µg/kg/day or approximately 0.3% of the maternal dose. This amount is too small to produce any clinical symptoms other than possible changes in gut flora.

T 1/2	2 h	MW	571 Da	PB	20%
Tmax	0.5 h	RID	0.3%	Vd	0.26 L/kg
Oral	Poor	M/P	0.8	pKa	

Adult Concerns: Headache, nausea, vomiting, diarrhea, elevation of liver enzymes, skin rash.

Adult Dose: 1-2 g IV every 8-12 hours.

Pediatric Concerns: None reported via milk.

Infant Monitoring: Vomiting, diarrhea, changes in gastrointestinal flora, and rash.

Alternatives:

References:
1. Pharmaceutical manufacturers prescribing information.
2. Sanders CC. Cefepime: the next generation? Clin Infect Dis. 1993;17(3):369-379.

CEFIDEROCOL

Trade: Fetroja

Category: Antibiotic, Cephalosporin

LRC: L3 - No Data-Probably Compatible

Cefiderocol is a new intravenous cephalosporin antibiotic Indicated for complicated urinary tract infections, including pyelonephritis, caused by susceptible gram-negative microorganisms in adults who have limited or no alternative treatment options. Cefiderocol has primarily shown efficacy against aerobic Gram-negative bacteria including *Escherichia coli*, *Klebsiella pneumoniae*, and *Pseudomonas aeruginosa*. At present there are no studies of the transfer of this cephalosporin antibiotic to human milk, although the transfer is unlikely in clinically relevant amounts. Observe for diarrhea, candida in breastfed infants.

T 1/2	2.8 h	MW	752.21 Da	PB	40%-60%
Tmax	1 h	RID		Vd	0.257 L/kg
Oral	Low	M/P		pKa	

Adult Concerns: Adverse reactions include diarrhea, constipation, nausea, vomiting, elevations in liver tests, rash, infusion site reactions, candidiasis, cough, headache, and hypokalemia. Observe for diarrhea in breastfed infants.

Adult Dose: 2 gram IV q 8 hours for 7-14 days.

Pediatric Concerns:

Infant Monitoring: Diarrhea, candida overgrowth.

Alternatives:

References:
1. Pharmaceutical manufacturers prescribing information.

CEFIXIME

Trade: Suprax

Category: Antibiotic, Cephalosporin

LRC: L2 - No Data-Probably Compatible

Cefixime is an oral, third generation cephalosporin used to treat common infections such as urinary tract infections.[1] It is poorly absorbed (40%-50%) by the oral route. In adults given a single 200 mg tablet, the average peak serum concentration was approximately 2 µg/mL (range 1 to 4 µg/mL); when given a single 400 mg tablet the average concentration was approximately 3.5 µg/mL (range 1.3 to 7.7 µg/mL).

Although there are no data on transfer to human milk, based on this drug's higher molecular weight (507 Da), low plasma concentrations in adult patients and poor oral bioavailability it is not anticipated to reach clinically significant levels in a breastfed infant. This antibiotic is commonly used in breastfeeding women with no reports of infant adverse effects at this time.

T 1/2	3-4 h	MW	507 Da	PB	65%
Tmax	2-6 h	RID		Vd	widely distributed L/kg
Oral	40%-50%	M/P		pKa	3.26

Adult Concerns: Dizziness, headache, dyspepsia, nausea, abdominal pain, diarrhea, skin rash.

Adult Dose: 400 mg once daily.

Pediatric Concerns: None reported via milk at this time.

Infant Monitoring: Vomiting, diarrhea, changes in gastrointestinal flora, and rash.

Alternatives:

References:
1. Pharmaceutical manufacturers prescribing information.

CEFOTAXIME

Trade: Claforan

Category: Antibiotic, Cephalosporin

LRC: L2 - Limited Data-Probably Compatible

Cefotaxime is a third generation cephalosporin antibiotic given intravenously or intramuscularly for bacterial infections. In a study of 12 women 3 days postpartum given a single 1 g IV cefotaxime dose, milk levels were obtained hourly for 6 hours postdose.[1] Milk levels peaked between 2-3 hours and averaged 0.26 mg/L at 1 hour, 0.32 mg/L at 2 hours, 0.30 mg/L at 3 hours, and 0.13 mg/L at 6 hours. The milk/serum ratios were 0.027, 0.092, and 0.17 at

1, 2, and 3 hours. A second publication reported similar findings in a few patients receiving 1 g IV, undetectable to trace amounts in milk 6 hours postdose.[2]

T 1/2	1-1.5 h	MW	455 Da	PB	30%-50%
Tmax	30 min	RID	0.14%-0.3%	Vd	0.22-0.29 L/kg
Oral	Poor	M/P	0.027-0.17	pKa	3.18

Adult Concerns: Nausea, vomiting, diarrhea, eosinophilia, rash.

Adult Dose: 1 g IV every 8 hours.

Pediatric Concerns: None reported via milk.

Infant Monitoring: Vomiting, diarrhea, changes in gastrointestinal flora, and rash.

Alternatives: Ceftriaxone(L1)

References:

1. Kafetzis DA, Lazarides CV, Siafas CA, Georgakopoulos PA, Papadatos CJ. Transfer of cefotaxime in human milk and from mother to foetus. J Antimicrob Chemother. 1980;6(suppl A):135-141.
2. Matsuda S. Transfer of antibiotics into maternal milk. Biol Res Pregnancy Perinatol. 1984;5(2):57-60.

CEFOTETAN

Trade: Apatef, Cefotan

Category: Antibiotic, Cephalosporin

LRC: L2 - Limited Data-Probably Compatible

Cefotetan is a second generation cephalosporin that is poorly absorbed orally and is only available in IM and IV injectable forms. The drug is distributed to human milk in low concentrations. Following a maternal dose of 1 g IM every 12 hours in five patients, breast milk concentrations ranged from 0.29 to 0.59 mg/L.[1] Plasma concentrations were almost 100 times higher. In a group of two to three women who received 1 g IV, the maximum average milk level reported was 0.2 mg/L at 4 hours with a milk/plasma ratio of 0.02.[2] In a study of seven women who received a 1 g dose IV, levels were undetectable in 2. In the remaining five, milk levels ranged from 0.22-0.34 mg/L. The mean peak level was 0.34 mg/L at 4 hours.[3]

T 1/2	3-4.6 h	MW	576 Da	PB	76%-90%
Tmax	1.5-3 h	RID	0.2%-0.3%	Vd	0.147 L/kg
Oral	Poor	M/P		pKa	4.06

Adult Concerns: Vomiting, diarrhea, changes in liver enzymes, rash.

Adult Dose: 1-2 g IV every 12 hours.

Pediatric Concerns: None reported via milk.

Infant Monitoring: Vomiting, diarrhea, changes in gastrointestinal flora, and rash.

Alternatives:

References:

1. Novelli A. The penetration of intramuscular cefotetan disodium into human extra-vascular fluid and maternal milk secretion. Chemoterapia. 1983;11(5):337-342.
2. Matsuda S. Transfer of antibiotics into maternal milk. Biol Res Pregnancy Perinatol. 1984;5(2):57-60.
3. Cho N, Fukunaga K, Kuni K. Fundamental and clinical studies on cefotetan (YM09330) in the field of obstetrics and gynecology. Chemotherapy. 1982;30(suppl 1):832-842.

CEFOXITIN

Trade: Mefoxin

Category: Antibiotic, Cephalosporin

LRC: L1 - Limited Data-Compatible

Cefoxitin is a second generation cephalosporin antibiotic. It is transferred to human milk in very low levels. In a study of 18 women receiving 2-4 g doses, only one breast milk sample contained cefoxitin (0.9 mg/L), the remaining were undetectable.[1]

In another study of two to three women who received 1 g IV, only trace amounts were reported in milk over 6 hours.[2] In a group of five women who received an IM injection of 2 g, the highest milk levels were reported at 4 hours after the dose.[3] The maternal plasma levels varied from 22.5 at 2 hours to 77.6 µg/mL at 4 hours. Maternal milk levels ranged from <0.25 to 0.65 mg/L.

In a group of 18 women, 25 milk samples were obtained following doses of 2-4 g IV.[4] In only one case was cefoxitin found in milk (0.9 mg/L). In another group of 15 women receiving 1 g IV 1 month postpartum, milk levels at 2 hours averaged 0.05 mg/L.[5]

T 1/2	0.7-1 h	MW	449.44 Da	PB	65%-79%
Tmax	20-30 min (IM)	RID	0.1%-0.3%	Vd	0.11-0.17 L/kg
Oral	Poor	M/P		pKa	3.59

Adult Concerns: Diarrhea, allergic rash, thrush.

Adult Dose: 1-2 g TID.

Pediatric Concerns: None reported via milk.

Infant Monitoring: Vomiting, diarrhea, changes in gastrointestinal flora, and rash.

Alternatives:

References:

1. Roex AJ, van Loenen AC, Puyenbroek JI, Arts NF. Secretion of cefoxitin in breast milk following short-term prophylactic administration in caesarean section. Eur J Obstet Gynecol Reprod Biol. 1987;25(4):299-302.
2. Matsuda S. Transfer of antibiotics into maternal milk. Biol Res Pregnancy Perinatol. 1984;5(2):57-60.
3. Dresse A, Lambotte R, Dubois M, Delapierre D, Kramp R. Transmammary passage of cefoxitin: additional results. J Clin Pharmacol. 1983;23(10):438-440.
4. Roex AJ, van Loenen AC, Puyenbroek JI, Arts NF. Secretion of cefoxitin in breast milk following short-term prophylactic administration in caesarean section. Eur J Obstet Gynecol Reprod Biol. August 1987;25(4):299-302.
5. Zhang Y, Zhang Q, Xu Z. [Tissue and body fluid distribution of antibacterial agents in pregnant and lactating women]. Zhonghua Fu Chan Ke Za Zhi. May 1997;32(5):288-292. Chinese.

CEFPODOXIME PROXETIL

Trade: Orelox, Vantin

Category: Antibiotic, Cephalosporin

LRC: L2 - Limited Data-Probably Compatible

Cefpodoxime is a third generation cephalosporin antibiotic that is used to treat many infections such as pneumonia, urinary tract infections, and skin infections.[1] Cefpodoxime is de-esterified in the GI tract to an active metabolite. Only 50% is orally absorbed. In a study of three lactating women, levels of cefpodoxime in human milk were 0%, 2%, and 6% of maternal serum levels at 4 hours following a 200 mg oral dose. At 6 hours postdose, levels were 0%, 9%, and 16% of concomitant maternal serum levels.

T 1/2	2-3 h	MW	558 Da	PB	21%-29%
Tmax	2-3 h	RID		Vd	0.15 L/kg
Oral	50%	M/P	0-0.16	pKa	3.22

Adult Concerns: Headache, nausea, vomiting, diarrhea, abdominal pain, rash.

Adult Dose: 100-400 mg every 12 hours.

Pediatric Concerns: None reported via milk. Pediatric indications down to 6 months of age are available.

Infant Monitoring: Vomiting, diarrhea, changes in gastrointestinal flora, and rash.

Alternatives:

References:

1. Pharmaceutical manufacturers prescribing information.

CEFPROZIL

Trade: Cefzil

Category: Antibiotic, Cephalosporin

LRC:

Cefprozil is a second generation cephalosporin antibiotic. Following an oral dose of 1 gram, the breast milk concentrations were 0.7, 2.5, and 3.5 mg/L at 2, 4, and 6 hours postdose, respectively. The peak milk concentration occurred at 6 hours and was lower thereafter.[1] Milk/plasma ratios varied from 0.05 at 2 hours to 5.67 at 12 hours. However, the milk concentration at 12 hours was small (1.3 µg/mL). Using the highest concentration found in breast milk (3.5 mg/L), an infant consuming 800 mL of milk daily would ingest about 2.8 mg of cefprozil daily. Because the dose used in this study is approximately twice that normally used, it is reasonable to assume that an infant would ingest less than 1.7 mg per day, an amount clinically insignificant.

T 1/2	1.3 h	MW		PB	36%
Tmax	1.5 h	RID	3.7%	Vd	0.23 L/kg
Oral	95%	M/P	0.05-5.67	pKa	3.53

Adult Concerns: Dizziness, nausea, vomiting, diarrhea, changes in liver enzymes, rash.

Adult Dose: 250-500 mg BID.

Pediatric Concerns: None reported via milk.

Infant Monitoring: Vomiting, diarrhea, changes in gastrointestinal flora, and rash.

Alternatives:

References:
1. Shyu WC, Shah VR, Campbell DA, et al. Excretion of cefprozil into human breast milk. Antimicrob Agents Chemother. 1992;36(5):938-941.

CEFTAROLINE FOSAMIL

Trade: Teflaro

Category: Antibiotic, Cephalosporin

LRC: L3 - No Data-Probably Compatible

Ceftaroline is a fifth-generation cephalosporin used in the treatment of acute bacterial skin infections and community-acquired pneumonia. This cephalosporin has a unique spectrum of activity which includes methicillin resistant *Staphylococcus aureus* (MRSA). While there are no data on the transfer of ceftaroline to human milk, cephalosporins rarely cause adverse effects in breastfed infants.

T 1/2	1.6-2.66 h	MW	744 Da	PB	20%
Tmax	1 hour	RID		Vd	0.29 L/kg
Oral		M/P		pKa	

Adult Concerns: Dizziness, convulsions, anemia, neutropenia, thrombocytopenia, diarrhea, urticaria, renal failure and anaphylaxis.

Adult Dose: 600 mg IV every 12 hours.

Pediatric Concerns: Safety and effectiveness in pediatric patients have not been established.

Infant Monitoring: Vomiting, diarrhea, changes in gastrointestinal flora, and rash.

Alternatives:

References:
1. Pharmaceutical manufacturers prescribing information.

CEFTAZIDIME

Trade: Ceftazidime, Ceptaz, Fortaz, Fortum, Tazidime

Category: Antibiotic, Cephalosporin

LRC: L1 - Limited Data-Compatible

Ceftazidime is a broad-spectrum, third generation cephalosporin antibiotic. It has poor oral absorption (<10%). In a group of 11 lactating women who received 2 g (IV) every 8 hours for 5 days, concentrations of ceftazidime in milk averaged 3.8 mg/L before the dose and 5.2 mg/L at 1 hour after the dose and 4.5 mg/L 3 hours after the dose.[1] There is, however, no progressive accumulation of ceftazidime in breast milk, as evidenced by the similar levels prior to and after seven doses. The therapeutic dose for neonates is 30-50 mg/kg every 12 hours.

T 1/2	1.4-2 h	MW	547 Da	PB	5%-24%
Tmax	60-90 min	RID	0.9%	Vd	0.23 L/kg
Oral	<10%	M/P		pKa	3.16

Adult Concerns: Diarrhea, changes in liver enzymes, eosinophilia, rash.

Adult Dose: 500-2000 mg every 8-12 hours.

Pediatric Concerns: None reported via milk at this time.

Infant Monitoring: Vomiting, diarrhea, changes in gastrointestinal flora, and rash.

Alternatives:

References:
1. Blanco JD, Jorgensen JH, Castaneda YS, Crawford SA. Ceftazidime levels in human breast milk. Antimicrob Agents Chemother. 1983;23(3):479-480.

CEFTIBUTEN

Trade: Cedax

Category: Antibiotic, Cephalosporin

LRC: L2 - No Data-Probably Compatible

Ceftibuten is a broad-spectrum, third generation oral cephalosporin antibiotic. No data are available on the transfer of ceftibuten to milk.[1] Due to the low protein binding and the small volume of distribution, small to moderate amounts may penetrate into milk. Cephalosporins rarely cause adverse effects in breastfed infants.

T 1/2	2.4 h	MW	446.43 Da	PB	65%
Tmax	2.6 h	RID		Vd	0.21 L/kg
Oral	75%-90%	M/P		pKa	3.68

Adult Concerns: Diarrhea, vomiting, loose stools, abdominal pain.

Adult Dose: 400 mg daily.

Pediatric Concerns: None reported via milk at this time; ceftibuten is indicated for pediatric use.[1,2]

Infant Monitoring: Vomiting, diarrhea, changes in gastrointestinal flora, and rash.

Alternatives:

References:
1. Pharmaceutical manufacturers prescribing information.
2. Barr WH, Affrime M, Lin CC, Batra V. Pharmacokinetics of ceftibuten in children. Pediatr Infect Dis J. 1995;14(7 suppl):S93-S101.

CEFTIZOXIME

Trade: Baxam, Cefizox

Category: Antibiotic, Cephalosporin

LRC: L1 - Limited Data-Compatible

Ceftizoxime is a third generation cephalosporin used to treat numerous types of infections (e.g., UTI). In a study of women given a single 1 g IV dose, milk levels of ceftizoxime 1-8 hours postdose were 0.32-0.52 mg/L.[1] In studies of five and seven women given 1 g IV, milk levels averaged 0.43 and 0.54 mg/L.[2,3] In a study of six women who received 1 g IV, milk levels of 0.25 mg/L were reported at 1 hour postdose.[4] In four studies, ceftizoxime produced only negligible levels in milk.

T 1/2	1.7 h	MW	405.38 Da	PB	30%
Tmax	<1 h	RID	0.3%-0.6%	Vd	0.4 L/kg
Oral	Minimal	M/P		pKa	3.13

Adult Concerns: Nausea, vomiting, diarrhea, skin rash.

Adult Dose: 1 g IV or IM every 8-12 h.

Pediatric Concerns: No known adverse reports in lactation.

Infant Monitoring: Vomiting, diarrhea, changes in gastrointestinal flora, and rash.

Alternatives: Ceftriaxone(L1)

References:

1. Matsuda S, Shimizu T, Ichinoe K, et al. [Pharmacokinetic and clinical studies of ceftizoxime in the perinatal period. The Chemotherapy Research Group for Mothers and Children]. Jpn J Antibiot. August 1988;41(8):1129-1141.
2. Cho N, Fukunaga K, Kunii K, Tezuka K, Kobayashi I. [Studies of ceftizoxime in perinatal period]. Jpn J Antibiot. August 1988;41(8):1142-1154.
3. Ito K, Izumi K, Takagi H, et al. [Pharmacokinetic and clinical studies of ceftizoxime in obstetrical and gynecological field (2)]. Jpn J Antibiot. August 1988;41(8):1155-1163.
4. Gerding DN, Peterson LR. Comparative tissue and extravascular fluid concentrations of ceftizoxime. J Antimicrob Chemother. November 1982;10(suppl C):105-116.

CEFTRIAXONE

Trade: Rocephin

Category: Antibiotic, Cephalosporin

LRC: L1 - Limited Data-Compatible

Ceftriaxone is a very popular third generation broad-spectrum cephalosporin antibiotic. Small amounts are transferred to milk (3%-4% of maternal serum level). Following a 1 g IM dose, breast milk levels were approximately 0.5-0.7 mg/L between 4-8 hours.[1,2] The estimated mean milk levels at steady state were 3-4 mg/L. Another source indicates that following a 2 g/day dose and at steady state, approximately 4.4% of dose penetrates into milk.[3] In this study, the maximum breast milk concentration was 7.89 mg/L after prolonged therapy (7 days). Poor oral absorption of ceftriaxone would further limit systemic absorption by the infant. The half-life of ceftriaxone in human milk varies from 12.8 to 17.3 hours (longer than maternal serum). Even at this high dose, no adverse effects were noted in the infant. Ceftriaxone levels in breast milk are probably too low to be clinically relevant, except for changes in gastrointestinal flora. Ceftriaxone is not commonly used in neonates due to worsening hyperbilirubinemia.

T 1/2	7.3 h	MW	555 Da	PB	95%
Tmax	1 h	RID	4.1%-4.2%	Vd	0.192 L/kg
Oral	Poor	M/P	0.03	pKa	3.96

Adult Concerns: Nausea, vomiting, diarrhea, changes in liver enzymes, eosinophilia, rash.

Adult Dose: 1-2 g every 12-24 hours depending on indication.

Pediatric Concerns: None reported via milk.

Infant Monitoring: Vomiting, diarrhea, changes in gastrointestinal flora, and rash.

Alternatives: Cefotaxime(L2)

References:

1. Kafetzis DA, Siafas CA, Georgakopoulos PA, Papadatos CJ. Passage of cephalosporins and amoxicillin into the breast milk. Acta Paediatr Scand. 1981;70(3):285-288.
2. Kafetzis DA, Brater DC, Fanourgakis JE, Voyatzis J, Georgakopoulos P. Ceftriaxone distribution between maternal blood and fetal blood and tissues at parturition and between blood and milk postpartum. Antimicrob Agents Chemother. 1983;23(6):870-873.
3. Bourget P, Quinquis-Desmaris V, Fernandez H. Ceftriaxone distribution and protein binding between maternal blood and milk postpartum. Ann Pharmacother. 1993;27(3):294-297.

CEFUROXIME

Trade: Ceftin, Kefurox, Zinacef, Zinnat

Category: Antibiotic, Cephalosporin

LRC: L2 - Limited Data-Probably Compatible

Cefuroxime is a broad-spectrum second generation cephalosporin antibiotic that is available orally and IV. The manufacturer states that it is secreted into human milk in small amounts, but the levels are not available.[1] In a study of 38 mothers who received a mean daily dose of 1000 mg of cefuroxime, 2.6% reported mild side effects that were not significantly different from controls (9%).[2] Following a single dose of 750 mg in five women, the mean peak level reported in milk was 370 µg/L.[3] In another group of eight women who received a single dose of 750 mg, milk levels at peak (8 hours) were 1.45 mg/L.[4] Cefuroxime has a very bitter taste. The IV salt form, cefuroxime sodium, is very poorly absorbed orally; only the axetil salt form is orally bioavailable.

T 1/2	1-2 h	MW	510 Da	PB	33%-50%
Tmax	2-3 h (oral); 2-3 min (IV)	RID	0.6%-2%	Vd	0.326 L/kg
Oral	30%-50%	M/P		pKa	3.15

Adult Concerns: Nausea, vomiting, diarrhea, increased lactate dehydrogenase, eosinophilia, rash.

Adult Dose: 250-500 mg BID.

Pediatric Concerns: None reported via milk.

Infant Monitoring: Vomiting, diarrhea, changes in gastrointestinal flora, and rash.

Alternatives:

References:
1. Pharmaceutical manufacturers prescribing information.
2. Benyamini L, Merlob P, Stahl B, et al. The safety of amoxicillin/clavulanic acid and cefuroxime during lactation. Ther Drug Monit. August 2005;27(4):499-502.
3. Takase Z, Shirofuji H, Uchida M. Fundamental and clinical studies of cefuroxime in the field of obstetrics and gynecology. Chemotherapy (Tokyo). 1979;27(suppl 6):600-602.
4. Voropaeva SD, Emelyanova AI, Ankirskaya AS, et al. Cefuroxime efficacy in obstetrics and gynecology. Antibiotiki. 1981;27:697-701.

CELECOXIB

Trade: Celebrex

Category: NSAID

LRC: L2 - Limited Data-Probably Compatible

Celecoxib is an NSAID that specifically blocks the cycyclooxygenase-2 (COX-2) enzyme. It is primarily used for arthritic or inflammatory pain. In a case report of a patient receiving 100 mg twice daily, the authors report a milk level of 133 and 101 ng/mL in left and right breasts 4.75 hours after the dose.[1] They estimated (using the C_{max} levels) the M/P ratio to be 0.27 to 0.59 and that the infant's exposure would be approximately 20 µg/kg/day. In data from our laboratories in five women receiving 200 mg once daily, the mean milk/plasma AUC ratio was 0.23.[2] The average concentration of celecoxib (AUC) in milk was 66 µg/L. The absolute infant dose averaged 9.8 µg/kg/day. Using this data, the relative infant dose was 0.30% of the maternal dose. Plasma levels of celecoxib in two infants studied were undetectable. In another study, blood and milk were sampled for 48 hours after celecoxib 200 mg orally in six lactating volunteers. The median infant dose was 0.23% of the maternal dose after adjusting for weight. Therefore, the authors suggest that the relative dose that infants are exposed to via milk is very low and breastfeeding would probably not be a threat to the infant.[3]

T 1/2	11 h	MW	381 Da	PB	97%
Tmax	2.8 h	RID	0.3%-0.7%	Vd	5.71 L/kg
Oral	99%	M/P	0.23-0.59	pKa	10.7

Adult Concerns: Headache, dizziness, high blood pressure, chest pain, asthma exacerbations, dyspepsia, nausea, abdominal pain, diarrhea, changes in renal function, bruising, thrombocytopenia, peripheral edema.

Adult Dose: 200 mg daily.

Pediatric Concerns: None reported via milk. Plasma levels in two infants were undetectable.

Infant Monitoring: Vomiting, diarrhea.

Alternatives: Ibuprofen(L1)

References:

1. Knoppert DC, Stempak D, Baruchel S, Koren G. Celecoxib in human milk: a case report. Pharmacotherapy. 2003;23(1):97-100.
2. Hale TW, McDonald R, Boger J. Transfer of celecoxib into human milk. J Hum Lact. November 2004;20(4):397-403.
3. Gardiner SJ, Doogue MP, Zhang M, Begg EJ. Quantification of infant exposure to celecoxib through breast milk. Br J Clin Pharmacol. 2006;61(1):101-104.

CEPHALEXIN

Trade: Keflex, Ceporex, Ibilex

Category: Antibiotic, Cephalosporin

LRC: L1 - Limited Data-Compatible

Cephalexin is a first generation cephalosporin antibiotic. Only minimal concentrations are secreted into human milk. Following a 1000 mg maternal oral dose, milk levels at 1, 2, 3, 4, and 5 hours ranged from 0.20, 0.28, 0.39, 0.50, and 0.47 mg/L, respectively.[1] Milk/serum ratios varied from 0.008 at 1 hour to 0.14 at 3 hours. These levels are probably too low to be clinically relevant. In a group of two to three patients who received 500 mg orally, milk levels averaged 0.7 mg/L at 4 hours although the average milk level was 0.36 mg/L over 6 hours.[2] The milk/plasma ratio was 0.25.

In another case report of a mother taking cephalexin 500 mg 4x/day along with probenecid 500 mg 4x/day (to prolong half-life of cephalexin), the baby had gastrointestinal adverse effects.[3] It was noted that while the mother was receiving IV cephalothin, her infant had a green liquid stool with severe diarrhea, discomfort, and crying. These symptoms continued when the mother was switched to oral cephalexin + probenecid. The infant did not have signs of dehydration; however, on day 13, the infant began supplementation with 15% of its daily intake as goat's milk formula. By day 20 the symptoms had resolved. The average milk concentration of probenecid and cephalexin was 964 μg/L and 745 μg/L, respectively. This corresponds to a relative infant dose of 0.7% for probenecid and 0.5% for cephalexin.

T 1/2	0.5-1.2 h	MW	365.41 Da	PB	6%-15%
Tmax	1 h	RID	0.39%-1.47%	Vd	0.25 L/kg
Oral	90%	M/P	0.008-0.25	pKa	4.5

Adult Concerns: Headache, dizziness, dyspepsia, nausea, vomiting, diarrhea, changes in liver function, eosinophilia, rash.

Adult Dose: 250-500 mg every 6 hours.

Pediatric Concerns: One case report of diarrhea in an infant exposed to IV cephalothin, then oral cephalexin + probenecid.[3]

Infant Monitoring: Vomiting, diarrhea, changes in gastrointestinal flora, and rash.

Alternatives:

References:

1. Kafetzis DA, Siafas CA, Georgakopoulos PA, Papadatos CJ. Passage of cephalosporins and amoxicillin into the breast milk. Acta Paediatr Scand. 1981;70(3):285-288.
2. Matsuda S. Transfer of antibiotics into maternal milk. Biol Res Pregnancy Perinatol. 1984;5(2):57-60.
3. Ilett K, Hackett P, Ingle B, Bretz PJ. Transfer of probenecid and cephalexin into breast milk. Ann Pharmacother. 2006;40:986-988.

CERTOLIZUMAB PEGOL

Trade: Cimzia

Category: Monoclonal Antibody

LRC: L2 - Limited Data-Probably Compatible

Certolizumab pegol is a pegylated, humanized monoclonal anti-TNF antigen binding fragment that blocks tumor necrosis factor-alpha (TNF-alpha).[1] Certolizumab is used for the treatment of rheumatoid arthritis, Crohn's disease, psoriatic arthritis, and ankylosing spondylitis.

A recent study of 17 breastfeeding women, more than 6 weeks postpartum, evaluated the use of certolizumab in lactation.[2] Sixteen women received certolizumab 200 mg every 2 weeks, and one received 400 mg every 4 weeks subcutaneously). Samples were collected at steady state every 2 days from day 0 to 14 and day 28 in the one patient receiving doses every 4 weeks. Breast milk samples from four of 17 women were undetectable throughout the dosing interval. Thirteen of 17 subjects had measurable levels in milk (peak 0.076 μg/mL) throughout the dosing interval. Fifty-six percent of all samples taken were below the limit of quantification. The estimated ADID ranged from 0 to 0.0104 mg/kg/day; median estimated ADID was 0.003503 mg/kg/day Using the Cave, the RID ranged from 0.04% to 0.35% while the median RID= 0.15%. Interestingly, certolizumab was below limit of quantitation in 56% of maternal milk samples. This study followed the breastfed infants for up to 5 weeks post maternal dose, and only one reported infant adverse event (nasopharyngitis), which was considered attributable to the medication. The milk levels found in this study are probably far too low to impact an infant.

In a separate study, plasma certolizumab pegol concentrations were collected 4 weeks after birth in nine breast-fed infants whose mothers had been currently taking Cimzia (regardless of being exclusively breastfed or not). Certolizumab pegol in infant plasma was not measurable i.e., below 0.032 mcg/mL.[1]

These levels in milk are probably too low to produce clinical effects in a breastfed infant.

T 1/2	14 days	MW	91,000 Da	PB	
Tmax	5.051 days	RID	0.04%-0.3%	Vd	0.09-0.11 L/kg
Oral	Low	M/P		pKa	

Adult Concerns: Headache, fever, dizziness, fatigue, changes in mood, seizures, hypertension, myocardial infarction, nausea, vomiting, changes in liver or renal function, peripheral neuropathy, anemia, pancytopenia, infection, malignancy, rash.

Adult Dose: Maintenance dose: 200 mg every 2 weeks or 400 mg every 4 weeks injected subcutaneously.

Pediatric Concerns: Nasopharyngitis has been reported in one breastfed infant.

Infant Monitoring: Fever, frequent infections, vomiting, poor feeding/poor weight gain. Based on clinical symptoms some infants may require monitoring of their hematology, liver, or renal function.

Alternatives:

References:
1. Pharmaceutical manufacturers prescribing information.
2. Clowse ME, Förger F, Hwang C, et al. Minimal to no transfer of certolizumab pegol into breast milk: results from CRADLE, a prospective, postmarketing, multicentre, pharmacokinetic study. Ann Rheum Dis. November 2017;76(11):1890-1896.

CETIRIZINE

Trade: Zyrtec, Reactine

Category: Antihistamine

LRC: L2 - No Data-Probably Compatible

Cetirizine is a popular new antihistamine useful for seasonal allergic rhinitis. It is a metabolite of hydroxyzine and is one of the most potent of the antihistamines. It is rapidly and extensively absorbed orally and due to a rather long half-life, is used only once daily. It penetrates the CNS poorly and therefore produces minimal sedation.[1] Studies in dogs suggests that only 3% of the dose is transferred to milk.

T 1/2	8 h	MW	389 Da	PB	93%
Tmax	1 h	RID		Vd	0.56 L/kg
Oral	70%	M/P		pKa	3.36

Adult Concerns: Sedation, fatigue, dry mouth.

Adult Dose: 5-10 mg daily.

Pediatric Concerns: None reported.

Infant Monitoring: Sedation, dry mouth, changes in feeding.

Alternatives: Loratadine(L1), Desloratadine(L2)

References:
1. Pharmaceutical manufacturers prescribing information.

CETUXIMAB

Trade: Erbitux

Category: Antineoplastic

LRC: L4 - No Data-Possibly Hazardous

Cetuximab is a recombinant, human/mouse chimeric monoclonal antibody that binds specifically to the human epidermal growth factor receptor, resulting in inhibition of cell growth, induction of apoptosis, and decreased matrix metalloproteinase and vascular endothelial growth factor production.[1] This monoclonal antibody is used to treat colorectal cancer. Although this medication has a long half-life with a mean of 112 hours (range 63-230 hours), and a volume of the distribution (Vd) which approximates the vascular space (2-3 L/m^2 or 0.05-0.08 L/kg), its very large molecular weight (152,000 Da) makes it unlikely to enter human milk.

Although the molecular weight of this medication is very large and the amount in breast milk is expected to be exceptionally low, there are no long-term data concerning the safety of using immune modulating medications in breastfeeding mothers. Further there are current data that suggest that some IgG drugs do transfer to milk, and perhaps the breastfed infant. Therefore, some caution is recommended and each woman should understand the benefits and risk of using this type of medication in lactation.

T 1/2	112 h (range 63-230 h)	MW	152,000 Da	PB	
Tmax		RID		Vd	0.05-0.08 L/kg
Oral		M/P		pKa	

Adult Concerns: Headache, fatigue, insomnia, anxiety, taste disturbances, stomatitis, dry mouth, dyspnea, nausea, constipation, diarrhea, changes in electrolytes, changes in renal failure.

Adult Dose: 400 mg/m^2 first dose, then 250 mg/m^2 weekly.

Pediatric Concerns:

Infant Monitoring: Avoid breastfeeding for approximately 60 days.

Alternatives:

References:
1. Pharmaceutical manufacturers prescribing information.

CEVIMELINE

Trade: Evoxac

Category: Cholinergic

LRC: L3 - No Data-Probably Compatible

Cevimeline is a cholinergic agonist agent, which binds to muscarinic receptors and can increase secretion of exocrine glands such as salivary and sweat glands, and increase tone in the gastrointestinal and urinary tracts. It is indicated for the treatment of patients with Sjrogren's syndrome.[1] This drug has a large volume of distribution, which suggests that most of the compound is stored in peripheral tissues, not the plasma compartment. Many such drugs produce lower milk levels. No data are available on its transfer to human milk. Due to its strong cholinergic effects, some caution is recommended in breastfeeding mothers.

T 1/2	3-5 h	MW	244 Da	PB	<20%
Tmax	1-2 h	RID		Vd	6 L/kg
Oral	Complete	M/P		pKa	

Adult Concerns: Insomnia, fatigue, vertigo, palpitations, coughing, nausea, abdominal pain, hot flashes, diaphoresis (excessive sweating), muscle cramps, rash.

Adult Dose: 30 mg TID.

Pediatric Concerns: No reports are available at this time.

Infant Monitoring: Excessive salivation, diarrhea, poor weight gain.

Alternatives: Pilocarpine(L3)

References:
1. Pharmaceutical manufacturers prescribing information.

CHAMOMILE, GERMAN

Trade:

Category: Herb

LRC: L3 - No Data-Probably Compatible

Chamomile has been used since Roman times, primarily for its anti-inflammatory, antispasmodic, carminative, mild sedative, and antiseptic properties.[1,2] It has been used for conditions such as insomnia, dyspepsia, diarrhea, and other gastrointestinal irritation. Reports of allergic reactions to chamomile include two cases of anaphylaxis, although this is probably rare.[3-5] The use of this product in lactation is controversial; some authors suggest this product should be avoided in pregnant and breastfeeding women, while others consider it suitable.[6-8] As with most herbal products, safety data in the infant are not well documented.

Adult Concerns: Allergic reactions, worsening asthma symptoms, hypotension, vomiting, hypoglycemia, increased risk of bleeding.

Adult Dose: 400-1200 mg daily in divided doses (variable based on product).

Pediatric Concerns: None reported via milk.

Infant Monitoring:

Alternatives:

References:
1. Berry M. The chamomiles. Pharm J. 1995;254:191-193.
2. Mann C, Staba EJ. The chemistry, pharmacology, and commercial formulations of chamomile. In: Simon JE, ed. Herbs, Spices, and Medicinal Plants: Recent Advances in Botany, Horticulture, and Pharmacology. vol 1. Arizona: Oryx Press; 1986.
3. Hausen BM. The sensitizing capacity of Compositae plants. Planta Med. 1984;50:229-234.
4. Casterline CL. Allergy to chamomile tea. JAMA. 1980;244(4):330-331.
5. Benner MH, Lee HJ. Anaphylactic reaction to chamomile tea. J Allergy Clin Immunol. 1973;52(5):307-308.
6. Habersang S, Leuschner F, Isaac O, Thiemer K. [Pharmacological studies with compounds of chamomile. IV. Studies on toxicity of (-)-alpha-bisabolol (author's transl)]. Planta Med. 1979;37(2):115-123.
7. Newall C, Anderson LA, Phillipson JD. Chamomile, German. In: Barnes J, Phillipson JD, Anderson LA, eds. Herbal medicine: a guide for the healthcare professionals. London, England: The Pharmaceutical Press; 1996.
8. The Complete German Commission E Monographs. Ed. M. Blumenthal Amer Botanical Council 1998.

CHLORAMBUCIL

Trade: Linfolysin, Leukeran

Category: Antineoplastic

LRC: L5 - No Data-Hazardous

Chlorambucil is a derivative of nitrogen mustard with molecular weight of 304.[1] When administered orally, it is fairly well absorbed (bioavailability >70%). It is eliminated rapidly with a half-life of 1-2 hours. Milk levels are unpublished, but probably low due to high protein binding, and amine structure.

Withhold breastfeeding for at least 24 hours.

T 1/2	1-1.9 h	MW	304.2 Da	PB	99%
Tmax	1 h	RID		Vd	0.3 L/kg
Oral	>70%; reduced with food	M/P		pKa	5.8

Adult Concerns: Agitation, ataxia, confusion, fever, oral ulcers, pulmonary fibrosis, vomiting, diarrhea, changes in liver function, amenorrhea, infertility, neutropenia, anemia, thrombocytopenia, bone marrow failure, muscular twitching, severe skin reactions.

Adult Dose: 0.1 mg/kg/day for 3-6 weeks or 0.4 mg/kg biweekly.

Pediatric Concerns:

Infant Monitoring: Withhold breastfeeding for at least 24 hours.

Alternatives:

References:
1. Grochow LB, Ames MM. A Clinician's Guide to Chemotherapy Pharmacokinetics and Pharmacodynamics. 1st ed. Baltimore, MD: Williams & Wilkins; 1998.

CHLORAMPHENICOL

Trade: Sopamycetin, Biocetin, Chloromycetin, Chloroptic, Chlorsig

Category: Antibiotic, Other

LRC: L4 - Limited Data-Possibly Hazardous

Chloramphenicol is a broad-spectrum antibiotic. In one study of five women receiving 250 mg chloramphenicol orally four times daily, the concentration of chloramphenicol in milk ranged from 0.54 to 2.84 mg/L.[1] In the same study, but in another group receiving 500 mg orally four times daily, the concentration of chloramphenicol in milk ranged from 1.75 to 6.1 mg/L.

In a published report documenting a group of patients being treated for typhus, information was found regarding the treatment of one lactating woman.[2] She had maternal plasma and milk levels quantified 2 days in a row; the plasma samples were 49 and 26 mg/L and the corresponding milk levels were 25 and 16 mg/L. Unfortunately, the timing of these levels and her daily dose was not reported clearly; however, the authors did report she received 7.2 g of chloramphenicol over 54 hours. In a study of 2-3 patients who received a single 500 mg oral dose, the average milk concentration at 4 hours was 4.1 mg/L.[3] The milk/plasma ratio at 4 hours was 0.84.

Safety in infants is controversial. Milk levels are most likely too low to produce overt toxicity in infants; however, chloramphenicol is generally considered contraindicated in nursing mothers. This antibiotic can be extremely toxic, particularly in neonates, and should not be used for trivial infections.[4]

T 1/2	4 h	MW	323 Da	PB	60%
Tmax	1 h	RID	2.98%-8.5%	Vd	0.5-1 L/kg
Oral	80%	M/P	0.5-0.6	pKa	5.5

Adult Concerns: Numerous blood dyscrasias, aplastic anemia, fever, skin rashes.

Adult Dose: 50-100 mg/kg daily divided every 6 hours.

Pediatric Concerns: None reported via milk. This medication has been associated with Gray baby syndrome, when administered directly to neonates.[4] This adverse effect is typically dose-related and occurs when levels are higher than 50 µg/mL. Symptoms include irregular breathing, cyanosis, circulatory collapse, abdominal distention, vomiting, flaccidity.

Infant Monitoring: Difficulty breathing, abdominal distention, vomiting, diarrhea, anemia, and rash.

Alternatives:

References:
1. Havelka J, Hejzlar M, Popov V, Viktorinova D, Prochazka J. Excretion of chloramphenicol in human milk. Chemotherapy. 1968;13(4):204-211.
2. Smadel JE, Woodward TE, Ley HL Jr, Lewthwaite R. Chloramphenicol in the treatment of tsutsugamushi disease. J Clin Invest. 1949;28:1196-1215.
3. Matsuda S. Transfer of antibiotics into maternal milk. Biol Res Pregnancy Perinatol. 1984;5(2):57-60.
4. Chin KG, McPherson CE, Hoffman M, et al. Use of anti-infective agents during lactation: part 2-aminoglycosides, macrolides, quinolones, sulfonamides, trimethoprim, tetracyclines, chloramphenicol, clindamycin, and metronidazole. J Hum Lact. 2001;17(1):54-65.

CHLORDIAZEPOXIDE

Trade: Libritabs, Librium, Medilium, Solium

Category: Antianxiety

LRC: L3 - No Data-Probably Compatible

Chlordiazepoxide is an older benzodiazepine. It is secreted in breast milk in moderate but unreported levels.[1] Chlordiazepoxide is metabolized to multiple active metabolites including desmethyldiazepam (long acting). Based on this medications long half-life and active metabolites other benzodiazepines are preferred in lactation (e.g., lorazepam).

T 1/2	6.6-28 h	MW	336.22 Da	PB	96%
Tmax	0.5-2 h	RID		Vd	3.3 L/kg
Oral	Complete	M/P		pKa	4.8

Adult Concerns: Sedation, dizziness, confusion, nervousness, blurred vision, syncope, and ataxia.

Adult Dose: 5-25 mg every 6-8 hours; varies by indication.

Pediatric Concerns: None reported via milk at this time.

Infant Monitoring: Sedation, slowed breathing rate, not waking to feed/poor feeding, and weight gain.

Alternatives: Lorazepam(L3)

References:
1. Pharmaceutical manufacturers prescribing information.

CHLORHEXIDINE

Trade: Hibiclens, Peridex, Periogard

Category: Antibiotic, Other

LRC: L4 - Limited Data-Possibly Hazardous

Chlorhexidine in various forms is a topical antimicrobial used in topical detergents, oral lozenges, and mouthwashes.[1] Pharmacokinetic studies with a 0.12% chlorhexidine gluconate oral rinse indicate approximately 30% of the active ingredient is retained in the oral cavity following rinsing. The drug retained in the oral cavity is slowly released into the oral fluids and swallowed. Studies conducted on human subjects and animals demonstrate chlorhexidine gluconate is poorly absorbed from the gastrointestinal tract.

In a study of 200 mothers in which 100 each received breast sprays containing water or 0.2% chlorhexidine in alcohol, the chlorhexidine/alcohol spray group showed greater compliance to breastfeeding and lower incidence of trauma and discomfort. No adverse effects occurred that could be attributed to the medications.[2] In another case report, a mother used chlorhexidine spray (430 μg/spray) on her breasts to prevent mastitis starting with the third feed when the baby was 12 hours old. After 48 hours, the baby developed bradycardia. Some episodes over the next 2 days required atropine therapy, which subsequently increased the heart rate. An electrocardiogram confirmed sinus bradycardia. The chlorhexidine spray was discontinued and the bradycardia became less severe and less frequent. By day 6, bradycardia was no longer present. Each spray of chlorhexidine contains 430 μg and over 24 hours the baby could have ingested 2.5 mg.[3]

The differences between the two studies could be attributed to the difference in the amount of chlorhexidine available to the infants or their age. Regardless, chlorhexidine should not be used on a breastfeeding mother's nipples. Its use topically on the skin (other than nipple), or in the mouth would not be contraindicated in breastfeeding mothers. The use of chlorhexidine on other skin surfaces is not contraindicated in breastfeeding women.

T 1/2	<4 h	MW	505 Da	PB	87%
Tmax	<12 h	RID		Vd	
Oral	Poor	M/P		pKa	10.8

Adult Concerns: Staining of teeth and dentures. Keep out of eyes. Changes in taste, increased plaque, staining of tongue.

Adult Dose: Swish 15 mL in mouth for 30 seconds and then spit. Do not swallow.

Pediatric Concerns: Bradycardia in one infant exposed to chlorhexidine on the nipple.

Infant Monitoring: Slow heart rate, staining of tongue.

Alternatives:

References:
1. Lacy C. Drug Information Handbook. Cleveland, OH: Lexi-Comp Inc.; 1996.
2. Herd B, Feeney JG. Two aerosol sprays in nipple trauma. Practicioner. 1986;230:31-38.
3. Quinn MW, Bini RM. Bradycardia associated with chlorhexidine spray. Arch Dis Child. 1989;64(6):892-893.

CHLOROQUINE

Trade: Aralen, Avloclor, Chlorquin, Avloquin

Category: Antimalarial

LRC: L2 - Limited Data-Probably Compatible

Chloroquine is an antimalarial agent used in the prevention and treatment of malaria. Following a single 600 mg base dose of chloroquine 11 breastfeeding women had their milk, saliva, and plasma sampled.[1] Five of these women had samples at 0, 3, and 24 hours postdose while the other six had samples taken more frequently for 48 hours and then randomly up to 7 days. The mean M/P ratio in five of the women was 6.6 for chloroquine and 1.5 for desethyl-chloroquine. The average maximum concentration of chloroquine in milk was 4.4 mg/L and the average half-life in milk was 8.8 days. Four neonates had urine samples at 12-24 hours; the samples had an average of 3.97 µg and 0.44 µg of chloroquine and desethylchloroquine, respectively. Using the maximum concentration in milk, we estimate the relative infant dose to be 7.7%. No neonatal adverse events were reported.

In five breastfeeding women, 2-2.5 months postpartum, milk and saliva samples were collected at the time of drug administration (300 mg chloroquine base) up to 168 hours postdose.[2] The average maximum concentration of chloroquine in milk was 3.97 µg/mL and the average concentration of chlororquine in milk was 1.57 µg/mL. The mean half-life in milk was 5.5 days. Women in this study withheld breast milk for 10-24 hours postdose to reduce infant exposure. Using the average concentration in milk, we estimated the RID to be 5.5%.

In a group of six women given 5 mg/kg chloroquine IM during delivery, and then again at 14 days postpartum, milk levels averaged 0.227 mg/L and ranged from 0.192 to 0.319 mg/L.[3] The milk/blood ratio ranged from 0.268 to 0.462. Based on these levels, the infant would consume approximately 34 µg/kg/day, an amount considered suitable for breastfeeding. The authors reported that if an infant consumed 500 mL/day of milk, it would receive an average of 113.5 µg/day of chloroquine.

In another study, three women were given a single oral dose of 12.5 mg pyrimethamine + 100 mg dapsone + 300 mg chloroquine base within 2-5 days of delivery.[4] Blood and milk samples were then collected over the next 9 days; if the three infants had been breastfed they would have received 400, 760, and 580 µg chloroquine over the study period of about 9 days if they each consumed about 1 L of milk a day. The authors estimated the relative infant dose to be 2.2%-4.2% of the maternal dose and the absolute infant dose to be 0.19 mg/kg over 9 days. The M/P ratio ranged from 1.96 to 4.26. None of the infants in this study were breastfed.

In a recent study, the milk samples of 16 women were collected on day 3, 4, 5, 10, and 18-22 following delivery and examined for the concentrations of chloroquine and its metabolite, desethylchloroquine.[5] These women were given 465 mg of chloroquine base on days 1-3 after delivery. The average concentration in milk during the sampling period was 167 µg/L for chloroquine and 54 µg/L for desethylchloroquine. The absolute infant doses were 34 µg/kg/day and 15 µg/kg/day for chloroquine and desethylchloroquine, respectively. The current recommended pediatric dose for prevention of malaria is 8.3 mg/kg/week, which exceeds that present in breast milk. The relative infant doses were 2.3% and 1% for chloroquine and desethylchloroquine, respectively. The authors suggested that chloroquine is compatible with breastfeeding.

The WHO considers chloroquine to be suitable for both prevention and treatment of malaria in lactation and pediatrics.[6]

T 1/2	72-120 h	MW	320 Da	PB	50%-65%
Tmax	1-2 h	RID	0.68%-7.71%	Vd	> 116-285 L/kg
Oral	Complete	M/P	0.268-6.6	pKa	8.4, 10.8

Adult Concerns: Headache, fatigue, insomnia, agitation, nervousness, hallucinations, confusion, depression, hearing and ocular changes including blindness, hypotension, arrhythmias, vomiting, diarrhea, anorexia, changes in liver enzymes, neutropenia, aplastic anemia, skin reactions.

Adult Dose: 300 mg base weekly for prophylaxis (varies by indication).

Pediatric Concerns: None reported via milk at this time.

Infant Monitoring: Irritability, insomnia, vomiting, diarrhea, decreased feeding/poor weight gain, weakness. If clinical signs of jaundice check liver enzymes or if ongoing infection check CBC. With prolonged exposure monitor vision and hearing.

Alternatives:

References:

1. Ogunbona FA, Onyeji CO, Bolaji OO, et al. Excretion of chloroquine and desethylchloroquine in human milk. Br J Clin Pharmac. 1987;23:473-476.
2. Ette EI, Essien EE, Ogonor JI, et al. Chloroquine in human milk. J Clin Pharmacol. 1987;27:499-502.

3. Akintonwa A, Gbajumo SA, Mabadeje AF. Placental and milk transfer of chloroquine in humans. Ther Drug Monit. 1988;10(2):147-149.
4. Edstein MD, Veenendaal JR, Newman K, Hyslop R. Excretion of chloroquine, dapsone and pyrimethamine in human milk. Br J Clin Pharmacol. 1986;22(6):733-735.
5. Law I, Ilett KF, Hackett LP, et al. Transfer of chloroquine and desethylchloroquine across the placenta and into milk in Melanesian mothers. Br J Clin Pharmacol. 2008;65(5):674-679.
6. World Health Organization (WHO). Malaria. In: International Travel and Health. 2010:chap 7. http://www.who.int/ith/ITH_chapter_7.pdf.

CHLOROTHIAZIDE

Trade: Chlotride, Diuril, Saluric

Category: Diuretic

LRC: L3 - Limited Data-Probably Compatible

Chlorothiazide is a typical thiazide diuretic. In one study of 11 lactating women, each receiving 500 mg of chlorothiazide, the concentrations in milk samples taken 1, 2, and 3 hours after the dose were all less than 1 mg/L with a milk/plasma ratio of 0.05.[1] Although thiazide diuretics are reported to produce thrombocytopenia in nursing infants, it is remote and unsubstantiated. Most thiazide diuretics are considered compatible with breastfeeding if doses are kept low and milk production is unaffected.

T 1/2	1.5 h	MW	296 Da	PB	95%
Tmax	1 h	RID	2.1%	Vd	0.3 L/kg
Oral	20%	M/P	0.05	pKa	9.1

Adult Concerns: Dizziness, headache, hypotension, anorexia, abdominal cramps, nausea, diarrhea, hematuria, changes in liver and renal function, changes in electrolytes, hyperglycemia, severe skin rashes.

Adult Dose: 500-2000 mg every 12-24 hours.

Pediatric Concerns: None reported.

Infant Monitoring: Observe for fluid loss, dehydration, lethargy.

Alternatives:

References:
1. Werthmann MW Jr, Krees SV. Excretion of chlorothiazide in human breast milk. J Pediatr. 1972;81(4):781-783.

CHLORPHENIRAMINE

Trade: Aller-Chlor, C.P.M., Chlor-Phen, Chlor-Trimeton Allergy, Teldrin HBP

Category: Antihistamine

LRC: L3 - No Data-Probably Compatible

Chlorpheniramine is a commonly used antihistamine. Although no data are available on secretion into breast milk, it has not been reported to produce side effects.[1]

T 1/2	12-43 h	MW	275 Da	PB	70%
Tmax	2-6 h	RID		Vd	5.9 L/kg
Oral	25%-45%	M/P		pKa	9.2

Adult Concerns: Headache, sedation, dizziness, dry mouth, urinary retention.

Adult Dose: 4 mg every 4-6 hours.

Pediatric Concerns: None reported.

Infant Monitoring: Sedation, changes in feeding.

Alternatives: Cetirizine(L2), Loratadine(L1)

References:
1. Paton DM, Webster DR. Clinical pharmacokinetics of H1-receptor antagonists (the antihistamines). Clin Pharmacokinet. 1985;10(6):477-497.

CHLORPROMAZINE

Trade: Chloractil, Chlorpromanyl, Largactil, Ormazine, Thorazine

Category: Antipsychotic, Typical

LRC: L3 - Limited Data-Probably Compatible

Chlorpromazine is a powerful CNS tranquilizer. Small amounts are known to be secreted into milk. Following a 1200 mg oral dose, samples were taken at 60, 120, and 180 minutes.[1] Breast milk concentrations were highest at 120 minutes and were 0.29 mg/L at that time. The milk/plasma ratio was less than 0.5. Ayd suggests that in one group of 16 women who took chlorpromazine during and after pregnancy, and while breastfeeding, the side effects were minimal and infant development was normal.[2] In a group of four breastfeeding mothers receiving unspecified amounts of chlorpromazine, milk levels varied from 7 to 98 µg/L.[3] Maternal serum levels ranged from 16 to 52 µg/L. Only the infant who ingested milk with a chlorpromazine level of 92 µg/L showed drowsiness and lethargy.

Chlorpromazine has a long half-life and is particularly sedating. Long-term use of this product in a lactating mother may be risky to the breastfed infant. There are consistent reports of phenothiazine products increasing the risk of apnea and SIDS; avoid if possible.

T 1/2	30 h	MW	319 Da	PB	95%
Tmax	1 h	RID	0.3%	Vd	10-35 L/kg
Oral	20%	M/P	<0.5	pKa	9.3

Adult Concerns: Sedation, dizziness, lethargy, seizure, apnea, hypotension, dry mouth, constipation, urinary retention, gynecomastia, extrapyramidal side effects, leukopenia, thrombocytopenia.

Adult Dose: 200 mg daily.

Pediatric Concerns: One report of lethargy and sedation.

Infant Monitoring: Sedation or irritability, apnea, not waking to feed/poor feeding, dry mouth, constipation, weight gain, and extrapyramidal symptoms.

Alternatives:

References:
1. Blacker KH, Weinstein BJ, Ellman GL. Mothers milk and chlorpromazine. Am J Psychol. 1962;114:178-179.
2. Ayd FJ. Excretion of psychotropic drugs in breast milk. Int Drug Ther Newslett. November-December 1973;8:33-40.
3. Wiles DH, Orr MW, Kolakowska T. Chlorpromazine levels in plasma and milk of nursing mothers. Br J Clin Pharmacol. 1978;5(3):272-273.

CHLORPROPAMIDE

Trade: Dibecon, Diabinese, Meldian

Category: Antidiabetic, Sulfonylurea

LRC: L3 - No Data-Probably Compatible

Chlorpropamide stimulates the secretion of insulin in some patients. Following one 500 mg dose, the concentration of chlorpropamide in milk after 5 hours was approximately 5 mg/L of milk.[1] This report by the manufacturer provided few details. May cause hypoglycemia in infants although effects are largely unknown and unreported.

T 1/2	33 h	MW	277 Da	PB	96%
Tmax	3-6 h	RID	10.5%	Vd	0.1-0.3 L/kg
Oral	Complete	M/P		pKa	4.8

Adult Concerns: Headache, dizziness, vomiting, diarrhea, anorexia, changes in liver function, and hypoglycemia.

Adult Dose: 250-500 mg daily.

Pediatric Concerns: None reported via breast milk at this time.

Infant Monitoring: Diarrhea, weight gain and signs of hypoglycemia- drowsiness, lethargy, pallor, sweating, tremor.

Alternatives: Metformin(L1)

References:
1. Pharmaceutical manufacturers prescribing information.

CHLORTHALIDONE

Trade: Hydone, Hygroton, Thalitone

Category: Diuretic

LRC: L4 - Limited Data-Possibly Hazardous

Chlorthalidone is a typical thiazide diuretic commonly used as an antihypertensive. In a group of seven women receiving 50 mg orally daily, milk levels 3 days postpartum ranged from 90 to 860 µg/L. The infant was estimated to have received approximately 180 µg per day.[1] The relative infant dose (RID) would range from 1.9%-18%, but the authors estimate the RID at 6%. Chlorthalidone has a long half-life, and clearance from the infant may be slow possibly leading to accumulation. Hydrochlorothiazide may be more appropriate in breastfeeding women, if a diuretic had to be used. When a child is exposed to chlorthalidone in pregnancy as well as through the mother's milk, the possibility for accumulation increases. The above study has estimated that a 3.5 kg infant would be born with about 250 µg of chlorthalidone in its blood if the mother was exposed to the drug throughout pregnancy. In the event that the child is also breastfed while the drug is present in the mother, an additional 180 µg per day may be administered. Due to the rapid accumulation that could occur in this situation, it may be appropriate to discontinue breastfeeding for a few days postpartum.[1]

T 1/2	40-60 h	MW	338 Da	PB	75%
Tmax	2-6 h	RID	1.9%-18.1%	Vd	3.9 L/kg
Oral	75%	M/P		pKa	9.22

Adult Concerns: Anorexia, photosensitivity, hypokalemia, epigastric pain, hypercalcemia, agranulocytosis, gout.

Adult Dose: 25-100 mg/day.

Pediatric Concerns: None reported via milk at this time.

Infant Monitoring: Observe for fluid loss, dehydration, lethargy; monitor maternal milk supply.

Alternatives: Hydrochlorothiazide(L2), Furosemide(L3)

References:
1. Mulley BA, Parr GD, Pau WK, Rye RM, Mould JJ, Siddle NC. Placental transfer of chlorthalidone and its elimination in maternal milk. Eur J Clin Pharmacol. May 17, 1978;13(2):129-131.

CHOLERA VACCINE

Trade: Cholera Vaccine, Dukoral

Category: Vaccine

LRC: L3 - No Data-Probably Compatible

Cholera vaccine is available in an oral preparation and a sterile injectable solution containing equal parts of phenol inactivated Ogawa and Inaba serotypes of Vibrio cholerae bacteria.

Maternal immunization with cholera vaccine significantly increases levels of anti-cholera antibodies (IgA, IgG) in their milk.[1] The vaccine is not contraindicated in nursing mothers. Breastfed infants are generally protected from cholera transmission. Immunization is approved from the age of 6 months and older.

Adult Concerns: Malaise, fever, headache, pain at injection site.

Adult Dose: Two doses of 0.5 mL injections (IM or SC) 1 week-1 month apart.

Pediatric Concerns: None reported.

Infant Monitoring:

Alternatives:

References:
1. Merson MH, Black RE, Sack DA, Svennerholm AM, Holmgren J. Maternal cholera immunization and secretory IgA in breast milk. Lancet. 1980;1(8174):931-932.

CHOLESTYRAMINE

Trade: Cholybar, Questran

Category: Gastrointestinal Agent

LRC: L2 - No Data-Probably Compatible

Cholestyramine is a bile salt chelating resin. Used orally in adults, it binds bile salts and prevents reabsorption of bile salts in the gut, thus reducing cholesterol levels.[1] This resin is not absorbed from the maternal gastrointestinal tract; therefore, it is highly unlikely to enter breast milk.

The only potential problem of using this product in breastfeeding mothers is the lowering of maternal plasma cholesterol levels, and the possible lowering of milk cholesterol levels. Milk cholesterol is particularly important in infant neurodevelopment.

T 1/2	6 min	MW		PB	
Tmax	21 days	RID		Vd	
Oral	0%	M/P		pKa	

Adult Concerns: Nausea, vomiting, constipation, vitamin deficiency and nutrient malabsorption, intestinal obstruction.

Adult Dose: 8-16 grams daily.

Pediatric Concerns: None reported via milk.

Infant Monitoring:

Alternatives:

References:
1. Pharmaceutical manufacturers prescribing information.

CHONDROITIN SULFATE

Trade:

Category: Antiarthritic

LRC: L3 - No Data-Probably Compatible

Chondroitin sulfate is a biological polymer that acts as a flexible connecting matrix between the protein filaments in cartilage. It is derived largely from natural sources such as shark or bovine cartilage and is chemically composed of a high-viscosity mucopolysaccharide (glycosaminoglycan) polymer found in most mammalian cartilaginous tissues.[1] Thus far, chondroitin has been found to be nontoxic. Its molecular weight averages 50,000 Da, which is far too large to permit its entry into human milk. Combined with a poor oral bioavailability and large molecular weight, it is unlikely to pose a problem for a breastfed infant.

T 1/2		MW	50,000 Da	PB	
Tmax		RID		Vd	
Oral	0%-13%	M/P		pKa	

Adult Concerns:

Adult Dose: 200-400 mg two or three times daily.

Pediatric Concerns: None reported via milk.

Infant Monitoring:

Alternatives:

References:
1. Review of Natural Products. St. Louis, MO: Facts and Comparisons; 1996.

CHROMIUM

Trade: Chromium Picrolinate

Category: Metals

LRC: L3 - Limited Data-Probably Compatible

Trace metal, required in glucose metabolism. Less than 1% is absorbed following oral administration. Chromium levels are depleted in multiparous women. Chromium levels in neonates are approximately 2.5 times that of maternal levels due to concentrating mechanism during gestation. Because chromium is difficult to measure, levels reported vary widely.

One article reports that breast milk levels are approximately 0.18 ng/mL, which is below the adequate daily intake of 0.2-5.5 µg/day for children 0-12 months of age.[1,2] Most importantly, breast milk levels are independent of maternal dietary intake and serum levels as chromium is thought to be secreted into breast milk by a well-controlled pumping mechanism.

T 1/2		MW	52 Da	PB	
Tmax		RID		Vd	
Oral	<1%	M/P		pKa	

Adult Concerns: Chromium poisoning if used in excess.

Adult Dose: 25-45 µg/day.

Pediatric Concerns: None reported.

Infant Monitoring: Chromium poisoning in overdose.

Alternatives:

References:
1. Anderson RA, Bryden NA, Patterson KY, Veillon C, Andon MB, Moser-Veillon PB. Breast milk chromium and its association with chromium intake, chromium excretion, and serum chromium. Am J Clin Nutr. 1993;57(4):519-523.
2. National Institutes of Health Office of Dietary Supplements [Internet]. Chromium dietary supplement fact sheet; November 2013 [July 25, 2016]. https://ods.od.nih.gov/factsheets/Chromium-HealthProfessional/#h3.

CICLESONIDE

Trade: Omnaris

Category: Corticosteroid

LRC: L3 - No Data-Probably Compatible

Ciclesonide is a nasal corticosteroid spray and inhaled corticosteroid used for allergic rhinitis and asthma.[1] Ciclesonide is a prodrug that is enzymatically hydrolyzed to a pharmacologically active metabolite des-ciclesonide. Ciclesonide and its active metabolite, des-ciclesonide, have negligible oral bioavailability (<1%) and high first-pass metabolism by the liver. While we have no data on its use in breastfeeding mothers, as with the other inhaled steroids, this product is expected to pose little risk.

T 1/2	6-7 h	MW	540 Da	PB	99%
Tmax	1.04 h	RID		Vd	12.1 L/kg
Oral	<1%	M/P		pKa	14.78

Adult Concerns: Headache, nose bleeds, nasopharyngitis, thrush.

Adult Dose: 100 µg/day in each nostril; 160-320 µg/day inhaled.

Pediatric Concerns: None reported via milk at this time.

Infant Monitoring: Feeding, growth, and weight gain.

Alternatives: Budesonide(L1), Fluticasone(L3), Mometasone(L3)

References:
1. Pharmaceutical manufacturers prescribing information.

CICLOPIROX OLAMINE

Trade: Loprox

Category: Antifungal

LRC: L3 - No Data-Probably Compatible

Ciclopirox is a broad-spectrum antifungal and is active in numerous species including tinea, Candida albicans, and trichophyton rubrum.[1] An average of 1.3% ciclopirox is absorbed when applied topically although only 0.01% of the dose is found in the urine. Topical application produces minimal systemic absorption; it is unlikely that topical use would expose the nursing infant to significant risks. The risk to a breastfeeding infant associated with application directly on the nipple is not known and it should not be used on the nipple.

T 1/2	1.7 h	MW	268 Da	PB	98%
Tmax	6 h	RID		Vd	
Oral		M/P		pKa	7.2

Adult Concerns: Pruritus and burning following topical therapy.

Adult Dose: Apply topically BID.

Pediatric Concerns: None via milk.

Infant Monitoring:

Alternatives: Fluconazole(L2), Miconazole(L2)

References:
1. Pharmaceutical manufacturers prescribing information.

CILASTATIN + IMIPENEM

Trade: Primaxin

Category: Antibiotic, Carbapenem

LRC: L3 - No Data-Probably Compatible

Imipenem/cilastatin is a combination drug product that is indicated for use in a variety of infections including infections of the bone or joint, skin and subcutaneous tissues, lower respiratory tract infections, and systemic bacterial infections.[1,2] Experience with this drug in breastfeeding women is limited; however, there is no evidence that the use of this drug will have adverse effects in the breastfed infant. Cilastatin is added to extend the half-life of an antibiotic called imipenem, structurally similar to penicillins. Both imipenem and cilastatin are poorly absorbed orally and must be administered IM or IV. Transfer to breast milk is probably minimal but no data are available at this time. At this time meropenem (another carbapenem) would be recommended if appropriate for treatment of the maternal condition as concentrations in milk are known to be very low.

T 1/2	60 min	MW	Imip/cila: 317/380 Da	PB	Imip/cila: 20%/40%
Tmax	Immediate (IV)	RID		Vd	Widely distributed L/kg
Oral	Poor	M/P		pKa	

Adult Concerns: Seizures, fever, dizziness, somnolence, hypotension, nausea, diarrhea, vomiting, abdominal pain, changes in liver function, pancytopenia.

Adult Dose: 500 mg IV q6h.

Pediatric Concerns: None reported via milk at this time; pediatric safety has been established in the neonatal and pediatric population.

Infant Monitoring: Vomiting, diarrhea, changes in gastrointestinal flora, and rash.

Alternatives: Meropenem(L3)

References:
1. Pharmaceutical manufacturers prescribing information.
2. McEvoy GE, ed. AFHS Drug Information. Bethesda, MD: American Society of Health-System Pharmacists; 2003.

CIMETIDINE

Trade: Cimbene, Cimedine, Tagamet

Category: Gastric Acid Secretion Inhibitor

LRC: L1 - Limited Data-Compatible

Cimetidine is an antisecretory, histamine-2 antagonist that reduces stomach acid secretion. Cimetidine is apparently actively transported to human milk as evidenced by a higher milk/plasma ratio. In a study of 12 women who received single oral doses of 100, 600, and 1200 mg cimetidine, the observed milk/serum ratios were 5.65, 5.84, and 5.83 respectively.[1] The reported maximum concentrations in milk were 2.5, 16.2, and 37.2 mg/L respectively.

In another study of one patient ingesting 600 mg daily, the reported milk level was 5.6 mg/L.[2] The maximum potential dose from lactation would be approximately 5.58 mg/kg/d, which is still quite small. The pediatric dose administered orally for therapeutic treatment of pediatric gastroesophageal reflux averages 20-40 mg/kg/day. However, other choices for breastfeeding mothers should preclude the use of this drug (see ranitidine, famotidine). Short-term use (days) would not be incompatible with breastfeeding.

T 1/2	2 h	MW	252 Da	PB	19%
Tmax	0.75-1.5 h	RID	9.8%-32.6%	Vd	1.3 L/kg
Oral	60%-70%	M/P	4.6-11.76	pKa	6.8

Adult Concerns: Headache, dizziness, somnolence, hypotension, bradycardia, gynecomastia, diarrhea, changes in liver and renal function, hemolytic anemia.

Adult Dose: 400 to 800 mg at bedtime.

Pediatric Concerns: None reported via milk; safety in pediatrics has been established.

Infant Monitoring:

Alternatives: Ranitidine(L2), Famotidine(L1)

References:
1. Oo CY, Kuhn RJ, Desai N, McNamara PJ. Active transport of cimetidine into human milk. Clin Pharmacol Ther. 1995;58(5):548-555.
2. Somogyi A, Gugler R. Cimetidine excretion into breast milk. Br J Clin Pharmacol. 1979;7(6):627-629.

CINACALCET

Trade: Sensipar

Category: Calcium Regulator

LRC: L3 - No Data-Probably Compatible

Cinacalcet is a calcium regulator/calcium-sensing receptor agonist used in the management of hypercalcemia when it occurs in the setting of parathyroid carcinoma, primary hyperparathyroidism and secondary hyperparathyroidism in dialysis patients.[1] There are no adequate and well-controlled studies or case reports in breastfeeding women. It is relatively large in molecular weight (357 Da) and has poor oral absorption (20%). Levels in milk are probably low.

T 1/2	30-40 h	MW	357 Da	PB	93%-97%
Tmax	2-6 h	RID		Vd	14.28 L/kg
Oral	20%-25%	M/P		pKa	8.72

Adult Concerns: Headache, depression fatigue, hypertension, nausea, vomiting, diarrhea, constipation, anorexia, hypocalcemia, hypercalcemia, dehydration, anemia, arthralgias, myalgias.

Adult Dose: 60 mg once to twice daily.

Pediatric Concerns:

Infant Monitoring: Vomiting, diarrhea or constipation, weight gain.

Alternatives:

References:
1. Pharmaceutical manufacturers prescribing information.

CINNARIZINE

Trade: Arlevert, Stugeron

Category: Antiemetic

LRC: L3 - No Data-Probably Compatible

Cinnarizine is an antiemetic used for motion sickness, and is not available in the United States.[1] It is an H1 histamine antagonist and calcium channel blocker. It is primarily used for vestibular disorders of the inner ear and the vomiting center of the hypothalamus. No data are available on its use in breastfeeding mothers.

T 1/2	3-6 h	MW	368 Da	PB	91%
Tmax	1-3 h	RID		Vd	
Oral		M/P		pKa	1.95, 7.5

Adult Concerns: Drowsiness, headache, dry mouth, sweating, abdominal pain, jaundice, weight gain.

Adult Dose: 25 mg three times a day.

Pediatric Concerns: Fatigue and slight hair loss have been reported from direct use of cinnarizine in children. No reports of complications via breast milk.

Infant Monitoring: Sedation or irritability, not waking to feed/poor feeding, weight gain, and extrapyramidal symptoms.

Alternatives:

References:
1. Pharmaceutical manufacturer prescribing information.

CIPROFLOXACIN

Trade: Ciloxan, Cipro, Ciproxin

Category: Antibiotic, Quinolone

LRC: L3 - Limited Data-Probably Compatible

Ciprofloxacin is a fluoroquinolone antibiotic primarily used for gram-negative coverage. Levels secreted into breast milk are variable, some reported levels exceed maternal concentrations. In a study of 10 women who received ciprofloxacin 750 mg every 12 hours for three doses the milk levels were ranged from 3.79 mg/L at 2 hours post third dose to 0.02 mg/L at 24 hours post third dose.[1] The maternal serum concentrations were lower, 2.06 mg/L at 2 hours post third dose to 0.02 mg/L at 24 hours post third dose.

In another study of a patient receiving 500 mg orally at bedtime, the concentrations about 11 hours postdose in maternal serum and breast milk on day 10 of therapy were 0.21 µg/mL and 0.98 µg/mL, respectively.[2] Plasma levels were undetectable (<0.03 µg/mL) in the infant. The dose to the 4-month-old infant was estimated to be 0.92 mg/day or 0.15 mg/kg/day. No adverse effects were noted in this infant.

In a patient 17 days postpartum, with acute kidney injury requiring dialysis, who received a 500 mg oral dose of ciprofloxacin, levels in milk were 3.02, 3.02, 3.02, and 1.98 mg/L at 4, 8, 12, and 16 hours postdose respectively.[3]

There has been one case of severe pseudomembranous colitis in an infant of a mother who self-medicated with ciprofloxacin for 6 days before the onset of the child's symptoms.[4] This 2-month-old girl had a history of necrotizing enterocolitis requiring a 14 day hospital admission. She presented with a 1 day history of decreased intake, fever, foul smelling diarrhea, and a distended and tender abdomen. She was found to have Clostridium difficile toxin positive stool and histopathologic confirmation of pseudomembranous colitis. After treatment for C. difficile, the infant was reported to be well.

Current studies seem to suggest that the amount of ciprofloxacin present in milk is quite low; however, if other oral antibiotic alternatives would be suitable to treat the maternal infection, this would be preferred as there is limited safety data in pediatric and breastfeeding patients. Ciprofloxacin is available in several ophthalmic preparations, where the absorption and clinical dose is minimal. As the absolute dose presented to the nursing mother is minimal, ophthalmic formulations would not be contraindicated in breastfeeding mothers.

T 1/2	4.1 h	MW	331 Da	PB	40%
Tmax	0.5-2.3 h	RID	0.44%-6.34%	Vd	2.1-2.7 L/kg
Oral	50%-85%	M/P	>1	pKa	7.1

Adult Concerns: Dizziness, restlessness, QTc prolongation, nausea, vomiting, diarrhea, abdominal cramps, gastrointestinal bleeding, changes in liver function. Several cases of tendon rupture have been noted.

Adult Dose: 500 mg BID.

Pediatric Concerns: Pseudomembranous colitis in one breastfed infant.[4] Tooth discoloration at 12-23 months of age was reported in two infants given the medication when less than 4 weeks of age.[5,6] The association of ciprofloxacin with tooth discoloration requires further evaluation.

Infant Monitoring: Vomiting, diarrhea, changes in gastrointestinal flora and rash.

Alternatives: Amoxicillin(L1), Cephalexin(L1), Nitrofurantoin(L2)

References:
1. Giamarellou H, Kolokythas E, Petrikkos G, Gazis J, Aravantinos D, Sfikakis P. Pharmacokinetics of three newer quinolones in pregnant and lactating women. Am J Med. 1989;87(5A):49S-51S.
2. Gardner DK, Gabbe SG, Harter C. Simultaneous concentrations of ciprofloxacin in breast milk and in serum in mother and breastfed infant. Clin Pharm. 1992;11(4):352-354.
3. Cover DL, Mueller BA. Ciprofloxacin penetration into human breast milk: a case report. DICP. 1990;24(7-8):703-704.

4. Harmon T, Burkhart G, Applebaum H. Perforated pseudomembranous colitis in the breast-fed infant. J Pediatr Surg. 1992;27(6):744-746.

5. Lumbiganon P, Pengsaa K, Sookpranee T. Ciprofloxacin in neonates and its possible adverse effect on the teeth. Pediatr Infect Dis J. 1991;10(8):619-620.

6. Ghaffar F, McCracken GH. Quinolones in pediatrics. In: Hooper DC, Rubinstein E, eds. Quinolone Antimicrobial Agents. Washington, DC: ASM Press; 2003:343-354.

CISAPRIDE

Trade: Prepulsid, Propulsid

Category: Stimulant, Gastrointestinal

LRC: L4 - Limited Data-Possibly Hazardous

Cisapride is a gastrointestinal stimulant used to increase lower esophageal sphincter pressure and increase the rate of gastric emptying. It is frequently used in gastroesophageal reflux.[1] It is often preferred over metoclopramide (Reglan) due to the lack of CNS side effects. CNS concentrations are generally two- or three-fold less than the serum levels. It is frequently used in pediatric patients and neonates.

Breast milk levels following a maternal dose of 60 mg/day for 4 days averaged 6.2 µg/L while maternal plasma levels averaged 137 µg/L.[2] The dose of cisapride absorbed in breastfeeding infants would be expected to be 600-800 times lower than the usual therapeutic dose. Manufacturers' internal data suggest that breast milk levels are less than 5% of maternal plasma levels (approximately 2.2 to 3.0 µg/L).[3]

T 1/2	7-10 h	MW	466 Da	PB	98%
Tmax	1-2 h	RID	0.1%	Vd	
Oral	35%-40%	M/P	0.045	pKa	14.58

Adult Concerns: Diarrhea, abdominal pain, cramping.

Adult Dose: 10 mg QID.

Pediatric Concerns: None reported via milk.

Infant Monitoring: D

Alternatives:

References:

1. McCallum RW, Prakash C, Campoli-Richards DM, Goa KL. Cisapride. A preliminary review of its pharmacodynamic and pharmacokinetic properties, and therapeutic use as a prokinetic agent in gastrointestinal motility disorders. Drugs. 1988;36(6):652-681.

2. Hofmeyr GJ, Sonnendecker EW. Secretion of the gastrokinetic agent cisapride in human milk. Eur J Clin Pharmacol. 1986;30(6):735-736.

3. Janssen Pharmaceuticals, personal communication. 1996.

CISATRACURIUM BESYLATE

Trade: Nimbex

Category: Skeletal Muscle Relaxant

LRC: L3 - No Data-Probably Compatible

Cisatracurium is a nondepolarizing skeletal muscle relaxant for intravenous administration. It acts to block cholinergic receptors, blocking neuromuscular transmission. The neuromuscular blockade produced by cisatracurium besylate is readily antagonized by anticholinesterase agents once recovery has started. In general, the more profound the neuromuscular block at the time of reversal, the longer the time required for recovery of neuromuscular function. Compared to other neuromuscular blocking agents, it is intermediate in its onset and duration of action. Due to its limited half-life and large molecular weight, its transmission to human milk is probably minimal. It is unlikely to be absorbed orally in an infant.

T 1/2	22-29 min	MW	1243.387 Da	PB	Unknown
Tmax		RID		Vd	145 L/kg
Oral	Nil	M/P		pKa	

Adult Concerns: Bradycardia, hypotension, flushing, bronchospasm, rash, weakness.

Adult Dose: Intravenous: 1-3 mcg/kg/minute but highly variable.

Pediatric Concerns:

Infant Monitoring: Bradycardia, hypotension, flushing, bronchospasm, rash, weakness.

Alternatives:

References:

1. Pharmaceutical manufacturers prescribing information.

CISPLATIN

Trade: Abiplatin, Bioplatino, C-Platin, Cis-Gry, Cisplatin, Placis

Category: Anticancer

LRC: L5 - Limited Data-Hazardous

Cisplatin is a platinum-containing anticancer agent. Platinum agents have high affinity for plasma proteins, approximately 90% of the platinum is bound to plasma proteins within 3 hours after a bolus injection.[1] Following administration of radioactive cisplatin, cisplatin levels were eliminated in a biphasic manner. T(alpha) was 25 to 49 minutes, T(beta) was 58 to 73 hours. Estimates of the terminal elimination half-life of total plasma platinum range between 36 to 47 days.[2] Platinum penetrates into tissues and is irreversibly bound to tissue proteins (highest concentration in kidney, liver, slightly less in bladder, muscles, pancreas and lowest in bowel, heart, lung, and brain). Platinum can be found in these tissues for up to 180 days.[2]

Plasma and breast milk samples were collected from a 24-year-old woman treated for 5 days with cisplatin (30 mg/m^2 infused IV over 4 h).[3] On the third day of cisplatin treatment, 30 minutes prior to chemotherapy, platinum levels in milk were 0.9 mg/L and plasma levels were 0.8 mg/L, giving a milk/plasma ratio of 1:1. In another study, no cisplatin was found in breast milk, following a dose of 100 mg/m^2.[4] Another case report suggests that milk levels are tenfold lower than serum levels in a 43-year-old woman, still breastfeeding 2 years postpartum, given 100 mg (60 mg/m^2; levels drawn after cycle 2 of 6; milk/plasma ratio-0.1).[5] Although these studies have variable results, they generally support the recommendation that mothers should not breastfeed while undergoing cisplatin therapy or withhold breastfeeding for many days (>20-30 days).

Eight women diagnosed with cervical cancer in their pregnancy were treated with cisplatin 20 mg/m^2; three samples of cisplatin in breast milk were obtained in the first few days postpartum.[6] The breast milk samples ranged from 0.2, 1.4, and 5.55 μg/L or 0.9, 2.3, and 9% of maternal blood concentrations. None of the infants were breastfed in this study due to the presence of the drug in breast milk.

In 2013, another case report was published that followed platinum until its disappearance in breast milk.[7] In this case, a 29-year-old woman had a c-section and radical hysterectomy at 37 weeks for stage IB1 adenocarcinoma of the uterine cervix (diagnosed at 20 weeks). She was given radiation plus weekly cisplatin 40 mg/m^2 starting at 6 weeks postpartum (cisplatin 70 mg IV weekly x 4 cycles + 1 additional dose). The patient had milk samples taken from both breasts at 4.25, 9.25, 13, 16.83, 21, 25, 28.67, 33.33, 40.75, 45.17, 48.58, 51.17, 57, 65.83, and 69.58 hours after the first dose. The patient pumped and dumped her milk for 1 week after her first dose and then discontinued breastfeeding after this point because of maternal side effects. The authors found that cisplatin was quantifiable for the first 13 hours postdose and remained above the limits of detection (2.5 μg/L) for up to 57 hours. The concentrations became undetectable at 66 and 70 hours postdose and were not measured after that. The authors calculated that an exclusively breastfed infant would receive 8.8 μg/day (range 7.3-10.3 μg/day); the relative infant dose was 0.29%-0.4%. The authors of this case report suggest that with repeated dosing cisplatin could accumulate in milk; however, they believe it is reasonable to withhold breast milk for 72 hours postdose and then resume breastfeeding.

Although the literature is highly variable, two options are suggested. One, the breast milk should be tested for platinum levels and not used as long as they are measurable. Or two, without measuring platinum levels, breastfeeding should be interrupted for at least 20 days for low doses as above, or much longer (permanently) for higher doses.

T 1/2	Cis: 0.5 h; plat: 36-47 days	MW	300 Da	PB	Platinum 90%
Tmax		RID	0.01%-39.71%	Vd	0.3-1.1 L/kg
Oral	poor	M/P		pKa	6.56

Adult Concerns: Encephalopathy, neuropathy, seizure, ototoxicity, tinnitus, nausea, vomiting, changes in liver or renal function, changes in electrolytes, myelosuppression, anemia, leukopenia, thrombocytopenia.

Adult Dose: Highly variable.

Pediatric Concerns: No case reports of infant adverse effects in lactation at this time (in lactation data thus far infants were not breastfed).

Infant Monitoring: General recommendation is to avoid breastfeeding; should patient resume breastfeeding 3-5 days after the last dose of maternal therapy, monitor the infant for difficulty swallowing/reflux, vomiting, diarrhea, constipation. Lab work could be drawn if clinical signs of liver or renal dysfunction, anemia, thrombocytopenia or an inability to fight infection.

Alternatives:

References:

1. DeConti RC, Toftness BR, Lange RC, et al. Clinical and pharmacological studies with cis-diamminedichloroplatinum (II). Cancer Res. 1973;33:1310-1315.
2. Pharmaceutical manufacturers prescribing information.
3. de Vries EGE, van der Zee AGJ, Uges DRA, et al. Excretion of cisplatin into breast milk. Lancet. 1989;1:497.
4. Egan PC, Costanza ME, Dodion P, et al. Doxorubicin and cisplatin excretion into human milk. Cancer Treat Rep. 1985;69:1387-1389.
5. Ben-Baruch G, Menczer J, Goshen R, et al. Cisplatin excretion in human milk. J Natl Cancer Inst. 1992;84:451-452.
6. Lanowska M, Kohler C, Oppelt P, et al. Addressing concerns about cisplatin application during pregnancy. J Perinat Med. 2001;39:279-285.
7. Hays K, Ryu RJ, Swisher EM, et al. Duration of cisplatin excretion in breast milk. J Hum Lact. 2013;29(4);469-472.

CITALOPRAM

Trade: Celexa, Cipram, Talohexal

Category: Antidepressant, SSRI

LRC: L2 - Limited Data-Probably Compatible

Citalopram is an SSRI antidepressant. SSRIs are the drugs of choice for use in depression and anxiety disorders during pregnancy and lactation. In general, these medications are more compatible with breastfeeding than tricyclic antidepressants.[1]

In one study of a 21-year-old patient receiving 20 mg citalopram per day, citalopram levels in milk peaked at 3-9 hours following administration.[2] Peak milk levels varied during the day, but the mean daily concentration was 298 nM (range 270-311 nM). The milk/serum ratio was approximately 3. The metabolite, desmethylcitalopram, was present in milk in low levels (23-28 nM). The concentration of metabolite in milk varied little during the day. Assuming a milk intake of 150 mL/kg, approximately 272 nM (88 μg or 16 ng/kg) of citalopram was passed to the baby each day. This amounts to only 0.4% of the dose administered to the mother. At 3 weeks, maternal serum levels of citalopram were 185 nM, compared to the infants plasma level of just 7 nM. No untoward effects were noted in this breastfed infant.

In another study, a milk/serum ratio of 1.16 to 1.88 was reported.[3] This study suggests the infant would ingest 4.3 μg/kg/day and a relative dose of 0.7% to 5.9% of the weight-adjusted maternal dose.

In another study of seven women receiving an average of 0.41 mg/kg/day citalopram, the average peak level (C_{max}) of citalopram was 154 μg/L and 50 μg/L for desmethylcitalopram (metabolite is eight times less potent than citalopram).[4] However, average milk concentrations (AUC) were lower and averaged 97 μg/L for citalopram and 36 μg/L for desmethylcitalopram during the dosing interval. The mean peak milk/plasma AUC ratio was 1.8 for citalopram. Low concentrations of citalopram (around 2-2.3 μg/L) were detected in only three of the seven infant plasmas. No adverse effects were found in any of the infants. The authors estimate the daily intake to be approximately 3.7% of the maternal dose.

In a study of a single patient starting citalopram 40 mg a day 4 weeks after delivery, the concentration in milk and serum were 205 μg/L and 98.9 ng/mL respectively.[5] Infant serum levels were 12.7 ng/mL. This infant was noted to have "uneasy" sleep patterns, which normalized upon lowering the maternal dose and using partial formula supplementation.

In a recent study of 31 women who were consuming citalopram while breastfeeding, no significant differences were noted in infant side effect profiles as compared to depressed and nondepressed control patients who were not consuming citalopram.[6] Of the side effects reported, one infant had colic, decreased feeding, and irritability/restlessness was reported and the other infant had irritability and restlessness. The authors recommend to continue breastfeeding while the mother is taking citalopram therapy.

Eleven mothers taking citalopram and their babies were monitored during pregnancy and lactation. Plasma and milk samples were taken that suggested citalopram and its metabolite concentrations in milk were 2-3 times higher than in maternal plasma, but infant plasma levels were very low or undetectable.[7]

In a case where an infant was exposed to citalopram 60 mg daily and ziprasidone 40 mg daily in utero and breast milk, the infant was reported to have no adverse effects from medication exposure in breast milk and the pediatrician reported that the infant had met all milestones by 6 months of age.[8] At 2, 9, and 18 weeks the pediatrician did not find symptoms of medication withdrawal or drug-related concerns from in-utero exposure. The mother breastfed for the first 6 months postnatally and no concerns with growth or development were noted by the pediatrician.

There is a case during which an infant exposed to citalopram in utero and through breast milk exhibited irregular breathing, apnea, abnormal sleep, and hypotonia starting on day 1 of life.[9] These symptoms resolved spontaneously after about 3 weeks; therefore, this infant may have been experiencing SSRI withdrawal, rather than side effects of breast milk exposure. These adverse effects have been associated with SSRI use in utero, and infants may need to be monitored if such effects occur after birth.

In a second case where an infant was reported to experience neonatal withdrawal syndrome after in utero exposure, the mother was taking 20-30 mg/day.[10] The symptoms started upon delivery, and the child was discharged at day 7 with no medical treatment needed. Measurements were taken in a breastfed infant at periodic intervals up to 53 days after delivery. Serum concentrations of citalopram were taken from both the infant and the mother and the ratios were compared. The infant's serum showed 1.4%-1.8% of the mother's citalopram concentrations, with absolute ranges of 3.7-7.1 nM. This analysis further showed that the concentrations of citalopram in breast milk were roughly twice that found in the mother's serum.

While the original anecdotal data suggested that symptoms such as somnolence, colic, and restlessness may occur in breastfed infants exposed to citalopram, the majority of new data suggest these symptoms are minimal and may not be associated with the use of this drug in lactation. However, recent data on escitalopram suggests it could be a better alternative.

T 1/2	36 h	MW	405 Da	PB	80%
Tmax	2-4 h	RID	3.56%-5.37%	Vd	12 L/kg
Oral	80%	M/P	1.16-3	pKa	9.59

Adult Concerns: Headache, dizziness, insomnia, anxiety, increased salivation, tachycardia, hypotension, flatulence, diarrhea, constipation, nausea, vomiting, and tremor. Doses higher than 40 mg have been reported to cause a prolonged QTc interval and a higher risk of developing Torsade de Pointes, especially when used in combination with other medications that can also prolong QTc.

Adult Dose: 20-40 mg daily.

Pediatric Concerns: There have been two cases of breastfed infants having had changes in sleep, breathing, and muscle tone. In one of these cases the adverse effects may have been due to withdrawal from in-utero exposure. The majority of studies show no or limited side effects in breastfed infants.

Infant Monitoring: Sedation or irritability, not waking to feed/poor feeding, and weight gain.

Alternatives: Sertraline(L2), Escitalopram(L2)

References:

1. Briggs G, Freeman RK, Yaffe SJ. Drugs in Pregnancy and Lactation: A Reference Guide to fetal and Neonatal Risk. 6th ed. Philadelphia, PA: Lippincott Williams & Wilkins; 2002.
2. Jensen PN, Olesen OV, Bertelsen A, Linnet K. Citalopram and desmethylcitalopram concentrations in breast milk and in serum of mother and infant. Ther Drug Monit. 1997;19(2):236-239.
3. Spigset O, Carieborg L, Ohman R, Norstrom A. Excretion of citalopram in breast milk. Br J Clin Pharmacol. 1997;44(3):295-298.
4. Rampono J, Kristensen JH, Hackett LP, Paech M, Kohan R, Ilett KF. Citalopram and demethylcitalopram in human milk; distribution, excretion and effects in breast fed infants. Br J Clin Pharmacol. 2000;50(3):263-268.
5. Schmidt K, Olesen OV, Jensen PN. Citalopram and breast-feeding: serum concentration and side effects in the infant. Biol Psychiatry. 2000;47(2):164-165.
6. Lee A, Woo J, Ito S. Frequency of infant adverse events that are associated with citalopram use during breast-feeding. Am J Obstet Gynecol. January 2004;190(1):218-221.
7. Heikkinen T, Ekblad U, Kero P, Ekblad S, Laine K. Citalopram in pregnancy and lactation. Clin Pharmacol Ther. 2002;72(2):184-191.
8. Werremeyer A. Ziprasidone and citalopram use in pregnancy and lactation in a woman with psychotic depression. Am J Psychiatry. 2009;166(11):1298.
9. Franssen EJ, Meijs V, Ettaher F, Valerio PG, Keessen M, Lameijer W. Citalopram serum and milk levels in mother and infant during lactation. Ther Drug Monit. February 2006;28(1):2-4.
10. Nordeng H, Lindemann R, Perminov KV, Reikvam A. Neonatal withdrawal syndrome after in utero exposure to selective serotonin reuptake inhibitors. Acta Paediatr. 2001;90:288-291.

CLADRIBINE

Trade: Leustat, Leustatin, Litak, Mavenclad

Category: Antineoplastic

LRC: L5 - No Data-Hazardous

Cladribine is a purine nucleoside analog used to treat various forms of leukemia and is currently under investigation for treatment of multiple sclerosis.[1] At this time there are no data regarding the entry of cladribine into human milk. Based on this medications small molecular weight (285 Da), and poor protein binding (20%), we anticipate this medication will enter milk.

Due to the potential for serious adverse effects with this medication, including myelosuppression, an increased risk of serious infection, and potential neuropathy with high doses this medication is not recommended for use in lactation. At this time, women should withhold breastfeeding for a minimum period of 48 hours after the last dose of medication. This recommended time period should be extended in those with poor renal function.

T 1/2	5.4-6.7 h	MW	285.7 Da	PB	20%
Tmax		RID		Vd	4.5-9 L/kg
Oral	37%-51%	M/P		pKa	13.89

Adult Concerns: Headache, fatigue, fever, nausea, vomiting, changes in renal function, anemia, neutropenia, thrombocytopenia, infection, severe rash.

Adult Dose: Varies by indication.

Pediatric Concerns:

Infant Monitoring: Withhold breastfeeding for a minimum period of 48 hours or longer if maternal renal dysfunction.

Alternatives:

References:
1. Pharmaceutical manufacturers prescribing information.

CLARITHROMYCIN

Trade: Biaxin, Klacid, Klaricid

Category: Antibiotic, Macrolide

LRC: L1 - Limited Data-Compatible

Clarithromycin is a macrolide antibiotic. In a study of 12 mothers receiving 250 mg twice daily, the C_{max} occurred at 2.2 hours and was reported to be 0.85 mg/L.[1] The estimated average dose of clarithromycin via milk was reported to be 150 µg/kg/day, or 2% of the maternal dose. Clarithromycin is probably compatible with breastfeeding.

T 1/2	5-7 h	MW	748 Da	PB	40%-70%
Tmax	1.7 h	RID	2.1%	Vd	3-4 L/kg
Oral	50%	M/P	>1	pKa	8.38, 12.46

Adult Concerns: Diarrhea, nausea, dyspepsia, abdominal pain, metallic taste.

Adult Dose: 250-500 mg BID.

Pediatric Concerns: None reported via milk. Pediatric indications are available.

Infant Monitoring: Vomiting, diarrhea, changes in gastrointestinal flora and rash.

Alternatives:

References:
1. Sedlmayr T, Peters F, Raasch W, Kees F. Clarithromycin, a new macrolide antibiotic. Effectiveness in puerperal infections and pharmacokinetics in breast milk. Geburtshilfe Frauenheilkd. July 1993;53(7):488-491.

CLEMASTINE

Trade: Dayhist Allergy, Tavist

Category: Antihistamine

LRC: L4 - Limited Data-Possibly Hazardous

Clemastine is a long-acting antihistamine. Following a maternal dose of 1 mg twice daily, a 10-week-old breastfeeding infant developed drowsiness, irritability, refusal to feed, and neck stiffness.[1] Levels in milk and plasma (20 hours post dose) were 5-10 µg/L (milk) and 20 µg/L (plasma) respectively.

T 1/2	10-12 h	MW	344 Da	PB	95%
Tmax	2-5 h	RID	5.2%	Vd	11.4 L/kg
Oral	100%	M/P	0.25-0.5	pKa	

Adult Concerns: Drowsiness, headache, fatigue, nervousness, appetite increase, depression.

Adult Dose: 1.34 to 2.68 mg BID or TID.

Pediatric Concerns: Drowsiness, irritability, refusal to feed, and neck stiffness in one infant. Increased risk of seizures.

Infant Monitoring: Drowsiness or irritability and changes in feeding.

Alternatives: Cetirizine, Loratadine(L1)

References:
1. Kok TH, Taitz LS, Bennett MJ, Holt DW. Drowsiness due to clemastine transmitted in breast milk. Lancet. 1982;1(8277):914-915.

CLIDINIUM BROMIDE

Trade:

Category: Anticholinergic

LRC: L3 - No Data-Probably Compatible

Clidinium bromide has anticholinergic properties giving pronounced antispasmodic and antisecretory effects on the gastrointestinal tract. In the United States, it is only available as an oral formulation in combination with chlordiazepoxide.

Clidinium is incompletely absorbed from the small intestine and is rapidly hydrolyzed in the liver to form its quaternary amino alcohol.[1] As a quaternary ammonium compound it is fully ionized, and as such has very limited lipid solubility. This in turn does not allow clidinium to cross the blood-brain barrier. High ionization does, however, cause it to exert a high nicotinic effect when compared to some other antimuscarinic agents.

It is currently unknown if clidinium is excreted into breast milk. Other antimuscarinic drugs have shown some data regarding transfer to milk, but so far no substantial evidence has been found to support that claim.

T 1/2	1.2/20 h, biphasic	MW	432.4 Da	PB	
Tmax		RID		Vd	
Oral	Incompletely absorbed	M/P		pKa	

Adult Concerns: Headache, drowsiness, nervousness, mental confusion, insomnia, dizziness, blurred vision, dry mouth, palpitations, constipation, urinary hesitancy, allergic urticaria, decreased sweating, lactation suppression, increased intraocular tension, cycloplegia, mydriasis.

Adult Dose: 2.5-5 mg three to four times daily.

Pediatric Concerns:

Infant Monitoring: Drowsiness or insomnia, dry mouth, constipation, urinary retention, weight gain.

Alternatives:

References:
1. McEvoy GE, ed. AHFS Drug Information. Bethesda, MD: American Society of Health-System Pharmacists, Inc.; 1959-2011, Selected Revisions May 2008.

CLINDAMYCIN

Trade: Cleocin, Clindacin

Category: Antibiotic, Other

LRC: L2 - Limited Data-Probably Compatible

Clindamycin hydrochloride is a broad-spectrum antibiotic frequently used for anaerobic infections. In one study of two nursing mothers given 600 mg IV every 6 hours, the concentration of clindamycin in breast milk was 3.1 to 3.8 mg/L at 0.2 to 0.5 hours after dosing.[1]

Following oral doses of 300 mg every 6 hours, the breast milk levels averaged 1 to 1.7 mg/L at 1.5 to 7 hours after dosing. In another study of two to three women who received a single oral dose of 150 mg, milk levels averaged 0.9 mg/L at 4 hours with a milk/plasma ratio of 0.47.[2]

There has been one case report of an infant with "two grossly bloody stools" on day 5 of maternal antibiotic therapy (antibiotic therapy ended hours before infants symptoms occurred).[3] The mother was receiving clindamycin 600 mg IV q6h and gentamicin 80 mg IV q8h for endometritis; however, it should be noted that the infant was also on

48 hours of ampicillin and gentamicin, while neonatal sepsis was ruled out, at the same time the mother was receiving her treatment. The infant temporarily stopped breastfeeding for 12 hours and symptoms resolved (8 month follow-up - no further concerns).

In a study by Steen in five breastfeeding patients who received 150 mg three times daily for 7 days, milk concentrations ranged from <0.5 to 3.1 mg/L with the majority of levels being <0.5 mg/L.[4]

In a study of 15 women who received 600 mg clindamycin intravenously, levels of clindamycin in milk averaged 1.03 mg/L at 2 hours following the dose.[5]

Lotions or ointments of clindamycin meant for topical application contain clindamycin phosphate equivalent to 10 mg/mL. Transcutaneous absorption is minimal (<1%-4%) and reported plasma levels are low to nil. Some does appear in urine of treated patients. Due to low maternal plasma levels, virtually none should be expected in breast milk and the amount in milk is unlikely to harm a breastfeeding infant.

T 1/2	2.4 h	MW	425 Da	PB	94%
Tmax	45-60 min	RID	0.9%-1.8%	Vd	2 L/kg
Oral	90%	M/P	0.47	pKa	7.45

Adult Concerns: Diarrhea, rash, pseudomembranous colitis, nausea, vomiting, gastrointestinal cramps.

Adult Dose: 150-450 mg every 6 hours.

Pediatric Concerns: One case of pseudomembranous colitis has been reported. Commonly used in pediatric anaerobic infections; the current pediatric dosage is 10-40 mg/kg/day divided every 6-8 hours.[6]

Infant Monitoring: Vomiting, diarrhea, changes in gastrointestinal flora, and rash.

Alternatives:

References:
1. Smith JA, Morgan JR, Rachlis AR, Papsin FR. Clindamycin in human breast milk. Can Med Assn J. 1975;112:806.
2. Matsuda S. Transfer of antibiotics into maternal milk. Biol Res Pregnancy Perinatol. 1984;5(2):57-60.
3. Mann CF. Clindamycin and breast-feeding. Pediatrics. 1980;66(6):1030-1031.
4. Steen B, Rane A. Clindamycin passage into human milk. Br J Clin Pharmacol. 1982;13(5):661-664.
5. Zhang Y, Zhang Q, Xu Z. Tissue and body fluid distribution of antibacterial agents in pregnant and lactating women. Zhonghua Fu Chan Ke Za Zhi. 1997;32:288-292.
6. Johnson KB, ed. The Harriet Lane Handbook. 13th ed. Maryland Heights, MO: Mosby Publishing; 1993.

CLINDAMYCIN TOPICAL

Trade: Cleocin T, Clinderm, ClindaMax, Clindagel, Clindatech, Dalacin T

Category: Antibiotic, Other

LRC: L2 - Limited Data-Probably Compatible

Clindamycin is a broad-spectrum antibiotic frequently used for anaerobic infections.[1] Lotions or ointments of clindamycin meant for topical application contain clindamycin phosphate equivalent to 10 mg/mL. Transcutaneous absorption is minimal (<1%-4%) and reported plasma levels are low to nil. Some does appear in urine of treated patients. Due to low maternal plasma levels, virtually none should be expected in breast milk. The amount in milk is unlikely to harm a breastfeeding infant.

T 1/2	1.5-2.6 h	MW		PB	
Tmax	10-14 h	RID		Vd	
Oral	None	M/P		pKa	

Adult Concerns: Headache, nausea, diarrhea, vomiting, abdominal pain, erythema, burning, itching, dryness, hypersensitivity.

Adult Dose: Apply topical twice daily.

Pediatric Concerns: One case of pseudomembranous colitis has been reported. It is unlikely the levels in breast milk would be clinically relevant. Commonly used in pediatric infections.

Infant Monitoring: Vomiting, diarrhea, changes in gastrointestinal flora and rash.

Alternatives:

References:
1. Pharmaceutical manufacturers prescribing information.

CLINDAMYCIN VAGINAL

Trade: Dalacin Vaginal Cream, Cleocin Vaginal

Category: Antibiotic, Other

LRC: L2 - Limited Data-Probably Compatible

Clindamycin is a broad-spectrum antibiotic frequently used for anaerobic infections. Clindamycin when administered intravenously has been found in breast milk. Only about 5% of clindamycin is absorbed into the maternal circulation, when applied vaginally (100 mg/dose), which would amount to approximately 5 mg clindamycin/day.[1] It is unlikely that clindamycin when administered via a vaginal gel would produce any significant danger to a breastfeeding infant.

T 1/2	2.9 h	MW	425 Da	PB	94%
Tmax	10-14 h	RID		Vd	
Oral	90%	M/P		pKa	

Adult Concerns: Diarrhea, rash, gastrointestinal cramps, colitis, rarely bloody diarrhea. Transient neutropenia (leukopenia), eosinophilia, agranulocytosis, and thrombocytopenia have been reported. No direct etiologic relationship to concurrent clindamycin therapy could be made in any of these reports.

Adult Dose: 100 mg intravaginally every HS for 3 days.

Pediatric Concerns: One case of pseudomembranous colitis has been reported. It is unlikely the levels in breastmilk would be clinically relevant. Commonly used in pediatric infections

Infant Monitoring: Vomiting, diarrhea, changes in gastrointestinal flora, and rash.

Alternatives:

References:
1. Pharmaceutical manufacturers prescribing information.

CLOBAZAM

Trade: Frisium, Onfi

Category: Sedative-Hypnotic

LRC: L3 - Limited Data-Probably Compatible

Clobazam is an older benzodiazepine primarily used as an adjunctive therapy to treat seizures.[1] The manufacturer reports that clobazam enters breast milk (no details provided). In a study of six women given clobazam 10 mg in the morning and 20 mg in the afternoon (milk was sampled at 2 hours postdose for 5 days), the average milk concentration on day 2 and 5 were 0.125 mg/L and 0.152 mg/L.[2,3] The maximum milk concentration was 0.33 mg/L on day 2. The average absolute infant dose reported on day 5 was 0.023 mg/kg/day (maximum infant dose 0.05 mg/kg/day). The M/P ratio of clobazam ranged from 0.13-0.36.[2] No infant data were provided in this study. Using the higher average milk concentration on day 5 we estimated the RID to be 5.3%. Please note this study was not available in English and has been summarized from other reviews.[3-5] Further, the assay was not specific for the parent (active) compound, but included the inactive metabolite.

Based on this data, short-term use of clobazam is probably compatible with breastfeeding.[3-5] Both the parent compound and its active metabolite both have rather long half-lives (36-42 hours parent drug; 71-82 hours desmethylclobazam), thus this medication has the potential to accumulate in a breastfeeding infant over time. If this medication is used, infants should be monitored for potential adverse events (e.g., sedation, poor feeding) throughout lactation.

T 1/2	36-42 h	MW	301 Da	PB	80%-90%
Tmax	0.5-4 h	RID	4.38%-5.33%	Vd	1.43 L/kg
Oral	87%	M/P	0.13-0.36	pKa	9

Adult Concerns: Sedation, drowsiness, confusion, weakness.

Adult Dose: 20-30 mg a day.

Pediatric Concerns: None reported via milk at this time.

Infant Monitoring: Sedation, slowed breathing rate, not waking to feed, poor feeding/poor sucking, and poor weight gain.

Alternatives: Lorazepam(L3), Clobazam(L3)

References:
1. Pharmaceutical manufacturers prescribing information.
2. Hajdu P, Wernicke OA. Untersuchung zur Uberprufung des Ubertritts von Frisium in die Muttermilch (Internal Report). Hoechst; 1978.
3. Bennett PN, ed. Drugs and Human Lactation. 2nd ed. Amsterdam, Netherlands: Elsevier; 1996:409-410.
4. Hagg S, Spigset O. Anticonvulsant use during lactation. Drug Saf. 2000;22(6):425-440.
5. Bar-Oz B, Nulman I, Koren G, Ito S. Anticonvulsants and breastfeeding. A critical review. Paediatr Drugs. 2000;2(2):113-126.

CLOBETASOL

Trade: Clobevate, Clobex, Cormax, Dermovate, Olux, Olux-E, Temovate, Temovate E

Category: Corticosteroid

LRC: L3 - No Data-Probably Compatible

Clobetasol propionate is a high potency topical corticosteroid used for the short-term relief of inflammation of moderate to severe corticosteroid responsive dermatoses, including psoriasis.[1] Because this is such a high potency steroid, oral absorption by an infant could be hazardous. There are reports of excretion of corticosteroids into breastmilk when administered systemically. When infants are exposed to corticosteroids through the milk there is a risk of growth suppression, though the risk for such an effect is greatest with prolonged use of high dose oral or IV corticosteroids. Do not use this on the nipple or areola of a breastfeeding mother and avoid use on large skin surfaces.

T 1/2		MW	467 Da	PB	
Tmax	2 months	RID		Vd	
Oral		M/P		pKa	13.6

Adult Concerns: Adrenal suppression, application site burning, cracking, dryness, irritation, and glucosuria.

Adult Dose: Apply twice daily.

Pediatric Concerns: Use is not recommended in children under 12 years of age. Do not use on the nipple or areola of the breast of a breastfeeding mother.

Infant Monitoring: Feeding, growth and weight gain.

Alternatives: Hydrocortisone, Mometasone(L3)

References:
1. Pharmaceutical manufacturers prescribing information.

CLOFAZIMINE

Trade: Lamprene

Category: Leprostatic

LRC: L3 - Limited Data-Probably Compatible

Clofazimine exerts a slow bactericidal effect on Mycobacterium leprae. In a study of eight female leprosy patients on clofazimine (50 mg/day or 100 mg on alternate days) for 1-18 months, blood samples were taken at 4-6 hours after the dose.[1] Average plasma and milk levels were 0.9 mg/L and 1.33 mg/L (range = 0.8 to 1.7 mg/L), respectively. The milk/plasma ratio varied from 1 to 1.7 with a mean of 1.48. A red tint and pigmentation has been reported in breastfed infants.[2,3]

T 1/2	70 days	MW	473 Da	PB	
Tmax	4-12 h	RID	14%-28.2%	Vd	High L/kg
Oral	45%-70%	M/P	1-1.7	pKa	8.37

Adult Concerns: Reversible red-brown discoloration of skin and eyes, nausea, vomiting, abdominal cramps, and pain. Splenic infarction, crystalline deposits of clofazimine in multiple organs and tissues.

Adult Dose: 100-200 mg daily.

Pediatric Concerns: Reddish discoloration of milk and infant may occur.

Infant Monitoring: Vomiting, changes in skin pigmentation.

Alternatives:

References:

1. Venkatesan K, Mathur A, Girdhar A, Girdhar BK. Excretion of clofazimine in human milk in leprosy patients. Lepr Rev. 1997;68(3):242-246.
2. Farb H, West DP, Pedvis-Leftick A. Clofazimine in pregnancy complicated by leprosy. Obstet Gynecol. 1982;59(1):122-123.
3. Freerksen E, Seydel JK. Critical comments on the treatment of leprosy and other mycobacterial infections with clofazimine. Arzneimittelforschung. 1992;42(10):1243-1245.

CLOMIPHENE

Trade: Clomid, Milophene, Serophene

Category: Gonadotropin

LRC: L4 - Limited Data-Possibly Hazardous

Clomiphene citrate is a selective estrogen receptor modulator. It appears to stimulate the release of the pituitary gonadotropins, follicle-stimulating hormone (FSH), and luteinizing hormone (LH), which result in development and maturation of the ovarian follicle, ovulation, and subsequent development and function of the corpus luteum. It has both estrogenic and anti-estrogenic effects. LH and FSH peak at 5-9 days after completing clomiphene therapy. It is closely related diethylstilbestrol, a known teratogen.

In a study of 60 postpartum women (1-4 days postpartum), clomiphene was effective in totally inhibiting lactation early postnatally and in suppressing established lactation (day 4).[1] Only 7 of 40 women receiving clomiphene to inhibit lactation had signs of congestion or discomfort. In the 20 women who received clomiphene to suppress established lactation (on day 4), a rapid amelioration of breast engorgement and discomfort was produced. After 5 days of treatment, no signs of lactation were present. In another study of 177 postpartum women, clomiphene was very effective at inhibiting lactation.[2]

Bromocriptine, stilboestrol, clomiphene, testosterone, and a placebo were given to 75 postpartum women for the suppression of puerperal lactation. An additional 15 women who breastfed their babies served as a control group.[3] Blood samples were taken for the determination of serum prolactin levels by a specific homologous double antibody radioimmunoassay. Concurrently, the clinical effectiveness of the various treatments was assessed. High levels of prolactin were found at the time of delivery. Bromocriptine effectively reduced serum prolactin and prevented lactation; stilboestrol increased serum prolactin and partially suppressed lactation; clomiphene citrate and testosterone propionate both lowered serum prolactin levels and partially suppressed lactation. The placebo showed almost no effect on serum prolactin.

Clomiphene appears in one study to be very effective in suppressing lactation when used up to 4 days postpartum. However, in another study of 10 puerperal women who received 100 mg of clomiphene orally for 7 days, beginning on day 1 postpartum, no change in maternal plasma prolactin or in milk production occurred in this group over the 7 days of the study.[4]

Its efficacy in reducing milk production in women, months after lactation is generally established, but it is believed to be minimal. However, the risk to a breastfed infant is not insignificant, particularly after prolonged exposure.

The half-life of clomiphene is prolonged, at least 5-7 days. The active isomers of clomiphene and include isomers such as Zuclomiphene and enclomiphene. These isomers peak rapidly within the first 24 hours, then decline to a prolonged but lower level which extends to many days and residues may be found in the bloodstream for up to 22 days and in stool samples even 6 weeks after intake.[5] Thus, the documented 5-7 day half-life may be much longer due to compartmental entrapment. The low but prolonged plasma levels could over time lead to significant exposure of the breastfed infant. While numerous teratologies have been reported in animal models, none thus far have been associated with its use in humans.[5] There is some evidence regarding a possible association of clomiphene exposure and fetal malformations, mainly neural tube defects and hypospadias, although these have yet to be confirmed.[6] There may be an increased risk of ovarian cancer and weight gain, although this risk seems low as well. Most of these untoward effects have yet to be confirmed.

Due to the prolonged half-life of this product, and the potential for repeated exposure over numerous cycles, breastfeeding of infants is not generally recommended.

T 1/2	5-7 days	MW	406 Da	PB	
Tmax	6 h	RID		Vd	>57 L/kg
Oral	Complete	M/P		pKa	9.31

Adult Concerns: Dizziness, insomnia, lightheadedness, hot flashes, ovarian enlargement, depression, headache, alopecia. May inhibit lactation early postpartum. This product has a long 5-7 day half-life and exposure to breastfeeding infants may be significant over many days. Breastfeeding following the use of this product is not recommended.

Adult Dose: 50 mg daily.

Pediatric Concerns: Transfer and effect on infant is unreported.

Infant Monitoring: May suppress lactation.

Alternatives:

References:
1. Masala A, Delitala G, Alagna S, Devilla L, Stoppelli I, Lo DG. Clomiphene and puerperal lactation. Panminerva Med. 1978;20(3):161-163.
2. Zuckerman H, Carmel S. The inhibition of lactation by clomiphene. J Obstet Gynaecol Br Commonw. 1973;80(9):822-823.
3. Weinstein D, Ben-David M, Polishuk WZ. Serum prolactin and the suppression of lactation. Br J Obstet Gynaecol. September 1976;83(9):679-682.
4. Canales ES, Lasso P, Soria J, Zarate A. Effect of clomiphene on prolactin secretion and lactation in puerperal women. Br J Obstet Gynaecol. October 1977;84(10):758-759.
5. Weller A, Daniel S, Koren G, Lunenfeld E, Levy A. The fetal safety of clomiphene citrate: a population-based retrospective cohort study. BJOG. October 2017;124(11):1664-1670. Epub May 15, 2017. PMID: 28334503.
6. Scaparrotta A, Chiarelli F, Verrotti A. Potential teratogenic effects of clomiphene citrate. Drug Saf. September 2017;40(9):761-769. Review. PMID: 28547654.

CLOMIPRAMINE

Trade: Anafranil, Placil

Category: Antidepressant, Tricyclic

LRC: L2 - Limited Data-Probably Compatible

Clomipramine is a tricyclic antidepressant frequently used for obsessive-compulsive disorder.[1] In one patient taking 125 mg/day, on the fourth and sixth day postpartum, milk levels were 342.7 and 215.8 µg/L respectively.[2] Maternal plasma levels were 211 and 208.4 µg/L at day 4 and 6 respectively. Milk/plasma ratios varied from 1.62 to 1.04 on day 4 to 6 respectively. Neonatal plasma levels continued to drop from a high of 266.6 ng/mL at birth to 127.6 ng/mL at day 4, to 94.8 ng/mL at day 6, to 9.8 ng/mL at 35 days.

In a study of four breastfeeding women who received doses of 75 to 125 mg/day, plasma levels of clomipramine in the breastfed infants were below the limit of detection, suggesting minimal transfer to the infant via milk.[3] No untoward effects were noted in any of the infants.

One small study that followed four groups of women prescribed TCAs throughout different stages of reproduction found no adverse events in the group of infants whose mothers were prescribed these medications in lactation.[4] This study included 21 women (1 on clomipramine) that initiated tricyclic antidepressant therapy at a mean of 10.3 weeks postpartum and breastfed on treatment for a mean of 12 weeks.

T 1/2	19-37 h	MW	315 Da	PB	96%
Tmax		RID	2.8%	Vd	17 L/kg
Oral	Complete	M/P	0.84-1.62	pKa	9.5

Adult Concerns: Drowsiness, fatigue, dry mouth, seizures, constipation, sweating, reduced appetite.

Adult Dose: 50 mg BID.

Pediatric Concerns: None reported in several studies.

Infant Monitoring: Sedation or irritability, dry mouth, not waking to feed/poor feeding, constipation, urinary retention, weight gain.

Alternatives: Sertraline(L2), Paroxetine(L2), Fluoxetine(L2)

References:
1. Pharmaceutical manufacturers prescribing information.
2. Schimmell MS, Katz EZ, Shaag Y, Pastuszak A, Koren G. Toxic neonatal effects following maternal clomipramine therapy. J Toxicol Clin Toxicol. 1991;29(4):479-484.
3. Wisner KL, Perel JM, Foglia JP. Serum clomipramine and metabolite levels in four nursing mother-infant pairs. J Clin Psychiatry. 1995;56(1):17-20.
4. Misri S, Sivertz K. Tricyclic drugs in pregnancy and lactation: a preliminary report. Int J Psychiatry Med. 1991;21:157-171.

CLONAZEPAM

Trade: Klonopin, Paxam, Rivotril

Category: Antianxiety

LRC: L3 - Limited Data-Probably Compatible

Clonazepam is a benzodiazepine anxiolytic and anticonvulsant. In one case report, milk levels varied between 11 and 13 µg/L (the maternal dose was omitted).[1] Milk/maternal serum ratio was approximately 0.33. In this report, the infant's serum level of clonazepam dropped from 4.4 µg/L at birth to 1 µg/L at 14 days while continuing to breast-feed, suggesting increasing clearance with time. In this case, excessive periodic breathing and apnea and cyanosis occurred in this infant (36 weeks gestation) at 6 hours until 10 days postpartum. The infant was exposed in utero as well as postpartum via breast milk.

In another study of a mother treated with 2 mg clonazepam twice daily, recorded peak milk concentrations of 10.7 µg/L at 4 hours postdose, and a maximum infant dose of 2.5% of the weight-adjusted maternal dose. The infant's serum level of clonazepam at days 2-4 was 4.7 µg/L.[2]

In a group of 11 mothers receiving 0.25 to 2 mg clonazepam daily, 10 of 11 breastfed infants had no detectable (limit of detection: 5-14 µg/L) clonazepam or metabolites in their serum.[3] One infant (1.9-weeks-old) had a serum concentration of 22 µg/L. Maternal dose was 0.5 mg daily.

In another study that included 124 breastfeeding women and their infants (aged 2-24 months), two infants (1.6%) were reported as having CNS depression.[4] The three most commonly taken benzodiazepines were lorazepam (52%), clonazepam (18%) and midazolam (15%). There was no correlation between infant sedation and maternal benzodiazepine dose or duration of use. The two mothers who reported infants with sedation were taking more medications that also cause similar CNS adverse effects than those without infant concerns (mean of 3.5 versus 1.7 medications).

These data suggest a low incidence of toxicity with this medication in breastfeeding infants.

T 1/2	18-50 h	MW	316 Da	PB	50%-86%
Tmax	1-4 h	RID	2.8%	Vd	1.5-4.4 L/kg
Oral	Complete	M/P	0.33	pKa	11.89

Adult Concerns: Sedation, dizziness, confusion, ataxia, apnea, hypotonia. Behavioral disturbances (in children) include aggressiveness, irritability, agitation.

Adult Dose: 0.5-1 mg TID.

Pediatric Concerns: Apnea, cyanosis, and hypotonia was reported in one infant at 6 hours postnatally to a woman consuming clonazepam throughout pregnancy. The infant had prolonged apnea, hypotonia, and repeated periodic breathing episodes up to 10 weeks of age (most likely due to in-utero exposure).[1] In another study of 11 mothers no infants had adverse events.[3]

Infant Monitoring: Sedation, slowed breathing rate, not waking to feed/poor feeding and weight gain.

Alternatives: Lorazepam(L3), Clobazam(L3)

References:
1. Fisher JB, Edgren BE, Mammel MC, Coleman JM. Neonatal apnea associated with maternal clonazepam therapy: a case report. Obstet Gynecol. 1985;66(3 suppl):34S-35S.
2. Soderman P, Matheson I. Clonazepam in breast milk. Eur J Pediatr. 1988;147(2):212-213.
3. Birnbaum CS, Cohen LS, Bailey JW, et al. Serum concentrations of antidepressants and benzodiazepines in nursing infants: a case series. Pediatrics. 1999;104:e11.
4. Kelly LE, Poon S, Madadi P, Koren G. Neonatal benzodiazepines exposure during breastfeeding. J Pediatr. 2012;161:448-451.

CLONIDINE

Trade: Catapres, Dixarit

Category: Antihypertensive

LRC: L3 - Limited Data-Probably Compatible

Clonidine is an antihypertensive that reduces sympathetic nerve activity from the brain. Clonidine is excreted in human milk minimally. In a study of nine nursing women receiving between 241.7 and 391.7 µg/day of clonidine, milk levels varied from approximately 1.8 µg/L to as high as 2.8 µg/L on postpartum day 10-14.[1] In another report following a maternal dose of 37.5 µg twice daily, maternal plasma was determined to be 0.33 ng/mL and milk level was 0.60 µg/L.[2] Clinical symptoms of neonatal toxicity are unreported and are unlikely in normal full-term infants.

Clonidine may reduce prolactin secretion and could conceivably reduce milk production early postpartum. Transdermal patches produce maternal plasma levels of 0.39, 0.84, and 1.12 ng/mL using the 3.5, 7, and 10.5 cm square patches respectively. The 3.7 square cm patch would produce maternal plasma levels equivalent to the 37.5 μg oral dose and would likely produce milk levels equivalent to the above study.

T 1/2	20-24 h	MW	230 Da	PB	20%-40%
Tmax	3-5 h	RID	0.9%-7.1%	Vd	3.2-5.6 L/kg
Oral	75%-100%	M/P	2	pKa	8.3

Adult Concerns: Headache, drowsiness, insomnia, dry mouth, hypotension, arrhythmias, constipation, changes in liver function, anorexia, urinary retention.

Adult Dose: 0.1-0.3 mg BID.

Pediatric Concerns: None reported via milk at this time.

Infant Monitoring: Drowsiness, lethargy, pallor, dry mouth, poor feeding, constipation, and weight gain; may reduce milk production by reducing prolactin secretion.

Alternatives:

References:
1. Hartikainen-Sorri AL, Heikkinen JE, Koivisto M. Pharmacokinetics of clonidine during pregnancy and nursing. Obstet Gynecol. 1987;69(4):598-600.
2. Bunjes R, Schaefer C, Holzinger D. Clonidine and breast-feeding. Clin Pharm. 1993;12(3):178-179.

CLOPIDOGREL

Trade: Plavix

Category: Platelet Aggregation Inhibitor

LRC: L3 - No Data-Probably Compatible

Clopidogrel selectively inhibits platelet adenosine diphosphate-induced platelet aggregation. It is used to prevent ischemic events in patients at risk (e.g., cardiovascular disease, strokes, myocardial infarction).

It is not known if clopidogrel transfers to human milk.[1] Although the plasma half-life is rather brief (6-8 hours), its metabolite (thiol derivative) covalently bonds to platelet receptors with a half-life of 11 days. Because it produces an irreversible inhibition of platelet aggregation, any present in milk could inhibit an infant's platelet function for a prolonged period. However, the thiol derivative of clopidogrel has but a 0.5-0.7 hour half-life. Thus patients could return to breastfeeding within 24 hours after stopping the use of clopidogrel.

T 1/2	8 h	MW	420 Da	PB	98%
Tmax	1 h	RID		Vd	
Oral	50%	M/P		pKa	5.3

Adult Concerns: Contraindicated in individuals with bleeding phenomenon.

Adult Dose: 75 mg daily.

Pediatric Concerns: None reported via milk at this time.

Infant Monitoring: Rare-bruising on the skin, blood in urine, vomit, or stool.

Alternatives:

References:
1. Pharmaceutical manufacturers prescribing information.

CLORAZEPATE

Trade: Tranxene, Tranxene-SD

Category: Antianxiety

LRC: L3 - Limited Data-Probably Compatible

Clorazepate is a typical benzodiazepine. The primary metabolite is nordiazepam. Clorazepate has a brief half-life of less than 2 hours, and is rapidly converted to the active drug, nordiazepam, and oxazepam. The active metabolite has a prolonged half-life.[1] In seven mothers who were breastfeeding early postnatally, and who received 20 mg IM clorazepate, levels of nordiazepam ranged from 7.5-15.5 µg/L 48 hours after the dose and 6-12 µg/L 4 days following the dose.[2]

T 1/2	20-160 h (metab)	MW	408 Da	PB	98%
Tmax	1 h	RID		Vd	1.7 L/kg
Oral	97%	M/P		pKa	3.32

Adult Concerns: Drowsiness, dizziness, confusion, blurred vision, dry mouth, headache, fatigue, ataxia, slurred speech.

Adult Dose: 15-60 mg/day.

Pediatric Concerns: None reported via milk at this time.

Infant Monitoring: Sedation, slowed breathing rate, not waking to feed/poor feeding, and weight gain.

Alternatives: Lorazepam(L3), Midazolam(L2)

References:
1. Pharmaceutical manufacturers prescribing information.
2. Rey E, Giraux P, d'Athis P, Turquais JM, Chavinie J, Olive G. Pharmacokinetics of the placental transfer and distribution of clorazepate and its metabolite nordiazepam in the feto-placental unit and in the neonate. Eur J Clin Pharmacol. April 17, 1979;15(3):181-185.

CLOTRIMAZOLE

Trade: Canesten, Clonea, Clotrimaderm, FemCare, Gyne-Lotrimin, Hiderm, Lotrimin AF, Trivagizole

Category: Antifungal

LRC: L2 - No Data-Probably Compatible

Clotrimazole is a broad-spectrum antifungal agent. It is generally used for candidiasis and various tinea species (athletes foot, ring worm). Clotrimazole is available in oral lozenges, topical creams, intravaginal tablets, and creams. No data are available on penetration into breast milk. However, after intravaginal administration, only 3%-10% of the drug is absorbed (peak serum level= 0.01 to 0.03 µg/mL) and even less by oral lozenge.[1] Hence, following vaginal administration it seems unlikely that levels absorbed by a breastfeeding infant would be high enough to produce untoward effects.

T 1/2	3.5-5 h	MW	345 Da	PB	
Tmax	3 h (oral)	RID		Vd	
Oral	Poor	M/P		pKa	4.7

Adult Concerns: Nausea, vomiting, changes in liver function, erythema, stinging, blistering, peeling, edema, pruritus, urticaria, burning, and general irritation of the skin. Contact dermatitis has been reported in breastfeeding women.

Adult Dose: Varies by indication.

Pediatric Concerns: None reported via milk. Limited oral absorption probably limits clinical relevance in breastfed infants.

Infant Monitoring: Vomiting, diarrhea.

Alternatives: Fluconazole(L2), Miconazole(L2)

References:
1. McEvoy GE, ed. AFHS Drug Information. Bethesda, MD: American Society of Health-System Pharmacists; 2003.

CLOXACILLIN

Trade: Alclox, Cloxapen, Kloxerate-DC, Orbenin, Tegopen

Category: Antibiotic, Penicillin

LRC: L2 - Limited Data-Probably Compatible

Cloxacillin is an oral penicillinase-resistant penicillin frequently used for peripheral (non-CNS) *Staphylococcus aureus* and *Staphylococcus epidermidis* infections, particularly mastitis. Following a single 500 mg oral dose of cloxacillin in lactating women, milk concentrations of the drug were zero to 0.2 mg/L 1 and 2 hours after the dose respectively and 0.2 to 0.4 mg/L after 6 hours.[1] Usual dose for adults is 250-500 mg four times daily for at least 10-14 days. As with most penicillins, it is unlikely these levels would be clinically relevant.

T 1/2	0.5 h	MW	475.9 Da	PB	94%
Tmax	1 h	RID	0.4%-0.8%	Vd	0.14 L/kg
Oral	50%	M/P		pKa	3.75

Adult Concerns: Rash, diarrhea, nephrotoxicity, fever, shaking, chills.

Adult Dose: 250-500 mg every 6 hours.

Pediatric Concerns: None reported but observe for gastrointestinal symptoms such as diarrhea.

Infant Monitoring: Vomiting, diarrhea, changes in gastrointestinal flora, and rash.

Alternatives:

References:
1. Matsuda S. Transfer of antibiotics into maternal milk. Biol Res Pregnancy Perinatol. 1984;5(2):57-60.

CLOZAPINE

Trade: Clozaril

Category: Antipsychotic, Atypical

LRC: L3 - Limited Data-Probably Compatible

Clozapine is an atypical antipsychotic, sedative drug somewhat similar to the phenothiazine family. In a study of one patient receiving 50 mg/day clozapine at delivery, the maternal and fetal plasma were reported to be 14.1 µg/L and 27 µg/L respectively.[1] After 24 hours postpartum, the maternal plasma level was 14.7 µg/L and maternal milk levels were 63.5 µg/L. On day 7 postpartum and receiving a dose of 100 mg/day clozapine, the maternal plasma and milk levels were 41.1 µg/L and 115.6 µg/L, respectively. From these data, it is apparent that clozapine concentrates in milk with a milk/plasma ratio of 4.3 at a dose of 50 mg/day and 2.8 at a dose of 100 mg/day. The change from day 1 to day 7 suggests that clozapine entry into mature milk is less.

T 1/2	8-12 h	MW	327 Da	PB	95%
Tmax	2.5 h	RID	1.33%-1.4%	Vd	5 L/kg
Oral	90%	M/P	2.8-4.3	pKa	7.6

Adult Concerns: Drowsiness, dizziness/vertigo, salivation, constipation, tachycardia, nausea, gastrointestinal distress, extrapyramidal symptoms, tardive dyskinesia, agranulocytosis.

Adult Dose: 300-600 mg daily.

Pediatric Concerns: None reported but use with great caution.

Infant Monitoring: Sedation or irritability, apnea, not waking to feed, poor feeding, extrapyramidal symptoms, and weight gain.

Alternatives:

References:
1. Barnas C, Bergant A, Hummer M, Saria A, Fleischhacker WW. Clozapine concentrations in maternal and fetal plasma, amniotic fluid, and breast milk. Am J Psychiatry. 1994;151(6):945.

COAGULATION FACTOR VIIa

Trade: NovoSeven RT, Niastase RT

Category: Hemostatic

LRC: L2 - No Data-Probably Compatible

Recombinant human coagulation factor VIIa (rFVIIa) is intended to promote coagulation by activating the extrinsic pathway of the coagulation cascade.[1] It is a vitamin K-dependent glycoprotein consisting of 406 amino acids and a molecular weight of 50,000 Da. The recombinant human coagulation factor VIIa is structurally similar to human plasma-derived Factor VIIa normally found in human plasma.

This is a large molecular weight protein that is very unlikely to enter milk. It is structurally similar to human plasma derived factor VIIa normally found in humans anyway.

T 1/2	1.7-2.7 h	MW	50,000 Da	PB	
Tmax		RID		Vd	0.103 L/kg
Oral	Nil	M/P		pKa	

Adult Concerns: Fever, allergic reaction, purpura, rash, hemorrhage, hemarthrosis, and hypertension.

Adult Dose: 90 µg/kg/2 hours until hemostasis is achieved.

Pediatric Concerns: None reported via milk. It is unlikely to enter milk.

Infant Monitoring:

Alternatives:

References:
1. Pharmaceutical manufacturers prescribing information.

COCAINE

Trade: Crack

Category: CNS Stimulant

LRC: L5 - Limited Data-Hazardous

Cocaine is a local anesthetic and a powerful central nervous system stimulant that increases dopamine in the brain.[1] It can be snorted, smoked, or injected and is known to have good absorption with a quick onset and brief effect because of redistribution out of the brain. It is also well known that with repeated use tolerance can develop.

Although the pharmacologic effects of cocaine are relatively brief (20-30 minutes), cocaine is metabolized and excreted over a prolonged period.[1] Urine samples can be positive for cocaine metabolites for 7 days or longer in adults. Even after the clinical effects of cocaine have subsided, breast milk contains significant quantities of Benzoylecgonine, the inactive metabolite of cocaine, so infants could test positive for cocaine metabolites in the urine for extended periods (days).[2]

Studies with exact estimates of cocaine transmission into breast milk have not been reported due to the difficulty of determining maternal dose and timing of milk samples; however, case reports demonstrating transmission of this drug and its metabolites into milk do exist. In the first case, a mother reported using 0.5 g of cocaine intranasally over 4 hours and breastfed her infant five times during this period.[2] The infant became irritable with vomiting/diarrhea, and had difficulty focusing on the mothers face with dilated pupils. Three hours after the last breastfeed the infant was brought to ER for increased irritability. On examination the infant was tremulous, irritable, tachycardic, tachypneic, and hypertensive with an increased startling response. The infants pupils were dilated with a poor response to light and reflexes were increased. The infant was treated with fluid and given formula, the symptoms resolved over 24-48 hours. The mothers milk had ~10 µg/L of cocaine and ~400 µg/L of benzoylecgonine at 12 hours postdose. Her milk samples were undetectable for both drug and metabolite by 36 hours after use. The infants urine contained ~120 µg/L of cocaine and ~875 µg/L of benzoylecgonine at 12 hours post maternal dose. The infants urine test was clear by 60 hours and the infant was discharged home with a normal neurological exam.

In a second case, a mother reported using cocaine 3 days prior to delivery, her milk was tested 6 days postdose and found to have 8 µg/L of cocaine. The authors of this report speculated that if the mother had used 0.5 g of cocaine the infant would have received about 0.48 mg/L of cocaine in milk or 1.62% of the maternal dose. [3]

In addition, an older case series tested the milk of two women known to use cocaine in pregnancy.[4] In the first case, the woman had used cocaine in the pregnancy and on day 13 postpartum her milk tested positive for cocaine and benzoylecgonine, subsequently a maternal urine test was sent (about 30 hours post milk sample) and was also positive. The authors were unable to report the timing of last use or quantify the amount of cocaine or its metabolite in milk. In their second case, the woman had a history of drug abuse and a positive urine drug screen the day prior to delivery. Her milk sample tested negative for cocaine 6 days after delivery.

A 2011 study that verified a method to quantify illicit substances in human milk obtained one milk sample from a woman using cocaine in lactation. Her milk sample contained 5 µg/L of cocaine, all of the metabolites were undetectable.[5] No details were provided regarding maternal dose, timing of use and milk sample or infant outcomes in this paper.

In a study of 11 mothers who admitted prior use of cocaine during pregnancy, cocaine was detected in six of the eleven milk samples taken as soon as possible after delivery.[6] The highest concentration of cocaine and its inactive metabolites in milk were provided from one woman who reported using cocaine 5 days prior to delivery. Her milk sample contained: cocaine 12.13 µg/mL, benzoylecgonine 4.07 µg/mL, norcocaine trace amounts, ecgonine methyl ester 0.119 µg/mL.

In addition, a mother of an 11-day-old infant applied cocaine powder to her nipples as an analgesic.[7] The woman initially bottle fed her infant but the infant vomited so she breastfed her son and put him to sleep. Three hours following breastfeeding, she discovered the infant choking, blue, and gasping for air. The infant had flexed limbs and his eyes "rolled back"; the father initiated CPR and the infant was taken to the ER. Upon examination the infant was in tachyarrhythmia, hypertensive, ashen, and cyanotic with irregular respirations. The infant was in status epilepticus by the time he was admitted to PICU. He required intubation and treatment of his seizures. Symptoms resolved and the infant was discharged about 5 days later. On follow-up he as reported to have normal development and growth at 6 months of age. Topical application to nipples is EXTREMELY dangerous and is contraindicated in lactation.

Breastfeeding mothers should avoid cocaine use. In those individuals who have used cocaine, a minimum pump and discard period of 24 hours is recommended before breastfeeding could be considered.[1-8] Additional concerns with cocaine use in lactation also need to be assessed prior to initiating breastfeeding such as risk factors for HIV and the potential for subsequent use.

T 1/2	5 min-1 h	MW	303 Da	PB	91%
Tmax	5-60 min	RID		Vd	1.6-2.7 L/kg
Oral	~35%	M/P		pKa	8.6

Adult Concerns: Agitation, nervousness, restlessness, euphoria, hallucinations, seizures, respiratory depression, hypertension, arrhythmias, cardia events, decreased appetite, nausea, vomiting, tremors.

Adult Dose:

Pediatric Concerns: Adverse effects have been reported with exposure from drug in breast milk and from drug used topically on the maternal nipple. Seizures, irritability, dilated pupils, choking, gasping, tachypnea, tachycardia, hypertension, vomiting, diarrhea, tremulousness, hyperactive startle reflex.[2,7]

Infant Monitoring: AVOID in lactation.

Alternatives:

References:

1. National Institute of Health. National Institute on Drug Abuse Drug Facts: cocaine; 2013. https://www.drugabuse.gov/publications/drugfacts/cocaine. Accessed March 25, 2016.
2. Chasnoff IJ, Douglas LE, Squires L. Cocaine intoxication in a breast-fed infant. Pediatrics. 1987;80:836-838.
3. Sarkar M, Djulus J, Koren G. When a cocaine-using mother wishes to breastfeed. Ther Drug Monit. 2005;27(1):1-2.
4. Dickson PH, Lind A, Studts P, et al. The routine analysis of breast milk for drugs of abuse in a clinical toxicology laboratory. J Forensic Sci. 1994;39(1):207-214.
5. Marchei E, Escuder D, Pallas CR, et al. Simultaneous analysis of frequently used licit and illicit psychoactive drugs in breast milk by liquid chromatography tandem mass spectrometry. J Pharm Biomed Anal. 2011;55:309–316.
6. Winecker RE, Goldberger BA, Tebbett IR, et al. Detection of cocaine and its metabolites in breast milk. J Forensic Sci. 2001;46:1221-1223.
7. Chaney NE, Franke J, Wadlington WB. Cocaine convulsions in a breast-feeding baby. J Pediatr. 1988;112(1):134-135.
8. Cressman AM, Koren G, Pupco A, Kim E, Ito S, Bozzo P. Maternal cocaine use during breastfeeding. Can Fam Physician. 2012;58:1218-1219.

CODEINE

Trade: Actacode, Codalgin, Empirin #3 # 4, Panadeine, Paveral, Penntuss, Tylenol # 3 # 4

Category: Analgesic

LRC: L3 - Limited Data-Probably Compatible

Codeine is considered a mild opiate analgesic whose action is due to its active metabolite morphine. The amount of codeine and morphine secreted into milk is dependent on the dose and maternal metabolism. The infants susceptibility to adverse events is higher during the neonatal period (first or second week). Tylenol #3 tablets contain 30 mg and Tylenol #4 tablets contain 60 mg of codeine in the United States.

Four cases of neonatal apnea have been reported following administration of 60 mg codeine every 4-6 hours to breastfeeding mothers, although codeine was not detected in serum of the infants tested.[1] Apnea resolved after discontinuation of maternal codeine.

In another study, following a dose of 60 mg, milk concentrations averaged 140 µg/L of milk with a peak of 455 µg/L at 1 hour.[2] Following 12 doses in 48 hours, the authors estimate the dose of codeine in milk (2000 mL milk) was 0.7 mg. There are few reported side effects following codeine doses of 30 mg, and it is believed to produce only minimal side effects in newborns.

In a study of seven mothers consuming 60 mg codeine, codeine and morphine levels were studied in breast milk of 17 samples, and neonatal plasma of 24 samples from 11 healthy, term neonates. Milk codeine levels ranged from 33.8 to 314 μg/L at 20 to 240 minutes after codeine; morphine levels ranged from 1.9 to 20.5 μg/L. Infant plasma samples one to four hours after feeding had codeine levels ranging from <0.8 to 4.5 μg/L; morphine ranged from <0.5 to 2.2 μg/L. The authors suggest that moderate codeine use during breastfeeding (< or = four 60 mg doses) is probably safe.[3]

The Sudden Infant Death Syndrome Institute reviewed all cases of infants referred for unexplained apnea, bradycardia and/or cyanosis in the first week of life (0.5-7 days) over a one year period (1984-1985).[4] The data demonstrated that opioids could have been a factor as 10 of the 12 infants were exposed to opioids and most of their mothers received more doses than the control group. In this review six mothers were taking codeine, four were taking propoxyphene and four were also given an intramuscular dose of meperidine.

An infant death was reported following the use of codeine (initially two tablets every 12 h, reduced to half that dose from day 2 to 2 weeks because of maternal somnolence and constipation) in the breastfeeding mother.[5] The infant was reported to have difficulty breastfeeding with lethargy on day 7 of life, grey color and decreased milk intake on day 11 of life and then was found cyanotic with absent vital signs on day 13 of life. Morphine levels in milk were reported to be 87 μg/L while the average reported milk levels in most mothers range from 1.9 to 20.5 μg/L at doses of 60 mg every 6 hours. Genotype analysis of this specific mother indicated that she was an ultra-rapid metabolizer of codeine. This genotype (which is very rare) leads to increased formation of morphine from codeine.

In 2012, a case series was published that added six new reports of neonatal concerns with codeine in breast milk.[6] In case one, the mother was discharged with a codeine prescription postpartum, the mother reported the infant appearing lethargic (sleeping all day, not opening eyes during feeds) and on day 8 (after a maternal codeine dose increase) the infant had respiratory arrest and required naloxone administration at the hospital. Maternal milk collected shortly after this hospital visit had a morphine concentration of 30 ng/mL. In case two, an infant was brought to hospital with dilated pupils and lethargy on day 7 of life. The infant's mother was taking codeine postpartum, based on this information the infant was given naloxone and the symptoms resolved. In case three, an infant was found hard to rouse on day 3 of life, the infant was going limp at the breast and post feeds would become sedated. After discontinuation of maternal codeine, the infants symptoms resolved. In this case, the mother was found to be a CYP2D6 extensive metabolizer. In case four, a 2-day-old infant had respiratory arrest and was felt to be too sedated to clear its airway. After breast milk was held and maternal codeine was stopped, symptoms resolved within 48 hours. In cases five and six, a 4 and 7 day old infant were both drowsy and hard to rouse, after discontinuation of maternal codeine and breast milk, symptoms resolved on their own.

Ultimately, each infant's response to codeine exposure in milk should be independently determined. In the vast majority of mothers, codeine taken in moderation and for a short duration was suitable for their breastfed infant. However, due to the inability to predict which infants will and will not tolerate codeine in lactation this product is not recommended for use in breastfeeding women. Any report of overt somnolence, apnea, poor feeding, grey skin, should be reported to the physician and could be associated with exposure to codeine in breast milk.

T 1/2	2.9 h	MW	299 Da	PB	7%
Tmax	0.5-1 h	RID	0.6%-8.1%	Vd	3.5 L/kg
Oral	Complete	M/P	1.3-2.5	pKa	8.2

Adult Concerns: Sedation, respiratory depression/apnea, nausea, vomiting, constipation, urinary retention, weakness.

Adult Dose: 15-60 mg every 4-6 h as needed.

Pediatric Concerns: Several cases of neonatal sedation, apnea, bradycardia and cyanosis have been reported in the literature and one death attributed to codeine use in lactation has occurred.[1,4-6] Other narcotics with no active metabolite and a lower relative infant dose are preferred.

Infant Monitoring: Sedation, slowed breathing rate/apnea, pallor, constipation, and appropriate weight gain.

Alternatives: Acetaminophen(L1), NSAIDs, Hydromorphone(L3)

References:

1. Davis JM, Bhutari VK. Neonatal apnea and maternal codeine use. Ped Res. 1985;19(4):170A. Abstract.
2. Findlay JW, DeAngelis RL, Kearney MF, Welch RM, Findlay JM. Analgesic drugs in breast milk and plasma. Clin Pharmacol Ther. 1981;29(5):625-633.
3. Meny RG, Naumburg EG, Alger LS, Brill-Miller JL, Brown S. Codeine and the breastfed neonate. J Hum Lact. December 1993;9(4):237-240.
4. Naumburg EG, Meny RG. Breast milk opioids and neonatal apnea. Pediatr Forum. 1998;142:11-12.
5. Koren G, Cairns J, Chitayat D, Gaedigk A, Leeder SJ. Pharmacogenetics of morphine poisoning in a breastfed neonate of a codeine-prescribed mother. Lancet. August 19, 2006;368(9536):704.
6. Lam J, Matlow JN, Ross CJ, et al. Postpartum maternal codeine therapy and the risk of adverse neonatal outcomes: the devil is in the details. Ther Drug Monit. 2012;34:378-380.

COENZYME Q10

Trade: CoQ10, Ubidecarenone, Ubiquinone

Category: Vitamin

LRC: L3 - No Data-Probably Compatible

Coenzyme Q10, also known as ubiquinone and ubidecarenone, is a cofactor in the mitochondrial electron-transport chain in the synthesis of ATP within the cell. It may also possess antioxidant and membrane-stabilizing properties. Although it is a naturally occurring cofactor, it is generally synthesized within the cell. Those cells that have the highest metabolic activity, such as the heart and the liver, have the highest CoQ10 concentrations.

The clinical uses of ubiquinone are quite interesting and include congestive heart disease, hypertension, periodontal disease, obesity, immune deficiencies, and angina.[1] Ubiquinone is slowly absorbed, requiring 5-10 hours to reach a peak. Following oral doses of 100 mg, peak blood levels of 1 µg/mL have been reported.[2] With doses of 300 mg/day, mean plasma levels were 5.4 µg/mL after 4 days.

No data are available on ubiquinone levels in milk. However, ubiquinone is very lipid soluble and has a long plasma half-life; transfer to milk is likely. If one were to assume a milk/plasma ratio of 1 and a significant maternal dose of 300 mg/d, then the average daily intake via milk in an infant would be approximately 16% of the weight-adjusted maternal dose. If these numbers are correct, it is not likely that this dose would be overtly toxic to an infant. Although ubiquinone is relatively nontoxic in adults, there are no data on the relative toxicity of this substance in infants. Most references suggest that pregnant and lactating women should avoid supplementation with this cofactor.

T 1/2	34 h	MW	863 Da	PB	
Tmax	5-10 h	RID		Vd	
Oral	Complete	M/P		pKa	

Adult Concerns: Nausea, epigastric pain, diarrhea, heartburn, appetite suppression.

Adult Dose: 50-100 mg daily.

Pediatric Concerns: None reported but high dose supplementation should be avoided.

Infant Monitoring: Vomiting, diarrhea, changes in feeding.

Alternatives:

References:
1. Gaby AR. Coenzyme Q10. In: Pizzorno JE, ed. Textbook of Natural Medicine. St. Louis, MO: Churchill Livingstone; 1999.
2. Greenberg S, Frishman WH. Co-enzyme Q10: a new drug for cardiovascular disease. J Clin Pharmacol. 1990;30(7):596-608.

COLCHICINE

Trade: Colchicine, Colcrys, Colgout

Category: Antigout

LRC: L3 - Limited Data-Probably Compatible

Colchicine is an old product primarily used to reduce pain associated with inflammatory gout; however, it has been used recently for some cardiac disorders associated with inflammation. Although it reduces the pain, it is not a true analgesic, it simply reduces the inflammation associated with uric acid crystals by inhibiting leukocyte and other cellular migration into the region. However, it is quite toxic; blood dyscrasias, hepatomegaly, and bone marrow depression are all possible adverse effects. Although the plasma half-life is only 20 minutes, it deposits in blood leukocytes and many other tissues, thereby extending the elimination half-life to over 60 hours.

No consistent data on colchicine concentrations in breast milk are available. In one published study, even the authors questioned the percent recovery in the breast milk, so the data must be considered questionable.[1,2] Nevertheless, the milk concentration varied from 1.2 to 2.5 µg/L (16-19 days postpartum) and there were no adverse events reported in the breastfed infant of a patient receiving 0.6 mg of colchicine twice daily.[1]

In another study of a mother taking 1 mg once daily, average milk concentrations were 30 µg/L in the 8 hours following maternal drug ingestion, leading to a daily maximum of 31% of the weight-adjusted maternal dose in the infant.[2] The authors of this study suggest that if a mother chooses to breastfeed, she should wait 8 hours postdose before feeding or pumping.

A third study of four women who took 1 mg of colchicine daily during pregnancy and lactation also found varying levels of colchicine in breast milk.[3] The maximum colchicine concentrations occurred within 3 hours in maternal serum and breast milk, and occurred by close to 1 hour for most of these women. The maximum breast milk concentrations ranged from 1.98 to 8.6 µg/L, the the serum concentrations were between 3.6 and 6.46 µg/L. By 6 hours the milk levels ranged between 0.87 to 2.57 µg/L and the serum levels were between 1.27 and 3.3 µg/L. The breastfed infants ranged from 4 to 58 days of life at the time of the study and no adverse events were reported during 10 months of follow up. In addition, these authors reported clinical data for an additional six women whom they cared for (prior to availability of the lab assay) that breastfed their infants for at least 3 months with no adverse effects during at least 2 years of follow-up.

A recent longitudinal study of 37 mother-infant pairs (one set of twins) who breastfed while taking colchicine found no increase in adverse developmental outcomes attributable to the drug.[4] The women were taking an average of 2.4 mg per day and breastfed for an average of 9.1 months. There were no neonatal side effects from colchicine exposure in breast milk (e.g., GI symptoms). When these infants were compared to a non-exposed cohort, no significant differences in growth or developmental/neurological problems were evident after 1-3 years of follow-up.

Colchicine is not a preferred medication in breastfeeding mothers as we have many other analgesics and anti-inflammatories that are superior in breastfeeding for the treatment of gouty symptoms. However, if this medication is required the infant should be monitored closely as relative infant doses vary from 2.1%-31%.

T 1/2	27-31 h	MW	399 Da	PB	34%-44%
Tmax	1-2 h	RID	2.1%-31.47%	Vd	5-8 L/kg
Oral	45%	M/P		pKa	15.06

Adult Concerns: Fatigue, headache, nausea, vomiting, diarrhea, abdominal pain, bone marrow suppression, myopathy.

Adult Dose: 0.5-0.6 mg one to four times a week.

Pediatric Concerns: None adverse effects have been reported in 50 breastfed infants.

Infant Monitoring: Vomiting, diarrhea.

Alternatives: Indomethacin(L3)

References:

1. Milunsky JM. Breast-feeding during colchicine therapy for familial Mediterranean fever. J Pediatr. 1991;119:164.
2. Guillonneau M, Aigrain EJ, Galliot M, Binet M, Darbois Y. Colchicine is excreted at high concentrations in human breast milk. Eur J Obstet Gynaecol Reprod Biol. 1995;61:177-178.
3. Ben-Chetrit E, Scherrmann J-M, Levy M. Colchicine in breast milk of patients with familial mediterranean fever. Arthritis Rheum. 1996;39(7):1213-1217.
4. Herscovici T, Merlob P, Stahl B, Laron-Kenet T, Klinger G. Colchicine use during breastfeeding. Breastfeed Med. 2015;10(2):92-95. doi:10.1089/bfm.2014.0086.

COLESEVELAM

Trade: WelChol

Category: Antihyperlipidemic

LRC: L2 - No Data-Probably Compatible

Colesevelam hydrochloride is a non-absorbed, polymeric, lipid-lowering agent that prevents the absorption of bile acids from the intestines.[1] As bile acids are the precursors for cholesterol production, hepatic cholesterol production is lowered. Colesevelam is almost totally unabsorbed from the gastrointestinal tract (only 0.05%) and is unlikely to enter milk at all (see cholestyramine).

The only potential problem of using this product in breastfeeding mothers is the lowering of maternal plasma cholesterol levels, and the possible lowering of milk cholesterol levels. Milk cholesterol is particularly important in infant neurodevelopment.

T 1/2		MW		PB	
Tmax		RID		Vd	
Oral	None	M/P		pKa	

Adult Concerns: Constipation, dyspepsia, and myalgia are the most commonly reported.

Adult Dose: 625 mg three to six times daily.

Pediatric Concerns: None reported via milk. It is totally unabsorbed, so none would penetrate milk.

Infant Monitoring: Weight gain, growth.

Alternatives: Cholestyramine(L2)

References:
1. Pharmaceutical manufacturers prescribing information.

COLESTIPOL

Trade: Colestid

Category: Antidiabetic, other

LRC: L2 - No Data-Probably Compatible

Colestipol is a bile acid sequestrant that is used to inhibit absorption of gastric bile acids, which are the precursors of plasma cholesterol.[1] Colestipol hydrochloride binds bile acids in the intestine, forming a complex that is excreted in the feces. As bile acids are the precursors for cholesterol production, hepatic cholesterol production is lowered. Colestipol is almost totally unabsorbed from the gastrointestinal tract and is unlikely to enter milk at all. Because this drug may significantly reduce plasma maternal cholesterol levels, milk cholesterol levels may be significantly reduced as well. Milk cholesterol from the mother is important for the growth and neurodevelopment of the infant. Colestipol is known to interfere with the absorption of fat-soluble vitamins A, D, E, and K. This may alter levels of these vitamins in human milk and have an effect on nursing infants.

T 1/2		MW	Very Large Da	PB	
Tmax		RID		Vd	
Oral	< 0.17%	M/P		pKa	

Adult Concerns: Constipation, abdominal discomfort, intestinal gas, indigestion, diarrhea, bloating.

Adult Dose: 1-6 five gram packets daily.

Pediatric Concerns: None expected.

Infant Monitoring: None likely.

Alternatives:

References:
1. Pharmaceutical manufacturers prescribing information.

COMFREY

Trade: Blackwort, Bruisewort, Knitbone, Russian comfrey, Slippery root

Category: Herb

LRC: L5 - No Data-Hazardous

Comfrey has been claimed to heal gastric ulcers, hemorrhoids, and suppress bronchial congestion and inflammation.[1] The product contains allantoin, tannin, and a group of dangerous pyrrolizidine alkaloids. Ointments containing Comfrey have been found to be anti-inflammatory, probably due to the allantoin content. Some of the topically applied pyrrolizidine alkaloids are absorbed transcutaneously.

However, when administered orally to animals, most members of this family (Boraginaceae) have been noted to induce severe liver toxicity, including elevated liver enzymes and liver tumors (hepatocellular adenomas).[2,3] Bladder tumors were noted at low concentrations. Russian Comfrey has been found to induce liver damage and pancreatic islet cell tumors.[4] A number of significant human toxicities have been reported, including several deaths, all associated with the ingestion of Comfrey teas or yerba mate tea.[5] Even when applied to the skin, pyrrolizidine alkaloids were noted in the urine of rodents. Lactating rats excreted pyrrolizidine alkaloids into breast milk.

Comfrey and members of this family are exceedingly dangerous and should not be used topically, ingested orally, or used in any form in breastfeeding or pregnant mothers.

T 1/2		MW		PB	
Tmax		RID		Vd	
Oral	Complete	M/P		pKa	

Adult Concerns: Liver toxicity, hepatic carcinoma, hepatocellular adenomas, hepatonecrosis.

Adult Dose:

Pediatric Concerns: Passes into animal milk. Absorbed topically. Too dangerous for breastfeeding mothers and infants in any form.

Infant Monitoring: Liver toxicity.

Alternatives:

References:

1. Review of Natural Products. St. Louis, MO: Facts and Comparisons; 1996.
2. Hirono I, Mori H, Haga M. Carcinogenic activity of symphytum officinale. J Natl Cancer Inst. 1978;61(3):865-869.
3. Yeong ML, Wakefield SJ, Ford HC. Hepatocyte membrane injury and bleb formation following low dose comfrey toxicity in rats. Int J Exp Pathol. 1993;74(2):211-217.
4. Yeong ML, Clark SP, Waring JM, Wilson RD, Wakefield SJ. The effects of comfrey derived pyrrolizidine alkaloids on rat liver. Pathology. 1991;23(1):35-38.
5. McGee J, Patrick RS, Wood CB, Blumgart LH. A case of veno-occlusive disease of the liver in Britain associated with herbal tea consumption. J Clin Pathol. 1976;29(9):788-794.

CONTRACEPTIVES - HORMONAL

Trade: Oral Contraceptives, Estradiol, Norethindrone, Copper Intra Uterine Devices, Levonorgestrel, Progesterone, Estrogen, Ethinyl Estradiol

Category: Contraceptive

LRC: L3 - Limited Data-Probably Compatible

There are dozens of hormonal contraceptive products on the market, as well as formulations that use the same/similar hormones for other medical purposes. All of them contain estrogen and/or progesterone analogs, although the specific compounds, dosages, and routes of administration vary (oral, injectable, intrauterine, etc.).

Hormonal contraceptives containing estrogens may interfere with milk production by decreasing the quantity and quality of milk production; although this hypothesis has been around for many years, the evidence to support this has been poorly documented. [1-4] Thus, it has been advisable to wait as long as possible postpartum prior to instituting therapy and to use a progesterone-only product to avoid reducing the milk supply.[5]

A study published in 1983 involving 330 women who used non-hormonal contraceptives (NHC), combined oral contraceptives (COCs), and Copper Intra Uterine Devices (Cu IUD) starting on day 30 postpartum, found more infants were weaned from breast milk at 6 and 8 months in the COC group (16.3% COC, 9% NHC, 4.7% Cu IUD at 6 months).[6] However, about 40% of women in all three groups were no longer breastfeeding by the end of one year. It was also noted that infants in the COC group were within the normal range for their weight but they did have significantly smaller weight gain at 6 and 12 months when compared to the NHC group.

In a double-blind randomized trial published in 2012, the effect of initiating progesterone-only contraceptives (0.35mg norethindrone) was compared to COCs (0.035mg ethinyl estradiol + 1 mg norethindrone) at 2 weeks postpartum.[7] In this study, there was no difference in continuation of breastfeeding between the two groups at 8 weeks (64.1% COCs vs. 63.5% progestin only) or 6 months. Women were more likely to stop breastfeeding if they supplemented with formula or had concerns with milk supply, regardless of which group they were in. Although no differences between changes in milk supply were found, this study lacked comparison with a placebo group (progestin effect on milk supply was not evaluated), and had potential for bias, as only the mother's perception of changes in milk volume, not actual volumes, were analyzed.

Several studies have demonstrated that levonorgestrel has limited, if any, effect on milk volume because the concentrations typically found with this product are very low (often in implants or IUDs).[8] In a study with 120 women who used progestin containing implants, no changes in breastfeeding at 5-6 weeks postpartum were identified.[9] In another study of 163 and 157 women who used levonorgestrel IUDs or Copper IUDs respectively, no change in breastfeeding, infant growth, and infant development was noted over 12 months.[10] Though the levonorgestrel data suggest minimal to no effect, we have received numerous reports at the Infantrisk center of milk suppression following insertion of the levonorgestrel IUD.

In light of such conflicting anecdotal evidence and less than rigorous data to date, when hormonal contraception is necessary, low-dose progesterone-only oral contraceptives should be recommended. If combined oral contraceptives are required a product with low estrogen is advised. The most sensitive time for changes in milk supply is early postpartum before lactation is established; therefore, waiting as long as possible (minimum 4 weeks) prior to use is advised.[5] All mothers who take hormonal contraception should be counseled of possible effects on milk supply and monitored for such.

It should also be noted that estrogen-containing products represent a serious health hazard to the mother in the early postpartum period as they further increase her risk of blood clots postpartum.[11] Both ACOG, WHO and the Centers for Disease Control and Prevention advise against using combination contraceptive products early postpartum in breastfeeding women.[12-18]

Estrogens and progestins are secreted into milk in minute quantities and do not appear to have clinically relevant effects on the infants health. Studies of these products in breastfeeding women have found typical RIDs to be less than 1% (RID < 1% for ethinylestradiol and 0.1% for progestogen).[19-20]

In a recent study of 259 mothers who received Mirena IUD immediately postpartum, no change in breastfeeding rates were noted.[21]

Adult Concerns: Headache, hypertension, nausea, vomiting, gallbladder disease, changes in liver function, abdominal cramps, bloating, breakthrough bleeding, spotting, amenorrhea, edema, thromboembolism (DVT, PE, stroke, MI). Potential suppression of milk supply.

Adult Dose:

Pediatric Concerns: Several cases of gynecomastia in infants have been reported but are extremely rare.

Infant Monitoring: Feminizing effects such as gynecomastia have been reported in the rare cases with male infants. Vaginal bleeding has been reported in female infants that may be associated with maternal use of progestins and estrogens.

Alternatives:

References:

1. Booker DE, Pahl IR. Control of postpartum breast engorgement with oral contraceptives. Am J Obstet Gynecol. 1967;98(8):1099–1101.
2. Booker DE, Pahl IR, Forbes DA. Control of postpartum breast engorgement with oral contraceptives II. Am J Obstet Gynecol. 1970;108(2):240–242.
3. Gambrell RDJ. Immediate postpartum oral contraception. Obstet Gynecol. 1970;36(1):101–106.
4. Kennedy KI, Short RV, Tully MR. Premature introduction of progestin-only contraceptive methods during lactation. Contraception. 1997;55(6):347-350.
5. Queenan J. Exploring contraceptive options for breastfeeding mothers. Obstet Gynecol. 2012;119(1):1-2.
6. Croxatto HB, Diaz S, Peralta O, et al. Fertility regulation in nursing women: IV. Long-term influence of a low-dose combined oral contraceptive initiated at day 30 postpartum upon lactation and infant growth. Contraception. 1983;27(1):13-25.
7. Espey E, Ogburn T, Leeman L, Singh R, Ostrom K, Schrader R. Effect of progestin compared with combined oral contraceptive pills on lactation. Obstet Gynecol. 2012;119(1):5-13.
8. Shaaban MM, Salem HT, Abdullah KA. Influence of levonorgestrel contraceptive implants, NORPLANT, initiated early postpartum upon lactation and infant growth. Contraception. 1985;32(6):623-635.
9. Shaaban MM. Contraception with progestogens and progesterone during lactation. J Steroid Biochem Mol Biol. 1991;40(4-6):705-710.
10. Shaamash AH, Sayed GH, Hussien MM, Shaaban MM. A comparative study of the levonorgestrel-releasing intrauterine system Mirena(R) versus the Copper T380A intrauterine device during lactation: breast-feeding performance, infant growth and infant development. Contraception. 2005;72(5):346-351.
11. de Bastos M, Stegeman BH, Rosendaal FR, et al. Combined oral contraceptives: venous thrombosis. Cochrane Database Syst Rev. 2014;3:CD010813.
12. ACOG Committee on Practice Bulletins-Gynecology. ACOG practice bulletin. No. 73: use of hormonal contraception in women with coexisting medical conditions. Obstet Gynecol. Jun 2006;107(6):1453-1472.
13. World Health Organization. Technical Consultation on Hormonal Contraceptive Use During Lactation and Effects on the Newborn: Summary Report. Geneva, Switzerland: World Health Organization; 2010.
14. Centers for Disease C, Prevention. Update to CDC's U.S. medical eligibility criteria for contraceptive use, 2010: revised recommendations for the use of contraceptive methods during the postpartum period. MMWR Morbid Mortal Weekly Rep. July 8, 2011;60(26):878-883.
15. ACOG Committee on Practice Bulletins-Gynecology. ACOG practice bulletin. No. 73: use of hormonal contraception in women with coexisting medical conditions. Obstet Gynecol. June 2006;107(6):1453-1472.
16. Cardiovascular disease and use of oral and injectable progestogen-only contraceptives and combined injectable contraceptives. Results of an international, multicenter, case-control study. World Health Organization Collaborative Study of Cardiovascular Disease and Steroid Hormone Contraception. Contraception. May 1998;57(5):315-324.
17. Heinemann LA, Assmann A, DoMinh T, Garbe E. Oral progestogen-only contraceptives and cardiovascular risk: results from the Transnational Study on Oral Contraceptives and the Health of Young Women. Eur J Contracept Reprod Health Care. June 1999;4(2):67-73.
18. Lidegaard O, Lokkegaard E, Jensen A, Skovlund CW, Keiding N. Thrombotic stroke and myocardial infarction with hormonal contraception. N Engl J Med. June 14, 2012;366(24):2257-2266.
19. Neville MC, McFadden TB, Forsyth I. Hormonal regulation of mammary differentiation and milk secretion. J Mammary Gland Biol Neoplasia. 2002;7(1):49-66.
20. World Health Organization. Technical Consultation on Hormonal Contraceptive use During Lactation and Effects on the Newborn: Summary Report. Geneva, Switzerland: World Health Organization; 2010.
21. Turok DK, Leeman L, Sanders JN, et al. Immediate postpartum levonorgestrel intrauterine device insertion and breast-feeding outcomes: a noninferiority randomized controlled trial. Am J Obstet Gynecol. December 2017;217(6):665.e1-665.e8.

CORONA VIRUS

Trade: COVID-19, SARS-CoV-2

Category: Infectious Disease

LRC: L4 - Limited Data-Possibly Hazardous

Below is from the CDC (March 2020)

There is enormous controversy concerning close contact and direct breastfeeding of an infant from a mother who is COVID-19 positive. At present, it is not clearly known if the infant can become infected with COVID-19 in utero, or during delivery, or during breastfeeding. Some recent evidence suggests that the viral particles can be found in mother's milk early postpartum.[1] But this case study was small, it is not certain the methodology was accurate, or that the virus in human milk is indeed infectious. In another case study, the newborn infant of a Covid-19-positive mother was not positive for COVID-19 at 24 hours post-delivery.[2]

At present, the CDC and other worldwide agencies (WHO) are providing somewhat inconsistent information about the risks to the infant and their advice concerning breastfeeding. Providing human milk to a newborn infant at this stage seems to be the most productive and medically advisable. Until we know more about the transfer of COVID-19 into human milk, and its ability to induce infection in the infant via milk, most authorities in this field advise that mothers continue to breastfeed or pump their milk and provide the milk to the infant.

WHO suggestions include[3]:

–Practice respiratory hygiene, including during feeding. If you have respiratory symptoms such as being short of breath, use a medical mask when near your child.

–Wash your hands thoroughly with soap or sanitizer before and after contact with your child.

–Routinely clean and disinfect any surfaces you touch.

–If you are severely ill with COVID-19 or suffer from other complications that prevent you from caring for your infant or continuing direct breastfeeding, express milk to safely provide breastmilk to your infant.

–If you are too unwell to breastfeed or express breastmilk, you should explore the possibility of relactation (restarting breastfeeding after a gap), wet nursing (another woman breastfeeding or caring for your child), or using donor human milk. Which approach to use will depend on cultural context, acceptability to you, and service availability.

Health facilities and their staff:

–If you are providing maternity and newborn services, you should not promote breastmilk substitutes, feeding bottles, teats, pacifiers or dummies in any part of your facilities, or by any of your staff.

–Enable mothers and infants to remain together and practice skin-to-skin contact, and rooming-in throughout the day and night, especially straight after birth during establishment of breastfeeding, whether or not the mother or child has suspected, probable, or confirmed COVID-19.

A number of laboratories are presently studying the transfer of this virus into human milk, and its ability to enter milk and to infect the infant. Seek more information from your healthcare advisor, pediatrician, or lactation consultant concerning the risk of breastfeeding during infection with this agent.

Adult Concerns:

Adult Dose:

Pediatric Concerns:

Infant Monitoring:

Alternatives:

References:

1. Tam PCK, Ly KM, Kernich ML, et al. Detectable severe acute respiratory syndrome coronavirus 2 (SARS-CoV-2) in human breast milk of a mildly symptomatic patient with coronavirus disease 2019 (COVID-19) [published online ahead of print, 2020 May 30]. Clin Infect Dis. 2020;ciaa673. doi:10.1093/cid/ciaa673
2. Lowe B, Bopp B. COVID-19 vaginal delivery - A case report [published online ahead of print, 2020 Apr 15]. Aust N Z J Obstet Gynaecol. 2020;10.1111/ajo.13173. doi:10.1111/ajo.13173
3. World Health Organization, 2020.

CORTICOTROPIN

Trade: ACT, ACTH, Acthar, Cortrosyn

Category: Pituitary Hormone

LRC: L3 - No Data-Probably Compatible

ACTH or adrenocorticotropic hormone is secreted by the anterior pituitary gland in the brain and stimulates the adrenal cortex to produce and secrete adrenocortical hormones (cortisol, hydrocortisone). Corticotropin is a sterile preparation of ACTH with pharmacological actions similar to that of endogenous ACTH.[1] As a peptide product, ACTH is easily destroyed in the infant's gastrointestinal tract. None would be absorbed by the infant.

ACTH stimulates the endogenous production of cortisol, which theoretically can transfer to the breastfed infant. However, the use of ACTH in breastfeeding mothers largely depends on the dose and duration of exposure and the risks to the infant. Brief exposures are probably not contraindicated. A synthetic ACTH called cosyntropin (Cortrosyn) is now available. It contains the first 24 of the 39 amino acids found in ACTH.

T 1/2	15 min	MW		PB	
Tmax		RID		Vd	
Oral	0%	M/P		pKa	

Adult Concerns: Hypersensitivity reactions, increased risk of infection, embryocidal effects, other symptoms of hypercorticalism.

Adult Dose: 80 units IM or SC (dose and frequency depends on indication).

Pediatric Concerns: None reported via milk.

Infant Monitoring: Increased risk of infection.

Alternatives:

References:
1. Pharmaceutical manufacturers prescribing information.

CRANBERRY EXTRACT

Trade:

Category: Herb

LRC: L3 - No Data-Probably Compatible

The primary use of cranberry extract and ingestion of large volumes of cranberry juice are for the prevention and treatment of urinary tract infections.[1,2] At this time there are no data regarding the transfer of cranberry extract to human milk or its safety in lactation. The use of cranberry supplements is not encouraged in lactation; however, there are no concerns with dietary intake.

Adult Concerns: Nausea, vomiting, diarrhea, kidney stones.

Adult Dose: Varies by indication.

Pediatric Concerns:

Infant Monitoring: Vomiting, diarrhea.

Alternatives:

References:
1. Cranberry. Natural Medicines Comprehensive Database [Internet Database]. Stockton, CA: Therapeutic Research Faculty; July 5, 2011.
2. Jean-Jacques D, Seely D, Perri D, et al. Safety and efficacy of cranberry (vaccinium macrocarpon) during pregnancy and lactation. Can J Clin Pharmacol. 2008;15(1):e80-e86.

CRITZOTINIB

Trade: Xalkori

Category: Anticancer

LRC: L5 - No Data-Hazardous

Critzotinib is an inhibitor of receptor tyrosine kinases. Highly toxic, this product has a huge volume of distribution, and elimination is delayed. While plasma half-life is 42 hours, its elimination from adipose and other lipid sinks is prolonged. Manufacturer recommends withdrawal from breastfeeding for 45 days following last dose.

T 1/2	42 h	MW	450.34 Da	PB	91%
Tmax		RID		Vd	25.31 L/kg
Oral	32%-66%	M/P		pKa	

Adult Concerns: Hepatotoxicity, vomiting, diarrhea, abdominal pain, Interstitial lung disease, prolonged QTc, bradycardia, severe visual loss, highly fetotoxic and teratogenic.

Adult Dose: 250 mg twice daily.

Pediatric Concerns:

Infant Monitoring: Extremely hazardous.

Alternatives:

References:
1. Pharmaceutical manufacturers prescribing information. 2017.

CROMOLYN SODIUM

Trade: Cromese, Gastrocrom, Intal, Nasalcrom, Opticrom, Rynacrom, Vistacrom

Category: Antiasthma

LRC: L2 - No Data-Probably Compatible

Cromolyn sodium is an extremely safe drug that is used clinically as an antiasthmatic, antiallergic, and to suppress mast cell degranulation and allergic symptoms. No data on penetration into human breast milk are available, based on its larger molecular weight minimal levels are expected.[1] Less than 0.001% of a dose was distributed into the milk of a monkey. No harmful effects have been reported in breastfeeding infants. Less than 1% of this drug is absorbed from the maternal (and probably the infant's) gastrointestinal tract, so it is unlikely to produce untoward effects in nursing infants. This product is frequently used in pediatric patients and poses little risk for an infant when used in a breastfeeding mother.

T 1/2	80-90 min	MW	512 Da	PB	
Tmax	<15 min	RID		Vd	
Oral	<1%	M/P		pKa	

Adult Concerns: Headache, drowsiness, insomnia, irritability, nasal congestion, sneezing, cough, wheezing, nausea, pancytopenia, myalgia, rash.

Adult Dose: 20 mg QID via inhalation.

Pediatric Concerns: None reported via milk.

Infant Monitoring: Irritability, insomnia, diarrhea or constipation, weight gain.

Alternatives:

References:
1. Pharmaceutical manufacturers prescribing information.

CYCLIZINE

Trade: Cyclivert

Category: Antiemetic

LRC: L3 - No Data-Probably Compatible

Cyclizine is an antihistamine commonly used to treat nausea and vomiting due to motion sickness.[1] There are no controlled studies in breastfeeding women, however, other studies of antihistamine medications suggest only low amounts were found in breast milk (see diphenhydramine).

T 1/2	20 h	MW	266 Da	PB	
Tmax		RID		Vd	
Oral		M/P		pKa	7.7

Adult Concerns: Dry mouth, drowsiness, headache, urinary retention, nausea.

Adult Dose: 50 mg TID prn.

Pediatric Concerns:

Infant Monitoring: Drowsiness, urinary retention.

Alternatives:

References:
1. Pharmaceutical manufacturers prescribing information.

CYCLOBENZAPRINE

Trade: Cycloflex, Flexeril

Category: Skeletal Muscle Relaxant

LRC: L3 - No Data-Probably Compatible

Cyclobenzaprine is a centrally acting skeletal muscle relaxant that is structurally and pharmacologically similar to the tricyclic antidepressants (e.g., amitriptyline).[1] Cyclobenzaprine is used short-term as an adjunct to rest and physical therapy for the relief of acute, painful musculoskeletal conditions.

In a recent case report of two patients, one received 5 mg cyclobenzaprine q 24 hours (case 1), and another receiving 10 mg twice daily (case 2), levels in milk were exceedingly low, with an average concentration of cyclobenzaprine less than 2.2 ng/mL and 10.3 ng/mL in milk, respectively.[2] Time to maximum concentration was 1 hour in the first case, and 2 hours in case 2. Based on these reported levels, levels in milk are far subclinical.

T 1/2	18 h (8-37 h)	MW	311 Da	PB	93%
Tmax	3-8 h	RID	0.46%-0.54%	Vd	High L/kg
Oral	33%-55%	M/P		pKa	8.47

Adult Concerns: Drowsiness, dizziness, unpleasant taste, dry mouth, nausea, vomiting. Rarely-tachycardia, hypotension, arrhythmias.

Adult Dose: 5-10 mg three times a day.

Pediatric Concerns: None reported, but caution is urged.

Infant Monitoring: Drowsiness/sedation, dry mouth, poor feeding, vomiting.

Alternatives:

References:
1. Pharmaceutical manufacturers prescribing information.
2. Burra B, Datta P, Rewers-Felkins K, Baker T, Hale TW. Transfer of cyclobenzaprine into human milk and subsequent infant exposure. J Hum Lact. 2019;35(3):559–562. doi:10.1177/0890334419843307.

CYCLOPENTOLATE

Trade: Cyclogyl, Cylate, Diopentolate, Minims Cyclopentolate, Ocu-Pentolate, Pentolair

Category: Mydriatic-Cycloplegic

LRC: L3 - No Data-Probably Compatible

Cyclopentolate is used to dilate the pupils to facilitate refraction, eye examinations and other diagnostic purposes in the eye.[1] Cyclopentolate is commonly used by ophthalmologists and optometrists because it works rapidly, and more brief than atropine. It is a potent anticholinergic and some is absorbed systemically. Children and particularly infants would be extremely susceptible to this agent. Several cases of pediatric seizures[2] and one case of necrotizing enterocolitis[3], has been reported following the ophthalmic use of this agent in children and an infant respectively. While no data are available on the transfer of this agent to human milk, it is rather unlikely that significant quantities would enter as maternal plasma levels are so low, and milk levels would be even lower.

Plasma levels are approximately 3000 times lower than ophthalmic levels. Only 3%-18% of muscarinic receptors were occupied after 55-124 minutes following administration. In healthy volunteers peak plasma concentration of cyclopentolate, 2.06 nM, occurred at 53 minutes, maximum receptor occupancy being 5.9%.[4] After topical application plasma receptor occupancy was not high enough to cause any significant changes in heart rate and in P-Q interval time. None of the subjects experienced subjectively or objectively adverse effects to be attributed to cyclopentolate. In another study, peak plasma drug concentrations of about 3 ng/mL occurred within 30 minutes after all formulations.[5] The mean elimination half-life of cyclopentolate was 111 minutes when all subjects and formulations were considered together.

Some caution is recommended with this product. A waiting period of perhaps 6 hours following its use would be sufficient to reduce risks.

T 1/2	111 min	MW	291 Da	PB	
Tmax	25-75 min	RID		Vd	
Oral		M/P		pKa	8.4

Adult Concerns: Seizures, sedation, blurred vision, fever, dry mouth, dry eye, urinary retention, constipation.

Adult Dose: 1-2 drops in each eye.

Pediatric Concerns: None via milk, but caution is recommended.

Infant Monitoring: A brief interruption of breastfeeding is advised to reduce risk.

Alternatives: Atropine(L3)

References:
1. Pharmaceutical manufacturers prescribing information.
2. Fitzgerald DA, Hanson RM, West C, Martin F, Brown J, Kilham HA. Seizures associated with 1% cyclopentolate eyedrops. J Paediatr Child Health. April 1990;26(2):106-107.
3. Bauer CR, Trottier MC, Stern L. Systemic cyclopentolate (Cyclogyl) toxicity inthe newborn infant. J Pediatr. March 1973;82(3):501-505.
4. Haaga M, Kaila T, Salminen L, Ylitalo P. Systemic and ocular absorption and antagonist activity of topically applied cyclopentolate in man. Pharmacol Toxicol. January 1998;82(1):19-22.
5. Lahdes K, Huupponen R, Kaila T, Monti D, Saettone MF, Salminen L. Plasma concentrations and ocular effects of cyclopentolate after ocular application of three formulations. Br J Clin Pharmacol. May 1993;35(5):479-483.

CYCLOPHOSPHAMIDE

Trade: Carloxan, Cycloblastin, Cytoxan, Endoxan, Endoxana, Neosar, Procytox

Category: Antineoplastic

LRC: L5 - No Data-Hazardous

Cyclophosphamide is a powerful and toxic antineoplastic drug, used in many treatments, including breast cancer. The oral bioavailability of CP is 75% and reaches a peak at 1 to 2 hours. The elimination half-life (T1/2 beta) is 7.5 hours.[1] The active metabolites stay in the plasma compartment with brief half-lives of four hours or less. Transport of CP and its metabolites into the CNS is exceedingly low. This would suggest milk levels will be low as well when they are ultimately determined. The kinetics of this agent are highly variable depending on renal function, creatinine clearance, liver function, etc.

A number of reports in the literature indicate that cyclophosphamide can transfer to human milk as evidenced by the production of leukopenia and bone marrow suppression in at least two breastfed infants. In one case of a mother who received 800 mg/week of cyclophosphamide, the infant was significantly neutropenic following 6 weeks of exposure via breast milk.[2] In another mother who was receiving 10 mg/kg intravenously daily for 7 days for a total of 3.5 g, major leukopenia was also reported in her breastfed infant.[3]

In a new study of a mother 6 months postpartum, who received 2.8 g cyclophosphamide daily for 4 days.[4] Low levels of cyclophosphamide were found in milk. Maximum concentrations of cyclophosphamide were observed on day 1 at 40.82 µg/mL, which peaked at 4 hours. At 24 hours, the levels gradually receded to minimum concentrations. Cyclophosphamide self-induces its on metabolism, thus levels in plasma and milk dropped over 4 days. The average relative infant dose (RID) for a period of 4 days varied from 4.7% at day 1 to 0.9% at day 4. Thus, cyclophosphamide is transferred into breast milk in low, but measurable quantities. However, great caution should be taken in counseling mothers regarding breastfeeding with this toxic drug.

T 1/2	7.5 h	MW	261 Da	PB	13%
Tmax	2-3 h	RID	0.9 – 4.7%	Vd	0.7 L/kg
Oral	75%	M/P		pKa	

Adult Concerns: Alopecia, mucositis, arrhythmias, diarrhea, anorexia, changes in liver function, hemorrhagic cystitis, leukopenia, neutropenia, anemia, infection.

Adult Dose: 1-5 mg/kg daily.

Pediatric Concerns: Leukopenia and bone marrow suppression in at least three breastfed infants.

Infant Monitoring: Withhold breastfeeding for a period of at least 72 hours.

Alternatives:

References:
1. Pharmaceutical manufacturers prescribing information.
2. Amato D, Niblett JS. Neutropenia from cyclophosphamide in breast milk. Med J Aust. 1977;1(11):383-384.
3. Durodola JI. Administration of cyclophosphamide during late pregnancy and early lactation: a case report. J Natl Med Assoc. 1979;71(2):165-166.
4. Fierro ME, Datta P, Rewers-Felkins K, Smillie C, Bresnahan A, Baker T, Hale T. Cyclophosphamide Use in Multiple Sclerosis: Levels Detected in Human Milk. Breastfeed Med. 2019;14(2):128-130. doi:10.1089/bfm.2018.0137

CYCLOSERINE

Trade: Closina, Cycloserine, Seromycin

Category: Antitubercular

LRC: L4 - Limited Data-Possibly Hazardous

Cycloserine is an antibiotic primarily used for treating tuberculosis. It is also effective against various staphylococcal infections. It is a small molecule with a structure similar to the amino acid, D-alanine and interferes with the bacterial cell wall synthesis. Following 250 mg oral dose given four times daily to mothers, milk levels ranged from 6 to 19 mg/L, an average of 13.4 mg/L.[1] This is approximately 2 mg/kg/day. The normal antitubercular dose in infants is 10-20 mg/kg/day. Levels of cycloserine in human milk may be significant. Mothers should probably withhold breastfeeding for 24 hours.

T 1/2	12 h	MW	102 Da	PB	Unbound
Tmax	4-8 h	RID	14.1%	Vd	
Oral	70%-90%	M/P	0.72	pKa	4.21

Adult Concerns: Drowsiness, confusion, dizziness, headache, lethargy, depression, seizures, arrhythmias, heart failure, vitamin B12 deficiency, changes in liver function, tremor.

Adult Dose: 250 mg BID.

Pediatric Concerns: None reported.

Infant Monitoring: Drowsiness, lethargy, poor feeding, and weight gain.

Alternatives:

References:
1. Charles E, McKenna MH, Morton RF. Studies on the absorption, diffusion, and excretion of cycloserine. Antibiot Annu. 1955;3:169-172.

CYCLOSPORINE

Trade: Neoral, Restasis, Sandimmune

Category: Immune Suppressant

LRC: L3 - Limited Data-Probably Compatible

Cyclosporine is an immunosuppressant used to reduce organ rejection following transplant and in autoimmune syndromes such as arthritis, etc. In a recent report of seven breastfeeding mothers treated with cyclosporine, the levels of cyclosporine in breast milk ranged from 50 to 227 µg/L. Corresponding plasma levels in the breastfed infants were undetectable (<30 ng/mL) in all infants. In this study, the infants received less than 300 µg per day via breast milk.[1]

In another study, following a dose of 320 mg/day, the milk level at 22 hours post dose was 16 µg/L and the milk/plasma ratio was 0.28.[2] In another report of a mother receiving 250 mg twice daily, the maternal plasma level of cyclosporine was measured at 187 µg/L, and the breast milk level was 167 µg/L.[3] None was detected in the plasma of the infant. In a study of a breastfeeding transplant patient who received 300 mg twice daily, maternal serum levels were 193, 273, and 123 ng/mL at 23 days, 6.5 and 9.7 weeks postpartum.[4] Corresponding milk cyclosporine levels were 160, 286, and 79 µg/L respectively. Using the higher milk level, an infant would receive less than 0.4% of the weight-adjusted maternal dose. In another mother receiving cyclosporine (3 mg/kg/day), the concentration of cyclosporine in milk averaged 596 µg/L, or a dose of about <0.1 mg/kg to the infant.[5] The infant's trough blood level was always <3 µg/L while the mother's was 260 µg/L. No untoward effects were noted in the infant.

In a more recent study of five patients receiving 5.3, 4.0, 5, 4.11, and 5 mg/kg/day cyclosporine respectively, the average concentration of cyclosporine in the mothers was 403 µg/L, 465 µg/L, 97.6 µg/L, 117.7 µg/L, and 84-144 µg/L (range) respectively.[6] Hind milk levels were much higher in one case, probably due to the high lipid content. In mother 1, the cyclosporine blood levels in the infant were 131 µg/L and 117 µg/L on two occasions, which were near a therapeutic trough. In none of the other infants, were blood levels of cyclosporine determinable (<25 μg/L). This study clearly suggests that some infants could potentially attain near-therapeutic levels from ingesting breast milk. From this data, the relative infant dose would be approximately 0.78% of the weight-normalized maternal dose.

In 2014, a case report was published of a women taking cyclosporine for psoriasis, she started taking 300 mg/day at 33 weeks gestational age and then continued during lactation on a lower dose of 200 mg/day.[7] The infant in this case report was exclusively breastfed for 6 months. Maternal blood and milk levels and infant blood levels were taken at day 10, 30, 40, and 50 postpartum. The maternal blood concentrations ranged from the lowest trough level taken just before her dose on day 40 at 62 μg/L to the highest level on day 50 at 462 μg/L taken 2 hours postdose. The milk levels also ranged from the lowest trough level taken just before her dose on day 10 at 128 μg/L to the highest level on day 50 at 364 μg/L taken 2 hours postdose. The infants levels were 30 μg/L on day 10 and then undetectable thereafter. Using the highest milk level on day 50, the RID is 1.9% and the infant dose is 0.055 mg/kg/day. No adverse events were reported in this infant and her growth and development were also reported as normal.

These studies together suggest cyclosporine transfer to milk is generally low, but one study suggests that some infants may receive more than what is expected. Therefore cyclosporine use in breastfeeding mothers should be followed by close observation of the infant for signs of toxicity and may include monitoring of the infants plasma levels.[8]

Restasis is the ophthalmic form of cyclosporine. Following 12 months of therapy, cyclosporine was not detectable in the plasma compartment, hence levels in the milk of breastfeeding mothers will be low to undetectable.

T 1/2	6-27 h	MW		PB	93%
Tmax	3.5 h	RID	0.05%-3%	Vd	3.1-4.3 L/kg
Oral	28% pediatric	M/P	0.28-0.4	pKa	9.3

Adult Concerns: Headache, hypertension, edema, gum hyperplasia, dyspepsia, vomiting, diarrhea, changes in liver and renal function, increased triglycerides, tremor, leg cramps, increased frequency of infection, hirsutism.

Adult Dose: 5-15 mg/kg daily, but highly variable.

Pediatric Concerns: In 14 reported cases, milk levels were low and infant plasma levels low to undetectable. However, one case of near-clinical levels in an infant have been reported.

Infant Monitoring: Vomiting, diarrhea, weight gain. If signs of liver dysfunction (yellowing of skin or whites of eyes) check liver enzymes and bilirubin; if signs of toxicity check drug level.

Alternatives:

References:

1. Nyberg G, Haljamae U, Frisenette-Fich C, Wennergren M, Kjellmer I. Breast-feeding during treatment with cyclosporine. Transplantation. 1998;65(2):253-255.
2. Flechner SM, Katz AR, Rogers AJ, Van Buren C, Kahan BD. The presence of cyclosporine in body tissues and fluids during pregnancy. Am J Kidney Dis. 1985;5(1):60-63.
3. K.D.T. Personal communication. 1997.
4. Munoz-Flores-Thiagarajan KD, Easterling T, Davis C, Bond EF. Breast-feeding by a cyclosporine-treated mother. Obstet Gynecol. 2001;97(5 pt 2):816-818.
5. Thiru Y, Bateman DN, Coulthard MG. Successful breast feeding while mother was taking cyclosporin. BMJ. 1997;315(7106):463.
6. Moretti ME, Sgro M, Johnson DW, et al. Cyclosporine excretion into breast milk. Transplantation. 2003;75(12):2144-2146.
7. Mazzuoccolo LD, Andrada R, Pellerano G, et al. Levels of cyclosporine in breast milk and passage into the circulation of the infant of a mother with psoriasis. Int J Dermatol. 2012;53:355-356.
8. American Academy of Pediatrics, Committee on Drugs. Transfer of drugs and other chemicals into human milk. Pediatrics. 2001;108(3):776-789.

CYPROHEPTADINE

Trade: Periactin

Category: Antihistamine

LRC: L3 - No Data-Probably Compatible

Cyproheptadine is a serotonin and histamine antagonist with anticholinergic and sedative effects. It has been used as an appetite stimulant in children and for rashes and pruritus (itching).[1] No data are available on its transfer to human milk. The main adverse effect to watch out for is sedation. Switching to a non-sedating antihistamine (loratadine, cetirizine) may be a suitable alternative.

T 1/2	16 h	MW	287 Da	PB	99%
Tmax		RID		Vd	
Oral		M/P		pKa	9.3

Adult Concerns: Sedation, nausea, vomiting, diarrhea, dizziness, blurred vision, constipation, dry mouth, throat, or nose, restlessness.

Adult Dose: 4 mg TID-QID.

Pediatric Concerns: None reported. Observe for sedation.

Infant Monitoring: Sedation, dry mouth, vomiting.

Alternatives: Hydroxyzine(L2), Cetirizine(L2), Loratadine(L1)

References:
1. Pharmaceutical manufacturers prescribing information.

CYTARABINE

Trade: Alexan, Arabine, Cytarabine, Cytosar, Cytosar-U, Tarabine PFS

Category: Antineoplastic

LRC: L5 - No Data-Hazardous

Cytosine arabinoside or Cytarabine is an antimetabolite and antineoplastic agent commonly used in the treatment of acute lymphoid leukemia in adults and children.[1] Cytarabine is rapidly metabolized by the liver and gastrointestinal mucosa, and it is not effective orally, less than 20% of the orally administered dose is absorbed from the gastrointestinal tract.

Following rapid intravenous injection of cytarabine, the disappearance from plasma is biphasic. There is an initial distributive phase with a half-life of about 10 minutes, followed by a second elimination phase with a half-life of about 1 to 3 hours.[1] After the distributive phase, more than 80% of the drug can be accounted for by the inactive metabolite 1-beta-D-arabinofuranosyluracil (ara-U). Cytarabine is essentially cleared from the body by conversion to ara-U. Within 24 hours about 80 percent of the administered drug is recovered in the urine, approximately 90 percent of which is excreted as ara-U. No data are available on its transfer to milk but levels would probably be quite low.

Withhold breastfeeding for at least 24-48 hours.

T 1/2	(beta) 1-3 h	MW	243.2 Da	PB	
Tmax		RID		Vd	0.6 L/kg
Oral	<20%	M/P		pKa	

Adult Concerns: Headache, dizziness, fever, mucositis, vomiting, diarrhea, anorexia, changes in liver and renal function, urinary retention, myelosuppression, leukopenia, neutropenia, anemia, rash.

Adult Dose: 100 mg/m² IV daily.

Pediatric Concerns:

Infant Monitoring: Withhold breastfeeding for at least 24-48 hours.

Alternatives:

References:
1. Pharmaceutical manufacturers prescribing information.

CYTOMEGALOVIRUS INFECTIONS

Trade: CMV, Human Cytomegalovirus

Category: Infectious Disease

LRC: L3 - Limited Data-Probably Compatible

Cytomegalovirus (CMV) is a double-stranded DNA herpesvirus that infects most of the world's population and is endemic to much of the United States. Infection is frequent and severe in immunosuppressed infants but infrequent in full-term neonates. CMV crosses the placenta, but infection is much more likely following peri- and post-natal exposure. Healthy infants generally exhibit minimal symptoms and suffer no sequelae from post-natal infection.[1] However, premature or otherwise immunocompromised infants may develop hepatitis, neurologic illness, or a diffuse interstitial pneumonitis.[2]

Vertical transmission of CMV can occur perinatally or via breast milk. Virtually all CMV positive women have PCR-detectable virus in their milk.[3] In healthy, full-term babies, the CMV found in breast milk is not overtly dangerous, and these mothers can breastfeed successfully.[4] The relative risk of contracting CMV is about the same in infants fed milk from seropositive mothers (5.7%) as those fed milk from seronegative mothers or formula (0%-11%).[5,6] However, a mother who seroconverts postpartum has a greater chance (up to 69%) of passing the infection to her baby.[6,7]

Premature infants ingesting CMV-positive breast milk appear to become infected more frequently than those fed milk from seronegative mothers or formula. However, the CMV infection seems not affect the rate of adverse clinical outcomes among preterm infants.[8] It is possible that this latter point is due to in-utero exposure or to a partial, passive immunity acquired through the milk. The American Academy of Pediatrics has stated that the benefits of milk from CMV positive mothers outweigh the risks of clinical disease from CMV transmission.[9]

Freezing milk is not effective in preventing transmission of CMV.[10] Pasteurization does prevent transmission but also destroys many of the benefits of the milk.[11] Fresh milk is preferred in all but the most severely immunocompromised patient.[9]

A new and excellent review of breast milk-associated CMV infections in premature infants suggests no new answers. CMV is essentially transferred via milk but the degree of transfer is low, and it is now known how the infection occurs.[12]

Adult Concerns: Asymptomatic to hepatosplenomegaly. Fever, fatigue, sore throat, swollen glands, decreased appetite, diarrhea, hepatitis.

Adult Dose:

Pediatric Concerns: CMV transfer into breast milk is known but apparently of low risk to infants born of CMV positive mothers. The incidence of postnatal transmission of CMV is apparently low.

Infant Monitoring: Fever, diarrhea, rash, if clinical symptoms arise (yellowing of skin or whites of eyes) check liver enzymes and bilirubin.

Alternatives:

References:

1. Kurath S, Halwachs-Baumann G, Muller W, Resch B. Transmission of cytomegalovirus via breast milk to the prematurely born infant: a systematic review. Clin Microbiol Infect. August 2010;16(8):1172-1178.
2. Rosenberg AA, Grover T. The newborn infant. In: Hay WW, Levin MJ, Deterding RR, Abzug MJ, eds. CURRENT Diagnosis & Treatment: Pediatrics, 22nd ed. New York, NY: McGraw-Hill; 2013.
3. Hotsubo T, Nagata N, Shimada M, Yoshida K, Fujinaga K, Chiba S. Detection of human cytomegalovirus DNA in breast milk by means of polymerase chain reaction. Microbiol Immunol. 1994;38(10):809-811.
4. Lawrence R. Breastfeeding: a guide for the medical profession. St. Louis, MO: Mosby Publishers; 1994.
5. Doctor S, Friedman S, Dunn MS, et al. Cytomegalovirus transmission to extremely low-birthweight infants through breast milk. Acta paediatrica. January 2005;94(1):53-58.
6. Miron D, Brosilow S, Felszer K, et al. Incidence and clinical manifestations of breast milk-acquired Cytomegalovirus infection in low birth weight infants. J Perinatol. May 2005;25(5):299-303.
7. Dworsky M, Yow M, Stagno S, Pass RF, Alford C. Cytomegalovirus infection of breast milk and transmission in infancy. Pediatrics. September 1983;72(3):295-299.
8. Schanler RJ. CMV acquisition in premature infants fed human milk: reason to worry? J Perinatol. May 2005;25(5):297-298.
9. American Academy of Pediatrics. Breastfeeding and the use of human milk. Pediatrics. March 2012;129(3):e827-e841.
10. Maschmann J, Hamprecht K, Weissbrich B, Dietz K, Jahn G, Speer CP. Freeze-thawing of breast milk does not prevent cytomegalovirus transmission to a preterm infant. Arch Dis Child Fetal Neonatal Ed. July 2006;91(4):F288-F290.
11. Hamprecht K, Maschmann J, Muller D, et al. Cytomegalovirus (CMV) inactivation in breast milk: reassessment of pasteurization and freeze-thawing. Pediatr Res. October 2004;56(4):529-535.
12. Schleiss MR. Breast milk-acquired cytomegalovirus in premature infants: uncertain consequences and unsolved biological questions. JAMA Pediatr. 2020;174(2):121-123. doi:10.1001/jamapediatrics.2019.4538.

DABIGATRAN ETEXILATE

Trade: Pradaxa

Category: Platelet Aggregation Inhibitor

LRC: L3 - No Data-Probably Compatible

Dabigatran is an inhibitor of platelet function and is used in the treatment of thromboembolic disorders.[1] There are no studies on the transfer of dabigatran to breast milk. The molecular weight is large (628 Da) and the oral bioavailability is low (6.5%); therefore, clinically relevant levels are not expected to occur in a breastfed infant.

T 1/2	12-17 h	MW	627.7 Da	PB	Low
Tmax	0.5-2 h	RID		Vd	0.71-1 L/kg
Oral	6.5%	M/P		pKa	

Adult Concerns: Dyspepsia, elevated liver enzymes, anemia, thrombocytopenia, hemorrhage (e.g., gastrointestinal bleeding, hematuria, etc.).

Adult Dose: 75 mg bid.

Pediatric Concerns:

Infant Monitoring: Rare-bruising on the skin, blood in urine, vomit, or stool.

Alternatives:

References:

1. Stangier J. Clinical pharmacokinetics and pharmacodynamics of the oral direct thrombin inhibitor dabigatran etexilate. Clin Pharmacokinet. 2008;47(5):285-295.

DACARBAZINE

Trade: Dacarbazine

Category: Anticancer

LRC: L5 - No Data-Hazardous

Dacarbazine is an anti-cancer agent that is administered intravenously. It is indicated for the treatment of metastatic malignant melanoma and Hodgkin's disease. The exact mechanism of action is still unknown. The transfer of Dacarbazine to human milk is still not known. Dacarbazine is widely distributed, exceeding the total body water content. When used in therapeutic doses, it is not significantly bound to plasma protein.[1] This product is very low in molecular weight (182 Da), with a brief half-life of 5 hours, and will probably enter milk easily, therefore mothers should be advised to withhold breastfeeding for at least 48 hours following exposure.

T 1/2	5 h	MW	182.19 Da	PB	0%-5%
Tmax		RID		Vd	1.49 L/kg
Oral		M/P		pKa	5.89

Adult Concerns: Alopecia, nausea, vomiting, anorexia, changes in liver enzymes and renal function, myelosuppression, leukopenia, anemia, thrombocytopenia.

Adult Dose: 2-4.5 mg/kg/day.

Pediatric Concerns: No data are available for breastfeeding mothers.

Infant Monitoring: Vomiting, diarrhea, weight gain, if clinical signs present, monitor liver function. Recommend to avoid breastfeeding for 48 hours.

Alternatives:

References:

1. Pharmaceutical manufacturers prescribing information.

DACLIZUMAB

Trade: Zinbryta

Category: Monoclonal Antibody

LRC: L3 - No Data-Probably Compatible

Daclizumab is used for the treatment of multiple sclerosis (MS), the potential mechanism by which it may treat relapsing MS is by inhibiting the IL-2 activation of lymphocytes by binding the CD25 subunit of the high affinity IL-2 receptor.[1] This medication is typically indicated in patients whom have had poor response to greater than two MS medications. At this time there are no data regarding the transfer of daclizumab to human milk; however, the manufacturer reports that this medication is known to enter the milk of monkeys.

Despite the fact that the molecular weight of this medication is very large and the amount in breast milk is expected to be exceptionally low, there are no long-term data concerning the safety of using immune modulating medications in breastfeeding mothers. Further there are current data that suggest that other immune modulating drugs (IgG) do transfer to milk in low levels, and may survive briefly in the intestine. Therefore, some caution is recommended, especially in the colostral phase. Until we know more about transfer of various IgG formulations in human milk, and their absorption and survival of IgG some caution is recommended.

T 1/2	21 days	MW	144,000 Da	PB	
Tmax	5-7 days	RID		Vd	0.09 L/kg
Oral		M/P		pKa	

Adult Concerns: Depression, seizure, colitis, changes in liver function, fever, infection, lymphadenopathy, leukopenia, autoimmune disease, anemia, acne, eczema, skin rash.

Adult Dose: 150 mg SC once monthly.

Pediatric Concerns: At this time there are no data in lactation or pediatric patients less than 17 years of age.

Infant Monitoring: Fever, frequent infections, poor feeding/poor weight gain, diarrhea. Based on clinical symptoms some infants may require monitoring their hematology, and/or liver function.

Alternatives:

References:
1. Pharmaceutical manufacturer product monograph, 2016.

DACTINOMYCIN

Trade: Actinomycin D, Cosmegen

Category: Antineoplastic

LRC: L5 - No Data-Hazardous

Dactinomycin is one of the actinomycins, a group of antibiotics produced by various species of Streptomyces, and it is used to treat Wilm's tumor, Ewing's sarcoma, and many other malignancies.[1] After single or multiple IV doses, dactinomycin is rapidly distributed into and extensively bound to body tissues. Results of a study with radioactive actinomycin D in patients with malignant melanoma indicate that dactinomycin is minimally metabolized, is concentrated in nucleated cells, and does not appreciably penetrate the blood-brain barrier (<10%). The terminal plasma half-life for for dactinomycin is approximately 36 hours. Dactinomycin is concentrated in nucleated cells; concentrations are highest in bone marrow and tumor cells relative to plasma. No data are available on its transfer to human milk; however, it is probably quite low as its molecular weight is high (1255 Da). That withstanding, it is extremely cytotoxic. Mothers should abstain from breastfeeding for at least 10 days.

T 1/2	36 h	MW	1255.4 Da	PB	
Tmax		RID		Vd	
Oral		M/P		pKa	11.1

Adult Concerns: Fatigue, fever, lethargy, alopecia, mucositis, vomiting, anorexia, changes in liver and renal function, hyperuricemia, hypocalcemia, agranulocytosis, anemia, edema, myalgia, severe rash.

Adult Dose: Do not exceed 15 µg/kg/day IV for five days per 2-week cycle.

Pediatric Concerns:

Infant Monitoring: Mothers should abstain from breastfeeding for at least 10 days.

Alternatives:

References:
1. Pharmaceutical manufacturers prescribing information.

DALBAVANCIN

Trade: Dalvance

Category: Antibiotic, Other

LRC: L3 - No Data-Probably Compatible

Dalbavancin is an intravenous lipoglycopeptide antibiotic indicated for the treatment of bacterial skin and soft tissue infections caused by susceptible gram-positive organisms including methicillin-resistant *Staphylococcus aureus* and *Enterococcus faecalis*.[1] At this time there are no data regarding the transfer of dalbavancin to human milk; however, based on its large molecular weight we anticipate very little should enter human milk. Structurally dalbavancin is a mixture of five similar homologs, each of which weigh 1802-1830 Da. In addition, this large molecular weight makes this drug unlikely to be absorbed in the infant's gastrointestinal tract should it enter human milk.

T 1/2	204 h	MW	1802-1830 Da	PB	93%
Tmax		RID		Vd	
Oral		M/P		pKa	

Adult Concerns: Headache, dizziness, flushing, nausea, vomiting, diarrhea, changes in liver function, anemia, leukopenia, neutropenia, thrombocytopenia.

Adult Dose: 1500 mg single dose by IV infusion.

Pediatric Concerns: No safety data in breastfed infants or pediatrics is available at this time.[1]

Infant Monitoring: Vomiting, diarrhea, changes in gastrointestinal flora, and rash; if clinical symptoms arise a CBC or liver function tests may be warranted.

Alternatives: Vancomycin, clindamycin.

References:
1. Pharmaceutical manufacturers prescribing information.

DALFOPRISTIN + QUINUPRISTIN

Trade: Synercid

Category: Antibiotic, Other

LRC: L3 - No Data-Probably Compatible

Dalfopristin and quinupristin is a combination product used to treat complicated infections of the skin and soft tissue.[1] It is a streptogramin antibacterial agent given intravenously to treat methicillin susceptible *Staphylococcus aureus* and *Streptococcus pyogenes*. It has been used to treat some cases of methicillin-resistant *Staphylococcus aureus* when other alternatives have failed. No data are available on its transfer to human milk; however, due to its large molecular weight, milk levels will probably be low.

T 1/2	Dalf/quin: 1 h/3 h	MW	Dalf/quin: 691/1022 Da	PB	Dalf/quin: 11%-26%/55%-78%
Tmax		RID		Vd	Dalf/quin: 0.24/0.45 L/kg
Oral	Dalf/quin: nil	M/P		pKa	

Adult Concerns: Headache, nausea, vomiting, diarrhea, hyperglycemia, increase in LDH and GGT, hyperbilirubinemia, anemia, arthralgia, myalgia, infusion site reactions.

Adult Dose: 7.5 mg/kg every 12 hours.

Pediatric Concerns: None reported via milk.

Infant Monitoring: Vomiting, diarrhea; if clinical symptoms check liver function.

Alternatives:

References:
1. Pharmaceutical manufacturers prescribing information.

DALTEPARIN SODIUM

Trade: Fragmin

Category: Anticoagulant

LRC: L2 - Limited Data-Probably Compatible

Dalteparin is a low molecular weight polysaccharide fragment of heparin (LMWH) used clinically as an anticoagulant. In a study of two patients who received 5,000-10,000 units of dalteparin, none was found in human milk.[1] In another study of 15 post-caesarian patients early postpartum (mean=5.7 days), blood and milk levels of dalteparin were determined 3-4 hours post-treatment.[2] Following subcutaneous doses of 2500 units, maternal plasma levels averaged 0.074 to 0.308 units/mL. Breast milk levels of dalteparin ranged from <0.005 to 0.037 IU/mL of milk. The milk/plasma ratio ranged from 0.025 to 0.224. Using this data, an infant ingesting 150 mL/kg/day of milk, would ingest approximately 5.5 units/kg/day. Due to the polysaccharide nature of this production, oral absorption is unlikely. Further, because this study was done early postpartum, it is possible that the levels in "mature" milk would be lower. The authors suggest that it appears highly unlikely that puerperal thromboprophylaxis with LMWH has any clinically relevant effect on the nursing infant.

T 1/2	2.3 h	MW	6000 Da	PB	
Tmax	2-4 h (SC)	RID		Vd	0.06 L/kg
Oral	None	M/P	0.025-0.224	pKa	

Adult Concerns: Bruising on the skin, hemorrhage, blood in urine or stool, thrombocytopenia and pain/bruising at injection site.

Adult Dose: 5,000 units sc daily for prophylaxis; 200 units/kg/day sc for treatment.

Pediatric Concerns: None reported via milk at this time.

Infant Monitoring: Rare-bruising on the skin, blood in urine, vomit or stool.

Alternatives: Enoxaparin(L2)

References:
1. Harenberg J, Leber G, Zimmermann R, Schmidt W. Prevention of thromboembolism with low-molecular weight heparin in pregnancy. Geburtshilfe Frauenheilkd. 1987; 47(1):15-18.
2. Richter C, Sitzmann J, Lang P, Weitzel H, Huch A, Huch R. Excretion of low molecular weight heparin in human milk. Br J Clin Pharmacol. 2001; 52(6):708-710.

DANAZOL

Trade: Azol, Cyclomen, Danocrine, Danol

Category: Androgen

LRC: L5 - No Data-Hazardous

Danazol suppresses the pituitary-ovarian axis by inhibiting ovarian steroidogenesis resulting in decreased secretion of estradiol and may increase androgens.[1] Danazol is believed to reduce plasma prolactin levels in individuals. The mechanisms through which Danazol treatment affects prolactin release has not been fully delineated, but it is probably due to the hypoestrogenic status resulting from the medication. Danazol is primarily used for treating endometriosis. Due to its effect on pituitary hormones and its androgenic effects, it may reduce the rate of breast milk production, although this has not been documented. No data on its transfer to human milk are available, however its use should be avoided in breastfeeding mothers.

T 1/2	4.5 h	MW	337 Da	PB	
Tmax	2 h	RID		Vd	
Oral	Complete	M/P		pKa	13.1

Adult Concerns: Breast size reduction, androgenic effects, hirsutism, acne, weight gain, edema, testicular atrophy, thrombocytopenia, thrombocytosis, hot flashes, breakthrough menstrual bleeding.

Adult Dose: 50-200 mg BID.

Pediatric Concerns: None reported, but caution is urged.

Infant Monitoring: Androgenic effects in the infant; may suppress prolactin production.

Alternatives:

References:
1. Pharmaceutical manufacturers prescribing information.

DANTROLENE

Trade: Dantrium

Category: Skeletal Muscle Relaxant

LRC: L4 - Limited Data-Possibly Hazardous

Dantrolene produces a direct skeletal muscle relaxation and is indicated for spasticity resulting from upper motor neuron disorders such as multiple sclerosis, cerebral palsy, etc.[1] It is not indicated for rheumatic disorders or musculoskeletal trauma.

In one study, a mother received IV dantrolene (160 mg) for symptoms of malignant hyperthermia, after the umbilical cord was clamped just after the delivery of her baby.[2] Concentrations of dantrolene in breastmilk ranged from

1.2 mg/L on day 2 to 0.05 mg/L on day 4. The relative infant dose is calculated at 7.9% of the maternal dose. The highest concentration in breast milk was detected 36 hours after the first IV bolus of dantrolene. Based on the elimination half-life determined in this study (9.02 hours), the authors suggest that breastfeeding is safe 2 days after discontinuation of IV dantrolene administration in the mother.

T 1/2	8.7 h	MW	314 Da	PB	
Tmax	5 h	RID	7.9%	Vd	
Oral	35%	M/P		pKa	9.23

Adult Concerns: Adverse effects are quite common and include weakness, dizziness, diarrhea, slurred speech, drooling, and nausea. Significant risk for hepatotoxicity. Visual and auditory hallucinations.

Adult Dose: 100 mg orally three times a day.

Pediatric Concerns: None reported, but caution is urged. A suitable waiting period for breastfeeding is recommended.

Infant Monitoring: Drowsiness, weakness, vomiting, diarrhea, liver toxicity (yellowing of the eyes or skin).

Alternatives:

References:
1. Pharmaceutical manufacturers prescribing information.
2. Fricker RM, Hoerauf KH, Drewe J, Kress HG. Secretion of dantrolene into breast milk after acute therapy of a suspected malignant hyperthermia crisis during cesarean section. Anesthesiology. 1998; 89(4):1023-1025.

DAPSONE

Trade: Aczone, Avlosulfon, Dapsone, Maloprim

Category: Antibiotic, Other

LRC: L4 - Limited Data-Possibly Hazardous

Dapsone is a sulfone antibiotic useful for treating leprosy, tuberculoid leprosy, dermatitis herpetiformis, brown recluse spider bites, and *Pneumocystis jiroveci* pneumonia (formerly known as P. carinii pneumonia or PCP).[1] In one case report of a mother consuming 50 mg daily while breastfeeding, both the mother and infant had symptoms of hemolytic anemia.[2] Plasma levels of dapsone in mother and infant were 1622 ng/mL and 439 ng/mL respectively. Breast milk levels were reported to be 1092 μg/L.

In another study, three women were given a single oral dose of 12.5 mg pyrimethamine + 100 mg dapsone + 300 mg chloroquine within 2-5 days of delivery.[3] Blood and milk samples were then collected over the next 9 days; the three infants were reported to receive about 590, 850 and 310 μg dapsone over the study period of about 9 days if they each consumed about 1 L of milk a day. The authors estimate the relative infant dose to be 14.3% of the maternal dose or 0.21 mg/kg over 9 days. No adverse effects were reported in any of the infants.

Dapsone gel 5% has just been released for the treatment of acne. After application twice daily for 14 days, the dapsone AUC 0-24 hours was 415 ng-h/mL for dapsone gel, 5%, whereas following a single 100 mg dose of oral dapsone the AUC was 52,641 ng-h/mL. Apparently, the transcutaneous absorption of dapsone is minimal.

Dapsone is one of those drugs which apparently has all the proper kinetic parameters to enter milk, high lipophilicity, low molecular weight, high volume of distribution, high pKa, etc. so it should be used very cautiously, if at all. Its topical use is probably of minimal risk to the infant.

T 1/2	28 h	MW	248 Da	PB	70%-90%
Tmax	4-8 h	RID	6.3%-22.5%	Vd	1-2 L/kg
Oral	86%-100%	M/P		pKa	1.3

Adult Concerns: Headache, fever, insomnia, psychosis, vertigo, blurred vision, tinnitus, tachycardia, vomiting, changes in liver and renal function, leukopenia, hemolytic anemia (particularly in G6PD deficient persons), methemoglobinemia, aplastic anemia, severe skin reactions.

Adult Dose: 100 mg daily.

Pediatric Concerns: Hemolytic anemia in one breastfed infant.

Infant Monitoring: Irritability, insomnia, vomiting, weight gain, if clinical symptoms check liver and renal function and CBC.

Alternatives:

References:
1. Pharmaceutical manufacturers prescribing information.
2. Sanders SW, Zone JJ, Foltz RL, Tolman KG, Rollins DE. Hemolytic anemia induced by dapsone transmitted through breast milk. Ann Intern Med. 1982; 96(4):465-466.
3. Edstein MD, Veenendaal JR, Newman K, Hyslop R. Excretion of chloroquine, dapsone and pyrimethamine in human milk. Br J Clin Pharmacol. 1986; 22(6):733-735.

DAPTOMYCIN

Trade: Cubicin

Category: Antibiotic, Other

LRC:

Daptomycin is used intravenously for the treatment of complicated skin infections caused by susceptible strains of *Staphylococcus aureus* (including methicillin-resistant or MRSA strains), *Streptococcus pyogenes, Streptococcus agalactiae, Streptococcus dysgalactiae,* and *Enterococcus faecalis.*[1]

In a mother 5 months postpartum who received 500 mg IV daily (6.7 mg/kg/day), the highest concentration measured in milk was 44.7 ng/mL at 8 hours following administration.[2] Reported levels in milk were 33.5, 44.7, 40.8, 39.3, and 29.2 ng/mL at 4, 8, 12, 16, and 20 hours respectively. The mother and infant received therapy for 4 weeks, and no adverse events were noted in the mother or infant. In addition, the daptomycin present in milk is poorly absorbed orally.

T 1/2	9 h	MW	1620 Da	PB	92%
Tmax	0.5 h	RID	0.06%-0.1%	Vd	0.1 L/kg
Oral	Nil	M/P	0.0012	pKa	5.3

Adult Concerns: Elevations of creatinine kinase have been reported suggesting skeletal muscle toxicity and blood tests are required weekly during treatment. Gastrointestinal disorders, injection site reactions, fever, headache, insomnia, dizziness, and rash have been infrequently reported.

Adult Dose: 4 mg/kg infusions once every 24 hours for 7-14 days.

Pediatric Concerns: None reported via milk in one case exposed for 4 weeks.

Infant Monitoring: Lethargy, vomiting, diarrhea, changes in gastrointestinal flora, and rash.

Alternatives:

References:
1. Pharmaceutical manufacturers prescribing information.
2. Buitrago MI, Crompton JA, Bertolami S, North DS, Nathan RA. Extremely low excretion of daptomycin into breast milk of a nursing mother with methicillin-resistant *Staphylococcus aureus* pelvic inflammatory disease. Pharmacotherapy. 2009 Mar;29(3):347-351.

DARBEPOETIN ALFA

Trade: Aranesp

Category: Hematopoietic

LRC: L3 - No Data-Probably Compatible

Darbepoetin alfa is used to treat anemia in patients with chronic renal failure and patients receiving chemotherapy. It stimulates erythropoiesis much the same way as endogenous erythropoietin. Administration can be either IV or subcutaneous, with peak serum levels following subcutaneous dosing occurring after 34 hours.[1] No data are available concerning levels in breast milk. However, this is a large molecular weight protein that is unlikely to enter the milk compartment, or be orally bioavailable to an infant.

T 1/2	21 h	MW	37,000 Da	PB	
Tmax		RID		Vd	0.06 L/kg
Oral	Nil	M/P		pKa	

Adult Concerns: Hypertension, hypotension, edema, fatigue, diarrhea, and infection.

Adult Dose: IV: 0.45 µg/kg once weekly; SQ: 2.25 µg/kg once weekly.

Pediatric Concerns: No data are available. Because of its large molecular weight, it is unlikely that this protein will enter breast milk.

Infant Monitoring:

Alternatives:

References:

1. Pharmaceutical manufacturers prescribing information.

DARIFENACIN

Trade: Enablex

Category: Renal-Urologic Agent

LRC: L3 - No Data-Probably Compatible

Darifenacin is an anticholinergic agent used for the treatment of overactive bladder with symptoms of urgent urinary incontinence, urgency, and frequency.[1] It is not known if darifenacin is transferred into human milk, although its chemistry would probably limit its transfer to milk. However, some caution is recommended as this is a strong anticholinergic muscarinic agent and could cause urinary retention, dry mouth, mydriasis, constipation, and other gastrointestinal symptoms in a breastfed infant.

T 1/2	12.3 h	MW	507 Da	PB	98%
Tmax	6.5 h	RID		Vd	2.3 L/kg
Oral	15%-19%	M/P		pKa	9.20

Adult Concerns: Typical anticholinergic symptoms: dry mouth, blurred vision, dry eyes, dyspepsia, abdominal pain, constipation, urinary retention, and heat exhaustion due to decreased sweating.

Adult Dose: 7.5 mg daily.

Pediatric Concerns: No data available at this time.

Infant Monitoring: Dry mouth, dry eyes, abdominal pain, constipation, urinary retention.

Alternatives:

References:

1. Pharmaceutical manufacturers prescribing information.

DASABUVIR+OMBITASVIR+PARITAPREVIR+RITONAVIR

Trade: Viekira Pak, Viekira XR, Holkira Pak

Category: Antiviral

LRC: L4 - Limited Data-Possibly Hazardous

This combination medication which contains dasabuvir, ombitasvir, paritaprevir and ritonavir is used for the treatment of chronic hepatitis C.[1] This medication combination may also be used in combination with ribavirin. The combination that includes ribavirin should not be used in breastfeeding mothers.

The transfer of dasabuvir, ombitasvir, paritaprevir to human milk is not known.[1] Ritonavir has been studied and is most commonly used to treat HIV.

A study that evaluated the safety of maternal antiretrovirals for prophylaxis against HIV transmission to the infant during lactation also reported the milk levels of ritonavir (n=23 samples).[2] This study tested maternal serum and breast milk on the day of delivery and at months 1, 3, and 6 postpartum. Infant levels were also taken at months 1, 3, and 6 of age. The median drug concentrations of ritonavir in maternal serum, breast milk and the infant were 422 ng/mL (160-982 ng/mL), 79 ng/mL (31-193 ng/mL) and 7 ng/mL (0-138 ng/mL), respectively. The milk to plasma ratio was 0.2. The relative infant dose that we calculated using the maternal dose of 100 mg twice a day and median milk level was 0.42%. This study also reported other infant adverse events (e.g., pneumonia, diarrhea, changes in liver function, neutropenia, thrombocytopenia), but was unable to determine which medication caused the effects based on drug levels, please see study for adverse event details.

In 2014, a study was published that looked at HIV RNA in milk and the pharmacokinetics of maternal medications in milk to prevent transmission of HIV to the infant during lactation.[3] In this study, 30 women were given one Combivir tablet twice a day (zidovudine 300 mg + lamivudine 150 mg/tab) with two tablets of Aluvia twice a day (lopinavir 200 mg + ritonavir 50 mg) starting post delivery until breastfeeding was stopped or 28 weeks. Samples were taken predose (time 0) and then at 2, 4, and 6 hours postdose when the women were enrolled at either 6, 12, or 24 weeks postpartum. The median drug concentrations of ritonavir in maternal serum, breast milk, and the infant were 364 ng/mL (280-489 ng/mL), 79 ng/mL (47-112 ng/mL) and undetectable, respectively. The milk to plasma ratio was 0.195. The RID that we calculated using the maternal dose of 100 mg twice a day and median milk level was 0.42%.

The decision to breastfeed while on the drug should be weighed against potential benefits and risks to both the mother and infant. Without more data, these products appear to be of moderate risk to the breastfed infant. Do not use if Ribavirin is added.

T 1/2	Das/omb/par/rit: 5.5-6 h/21-25 h/5.5 h/4 h	MW	Das/omb/par/rit: 2874.539 Da	PB	Das/omb/par/rit: >99.5%/99.9%/97%-98.6%/>99%
Tmax	Das/omb/par/rit: 4 h/5 h/4-5 h/4-5 h	RID		Vd	Das/omb/par/rit: 2.129/2.471/1.471/.307 L/kg
Oral	Das/omb/par/rit: 70%/485/53%/NA	M/P		pKa	

Adult Concerns: Viekira Pak with ribavirin: Fatigue, nausea, pruritus, other skin reactions, insomnia, and asthenia. Viekira Pak without ribavirin: Nausea, pruritus, and insomnia.

Adult Dose: Two ombitasvir, paritaprevir, ritonavir tablets once daily and one dasabuvir tablet twice daily.

Pediatric Concerns:

Infant Monitoring: This combination product is basically unstudied in breastfeeding mothers and should probably not be used until more data are available on the individual components in the combination product.

Alternatives:

References:
1. Pharmaceutical manufacturers prescribing information.
2. Palombi L, Pirillo MF, Andreotti M, et al. Antiretroviral prophylaxis for breastfeeding transmission in Malawi: drug concentrations, virological efficacy and safety. Antivir Ther. 2012;17:1511-1519.
3. Corbett AH, Kayira D, White NR, et al. Antiretroviral pharmacokinetics in mothers and breastfeeding infants from 6 to 24 weeks postpartum: results of the BAN study. Antivir Ther. 2014;19(6):587-595.

DAUNORUBICIN

Trade: Cerubidin, Cerubidine, DaunoXome, Daunoblastin, Daunoblastina

Category: Antineoplastic

LRC: L5 - No Data-Hazardous

This is a typical anthracycline agent used in many forms of cancer, including acute myelogenous, and lymphocytic leukemias, and others. As with doxorubicin, it is widely distributed to many body tissues. It is eliminated from the plasma compartment with a triphasic elimination curve. Its last elimination T1/2 (gamma) ranges from 11.2 to 47.4 hours, depending on the dose. It is rapidly metabolized to daunorubicinol, which achieves a C_{max} at 24 hours.[1] Daunorubicinol has a half-life of approximately 27 hours. No data are available on the transfer of this anthracycline to human milk. However, a close congener, doxorubicin, has been measured in milk, and the levels are low, but prolonged. Withhold breastfeeding for a minimum of 7 to 10 days.

T 1/2	18.5 h; 27h daunorubicinol	MW	563.99 Da	PB	97%
Tmax		RID		Vd	
Oral		M/P		pKa	9.53

Adult Concerns: Alopecia, arrhythmias, heart failure, stomatitis, vomiting, diarrhea, discoloration of urine and saliva and sweat and tears, myelosuppression, leukopenia, neutropenia, anemia, thrombocytopenia.

Adult Dose: 45-100 mg/m²/day IV.

Pediatric Concerns: None reported at this time.

Infant Monitoring: Withhold breastfeeding for a minimum of 7 to 10 days.

Alternatives:

References:
1. Pharmaceutical manufacturers prescribing information.

DEET

Trade: 6-12 Plus, Cutter Insect Repellent, DEET, Deep Woods Off!, Diethyl-m-Toluamide, Diethyltoluamide, Muskol, Off!

Category: Insect Repellant

LRC: L3 - No Data-Probably Compatible

N,N-Diethyl-meta-toluamide (DEET) is used worldwide as an insect repellant.[1-4] The US EPA estimates that 30% of the US population applies DEET every year. DEET is available in numerous concentrations as the protection time provided by topical use is concentration dependent. This product has been in use for more than 45 years and the reports of adverse effects in humans have been relatively rare. While there are reports of DEET toxicity, most involve the use of concentrated solutions over large body areas, or oral ingestion. Most case reports of toxicity with topical use were not serious; however, some cases of seizure have occurred with topical use and death with oral ingestion.

Skin absorption is significant and generally occurs within 2 hours of application.[1] DEET is very lipophilic and has a large volume of distribution (2.7-6.21 L/kg) and remains in the skin and adipose tissue for long periods, slowly leaking into the plasma compartment and being eliminated. Between 9% and 56% of an applied dose is absorbed in 6 hours, and most is eliminated from the plasma compartment within 4 hours via hepatic metabolism and excretion in urine.

No data are available on the transfer of DEET to human milk, but due to its lipophilicity, some probably enters the milk compartment.[3-5] Avoid the use of concentrated solutions (>30%) over large surface areas of the body if you are breastfeeding. A brief waiting period of 4 hours or more may be useful in avoiding transfer of high levels to milk, but this is probably unnecessary under conditions of normal use. Mothers should avoid chronic use over large body surface areas, and use the lowest concentration possible (depending on protection time required).

T 1/2	2.5 h	MW	191 Da	PB	
Tmax	1-2 h	RID		Vd	
Oral	Complete; 9%-56% cutaneous	M/P		pKa	

Adult Concerns: Disorientation, seizures, ataxia, depression, hypotension, dyspnea, hypersalivation, tremors, contact dermatitis, pruritus.

Adult Dose:

Pediatric Concerns: No data in lactation at this time. The American Academy of Pediatrics (AAP) recommends the use of topical DEET (10%-30%) for children greater than 2 months of age.[4]

Infant Monitoring: Seizures, dyspnea, tremors.

Alternatives:

References:

1. Robbins PJ, Cherniack MB. Review of the biodistribution and toxicity of the insect repellent N,N-diethyl-m-toluamide (DEET). J Toxicol Environ Health. 1986;18:502-525.
2. Selim S, Hartnagel RE Jr, Osimitz TG, Gabriel KL, Schoenig GP. Absorption, metabolism, and excretion of N,N-diethyl-m-toluamide: following dermal application to human volunteers. Fundam Appl Toxicol. 1995;25 (1):95-100.
3. Koren G, Matsui D, Bailey B. DEET-based insect repellents: safety implications for children and pregnant and lactation women. CMAJ. 2003;169(3):209-212.
4. American Academy of Pediatrics (AAP). 2015 Summer Safety Tips: Bug Safety. https://www.aap.org
5. Katz TM, Miller JH, Hebert AA, et al. Insect repellents: historical perspectives and new developments. J Am Acad Dermatol. 2008;58:865-871.

DEFERASIROX

Trade: Exjade

Category: Heavy Metal Chelator

LRC: L3 - No Data-Probably Compatible

Deferasirox is an orally bioavailable chelating agent that is selective for iron. It forms a complex with the iron that is unabsorbed and subsequently excreted in the feces. While deferasirox has a very low affinity for other metals such as zinc and copper, it still decreases serum concentrations of these metals. It is used in chronic iron overload due to blood transfusions.[1] No data are available on the concentrations in the breast milk compartment; however, it is unlikely that high concentrations would be in breast milk due to its high protein binding. Should the mother breast-feed, the infant's ferritin and iron levels should be monitored.

T 1/2	8-16 h	MW	373 Da	PB	99%
Tmax	2-4 h	RID		Vd	14.4 L/kg
Oral	70%	M/P		pKa	8.41

Adult Concerns: Headache, fever, dizziness, changes in vision, vomiting, diarrhea, changes in liver and renal function, leukopenia, thrombocytopenia.

Adult Dose: 20 mg/kg daily.

Pediatric Concerns: No data available in infants.

Infant Monitoring: Vomiting, diarrhea; may test infant ferritin and iron levels and supplement with iron drops if necessary.

Alternatives: Deferoxamine(L3)

References:
1. Pharmaceutical manufacturers prescribing information.

DEFEROXAMINE

Trade: Desferal, Desferrioxamine

Category: Heavy Metal Chelator

LRC: L3 - No Data-Probably Compatible

Deferoxamine is an iron-chelating agent, commonly used to facilitate the increased clearance of iron from the plasma compartment. It is indicated for the treatment of acute iron intoxication and of chronic iron overload due to transfusion-dependent anemias.[1] No data are available on its transfer into human milk, but levels in milk are likely low. Further, oral bioavailability of this product is virtually nil.

T 1/2	3-6 h	MW	656 Da	PB	
Tmax		RID		Vd	1.33 L/kg
Oral		M/P		pKa	8.39

Adult Concerns: Headache, fever, dizziness, seizure, flushing, changes in vision, hypotension, vomiting, diarrhea, urine discoloration, changes in liver and renal function, leukopenia, thrombocytopenia.

Adult Dose: 1 g then 500 mg every 4 hours for two doses (variable).

Pediatric Concerns: None reported via milk, but no studies are available.

Infant Monitoring: Vomiting, diarrhea; may test infant ferritin and iron levels.

Alternatives:

References:
1. Pharmaceutical manufacturers prescribing information.

DEHYDROEPIANDROSTERONE (DHEA)

Trade: DHEA

Category: Dietary Supplement

LRC: L5 - Limited Data-Hazardous

Dehydroepiandrosterone (DHEA) is a metabolic precursor to testosterone and estrogen. The use of DHEA-S for labor induction has been associated with a decrease in milk production postpartum with no changes in prolactin levels.[1] This may be due to the biotransformation of DHEA-S to estrogens. The use of DHEA during lactation is not recommended due to possible androgen effects.

T 1/2		MW	288.4 Da	PB	
Tmax		RID		Vd	
Oral		M/P		pKa	

Adult Concerns: Acne, hirsutism, decreased HDL, insomnia, headache, irregular menses.

Adult Dose:

Pediatric Concerns:

Infant Monitoring:

Alternatives:

References:
1. Aisaka K, Ando S, Kokubo K, Sasaki S, Yoshida K. Comprehensive approach to the clinical study of the administration of dehydro-epiandrosterone-sulfate (DHA-S) during the induction of labor. Nippon Sanka Fujinka Gakkai Zasshi. 1986;38:1605-1612.

DELAVIRDINE

Trade: Rescriptor

Category: Antiviral

LRC: L5 - No Data-Hazardous if Maternal HIV infection

Delavirdine is an antiretroviral agent that is commonly used in the treatment of human immunodeficiency virus (HIV). Currently, there are no studies regarding drug transfer to human milk or case reports in breastfeeding women. Maternal milk levels are expected to be low as delavirdine is a large drug molecule (553 Da) and has high protein binding (98%). Breastfeeding is not recommended in mothers who have HIV.[1,2]

Note: This medication is an L5 to highlight the contraindication of breastfeeding when the mother is known to be infected with HIV; this medication is not an L5 based on its risk to the infant in breast milk (no data available at this time). The Centers for Disease Control and Prevention recommend that HIV-1 infected mothers do not breastfeed their infants to avoid postnatal transmission of HIV-1.

T 1/2	5.8 h	MW	553 Da	PB	98%
Tmax	1 h	RID		Vd	
Oral	85%-100%	M/P		pKa	

Adult Concerns: Fever, headache, nausea, vomiting, diarrhea, rash, symptoms of depression, elevated liver enzymes, anxiety, bronchitis, abdominal pain, increased prothrombin time, Steven-Johnson syndrome, acute renal failure.

Adult Dose: 400 mg three times daily.

Pediatric Concerns:

Infant Monitoring: Breastfeeding is not recommended in mothers who have HIV.

Alternatives:

References:
1. World Health Organization. Global Programme on AIDS. Consensus Statement from the WHO/UNICEF Consultation on HIV Transmission and Breast-feeding. Geneva, Switzerland: WHO; 1992.
2. Latham MC, Greiner T. Breastfeeding versus formula feeding in HIV infection. Lancet. 1998;352:737.

DENOSUMAB

Trade: Prolia, Xgeva

Category: Calcium Regulator

LRC: L4 - No Data-Possibly Hazardous

Denosumab is a monoclonal antibody used in the treatment of postmenopausal osteoporosis and to prevent osteopenia in those on breast cancer and prostate cancer therapy. Also used to prevent bone metastasis. Denosumab is an IgG2 monoclonal antibody that inhibits the human RANKL (receptor activator of nuclear factor kappa-B ligand), thereby interfering with the action of the bone-resorbing osteoclasts.[1] Pregnancy studies done in mice have shown that the removal of the gene for RANKL, and subsequent absence of RANKL in pregnant mice resulted in impaired mammary gland development and absence of postpartum milk production. There are currently no studies available on the transfer of denosumab to human breast milk. The manufacturer advises against its use in nursing mothers.

Although the molecular weight of this medication is very large and the amount in breast milk is expected to be exceptionally low, there are no long-term data concerning the safety of using immune modulating medications in breastfeeding mothers. Further there are current data that suggest that some monoclonal antibody drugs do transfer to milk, and perhaps the breastfed infant. Therefore, some caution is recommended, and each woman should understand the benefits and risk of using this type of medication in lactation.

T 1/2	25.4-28 days	MW	147,000 Da	PB	
Tmax	10 days	RID		Vd	
Oral	62% sc	M/P		pKa	

Adult Concerns: Hypercholesterolemia, nausea, vomiting, arthralgia, cystitis, upper respiratory tract infections. Serious but rare side effects include rash, pancreatitis, hypocalcemia, hypophosphatemia, dyspnea, aseptic necrosis of jawbone. Contraindicated in hypocalcemia.

Adult Dose: 60 mg every 6 months, subcutaneous.

Pediatric Concerns:

Infant Monitoring: Fever, frequent infections, poor feeding/poor weight gain.

Alternatives:

References:
1. Pharmaceutical manufacturers prescribing information.

DESIPRAMINE

Trade: Norpramin, Pertofran

Category: Antidepressant, Tricyclic

LRC: L2 - Limited Data-Probably Compatible

Desipramine is a prototypic tricyclic antidepressant. In one case report, a mother taking 200 mg of desipramine at bedtime had milk/plasma ratios of 0.4 to 0.9 with milk levels ranging between 17-35 µg/L.[1] Desipramine was not found in the infant's blood although these levels are probably too low to measure.

In another study of a mother consuming 300 mg of desipramine daily, the milk levels were 30% higher than the maternal serum.[2] The milk concentrations of desipramine were reported to be 316 to 328 µg/L with peak concentrations occurring at 4 hours postdose. Assuming an average milk concentration of 280 µg/L, an infant would receive approximately 42 µg/kg/day.

One small study that followed four groups of women prescribed TCAs throughout different stages of reproduction found no adverse events in the group of infants whose mothers were prescribed these medications in lactation.[3] This study included 21 women (one on desipramine) that initiated tricyclic antidepressant therapy at a mean of 10.3 weeks postpartum and breastfed on treatment for a mean of 12 weeks.

T 1/2	7-60 h	MW	266 Da	PB	82%
Tmax	4-6 h	RID	0.3%-0.9%	Vd	22-59 L/kg
Oral	90%	M/P	0.4-0.9	pKa	9.5

Adult Concerns: Anticholinergic side effects, such as drying of secretions, dilated pupils, sedation, constipation, fatigue, peculiar taste.

Adult Dose: 100-200 mg daily.

Pediatric Concerns: None reported at this time.

Infant Monitoring: Sedation or irritability, dry mouth, not waking to feed/poor feeding, constipation, urinary retention, weight gain.

Alternatives: Amoxapine(L2), Imipramine(L2), Sertraline(L2)

References:
1. Sovner R, Orsulak PJ. Excretion of imipramine and desipramine in human breast milk. Am J Psychiatry. 1979;136(4A):451-452.
2. Stancer HC, Reed KL. Desipramine and 2-hydroxydesipramine in human breast milk and the nursing infant's serum. Am J Psychiatry. 1986;143(12):1597-1600.
3. Misri S, Sivertz K. Tricyclic drugs in pregnancy and lactation: a preliminary report. Int J Psychiatry Med. 1991;21:157-171.

DESLORATADINE

Trade: Clarinex

Category: Antihistamine

LRC: L2 - Limited Data-Probably Compatible

Desloratadine is the active metabolite of loratadine and its half-life is longer than the parent compound. While we do not have specific data on desloratadine, we do have a good report on the prodrug loratadine.

Six women 1-12 months postpartum were given a single 40 mg dose of loratadine and instructed not to breastfeed their infant postdose.[1] Maternal blood and milk samples were drawn at multiple time points from 0-48 hours postdose. The peak maternal plasma concentrations of loratadine and its active metabolite descarboethoxyloratadine were 30.5 ng/mL and 18.6 ng/mL, respectively. This produced peak milk concentrations of 29.2 ng/mL and 16 ng/mL of loratadine and its metabolite, respectively. Therefore, the total peak milk concentrations of loratadine and its metabolite following a 40 mg maternal dose is 45.2 ng/mL. Over 48 hours, the amount of loratadine transferred via milk was 4.2 µg, which was 0.01% of the maternal dose. Through 48 hours, only 6 µg of descarboethoxyloratadine (7.5 µg loratadine equivalents) was excreted into breast milk, which was 0.019% of the maternal dose. This amounts to a total of 11.7 µg or 0.029% of the administered dose of loratadine and its active metabolite transferred into milk over 48 hours. According to the authors, a 4 kg infant would receive only 2.9 µg/kg of loratadine.

T 1/2	27 h	MW	310 Da	PB	87%
Tmax	3 h	RID	0.03%	Vd	
Oral	Good	M/P		pKa	9.73

Adult Concerns: Sedation, dry mouth, fatigue, nausea, tachycardia, palpitations.

Adult Dose: 5 mg daily.

Pediatric Concerns: None reported via milk. Levels of loratadine have been reported and are low. No adverse effects have been reported in breastfeeding infants with loratadine or desloratadine.

Infant Monitoring: Sedation.

Alternatives: Loratadine(L1), Cetirizine(L2)

References:
1. Pharmaceutical manufacturers prescribing information.

DESMOPRESSIN ACETATE

Trade: DDAVP, Desmospray, Minirin, Rhinyle, Stimate

Category: Vasopressor

LRC: L2 - Limited Data-Probably Compatible

Desmopressin acetate (DDAVP) is a small synthetic octapeptide antidiuretic hormone.[1] Desmopressin increases reabsorption of water by the collecting ducts in the kidneys resulting in decreased urinary flow (ADH effect). Generally used in patients who lack pituitary vasopressin, it is primarily used intranasally or intravenously. Unlike natural vasopressin, desmopressin has no effect on growth hormone, prolactin, or luteinizing hormone. Following intranasal administration, less than 10%-20% is absorbed through the nasal mucosa. This peptide has been used in lactating women without effect on nursing infants.[2,3]

In a study of one breastfeeding mother receiving 10 µg twice daily of DDAVP (desmopressin), maternal plasma levels peaked at 40 minutes after the dose at approximately 7 ng/L, while milk levels were virtually unchanged at 1-1.5 ng/L.[4] Because DDAVP is easily destroyed in the gastrointestinal tract by trypsin, the oral absorption of these levels in milk would be nil.

T 1/2	75.5 min	MW	1069 Da	PB	
Tmax	40 min	RID	0.08%	Vd	
Oral	0.16%	M/P	0.2	pKa	4.8

Adult Concerns: Reduced urine production, edema, fluid retention.

Adult Dose: 10-40 µg intranasally daily.

Pediatric Concerns: None reported. It is probably not absorbed orally.

Infant Monitoring:

Alternatives:

References:
1. Pharmaceutical manufacturers prescribing information.
2. Hime MC, Richardson JA. Diabetes insipidus and pregnancy. Case report, incidence and review of literature. Obstet Gynecol Surv. 1978;33(6):375-379.

3. Hadi HA, Mashini IS, Devoe LD. Diabetes insipidus during pregnancy complicated by preeclampsia. A case report. J Reprod Med. 1985;30(3):206-208.

4. Burrow GN, Wassenaar W, Robertson GL, Sehl H. DDAVP treatment of diabetes insipidus during pregnancy and the post-partum period. Acta Endocrinol (Copenh). 1981;97(1):23-25.

DESOGESTREL

Trade:

Category: Progestin

LRC: L3 - Limited Data-Probably Compatible

Desogestrel is a potent progestin used in hormonal contraceptives. Progesterone is a naturally occurring steroid (progestin) that is secreted by the ovary, placenta, and adrenal gland. Oral administration is hampered by rapid and extensive intestinal and liver metabolism leading to poorly sustained serum concentrations and poor bioavailability.[1] As progesterone is virtually unabsorbed orally, the vaginal route has become the most established way to deliver natural progesterone because it is easily administered, avoids liver first-pass metabolism, and has no systemic side effects. Absorption through the vagina produces higher uterine levels and is called the uterine first-pass effect. A study by Levine[2] suggests the area under the curve is about 38 times less with oral administration as with progesterone vaginal gel. Thus, fewer systemic effects are noted.

With the use of progesterone in breastfeeding mothers, two principles are of paramount interest. What effect does it have on milk production and the components of milk? Does it transfer into milk in high enough levels to affect the infant directly? In general, there is significant confusion in the literature as to the effect of progestins on milk composition, but the compositional changes do not appear major, volume is normal or higher, and some authors report minor changes in lipid and protein content.[3-5] However, the majority of the studies are with other progestins (e.g., medroxyprogesterone). Shaaban studied the effect of an intravaginal progesterone ring (10 mg/d) in 120 women and found no changes in growth and development of the infant or breastfeeding performance of the study participants.[6] The author suggests the ring adds a measure of safety because the amount of steroid present in milk would be effectively absorbed from the infant's gut. Another new study also suggests no impact on breastfeeding from the intravaginal progesterone ring.[7]

The effect of progestins on milk production is poorly studied. Early postpartum, while progestin receptors are still present in the breast, administering progestins may actually suppress milk production just as it does in the pregnant women. This has been seen occasionally in patients early postpartum. Several days to a week later, most progestin receptors disappear from the lactocyte and breast tissues become relatively immune to the effects of progestins. Thus, it is advisable to wait as long as possible postpartum prior to instituting therapy with progesterone to avoid reducing the milk supply.

The direct effect of progesterone therapy on the nursing infant is generally unknown, but it is believed minimal to none as natural progesterone is poorly bioavailable to the infant via milk. Several cases of gynecomastia in infants have been reported but are extremely rare.

T 1/2	13-18	MW	314 Da	PB	99%
Tmax	6 h	RID		Vd	
Oral	Low	M/P		pKa	13.04

Adult Concerns: Headache, hypertension, nausea, vomiting, gallbladder disease, changes in liver function, abdominal cramps, bloating, breakthrough bleeding, spotting, amenorrhea, edema, thromboembolism (DVT, PE, stroke, MI). Potential suppression of milk supply.

Adult Dose:

Pediatric Concerns: None reported, not bioavailable.

Infant Monitoring: Small amounts are present in human milk. Possible suppression of milk production early postpartum is reported. Used in combination with ethinyl estradiol.

Alternatives:

References:

1. Levy T, Gurevitch S, Bar-Hava I, et al. Pharmacokinetics of natural progesterone administered in the form of a vaginal tablet. Hum Reprod. 1999;14(3):606-610.

2. Naqvi HM, Baseer A. Milk composition changes--a simple and non-invasive method of detecting ovulation in lactating women. J Pak Med Assoc. 2001;51(3):112-115.

3. Rodriguez-Palmero M, Koletzko B, Kunz C, Jensen R. Nutritional and biochemical properties of human milk: II. Lipids, micronutrients, and bioactive factors. Clin Perinatol. 1999;26(2):335-359.

4. Costa TH, Dorea JG. Concentration of fat, protein, lactose and energy in milk of mothers using hormonal contraceptives. Ann Trop Paediatr. 1992;12(2):203-209.

5. Sas M, Gellen JJ, Dusitsin N, et al. An investigation on the influence of steroidal contraceptives on milk lipid and fatty acids in Hungary and Thailand. WHO special programme of research, development and research training in human reproduction. Task force on oral contraceptives. Contraception. 1986;33(2):159-178.
6. Shaaban MM. Contraception with progestogens and progesterone during lactation. J Steroid Biochem Mol Biol. 1991;40(4-6):705-710.
7. Massai R, Quinteros E, Reyes MV, et al. Extended use of a progesterone-releasing vaginal ring in nursing women: a phase II clinical trial. Contraception. 2005 Nov;72(5):352-357.

DESONIDE

Trade: DesOwen, Desocort, Desonate, LoKara, Verdeso

Category: Corticosteroid

LRC: L3 - Limited Data-Probably Compatible

Corticosteroids when systemically absorbed are poorly excreted in the breastmilk. Absorption varies when applied topically, depending on potency.[1] Low potency agents are generally preferred for infants due to high body surface area to weight ratio. No studies are available to show whether topical corticosteroids are distributed in detectable quantities in human milk. Systemic adverse effects may occur when applied on large areas of the body, used for prolonged periods of time, and used with occlusive dressings. Apply sparingly and caution should be used when breastfeeding.[2,3]

In one case report, daily topical administration of a corticosteroid with a high mineralocorticoid activity to the mother's nipples since birth resulted in a prolonged QTc interval, hypokalemia, hypertension, and decreased growth in the 2-month-old infant. Infant's blood pressure remained high for 6 months, but normalized after a year.[4]

T 1/2		MW	416.5 Da	PB	
Tmax		RID		Vd	
Oral		M/P		pKa	13.74

Adult Concerns: Serious systemic reactions - Adrenocortical suppression, Cushing syndrome, hyperglycemia. Common side effects are dry skin, pruritus, stinging of skin, and burning sensation.

Adult Dose: 0.05%.

Pediatric Concerns: Adrenocortical suppression, Cushing's syndrome, intracranial hypertension.

Infant Monitoring: Feeding, growth, and weight gain.

Alternatives:

References:
1. Lexi-Comp OnlineTM. Lexi-Drugs OnlineTM. Hudson, Ohio: Lexi-Comp, Inc.; 2007; May 26, 2011.
2. AHFS drug information 2007. In: McEvoy GK, ed. Desonide. Bethesda, MD: American Society of Health-Systems Pharmacists; 2007:3529-3530.
3. AHFS drug information 2007. In: McEvoy GK, ed. Topical corticosteroids general statement. Bethesda, MD: American Society of Health-System Pharmacists; 2005:3423-3425.
4. De Stefano B, Bongo IG, Borgna-Pignatti C, et al. Factitious hypertension with mineralocorticoid excess in an infant. Helv Paediatr Acta. 1983;38:185-189.

DESVENLAFAXINE

Trade: Pristiq

Category: Antidepressant, other

LRC: L3 - Limited Data-Probably Compatible

Desvenlafaxine (O-desmethylvenlafaxine) is an active metabolite of venlafaxine with similar antidepressant activity. There are some data on the transmission of desvenlafaxine to human milk following the use of its precursor, venlafaxine.[1,2] In a study of six women receiving an average of 244 mg/day venlafaxine, the mean maximum concentration of desvenlafaxine in milk was 796 ng/mL. Desvenlafaxine was detected in the plasma of four of the infants ranging from 3 to 38 ng/mL.[1] All the infants were healthy and unaffected. The milk/plasma ratio for venlafaxine and desvenlafaxine were 2.5 and 2.7 respectively. In a group of 13 women who consumed from 37.5 to 300 mg/day (mean=194.3 mg/day) of venlafaxine, levels of desvenlafaxine in milk ranged from 318 to 1912.7 ng/mL with a mean of 919 ng/mL.[2] The relative infant dose for desvenlafaxine using the highest levels reported (Cmax) ranged from 6.8% to 9.3%.

A recent literature review revealed a few reports of milk levels following desvenlafaxine therapy; these are briefed below. The milk levels of desvenlafaxine were measured in a 35-year-old breastfeeding mother who had been on

250 mg desvenlafaxine daily for 2 months prior to the initiation of this study.[3] Assuming a milk ingestion of 0.15 L/kg/day, the absolute infant dose was found to be 294 µg/kg/day and the relative infant dose was calculated to be 7.8%. No untoward effects were noted or reported in the breastfed infant. Yet in another study, the transfer of desvenlafaxine to human milk was studied in 10 women who were being treated with 50-150 mg daily dose of desvenlafaxine for postpartum depression.[4] The mean relative infant dose in this study was calculated to be 6.8% (5.5%-8.1%), with a mean milk/plasma ratio of 2.24. Interestingly, in this study, it was found that the peak concentrations (C_{max}) in milk occurred at 3.28 hours, which did not parallel with the C_{max} in maternal plasma which is 7.5 hours. This suggests that milk concentration kinetics do not always co-relate with plasma concentration kinetics. The authors of this study suggest that the relative infant dose of desvenlafaxine remains almost the same, whether received from direct desvenlafaxine therapy or as an active metabolite of venlafaxine therapy; but desvenlafaxine therapy may be preferable since the absolute infant dose of total antidepressant activity following desvenlafaxine therapy only is 41%-45% of that following venlafaxine therapy.

Therefore, desvenlafaxine does enter the milk in moderate amounts; however, no side effects have been reported following its lactational exposure. The total antidepressant dose to the infant following desvenlafaxine therapy is only 41%-45% of that following venlafaxine therapy, and may therefore be preferred over venlafaxine for the treatment of postpartum depression.

T 1/2	11 h	MW	263 Da	PB	30%
Tmax	7.5 h	RID	5.9%-9.3%	Vd	3.4 L/kg
Oral	80%	M/P	2.7	pKa	10.11

Adult Concerns: Headache, somnolence, dizziness, insomnia, dry mouth, hypertension (at higher doses), nausea/vomiting, weakness.

Adult Dose: 50-100 mg/day.

Pediatric Concerns: None reported via milk at this time.

Infant Monitoring: Sedation or irritability, not waking to feed/poor feeding, and weight gain.

Alternatives: Sertraline(L2), Fluoxetine(L2)

References:

1. Ilett KF, Hackett LP, Dusci LJ, et al. Distribution and excretion of venlafaxine and O-desmethylvenlafaxine in human milk. Br J Clin Pharmacol. 1998;45(5):459-462.
2. Newport DJ, Ritchie JC, Knight BT, Glover BA, Zach EB, Stowe ZN. Venlafaxine in human breast milk and nursing infant plasma: determination of exposure. J Clin Psychiatry. 2009 Sep;70(9):1304-1310.
3. Ilett KF, Watt F, Hackett LP, Kohan R, Teoh S. Assessment of infant dose through milk in a lactating woman taking amisulpride and desvenlafaxine for treatment-resistant depression. Ther Drug Monit. 2010 Dec;32(6):704-707.
4. Rampono J, Teoh S, Hackett LP, Kohan R, Ilett KF. Estimation of desvenlafaxine transfer into milk and infant exposure during its use in lactating women withpostnatal depression. Arch Womens Ment Health. 2011 Feb;14(1):49-53.

DEXAMETHASONE

Trade: Decadron, Maxidex, Dexycu

Category: Corticosteroid

LRC: L3 - No Data-Probably Compatible

Dexamethasone is a long-acting corticosteroid, similar in effect to prednisone, although more potent. Dexamethasone 0.75 mg is equivalent to a 5 mg dose of prednisone.[1] While the elimination half-life is brief, only 3-6 hours in adults, its metabolic effects last for up to 72 hours. No data are available on the transfer of dexamethasone to human milk. It is likely similar to that of prednisone, which is extremely low. Doses of prednisone as high as 120 mg fail to produce clinically relevant milk levels. This product is commonly used in pediatrics for treating immune syndromes such as arthritis and, particularly, acute onset asthma or other bronchoconstrictive diseases. It is not likely that the amount in milk would produce clinical effects unless used in high doses over prolonged periods.

Dexycu is an intraocular formulation used following eye surgery. Plasma levels are low and exposure of infant should be minimal to nil.

Studies have shown that large doses of similar steroids in joints have resulted in suppressed lactation in some individuals.[3,4] This effect has not been demonstrated one way or the other with dexamethasone.

T 1/2	3.3 h	MW	392 Da	PB	
Tmax	1-2 h	RID		Vd	2 L/kg
Oral	78%	M/P		pKa	12.42

Adult Concerns: In pediatrics: shortened stature, gastrointestinal bleeding, gastrointestinal ulceration, edema, osteoporosis, glaucoma, and other symptoms of hyperadrenalism.

Adult Dose: 0.5-9 mg daily.

Pediatric Concerns: None reported via milk. Avoid high doses over prolonged periods of time.

Infant Monitoring: Feeding, growth and weight gain.

Alternatives: Prednisone(L2)

References:
1. Pharmaceutical manufacturers prescribing information.
2. McGuire E . Sudden loss of milk supply following high-dose triamcinolone (Kenacort) injection. Breastfeed Rev. 2012;20:32-34.
3. Babwah TJ, Nunes P, Maharaj RG. An unexpected temporary suppression of lactation after a local corticosteroid injection for tenosynovitis. Eur J Gen Pract. 2013;19:248-250.

DEXBROMPHENIRAMINE

Trade: Ala-Hist IR

Category: Antihistamine

LRC: L3 - No Data-Probably Compatible

Dexbrompheniramine is a first-generation antihistamine with anticholinergic properties. Due to the fact that dexbrompheniramine is well-absorbed and has a long half-life, it is likely secreted into human milk. One case report of a 3-month-old nursing infant suggests that it causes irritability, excessive crying, and difficulty sleeping; symptoms resolved after discontinuation of dexbrompheniramine 6 mg.[1] Since there are also anticholinergic effects, milk production may be impacted adversely. However, there have been no reports of decreased milk production in the literature.

T 1/2	25 h	MW		PB	
Tmax	5 h	RID		Vd	
Oral	Well absorbed	M/P		pKa	3.59, 9.12

Adult Concerns: Maculopapular rash, dry mouth, drowsiness, dizziness, nervousness, insomnia.

Adult Dose:

Pediatric Concerns: Irritability, excessive crying, disrupted sleep patterns.

Infant Monitoring: Drowsiness or excitement, irritability, dry mouth, constipation.

Alternatives: Diphenhydramine(L2), Loratadine(L1), Cetirizine(L2)

References:
1. Mortimer EA Jr. Drug toxicity from breast milk? Pediatrics. 1977;60(5):780-781.

DEXCHLORPHENIRAMINE

Trade: Polaramine

Category: Antihistamine

LRC: L3 - No Data-Probably Compatible

Dexchlorpheniramine is structurally similar to chlorpheniramine but is the pharmacologically active dextrorotatory isomer of chlorpheniramine. Chlorpheniramine is a commonly used antihistamine in over-the-counter medications. Although no data are available on its secretion into breast milk, it has not been reported to produce side effects. Sedation is main side effect.[1] Use non-sedating antihistamines if at all possible. See alternatives.

T 1/2	3-6 h	MW		PB	72%
Tmax	1 hr	RID		Vd	
Oral	Complete	M/P		pKa	9.2

Adult Concerns: Sedation, dry mouth.

Adult Dose:

Pediatric Concerns: No reported complications, but we suggest you use non-sedating antihistamines if at all possible.

Infant Monitoring: Sedation, dry mouth, constipation.

Alternatives: Cetirizine(L2), Loratadine(L1)

References:

1. Paton DM, Webster DR. Clinical pharmacokinetics of H1-receptor antagonists (the antihistamines). Clin Pharmacokinet. 1985;10(6):477-497.

DEXLANSOPRAZOLE

Trade: Dexilant, Kapidex

Category: Gastric Acid Secretion Inhibitor

LRC: L2 - No Data-Probably Compatible

Dexlansoprazole is a proton pump inhibitor and is the active metabolite of lansoprazole. Due to poor stability at acidic pH and short half-life, these products are encased in prolonged release formulations that open in the small intestine over a prolonged period of time. Structurally similar to omeprazole and lansoprazole, it is very unstable in stomach acid and to a large degree would be denatured by acidity of the infant's stomach.[1] A new study shows milk levels of omeprazole in milk are minimal (see omeprazole) and it is likely milk levels of dexlansoprazole are low as well. Although there are no studies of dexlansoprazole in breastfeeding mothers, transfer to milk and infant oral absorption (via milk) is expected to be minimal.

T 1/2	1-2 h	MW	369 Da	PB	99%
Tmax	1-2 h	RID		Vd	0.58 L/kg
Oral	Poor	M/P		pKa	

Adult Concerns: Nausea, vomiting, diarrhea, abdominal pain, flatulence, changes in liver and renal function.

Adult Dose: 30-60 mg daily.

Pediatric Concerns: None reported via milk.

Infant Monitoring: Unlikely to be absorbed while dissolved in milk due to instability in acid.

Alternatives: Omeprazole(L2), Lansoprazole(L2), Famotidine(L1), Ranitidine(L2)

References:

1. Pharmaceutical manufacturers prescribing information.

DEXMEDETOMIDINE HYDROCHLORIDE

Trade: Dexdor, Precedex

Category: Adrenergic

LRC: L4 - No Data-Possibly Hazardous

Dexmedetomidine is a selective alpha-2 adrenergic agonist used for sedation of initially intubated and mechanically ventilated patients in the intensive care unit and sedation of non-intubated patients prior to and/or during procedures.[1]

It has sedative, analgesic, sympathetic, and anxiolytic effects that decrease many of the cardiovascular responses in the perioperative period. It reduces the requirements for volatile anesthetics, sedatives, and analgesics without causing significant respiratory depression. It is metabolized in the liver to inactive metabolites and excreted in urine. It is not known if it is excreted in human milk. Radio-labeled dexmedetomidine administered subcutaneously to lactating female rats was excreted in milk. Caution should be exercised when it is administered to a nursing woman.

T 1/2	2 h	MW	236.7 Da	PB	94%
Tmax		RID		Vd	1.64 L/kg
Oral	16%-82%	M/P		pKa	7.1

Adult Concerns: Hypotension, bradycardia, and dry mouth are most common. If used for more than 24 hours, there is an increased risk of acute respiratory distress syndrome (ARDS), respiratory failure and agitation.

Adult Dose: 1 μg/kg over 10 minutes, then 0.2 to 0.7 μg/kg/hour (max 24 hours).

Pediatric Concerns: No data available for exposure via milk at this time.

Infant Monitoring: Observe for excitement or irritability, poor sleep, tremors, and weight gain.

Alternatives:

References:

1. Pharmaceutical manufacturers prescribing information.
2. Anttila M, Penttila J, Helminen A, Vuorilehto L, Scheinin H. Bioavailability of dexmedetomidine after extravascular doses in healthy subjects. Br J Clin Pharmacol. 2003;56(6):691–693.

DEXMETHYLPHENIDATE

Trade: Focalin

Category: CNS Stimulant

LRC: L3 - No Data-Probably Compatible

Dexmethylphenidate hydrochloride, the more pharmacologically active d-enantiomer of racemic methylphenidate, is a CNS stimulant that is used mainly in the treatment of ADHD. It is available in extended release formulations, which would extend its biological half-life.[1] In a study of three women receiving an average of 52 (35-80) mg/day of methylphenidate, the average drug in milk was 19 (13-28) µg/L.[2] The milk/plasma ratio averaged 2.8 (2-3.6). The absolute infant dose averaged 2.9 (2-4.25) µg/kg/day. The average relative infant dose was 0.9% (0.7-1.1). In the one infant studied, plasma levels were <1 µg/L. These levels are probably too low to be clinically relevant. Another case reported a mother taking 15 mg/day with breast milk concentrations averaging 2.5 ng/mL. The daily infant dose was estimated at 0.38 µg/kg, which corresponds to 0.16% of the maternal dose.[3] No drug was detected in breast milk 20-21 hours after the maternal dose.

A mother taking 80 mg/day was determined to have a milk-to-plasma ratio of 2.7, giving an absolute infant dose of 2.3 µg/kg/day, or 0.2% of the maternal dose. Methylphenidate was not detected in the infant's plasma.[4] No adverse effects were noted in any of the infants.

While we do not have individual studies with dexmethylphenidate, one should assume they will be similar to the above studies with methylphenidate. These levels are significantly less than for dextroamphetamine. Infants should be observed for agitation, and reduced weight gain, although these are quite unlikely at these levels.

T 1/2	2-4.5 h	MW	270 Da	PB	
Tmax	1-1.5 h	RID		Vd	1.54-3.76 L/kg
Oral	22%-25%	M/P		pKa	8.9

Adult Concerns: Dizziness, headache, restlessness, anxiety, xerostomia.

Adult Dose: 20-40 mg per day.

Pediatric Concerns: None yet reported via milk; however, observe for excitation, poor feeding and appetite, insomnia.

Infant Monitoring: Agitation, hyperactivity, insomnia, decreased appetite, weight gain, tremor.

Alternatives: Methylphenidate(L2)

References:

1. Pharmaceutical manufacturers prescribing information.
2. Hackett LP, Ilett KF, Kristensen JH, Kohan R, Hale TW. Infant dose and safety of breastfeeding for dexamphetamine and methylphenidate in mothers with attention deficit hyperactivity disorder. Proceedings of the 9th International Congress of Therapeutic Drug Monitoring and Clinical Toxicology; April 23-28, 2005; Louisville, USA; Ther Drug Monit. 2005;27:220. (Abstract # 40).
3. Spigset O, Brede WR, Zahlsen K. Excretion of methylphenidate in Breast Milk. Am J Psychiatry. 2007;164(2):348.
4. Hackett LP, Kristensen JH, Hale TW, Paterson R, Ilett KF. Methylphenidate and breast-feeding. Ann Pharmacother. 2006;40(10):1890-1891.

DEXTROAMPHETAMINE

Trade: Adderall, Adderall XR, Amphetamine, Dexamphetamine, Dexedrine, Dexten, Dextrostat, Liquadd, Oxydess, ProCentra, Adzenys XR

Category: Adrenergic Stimulant

LRC: L3 - Limited Data-Probably Compatible

Dextroamphetamine is a potent and long-acting amphetamine. In a study of four mothers who received 15-45 mg/day dextroamphetamine, the median maximum concentration in milk was 219 µg/L and the mean of the average milk concentrations for each patient was 140 µg/L.[1] The median absolute infant dose was 21 (11-39) µg/kg/day. The authors suggest the median relative infant dose was 5.7% (4-10.6). Plasma levels were measured in three of the four infants and were undetectable, 2 µg/L and 18 µg/L, respectively. No untoward effects were noted in any of the four infants.

An older case report from 1978 describes the transmission of racemic amphetamine into breast milk on day 10 and 42 postpartum.[2] In this case, the mother was taking 5 mg of oral amphetamine four times a day (10 am, noon, 2 pm, and 4 pm) to treat narcolepsy. The authors found the M/P ratios were high, 3 on day 10 and 7 on day 42. The concentrations of amphetamine in milk on day 10 were 55 ng/mL when pumped 20 minutes pre 10 am dose and 118 ng/mL when pumped immediately before the 2 pm dose. The concentrations of amphetamine in milk on day 42 were 68 ng/mL when pumped 20 minutes pre 10 am dose and 138 ng/mL when pumped immediately before the 2 pm dose. The absolute infant dose was about 10-20 µg/kg/day and the RID ranged from 2.9-7%. The infant was followed for 24 months, with no adverse effects reported.

In 2015, another case report was published that described the transmission of racemic amphetamine to breast milk.[3] In this case, the woman was taking 35 mg of amphetamine to treat narcolepsy. Blood and breast milk samples were taken prior to the morning dose at 2, 5, and 9 weeks postpartum. The milk sample concentrations ranged from 74-82.3 ng/mL and the average M/P ratio was 3.02. The infant's plasma concentrations ranged from 1.4 to 3.1 ng/mL. The absolute infant dose and RID estimated using the highest milk concentration were 12.4 µg/kg/day and 2.4%, respectively. This mother exclusively breastfed her infant for 6 months and then partially breastfed her infant until 10 months of age and no adverse events or concerns with development were reported.

The above data suggest that with normal therapeutic doses, the dose of dextroamphetamine in milk is probably subclinical. However, abuse of this medication is common. Doses are unknown and sometimes extraordinarily high. Thus, mothers should be strongly advised to withhold breastfeeding for 24 hours following the non-clinical use of dextroamphetamine.

This drug is also available as continuous release formulations (Adderall XR). With continuous release formulations, plasma levels are virtually identical to the twice daily dosing system. Thus, if a patient is using XR 20 mg, plasma levels are identical to the 10 mg twice daily.

This medication is considered an L3 when used in clinical doses; however, should this medication be abused the risk would increase to an L5 based on potential increased dose ingested and potential lack of infant monitoring.

T 1/2	9.77 to 11 h	MW	368 Da	PB	16%-20%
Tmax	1-2 h	RID	2.46%-7.25%	Vd	3.2-5.6 L/kg
Oral	Complete	M/P	2-5.2	pKa	9.9

Adult Concerns: Nervousness, insomnia, anorexia, hyperexcitability.

Adult Dose: 5-60 mg daily.

Pediatric Concerns: Possible insomnia, irritability, anorexia, reduced weight gain, or poor sleeping patterns in infants. However, in these studies, none of the infants were affected.

Infant Monitoring: Agitation, hyperactivity, insomnia, decreased appetite, weight gain, tremor.

Alternatives: Methylphenidate(L2)

References:
1. Ilett KF, Hackett LP, Kristensen JH, Kohan R. Transfer of dexamphetamine into breast milk during treatment for attention deficit hyperactivity disorder. Br J Clin Pharmacol. 2006;63(3):371-375.
2. Steiner E, Villen T, Hallberg M, et al. Amphetamine secretion in breast milk. Eur J Clin Pharmacol. 1984;27(1):123-124.
3. Ohman I, Norstedt Wikner B, Beck O, et al. Narcolepsy treated with racemic amphetamine during pregnancy and breastfeeding. J Hum Lact. 2015;31(3):374-376.

DEXTROMETHORPHAN

Trade: Babee Cof Syrup, Creomulsion, Dexalone, Hold DM, Robitussin, Vicks 44 Cough Relief

Category: Antitussive

LRC: L3 - No Data-Probably Compatible

Dextromethorphan is a weak antitussive commonly used in adults. It is a congener of codeine and appears to elevate the cough threshold in the brain. It does not have addictive, analgesic, or sedative actions, and it does not produce respiratory depression at normal doses.[1] No data on its transfer to human milk are available. It is very unlikely that enough would transfer via milk to provide clinically significant levels in a breastfed infant.

Note: Although non-drug measures are preferred, this cough suppressant could be considered as other products such as codeine and benzonatate are not recommended for cough suppression in lactation.

T 1/2	<4 h	MW	271 Da	PB	
Tmax	2-3 h	RID		Vd	
Oral	Complete	M/P		pKa	9.85

Adult Concerns: Drowsiness, dizziness, confusion, irritability, nausea, vomiting.

Adult Dose: 10-20 mg every 4 hours.

Pediatric Concerns: None reported.

Infant Monitoring: Sedation.

Alternatives:

References:
1. Pender ES, Parks BR. Toxicity with dextromethorphan-containing preparations: a literature review and report of two additional cases. Pediatr Emerg Care. 1991;7(3):163-165.

DIATRIZOATE

Trade: Angiovist, Cardiografin, Cystografin, Gastrografin, Hypaque, Reno-M, Renografin, Retrografin, Urovist, Sinografin

Category: Diagnostic Agent, Radiological Contrast Media

LRC: L2 - Limited Data-Probably Compatible

Diatrizoate is an iodinated radiopaque medium used in a wide variety of X-rays. These radiocontrast agents contain iodine in the range of 8.5% to 59.87% iodine.[1] However, the iodine is covalently bound to the molecule and is poorly released after injection, most being eliminated rapidly in the urine. Reported levels in breast milk are very low. In a study of a single patient who received 18.5 grams of iodine in the form of sodium and meglumine salts of diatrizoate, diatrizoate levels were undetectable (Level of Detection <2 mg/L).[2] In another woman who received 93 grams of Iodine as diatrizoate, total iodine transferred into breast milk in the first 24 hours was 0.03% or 31 mg.[3] Based on kinetic data, the American College of Radiology suggests that it is safe for mothers to continue breastfeeding after receiving iodinated X-ray contrast media.[4]

T 1/2	120 min	MW	614 Da	PB	0%-10%
Tmax		RID		Vd	
Oral	0.04%-1.2 %	M/P		pKa	2.17

Adult Concerns: Pain at injection site, flushing, nephrosis, taste alteration, nausea, vomiting, dizziness, cough, paresthesia, hypersensitivity, edema.

Adult Dose:

Pediatric Concerns: None reported via breast milk.

Infant Monitoring:

Alternatives:

References:
1. Pharmaceutical manufacturers prescribing information.
2. Fitz John TP, Williams DG, Laker MF, Owen JP. Intravenous urography during lactation. Br J Radiol. 1982;55(656):603-605.
3. Texier F, Roque DO, Etling N. Stable iodine level in human milk after pulmonary angiography. Presse Med. 1983;12(12):769.
4. American College of Radiology. Manual on Contrast Media, Version 10.3, 2018.

DIAZEPAM

Trade: Antenex, Azepan, Vivol, Sedapam, Valium

Category: Antianxiety

LRC: L3 - Limited Data-Probably Compatible

Diazepam is a powerful CNS depressant and anticonvulsant. Published data on milk and plasma levels are highly variable and many are poor studies. In three mothers receiving 10 mg three times daily for up to 6 days, the maternal plasma levels of diazepam averaged 491 ng/mL (day 4) and 601 ng/mL (day 6).[1] Corresponding milk levels were 51 ng/mL (day 4) and 78 ng/mL (day 6). The milk/plasma ratio was approximately 0.1. In a case report of a patient taking 6-10 mg of diazepam daily, her milk levels varied from 7.5 to 87 µg/L.[2]

In a study of nine mothers receiving diazepam postpartum, milk levels of diazepam varied from approximately 0.01 to 0.08 mg/L.[3] Other reports suggest slightly higher values. Taken together, most results suggest that the dose of diazepam and its metabolite, desmethyldiazepam, to a suckling infant will be on average 0.78%-9.1% of the weight-adjusted maternal dose of diazepam.[4] The active metabolite, desmethyldiazepam, in general has a much longer half-life in adults and pediatric patients and may tend to accumulate on longer therapy.

The excretion of diazepam, N-desmethyldiazepam, temazepam, and oxazepam in breast milk was studied during withdrawal of a 22-year-old patient from combined high dose of 80 mg diazepam and 30 mg oxazepam therapy.[5] The mean milk/plasma ratio of diazepam and its metabolite Desmethyldiazepam was found to be 0.2 and 0.13 respectively. The milk concentration of diazepam during therapy ranged between 67-307 μg/L and that of desmethyldiazepam was 42-141 μg/L; with the milk concentrations being barely 6 μg/L 8 days following cessation of therapy. No diazepam was detected in infant's plasma and only low levels of desmethyldiazepam were present in infant's plasma. No untoward effects were reported in the breastfed infant. The authors conclude that very low levels of benzodiazepines get transferred into breast milk and are unlikely to be clinically relevant in the breastfed infant.

Some reports of lethargy, sedation, and poor suckling have been found. The acute use such as in surgical procedures is not likely to lead to significant accumulation. Long-term, sustained therapy may prove troublesome. The benzodiazepine family, as a rule, is not ideal for breastfeeding mothers due to relatively long half-lives and the development of dependence. However, it is apparent that the shorter-acting benzodiazepines (lorazepam, alprazolam) are safest during lactation provided their use is short-term or intermittent and low dose.[10]

T 1/2	43 h	MW	285 Da	PB	99%
Tmax	1-2 h	RID	0.88%-7.14%	Vd	0.7-2.6 L/kg
Oral	Complete	M/P	0.2-2.7	pKa	3.4

Adult Concerns: Drowsiness, dizziness, confusion, blurred vision, dry mouth, headache, fatigue, ataxia, slurred speech.

Adult Dose: 2-10 mg two to four times per day as needed.

Pediatric Concerns: Some reports of lethargy, sedation, poor suckling have been found.

Infant Monitoring: Sedation, slowed breathing rate, not waking to feed/poor feeding, and weight gain.

Alternatives: Lorazepam(L3), Midazolam(L2)

References:
1. Erkkola R, Kanto J. Diazepam and breast-feeding. Lancet. 1972;1(7762):1235-1236.
2. Wesson DR, Camber S, Harkey M, Smith DE. Diazepam and desmethyldiazepam in breast milk. J Psychoactive Drugs. 1985;17(1):55-56.
3. Cole AP, Hailey DM. Diazepam and active metabolite in breast milk and their transfer to the neonate. Arch Dis Child. 1975;50(9):741-742.
4. Spigset O. Anaesthetic agents and excretion in breast milk. Acta Anaesthesiol Scand. 1994;38(2):94-103.
5. Dusci LJ, Good SM, Hall RW, Ilett KF. Excretion of diazepam and its metabolites in human milk during withdrawal from combination high dose diazepam and oxazepam. Br J Clin Pharmacol. 1990 Jan;29(1):123-126.
6. Maitra R, Menkes DB. Psychotropic drugs and lactation. N Z Med J. 1996;109(1024):217-218.

DIBUCAINE

Trade: Nupercainal

Category: Anesthetic, Local

LRC: L3 - No Data-Probably Compatible

Dibucaine is a long-acting local anesthetic generally used topically. It is primarily used topically in creams and ointments, and due to toxicity, has been banned in the United States for IV or IM injections.[1] No data are available on transfer to breast milk. Dibucaine is effective for sunburn, topical burns, rash, rectal hemorrhoids, and other skin irritations. Long-term use and use over large areas of the body are discouraged. Although somewhat minimal, some dibucaine can be absorbed from irritated skin. Do not use dibucaine ointment on the nipple. Two toddlers developed seizures following a dose of 15 mg/kg of 1% dibucaine ointment.

T 1/2		MW	379 Da	PB	
Tmax		RID		Vd	
Oral		M/P		pKa	8.8

Adult Concerns: Rash. burning or allergic symptoms.

Adult Dose:

Pediatric Concerns: None reported via milk. Two toddlers developed seizures following a dose of 15 mg/kg of 1% dibucaine ointment.

Infant Monitoring: Do not use dibucaine ointment on the nipple.

Alternatives:

References:
1. Pharmaceutical manufacturers prescribing information.

DICLOFENAC

Trade: Cambia, Cataflam, Fenac, Flector patch, Pennsaid, Voltaren, Voltarol, Zipsor

Category: NSAID

LRC: L2 - Limited Data-Probably Compatible

Diclofenac is a typical nonsteroidal analgesic (NSAID). Diclofenac is available in both sustained release formulations (Voltaren), as well as in immediate release formulations (Cataflam). In one study of six postpartum mothers receiving three 50 mg doses on day 1, followed by two 50 mg doses on day 2, the levels of diclofenac in breast milk were approximately 5 μg/L of milk, although the limit of detection was reported as <19 ng/mL.[1]

In another patient on long-term treatment with diclofenac, milk levels of 0.1 μg/mL milk were reported, which would amount to 0.015 mg/kg/day ingested.[2] These amounts are probably far too low to affect an infant.

T 1/2	1.1 h	MW	318 Da	PB	99.7%
Tmax	1 h (Cataflam)	RID		Vd	0.55 L/kg
Oral	Complete	M/P		pKa	4

Adult Concerns: Headache, dizziness, high blood pressure, asthma exacerbations, dyspepsia, peptic ulcer/GI bleed, nausea, abdominal pain, diarrhea, changes in liver and renal function, bruising, thrombocytopenia, anemia, peripheral edema.

Adult Dose: 50 mg every 8-12 h.

Pediatric Concerns: None reported via milk. Milk levels are extremely low.

Infant Monitoring: Vomiting, diarrhea.

Alternatives: Ibuprofen(L1)

References:
1. Sioufi A, et al. Recent findings concerning clinically relevant pharmacokinetics of diclofenac sodium. In: Kass, ed. Voltaren-new Findings. Bern: Hans Huber Publishers; 1982.
2. Pharmaceutical manufacturers prescribing information.

DICLOXACILLIN

Trade: Diclocil, Dicloxsig, Dycill, Dynapen, Pathocil

Category: Antibiotic, Penicillin

LRC: L2 -Significant Data-Compatible

Dicloxacillin is an oral penicillinase-resistant penicillin frequently used for peripheral (non CNS) infections caused by *Staphylococcus aureus* and *Staphylococcus epi*dermidis infections, particularly mastitis. Following oral administration of a 250 mg dose, milk concentrations of the drug were zero, 0.2-0.3, and a trace to 0.3 mg/L at 1, 2, and 4 hours after the dose respectively.[1] Levels were undetectable at 1 and 6 hours. Compatible with breastfeeding.

T 1/2	0.6-0.8 h	MW	470 Da	PB	96%
Tmax	0.5-2 h	RID	0.6%-1.4%	Vd	
Oral	35%-76%	M/P		pKa	3.75

Adult Concerns: Elimination is delayed in neonates. Rash, diarrhea.

Adult Dose: 125-250 mg every 6 hours.

Pediatric Concerns: None reported via milk.

Infant Monitoring: Vomiting, diarrhea, changes in gastrointestinal flora, and rash.

Alternatives: Amoxicillin(L1), Cephalexin(L1)

References:

1. Matsuda S. Transfer of antibiotics into maternal milk. Biol Res Pregnancy. 1984;5:57-60.

DICYCLOMINE

Trade: Antispas, Bentyl, Bentylol, Formulex, Lomine, Merbentyl, Spasmoject

Category: Cholinergic Antagonist

LRC: L4 - Limited Data-Possibly Hazardous

Dicyclomine is a tertiary amine antispasmodic. It belongs to the family of anticholinergics such as atropine and the belladonna alkaloids. It was previously used for infant colic but due to overdoses and reported apnea, it is seldom recommended for this use. Infants are exceedingly sensitive to anticholinergics, particularly in the neonatal period. Following a dose of 20 mg in a lactating woman, a 12-day-old infant reported severe apnea. The manufacturer reports milk levels of 131 µg/L with corresponding maternal serum levels of 59 µg/L.[1] The reported milk/plasma level was 2.22.

T 1/2	9-10 h	MW	345 Da	PB	
Tmax	1-1.5 h	RID	6.9%	Vd	
Oral	67%	M/P	2.22	pKa	9

Adult Concerns: Apnea, dry secretions, urinary hesitancy, dilated pupils.

Adult Dose: 20-40 mg QID.

Pediatric Concerns: Severe apnea in one 12-day-old infant. Observe for anticholinergic symptoms, drying, constipation, rapid heart rate.

Infant Monitoring: Sedation or irritability, drying of oral and ophthalmic secretions, urinary retention, constipation.

Alternatives:

References:

1. Pharmaceutical manufacturers prescribing information.

DIDANOSINE

Trade: Videx

Category: Antiviral

LRC: L5 - No Data-Hazardous if Maternal HIV infection

Didanosine is an anti-retroviral agent used for the treatment of HIV infection. Currently, there are no studies regarding drug transfer in human milk or case reports in breastfeeding women. This medication is expected to enter maternal milk as didanosine is a small drug molecule (236 Da) with very low protein binding (<5 %). Breastfeeding is generally not recommended in mothers who have HIV.[1,2]

Note: This medication is an L5 to highlight the contraindication of breastfeeding when the mother is known to be infected with HIV; this medication is not an L5 based on its risk to the infant in breast milk (no data available at this time). The Centers for Disease Control and Prevention recommend that HIV-1 infected mothers do not breastfeed their infants to avoid postnatal transmission of HIV-1.

T 1/2	1.3-1.5 h	MW	236 Da	PB	<5%
Tmax	0.67-2 h	RID		Vd	0.8-1 L/kg
Oral	21%-43%	M/P		pKa	9.13

Adult Concerns: Abdominal pain, diarrhea, rash, nausea, vomiting, peripheral neuropathy, headache, elevated liver enzymes, pancreatitis, arrhythmia, increased risk of heart attack, nephrotoxicity, hypersensitivity, hepatitis, leucopenia, anemia, arthralgia, myalgia, hyperuricemia, increased or decreased blood sugar.

Adult Dose:

Pediatric Concerns:

Infant Monitoring: Breastfeeding is not recommended in mothers who have HIV.

Alternatives:

References:
1. World Health Organization. Global Programme on AIDS. Consensus Statement from the WHO/UNICEF Consultation on HIV Transmission and Breast-Feeding. Geneva, Switzerland: WHO; 1992.
2. Latham MC, Greiner T. Breastfeeding versus formula feeding in HIV infection. Lancet. 1998;352:737.

DIETHYLPROPION

Trade: Dospan, Tenuate, Tepanil

Category: Antiobesity Agent

LRC: L5 - No Data-Hazardous

Diethylpropion belongs to the amphetamine family and is typically used to reduce food intake. No data or literature reports are available of the transfer of this drug to human milk. Manufacturer states that this medication is secreted to breast milk.[1] Diethylpropion's structure is similar to amphetamines. Upon withdrawal, significant withdrawal symptoms have been reported in adults. Such symptoms could be observed in breastfeeding infants of mothers using this product. The use of this medication during lactation is simply unrealistic and not justified. Weight-loss medications are generally not recommended for breastfeeding women since this may interfere with the nutritive properties of the breast milk provided to the infant.[2]

T 1/2	8 h	MW	205 Da	PB	
Tmax	2 h	RID		Vd	
Oral	70%	M/P		pKa	8.2

Adult Concerns: Overstimulation, insomnia, anorexia, jitteriness, rapid heart rate, elevated blood pressure.

Adult Dose: 25 mg TID.

Pediatric Concerns: None reported, but observe for anorexia, agitation, insomnia.

Infant Monitoring: Not recommended in lactation.

Alternatives:

References:
1. Pharmaceutical manufacturers prescribing information.
2. Schaefer C. Drugs During Pregnancy and Lactation. Amsterdam, The Netherlands: Elsevier Science B.V.; 2001.

DIFLUNISAL

Trade: Dolobid

Category: NSAID

LRC: L3 - Limited Data-Probably Compatible

Diflunisal is a derivative of salicylic acid. It is a nonsteroidal anti-inflammatory agent (NSAID).[1] Diflunisal is excreted into human milk in concentrations 2%-7% of the maternal plasma levels following 7 days of treatment with 125-250 mg twice daily, although specific milk levels were not reported. Thus, levels in the infant would probably be quite low to undetectable. This product is potentially a higher risk NSAID and other NSAIDs with more data in lactation are preferred such as ibuprofen and naproxen.

T 1/2	8-12 h	MW	250 Da	PB	99%
Tmax	2-3 h	RID	7.8%-11.5%	Vd	0.11 L/kg
Oral	Complete	M/P		pKa	

Adult Concerns: Headache, dizziness, insomnia, dyspepsia, ulcers, nausea, vomiting, diarrhea, changes in renal function, thrombocytopenia, anemia.

Adult Dose: 500 mg BID or TID.

Pediatric Concerns: None reported, but alternatives with more lactation data are preferred.

Infant Monitoring: Vomiting, diarrhea.

Alternatives: Ibuprofen(L1), Naproxen(L3)

References:
1. Steelman SL, Breault GO, Tocco D. Pharmacokinetics of MK-647, a novel salicylate. Clin Pharmacol Ther. 1975;17:245. Abstract.

DIFLUPREDNATE

Trade: Durezol, Epitopic, Myser

Category: Corticosteroid

LRC: L3 - No Data-Probably Compatible

Difluprednate is an adrenal glucocorticoid ophthalmic solution used as an anti-inflammatory agent after ophthalmic surgery. The medication comes in 0.01% and 0.05% strengths. There is limited systemic absorption. One study found no metabolites in the urine of patients using the ophthalmic solution daily for 1 week.[1] Clinical pharmacokinetic studies of difluprednate after repeat ocular instillation of 2 drops of difluprednate (0.01% or 0.05%) QID for 7 days showed that DFB levels in blood were below the quantification limit (50 ng/mL) at all time points for all subjects, indicating the systemic absorption of difluprednate after ocular instillation of Durezol is limited. Due to the limited systemic absorption, levels of difluprednate in milk are probably minimal to nil.

T 1/2		MW	508.6 Da	PB	
Tmax		RID		Vd	
Oral		M/P		pKa	

Adult Concerns: Blepharitis, anterior chamber flare, corneal edema, blepharitis, pain, photophobia, conjunctiva edema, posterior capsule opacification, ocular hyperemia, constipation.

Adult Dose: Instill one drop four times a day.

Pediatric Concerns:

Infant Monitoring: Feeding, growth and weight gain.

Alternatives:

References:
1. Pharmaceutical manufacturers prescribing information.

DIGOXIN

Trade: Lanoxicaps, Lanoxin

Category: Cardiac Glycoside

LRC: L2 - Limited Data-Probably Compatible

Digoxin is a cardiac stimulant used primarily to strengthen the contractile process. In one mother receiving 0.25 mg digoxin daily, the amount found in breast milk ranged from 0.96 to 0.61 µg/L at 4 and 6 hours postdose respectively.[1] Mean peak breast milk levels varied from 0.78 µg/L in one patient to 0.41 µg/L in another. Plasma levels in the infants were undetectable.

In another study of five women receiving digoxin therapy, the average breast milk concentration was 0.64 µg/L.[2] From these studies, it is apparent that a breastfeeding infant would receive less than 1 µg/day of digoxin, too low to be clinically relevant. The small amounts secreted into breast milk have not produced problems in nursing infants. Poor and erratic gastrointestinal absorption could theoretically reduce absorption in nursing infants.

Digoxin immune fab (ovine) is composed of antigen binding fragments made from anti-digoxin antibodies. It is used for life-threatening digoxin toxicity or overdose. The molecular weight of these fragments is approximately 46,000 Da, and thus would not be able to transfer into the milk compartment.[3]

T 1/2	36-48 h	MW	781 Da	PB	25%
Tmax	1-3 h	RID	2.7%-2.8%	Vd	6-7 L/kg
Oral	60%-80%	M/P	<0.9	pKa	7.15

Adult Concerns: Headache, dizziness, confusion, blurred or yellow vision, arrhythmias, abdominal pain, diarrhea, anorexia, and rash.

Adult Dose: 0.125-0.5 mg daily.

Pediatric Concerns: None reported in via milk in several studies.

Infant Monitoring: Drowsiness, lethargy, cardiac arrhythmias, pallor, poor feeding, and weight gain

Alternatives:

References:
1. Loughnan PM. Digoxin excretion in human breast milk. J Pediatr. 1978 Jun;92(6):1019-1020.
2. Levy M, Granit L, Laufer N. Excretion of drugs in human milk. N Engl J Med. 1977 Oct;297(14):789.
3. Pharmaceutical manufacturers prescribing information.

DILTIAZEM

Trade: Adizem, Britiazim, Cardcal, Cardizem, Dilzem, Tildiem, Cartia XT, Coras, Dilacor-XR

Category: Calcium Channel Blocker

LRC: L3 - Limited Data-Probably Compatible

Diltiazem hydrochloride is an typical calcium channel blocker antihypertensive.[1] In a report of a single patient receiving 240 mg/day on day 14 postpartum, levels in milk were parallel to those of serum (milk/plasma ratio is approximately 1).[2] Peak level in milk (and plasma) was slightly higher than 200 µg/L and occurred at 8 hours. Nifedipine is probably a preferred choice for a calcium channel blocker because of our experience with it, the relative infant dose with this agent is quite small and it is not likely to be problematic.

T 1/2	3.5-6 h	MW	433 Da	PB	78%
Tmax	2-3 h	RID	0.87%	Vd	1.7 L/kg
Oral	40%-60%	M/P	1	pKa	7.7

Adult Concerns: Headache, dizziness, hypotension, arrhythmias, constipation, peripheral edema.

Adult Dose: 120-240 mg daily extended release.

Pediatric Concerns: None reported via milk at this time.

Infant Monitoring: Drowsiness, lethargy, pallor, poor feeding, and weight gain.

Alternatives: Nifedipine(L2), Labetalol(L2), Verapamil(L2)

References:
1. Pharmaceutical manufacturers prescribing information.
2. Okada M, Inoue H, Nakamura Y, Kishimoto M, Suzuki T. Excretion of diltiazem in human milk. N Engl J Med. 1985;312(15):992-993.

DIMENHYDRINATE

Trade: Dramamine, Driminate, Hydrate, Triptone

Category: Antihistamine

LRC: L2 - Limited Data-Probably Compatible

Dimenhydrinate is an antihistamine and an antiemetic agent used for the treatment and prevention of motion sickness. Consists of 55% diphenhydramine and 45% 8-chlorotheophylline. Diphenhydramine is considered to be the active ingredient. Small but unreported levels of diphenhydramine are thought to be secreted into breast milk. In one study following an IM dose of 100 mg, drug levels in milk were undetectable in two individuals, and ranged from 42 to 100 µg/L in two subjects.[1] While these levels are low, this sedating antihistamine should only be used for a short duration in breastfeeding mothers. There are anecdotal reports that diphenhydramine suppresses milk production. There are no data to support this theory.

T 1/2	8.5 h	MW	470 Da	PB	78%
Tmax	1-2 h	RID		Vd	
Oral		M/P		pKa	

Adult Concerns: Sedation, dry mouth, constipation.

Adult Dose: 50-100 mg every 4-6 hours.

Pediatric Concerns: None reported via milk. See diphenhydramine.

Infant Monitoring: Sedation, dry mouth.

Alternatives:

References:
1. Rindi V. La eliminazione degli antistaminici di sintesi con il latte e l'azione latto-goga de questi. Riv Ital Ginecol. 1951;34:147-157.

DIMETHICONE

Trade:

Category: Dermatologic Agents

LRC: L3 - No Data-Probably Compatible

Dimethicone is a silicone compound mainly used in topical creams.[1] There are no adequate and well-controlled studies or case reports in breastfeeding women. Because the drug is not absorbed, the risk to a nursing infant from maternal use of dimethicone is thought to be negligible.

Adult Concerns: Rash due to hypersensitivity reactions to ingredient.

Adult Dose:

Pediatric Concerns:

Infant Monitoring:

Alternatives:

References:
1. Pharmaceutical manufacturers prescribing information.

DIMETHYL FUMARATE

Trade: Tecfidera

Category: Immune Suppressant

LRC: L2 - Limited Data-Probably Compatible

Dimethyl fumarate has been recently introduced for the treatment of multiple sclerosis. The mechanism by which dimethyl fumarate exerts its therapeutic effect in multiple sclerosis is unknown. Dimethyl fumarate is rapidly metabolized to monomethyl fumarate, which produces brief plasma levels. Taken twice daily at 240 mg, maternal plasma levels produced a C_{max} of 1.87 mg/L and AUC was 8.21 mg.hr/L in MS patients. The active drug component (monomethyl fumarate) has a low molecular weight of only 129 Da and low protein binding (27-45%).[1] This product will probably enter milk but preliminary unpublished data suggests levels are exceedingly low.

T 1/2	1 h	MW	129 (metabolite MMF) Da	PB	27%-45%
Tmax	2-2.5 h	RID		Vd	0.75-1.04 L/kg
Oral		M/P		pKa	

Adult Concerns: Flushing, dyspepsia, nausea, abdominal pain, diarrhea, changes in liver function, proteinuria, lymphocytopenia, rash.

Adult Dose: 120-240 mg twice daily.

Pediatric Concerns: None reported.

Infant Monitoring: Vomiting, diarrhea.

Alternatives: Glatiramer(L3), beta interferon.

References:
1. Pharmaceutical manufacturers prescribing information.

DIMETHYL SULFOXIDE

Trade: DMSO, DMSO2, MSM, Rimso-50, Dimethyl sulfoxide

Category: Renal-Urologic Agent

LRC: L4 - Limited Data-Possibly Hazardous

Dimethyl sulfoxide (DMSO) is a solvent that has been found useful for musculoskeletal inflammation and injury, and interstitial cystitis. It has been used topically, orally, and intravenously. DMSO is relatively nontoxic, requiring rather large intravenous doses to induce toxicity (20 gm). Following dermal application of 1 gm/kg (640 mL/70 kg), reported serum concentrations were 560 mg/L within 4-8 hours. By 48 hours, only traces were detectable.[1] Daily oral doses of 32 mL/70 kg for 14 days produced peak serum levels of 1850 mg/L.

One mother with a 4-month-old infant, was diagnosed with interstitial cystitis and received a single treatment of RIMSO (50/50 dilution of DMSO, 50 mL, 0.54 g/mL, 27.0 g total) instilled into the bladder, which was held for 15 minutes and then voided. She collected milk samples at 0, 5, 11, 19, 24, 27, 32, and 36 hours after the treatment. The C_{max} of DMSO in milk at 1 hour was 34.5 µg/mL, and C_{ave} was 13.42 µg/mL. Reported levels in milk were 34.49 µg/mL at 1 hour, 12.94 µg/mL at 11 hours, 5.39 µg/mL at 19 hours, and 0.21µg/mL after 36 hours. The relative infant dose derived from the C_{ave} was 0.457. The estimated infant dose an infant would receive per treatment was determined to be approximately 2.01 mg/kg/day

Milk should probably be pumped and discarded for at least 24 hours. Although the overall toxicity of this compound is quite minimal, exposing an infant to this agent is probably not justified.

Methylsulfonylmethane (DMSO2, MSM, "Crystalline DMSO") is the normal oxidation product of DMSO. No data are available on this product, but it is probably distributed and eliminated the same as DMSO above.

T 1/2	11-14 h (dermal)	MW	78.13 Da	PB	
Tmax	4-8 h (topically)	RID		Vd	0.53 L/kg
Oral	Complete	M/P		pKa	

Adult Concerns: DMSO imparts a garlic-like breath, taste, and body odor to all users. Sedation, dizziness, headache, nausea, vomiting, changes in liver function, neuropathy, dermatologic rash. Neurologic concerns due to liver toxicity has been reported in two elderly patients receiving IV infusions of 100 g of 20% DMSO.

Adult Dose: Variable.

Pediatric Concerns: None reported. This agent is not particularly effective, therefore the risks do not justify its use in breastfeeding mothers.

Infant Monitoring: Garlic-like breath, body odor, vomiting, diarrhea.

Alternatives:

References:

1. Baselt RC. Disposition of Toxic Drugs and Chemicals in Man. Foster City, CA: Chemical Toxicology Institute; 2000:282-283.
2, Rewers-Felkins K, Ella Speck BS, Palika D, Teresa B, Hale TW. Bladder to Breastmilk – DMSO Treatment of Interstitial Cystitis. In Publication. 2020.

DINOPROSTONE

Trade: Cervidil, Prepidil, Propess, Prostin E2

Category: Prostaglandin

LRC: L3 - No Data-Probably Compatible

Dinoprostone is a naturally occurring prostaglandin E2 that is primarily used for induction of labor, for cervical ripening, as an abortifacient, for postpartum bleeding, and for uterine atony.[1] Available as a vaginal gel or insert, it is slowly absorbed into the plasma where it is rapidly cleared and metabolized by most tissues and the lung. Its half-life is brief 2.5 to 5 minutes although absorption from the vaginal mucosa is slow. The amount of dinoprostone entering milk is unknown.

Dinoprostone has been used to suppress lactation. When used orally (2 mg orally/day on day 3 and 4; then 6 mg/day thereafter) it has been found to significantly suppress milk production.[2,3] However, the use of prostaglandin E2 products for cervical ripening (during delivery) is generally brief and probably does not clinically impact the production of breast milk many hours or days later.

T 1/2	2.5-5 min	MW	352.5 Da	PB	High
Tmax	0.5-1 h	RID		Vd	
Oral		M/P		pKa	4.9

Adult Concerns: Side effects of vaginal dinoprostone are numerous and include abortion, labor induction, blood loss, hypotension, syncope, tachycardia, dizziness, hyperthermia, nausea, vomiting, diarrhea, and taste disorders.

Adult Dose: Varies by indication.

Pediatric Concerns: None reported via milk, but a washout period is suggested.

Infant Monitoring: Vomiting, diarrhea, flushing.

Alternatives:

References:
1. Pharmaceutical manufacturers prescribing information.
2. Caminiti F, De Murtas M, Parodo G, Lecca U, Nasi A. Decrease in human plasma prolactin levels by oral prostaglandin E2 in early puerperium. J Endocrinol. 1980;87(3):333-337.
3. Nasi A, De Murtas M, Parodo G, Caminiti F. Inhibition of lactation by prostaglandin E2. Obstet Gynecol Surv. 1980;35(10):619-620.

DIPHENHYDRAMINE

Trade: Benadryl

Category: Antihistamine

LRC: L2 - Limited Data-Probably Compatible

Diphenhydramine is an antihistamine used for allergic conditions. It is also used as a sleep aid and as an antiemetic agent for the prevention of motion sickness. Small but unreported levels are thought to be secreted into breast milk. In one study following an IM dose of 100 mg, drug levels in milk were undetectable in two individuals, and ranged from 42 to 100 µg/L in two subjects.[1] While these levels are low, this sedating antihistamine should only be used for a short duration in breastfeeding mothers. Non-sedating antihistamines are generally preferred. There are anecdotal reports that diphenhydramine suppresses milk production. There are no data to support this theory.

T 1/2	4.3 h	MW	255 Da	PB	78%
Tmax	2-3 h	RID	0.7%-1.4%	Vd	3-4 L/kg
Oral	43%-61%	M/P		pKa	8.3

Adult Concerns: Sedation, drowsiness.

Adult Dose: 25-50 mg every 4-6 hours.

Pediatric Concerns: None reported, but observe for sedation. Some suggestions of reduced milk supply but these are unsubstantiated.

Infant Monitoring: Sedation, dry mouth, constipation.

Alternatives: Cetirizine(L2), Loratadine(L1)

References:
1. Rindi V. La eliminazione degli antistaminici di sintesi con il latte e l'azione latto-goga de questi. Riv Ital Ginecol. 1951;34:147-157.

DIPHENOXYLATE

Trade: Lomotil

Category: Antidiarrheal

LRC: L3 - No Data-Probably Compatible

Diphenoxylate is an antidiarrheal drug chemically similar to meperidine. When combined with atropine, it is marketed as Lomotil. This drug slows gut transit time in a manner similar to other opiates. Diphenoxylate has no analgesic properties at clinical doses.[1]

No studies examining diphenoxylate secretion into breast milk have been published. Pharmacokinetic data are also sparse, but pre-marketing testing suggests that the majority of the drug remains in the intestine.[1] This drug is likely to be secreted in breast milk in very small quantities, but unlikely to be clinically relevant to the baby.

T 1/2	12-14 h	MW	453 Da	PB	22%
Tmax	2 h	RID		Vd	3.8 L/kg
Oral	90%	M/P		pKa	7.1

Adult Concerns:

Adult Dose: 5-20 mg/day.

Pediatric Concerns:

Infant Monitoring:

Alternatives:

References:
1. Pharmaceutical manufacturer prescribing information.

DIPHTHERIA + TETANUS + PERTUSSIS VACCINE (DTaP/Tdap/DTP)

Trade: Acel-Imune(DTaP), Adacel (Tdap), Boostrix (Tdap), DTP, DTaP, Daptacel (DTaP), Infanrix (DTaP), Tdap, Tripedia (DTaP), Triple Antigen (DTP)

Category: Vaccine

LRC: L2 - No Data-Probably Compatible

This is a combination vaccine containing the diphtheria and tetanus toxoids, along with acellular pertussis adsorbed vaccine.[1] Those currently licensed for use in the United States by the FDA are DTaP and Tdap. The primary difference between these is that Tdap contains reduced diphtheria toxoid making it suitable for use in adults and those more than 10 years of age. DTaP is used only in those between 6 weeks and 6 years of age. DTP vaccines which contain diphtheria and tetanus toxoids, along with whole-cell pertussis vaccines are used in some countries, but is not licensed for use in the United States due to higher risk of severe adverse reactions, such as seizures, attributed to the whole-cell pertussis content of this vaccine. DTaP is generally recommended at 2, 4, and 6 months of age with boosters at 15-20 months and at 4-6 years of age. Tdap is given as a single booster dose after the age of 10 years and is recommended for all adults who are, or anticipate being, in close contact with an infant of less than 12 months of age, if not previously immunized with Tdap.[2]

Diphtheria vaccine contains diphtheria toxoid, which is a formalin-inactivated form of diphtheria toxin. Currently, no data are available on the transfer of diphtheria toxoid in to human milk. However, diphtheria toxoid is considered compatible with breastfeeding.[3,4] The diphtheria toxoid is a large molecular weight protein toxoid. It is extremely unlikely that proteins of this size would transfer to breast milk.

There are two types of pertussis vaccines, whole cell and acellular. Whole cell pertussis vaccine is made form inactivated B. pertussis cells. Acellular pertussis vaccines are made from inactivated components of B. pertussis cells. Because pertussis vaccine is an inactivated bacterial product, there is no specific contraindication in breastfeeding following injection with this vaccine. It is extremely unlikely proteins of this size would be secreted in breast milk.

Tetanus vaccine is made from inactivated tetanus toxoid by formaldehyde.[5] Because tetanus vaccine is an inactivated bacterial product, there is no specific contraindication in breastfeeding following injection with this vaccine. It is extremely unlikely proteins of this size would be secreted in breast milk.

Because this is an inactivated bacterial product, there is no specific contraindication in breastfeeding following injection with these vaccines.

Adult Concerns: Headache, drowsiness, anorexia, vomiting, swelling, redness, tenderness at the site of injection. Hypersensitivity reactions to any component of the vaccine. Avoid during ongoing acute illness. Guillain-Barre syndrome may occur within 6 weeks of receipt of a tetanus-toxoid containing vaccine.

Adult Dose: 0.5 mL injection (IM).

Pediatric Concerns: None reported via breast milk exposure.

Infant Monitoring:

Alternatives:

References:
1. Pharmaceutical manufacturers prescribing information.
2. Centers for Disease Control and Prevention. Guidelines for Vaccinating Pregnant Women. March 2014. http://www.cdc.gov/vaccines/pubs/preg-guide.htm, 2014.
3. Advisory Committee on Immunization Practice. Resource materials: general recommendations on immunization. Am J Prev Med. 1994;10(suppl):60-82.
4. Schaefer CS, Chaefer C. Drugs During Pregnancy and Lactation. Amsterdam, the Netherlands: Elsevier Science B.V.; 2001.
5. Atkinson W, Wolfe S, Hamborsky J, eds. Tetanus. "Centers for Disease Control and Prevention. Epidemiology and Prevention of Vaccine-Preventable Diseases". 12th ed. Washington, DC: Public Health Foundation; 2011.

DIPHTHERIA + TETANUS VACCINE (DT/Td)

Trade: ADT (Td), ADT TM (DT), CDT TM (DT), DT, Decavac (Td), Diftavax (Td), Td

Category: Vaccine

LRC: L2 - No Data-Probably Compatible

This is a combination vaccine containing both the diphtheria and tetanus toxoids. It is indicated for prevention of diphtheria and tetanus. Those currently licensed for use in the United States are DT and Td. The primary difference between these is that Td contains reduced diphtheria toxoid, making it suitable for use in adults and those more than 7 years of age. DT is recommended for those up to 7 years of age.

Diphtheria vaccine contains diphtheria toxoid, which is a formalin-inactivated form of diphtheria toxin. Diphtheria toxoid is almost always administered along with other vaccines such as tetanus toxoid vaccine and pertussis vaccine. Currently, no data are available on the transfer of diphtheria toxoid in human milk. However, diphtheria toxoid is considered compatible with breastfeeding.[1-3] The diphtheria toxoid is a large molecular weight protein toxoid. It is extremely unlikely that proteins of this size would transfer to breast milk.

Tetanus toxoid vaccine contains a large molecular weight protein. It is always given in combination with diphtheria toxoid. Tetanus vaccine is made from inactivated tetanus toxoid by formaldehyde.[4] Tetanus vaccine is part of Tdap, DT, Td, DTaP, Pediarix, Pentacel, and DTP vaccines. Because tetanus vaccine is an inactivated bacterial product, there is no specific contraindication in breastfeeding following injection with this vaccine. It is extremely unlikely proteins of this size would be secreted in breast milk.

The diphtheria toxoid + tetanus toxoid vaccine combination (Td) is considered compatible with breastfeeding.

Adult Concerns: Headache, drowsiness, anorexia, vomiting, swelling, redness, tenderness at the site of injection. Hypersensitivity reactions to any component of the vaccine. Avoid during ongoing acute illness. Guillain-Barre syndrome may occur within 6 weeks of receipt of a tetanus-toxoid containing vaccine.

Adult Dose: 0.5 ml injection intramuscular.

Pediatric Concerns: None reported via breast milk exposure.

Infant Monitoring:

Alternatives:

References:

1. Advisory Committee on Immunization Practice. Resource materials: general recommendations on immunization. Am J Prev Med. 1994;10(suppl):60-82.
2. Schaefer C, Schaefer C. Drugs During Pregnancy and Lactation. Amsterdam, the Netherlands: Elsevier Science B.V.; 2001.
3. Product Information: Infanrix(R), Diphtheria and Tetanus Toxoids and a Cellular Pertussis Vaccine Adsorbed. Research Triangle Park, NC: GlaxoSmithKline Biologicals; 2003.
4. Atkinson W, Wolfe S, Hamborsky J, eds. Tetanus. "Centers for Disease Control and Prevention. Epidemiology and Prevention of Vaccine-Preventable Diseases". 12th ed. Washington, DC: Public Health Foundation; 2011.

DIPHTHERIA VACCINE

Trade: Diphtheria vaccine

Category: Vaccine

LRC: L2 - No Data-Probably Compatible

Diphtheria vaccine contains diphtheria toxoid, which is a formalin-inactivated form of diphtheria toxin. Diphtheria toxoid, when injected, induces an immunological response against diphtheria toxin by producing anti-diphtheria antibodies. Adequate titers of anti-diphtheria antibodies in the serum protects the individual from subsequent diphtheria infection. Diphtheria toxoid is almost always administered along with other vaccines such as tetanus toxoid vaccine and pertussis vaccine. The use of diphtheria toxoid alone is not recommended, especially in those 7 years of age and older, due to the risk of adverse reactions. Diphtheria toxoid, alone however, is reserved for use in those pediatric patients in whom the use of tetanus toxoid and/or pertussis vaccine is contraindicated.

Currently, no data are available on the transfer of diphtheria toxoid into human milk. However, diphtheria toxoid is considered compatible with breastfeeding.[1,2] The diphtheria toxoid is a large molecular weight protein toxoid. It is extremely unlikely that proteins of this size would transfer into breast milk. Remember, the use of combination vaccines of diphtheria, tetanus toxoid, and pertussis (adsorbed DTP/DTaP), is contraindicated in adults and those older than 7 years of age due to increased risk of adverse reactions.[3] But the combination of diphtheria and tetanus toxoid (Td) may be safely used in all adults, including breastfeeding women.

Adult Concerns: Redness, tenderness, and induration at the site of injection.

Adult Dose:

Pediatric Concerns:

Infant Monitoring:

Alternatives:

References:
1. Advisory Committee on Immunization Practice. Resource materials: general recommendations on immunization. Am J Prev Med. 1994;10(suppl):60-82.
2. Schaefer C, Schaefer C. Drugs During Pregnancy and Lactation. Amsterdam, The Netherlands: Elsevier Science B.V.; 2001.
3. Product Information: Infanrix(R), diphtheria and tetanus toxoids and acellular pertussis vaccine adsorbed. Research Triangle Park, NC: GlaxoSmithKline Biologicals; 2003.

DIPIVEFRIN

Trade: Propine

Category: Antiglaucoma

LRC: L2 - No Data-Probably Compatible

Dipivefrin is a synthetic prodrug that is metabolized to epinephrine although it is only used topically in the eye. Because of its structure, it is more lipophilic and better absorbed into the eye; hence, it is more potent.[1] Following absorption into the eye, dipivefrin reduces intraocular pressure. It is not known if dipivefrin enters milk, but small amounts may be present. It is unlikely that any dipivefrin or epinephrine present in milk would be orally bioavailable to the infant.

T 1/2		MW		PB	
Tmax	1 h	RID		Vd	
Oral	Minimal	M/P		pKa	

Adult Concerns: Burning, itching, tearing, hyperemia of eyes, redness of the eyes, burning and stinging have been reported. Infrequently, tachycardia, arrhythmias, hypertension have occurred with intraocular epinephrine.

Adult Dose: 1 drop in affected eye every 12 hours.

Pediatric Concerns: None via milk.

Infant Monitoring:

Alternatives:

References:
1. Pharmaceutical manufacturers prescribing information.

DIPYRIDAMOLE

Trade: Persantin, Persantine

Category: Platelet Aggregation Inhibitor

LRC: L3 - No Data-Probably Compatible

Dipyridamole is most commonly used in addition to coumarin anticoagulants to prevent thromboembolic complications after cardiac valve replacement.[1] According to the manufacturer this medication is excreted in human milk, although concentrations in milk were not reported. Based on this medication's large molecular weight and high protein binding levels in milk are expected to be low.

T 1/2	10-12 h	MW	505 Da	PB	91%-99%
Tmax	2-2.5 h	RID		Vd	2-3 L/kg
Oral	Poor	M/P		pKa	14.97

Adult Concerns: Headache, dizziness, hypotension, arrhythmias, nausea, vomiting, diarrhea, changes in liver function, thrombocytopenia.

Adult Dose: 75-100 mg QID.

Pediatric Concerns: No adverse effects have been reported at this time.

Infant Monitoring: Rare-bruising on the skin, blood in urine, vomit, or stool.

Alternatives:

References:
1. Pharmaceutical manufacturers prescribing information.

DISOPYRAMIDE

Trade: Isomide, Napamide, Norpace, Rythmodan

Category: Antiarrhythmic

LRC: L2 - Limited Data-Probably Compatible

Disopyramide is used for treating cardiac arrhythmias similar to quinidine and procainamide. Small levels are secreted into milk. Following a maternal dose of 450 mg every 8 hours for 2 weeks, the milk/plasma ratio was approximately 1.06 for disopyramide and 6.24 for its active metabolite.[1] Although no disopyramide was measurable in the infant's plasma, the milk levels were 2.6-4.4 mg/L (disopyramide), and 9.6-12.3 mg/L (metabolite). Infant urine collected over an 8-hour period contained 3.3 mg/L of disopyramide. Such levels are probably too small to affect an infant. No side effects were reported.

In another study, in a woman receiving 100 mg five times daily, the maternal serum level was 10.3 µmol/L and the breast milk level was 4.0 µmol/L, giving a milk/serum ratio of 0.4.[2] From these levels, an infant ingesting 1 liter of milk would receive only 1.5 mg per day. Lowest milk levels are at 6-8 hours postdose.

T 1/2	8.3-11.65 h	MW	339 Da	PB	50%
Tmax	2.3 h	RID	3.4%	Vd	0.6-1.3 L/kg
Oral	60%-83%	M/P	0.4-1.06	pKa	8.4

Adult Concerns: Dry mouth, constipation, edema, hypotension, nausea, vomiting, diarrhea.

Adult Dose: 150 mg every 6 hours.

Pediatric Concerns: None reported.

Infant Monitoring: Drowsiness, lethargy, pallor, arrhythmias, heart failure, poor feeding, weight gain.

Alternatives:

References:
1. MacKintosh D, Buchanan N. Excretion of disopyramide in human breast milk. Br J Clin Pharmacol. 1985;19(6):856-857.
2. Ellsworth AJ, Horn JR, Raisys VA, Miyagawa LA, Bell JL. Disopyramide and N-monodesalkyl disopyramide in serum and breast milk. DICP. 1989;23(1):56-57.

DOBUTAMINE

Trade: Dobutrex

Category: Adrenergic

LRC: L2 - No Data-Probably Compatible

Dobutamine is an isoproterenol derivative that stimulates beta receptors in the heart to increase cardiac output and provide short-term treatment of severe cardiac decompensation (e.g., heart failure, severe hypotension, shock).[1] This medication is administered intravenously as it is rapidly destroyed in the gastrointestinal tract. It is not known if dobutamine transfers to human milk.

T 1/2	2 min	MW	337.85 Da	PB	
Tmax		RID		Vd	0.2 L/kg
Oral		M/P		pKa	10.14

Adult Concerns: Headache, arrhythmias, hypertension, tachycardia, hypotension, chest pain, dyspnea, nausea, hypokalemia, thrombocytopenia, paresthesia.

Adult Dose: 2.5-20 µg/kg/min IV.

Pediatric Concerns:

Infant Monitoring: Irritability, lethargy, not waking to feed/poor feeding.

Alternatives:

References:
1. Pharmaceutical manufacturers prescribing information.

DOCETAXEL

Trade: Taxotere

Category: Antineoplastic

LRC: L5 - No Data-Hazardous

Docetaxel is an antineoplastic agent derived from the yew plant. It has a large molecular weight of 861 Da and acts by disrupting the mitotic and interphase cellular functions. Docetaxel's pharmacokinetic profile is consistent with a three-compartment kinetic model, with half-lives for the alpha, beta, and gamma of 4 minutes, 36 minutes, and 11.1 hours, respectively. Oral bioavailability is just 8%. The initial rapid decline represents distribution to the peripheral compartments, and the late (terminal) phase is due, in part, to a relatively slow efflux of docetaxel from the peripheral compartment. Mean value for steady state volume of distribution is 113 L.[1] Within 7 days, urinary and fecal excretion accounted for approximately 6% and 75% of the administered radioactivity, respectively. About 80% of the radioactivity recovered in feces is excreted during the first 48 hours, as metabolites with very small amounts (less than 8%) of unchanged drug. No data are available on its transfer into human milk. Due to its large molecular weight and high protein binding, milk levels are probably quite low. Withhold breastfeeding for a minimum of 4 to 5 days.

T 1/2	11.1 h (gamma)	MW	807.9 Da	PB	95%
Tmax		RID		Vd	1.6 L/kg
Oral		M/P		pKa	10.96

Adult Concerns: Alopecia, neuropathy, fever, stomatitis, vomiting, diarrhea, changes in liver function, leukopenia, neutropenia, anemia, weakness.

Adult Dose:

Pediatric Concerns:

Infant Monitoring: Withhold breastfeeding for a minimum of 4 to 5 days.

Alternatives:

References:
1. Pharmaceutical manufacturers prescribing information.

DOCOSAHEXAENOIC ACID (DHA)

Trade: DHA

Category: Vitamin

LRC: L3 - No Data-Probably Compatible

Docosahexaenoic Acid (DHA) is a N-3 fatty acid that is produced from alpha linolenic acid. Fish that live in cold water are high in DHA content. The central nervous system and retina contain high amounts of DHA. DHA accumulation in the brain is thought to be most rapid during the last trimester of pregnancy and the first year of life. The first year of life is thought to have critical windows when DHA is most important to infant development.

Animal studies with nonhuman primates suggest that DHA enhances the development of the brain's neurotransmitter systems such as the dopaminergic and serotonergic systems. However, research in humans has so far failed to provide strong evidence for or against the efficacy of DHA supplementation in pregnancy and lactation.[1-3]

It is not known whether omega-3-acid ethyl esters are excreted in human milk, but we do know that docosahexaenoic acid (DHA) is a common lipid in human milk. DHA is in varying levels depending on maternal diet; thus, high dose supplementation could be hazardous.

The American Academy of Pediatrics (AAP) recommends that breastfeeding women have an average of 200-300 mg per day of omega-3 long chain polyunsaturated fatty acids (docosahexaenoic acid [DHA]).[4-6] Both the AAP and the Dietary Guidelines for Americans encourage dietary sources such as consumption of one or two portions or 8-12 ounces of fish per week.[4-6]

T 1/2	20 h	MW	328 Da	PB	
Tmax		RID		Vd	
Oral	Complete	M/P		pKa	

Adult Concerns: Fishy taste, belching, nausea, flatulence, diarrhea, increase in ALT, prolonged bleeding time.

Adult Dose: 250-500 mg DHA + EPA per day.

Pediatric Concerns:

Infant Monitoring: Diarrhea.

Alternatives:

References:

1. Makrides M, Gould JF, Gawlik NR, et al. Four-year follow-up of children born to women in a randomized trial of prenatal DHA supplementation. JAMA. 2014;311(17):1802-1804.
2. Gould JF, Smithers LG, Makrides M. The effect of maternal omega-3 (n-3) LCPUFA supplementation during pregnancy on early childhood cognitive and visual development: a systematic review and meta-analysis of randomized controlled trials. Am J Clin Nutr. 2013 Mar;97(3):531-544.
3. Carlson SE. Docosahexaenoic acid supplementation in pregnancy and lactation. Am J Clin Nutr. 2009 Feb;89(2):678S-684S. Epub 2008 Dec 30.
4. Johnston M, Landers S, Noble L, et al. Breastfeeding and the use of human milk. Pediatrics. 2012;129:e827-e841.
5. U.S. Department of Agriculture and U.S. Department of Health and Human Services. Dietary Guidelines for Americans, 2010. 7th ed. Washington, DC: U.S. Government Printing Office, December 2010. [Online] http://www.health.gov/dietaryguidelines/dga2010/DietaryGuidelines2010.pdf. Accessed May 7, 2016.
6. Vannice G, Rasmussen H. Position of the academy of nutrition and dietetics: dietary fatty acids for healthy adults. J Acad Nutr Diet. 2014;114(1):136-153.

DOCOSANOL

Trade: Abreva

Category: Antiviral

LRC: L3 - No Data-Probably Compatible

Docosanol, also called behenyl alcohol, is a fatty alcohol use in cosmetics as a thickener, emulsifier, and an emollient. It is also approved as an antiviral agent for treatment of oral-facial herpes simplex only. It should not be used in the eyes or on the genitalia. It inhibits lipid-enveloped viruses from entering the cell by fusion between the plasma membrane and the viral envelope.[1] There have been no studies on docosanol in breast milk, however it is not orally absorbed and therefore probably poses little threat to a nursing infant.

T 1/2		MW	327 Da	PB	
Tmax		RID		Vd	
Oral	0%	M/P		pKa	

Adult Concerns: Headache, rash, increased redness.

Adult Dose: Apply topically five times daily to lesions until healed.

Pediatric Concerns: No data are available at this time.

Infant Monitoring: Poor oral absorption in the infant; adverse effects unlikely.

Alternatives:

References:

1. Pharmaceutical manufacturers prescribing information.

DOCUSATE

Trade: Colace, Dulcolax Stool Softener

Category: Laxative

LRC: L2 - No Data-Probably Compatible

Docusate is a detergent commonly used as a stool softener. The degree of oral absorption is poor, but some is known to be absorbed and re-secreted in the bile. Although some drug is absorbed by mother via her gastrointestinal tract, transfer into breast milk is unknown but probably minimal. Watch for loose stools in infant. It is not likely this would be overly detrimental to a breastfed infant.

T 1/2		MW	444 Da	PB	
Tmax		RID		Vd	
Oral	Poor	M/P		pKa	

Adult Concerns: Nausea, diarrhea.

Adult Dose: 50-200 mg daily.

Pediatric Concerns: None reported.

Infant Monitoring: Diarrhea.

Alternatives:

References:
1. Pharmaceutical manufacturers prescribing information.

DOLASETRON

Trade: Anzemet

Category: Antiemetic

LRC: L3 - No Data-Probably Compatible

Dolasetron mesylate and its active metabolite, hydrodolasetron, are selective serotonin 5-HT3 receptor antagonists, primarily in the chemoreceptor trigger zone responsible for control of nausea and vomiting. It is believed that chemotherapeutic agents release serotonin in the gastrointestinal tract that then activate the 5-HT3 receptors on the vagus nerve that initiates the vomiting reflex. This product is used prior to treatment with cancer chemotherapeutic agents, or prior to surgery and general anesthesia.[1]

No data are available on its transfer to milk. The maximum concentration in maternal plasma would be 556 ng/mL, which is quite low. At this plasma level and assuming a 1:1 milk/plasma ratio, an infant would likely receive far less than a milligram daily. It has been safely used in children 2 years of age at doses of 1.2 mg/kg.

T 1/2	8.1 h	MW	438 Da	PB	77%
Tmax	1 h	RID		Vd	5.8 L/kg
Oral	75%	M/P		pKa	

Adult Concerns: Headache, fatigue, dizziness, bradycardia, arrhythmias (e.g., QTc prolongation), abdominal pain, dyspepsia, diarrhea, hyperbilirubinemia, changes in liver and renal function.

Adult Dose: 100 mg orally.

Pediatric Concerns: None reported via milk.

Infant Monitoring: Drowsiness, lethargy, diarrhea.

Alternatives: Ondansetron(L2)

References:
1. Pharmaceutical manufacturers prescribing information.

DOLUTEGRAVIR

Trade: Tivicay

Category: Antiviral

LRC: L3 - Limited Data-Probably Compatible

Dolutegravir is used for the treatment of HIV-1, in combination with other HIV drugs. It is a member of the integrase inhibitor class of HIV drugs and can be used with other anti-retroviral agents in both adults and children who weigh at least 30 kg (66.1 lbs).[1] It can also be used in combination with rilpivirine (a second generation HIV medication) as a complete HIV regimen in adults if the prescribed patient has: 1) a viral load < 50/mL, 2) been on a stable antiretroviral regimen for at least 6 months, 3) no history of treatment failure, and 4) no previous history of resistance to either rilpivirine or dolutegravir.[1] Like other HIV medications, dolutegravir cannot cure HIV, but it can prolong the length and enhance the quality of life. It can also reduce the risk of HIV transmission. [1]

In the United States and other developed countries, to reduce the risk of transmitting HIV to their infants, mothers living with HIV are NOT recommended to breastfeed even if they are on anti-retroviral therapy (ART). [2] However, if there are no acceptable alternatives to breastfeeding (usually only in developing countries), the World Health Organization (WHO) recommends that the mother exclusively breastfeed for 6 months, regardless of her HIV positive status.[3] The same recommendation holds true for HIV-infected mothers in the United States and other developed countries who choose to breastfeed despite medical advisory against it.[2] In such cases, if a mother is treated with an HIV regimen that contains dolutegravir, there is limited data on the transfer of this drug to human milk and its effects on the infant. Only one case report thus far has reported dolutegravir levels in breast milk and in maternal and infant plasma.[4]

The case report follows a 35-year-old HIV-1 positive mother over 10 months. While breastfeeding, the mother took daily doses of Triumeq (contains 50 mg dolutegravir, 600 mg abacavir, and 300 mg lamivudine). Due to ethical reasons, maternal plasma sampling was limited and only one plasma sample was obtained at about 28 weeks post-partum. The maternal plasma dolutegravir levels in this sample were measured 11 hours after dosing and amounted to 4.48 mg/L. Breast milk samples were obtained three times over the 10-month period and the average dolutegravir concentration in the samples amounted to 0.1 mg/L at 11 hours after the dose. Using this data, the milk-to-plasma ratio (M/P ratio) was calculated to be 0.02. The authors note that this M/P ratio was higher than expected, as pharmacokinetic studies have shown that dolutegravir has a plasma protein binding rate of almost 99%, which should severely limit the drug's transfer rate to human milk. The authors suspect that the unexpectedly high transfer rate of dolutegravir to human milk may be due to active transport mechanisms. The authors also estimated the daily infant dolutegravir dose to be 0.015 mg/kg. In addition, the infant's dolutegravir plasma concentrations were measured three times during the 10-month period and averaged to about 0.10 mg/L. No significant side effects were observed in the infant.[4]

In conclusion, only limited data exists on the transfer of dolutegravir to human milk. Based on the case report described, it would seem that dolutegravir has an unexpectedly high transfer rate to breast milk. Despite this high transfer rate, the relative infant dose (RID) was only 2.1%, which is significantly below the RID 10% cutoff that is used to determine safe levels of infant drug exposure. Regardless, the primary recommendation for women in developed countries living with HIV is to NOT breastfeed their infants.[2]

T 1/2	14 h	MW	419.385 Da	PB	98.9%
Tmax	2-3 h	RID	2.1%	Vd	0.248 L/kg
Oral		M/P	0.02	pKa	8.2

Adult Concerns: Fever, ill feeling, tiredness, muscle and joint pains, blisters and sores of mouth.

Adult Dose: 50 mg daily.

Pediatric Concerns:

Infant Monitoring: Rash, liver injury.

Alternatives:

References:
1. Pharmaceutical manufacturers prescribing information.
2. Panel on Treatment of Pregnant Women with HIV Infection and Prevention of Perinatal Transmission. Recommendations for Use of Antiretroviral Drugs in Transmission in the United States. http://aidsinfo.nih.gov/contentfiles/lvguidelines/PerinatalGL.pdf. Accessed 15 May 2018. F-1-F-5.
3. World Health Organization. Guideline: Updates on HIV and Infant Feeding: The Duration of Breastfeeding and Support from Health Services to Improve Feeding Practices Among Mothers Living with HIV. Geneva: WHO; 2016.
4. Kobbe R, Schalkwijk S, Dunay G, et al. Dolutegravir in breast milk and maternal and infant plasma during breastfeeding. AIDS.2016 Nov;30(17):2731-2733.

DOMPERIDONE

Trade: Motilidone, Motilium

Category: Dopamine Antagonist

LRC: L3 - Limited Data-Probably Compatible

Domperidone is a peripheral dopamine antagonist (similar to metoclopramide) generally used for controlling nausea and vomiting, dyspepsia, and gastric reflux. It blocks peripheral dopamine receptors in the gastrointestinal wall and in the CRTZ (nausea center) in the brain stem and is currently used in Canada as an antiemetic.[1] Unlike metoclopramide, it does not enter the brain compartment and thus has fewer CNS effects.

It is also known to produce significant increases in prolactin levels and has proven useful as a galactagogue. Serum prolactin levels have been found to increase from 8.1 ng/mL to 124.1 ng/mL in non-lactating women after one 20 mg dose.[2] Concentrations of domperidone reported in milk vary according to dose. But following a dose of 10 mg three times daily, the average concentration in milk was only 2.6 µg/L.[3]

A small study published in 1985 enrolled both women with a history of lactation failure and those with poor milk supply.[4] In this study 8 of 15 women with a history of poor milk supply with a previous infant were given domperidone 10 mg tid on days 2-5 postpartum and the others were given placebo and 9 of 17 women with low milk supply 2 weeks postpartum (1st infant, milk supply 30% less than normal) were given domperidone 10 mg tid for 10 days and the others were given placebo. In both groups of women given domperidone, an increase in prolactin and milk supply was reported when compared to placebo. In addition, all women given domperidone had adequate milk supply at 1 month postpartum where numerous women in the placebo group did not.

In a study by da Silva, 16 mothers with premature infants and low milk production (mean = 112.8 mL/day in domperidone group; 48.2 mL/day in placebo group) were randomly chosen to receive placebo (n = 9) or domperidone (10 mg TID) (n = 7) for 7 days.[5] Milk volume increased from 112.8 to 162.2 mL/day in the domperidone group and 48.2 to 56.1 mL/day in the placebo group. Prolactin levels increased from 12.9 to 119.3 µg/L in the domperidone group and 15.6 to 18.1 µg/L in the placebo group. On day 5, the mean domperidone concentrations in the treatment group were 6.6 ng/mL in plasma and 1.2 µg/L in breast milk (n = 6). No adverse effects were reported in infants or mothers.

In a 2008 study, a group of six breastfeeding women were placed in a double blind randomized crossover trial to compare doses of domperidone.[6] In this trial, mothers were studied in a run-in phase (no drug treatment), 30 mg, or 60 mg domperidone per day (10 or 20 mg every 8 hours). Milk volume created per hour and plasma prolactin levels were monitored. Two mothers did not respond to domperidone treatment and had no change in milk production. Four mothers showed a significant increase from 8.7 g/hour in the run-in phase to 23.6 g/hour for the 30 mg/day dose, to 29.4 g/hour for the 60 mg/day dose. While plasma prolactin levels were increased by domperidone treatment, there was only a slight increase in milk production at the 60 mg/day dose. Median domperidone concentrations in milk were 0.28 µg/L and 0.49 µg/L for the 30 mg and 60 mg daily doses, respectively. The mean RID was 0.012% at 30 mg/day and 0.009% at 60 mg/day. The authors suggest that milk production increased at both doses and there was a small trend for a dose-response.

Forty-six mothers who delivered infants at <31 weeks' gestation, and also experienced lactation failure, were randomly assigned to receive domperidone 10 mg TID or placebo for 14 days.[7] Protein, energy, fat, carbohydrate, sodium, calcium, and phosphate levels in breast milk were measured on days 0, 4, 7, and 14, serum prolactin levels were measured on days 0, 4, and 14, and total milk production was recorded daily. By day 14, breast milk volumes had increased by 267% in the domperidone group and by 18.5% in the placebo group. Serum prolactin increased by 97% in the domperidone group and by 17% in the placebo group. Mean breast milk protein declined by 9.6% in the domperidone group and increased by 3.6% in the placebo group. There were no changes in caloric content, fat, carbohydrate, sodium, or phosphate content. Significant increases in milk carbohydrate (2.7% vs. -2.7%) and calcium (61.8% vs. -4.4%) were noted in the domperidone group. No adverse effects were observed in infants or mothers. The authors concluded that domperidone increases the volume of breast milk of preterm mothers experiencing lactation failure, without substantially altering the nutrient composition.

In 2013, a study was published that compared the efficacy of two different domperidone doses.[8] Patients were randomized to two treatment regimens, 10 or 20 mg three times daily for 4 weeks, followed by a titration off of therapy (twice daily therapy for 1 week, then once daily for 1 week and then off). Over a 1 month period, there was a significant increase in daily milk volumes within each group. Breast milk concentrations were measured an average of 3 hours after the domperidone dose on the same day between days 10-15 of therapy. The median concentrations of domperidone in breast milk at this time were 3.4 µg/L in the 10 mg (n = 4) and 6.9 µg/L in the 20 mg (n = 3) groups, respectively. The median AUCs were 15.8 µg.h/L and 31.9 µg.h/L, in the 10 mg and 20 mg groups, respectively. In this study, the higher domperidone dose of 20 mg three times daily was not associated with a statistically significant increase in milk production; however, the authors report a clinically significant increase in milk production in this higher dose group.

Thus far only one study has been published which focused on the effect of stopping domperidone on subsequent milk production.[9] Twenty-five women who initially received domperidone (20 mg QID) were gently withdrawn off the medication over a 2-4 week period, from 20 mg QID to 10 mg QID to no therapy. Formula use was reported during this duration. Twenty three of twenty five cases (93%) reported no significant increase in formula use after stopping domperidone. Normal infant growth was reported in all cases. The authors concluded that following a slow withdrawal from domperidone, there is no significant increase in formula supplementation. This clearly suggests that once sufficient milk production is established, it is maintained even without the use of domperidone.

When metoclopramide and domperidone were compared in a 2012 randomized controlled trial, both medications were found to increase milk supply with similar efficacy.[10] Sixty-five women were given 10 mg TID of either domperidone or metoclopramide for 10 days. These women had given birth to preterm infants (average gestation at birth= 28 weeks) and started this medication if they were unable to produce 160 mL/kg/day of milk; most women in this trial started drug therapy about 4 weeks postpartum. Women in the domperidone and metoclopramide groups increased their milk supply by 96.3% and 93.7%, respectively. More women in the metoclopramide group reported adverse effects (7 vs. 3) such as headache, mood swings, dry mouth, change in appetite, and diarrhea.

In a study that evaluated the use of domperidone in women with preterm infants, 32 women were randomized to domperidone or placebo after 7-14 days postpartum with poor milk supply.[11] The median milk increase was 186 mL/day (range 126.5-240 mL/day) versus 70 mL/day (49.5-97 mL/day) in the domperidone group compared to the placebo group at day 7 of therapy. The median increase in serum prolactin from day 1 to 8 was not significant in the domperidone 18.7 µg/L (-39.5-55.6 µg/L) versus placebo group 11.9 µg/L (-8.3-37.5 µg/L). In addition, this study reported no difference in the infants weight gain and no maternal adverse events. The authors of this study report that domperidone should be offered only after non-drug measures have been exhausted to increase milk supply.

The most recently published multi-center randomized trial included 90 women and their 109 preterm infants (mean 27 weeks).[12] In this study, group A received domperidone 10 mg TID for 28 days and grouped B received placebo TID 14 days, then domperidone 10 mg TID for 14 days. There were no differences in mean milk volume on day 14 (group A 267 mL/day vs. group B 217 mL/day) or day 28 (group A 290 mL/day vs. group B 302 mL/day). There were more women with a > 50% increase in milk volume on day 14 in group A compared to group B (group A 77.8%, group B 57.78%); however, this difference was no longer significant on day 28 when both groups were on domperidone. The authors report there were no appreciable increases in milk volume with the longer course of therapy (28 days). The main maternal side effects were headache and gastrointestinal. There were two maternal reports of cardiac symptoms, one of which was a report of palpitations with a normal ECG and the other was a low-lying ectopic atrial rhythm (benign variant). In this study, 86% of the women had ECGs completed at entry and 73% at end of week 4. In addition, 92% of the infants had ECGs completed at entry and 75% at end of week 4. Five infants had ECGs with QTc > 500 ms; all infants were asymptomatic and no interventions were needed (authors unable to rule out other causes such as prematurity). Other neonatal adverse events reported included gastrointestinal symptoms, neurological symptoms and other events that were more likely due to prematurity and delivery (e.g., pulmonary, infection, genitourinary). Please note that enrollment in this study was stopped early (target n=560) due to low recruitment, the authors of this study speculated that the country's recent government health warnings regarding QTc prolongation may have contributed to this.

Most of these studies demonstrated that domperidone 10 mg three times daily modestly increased milk production in women with premature infants.[1-12] Doses higher than this should be avoided in breastfeeding mothers as the US FDA and Health Canada have issued warnings that domperidone can induce life-threatening cardiac arrhythmias and that this effect is most likely dose related.[13,14] The medication is not recommended in patients with a preexisting arrhythmia, history of cardiac disease or those taking other medications which can also prolong the QTc interval.

In summary, the recommended domperidone dose is 10-20 mg three times a day. There is no evidence that higher doses are more effective, but may dramatically increase the risk of QTc prolongation.

Warning: The InfantRisk center has now received numerous reports of withdrawal-like symptoms in mothers consuming large doses of domperidone (> 90 mg daily) to stimulate milk production. In one case report, these included insomnia, rigors, severe psychomotor agitations, and panic attacks.[15] In other cases, severe muscle pain, and gastric symptoms were reported. Apparently, the only treatment for these symptoms is too reinstate the same dose of domperidone(or one that controls the symptoms) and proceed to reduce the dose over a month or longer.

T 1/2	7-14 h	MW	426 Da	PB	93%
Tmax	30 min	RID	0.01%-0.35%	Vd	
Oral	13%-17%	M/P	0.25	pKa	7.9

Adult Concerns: Headache, drowsiness, dizziness, changes in mood, seizures (rare), arrhythmias (QTc prolongation), dry mouth, abdominal cramps, diarrhea, extrapyramidal symptoms (rare). Withdrawal symptoms following high doses.

Adult Dose: 10 mg three times daily.

Pediatric Concerns: In a lactation study published in 2017, five infants exposed to domperidone in milk had ECGs with QTc > 500 ms; all infants were asymptomatic and no interventions were needed (authors were unable to rule out other causes such as prematurity).[12] Other neonatal adverse events reported in this study included gastrointestinal symptoms, neurological symptoms and events that were more likely due to prematurity and delivery (e.g., infection).

Infant Monitoring: Diarrhea.

Alternatives: Metoclopramide(L2)

References:
1. Hofmeyr GJ, van Iddekinge B. Domperidone and lactation. Lancet. 1983;1(8325):647.
2. Brouwers JR, Assies J, Wiersinga WM, Huizing G, Tytgat GN. Plasma prolactin levels after acute and subchronic oral administration of domperidone and of metoclopramide: a cross-over study in healthy volunteers. Clin Endocrinol (Oxf). 1980;12(5):435-440.
3. Hofmeyr GJ, van Iddekinge B, Blott JA. Domperidone: secretion in breast milk and effect on puerperal prolactin levels. Br J Obstet Gynaecol. 1985;92(2):141-144.
4. Petraglia F, De Leo V, Sardelli S, et al. Domperidone in defective and insufficient lactation. Eur J Obstet Gynecol Reprod Biol. 1985;19:281-287.
5. da Silva OP, Knoppert DC, Angelini MM, Forret PA. Effect of domperidone on milk production in mothers of premature newborns: a randomized, double-blind, placebo-controlled trial. CMAJ. 2001;164(1):17-21.

6. Wan E WX, Davey K, Page-Sharp M, Hartmann PE, Simmer K, Ilett KF. Dose-effect study of domperidone as a galactagogue in preterm mothers with insufficient milk supply, and its transfer into milk. Br J Clin Pharmacol. 2008;66(2):283-289.

7. Campbell-Yeo ML, Allen AC, Joseph KS, et al. Effect of domperidone on the composition of preterm human breast milk. Pediatrics. 2010 Jan;125(1):e107-e114. Epub 2009 Dec 14.

8. Knoppert DC, Page A, Warren J, et al. The effect of two different domperidone doses on maternal milk production. J Hum Lact. 2013 Feb;29(1):38-44.

9. Livingston V, Blaga Stancheva L, Stringer J. The effect of withdrawing domperidone on formula supplementation. Breastfeed Med. 2007;2:278, Abstract 3.

10. Ingram J, Taylor H, Churchill C, et al. Metoclopramide or domperidone for increasing maternal breast milk output: a randomized controlled trial. Arch Dis Child Fetal Neonatal Ed. 2012:97:F241-F245.

11. Rai R, Mishra N, Singh DK. Effect of domperidone in 2nd week postpartum on milk output in mothers of preterm infants. Indian J Pediatr. 2016;83(8):894-895.

12. Asztalos EV, Campbell-Yao M, da Silva OP, et al. Enhancing human milk production with domperidone in mothers of preterm infants: results from the EMPOWER Trial. J Hum Lact. 2017;22(1):181-187.

13. Osborne RJ, Slevin ML, Hunter RW, Hamer J. Cardiac arrhythmias during cytotoxic chemotherapy: role of domperidone. Hum Toxicol. 1985 Nov;4(6):617-626.

14. Health Canada. Summary Safety Review- Domperidone- Serious abnormal heart rhythms and sudden death (cardiac arrest). Jan 2015 [Online].

15. Doyle M, Grossman M. Case report: domperidone use as a galactagogue resulting in withdrawal symptoms upon discontinuation. Arch Womens Ment Health. 2018;21(4):461-463. doi:10.1007/s00737-017-0796-8

DONEPEZIL

Trade: Aricept

Category: Cholinergic

LRC: L4 - No Data-Possibly Hazardous

Donepezil is a reversible inhibitor of acetylcholinesterase that ultimately increases synaptic levels of acetylcholine by inhibition of its breakdown. It is believed to improve mild to moderate dementia and cognitive function in patients with Alzheimer's disease. While this agent is only "cleared" for treatment of patients with Alzheimer's disease, other applications may exist. No data are available on its transfer to human milk. Due to its long half-life, and its ability to affect cholinergic function in all mammals, some caution is recommended in breastfeeding women until data are available.

T 1/2	70 h	MW	415 Da	PB	96%
Tmax	3-4 h	RID		Vd	12 L/kg
Oral	100%	M/P		pKa	9.1

Adult Concerns: Headache, fatigue, insomnia, agitation, seizures, bradycardia, nausea, increased gastric acid secretion, diarrhea, weight loss, muscle cramps.

Adult Dose: 5-10 mg daily.

Pediatric Concerns: None reported via milk at this time.

Infant Monitoring: Not commonly used in lactation - Poor sleep, irritability, vomiting, diarrhea, poor weight gain.

Alternatives:

References:
1. Pharmaceutical manufacturers prescribing information.

DOPAMINE

Trade: Intropin, Revimine

Category: Adrenergic

LRC: L2 - No Data-Probably Compatible

Dopamine is a catecholamine pressor agent used in shock and severe hypotension.[1] It is rapidly destroyed in the gastrointestinal tract and is only used IV. It is not known if it transfers into human milk, but the half-life is so short they would not last long. Dopamine, while in the plasma, significantly (>60%) inhibits prolactin secretion and would likely inhibit lactation while being used.

T 1/2	2 min	MW	189 Da	PB	
Tmax	5 min	RID		Vd	
Oral		M/P		pKa	8.93

Adult Concerns: Stimulation, agitation, tachycardia.

Adult Dose: 1-50 µg/kg/min IV.

Pediatric Concerns: None reported. No gastrointestinal absorption.

Infant Monitoring: Irritability, not waking to feed/poor feeding, and tremor.

Alternatives:

References:

1. McEvoy GE, ed. AFHS Drug Information. New York, NY: McGraw-Hill; 2003.

DORIPENEM

Trade: Doribax

Category: Antibiotic, Carbapenem

LRC: L3 - No Data-Probably Compatible

Doripenem is a new carbapenem antibiotic similar in structure to the penicillins.[1] Doripenem is resistant to most beta-lactamases produced by gram-positive and gram-negative bacteria and is used to treat multi-drug resistant bacteria. At this time there are no data regarding the transfer of this medication into human milk. Based on this medication's small volume of distribution and low protein binding some drug is expected to enter human milk; however, the oral bioavailability of this medication is low. At this time meropenem (another carbapenem) would be recommended if appropriate for treatment of the maternal condition as concentrations in milk are known to be very low.

T 1/2	1 h	MW	438 Da	PB	8%-9%
Tmax	1 h	RID		Vd	0.24 L/kg
Oral	Poor	M/P		pKa	2.8, 7.9

Adult Concerns: Headache, phlebitis, nausea, diarrhea, changes in liver function, anemia, severe skin rashes.

Adult Dose: 500 mg IV every 8 hours.

Pediatric Concerns: None reported via milk at this time.

Infant Monitoring: Vomiting, diarrhea, changes in gastrointestinal flora, and rash.

Alternatives: Meropenem(L3)

References:

1. Pharmaceutical manufacturers prescribing information.

DORNASE

Trade: Pulmozyme

Category: Mucolytic

LRC: L3 - No Data-Probably Compatible

Dornase is a mucolytic enzyme used in the treatment of cystic fibrosis. It is a large molecular weight peptide (260 amino acids, 37,000 Da) that selectively digests DNA.[1] It is poorly absorbed by the pulmonary tissues. Serum levels are undetectable. Even if it were to reach the milk, it would not be orally bioavailable in the infant.

T 1/2		MW	37,000 Da	PB	
Tmax		RID		Vd	
Oral	None	M/P		pKa	

Adult Concerns: Hoarseness, sore throat, facial edema.

Adult Dose: 2.5 mg via inhalation.

Pediatric Concerns: None reported.

Infant Monitoring:

Alternatives:

References:
1. Pharmaceutical manufacturers prescribing information.

DORZOLAMIDE

Trade: Trusopt

Category: Antiglaucoma

LRC: L3 - No Data-Probably Compatible

Dorzolamide is a carbonic anhydrase inhibitor used to treat conditions such as intraocular hypertension and open angle glaucoma.[1] It is a unique formulation that exerts its effects directly in the eye. No data are available on its transfer into human milk. However, this product would only be slightly absorbed by the mother. This agent is stored for long periods in the red blood cell, although plasma levels are exceedingly low. Milk levels are expected to be low to undetectable.

T 1/2		MW	361 Da	PB	33%
Tmax	2 h	RID		Vd	
Oral		M/P		pKa	8.18

Adult Concerns: Vertigo, dizziness, bitter or unusual taste, contact dermatitis in the throat, allergic reactions.

Adult Dose: One drop in eye three times daily.

Pediatric Concerns: No data in lactation at this time.

Infant Monitoring:

Alternatives:

References:
1. Pharmaceutical manufacturers prescribing information.

DOXAZOSIN

Trade: Cardura, Carduran

Category: Alpha-Adrenergic Blocker

LRC: L3 - Limited Data-Probably Compatible

Doxazosin mesylate is an alpha-1 adrenergic receptor blocker indicated for use in hypertension. In a case report of a single patient (58 kg) who received 4 mg daily for 2 days, the average and maximum milk concentrations were 2.9 and 4.2 µg/L.[1] The authors suggest this provides a relative infant dose of 0.06% and 0.09%, respectively. Our relative infant dose calculations based on these milk concentrations were slightly higher, 0.58%-0.87%.

T 1/2	9-22 h	MW	451 Da	PB	98%
Tmax	2 h	RID	0.58%-0.87%	Vd	
Oral	62%-69%	M/P	20	pKa	6.93

Adult Concerns: Headache, dizziness, fatigue, insomnia, flushing, hypotension, arrhythmias, dry mouth, dyspepsia, polyuria, edema.

Adult Dose: 2-4 mg daily.

Pediatric Concerns: None reported via milk at this time.

Infant Monitoring: Drowsiness, low blood pressure, lethargy, pallor, poor feeding, and weight gain.

Alternatives: Propranolol(L2), Metoprolol(L2)

References:
1. Jensen BP, Dalrymple JM, Begg EJ. Transfer of doxazosin into breast milk. J Hum Lact. 2013 May;29(2):150-153.

DOXEPIN

Trade: Adapin, Deptran, Silenor, Sinequan

Category: Antidepressant, Tricyclic

LRC: L5 - Limited Data-Hazardous

Doxepin is a tricyclic antidepressant used in the treatment of depression, anxiety, insomnia, and depressive disorders with psychotic features.[1] There are numerous alternatives to doxepin to treat these conditions that should be considered in lactation as doxepin has been associated with two cases of serious CNS depression from medication exposure in milk.

In the first case a woman started taking doxepin 10 mg daily 2 weeks postpartum.[2] Four days before her infant had significant CNS depression her dose was increased to 25 mg three times a day. Her 8-week-old daughter was found to be pale, limp, and barely breathing. After resuscitation her skin color improved but within 30 minutes she returned to her original state. All other causes were ruled out and the episode was attributed to doxepin exposure in breast milk as her symptoms resolved 24 hours after breast milk was withheld. The peak concentrations of doxepin in milk were 27-29 µg/L at 4-6 hours postdose (RID of 0.3%). The average concentration of the active metabolite, n-desmethyldoxepin, was 9 µg/L; the authors estimated this infant would have consumed about 14 µg of doxepin and 7 µg of the metabolite daily. Plasma levels of the metabolite were found to be similar to the mothers (58 and 66 µg/L); the high concentration was most likely due to accumulation of the metabolite as the young infant was most likely unable to readily eliminate the medication.

In the second case, a woman was started on doxepin 75 mg in 3rd trimester; the dose was gradually reduced during the last weeks of pregnancy and the patient was maintained on 35 mg daily postpartum.[3] At 9 days of life, the infant was re-admitted to hospital for poor sucking, swallowing, poor muscle tone, vomiting weight loss, and jaundice. Although the jaundice resolved with phototherapy, the drowsiness and vomiting persisted. At this time, the breast milk was withheld and within 24 hours the infant was lively and active. Both doxepin and its metabolite were found to have levels below the level of detection in the infant; however, milk levels were found to be between 60-100 µg/L for doxepin and its metabolite. The authors estimate the infant would receive about 10-20 µg/kg of doxepin and its metabolite per day in milk, with an RID of about 3%.

In a third case report a woman was started on doxepin 150 mg daily thirty days postpartum.[4] Maternal blood and milk samples were taken eight times over 99 days of treatment and an infant blood sample was taken on day 43. The mean maternal milk sample of doxepin and its metabolite were 60 µg/L and 111 µg/L; the authors estimated the infant would receive about 71 µg of doxepin and 131 µg of its metabolite daily (RID 2.2%). The infant's level on day 43 was undetectable for doxepin and 15 µg/L for the metabolite. In this case, the infant had no adverse effects from the medication in milk

It has been hypothesized that infants less than 10 weeks of age may be at greatest risk of adverse effects due to their limited ability to metabolize this medication; full-term infants have very limited metabolism prior to 15 days of life, this capacity increases by about 2-3 months of age.[5]

The decision to use this drug during lactation must involve careful consideration of the risks and benefits to both mother and baby; numerous other therapies such as SSRIs, antipsychotics, and short acting benzodiazepines should be considered first.

T 1/2	15 h doxepin; 31 h active metabolite	MW	315.8 Da	PB	80%
Tmax	3.5 h	RID	0.32%-3%	Vd	20.2 L/kg
Oral	30%	M/P	1.08-1.66	pKa	8.96, 9.75

Adult Concerns: Headache, dizziness, sedation, confusion, hallucinations, dry mouth, changes in blood pressure, tachycardia, nausea, vomiting, constipation or diarrhea, anorexia, urinary retention, tremor, rash.

Adult Dose: 75-150 mg daily.

Pediatric Concerns: One report of dangerous sedation and respiratory arrest in an infant.[2] Poor sucking and swallowing, muscle hypotonia, vomiting, drowsiness, and jaundice reported in a second infant.[3]

Infant Monitoring: Sedation or irritability, dry mouth, difficulty breathing, not waking to feed/poor feeding, constipation, urinary retention, weight gain.

Alternatives: Amitriptyline(L2), Sertraline(L2), Citalopram(L2), Escitalopram(L2)

References:

1. Pharmaceutical manufacturers prescribing information.
2. Matheson I, Pande H, Alertsen AR. Respiratory depression caused by N-desmethyldoxepin in breast milk. Lancet. 1985 Nov;2(8464):1124.

3. Frey OR, Scheidt P, von Brenndorff AI. Adverse effects in a newborn infant breast-fed by a mother treated with doxepin. Ann Pharmacother. 1999 Jun;33(6):690-693.
4. Kemp J, Ilett KF, Booth J, Hackett LP. Excretion of doxepin and N-desmethyldoxepin in human milk. Br J Clin Pharmacol. 1985 Nov;20(5):497-499.
5. Wisner KL, Perel JM, Findling RL. Antidepressant treatment during breast-feeding. Am J Psychiatry. 1996 Sep;153(9):1132-1137.

DOXEPIN CREAM

Trade: Prudoxin cream, Zonalon cream

Category: Antipruritic

LRC: L4 - Limited Data-Possibly Hazardous

Doxepin cream is an antihistamine-like cream used to treat severe itching. In one study of 19 women, plasma levels ranged from zero to 47 µg/L following transcutaneous absorption.[1] Target therapeutic ranges in doxepin antidepressant therapy is 30-150 µg/L. Small but significant amounts are secreted in milk. Two published reports indicate absorption by infant varying from significant to modest but only in mothers consuming oral doses.[2,3] This product is not recommended for use in breastfeeding mothers.

T 1/2	15 h doxepin; 31 h active metabolite	MW	315.8 Da	PB	80%
Tmax	3.5 h	RID		Vd	20.2 L/kg
Oral	30%	M/P	1.08, 1.66	pKa	

Adult Concerns: Headache, dizziness, sedation, confusion, hallucinations, dry mouth, rash, burning, stinging, and application site reactions.

Adult Dose: 5% cream used three times a day for up to 8 days for itch.

Pediatric Concerns: Sedation, respiratory arrest have been reported following oral administration.

Infant Monitoring: Sedation or irritability, dry mouth, difficulty breathing, not waking to feed/poor feeding, constipation, urinary retention, weight gain.

Alternatives: Diphenhydramine(L2)

References:
1. Drug Facts and Comparisons 2017.
2. Kemp J, Ilett KF, Booth J, Hackett LP. Excretion of doxepin and N-desmethyldoxepin in human milk. Br J Clin Pharmacol. 1985;20(5):497-499.
3. Matheson I, Pande H, Alertsen AR. Respiratory depression caused by N-desmethyldoxepin in breast milk. Lancet. 1985;2(8464):1124.

DOXERCALCIFEROL

Trade: Hectoral, Hectorol

Category: Vitamin

LRC: L3 - No Data-Probably Compatible

Doxercalciferol is a vitamin D analog that following metabolic activation becomes 1,25-dihydroxyvitamin D2. Doxercalciferol is indicated for the treatment of hyperparathyroidism associated with chronic renal failure in patients undergoing hemodialysis. Excessive doses may lead to dangerously elevated plasma calcium levels. No data are available on its transfer to human milk. It is not likely that normal doses would lead to clinically relevant levels in human milk, particularly since vitamin D transfers only minimally to human milk. While plasma levels of vitamin D are normally quite low in human milk (<20 IU/L), at least one study now suggests that supplementing a mother with extremely high levels of vitamin D2 can significantly elevate milk levels, and subsequently lead to hypercalcemia in a breastfed infant.[1] Some caution with these highly active forms of vitamin D is recommended.

T 1/2	32-37 h	MW		PB	99%
Tmax	8 h	RID		Vd	
Oral	Complete	M/P		pKa	

Adult Concerns: Adverse events include hypercalcemia, hyperphosphatemia, and over suppression of parathyroid hormone. Additional side effects include edema, headache, malaise, dizziness, pruritus, and constipation.

Adult Dose: 4 µg three times weekly.

Pediatric Concerns: None reported via milk, but caution is recommended in breastfeeding mothers.

Infant Monitoring: Constipation.

Alternatives: Vitamin d(L1)

References:

1. Greer FR, Hollis BW, Napoli JL. High concentrations of vitamin D2 in human milk associated with pharmacologic doses of vitamin D2. J Pediatr. 1984;105(1):61-64.

DOXORUBICIN

Trade: Adriamycin, Adriblastina, Caelyx

Category: Anthracycline

LRC: L5 - Limited Data-Hazardous

Doxorubicin is an anticancer agent. Doxorubicin and its metabolite are secreted in significant amounts in breast milk. Following a dose of 70 mg/m^2, peak milk levels of doxorubicin and metabolite occurred at 24 hours and were 128 and 111 µg/L respectively.[1] The highest milk/plasma ratio was 4.43 at 24 hours.

A classic anthracycline, doxorubicin is one of a number of anthracyclines in this family. Doxorubicin when administered reaches a rapid C_{max} and disappears from the plasma compartment with a 3-exponential decay characterized by three differing half-lives, 3-5 minutes, 1-2 hours, and 24-36 hours.[2] A fourth curve has been identified with a half-life of 110 hours which accounts for approximately 30% of the total AUC. The last two elimination curves are probably due to this product's high volume of distribution. In essence, it is distributed and stored in sites remote from the plasma compartment and leaks into the plasma over many days thereafter. However, the peak in milk occurred at 24 hours. Because this product is detectable in plasma (and milk) for long periods, a waiting period of approximately 7-10 days is recommended. The kinetics of this agent are highly variable, depending on renal function, creatinine clearance, liver function, etc. Waiting periods before returning to breastfeeding should be adjusted for this factor. Withhold breastfeeding for at least 7 to 10 days.

In mothers whose infants are receiving doxorubicin, some caution is recommended for breastfeeding. The infant's saliva may contain significant levels of doxorubicin and may prove damaging to the nipple mucosa. At least a 3-day withholding of direct breastfeeding is recommended to reduce the risk of damage to the mothers' nipple. Mothers should wash their nipple with soap and water following breastfeeding.

T 1/2	24-36 h	MW	579.99 Da	PB	85%
Tmax	24 h	RID	2.44%	Vd	25 L/kg
Oral	Poor	M/P	4.43	pKa	9.53

Adult Concerns: Bone marrow suppression, cardiac toxicity, arrhythmias, nausea, vomiting, stomatitis, liver toxicity.

Adult Dose: 20-75 mg/m^2 IV.

Pediatric Concerns: This product could be extremely toxic to a breastfeeding infant and is not recommended.

Infant Monitoring:

Alternatives:

References:

1. Egan PC, Costanza ME, Dodion P, Egorin MJ, Bachur NR. Doxorubicin and cisplatin excretion into human milk. Cancer Treat Rep. 1985;69(12):1387-1389.
2. Grochow LB, Ames MM. A Clinician's Guide to Chemotherapy Pharmacokinetics and Pharamcodynamics. 1st ed. Baltimore, MD: Williams & Wilkins; 1998.
3. American Academy of Pediatrics, Committee on Drugs. Transfer of drugs and other chemicals into human milk. Pediatrics. 2001;108(3):776-789.

DOXYCYCLINE

Trade: Doryx, Doxychel, Doxycin, Doxylar, Doxylin, Periostat, Vibra-Tabs, Vibramycin

Category: Antibiotic, Tetracycline

LRC: L3 - Limited Data-Probably Compatible

Doxycycline is a long half-life tetracycline antibiotic. In a study of 15 subjects, the average doxycycline level in milk was 0.77 mg/L following a 200 mg oral dose.[1] One oral dose of 100 mg was administered 24 hours later, and the breast milk levels were 0.38 mg/L. Following a dose of 100 mg daily in 10 mothers, doxycycline levels in milk on day 2 averaged 0.82 mg/L (range 0.37-1.24 mg/L) at 3 hours after the dose, and 0.46 mg/L (range 0.3-0.91 mg/L) 24 hours after the dose.[2] The relative infant dose in an infant would be < 6% of the maternal weight-adjusted dosage.

Following a single dose of 100 mg in three women or 200 mg in 3 women, peak milk levels occurred between 2 and 4 hours following the dose. The average peak milk levels were 0.96 mg/L (100 mg dose) or 1.8 mg/L (200 mg dose). After repeated dosing for 5 days, milk levels averaged 3.6 mg/L at doses of 100 mg twice daily.[3] In another study of 13 women receiving 100-200 mg doses of doxycycline, peak levels in milk were 0.6 mg/L (n=3 at 100 mg dose) and 1.1 mg/L (n=11 at 200 mg dose).[4]

Tetracyclines administered orally to infants are known to bind in teeth, producing discoloration and inhibit bone growth, although doxycycline and oxytetracycline stain teeth the least severely. Although most tetracyclines secreted into milk are generally bound to calcium, thus inhibiting their absorption, doxycycline is the least bound (20%), and may be better absorbed in a breastfeeding infant than the older tetracyclines. While the absolute absorption of older tetracyclines may be dramatically reduced by calcium salts, the newer doxycycline and minocycline analogs bind less and their overall absorption while slowed, may be significantly higher than earlier versions. Prolonged use (months) could potentially alter gastrointestinal flora, and induce dental staining although doxycycline produces the least dental staining. Short-term use (3-4 weeks) is not contraindicated and has not be found to produce dental staining according to a recent study from the CDC.[5] No harmful effects have yet been reported in breastfeeding infants but prolonged use is not advised. For prolonged administration such as for exposure to anthrax, check the CDC web site as they have published specific dosing guidelines.

T 1/2	15-25 h	MW	462 Da	PB	90%
Tmax	1.5-4 h	RID	4.2%-13.3%	Vd	
Oral	90%-100%	M/P	0.3-0.4	pKa	4.79

Adult Concerns: Abdominal cramps, vomiting, diarrhea, anorexia, changes in liver and renal function, photosensitivity.

Adult Dose: 100 mg daily.

Pediatric Concerns: None reported.

Infant Monitoring: Vomiting, diarrhea, changes in gastrointestinal flora, rash; prolonged exposure may lead to dental staining, and decreased bone growth.

Alternatives:

References:
1. Morganti G, Ceccarelli G, Ciaffi G. Comparative concentrations of a tetracycline antibiotic in serum and maternal milk. Antibiotica. 1968;6(3):216-223.
2. Lutziger H. Konzentrationsbestimmungen und klinisch wirksamkeit von doxycyclin (Vibramycin) in uterus, adnexen und muttermilch. Ther Umsch. 1969;26:476-480.
3. Tokuda G, Yuasa M, Mihara S, et al. Clinical study of doxycycline in obstetrical and gynecological fields. Chemotherapy (Tokyo). 1969;17:339-344.
4. Borderon E, Soutoul JH, Borderon JC, et al. Excretion of antibiotics in human milk. Med Mal Infect. 1975;5:373-376.
5. Todd S, Dahlgren F, Traeger M, et al. No evidence of tooth staining following doxycycline administration in children for treatment of Rocky Mountain spotted fever. J Pediatr. 2015;166:1246-1251.

DOXYLAMINE

Trade: Aldex AN, Unisom

Category: Antihistamine

LRC: L3 - No Data-Probably Compatible

Doxylamine is an antihistamine with strong sedative properties, it is primarily used in over-the-counter sleep aids and in a combination prescription medication for nausea and vomiting of pregnancy.[1] Based on this medications small molecular weight, and long half-life it is anticipated that some of this medication will enter milk; however, the extent of drug entry is unknown at this time. A manufacturer reports that excitement, irritability and sedation has occurred in breastfed infants with maternal use of doxylamine. Thus, caution is recommended, particularly in premature or term neonates and in those with a history of apneas or other respiratory syndromes.

T 1/2	10-12 h	MW	388.46 Da	PB	
Tmax	2.4 h	RID		Vd	2.6 L/kg
Oral		M/P		pKa	9.3

Adult Concerns: Headache, sedation, dizziness, paradoxical CNS stimulation, agitation, tachycardia, urinary retention, constipation.

Adult Dose: 25-50 mg orally for insomnia.

Pediatric Concerns: None reported via milk, but observe for sedation and paradoxical CNS stimulation. Do not use in infants with apnea.

Infant Monitoring: Sedation or irritability, apneas, urinary retention, constipation.

Alternatives: Diphenhydramine(L2), Dimenhydrinate(L2)

References:
1. Pharmaceutical manufacturer prescribing information.

DOXYLAMINE + PYRIDOXINE

Trade: Diclectin (Canada), Diclegis, Bonjesta

Category: Antiemetic

LRC: L3 - No Data-Probably Compatible

Doxylamine + pyridoxine is a combination drug product used to treat nausea and vomiting of pregnancy.[1,2] Doxylamine is an antihistamine with strong sedative properties, it is primarily used in over-the-counter sleep aids. Based on this medications small molecular weight, and long half-life it is anticipated that some of this medication will enter milk; however, the extent of drug entry is unknown at this time. The manufacturer reports that excitement, irritability and sedation has occurred in breastfed infants with maternal use of doxylamine.[1] Thus caution is recommended, particularly in premature infants and in those with a history of apneas or other respiratory syndromes.

The recommended daily allowance of pyridoxine (vitamin B6) for non-pregnant women is 1.3 mg/day.[3] Pyridoxine is required in slight excess during pregnancy (1.9 mg/day) and lactation (2 mg/day) and most prenatal vitamin supplements contain 10 mg/day.[4]

Pyridoxine is secreted in milk in direct proportion to maternal intake.[5] In a study of 20 women breastfeeding term infants, 14 women were supplemented with a prenatal vitamin (2 mg/day pyridoxine) and six were supplemented with 27 mg/day of pyridoxine. Maternal blood and milk were collected on day 0, 7, 14, and 28 days after birth. In this study, total vitamin B6 concentrations in milk ranged from 75-120 ng/mL (450-700 nmol/L) in the 2 mg/day group and from 390-525 ng/mL (2300-3100 nmol/L) in the 27 mg/day group. It should be noted that vitamin B6 levels in the infants were 10 ng/mL in the maternal prenatal vitamin group and 49 ng/mL in the maternal 27 mg/day group on day 28. It was also reported that in this study milk volumes were higher on day 28 in the 2 mg/day maternal supplement group.

In one study, which compared pyridoxine (600 mg/day x 6 days) to stilboestrol and placebo for cessation of lactation in women 2-3 days postpartum, pyridoxine was found to be superior.[6] More women were symptom free within 10-12 hours of starting therapy and 93% of women ceased producing milk within 1 week of starting therapy. A second study that administered a combination tablet of Vitamin B1, B6, and B12 to postpartum women starting on the day of delivery reported that pyridoxine (300 mg/day x 7 days) inhibited lactation in 96% of patients given the vitamin compared to 76.5% of those given placebo when started before lactation was established.[7]

However, these data have been refuted in two studies where high doses of pyridoxine failed to suppress prolactin levels and lactation.[8,9] In the first study, pyridoxine (600 mg/day x 7 days) was given to nine women starting immediately postpartum. The prolactin levels of these women were compared to nine women who were breastfeeding their infants.[8] There were no differences in the serum prolactin levels at baseline and on day 5 when the treatment group had prolactin levels that were 53% of their baseline level and the control group had prolactin levels that were 68% of their baseline level. In addition, lactation was not suppressed in the treatment group. In the second study, 14 women given pyridoxine (450 mg/day x 7 days) starting on the day of delivery were compared to 20 women given bromocriptine (7.5 mg/day x 7 days).[9] In this study, pyridoxine had no effect on prolactin levels or engorgement when compared to bromocriptine.

In summary, one study clearly indicates that pyridoxine readily transfers to breast milk and that levels in milk correlate closely with maternal intake, thus excessive maternal doses of pyridoxine in lactation are not recommended.[5] At this time, the use of this combination product with typical dosing (doxylamine 10 mg + pyridoxine 10 mg - one tablet in the morning and afternoon and two tablets at bedtime) would seem reasonable in lactation if the infant is monitored for antihistamine side effects and has no other contraindications to its use.

T 1/2	Dox/Pyr: 12 h/0.5 h (active metabolite days)	MW	Dox/Pyr: 388/205 Da	PB	Pyridoxine is highly protein bound.
Tmax	Dox/Pyr: 7.8 h/5.6 h	RID		Vd	Dox/Pyr: 2.6/ L/kg
Oral	Dox/Pyr: /Well absorbed	M/P		pKa	Dox/Pyr: 9.3/9.4

Adult Concerns: Headache, sedation, dizziness, ataxia, paradoxical CNS stimulation, agitation, tachycardia, nausea, changes in liver enzymes, urinary retention, constipation, diarrhea, paresthesia. Note: seizures can occur with high IV doses pyridoxine.

Adult Dose: doxylamine 10 mg + pyridoxine 10 mg - one tablet in the morning and afternoon and two tablets at bedtime.

Pediatric Concerns: None reported via milk, but observe for sedation and paradoxical CNS stimulation. Do not use in infants with apnea.

Infant Monitoring: Sedation or irritability, apneas, vomiting, urinary retention, constipation.

Alternatives: Dimenhydrinate(L2), Metoclopramide(L2)

References:

1. Pharmaceutical manufacturer prescribing information.
2. Gill SK, Garcia –Bournissen F, Koren G. Systemic bioavailability and pharmacokinetics of the doxylamine-pyridoxine delayed-release combination (Diclectin). Ther Drug Monit. 2011;33(1):115-119.
3. 2015 Dietary Guidelines Advisory Committee. Appendix 7: Nutritional Goals for Age-Sex Groups Based on Dietary Reference Intakes and Dietary Guidelines Recommendations. Dietary Guidelines for Americans 2015-2020. 8th Ed. https://health.gov/dietaryguidelines/2015/guidelines/appendix-7/
4. National Institutes of Health (NIH) Office of Dietary Supplements. Vitamin B6 Dietary Supplement Fact Sheet (last updated Feb 2016). https://ods.od.nih.gov/factsheets/VitaminB6-HealthProfessional/#disc
5. Kang-Yoon SA, Kirksey A, Giacoia G, West K. Vitamin B-6 status of breast-fed neonates: influence of pyridoxine supplementation on mothers and neonates. Am J Clin Nutr. 1992;56(3):548-558.
6. Foukas MD. An antilactogenic effect of pyridoxine. J Obstet Gynaecol Br Commonw. 1973;80(8):718-720.
7. Marcus RG. Suppression of lactation with high doses of pyridoxine. S Afr Med J. 1975; 49(52):2155-2156.
8. de Waal JM, Steyn AF, Harms JHK, Slabber CF, Pannall PR. Failure of pyridoxine to suppress raised serum prolactin levels. S Afr Med J. 1978;53(8):293-294.
9. Canales ES, Soria J, Zarate A, Mason M, Molina M. The influence of pyridoxine on prolactin secretion and milk production in women. Br J Obstet Gynaecol. 1976;83(5):387-388.

DRONABINOL

Trade: Marinol, Elevat

Category: Antiemetic

LRC: L4 - No Data-Possibly Hazardous

Dronabinol (delta-9-THC) is a cannabinoid that is used for the treatment of chemotherapy-induced nausea and vomiting (resistant to other therapies) and the management of weight loss and decreased appetite in patients with AIDS.[1] Dronabinol, structurally is similar to a naturally occurring active component of the plant Cannabis sativa (marijuana).

Its oral bioavailability is 10%-20% with a high protein binding of 97%. It has high lipid solubility and a high volume of distribution with a prolonged half-life; therefore, it is widely distributed in the body and both the drug and its metabolites may be excreted in low levels for an extended period of time.[1] Following single doses, metabolites (e.g., 11-OH-THC) have been found in the urine and feces for at least 5 weeks.

Adequate data on the transfer of dronabinol in human milk are currently unavailable.[1] However, there are data on the transfer of delta-9-THC into breast milk after marijuana use. In one report of a mother who smoked marijuana once daily for 7 months, up to 105 µg/L of THC was quantified in her milk.[2] Her infant had negative urine samples and was reported to have normal development by the pediatrician. Another mother who used the drug seven times per day for 8 months was found to have 340 µg/L of THC and 4.2 µg/L of 11-OH-THC (active metabolite) in her first milk sample. In her second milk sample, she had 60.3 µg/L of THC, 1.1 µg/L of 11-OH-THC and 1.6 µg/L 9-carboxy-THC (inactive metabolite). In this case, the mother had eight times more THC in her milk than plasma. Her infant had negative urine samples but positive fecal samples for 347 ng of THC, 67 ng of 11-OH-THC and 611 ng 9-carboxy-THC. This infant was also reported to have normal development by the pediatrician.

A 2011 study that verified a method to quantify illicit substances in human milk obtained one milk sample from a woman using cannabis in lactation. Her milk sample contained 86 µg/L of THC and 5 µg/L of 11-OH-THC.[3] No details were provided regarding maternal use, timing of milk sample, or infant outcomes in this paper. In addition, numerous animal studies have also reported the transfer of THC into milk.[4,5]

At this time, safety data for maternal marijuana use in lactation is lacking for both short- and long-term infant outcomes. In addition, most of the data is limited by small sample sizes, shortcomings in study design, poor dose characterization, in-utero exposure, and other concomitant maternal medications.

In one study comparing 27 women who smoked marijuana routinely during breastfeeding to 35 non-marijuana smoking women, no differences were noted in their children's growth, mental, and motor development.[6] A 1990 prospective study evaluated the motor and mental abilities of infants exposed to marijuana via milk.[7] This study used participants from a previous study, which evaluated diet, alcohol, and smoking in lactation and their influence on infant growth and development. Of these participants, 68 women used marijuana in lactation (largely first and third month). When matched to 68 women with similar exposures in pregnancy that did not use marijuana in lactation, it was found that those infants with higher marijuana exposure in first trimester or the first month of lactation had significantly lower psychomotor development index scores than infants with no exposure in these periods at 1 year of age. No differences in mental development were noted.

The peak plasma concentrations of THC following use of dronabinol in clinical doses ranges from 1.32 to 7.88 ng/mL.[1] This appears to be similar to what was found in one case report where maternal blood samples were drawn at the time of milk sampling (unsure if peak sample) and reported maternal levels of 7.2 ng/mL of THC and 2.5 ng/mL of 11-OH-THC.[2]

Although this medication has low oral bioavailability, high protein binding and a large volume of distribution, we expect this medication will enter milk based on marijuana data. Until more data are available for short-term and chronic long-term effects of delta-9-THC exposure in breastfed infants, it is best advised that long-term use of dronabinol in breastfeeding mothers should be avoided and alternative therapies to treat the maternal health condition should be offered. This product is not recommended in breastfeeding mothers.

T 1/2	25-36 h	MW	314.47 Da	PB	97%
Tmax	2-4 h	RID		Vd	10 L/kg
Oral	10%-20%	M/P	8	pKa	10.6

Adult Concerns: Seizures, sedation, euphoria, mood disturbances, hallucinations, changes in blood pressure, palpitations, syncope, tachycardia, nausea, vomiting, diarrhea, abdominal pain. Contraindicated in those with allergies to cannabinoid or sesame seed oil.

Adult Dose: 2.5-20 mg per day.

Pediatric Concerns: Very limited information with delta-9-THC in lactation and pediatrics at this time.

Infant Monitoring: Sedation, not waking to feed/poor feeding, weight gain, potential neurobehavioral or psychomotor delays.

Alternatives:

References:

1. Pharmaceutical manufacturers prescribing information.
2. Perez-Reyes M, Wall ME. Presence of delta9-tetrahydrocannabinol in human milk. N Engl J Med. 1982;307(13):819-820.
3. Marchei E, Escuder D, Pallas CR, et al. Simultaneous analysis of frequently used licit and illicit psychoactive drugs in breast milk by liquid chromatography tandem mass spectrometry. J Pharm Biomed Anal. 2011;55:309–316.
4. Ahmad GR, Ahmad N. Passive consumption of marijuana through milk: a low level chronic exposure to delta-9-tetrahydrocannabinol (THC). J Toxicol Clin Toxicol. 1990;28(2):255-260.
5. Chao FC, Green DE, Forrest IS, Kaplan JN, Winship-Ball A, Braude M. The passage of 14C-delta-9-tetrahydrocannabinol into the milk of lactating squirrel monkeys. Res Commun Chem Pathol Pharmacol. 1976;15(2):303-317.
6. Tennes K, Avitable N, Blackard C, et al. Marijuana: prenatal and postnatal exposure in the human. NIDA Res Monogr. 1985;59:48-60.
7. Astley SJ, Little RE. Maternal marijuana use during lactation and infant development at one year. Neurotoxicol Teratol. 1990;12:161-168.

DRONEDARONE

Trade: Dronedarone Sanofi, Dronedarone Winthrop, Multaq

Category: Antiarrhythmic

LRC: L3 - No Data-Probably Compatible

Dronedarone was developed as an anti-arrhythmic agent for the first line treatment of atrial fibrillation and atrial flutter. It is structurally related to amiodarone but lacks the iodine component.[1] It is not known whether dronedarone is excreted in human breastmilk. Animal studies have shown excretion of dronedarone and its metabolites in breast milk. A study of rats suggests maternal dronedarone administration was associated with minor reduced body-weight gain in the offspring.[1] It is poorly absorbed orally, so clinically significant plasma levels in the infant are not expected via breast milk exposure.

T 1/2	13-19 h	MW	566.8 Da	PB	>98%
Tmax	3-6 h	RID		Vd	20 L/kg
Oral	15%	M/P		pKa	9.40

Adult Concerns: Bradycardia, prolonged QT interval, heart failure, decreased renal function, changes in liver function, diarrhea, nausea, or weakness.

Adult Dose: 400 mg twice daily.

Pediatric Concerns: None reported via milk at this time.

Infant Monitoring: Drowsiness, lethargy, pallor, arrhythmias, changes in liver function, poor feeding, weight gain.

Alternatives:

References:
1. Pharmaceutical manufacturers prescribing information.

DROPERIDOL

Trade: Droleptan, Inapsine

Category: Antiemetic

LRC: L3 - No Data-Probably Compatible

Droperidol is a powerful tranquilizer. It is sometimes used as a preanesthetic medication in labor and delivery because of fewer respiratory effects in neonates. In pediatric patients 2-12 years of age, it is sometimes used as an antiemetic (0.01-0.015 mg/kg IV).[1,2] There are no data available on secretion into breast milk. Due to the potent sedative properties of this medication, caution is urged.

T 1/2	2.2 h	MW	379 Da	PB	85%-90%
Tmax	10-30 min (IM)	RID		Vd	1.5 L/kg
Oral		M/P		pKa	7.46

Adult Concerns: Sedation, hypotension, dizziness, unusual ocular movements, extrapyramidal symptoms, chills, shivering.

Adult Dose: 0.625-1.25 mg IM or IV.

Pediatric Concerns: None reported via milk at this time.

Infant Monitoring: Sedation, irritability, not waking to feed/poor feeding, weight gain, and extrapyramidal symptoms.

Alternatives: Haloperidol(L3)

References:
1. McEvoy GE, ed. AFHS Drug Information. Bethesda, MD: American Society of Health-System Pharmacists; 1992.
2. Pharmaceutical manufacturers prescribing information.

DULAGLUTIDE

Trade: Trulicity

Category: Antidiabetic, other

LRC: L4 - No Data-Possibly Hazardous

Dulaglutide is glucagon-like peptide 1 receptor agonist covalently linked to an IgG4 fragment.[1] Used in type II diabetes to lower blood sugar, there are no data on its use in breastfeeding mothers. It is a large peptide with a molecular weight of 59,669 Da and it is rather unlikely that it would penetrate the milk compartment after the first week following birth. However, caution is recommended until we have more data on milk levels following the use of this hypoglycemic agent.

T 1/2	5 days	MW	59,669.81 Da	PB	N/A
Tmax	24-72 h (median 48 h)	RID		Vd	0.27 L/kg
Oral		M/P		pKa	

Adult Concerns: Observe for: nausea, diarrhea, vomiting, abdominal pain, decreased appetite, dyspepsia, fatigue, sinus tachycardia constipation, flatulence, abdominal distension, gastroesophageal reflux disease, eructation, GI adverse reactions, hypoglycemia, heart rate increase, immunogenicity, hypersensitivity, injection-site reactions, amylase and lipase activity

Adult Dose: 0.75 mg QD; may be increased to 1.5 mg daily

Pediatric Concerns:

Infant Monitoring: Observe for hypoglycemia.

Alternatives:

References:
1. Pharmaceutical manufacturers prescribing information.

DULOXETINE

Trade: Ariclaim, Cymbalta, Duceten, Xeristar, Yentreve

Category: Antidepressant, other

LRC: L3 - Limited Data-Probably Compatible

Duloxetine is a selective serotonin and norepinephrine reuptake inhibitor (SNRI) that is indicated for depression and for patient with neuropathic pain.[1] The primary role of SNRIs is as an alternative in patients with major depressive disorder who have responded poorly to other agents (e.g., tricyclics or SSRIs).

The transfer of duloxetine to breast milk was studied in six women who were at least 12 weeks postpartum and taking 40 mg twice daily for 3.5 days.[2] Paired blood and breast milk samples were taken at 0, 1, 2, 3, 6, 9, and 12 hours post-dose. The milk/plasma ratio was reported to be about 0.267. The daily dose of duloxetine was estimated to be 7 µg/day (range = 4-15 µg/day). According to the manufacturer, the weight-adjusted infant dose would be approximately 0.141% of the maternal dose. Further, even this is unlikely absorbed, as duloxetine is unstable under acid conditions of the infant's stomach. In a more recent study in a mother consuming duloxetine (60 mg daily), levels in milk were 31 µg/L and 64 µg/L at trough and peak respectively.[3] The milk/plasma ratios were 1.29 (trough) and 1.21 (peak). These authors suggest a relative infant dose of 0.14%.

An investigation was undertaken to study the transfer of duloxetine across placenta as well as breast milk in a 31-year-old mother who received 60 mg duloxetine daily throughout her pregnancy and continued it during lactation.[4] An assessment of maternal and cord blood concentrations immediately at birth revealed that the placental transfer for duloxetine is low. No withdrawal symptoms or malformations occurred in the infant. Breast milk samples were obtained at 18 days post-delivery. The first milk sample was obtained just prior to the morning dose, and subsequently eight more milk samples were obtained over a period of 22.5 hours following the morning dose. A mean milk concentration of 51 µg/L rendered a mean relative infant dose (RID) of 0.81%. This RID for duloxetine is low as compared to some of other commonly used SSRIs/SNRIs such as venlafaxine, desvenlafaxine, citalopram, mirtazepine, fluoxetine. Further, it was found that the concentration of duloxetine in hindmilk was 1.5-2 times that in foremilk, suggesting a lipid co-transport for duloxetine. The authors of this study concluded that the placental and milk transfer of duloxetine is low as compared to a few other SSRIs/SNRIs commonly used. No untoward effects were reported in the infant.

In another case study of a woman who consumed duloxetine (60 mg daily) during pregnancy and postpartum, at day 6 postpartum, the concentration of duloxetine was 23.6 ng/mL in the foremilk and 14.3 ng/mL in the hindmilk (authors estimated RID at 0.4% and 0.2%, respectively).[5] At week 6 postpartum, the concentration was 25.2 ng/mL in the fore milk and 29.3 ng/mL in the hind milk (RID of 0.4% and 0.4%, respectively).

T 1/2	12 h	MW	333 Da	PB	>90%
Tmax	6 h	RID	0.12%-1.12%	Vd	23.4 L/kg
Oral	>70%	M/P	0.267-1.29	pKa	9.5

Adult Concerns: Fatigue, dizziness, somnolence, insomnia, blurred vision, dry mouth, nausea, vomiting, constipation, diarrhea, decreased appetite, changes in liver function, tremor, sweating, erectile dysfunction.

Adult Dose: 40-60 mg/day.

Pediatric Concerns: None reported via milk at this time.

Infant Monitoring: Sedation or irritability, not waking to feed/poor feeding, and weight gain.

Alternatives: Venlafaxine(L2), Sertraline(L2), Citalopram(L2)

References:
1. Pharmaceutical manufacturers prescribing information, 2005.
2. Lobo ED, Loghin C, Knadler MP, et al. Pharmacokinetics of duloxetine in breast milk and plasma of healthy postpartum women. Clin Pharmacokinet. 2008;47:103-109.
3. Briggs GG, Ambrose PJ, Ilett KF, Hackett LP, Nageotte MP, Padilla G. Use of duloxetine in pregnancy and lactation. Ann Pharmacother. 2009 Nov;43(11):1898-1902.

4. Boyce PM, Hackett LP, Ilett KF. Duloxetine transfer across the placenta duringpregnancy and into milk during lactation. Arch Womens Ment Health. 2011;14(2):169-172.
5. Collin-Lévesque L, El-Ghaddaf Y, Genest M, et al. Infant exposure to methylphenidate and duloxetine during lactation. Breastfeed Med. 2018 Apr;13(3):221-225. PubMed PMID: 29485905.

ECHINACEA

Trade:

Category: Herb

LRC: L3 - No Data-Probably Compatible

Echinacea is a popular herbal remedy in the central US and has been traditionally used topically to stimulate wound healing and internally to stimulate the immune system. The plant contains a complex mixture of compounds and, thus far, no single component appears responsible for its immunostimulant properties. A number of in vitro and animal studies have documented the activation of immunologic properties although most of these are via intraperitoneal injections, not orally. Three recent studies have reported echinacea may not be a active against the common cold.[1-3] but more studies are presently underway. Thus far, little is known about the toxicity of this plant although its use has been widespread for many years. Apparently, purified Echinacea extract is relatively non-toxic even at high doses.[3,4] No data are available on its transfer into human milk or its effect on lactation.[4]

Adult Concerns: Dizziness, nausea, rash.

Adult Dose:

Pediatric Concerns: None reported via milk.

Infant Monitoring:

Alternatives:

References:

1. Turner RB, Bauer R, Woelkart K, Hulsey TC, Gangemi JD. An evaluation of Echinacea angustifolia in experimental rhinovirus infections. N Engl J Med. 2005;353(4):341-348.
2. Taylor JA, Weber W, Standish L, et al. Efficacy and safety of echinacea in treating upper respiratory tract infections in children: a randomized controlled trial. JAMA. 2003;290(21):2824-2830.
3. Barrett BP, Brown RL, Locken K, Maberry R, Bobula JA, D'Alessio, D. Treatment of the common cold with unrefined echinacea. A randomized, double-blind, placebo-controlled trial. Ann Intern Med. 2002;137(12):939-946.
4. Blumenthal M, Busse WR, Goldberg A, et al; eds. The Complete German Commission E Monographs. Austin, TX: American Botanical Council; 1998.

ECONAZOLE

Trade: Spectazole

Category: Antifungal

LRC: L3 - No Data-Probably Compatible

Econazole nitrate is a typical azole antifungal and is indicated for topical application in the treatment of tinea pedis, tinea cruris, and tinea corporis.[1] Absorption following topical administration is minimal to nil, less than 1% of the applied dose was recovered in the urine and feces of humans. It is not known whether econazole nitrate is excreted in human milk, but the levels here are probably far subclinical if even detectable.

T 1/2		MW	381.7 Da	PB	
Tmax		RID		Vd	
Oral		M/P		pKa	6

Adult Concerns: Erythema, burning sensation, stinging, pruritus.

Adult Dose: Apply topically 1-2 times daily.

Pediatric Concerns:

Infant Monitoring: Vomiting, diarrhea.

Alternatives: Miconazole(L2)

References:

1. Pharmaceutical manufacturers prescribing information.

ECULIZUMAB

Trade: Soliris

Category: Monoclonal Antibody

LRC: L3 - No Data-Probably Compatible

Eculizumab is a large monoclonal antibody used in the treatment of paroxysmal nocturnal hemoglobinuria to reduce hemolysis, and the need for RBC transfusions.[1] It is a monoclonal antibody with high affinity to complement protein C5. It is extremely unlikely that this antibody would be transported into human milk after the colostral period, and due to its size, it would be largely unable to penetrate the milk compartment after the first week postpartum. Oral bioavailability would be nil.

Although the molecular weight of this medication is very large and the amount in breast milk is expected to be exceptionally low, there are no long-term data concerning the safety of using immune modulating medications in breastfeeding mothers. Further there are current data that suggest that some monoclonal antibody drugs do transfer into milk, and perhaps the breastfed infant. Therefore, some caution is recommended, and each woman should understand the benefits and risk of using this type of medication in lactation.

T 1/2	272 h	MW	148,000 Da	PB	
Tmax		RID		Vd	7.7 L/kg
Oral		M/P		pKa	

Adult Concerns: Headache, nasopharyngitis, back pain, nausea, and fatigue.

Adult Dose: Variable.

Pediatric Concerns: None reported via milk.

Infant Monitoring: Fever, frequent infections, poor feeding/poor weight gain.

Alternatives:

References:
1. Pharmaceutical manufacturers prescribing information.

EDROPHONIUM

Trade: Enlon, Reversol, Tensilon

Category: Cholinergic

LRC: L3 - No Data-Probably Compatible

Edrophonium is used to diagnose myasthenia gravis, to differentiate cholinergic crises from myasthenia crises, and to reverse neuromuscular blockers.[1] It inhibits acetylcholinesterase and thus prevents the metabolism of acetylcholine. This product is only used for acute episodes or for diagnosis, as its effects last only briefly (10 minutes) before it is rapidly redistributed to peripheral tissues. It also has a unique structure that would largely preclude its entry into human milk. A brief waiting period of a few hours would reduce any possible risk from this medication in breastfed infants.

T 1/2	1.2-2.4 h	MW	166 Da	PB	
Tmax		RID		Vd	1.1 L/kg
Oral		M/P		pKa	

Adult Concerns: Headache, dizziness, flushing, arrhythmias, bronchospasm, salivation, nausea, stomach cramps, diarrhea, urinary urgency, weakness.

Adult Dose: 10 mg IM, or 2 mg IV.

Pediatric Concerns: Can be used in infants and in children.

Infant Monitoring: Breathing difficulty, weakness.

Alternatives:

References:
1. Pharmaceutical manufacturers prescribing information.

EFAVIRENZ

Trade: Atripla, Sustiva

Category: Antiviral

LRC: L5 - Limited Data-Hazardous if Maternal HIV Infection

Efavirenz is an antiretroviral agent used in the treatment of HIV infection.[1] In 2008, a study of 13 mothers who were taking efavirenz (600 mg/day) while breastfeeding were followed for 6 months.[2] Schneider et al. found that infant efavirenz plasma concentrations were on average about 13.1% of the maternal plasma concentrations. Efavirenz concentrations were 6.55 mg/L in maternal plasma, 3.51 mg/L in skim breast milk, and 0.85 mg/L in infant plasma. The milk plasma (M/P) ratio was 0.54. The infants were followed for 6 months and no adverse effects of the medication were reported, infant growth and development were reported as normal. Breastfeeding in developed countries is generally not recommended in mothers who have HIV.[3,4]

Note: This medication is an L5 to highlight the contraindication of breastfeeding when the mother is known to be infected with HIV, this medication is not an L5 based on its risk to the infant in breast milk. The Centers for Disease Control and Prevention recommend that HIV-1 infected mothers do not breastfeed their infants to avoid postnatal transmission of HIV-1.

T 1/2	40-55 h	MW	315.68 Da	PB	99 %
Tmax	3-5 h	RID	6.13%	Vd	3.6 L/kg
Oral	42%	M/P		pKa	12.52

Adult Concerns: Fatigue, dizziness, headache, depression, anxiety, fever, cough, vomiting, diarrhea, elevated liver enzymes, elevated total cholesterol and triglycerides, neutropenia, rash, and itching.[4].

Adult Dose: 600 mg once daily.

Pediatric Concerns: No adverse effects via breast milk have been reported in 13 infants.[1]

Infant Monitoring: Breastfeeding is not recommended in mothers who have HIV.

Alternatives:

References:

1. Pharmaceutical manufacturers prescribing information.
2. Schneider S, Peltier A, Gras A, et al. Efavirenz in human breast milk, mothers', and newborns' plasma. J Acquir Immune Defic Syndr. 2008;48(4):450-454.
3. World Health Organization. Global Programme on AIDS. Consensus Statement from the WHO/UNICEF Consultation on HIV Transmission and Breast-Feeding. Geneva: WHO; 1992.
4. Latham MC, Greiner T. Breastfeeding versus formula feeding in HIV infection. Lancet. 1998;352(9129):737.

EFINACONAZOLE

Trade: Jublia, Clenafin

Category: Antifungal

LRC: L3 - No Data-Probably Compatible

Efinaconazole is an azole antifungal indicated for the topical treatment of fungal infections of the toenails due to Trichophyton rubrum and Trichophyton mentagrophytes.[1] At this time there are no data in human milk; however, after several subcutaneous applications this drug was detected in rodent milk.

In a study of 18 adults with severe toenail fungal infections, systemic absorption from topical application of efinaconazole appeared to be low.[1] The mean peak plasma concentration on Day 28 of topical application was 0.67 ± 0.37 ng/mL. Thus, based on the low plasma concentration significant levels of efinaconazole in human milk are not expected.

T 1/2	29.9 h	MW	348 Da	PB	95.8% - 96.5% (in vitro data)
Tmax		RID		Vd	
Oral		M/P		pKa	

Adult Concerns: Ingrown nail, application site dermatitis, vesicles, and pain.

Adult Dose: Applied to affected toenail(s) once daily for 48 weeks.

Pediatric Concerns: No data available in lactation at this time.

Infant Monitoring:

Alternatives:

References:
1. Pharmaceutical manufacturer prescribing information.
2. National Center for Biotechnology Information. PubChem Compound Database; CID=489181, https://pubchem.ncbi.nlm.nih.gov/compound/489181

EFLORNITHINE HYDROCHLORIDE

Trade: Vaniqa

Category: Hair Growth Retardant

LRC: L3 - No Data-Probably Compatible

Eflornithine hydrochloride is used topically to remove unwanted facial hair in women.[1] Eflornithine hydrochloride is an inhibitor of ornithine decarboxylase; inhibition of this enzyme leads to decreased hair growth. No data are available on the transfer of eflornithine into human milk; however, when used topically on the face, this medication is minimally absorbed and produces steady state plasma levels of 5-10 ng/mL. These maternal concentrations after topical use are likely far too low to produce clinically relevant levels in milk.

Even though the risks are probably quite low, until human lactation data is available the risk-benefit assessment of this product does not necessarily suggest the benefits are worth the risks for a breastfed infant.

T 1/2	8 h (topical); 3-3.5 h (IV)	MW	218 Da	PB	None
Tmax		RID		Vd	0.3 - 0.35 L/kg
Oral		M/P		pKa	

Adult Concerns: Headache, dizziness, dyspepsia, anorexia, acne, pseudofolliculitis barbae, stinging, itching, and tingling skin.

Adult Dose: 0.5 g applied topically twice a day.

Pediatric Concerns: No data are available.

Infant Monitoring:

Alternatives:

References:
1. Pharmaceutical manufacturers prescribing information.

EICOSAPENTAENOIC ACID (EPA)

Trade: EPA

Category: Dietary Supplement

LRC: L3 - Limited Data-Probably Compatible

Eicosapentaenoic acid (EPA) is an omega-3 fatty acid which is usually found in fish or fish oil and usually used in combination with docosahexaenoic acid (DHA).[1-3] Eicosapentaenoic acid is a polyunsaturated lipid commonly found in human milk. In one study, cod liver oil supplementation increased breast milk composition of EPA by 0.15% (wt %) and DHA by 0.36% (wt %).[1] Another study suggested that infant serum EPA increased from 0.11% to 0.7% after breastfeeding women were given fish oil supplementation consisting of 3,092 mg/day of total omega-3 fatty acid which contain 2,006 mg of very long-chain omega-3 fatty acid (>C18).[2]

The American Academy of Pediatrics (AAP) recommends that breastfeeding women have an average of 200-300 mg per day of omega-3 long chain polyunsaturated fatty acids (docosahexaenoic acid [DHA]).[4-6] Both the AAP and the Dietary Guidelines for Americans encourage dietary sources such as consumption of 1-2 portions or 8-12 ounces of fish per week.[4-6]

T 1/2		MW	302 Da	PB	
Tmax		RID		Vd	
Oral		M/P		pKa	

Adult Concerns: Fishy taste, belching, nausea, flatulence, diarrhea, increase in ALT, prolonged bleeding time.

Adult Dose: 250-500 mg DHA + EPA per day.

Pediatric Concerns:

Infant Monitoring:

Alternatives:

References:

1. Helland IB, Saarem K, Saugstad OD, Drevon CA. Fatty acid composition in maternal milk and plasma during supplementation with cod liver oil. Eur J Clin Nutr. 1998 Nov;52(11):839-845.
2. Henderson RA, Jensen RG, Lammi-Keefe CJ, Ferris AM, Dardick KR. Effect of fish oil on the fatty acid composition of human milk and maternal and infant erythrocytes. Lipids. 1992 Nov;27(11):863-869.
3. FDA News Release. FDA announces qualified health claims for mega-3 fatty acids; September 2004. [Online] http://www.fda.gov/SiteIndex/ucm108351.htm. Accessed May 7, 2016.
4. Johnston M, Landers S, Noble L, et al. Breastfeeding and the use of human milk. Pediatrics. 2012;129:e827-e841.
5. U.S. Department of Agriculture and U.S. Department of Health and Human Services. Dietary Guidelines for Americans, 2010. 7th ed. Washington, DC: U.S. Government Printing Office; December 2010. [Online]http://www.health.gov/dietaryguidelines/dga2010/DietaryGuidelines2010.pdf. Accessed May 7, 2016.
6. Vannice G, Rasmussen H. Position of the academy of nutrition and dietetics: dietary fatty acids for healthy adults. J Acad Nutr Diet. 2014;114(1):136-153.

ELAGOLIX

Trade: Orilissa

Category: Gonadotropin Releasing Hormone Antagonist

LRC: L4 - No Data-Possibly Hazardous

Elagolix is a gonadotropin-releasing hormone (GnRH) receptor antagonist indicated for the management of moderate to severe pain associated with endometriosis. Elagolix is an orally administered, nonpeptide small molecule gonadotropin-releasing hormone (GnRH) receptor antagonist that inhibits endogenous GnRH signaling by binding competitively to GnRH receptors in the pituitary gland.

Elagolix results in dose-dependent suppression of luteinizing hormone (LH) and follicle-stimulating hormone (FSH), leading to decreased blood levels of the ovarian sex hormones, estradiol and progesterone. Elagolix causes a dose-dependent decrease in bone mineral density (BMD). BMD loss is greater with increasing duration of use and may not be completely reversible after stopping treatment.

As milk production is dependent on at least minimal levels of estrogen, this product may reduce milk production.

T 1/2	4-6 h	MW	653.58 Da	PB	80%
Tmax	1 h	RID		Vd	23.91 L/kg
Oral		M/P		pKa	

Adult Concerns: Elagolix causes a dose-dependent decrease in bone mineral density (BMD). Common adverse reactions of elagolix include hot flush, headache, nausea, insomnia, mood alterations, amenorrhea, depression, anxiety, arthralgia, bone loss, changes in menstrual bleeding patterns, suicidal ideation and behavior, exacerbation of existing mood disorders, and/or hepatic transaminase elevations.

Adult Dose: 150-200 mg daily.

Pediatric Concerns:

Infant Monitoring: Inform patients that estrogen containing contraceptives are expected to reduce the efficacy of Elagolix. Inform patients about the risk of bone loss. Advise adequate intake of calcium and vitamin D. Patients should seek immediate medical attention for suicidal ideation, or new onset or worsening depression, anxiety, or other mood changes.

Alternatives:

References:

1. Manufacturers prescribing information, 2019.

ELBASVIR + GRAZOPREVIR

Trade: Zepatier

Category: Antiviral

LRC: L3 - No Data-Probably Compatible

Zepatier is a fixed-dose combination product containing elbasvir, a hepatitis C virus (HCV) NS5A inhibitor, and grazoprevir, an HCV NS3/4A protease inhibitor. It is indicated for treatment of chronic HCV genotype 1 or 4 infection in adults. These two agents are very specific for enzymes in the hepatitis C virus, and therefore have little impact on the human system. Side effects are few.

While there is no information available on its transfer into human milk, levels are probably going to be minimal. Be advised, that this product is sometimes used with Ribavirin, which should not be used in breastfeeding mothers.

T 1/2	24 h / 31 h	MW	882.02 / 766.90 Da	PB	99.8% / 98.8%
Tmax	3 h/ 2 h	RID		Vd	9.7 / 17.85 L/kg
Oral	32% / 27%	M/P		pKa	

Adult Concerns: Fatigue, headache, and nausea.

Adult Dose: One dose daily of combination pill.

Pediatric Concerns:

Infant Monitoring: Observe for fatigue and nausea.

Alternatives:

References:
1. Pharmaceutical manufacturers prescribing information.

ELETRIPTAN

Trade: Relpax

Category: Antimigraine

LRC: L3 - Limited Data-Probably Compatible

Eletriptan is a serotonin receptor agonist used to treat migraine headaches.[1] Activating these receptors is believed to constrict cranial blood vessels and block the release of pro-inflammatory neuropeptides from the trigeminal nerve. Although the oral bioavailability of eletriptan is about 3 times greater than sumatriptan, this medication has much higher protein binding.

The manufacturer reports that in a study of 8 women given a single 80 mg dose of eletriptan, the mean total amount of drug in breast milk was approximately 0.02% of the administered dose over 24 hours. The milk/plasma ratio was 0.25 but there was great variability. The concentration-time profile in milk was similar to plasma over 24 hours, with very low concentrations of drug (mean 1.7 ng/mL) still present in milk 18-24 hours post dose. It is unlikely that a breastfeeding infant would be harmed by this amount of drug.

T 1/2	4 h	MW	463 Da	PB	85%
Tmax	1.5 h	RID	0.02%	Vd	1.97 L/kg
Oral	50%	M/P	0.25	pKa	

Adult Concerns: Dizziness, drowsiness, dry mouth, chest pain, feeling of heaviness, nausea, abdominal pain, weakness, paresthesia.

Adult Dose: 20-40 mg initially, may repeat in 2 hours if needed.

Pediatric Concerns: None reported via milk in one study.

Infant Monitoring: Drowsiness, vomiting, poor feeding.

Alternatives: Sumatriptan(L3), NSAIDs, Acetaminophen(L1)

References:
1. Pharmaceutical manufacturers prescribing information.

EMTRICITABINE

Trade: Emtriva

Category: Antiviral

LRC: L5 - Limited Data-Hazardous if Maternal HIV Infection

Emtricitabine is a cytosine analog that acts as a reverse transcriptase inhibitor, which is used in the treatment of HIV infection with at least two other antiretroviral agents.[1]

In 2011, a study was published that determined the concentrations of tenofovir and emtricitabine in breast milk when given in labor and postpartum to prevent resistance after nevirapine is given in labor for prevention of maternal to child transmission of HIV.[2] These women were treated with tenofovir 600 mg/emtricitabine 400 mg at the time of delivery, followed by tenofovir 300 mg/emtricitabine 200 mg daily for 7 days postpartum. In this study, milk samples were collected on days 1, 2, 3, and 7 postpartum (10 min to 21 hours postdose). The maximum milk concentrations occurred 4-5 hours postdose and the lowest concentration was about 19 hours postdose. The median maximum and minimum emtricitabine concentrations in milk were 679 ng/mL (658-743 ng/mL) and 177 ng/mL (105-253.5 ng/mL). The authors of this study estimated the infant dose to be 126 µg/day (2% of an infant dose) based on the median of the maximum and minimum levels and a daily infant intake of 500 mL. The infant intake of emtricitabine in milk correlated to levels 3.2 to 12 times the IC50 and 3.2 to 12 times lower than the C_{min} for this medication. The authors of this study comment that subtherapeutic exposure of emtricitabine in breast milk could put an HIV positive infant at risk of developing resistance.

Note: This medication is an L5 to highlight the contraindication of breastfeeding when the mother is known to be infected with HIV, this medication is not an L5 based on its risk to the infant in breast milk. The Centers for Disease Control and Prevention recommend that HIV infected mothers do not breastfeed their infants to avoid postnatal transmission of HIV.

T 1/2	10 h	MW	247 Da	PB	<4%
Tmax	1-2 h	RID	0.93% - 3.57%	Vd	
Oral	93%	M/P		pKa	2.65

Adult Concerns: Dizziness, insomnia, abnormal dreams, rash, nausea, vomiting, diarrhea, abdominal pain, weakness, headache, depression, dyspepsia. Emtricitabine is known to cause lactic acidosis and severe hepatomegaly with steatosis.

Adult Dose: 200 mg daily.

Pediatric Concerns: Fever, hyperpigmentation of palms and/or soles, nausea, vomiting, diarrhea, gastroenteritis, otitis media, cough, rhinitis, pneumonia, infection.

Infant Monitoring: Breastfeeding is not recommended in mothers who have HIV.

Alternatives:

References:

1. Pharmaceutical manufacturers prescribing information.
2. Benaboud S, Pruvost A, Coffie PA, et al. Concentrations of tenofovir and emtricitabine in breast milk of HIV-1-infected women in Abidjan, Cote d'Ivoire, in the ANRS 12109 TEmAA Study, Step 2. Antimicrob Agents Chemother. 2011; 55(3):1315-1317.

ENALAPRIL

Trade: Amprace, Innovace, Renitec, Vasotec

Category: ACE Inhibitor

LRC: L2 - Limited Data-Probably Compatible

Enalapril maleate is an ACE inhibitor used to treat hypertension. Upon absorption, it is rapidly metabolized by the adult liver to enalaprilat, the biologically active metabolite. In one study of 5 lactating mothers who received a single 20 mg dose, the mean maximum milk concentration of enalapril and enalaprilat was only 1.74 µg/L and 1.72 µg/L respectively.[1] The author suggests that an infant consuming 850 mL of milk daily would ingest less than 2 µg of enalapril daily. The milk/plasma ratios for enalapril and enalaprilat averaged 0.013 and 0.025 respectively. However, this was only a single dose study, and the levels transferred into milk at steady state may be slightly higher.

In a study by Rush of a patient receiving 10 mg/day, the total amount of enalapril and enalaprilat measured in milk during the 24 hour period was 81.9 ng and 36.1 ng respectively or 1.44 µg/L and 0.63 µg/L of milk respectively.[2] Some caution is recommended in using ACE inhibitors in mothers with premature infants due to possible renal toxicity.

Both the ACE inhibitor family and the specific Angiotensin II receptor blockers are contraindicated in pregnancy and thus should be used with caution in women who are planning a subsequent pregnancy in the near future.

T 1/2	35 h (metabolite)	MW	492 Da	PB	60%
Tmax	0.5-1.5 h	RID	0.07% - 0.2%	Vd	
Oral	60%	M/P		pKa	3.67

Adult Concerns: Headache, dizziness, fatigue, hypotension, abnormal taste, cough, nausea, diarrhea, constipation, changes in renal function/urine output, hyperkalemia, rash.

Adult Dose: 10-40 mg daily.

Pediatric Concerns: None reported via milk at this time.

Infant Monitoring: Drowsiness, lethargy, pallor, poor feeding, and weight gain.

Alternatives: Captopril(L2), Benazepril(L2)

References:

1. Redman CW, Kelly JG, Cooper WD. The excretion of enalapril and enalaprilat in human breast milk. Eur J Clin Pharmacol. 1990;38(1):99.
2. Rush JE, Snyder BA, Barrish A, et al. Comment. Clin Nephrol. 1991;35:234.

ENOXAPARIN

Trade: Clexane, Lovenox

Category: Anticoagulant

LRC: L2 - Limited Data-Probably Compatible

Enoxaparin is a low molecular weight fraction of heparin used clinically as an anticoagulant. In a study of 12 women receiving 20-40 mg of enoxaparin daily for up to 5 days postpartum for venous pathology (n= 4) or cesarean section (n= 8), no change in anti-Xa activity was noted in the in the 12 breastfed infants.[1] Because it is a peptide fragment of heparin, its molecular weight is large (2,000-8,000 Da). The size alone would largely preclude its entry into human milk at levels clinically relevant. Due to minimal oral bioavailability, any present in milk would not be orally absorbed by the infant. A similar compound, dalteparin, has been studied and milk levels are extremely low as well. See the dalteparin monograph for more information.

T 1/2	4.5-7 h	MW	8,000 Da	PB	
Tmax	3-5 h	RID		Vd	0.06 L/kg
Oral	None	M/P		pKa	

Adult Concerns: Bruising on the skin, hemorrhage, blood in urine or stool, thrombocytopenia, and pain/bruising at injection site.

Adult Dose: 30 mg BID.

Pediatric Concerns: No change in clotting factors of 12 infants and no adverse events reported via milk at this time.

Infant Monitoring: Rare bruising on the skin, blood in urine, vomit, or stool.

Alternatives: Dalteparin(L2)

References:

1. Guillonneau M, de Crepy A, Aufrant C, Hurtaud-Roux MF, Jacqz-Aigrain E. Breast-feeding is possible in case of maternal treatment with enoxaparin. Arch Pediatr. 1996 May;3(5):513-514.

ENTECAVIR

Trade: Baraclude

Category: Antiviral

LRC: L4 - No Data-Possibly Hazardous

Entecavir is an oral antiviral used to treat chronic infections of hepatitis B.[1] This medication works by inhibiting hepatitis B viral polymerase which blocks the reverse transcriptase and reduces viral DNA synthesis. There is currently no information available regarding the transfer of entecavir into human milk; however, it can be found in rodent milk. Due to this medication's long half-life, small molecular weight, and good oral absorption, the use of this medication in breastfeeding is cautioned.

T 1/2	128–149 h	MW	295.3 Da	PB	13%
Tmax		RID		Vd	High L/kg
Oral	100%	M/P		pKa	

Adult Concerns: Alopecia, headache, fatigue, dizziness, fever, nausea, increase in lipase, changes in liver and renal function, ascites, lactic acidosis, hyperglycemia, hematuria, peripheral edema, and rash.

Adult Dose: 0.5-1 mg once daily.

Pediatric Concerns: No safety data in pediatrics at this time.

Infant Monitoring: Caution is recommended in lactation.

Alternatives:

References:
1. Pharmaceutical manufacturers prescribing information.

ENTEROVIRUS

Trade: Coxsackievirus, Echovirus, Hand Foot Mouth Disease, Poliovirus

Category: Infectious Disease

LRC: L3 - Limited Data-Probably Compatible

The enterovirus are genus of (+)ssRNA viruses. On the basis of their pathogenesis, they are classified into four groups, polioviruses, Coxsackie A viruses (CA), Coxsackie B viruses (CB), and echoviruses. They spread through fecal-oral route and can result in wide variety of symptoms such as common cold, hand, foot and mouth disease, acute hemorrhagic conjunctivitis, aseptic meningitis, myocarditis, acute flaccid paralysis, and severe neonatal sepsis.[1]

Coxsackievirus: Coxsackie A viruses are associated with hand, foot and mouth disease. Herpangina is caused by Coxsackie A virus, and causes a vesicular rash in the oral cavity and on the pharynx, along with high fever, sore throat, malaise, and often dysphagia, loss of appetite, back pain, and headache. It is also self-limiting, with symptoms typically ending in 3–4 days. Coxsackie B viruses cause mild symptoms of cold and can lead to myocarditis, pericarditis, meningitis, and pancreatitis. Echovirus are the cause of many non-specific viral infections. They are found in the intestine and can cause nervous disorders.

Poliovirus: Poliovirus have three serotypes PV1, PV2, PV3. All three forms are extremely infectious and affect spinal cord and cause poliomyelitis.

The protective benefits of breast milk in fighting against enterovirus infection in the infant has been well established. Maternal immunity is transferred to the infant by antibodies. Both transplacentally transported maternal IgG as well as breast milk IgA, can protect the child against infections by neutralizing the infectivity of enterovirus. Therefore, infants with enterovirus illness are encouraged to breastfeed.[2,3] However, a study has detected Coxsackie B3 in maternal milk, a report was presented in which viral RNA was present in maternal milk and two neonates were severely infected. However, after 12 to 14 days of onset of symptoms Coxsackie B3 could not be detected in breast milk of symptomatic mothers.[4] Therefore the chance of transmission of this virus is most likely during acute viremia stage; however it is not known if viral transmission via milk leads to any serious danger to infant.

Enterovirus infections late in pregnancy are common. Maternal echovirus or Coxsackie B virus infections are not associated with an increased risk of spontaneous abortions, but stillbirths late in pregnancy and a slightly increased risk for congenital heart defects and urogenital anomalies have been reported for the offspring of women with the group B Coxsackie virus infection during pregnancy.

Transmission of enteroviruses from mother to infant is relatively common and may occur through contact with maternal secretions during vaginal delivery, blood, or upper respiratory tract secretions.[1] One study documented the transplacental transfer of coxsackievirus from mother to fetus. Fever occurred in this baby immediately after birth by cesarean section, suggesting the presence of transplacental virus transmission, as confirmed by culture of the virus from the patient's throat and rectal swab and from his mother's throat.[2] Another report found Coxsackie B3 in the blood of a neonate with congenital myocarditis, and serological evidence of enterovirus infection in mother was documented.[3,4]

Infants diagnosed with enterovirus or Hand, Foot, and Mouth disease should continue to breastfeed.

Adult Concerns: Myopericarditis, acute hemorrhagic conjunctivitis, aseptic meningitis, herpangina, and encephalitis. Paralytic polio by polio virus, pleurodynia which consists of sudden onset of fever accompanied by muscular pain in the chest and abdomen and hand-foot-and-mouth disease by coxsackieviruses.

Coxsackievirus notoriously replicates in the pharynx (herpangina), the skin (hand-foot-mouth disease), the myocardium (myocarditis), and meninges (aseptic meningitis). It can also involve the adrenal glands, pancreas, liver, pleura, and lung. Coxsackie A viruses are associated with hand, foot and mouth disease, herpangina is caused by Coxsackie A virus, and causes a vesicular rash in the oral cavity and on the pharynx, along with high fever, sore throat, malaise, and often dysphagia, loss of appetite, back pain, and headache. It is also self-limiting, with symptoms typically ending in 3–4 days, while Coxsackie B viruses cause mild symptoms of cold and can lead to myocarditis, pericarditis, meningitis, and pancreatitis.

Echovirus can replicate in the liver (hepatic necrosis), the myocardium, the skin (viral exanthems), the meninges (aseptic meningitis), the lungs, and the adrenal glands. They are cause of many nonspecific viral infections, they are found in intestines and can cause nervous disorders.

Poliovirus replicates in the oropharynx and GI tissue. Following this replication, polio advances, to the spinal cord and an progress to other CNS regions causing death of neurons and paralysis. Neuropathy occurs due to direct cellular destruction and leads to paralysis.

Adult Dose:

Pediatric Concerns: Same as in adults, and congenital myocarditis and diabetes mellitus can occur from maternal transplacental transmission.

Infant Monitoring: Maternal-fetal and maternal-infant transmission is possible. Use caution.

Alternatives:

References:

1. Oberste MS, Maher K, Kilpatrick DR, Pallansch MA. Molecular evolution of the human enteroviruses: correlation of serotype with VP1 sequence and application to picornavirus classification. J Virol. 1999;73(3):1941-1948. PMC 104435. PMID 9971773.
2. Newburg DS, Ruiz-Palacios GM, Morrow AL. Human milk glycans protect infants against enteric pathogens. Annu Rev Nutr. 2004;25:37-58.
3. Orsi N. The antimicrobial activity of lactoferrin: current status and perspectives. Biometals. 2004;17:189-196.
4. http://journals.lww.com/pidj/pages/articleviewer.aspx?year=2006&issue=10000&article=00025&type=abstract

EPHEDRINE

Trade: Adalixin, Amsec, Anestan, Anodesyn, Bethal, Cam, Vatronol Nose Drops, Primatene

Category: Adrenergic

LRC: L4 - Limited Data-Possibly Hazardous

Ephedrine is a mild stimulant that belongs to the adrenergic family and functions similar to the amphetamines. Small amounts of d-isoephedrine, a close congener of ephedrine, is believed to be secreted into milk although no data is available on ephedrine itself.[1] This product is commonly used to support blood pressure of parturients during delivery. On an acute basis, it is not likely to harm a breastfeeding infant. However, it should not be used regularly by breastfeeding mothers.

T 1/2	3-5 h	MW	165 Da	PB	
Tmax	15-60 min	RID		Vd	
Oral	85%	M/P		pKa	9.6

Adult Concerns: Anorexia, tachycardia, arrhythmias, agitation, insomnia, hyperstimulation.

Adult Dose: 5-25 mg/dose IV slow push, 25-50 mg orally TID.

Pediatric Concerns: None reported via milk at this time.

Infant Monitoring: Irritability, insomnia, changes in feeding, poor weight gain, tremors.

Alternatives:

References:

1. Mortimer EA, Jr. Drug toxicity from breast milk? Pediatrics. 1977;60(5):780-781.

EPINASTINE HYDROCHLORIDE

Trade: Epinastine

Category: Antihistamine

LRC: L3 - No Data-Probably Compatible

Epinastine hydrochloride is an ophthalmic solution that is a direct H1 receptor antagonist, and inhibits the release of histamine from mast cells. It is indicated for the treatment of itching with allergic conjunctivitis. Epinastine does not penetrate the blood-brain barrier, plasma levels are exceedingly low, and no CNS side effects are expected. The transfer of epinastine into human milk is still not known but unlikely following ophthalmic administration[1].

T 1/2	12 h	MW	249.3 Da	PB	64%
Tmax	2 h	RID		Vd	
Oral		M/P		pKa	

Adult Concerns: Burning sensation in the eye, folliculosis, hyperemia, and pruritus.

Adult Dose: One drop per eye BID.

Pediatric Concerns: No data are available for breastfeeding mothers.

Infant Monitoring:

Alternatives:

References:
1. Pharmaceutical manufacturers prescribing information.

EPINEPHRINE

Trade: Adrenalin, Adrenutol, Bronkaid, Epi-pen, Medihaler, Primatene, Simplene

Category: Adrenergic

LRC: L2 - Limited Data-Probably Compatible

Epinephrine is a powerful adrenergic stimulant. Although likely to be secreted in milk, it is almost instantly destroyed in the gastrointestinal tract. It is unlikely that any would be absorbed by the infant unless in the early neonatal period. In addition, it has a half-life of only 2 minutes.

T 1/2	2 min	MW	183 Da	PB	
Tmax	<1-10 min	RID		Vd	
Oral	Poor	M/P		pKa	9.69

Adult Concerns: Nervousness, tremors, agitation, tachycardia.

Adult Dose: 0.3 mg IM or SC for anaphylaxis, can also be given IV for cardiac conditions.

Pediatric Concerns: None reported but observe for brief stimulation.

Infant Monitoring: Observe for excitement, poor sleep, and tremors.

Alternatives:

References:

EPIRUBICIN

Trade: Ellence, Epi-Cell, Farmorubicina, Pharmarubicin, Rubina

Category: Anticancer

LRC: L5 - No Data-Hazardous

Epirubicin is an anthracycline similar to but less cardiotoxic than doxorubicin. It is used for the treatment of breast, lung, and bladder cancer. The terminal T1/2 is 33 hours, even though the plasma levels are much lower than doxorubicin.[1,2] The volume of distribution for epirubicin is variable in the literature, it may be similar or if not higher than doxorubicin. No data are available on its transfer to milk, but it is probably as low if not lower than doxorubicin. Mothers should be advised to discontinue breastfeeding for at least seven to ten days following the use of this product.

T 1/2	33 h	MW	579.95 Da	PB	77%
Tmax		RID		Vd	21-27 L/kg
Oral		M/P		pKa	9.53

Adult Concerns: Lethargy, alopecia, fever, hot flashes, arrhythmias, mucositis, nausea, vomiting, diarrhea, anorexia, leukopenia, neutropenia, thrombocytopenia, anemia.

Adult Dose:

Pediatric Concerns: Potentially hazardous chemotherapeutic agent.

Infant Monitoring: Drowsiness, pallor, vomiting, diarrhea, weight gain. Recommend to avoid breastfeeding for at least seven to ten days following use.

Alternatives:

References:
1. Grochow LB, Ames MM. A Clinician's Guide to Chemotherapy Pharmacokinetics and Pharmacodynamics. 1st ed. Baltimore, MD: Williams & Wilkins; 1998.
2. Pharmaceutical manufacturers prescribing information.

EPLERENONE

Trade: Inspra

Category: Diuretic

LRC: L3 - No Data-Probably Compatible

Eplerenone blocks the binding of aldosterone by competitively inhibiting the aldosterone receptor and regulating blood pressure as a result. It is similar in structure to spironolactone, but has a lower affinity to steroid receptors, and thus has fewer adverse reactions.[1] It is used to improve survival of stable patients with left ventricular systolic dysfunction (ejection fraction <=40%) and clinical evidence of congestive heart failure after an acute myocardial infarction. No data are currently available on the transfer on eplerenone into human milk. Until more is known about this drug, caution is urged while administering in breastfeeding women.

T 1/2	4-6 h	MW	414 Da	PB	50%
Tmax	1.5 h	RID		Vd	1.28 L/kg
Oral	69%	M/P		pKa	

Adult Concerns: Headache, cough, angina, heart attack, diarrhea, hyperkalemia.

Adult Dose: 25 mg once to twice daily.

Pediatric Concerns: No data are available.

Infant Monitoring: Dehydration, lethargy.

Alternatives: Spironolactone(L2)

References:
1. Pharmaceutical manufacturers prescribing information.

EPOETIN ALFA

Trade: Epogen

Category: Hematopoietic

LRC: L3 - No Data-Probably Compatible

Epoetin alfa is a glycoprotein which stimulates red blood cell production.[1] Structurally similar to the natural erythropoietin, it consists of 165 amino acids manufactured by recombinant DNA technology. It has a molecular weight of 30,400 Da. Large molecular weight proteins in general are poorly transferred into human milk after the first week postpartum. Due to its protein nature, it would not likely be absorbed orally to any degree by the infant.

T 1/2	4-13 h	MW	30,400 Da	PB	
Tmax	5-24 h	RID		Vd	
Oral	Nil	M/P		pKa	4.5-5.5

Adult Concerns: Headache, hypertension, arthralgias, nausea, edema, vomiting, and chest pain have been reported in adults.

Adult Dose: 50-100 units/kg three times a week.

Pediatric Concerns: None reported via milk.

Infant Monitoring:

Alternatives:

References:
1. Pharmaceutical manufacturers prescribing information.

EPOPROSTENOL

Trade: Flolan, Caripul, Veletri, Dynovase

Category: Prostaglandin

LRC: L3 - No Data-Probably Compatible

Epoprostenol (Prostacyclin; PGX; PGI-2) is a naturally occurring prostaglandin that is a potent inhibitor of platelet aggregation and a vasodilator. It is commonly used to treat primary pulmonary hypertension. It is rapidly metabolized in plasma to two active metabolites and multiple inactive metabolites with a half-life of only a few minutes.[1] At this time there is no assay that can assess the pharmacokinetics of epoprostenol in humans. In animals epoprostenol had a small volume of distribution (0.375 L/kg) and short half-life (2.7 min).

Prostaglandins are known to be transferred into human milk, but they are believed to be derived from mammary tissue and synthesized with cellular components of breast milk.[2] With the extraordinarily short half-life of this product, it is unlikely any would penetrate into milk, be retained for very long, or be stable in the infant's gut. Oral absorption by the infant is unlikely.[1-2]

T 1/2	6 min	MW	374 Da	PB	
Tmax		RID		Vd	
Oral	Nil	M/P		pKa	

Adult Concerns: Flushing, headache, dizziness, anxiety, hypotension, chest pain, bradycardia or tachycardia, pulmonary edema, nausea, vomiting, abdominal pain, anorexia, thrombocytopenia, arthralgia, myalgia, severe skin rashes.

Adult Dose: Start with 2 ng/kg/min then increase by 1-2 ng/kg/min every 15 min to effect or dose-limiting side effects (typically 25-40 ng/kg/min).

Pediatric Concerns: None reported, unlikely to be absorbed.

Infant Monitoring: Lethargy, flushing, vomiting, diarrhea.

Alternatives:

References:
1. Pharmaceutical manufacturers prescribing information.
2. Friedman Z. Prostaglandins in breast milk. Endocrinol Exp. 1986;20(2-3):285-291.

EPROSARTAN

Trade: Teveten

Category: Antihypertensive

LRC: L3 - No Data-Probably Compatible

Eprosartan is an angiotensin receptor blocker (ARB) used in the treatment of hypertension.[1] No data are available on its use in breastfeeding mothers. Its use in mothers breastfeeding premature infants or even infants less than 4 months should be cautioned due to possible renal toxicity. There are other antihypertensives with more data in lactation that should be considered (e.g. captopril, enalapril, labetalol, nifedipine etc.).

T 1/2	20 h	MW	520 Da	PB	98%
Tmax	1-2 h	RID		Vd	4.4 L/kg
Oral	13%	M/P		pKa	4.38

Adult Concerns: Headache, dizziness, fatigue, hypotension, nausea, diarrhea, constipation, changes in renal function/urine output, hyperkalemia.

Adult Dose: 400-800 mg/day.

Pediatric Concerns: None reported via milk at this time.

Infant Monitoring: Drowsiness, lethargy, pallor, poor feeding and weight gain.

Alternatives: Captopril(L2), Enalapril(L2), Ramipril(L3), Labetalol(L2), Nifedipine(L2)

References:
1. Pharmaceutical manufacturers prescribing information.

EPSTEIN-BARR VIRUS

Trade: EBV, Mononucleosis

Category: Infectious Disease

LRC: L3 - Limited Data-Probably Compatible

The Epstein-Barr virus (EBV) is one of the causes of infectious mononucleosis. EBV belongs to the herpesvirus family. Symptoms include fever, exudative pharyngitis, lymphadenopathy, hepatosplenomegaly, and atypical lymphocytosis. Close personal contact is generally required for transmission and it is not known if EBV is secreted into human milk, although it is likely. Studies by Kusuhara[1] indicate that the seroprevalence of EBV at 12-23 months was the same in bottle-fed and in breastfed infants. This data suggests that breastmilk is not a significant source of early EBV infections. That said other data clearly show the transmission is significant. One study found that the prevalence of EBV DNA and the mean EBV load were significantly higher at 6 weeks and decreased through postpartum week 18 in mothers who were infected with malaria at birth.[2] To determine whether viral DNA was encapsulated, breast milk samples were treated with DNase before DNA extraction. Sixty percent of samples were DNase resistant, suggesting that the viral DNA in breast milk was encapsulated, and infectious. This data suggests that breast milk contains infectious EBV and is a potential source of viral transmission to infants living in malaria-endemic regions.

Adult Concerns: Symptoms include fever, exudative pharyngitis, lymphadenopathy, hepatosplenomegaly, and atypical lymphocytosis.

Adult Dose:

Pediatric Concerns:

Infant Monitoring: Fever, lymph node enlargement.

Alternatives:

References:
1. Kusuhara K, Takabayashi A, Ueda K, et al. Breast milk is not a significant source for early Epstein-Barr virus or human herpesvirus 6 infection in infants: a seroepidemiologic study in 2 endemic areas of human T-cell lymphotropic virus type I in Japan. Microbiol Immunol. 1997;41(4):309-312.
2. Daud II, Coleman CB, Smith NA, et al. Breast milk as a potential source of Epstein-Barr virus transmission among infants living in a malaria-endemic region of Kenya. J Infect Dis. 2015 Dec;212(11):1735-1742. PMID: 4633760.

EPTIFIBATIDE

Trade: Integrilin

Category: Platelet Aggregation Inhibitor

LRC: L3 - No Data-Probably Compatible

Eptifibatide is used in the treatment of acute coronary syndrome. It works by blocking the platelet glycoprotein IIb/IIIa receptor, and thus inhibits platelet aggregation.[1] It is a small peptide of approximately 831 Da and is probably poorly absorbed orally if at all. No data are available on the transfer into human milk, however, due to the large molecular weight of eptifibatide and its poor bioavailability as a peptide, it is unlikely that it would pass into the milk compartment or be absorbed orally by the infant.

T 1/2	2.5 h	MW	832 Da	PB	25%
Tmax		RID		Vd	0.2 L/kg
Oral	Nil	M/P		pKa	

Adult Concerns: Hypotension, thrombocytopenia, major and minor bleeding, injection site reactions.

Adult Dose: 180 µg/kg bolus, then 2 µg/kg/min IV.

Pediatric Concerns: No data are available at this time in lactation. Pediatric data also unavailable at this time.

Infant Monitoring: Rare- bruising on the skin, blood in urine, vomit or stool.

Alternatives:

References:
1. Pharmaceutical manufacturers prescribing information.

ERENUMAB-AOOE

Trade: Aimovig

Category: Calcitonin Gene-related Peptide (CGRP) Antagonists

LRC: L3 - No Data-Probably Compatible

Erenumab-aooe is a human monoclonal antibody that binds to the calcitonin gene-related peptide (CGRP) receptor and antagonizes CGRP receptor function. It is administered IM once monthly. Erenumab-aooe is a human immunoglobulin G2 (IgG2) monoclonal antibody that binds to the calcitonin gene-related peptide receptor. As an IgG2 antibody, it is not transported into human milk. Levels in milk are likely minimal. Any present in milk is unlikely to absorbed orally by the infant, or to survive the metabolic enzymes in the stomach of the infant.

T 1/2	28 days	MW	150,000 Da	PB	
Tmax		RID		Vd	
Oral		M/P		pKa	

Adult Concerns: Area injection site irritation. Rare constipation.

Adult Dose: Administered subcutaneously at 70 mg once monthly or 140 mg monthly.

Pediatric Concerns:

Infant Monitoring: Unlikely to be orally absorbed. Constipation is seen in adults.

Alternatives:

References:
1. Manufacturers prescribing information, 2018.

ERGONOVINE

Trade: Ergotrate, Syntometrine

Category: Pituitary Hormone

LRC: L3 - Limited Data-Probably Compatible

Ergonovine maleate and its close congener, methylergonovine maleate, directly stimulate uterine contraction and are given intramuscularly at the time of delivery to prevent/treat postpartum hemorrhage. At this time there are no data regarding the transfer of ergonovine into milk; however, there are numerous studies reviewing the transfer of methylergonovine. In a group of eight postpartum women receiving 125 µg three times daily for 5 days, the concentration of methylergonovine in plasma and milk were studied on the morning of day 5 after a 250-µg dose.[1] The milk concentrations ranged from <0.5 µg/L to 1.3 µg/L at one hour postdose and <0.5 µg/L to 1.2 µg/L at 8 hours postdose. In this study, only 5 of 16 milk samples had detectable methylergonovine levels. Using a dose of 1.3 µg/L of milk, an infant would only consume approximately 0.2 µg/kg/day, which is incredibly low compared to the maternal dose given in this study. The milk/plasma ratio averaged about 0.3.

In a 2004 prospective study following a maternal oral dose of 250 µg in 10 lactating women, the mean time to peak and peak milk concentration of methylergonovine occurred at 1.8 hours and was about 0.657 µg/L (range 410-830 µg/L).[2] The mean milk/plasma ratio was 0.18 at 1 hour and 0.17 at 2 hours postdose. We estimate that the infant would receive about 0.098 µg/kg/day or 2.7% of the maternal dose.

In a 2012 study, 12 lactating women were given methylergonovine 0.125 mg three times a day for 5 days.[3] Milk samples were collected on day 1 of therapy after the first dose. The peak concentration was 0.437 µg/L at 2 and declined to 0.086 µg/L by 5 hours. We used both of these concentrations to estimate an infant would receive between 0.7-3.6% of the maternal dose.

In a study of 10 women given methylergonovine 0.2 mg orally three times a day for one week compared to 10 lactating women given no therapy, no difference in maternal prolactin levels or breast milk volume were reported.[4]

However, studies have shown a suppression in prolactin and milk production. One study suggested a 50% decrease in prolactin levels 30 to 75 minutes after a 0.2 mg intramuscular injection of methylergonovine in women 3 days postpartum.[5] Prolactin levels were reported to increase 180 to 240 min after the injection. In a study of 30 lactating women receiving 0.6 mg orally from day 1 to day 7 postpartum, prolactin levels were significantly lower at day 7, while milk production was significantly reduced at days 3 and 7 when compared to untreated women.[6] In a study of 14 postpartum women who received 0.2 mg intramuscularly, plasma prolactin concentrations were lower (141 µg/L) as compared to 15 control subjects (266 µg/L) at 1.5 hours postpartum.[7] The authors did comment that in both groups the mothers were separated from their infants after delivery. No further information regarding breastfeeding status was given.

Another prolactin study with 10 women given ergonovine 0.2 mg orally three times a day from days 1 to 7 after a vaginal delivery reported lower prolactin levels compared to six postpartum women separated from their infants.[8] The initial prolactin concentration was 537 µg/L before drug administration and 89.7 µg/L on day 7. The initial prolactin concentration was 562 µg/L in the control group and 218 µg/L on day 7. None of these patients breastfed their infants. The authors also reported one woman post c-section given ergonovine 0.2 mg intravenously to have lower prolactin levels. Furthermore, two breastfeeding women given ergonovine intravenously on day 5 postpartum demonstrated a blunted prolactin response to suckling.

In a randomized controlled trial of 1429 women given ergonovine 0.5 mg intravenously for active management of the third stage of labor a small sub-analysis of 126 women found the post-suckling peak prolactin levels (48-72 h postpartum) to be no different than those in the control group.[9] The authors did report that women who did not receive the medication were more likely to continue breastfeeding beyond 4 weeks; however, there were numerous limitations when studying this last finding.

Short-term use of these agents when clinically indicated does not appear to pose problems in nursing infants. The prolonged use of ergot alkaloids should be avoided as they may negatively affect milk production.

T 1/2	0.5-2 h	MW	441 Da	PB	
Tmax	30-180 min	RID	2.73% - 5.46%	Vd	
Oral	>60%	M/P		pKa	15

Adult Concerns: Headache, dizziness, vertigo, hypertension, bradycardia, angina, MI, thrombophlebitis, shortness of breath, vomiting, diarrhea.

Adult Dose: 0.2 mg IM every 2-4 hours (max 5 doses).

Pediatric Concerns: None reported in milk at this time.

Infant Monitoring:

Alternatives: Methylergonovine(L2)

References:

1. Erkkola R, Kanto J, Allonen H, Kleimola T, Mantyla R. Excretion of methylergometrine (methylergonovine) into the human breast milk. Int J Clin Pharmacol Biopharm. 1978;16(12):579-580.
2. Vogel D, Burkhardt T, Rentsch K, et al. Misoprostol versus methylergometrine: pharmacokinetics in human milk. Am J Obstet Gynecol. 2004 Dec;191(6):2168-2173.
3. Nakamichi T, Yawata A, Hojo H, et al. Monitoring of methylergonovine in human breast milk by solid-phase extraction and high-performance liquid chromatography with fluorimetric detection. Pharmazie. 2012;67:482-484.
4. Del Pozo E, Brun DR, Hinselmann M. Lack of effect of methyl-ergonovine on postpartum lactation. Am J Obstet Gynecol. 1975;123(8):845-846.
5. Perez-Lopez FR, Delvoye P, Denayer P, L'Hermite M, Roncero MC, Robyn C. Effect of methylergobasine maleate on serum gonado-trophin and prolactin in humans. Acta Endocrinol (Copenh). 1975;79(4):644-657.
6. Peters F, Lummerich M, Breckwoldt M. Inhibition of prolactin and lactation by methylergometrine hydrogenmaleate. Acta Endocrinol (Copenh). 1979;91(2):213-216.
7. Weiss G, Klein S, Shenkman L, Kataoka K, Hollander CS. Effect of methylergonovine on puerperal prolactin secretion. Obstet Gynecol. 1975;46(2):209-210.
8. Canales ES, Garrido JT, Zarate A, Mason M, Soria J. Effect of ergonovine on prolactin secretion and milk let-down. Obstet Gynecol. 1976;48(2):228-229.
9. Begley CM. The effect of ergometrine on breast feeding. Midwifery. 1990;6:60-72.

ERGOTAMINE

Trade: Cafergot, DHE-45, Ergodryl, Ergomar, Ergostat, Gynergen, Lingraine, Migral, Wigraine

Category: Antimigraine

LRC: L4 - Limited Data-Possibly Hazardous

Ergotamine tartrate is a potent vasoconstrictor generally used in acute phases of migraine headache. It is never used chronically for prophylaxis of migraine. Although early reports suggest ergotamine compounds are secreted in breast milk[1] and cause symptoms of ergotism (vomiting, and diarrhea) in infants, other authors[2] suggest that the short-term use of ergotamine (0.2 mg postpartum) generally presents no problem to a nursing infant. This is likely, due to the fact that less than 5% of ergotamine is orally absorbed in adults. However, excessive dosing and prolonged administration may inhibit prolactin secretion and hence lactation. Although the initial plasma half-life is only 2 hours, ergotamine is stored for long periods in various tissues producing long-lasting effects (terminal half-life= 21 hours). Prolonged use during lactation should be strongly discouraged. Single use is probably OK due to low oral bioavailability. Major concern is hypoprolactinemia.

T 1/2	21 h	MW	581 Da	PB	
Tmax	0.5-3 h	RID		Vd	
Oral	<5%	M/P		pKa	9.7

Adult Concerns: Ergotism, peripheral artery insufficiency, nausea, vomiting, paresthesia, cold skin temperatures, headache.

Adult Dose: 2 mg every 30 minutes (max 3 doses).

Pediatric Concerns: One case of ergotism reported and included symptoms such as vomiting and diarrhea. Long-term exposure is contraindicated.

Infant Monitoring:

Alternatives: Sumatriptan(L3), NSAIDs, Acetaminophen(L1)

References:
1. Fomina PI. Untersuchungen uber den ubergang des aktiven Agens des Mutterkorns in die milch stillender Mutter. Arch Gynakol. 1934;157:275-285.
2. White G, White M. Breastfeeding and drugs in human milk. Vet Hum Toxicol. 1984;26(supplement 1):3.

ERLOTINIB

Trade: Tarceva

Category: Antineoplastic

LRC: L5 - No Data-Hazardous

Erlotinib is a human epidermal growth factor receptor inhibitor. It is an antineoplastic used for the treatment and maintenance therapy of advanced non-small cell lung cancer after the failure of other chemotherapy treatment. It is also used in conjunction with gemcitabine to treat cancer of the pancreas.

Erlotinib is about 60% absorbed after oral administration, and its bioavailability is substantially increased by food to almost 100%.[1] Its half-life is about 36 hours. Bioavailability of erlotinib following a 150 mg oral dose is about 60%, and peak plasma levels occur four hours after dosing. Following absorption, erlotinib is approximately 93% protein bound to albumin and alpha-1 acid glycoprotein (AAG). Erlotinib has an apparent volume of distribution of 232 liters (3.3 L/kg).

No data are available on its transfer to human milk. While administering in breastfeeding women, weigh the potential benefits against the potential risks. Because this drug is a inhibitor of epidermal growth factor, it could have profound effects on a rapidly growing infant. Its entry into milk is likely minimal due to its size and pKa, but because of its enormous volume of distribution, mothers should withhold breastfeeding for a minimum of 10-15 days.

T 1/2	36 h	MW	429.9 Da	PB	93%
Tmax	4 h	RID		Vd	3.3 L/kg
Oral		M/P		pKa	5.42

Adult Concerns: Fatigue, dizziness, fever, chest pain, cough, dyspnea, mucositis, dry mouth, stomatitis, diarrhea, anorexia, urinary tract infections, leukopenia, thrombocytopenia, anemia, weakness, arthralgias, peripheral edema, infection.

Adult Dose: 100-150 mg per day.

Pediatric Concerns:

Infant Monitoring: Withhold breastfeeding for a minimum of 10-15 days.

Alternatives:

References:
1. Pharmaceutical manufacturers prescribing information.

ERTAPENEM

Trade: Invanz

Category: Antibiotic, Carbapenem

LRC: L2 - Limited Data-Probably Compatible

Ertapenem is an antibiotic indicated for treatment of complicated infections of the skin/subcutaneous tissues, urinary tract and respiratory tract. The manufacturer reports the concentration of ertapenem in breast milk from five lactating women with pelvic infections (5 to 14 days postpartum). The breast milk samples were measured at random time points each day for 5 consecutive days following the last 1 gram dose of intravenous therapy (3-10 days of therapy). The concentration of ertapenem in breast milk within 24 hours of the last dose of therapy in all five women ranged from <0.13 (lower limit of quantitation) to 0.38 mg/L; peak concentrations were not assessed unfortunately. By day 5 after discontinuation of therapy, the level of ertapenem was undetectable in the breast milk of four women and below the lower limit of quantitation (<0.13 μg/mL) in one woman.[1]

The above data does not report C_{max} concentrations in milk nor the time samples were collected, so it is virtually worthless for determining infant exposure to the medication during the day and following the administration.

Using the above data and an assumed average weight of 70 kg, the mothers received about 14.28 mg/kg/day. After 24 hours, the infant would ingest about 57 μg/kg/day. The relative infant dose would be 0.4% of the maternal dose at this time. Without good data it is not possible to estimate clinical dose to the infant, but it is likely small and its oral bioavailability is poor. Almost all the penicillins and the carbapenems are suitable for use in breastfeeding mothers.

T 1/2	4 h	MW	497 Da	PB	95%
Tmax	2 h	RID		Vd	0.11 L/kg
Oral	Poor	M/P		pKa	4.05

Adult Concerns: Diarrhea, infused vein complications, nausea, headache, vaginitis in females, thrombophlebitis, vomiting, fever, abdominal pain. Do not use if penicillin allergic. Seizures, altered mental status.

Adult Dose: 1 gram IV/IM daily.

Pediatric Concerns: None reported via milk.

Infant Monitoring: Vomiting, diarrhea, changes in gastrointestinal flora, and rash.

Alternatives: Imipenem(L3), Meropenem(L3)

References:
1. Pharmaceutical manufacturers prescribing information.

ERYTHROMYCIN

Trade: Ceplac, E-Mycin, Ilotycin, EES, Emu-V E, Ery-Tab, Eryc, Erycin, Erythrocin, Erythromide, Ilosone

Category: Antibiotic, Macrolide

LRC: L3 - Limited Data-Probably Compatible

Erythromycin is an older, macrolide antibiotic. In one study of patients receiving 400 mg three times daily, milk levels varied from 0.4 to 1.6 mg/L.[1] Doses as high as 2 g per day produced milk levels of 1.6 to 3.2 mg/L. One case of hypertrophic pyloric stenosis apparently linked to erythromycin administration has been reported.[2] In a study of 2-3 patients who received a single 500 mg oral dose, milk levels at 4 hours ranged from 0.9 to 1.4 mg/L with a milk/plasma ratio of 0.92.[3]

At this time, there is some controversy regarding the use of macrolide antibiotics for treatment of neonatal infections, especially in infants less than two weeks of age because of a potential increased risk of hypertrophic pyloric stenosis. A 2003 study investigating the risk of infantile hypertrophic pyloric stenosis in infants exposed to macrolide antibiotics through breast milk did not demonstrate a strong association.[4] One subgroup analysis of female infants exposed within 70 days post-delivery found a statistically significant increased risk of infantile hypertrophic pyloric stenosis. The association in all other infants exposed within 42, 56, 70, and 90 days after delivery was found to be non-significant. In 2009, a small study prospectively assessed the neonatal risk of adverse effects from macrolide exposure via breast milk and found that rates and types (diarrhea, rash etc.) of adverse reactions were similar to amoxicillin exposure in milk.[5] This study was too small to assess for risk of hypertrophic pyloric stenosis.

T 1/2	1.5-2 h	MW	734 Da	PB	84%
Tmax	2-4 h	RID	1.4% - 1.7%	Vd	
Oral	Variable	M/P	0.92	pKa	12.44

Adult Concerns: Seizure, hearing loss, QTc prolongation, arrhythmias, nausea, vomiting, abdominal cramping diarrhea, hepatitis, cholestatic jaundice (common with estolate), and severe rashes.

Adult Dose: 250-500 mg base every 6-12 hours; 400-800 mg ethylsuccinate every 6-12 hours (max 4 g/day).

Pediatric Concerns: Pyloric stenosis has been associated with the use of erythromycin in neonates and via breast milk exposure.[4]

Infant Monitoring: Vomiting, diarrhea, changes in gastrointestinal flora, and rash.

Alternatives: Azithromycin(L2), Clarithromycin(L1)

References:

1. Knowles JA. Drugs in milk. Pediatr Currents. 1972;1:28-32.
2. Stang H. Pyloric stenosis associated with erythromycin ingested through breastmilk. Minn Med. 1986;69(11):669-670, 682.
3. Matsuda S. Transfer of antibiotics into maternal milk. Biol Res Pregnancy Perinatol. 1984;5(2):57-60.
4. Sorensen HT, Skriver MV, Pedersen L, Larsen H, Ebbesen F, Schonheyder HC. Risk of infantile hypertrophic pyloric stenosis after maternal postnatal use of macrolides. Scand J Infect Dis. 2003;35(2):104-106.
5. Goldstein LH, Berlin M, Tsur L, et al. The safety of macrolides during lactation. Breastfeed Med. 2009;4(4):197-200.

ESCITALOPRAM

Trade: Lexapro

Category: Antidepressant, SSRI

LRC: L2 - Limited Data-Probably Compatible

Escitalopram is a selective serotonin reuptake inhibitor (SSRI) used in the treatment of depression. It is the active S(+) enantiomer of citalopram (Celexa). While this agent is very specific for the serotonin receptor site, it does apparently have a number of other side effects which may be related to activities at other receptors. Antagonism of muscarinic, histaminergic, and adrenergic receptors has been hypothesized to be associated with various anticholinergic, sedative, and cardiovascular side effects.

In a case report of a 32-year-old mother taking escitalopram (5 mg/day) while breastfeeding her newborn, the reported milk level was 24.9 ng/mL at 1 week postpartum.[1] The infant's daily dose was estimated to be 3.74 µg/kg. At 7.5 weeks of age, the mother was taking 10 mg/day and the milk concentration level was 76.1 ng/mL. The infant daily dose was 11.4 µg/kg. There were no adverse events reported in the infant.

In a recent study of eight breastfeeding women taking an average of 10 mg/day, the total relative infant dose of escitalopram and its metabolite was reported to be 5.3% of the mothers' dose.[2] The mean M/P ratio (AUC) was 2.2 for escitalopram and 2.2 for demethylescitalopram. Absolute infant doses were 7.6 µg/kg/day for escitalopram and 3 µg/kg/day for demethylescitalopram. The drug and its metabolite were undetectable in most of the infants tested. No adverse events in the infants were reported.

Two of seven women in a case series that followed pregnant women taking escitalopram breastfed.[3] The seven mother-infant pairs were followed for up to 6 months postpartum and no adverse events reported in the two breastfed infants.

T 1/2	27-32 h	MW	414 Da	PB	56%
Tmax	5 h	RID	5.2% - 7.9%	Vd	20 L/kg
Oral	80%	M/P	2.2	pKa	9.5

Adult Concerns: Headache, insomnia, somnolence, diarrhea, and nausea. This medication has also been found to cause a prolonged QTc interval and a higher risk of developing Torsades de Pointes, especially when other medications that can also prolong QTc are used in combination with this product.

Adult Dose: 10-20 mg daily.

Pediatric Concerns: There is one case report of an infant exposed to escitalopram in pregnancy and lactation who developed necrotizing enterocolitis (NEC). The authors of this report propose multiple mechanisms for SSRIs potentially increasing the risk of NEC including: withdrawal of SSRI leading to a hypercoaguable state, vasoconstriction on smooth muscle in the gastrointestinal tract and inhibiting nitric oxide production. In this case report the infant was exposed to the medication in utero and via milk, had a 3-day admission to NICU for respiratory distress and then the adverse event occurred on day 5 of life. Other potential causes and in utero exposure also need to be considered in this case.[4]

Infant Monitoring: Sedation or irritability, not waking to feed/poor feeding, and weight gain.

Alternatives: Sertraline(L2), Fluoxetine(L2)

References:

1. Castberg I, Spigset O. Excretion of escitalopram in breast milk. J Clin Psychopharm. 2006;26(5):536-538.
2. Rampono J, Hackett LP, Kristensen JH, Kohan R, Page-Sharp M, Ilett KF. Transfer of escitalopram and its metabolite demethylescitalopram into breastmilk. Br J Clin Pharmacol. 2006;62(3):316-322.
3. Bellantuono C, Bozzi F, Orsolini L. Safety of escitalopram in pregnancy: a case series. Neuropsychiatr Dis Treat. 2013;9:1333-1337.
4. Potts AL, Young KL, Carter BS, Shenai JP. Necrotizing enterocolitis associated with in utero and breast milk exposure to the selective serotonin reuptake inhibitor, escitalopram. J Perinatol. 2007;27:120-122.

ESKETAMINE

Trade: Spravato

Category: Antidepressant, other

LRC: L3 - No Data-Probably Compatible

Esketamine is the S-enantiomer of racemic ketamine. It is a non-selective, non-competitive N methyl-D-aspartate (NMDA) receptor antagonist (NMDA). The mechanism by which esketamine exerts its antidepressant effect is not fully understood. It is presently indicated for treatment of treatment-resistant depression. At present, there are no available data on the transmission of ketamine or esketamine into human milk.[1]

T 1/2	7-12 h	MW	274.2 Da	PB	45%
Tmax	20-40 min	RID		Vd	10.12 L/kg
Oral	48% intranasal	M/P		pKa	

Adult Concerns: Dissociation, dizziness, nausea, sedation, vertigo, hypoesthesia, anxiety, lethargy, blood pressure increased, vomiting, and feeling drunk

Adult Dose: 28 mg via intranasal device.

Pediatric Concerns:

Infant Monitoring: Observe for nausea, sedation, vomiting.

Alternatives:

References:
1. Pharmaceutical manufacturers prescribing information.

ESMOLOL

Trade: Brevibloc

Category: Beta Adrenergic Blocker

LRC: L3 - No Data-Probably Compatible

Esmolol is an ultra-short-acting beta blocker agent (T1/2= 9 minutes) with low lipid solubility. It is of the same family as propranolol. It is primarily used for treatment of supraventricular tachycardia. It is only used IV and has an extremely short half-life. It is almost completely hydrolyzed in 30 minutes.[1] No data are available on its use in breastfeeding mothers.

T 1/2	9 min	MW	295 Da	PB	55%
Tmax	15 min	RID		Vd	
Oral	Poor	M/P		pKa	9.5

Adult Concerns: Headache, dizziness, insomnia, depression, fatigue, chest pain, bradycardia, hypotension, heart failure, wheezing, vomiting, constipation, myalgia, infusion reactions.

Adult Dose: 100 µg/kg/minute.

Pediatric Concerns: None reported via milk at this time.

Infant Monitoring: Drowsiness, lethargy, pallor, poor feeding, and weight gain.

Alternatives: Propranolol(L2), Metoprolol(L2)

References:
1. DrugBank, Esmolol, 2019.

ESOMEPRAZOLE

Trade: Nexium

Category: Gastric Acid Secretion Inhibitor

LRC: L2 - Limited Data-Probably Compatible

Esomeprazole is the S-isomer of omeprazole (Prilosec) and is essentially identical to omeprazole.[1] Omeprazole is a potent inhibitor of gastric acid secretion. In a study of one patient receiving 20 mg omeprazole daily, the maternal serum concentration was negligible until 90 minutes after ingestion and then reached 950 nM at 240 min[2] The breast milk concentration of omeprazole began to rise minimally at 90 minutes after ingestion and peaked after 180 minutes at only 58 nM, or less than 7% of the highest serum level. This would indicate a maximum dose of 3 µg/kg/day in a breastfed infant. Omeprazole milk levels were essentially flat over 4 hours of observation. Omeprazole is extremely acid labile with a half-life of 10 minutes at pH values below 4.[3] Virtually all omeprazole ingested via milk would probably be destroyed in the stomach of the infant prior to absorption. Esomeprazole is probably compatible with breastfeeding.

T 1/2	1-1.5 h	MW	767.2 Da	PB	97%
Tmax	1.5 h	RID		Vd	0.23 L/kg
Oral	90%	M/P		pKa	9.68

Adult Concerns: Headache, dizziness, dry mouth, nausea, diarrhea, constipation, flatulence, abdominal pain, changes in liver and renal function, anemia.

Adult Dose: 20-40 mg daily.

Pediatric Concerns: None reported via milk at this time.

Infant Monitoring: Unlikely to be absorbed while dissolved in milk due to instability in acid.

Alternatives: Omeprazole(L2), Ranitidine(L2), Famotidine(L1)

References:
1. Pharmaceutical manufacturers prescribing information.
2. Marshall JK, Thompson AB, Armstrong D. Omeprazole for refractory gastroesophageal reflux disease during pregnancy and lactation. Can J Gastroenterol. 1998;12(3):225-227.
3. Pilbrant A, Cederberg C. Development of an oral formulation of omeprazole. Scand J Gastroenterol Suppl. 1985;108:113-120.

ESTAZOLAM

Trade: Prosom

Category: Sedative-Hypnotic

LRC: L3 - No Data-Probably Compatible

Estazolam is a benzodiazepine sedative hypnotic. Estazolam, like other benzodiazepines, is secreted into rodent milk although the levels are unpublished.[1] No data are available on human milk levels. It is likely that some is secreted in human milk as well. Other benzodiazepines with more data in lactation should be considered instead (e.g. lorazepam).

T 1/2	10-24 h	MW	295 Da	PB	93%
Tmax	0.5-3 h	RID		Vd	
Oral	Complete	M/P		pKa	9

Adult Concerns: Sedation.

Adult Dose: 1-2 mg daily.

Pediatric Concerns: None reported via milk, but observe for sedation, apnea.

Infant Monitoring: Sedation, slowed breathing rate, not waking to feed/poor feeding, and weight gain.

Alternatives: Lorazepam(L3), Midazolam(L2)

References:
1. Pharmaceutical manufacturers prescribing information.

ESTROGENS, CONJUGATED

Trade: Premarin

Category: Estrogen

LRC: L3 - Limited Data-Probably Compatible

Conjugated estrogens consist primarily of estrone (>50%), equilin (15-25%) and equilenin. In this form the estrogen molecules are conjugated or attached to hydrophilic side groups such as sulfates. These are commonly found in the product, Premarin. Although small amounts may pass into breast milk, the effects of estrogens on the infant appear minimal. Early postpartum use of estrogens may reduce volume of milk produced and the protein content, but it is variable and depends on dose and the individual.[1-4] Breastfeeding mothers should attempt to wait until lactation is firmly established (6-8 weeks) prior to use of estrogen-containing oral contraceptives. In one study of six lactating women who received 50 or 100 mg vaginal suppositories of estradiol, the plasma levels peaked at 3 hours.[5] These doses are extremely large and are not used clinically. In another study of 11 women, the mean concentration of estradiol in breast milk was found to be 113 picograms/mL.[6] This is very close to that seen when the woman begins ovulating during lactation. If oral contraceptives are used during lactation, the transfer of estradiol to human milk will be low and will not exceed the transfer during physiologic conditions when the mother has resumed ovulation. However, suppression of lactation is still the major concern with the use of these products in breastfeeding mothers. If at all possible, do not use in breastfeeding mothers. See oral contraceptives.

T 1/2	60 min	MW	272 Da	PB	98%
Tmax	Rapid	RID		Vd	
Oral	Complete, vaginal 77%	M/P	0.08	pKa	19.38

Adult Concerns: Headache, hypertension, increased breast size, dysmenorrhea, uterine or fibroid growth, bloating, edema, thromboembolism, chloasma. Possible suppression of milk production.

Adult Dose: 10 mg TID.

Pediatric Concerns: None reported. Infantile feminization is unlikely at normal dosages.

Infant Monitoring: Small amounts are present in human milk. Possible suppression of milk production early postpartum is reported.

Alternatives: Norethindrone.

References:
1. Booker DE, Pahl IR. Control of postpartum breast engorgement with oral contraceptives. Am J Obstet Gynecol. 1967;98(8):1099-1101.
2. Kamal I, Hefnawi F, Ghoneim M, Abdallah M, Abdel RS. Clinical, biochemical, and experimental studies on lactation. V. Clinical effects of steroids on the initiation of lactation. Am J Obstet Gynecol. 1970;108(4):655-658.
3. Kora SJ. Effect of oral contraceptives on lactation. Fertil Steril. 1969;20(3):419-423.
4. Koetsawang S, Bhiraleus P, Chiemprajert T. Effects of oral contraceptives on lactation. Fertil Steril. 1972;23(1):24-28.
5. Laukaran VH. The effects of contraceptive use on the initiation and duration of lactation. Int J Gynaecol Obstet. 1987;25 Suppl:129-142.
6. Nilsson S, Nygren KG, Johansson ED. Transfer of estradiol to human milk. Am J Obstet Gynecol. 1978;132(6):653-657.

ESZOPICLONE

Trade: Lunesta

Category: Sedative-Hypnotic

LRC: L3 - No Data-Probably Compatible

Eszopiclone is a non-benzodiazepine hypnotic-sedative drug, although they both interact at the same GABA receptor.[1] Used as a nighttime sedative, its transfer into human milk has not yet been reported. However, a derivative which is virtually identical, zopiclone, has been studied (see zopiclone) and 1.5% of the maternal dose transferred into milk. Therefore, due to the structural similarity, one should expect a similar RID with eszopiclone. The use of eszopiclone in mothers with premature infants or newborns, and particularly those with infants subject to apnea, should be cautioned. Use in healthy older infants is probably suitable.

T 1/2	6 h	MW	388 Da	PB	59%
Tmax	1 h	RID		Vd	
Oral	>75%	M/P		pKa	5.35

Adult Concerns: Headache, somnolence, dizziness, anxiety, dry mouth, unpleasant taste, dyspepsia, vomiting, diarrhea.

Adult Dose: 2-3 mg at bedtime.

Pediatric Concerns: None reported via milk at this time.

Infant Monitoring: Sedation, slowed breathing rate, dry mouth, not waking to feed/poor feeding, and weight gain.

Alternatives: Zopiclone(L2)

References:
1. Pharmaceutical manufacturer package insert.

ETANERCEPT

Trade: Enbrel

Category: Monoclonal Antibody

LRC: L2 - Limited Data-Probably Compatible

Etanercept is a dimeric fusion protein consisting of the extracellular ligand-binding portion of tumor necrosis factor bound to human IgG1. Etanercept binds specifically to tumor necrosis factor (TNF) and blocks its inflammatory and immune activity in rheumatoid arthritis patients.[1] Elevated levels of TNF are found in the synovial fluid of arthritis patients.

In a recent study of a non-breastfeeding mother who received 25 mg twice weekly, etanercept was measured in the milk retained in the breast.[2] This mother was not breastfeeding but retained some milk in the breast after 30 days. The author reported milk levels of 75 ng/mL on the day after injection. While this data is interesting, measuring drug transfer in residual breast milk following involution of alveolar tissues is simply not clinically relevant. After involution, the alveolar system would be totally open to drug transfer due to the breakdown of the tight intercellular junctions between lactocytes.

In a study of a single patient receiving etanercept first 25 mg twice weekly, then 50 mg once weekly at 3 months postpartum, levels ranged from 4.48 ng/mL at 24 hours following a 25 mg dose, to 7.5 ng/mL at 72 hours following a 50 mg dose.[3]

In another study, one patient received 25 mg twice weekly during pregnancy. Following delivery, the infant plasma levels dropped quickly.[4] Breast milk levels at 12 weeks postpartum were only 3.5 ng/mL while the maternal plasma levels were 2872 ng/mL. None was detectable in the infant's plasma compartment. Due to its enormous molecular weight (150,000 Da), it is extremely unlikely that clinically relevant amounts would transfer into milk in actively breastfeeding mothers. In addition, due to its protein structure, it would not be orally bioavailable in an infant. Infliximab is somewhat similar and is apparently not secreted into human milk (see infliximab).

T 1/2	115 h	MW	150,000 Da	PB	
Tmax	72 h	RID	0.07% - 0.2%	Vd	0.24 L/kg
Oral	Nil	M/P		pKa	

Adult Concerns: Headache, dizziness, fever, dyspepsia, vomiting, diarrhea, anorexia, weakness, increased frequency of infection, injection site reactions.

Adult Dose: 25 mg twice weekly.

Pediatric Concerns: None reported via milk.

Infant Monitoring:

Alternatives: Infliximab(L3)

References:
1. Pharmaceutical manufacturers prescribing information.
2. Ostensen M, Eigenmann GO. Etanercept in breast milk. J Rheumatol. 2004 May;31(5):1017-1018.
3. Keeling S, Wolbink GJ. Measuring multiple etanercept levels in the breast milk of a nursing mother with rheumatoid arthritis. J Rheumatol. 2010 Jul;37(7):1551.
4. Murashima A, Watanabe N, Ozawa N, Saito H, Yamaguchi K. Etanercept during pregnancy and lactation in a patient with rheumatoid arthritis: drug levels in maternal serum, cord blood, breast milk and the infant's serum. Ann Rheum Dis. 2009 Nov;68(11):1793-1794.

ETHACRYNIC ACID

Trade: Edecrin

Category: Diuretic

LRC: L3 - No Data-Probably Compatible

Ethacrynic acid is a potent, short-acting loop diuretic similar to Lasix. A significant decrease in maternal blood pressure or blood volume may reduce milk production although this is speculative. No data on transfer into human milk are available.[1]

T 1/2	2-4 h	MW	303 Da	PB	90%
Tmax	2 h (oral)	RID		Vd	
Oral	100%	M/P		pKa	3.5

Adult Concerns: Diuresis, hypotension, diarrhea.

Adult Dose: 50-200 mg daily.

Pediatric Concerns: None reported.

Infant Monitoring: Observe for fluid loss, dehydration, lethargy.

Alternatives: Furosemide(L3)

References:
1. Pharmaceutical manufacturers prescribing information.

ETHAMBUTOL

Trade: Ethambutol, Etibi, Myambutol

Category: Antitubercular

LRC: L3 - Limited Data-Probably Compatible

Ethambutol is an antimicrobial used for tuberculosis. Small amounts are secreted in milk although no studies are available which clearly document levels. In one unpublished study, the mother had an ethambutol plasma level of 1.5 mg/L 3 hours after a dose of 15 mg/kg daily. Following a similar dose in the same patient, the concentration in milk was 1.4 mg/L.[1] In another patient, the maternal plasma level was 4.62 mg/L and the corresponding milk concentration was 4.6 mg/L (no dose available).[1]

T 1/2	3.1 h	MW	204 Da	PB	8-22%
Tmax	2-4 h	RID	1.5%	Vd	
Oral	80%	M/P	1.0	pKa	6.6, 9.5

Adult Concerns: Headache, dizziness, malaise, changes in vision, vomiting, anorexia, changes in liver function, hyperuricemia, arthralgias, peripheral neuropathy, and rash.

Adult Dose: 15-25 mg/kg daily.

Pediatric Concerns: None reported, but caution is recommended.

Infant Monitoring: Drowsiness, lethargy, vomiting and weight gain. If clinical symptoms arise (e.g. yellowing of the skin or eyes) check liver function tests.

Alternatives:

References:
1. Snider DE Jr, Powell KE. Should women taking antituberculosis drugs breast-feed? Arch Intern Med. 1984;144(3):589-590.

ETHANOL

Trade: Alcohol

Category: Drugs of Abuse

LRC: L4 - Limited Data-Possibly Hazardous

Alcohol transfers into human milk readily, with an average milk/plasma ratio of about 1. This does not necessarily mean that the dose of alcohol in milk is high, only that the levels in plasma correspond closely with those in milk. The absolute amount (dose) of alcohol transferred into milk is generally low and is a function of the maternal level. Older studies, some in animals, suggested that beer (or more likely, barley) may stimulate prolactin levels.[1-4] While this may be true, we now know clearly that alcohol is a profound inhibitor of oxytocin release, and inevitably reduces milk letdown and the amount of milk delivered to the infant. Thus beer should not be considered a galactagogue.

In a study of 12 breastfeeding mothers who ingested 0.3 g/kg of ethanol in orange juice (equivalent to 1 can of beer for the average-sized woman), the mean maximum concentration of ethanol in milk was 320 mg/L.[5] This report suggests a 23% reduction (156 to 120 mL) in breast milk production following ingestion of beer and an increase in milk odor as a function of ethanol content. In another group of five women, who consumed 0.4 g/kg at one setting, milk and maternal plasma levels were similar. Levels of alcohol in milk averaged 0.44 g/L at peak and fell to 0.09 g/L at 180 minutes.[6] In an interesting study of the effect of alcohol on milk ingestion by infants, the rate of milk consumption by infants during the 4 hours immediately after exposure to alcohol (0.3 g/kg) in 12 mothers was significantly less.[7] Compensatory increases in intake were then observed during the 8-16 hours after exposure when mothers refrained from drinking. Excess levels may lead to drowsiness, deep sleep, weakness, and decreased linear growth in infant. Maternal blood alcohol levels must attain 300 mg/dL before significant side effects are reported in the infant. Reduction of letdown is apparently dose-dependent and requires alcohol consumption of 1.5 to 1.9 g/kg.[8] Other studies have suggested psychomotor delay in infants of moderate drinkers (2+ drinks daily). Avoid breastfeeding during and for at least 2 hours after drinking alcohol (moderate). Heavy drinkers should wait longer.

A new study suggests that the state of lactation metabolically changes the rate of alcohol bioavailability.[9] In this study, blood alcohol levels were significantly lower in lactating women as compared to non-lactating women. The reduced AUC levels for alcohol suggest that the metabolism of ethanol is higher in lactating women. However, the subjective effects of alcohol were still similar. Another study reported one infant that developed pseudo-Cushing syndrome as a result of exposure to alcohol in breast milk. The mother consumed at least 50 12-ounce beers weekly in addition to other concentrated alcoholic beverages. She had stopped drinking while pregnant, and resumed postpartum. The infant showed signs of Cushing syndrome at age 8 weeks. When the mother stopped drinking while breastfeeding, the baby's appearance gradually returned to normal.[10]

Adult metabolism of alcohol is approximately 1 oz of pure ethanol in 3 hours, so mothers who ingest alcohol in moderate amounts can generally return to breastfeeding as soon as they feel neurologically normal. A good rule is 2 hours for each drink consumed. Chronic or heavy consumers of alcohol should not breastfeed. Readers are urged to consult Koren's excellent nomogram on counseling women concerning alcohol consumption.[11] Remember, this nomogram calculates, as a function of body weight and amount of alcohol consumed, the time to "zero" plasma levels in the mother.

T 1/2	0.24 h	MW	46 Da	PB	0%
Tmax	30-90 min (oral)	RID	16%	Vd	0.53 L/kg
Oral	100%	M/P	1.0	pKa	16

Adult Concerns: Sedation, decreased milk supply, altered milk taste.

Adult Dose:

Pediatric Concerns: One infant developed pseudo-Cushing syndrome as a result of exposure to alcohol in breast milk. The mother consumed at least 50 12-ounce beers weekly in addition to other concentrated alcoholic beverages. She had stopped drinking while pregnant, and resumed postpartum. The infant showed signs of Cushing syndrome at age 8 weeks. When the mother stopped drinking while breastfeeding, the baby's appearance gradually returned to normal.[10] In another case report of a heavy user, the infant was restless and insomniac for several days then exhibited violent fits and tonic-clonic seizures.[12] After removal from this mother's breast, the infant calmed. Other studies suggest changes in behavioral state such as shorter periods of sleep, crying more often, and heightened startling reflexes after exposure to alcohol.

Infant Monitoring: Use with caution, not recommended. Sedation, poor feeding, decreased milk supply, altered milk taste.

Alternatives:

References:

1. Marks V, Wright JW. Endocrinological and metabolic effects of alcohol. Proc R Soc Med. 1977;70(5):337-344.
2. De Rosa G, Corsello SM, Ruffilli MP, Della CS, Pasargiklian E. Prolactin secretion after beer. Lancet. 1981;2(8252):934.
3. Carlson HE, Wasser HL, Reidelberger RD. Beer-induced prolactin secretion: a clinical and laboratory study of the role of salsolinol. J Clin Endocrinol Metab. 1985;60(4):673-677.
4. Koletzko B, Lehner F. Beer and breastfeeding. Adv Exp Med Biol. 2000;478:23-28.
5. Mennella JA, Beauchamp GK. The transfer of alcohol to human milk. Effects on flavor and the infant's behavior. N Engl J Med. 1991;325(14):981-985.
6. da-Silva VA, Malheiros LR, Moraes-Santos AR, Barzano MA, McLean AE. Ethanol pharmacokinetics in lactating women. Braz J Med Biol Res. 1993 Oct;26(10):1097-1103.
7. Mennella JA. Regulation of milk intake after exposure to alcohol in mothers' milk. Alcohol Clin Exp Res. 2001;25(4):590-593.
8. Cobo E. Effect of different doses of ethanol on the milk-ejecting reflex in lactating women. Am J Obstet Gynecol. 1973;115(6):817-821.
9. Pepino MY, Steinmeyer AL, Mennella JA. Lactational state modifies alcohol pharmacokinetics in women. Alcohol Clin Exp Res. 2007 Jun;31(6):909-918.
10. Binkiewicz A, Robinson MJ, Senior B. Pseudo-cushing syndrome caused by alcohol in breast milk. J Pediatr. 1978 Dec;93(6):965-967.
11. Ho E, Collantes A, Kapur BM, Moretti M, Koren G. Alcohol and breast feeding: calculation of time to zero level in milk. Biol Neonate. 2001;80(3):219-222.
12. Budin P. Lecture VI. In: The Nursling: The Feeding and Hygiene of Premature and Full-Term Infants. London: Caxton Publishing Company; 1907:85-101.

ETHINYL ESTRADIOL

Trade: Activelle, Adgyn Estro, Aerodiol

Category: Estrogen

LRC: L3 - Limited Data-Probably Compatible

Ethinyl estradiol is an estrogenic agent. Although small amounts of estrogens may pass into breast milk, the effects of estrogens on the infant appear minimal. In one study, ethinyl estradiol was not detected in breast milk after administration of 50 µg/day.[1] After administration of 500 µg/day, the level in breast milk was approximately 300 pg/mL.[1]

Early postpartum use of estrogens may reduce volume of milk produced and the protein content, but it is variable, controversial, and depends on dose and the individual.[2-5] Breastfeeding mothers should attempt to wait until lactation is firmly established (6-8 weeks) prior to use of estrogen-containing oral contraceptives. Progestin-only birth control products are preferred in breastfeeding mothers.

T 1/2	36 h	MW	296 Da	PB	97%
Tmax		RID		Vd	
Oral	Complete	M/P	1:4	pKa	17.6

Adult Concerns: Headache, hypertension, increased breast size, dysmenorrhea, uterine or fibroid growth, bloating, edema, thromboembolism, chloasma. Possible suppression of milk production.

Adult Dose:

Pediatric Concerns: Reduced milk supply is possible. Do not use early postpartum.

Infant Monitoring: Small amounts are present in human milk. Possible suppression of milk production early postpartum is reported.

Alternatives:

References:
1. Nilsson S, Nygren KG, Johansson ED. Ethinyl estradiol in human milk and plasma after oral administration. Contraception. 1978 Feb;17(2):131-139.
2. Booker DE, Pahl IR. Control of postpartum breast engorgement with oral contraceptives. Am J Obstet Gynecol. 1967;98(8):1099-1101.
3. Kamal I, Hefnawi F, Ghoneim M, Abdallah M, Abdel RS. Clinical, biochemical, and experimental studies on lactation. V. Clinical effects of steroids on the initiation of lactation. Am J Obstet Gynecol. 1970;108(4):655-658.
4. Kora SJ. Effect of oral contraceptives on lactation. Fertil Steril. 1969;20(3):419-423.
5. Koetsawang S, Bhiraleus P, Chiemprajert T. Effects of oral contraceptives on lactation. Fertil Steril. 1972;23(1):24-28.

ETHOSUXIMIDE

Trade: Zarontin

Category: Anticonvulsant

LRC: L4 - Limited Data-Possibly Hazardous

Ethosuximide is an anticonvulsant used in epilepsy. Rane's data suggest that although significant levels of ethosuximide are transferred into human milk, the plasma level in the infant is quite low.[1] A peak milk concentration of approximately 55 mg/L was reported at 1 month postpartum in a mother consuming 250 mg twice daily. Milk/plasma ratios were reported to be 1.03 on day 3 postpartum and 0.8 during the first 3 months of therapy. The infant's plasma reached a peak (2.9 mg/dL) at approximately 1.5 months postpartum and then declined significantly over the next 3 months suggesting increased clearance by the infant. Although these levels are considered subtherapeutic, it is suggested that the infant's plasma levels be occasionally tested.

In another study of a women receiving 500 mg twice daily, her milk levels, as estimated from a graph, averaged 60-70 mg/L.[2] A total daily exposure to ethosuximide of 3.6-11 mg/kg as a result of nursing was predicted.

In a study by Kuhnz of 10 epileptic breastfeeding mothers (and 13 infants) receiving 3.5 to 23.6 mg/kg/day, the breast milk concentrations were similar to those of the maternal plasma (milk/serum: 0.86) and the breastfed infants maintained serum levels between 15 and 40 µg/mL.[3] Maximum milk concentration reported was 77 mg/L although the average was 49.54 mg/L. Neonatal behavior complications such as poor suckling, sedation, and hyperexcitability occurred in seven of the 12 infants. Interestingly, one infant who was not breastfed, exhibited severe withdrawal symptoms such as tremors, restlessness, insomnia, crying, and vomiting which lasted for 8 weeks causing a slow weight gain. Thus, the question remains: is it safer to breastfeed and avoid these severe withdrawal reactions?

These studies clearly indicate that the amount of ethosuximide transferred to the infant is significant. With milk/plasma ratios of approximately 0.86-1 and relatively high maternal plasma levels, the maternal plasma levels are a good indication of the dose transferred to the infant. Milk levels are generally high. Caution is recommended.

T 1/2	30-60 h	MW	141 Da	PB	0%
Tmax	4 h	RID	31.4% - 73.5%	Vd	0.72 L/kg
Oral	Complete	M/P	0.94	pKa	9.3

Adult Concerns: Drowsiness, ataxia, nausea, vomiting, anorexia, rash.

Adult Dose: 250-750 mg BID.

Pediatric Concerns: Neonatal behavior complications such as poor suckling, sedation, and hyperexcitability occurred in 7 of 12 infants in one study. Milk levels are significant. Caution is recommended.

Infant Monitoring: Sedation or irritability, not waking to feed/poor feeding and weight gain. Based on clinical symptoms some infants may require monitoring of liver enzymes.

Alternatives:

References:

1. Rane A, Tunell R. Ethosuximide in human milk and in plasma of a mother and her nursed infant. Br J Clin Pharmacol. 1981;12(6):855-858.
2. Koup JR, Rose JQ, Cohen ME. Ethosuximide pharmacokinetics in a pregnant patient and her newborn. Epilepsia. 1978;19(6):535-539.
3. Kuhnz W, Koch S, Jakob S, Hartmann A, Helge H, Nau H. Ethosuximide in epileptic women during pregnancy and lactation period. Placental transfer, serum concentrations in nursed infants and clinical status. Br J Clin Pharmacol. 1984;18(5):671-677.

ETHOTOIN

Trade: Peganone

Category: Anticonvulsant

LRC: L3 - No Data-Probably Compatible

Ethotoin is a typical phenytoin-like anticonvulsant.[1] Although no data is available on concentrations in breast milk, its similarity to phenytoin would suggest that some is secreted via breast milk. No specific data for ethotoin are available.

Phenytoin is an old and efficient anticonvulsant. It is secreted in small amounts into breast milk. The effect on infant is generally considered minimal if the levels in the maternal circulation are kept in low-normal range (10 μg/mL). Phenytoin levels peak in milk at 3.5 hours.

In one study of six women receiving 200-400 mg/day of phenytoin, plasma concentrations varied from 12.8 to 78.5 μmol/L, while their milk levels ranged from 1.61 to 2.95 mg/L.[2] The milk/plasma ratios were low, ranging from 0.06 to 0.18. In only two of these infants were plasma concentrations of phenytoin detectable (0.46 and 0.72 μmol/L). No untoward effects were noted in any of these infants. Others have reported milk levels of 6 μg/mL[3], or 0.8 μg/mL.[4] Although the actual concentration in milk varies significantly between studies, the milk/plasma ratio appears relatively similar at 0.13 to 0.45. Breast milk concentrations varied from 0.26 to 1.5 mg/L depending on the maternal dose. In a mother receiving 250 mg twice daily, milk levels were 0.26 mg/L and the milk/plasma ratio was 0.45.[5] The maternal plasma level was phenytoin was 0.58. In another study of two patients receiving 300-600 mg/d, the average milk level was 1.9 mg/L.[6] The maximum observed milk level was 2.6 mg/L.

The neonatal half-life of phenytoin is highly variable for the first week of life. Monitoring of the infants' plasma may be useful although it is not definitely required. All of the current studies indicate rather low levels of phenytoin in breast milk and minimal plasma levels in breastfeeding infants.

T 1/2	3-9 h	MW	204 Da	PB	41%
Tmax	1-2 h	RID		Vd	
Oral	Complete	M/P		pKa	11.29

Adult Concerns: Drowsiness, dizziness, insomnia, headache, blood dyscrasia.

Adult Dose: 1 g per day initially, increased to 2-3 g daily.

Pediatric Concerns: None reported, but see phenytoin.

Infant Monitoring: Sedation or irritability, not waking to feed/poor feeding, and weight gain. Based on clinical symptoms some infants may require monitoring of liver enzymes.

Alternatives:

References:
1. DrugBank, 2019.
2. Steen B, Rane A, Lonnerholm G, Falk O, Elwin CE, Sjoqvist F. Phenytoin excretion in human breast milk and plasma levels in nursed infants. Ther Drug Monit. 1982;4(4):331-334.
3. Svenmark O, Schiller PJ, Buchthal F. 5, 5-Diphenylhydantoin (dilantin) blood levels after oral or intravenous dosage in man. Acta Pharmacol Toxicol (Copenh). 1960;16:331-346.
4. Kaneko S, Sato T, Suzuki K. The levels of anticonvulsants in breast milk. Br J Clin Pharmacol. 1979;7(6):624-627.
5. Rane A, Garle M, Borga O, Sjoqvist F. Plasma disappearance of transplacentally transferred diphenylhydantoin in the newborn studied by mass fragmentography. Clin Pharmacol Ther. 1974;15(1):39-45.
6. Mirkin BL. Diphenylhydantoin: placental transport, fetal localization, neonatal metabolism, and possible teratogenic effects. J Pediatr. 1971;78(2):329-337.

ETIDRONATE

Trade: Didronel

Category: Calcium Regulator

LRC: L3 - No Data-Probably Compatible

Etidronate is a bisphosphonate that slows the dissolution of hydroxyapatite crystals in the bone, thus reducing bone calcium loss in certain syndromes such as Paget's syndrome.[1] Etidronate also reduces the remineralization of bone and can result in osteomalacia over time. It is not known how the administration of this product during active lactation would affect the maternal bone porosity. It is possible that milk calcium levels could be reduced although this has not been reported. Etidronate is poorly absorbed orally (1%) and must be administered in between meals on an empty stomach. Its penetration into milk is possible due to its small molecular weight, but it has not yet been reported. However, due to the presence of fat and calcium in milk, its oral bioavailability in infants would be exceedingly low. Whereas the plasma half-life is approximately 6 hours, the terminal elimination half-life (from bone) is >90 days.

T 1/2	6 h (plasma)	MW	206 Da	PB	
Tmax	2 h	RID		Vd	1.37 L/kg
Oral	1-2.5%	M/P		pKa	1.46

Adult Concerns: Headache, abdominal pain, nausea, diarrhea, osteomalacia, bone pain. There are reports of osteonecrosis of the jaw, esophagitis and esophageal ulceration in patients taking etidronate.

Adult Dose: 5-10 mg/kg daily.

Pediatric Concerns: None reported via milk.

Infant Monitoring: Vomiting, reflux, diarrhea.

Alternatives:

References:
1. Pharmaceutical manufacturers prescribing information.

ETODOLAC

Trade: Etodolac, Lodine, Ultradol

Category: NSAID

LRC: L3 - No Data-Probably Compatible

Etodolac is a prototypical nonsteroidal anti-inflammatory agent (NSAID) with analgesic, antipyretic, and anti-inflammatory properties.[1] Thus far no data are available regarding its secretion into human breastmilk. As with most NSAIDs, milk levels are likely minimal. Shorter half-life medications are preferred and there are many NSAIDs with established data in lactation that should be considered as alternatives (e.g. ibuprofen).

T 1/2	7.3 h	MW	287 Da	PB	95-99%
Tmax	1-2 h	RID		Vd	0.4 L/kg
Oral	80-100%	M/P		pKa	4.7

Adult Concerns: Dizziness, depression, nervousness, chills/fever, tinnitus, dyspepsia, nausea, vomiting, abdominal cramps, diarrhea, gastrointestinal bleeding, changes in renal function, polyuria, weakness.

Adult Dose: 200-400 mg every 6-8 hours.

Pediatric Concerns: None reported via milk, but observe for nausea, diarrhea, indigestion. Ibuprofen probably preferred at this time.

Infant Monitoring: Vomiting, diarrhea.

Alternatives: Ibuprofen(L1), Diclofenac(L2)

References:
1. Pharmaceutical manufacturers prescribing information.

ETOPOSIDE

Trade: Abiposid, Celltop, Eposid, Eposin, Etopofos, Etopophos, Toposar, VP-16

Category: Antineoplastic

LRC: L5 - Limited Data-Hazardous

Etoposide is an inhibitor of mitosis. It is commonly used to treat testicular, lung, and other cancers, and in bone marrow transplant.[1] Oral bioavailability ranges from 50% to higher, and it is apparently associated with the dose, with lesser absorption at higher doses. Etoposide is approximately 95% bound to plasma proteins. On intravenous administration, the disposition of etoposide is best described as a biphasic process, with a distribution phase half-life of about 1.5 hours and terminal elimination half-life ranging from 4 to 11 hours.

In a 28-year-old female receiving mitoxantrone, behenoyl cytosine arabinoside, and etoposide (80 mg/m^2) for treatment of acute promyelocytic leukemia, etoposide breast milk levels were found to peak just after administration and then rapidly decrease to undetectable levels within 24 hours.[2] Against the research team's advice, the patient breastfed her infant starting 3 weeks after completion of therapy; the infant was followed without report of adverse effects up to 16 months of age.

Mothers should withhold breastfeeding for at least two to three days following exposure to this agent.

T 1/2	4-11 h	MW		PB	94-97%
Tmax	1-1.5 h	RID		Vd	0.25-0.41 L/kg
Oral	25-75%	M/P		pKa	9.33

Adult Concerns: Alopecia, stomatitis, hypotension, nausea, vomiting, diarrhea, mucositis, changes in liver function, metabolic acidosis, leukopenia, thrombocytopenia, anemia, peripheral neuropathy, severe skin reactions.

Adult Dose:

Pediatric Concerns:

Infant Monitoring: Withhold breastfeeding for two to three days.

Alternatives:

References:
1. Pharmaceutical manufacturers prescribing information.
2. Azuno Y, Kaku K, Fujita N, Okubo M, Kaneko T, Matsumoto N. Mitoxantrone and etoposide in breast milk. Am J Hematol. 1995 Feb;48(2):131-132.

ETRAVIRINE

Trade: Intelence

Category: Antiviral

LRC: L5 - No Data-Hazardous if Maternal HIV Infection

Etravirine is an antiretroviral agent used for the treatment of HIV infection. Etravirine is an NNRTI of human immunodeficiency virus type 1 (HIV-1). Etravirine binds directly to reverse transcriptase (RT) and blocks the RNA-dependent and DNA-dependent DNA polymerase activities by causing a disruption of the enzyme's catalytic site. Etravirine does not inhibit the human DNA polymerases α, β, and γ.

There are no adequate and well-controlled studies or case reports in breastfeeding women. Breastfeeding is not recommended in mothers who have HIV.[1,2]

T 1/2	41 h	MW	435.28 Da	PB	99.9
Tmax	2.5-4 h	RID		Vd	
Oral		M/P		pKa	<3

Adult Concerns: Nausea, rash, hyperlipidemia, hyperglycemia, elevated liver enzymes, elevated serum creatinine, peripheral neuropathy, hypersensitivity, myocardial infarction.

Adult Dose: 200 mg twice daily.

Pediatric Concerns:

Infant Monitoring: Breastfeeding is not recommended in mothers who have HIV.

Alternatives:

References:

1. World Health Organization. Global Programme on AIDS. Consensus Statement from the WHO/UNICEF Consultation on HIV Transmission and Breast-Feeding. Geneva: WHO; 1992.
2. Latham MC, Greiner T. Breastfeeding versus formula feeding in HIV infection. Lancet. 1998;352:737.

EUCALYPTUS

Trade:

Category: Decongestant

LRC: L3 - No Data-Probably Compatible

There are many compounds contained in eucalyptus extract such as eucalyptol, cineole, and hydrocyanic acid. Antimicrobial, hypoglycemic, analgesic, and anti-inflammatory effects have been observed in animal studies.[1-3] Eucalyptus leaf has been traditionally used orally for treating fever, cough, infection, and dyspepsia. Eucalyptus oil also has been used topically for respiratory tract inflammation, nasal congestion, and rheumatoid arthritis.[4] There are no adequate or well-controlled studies or case reports of the use of eucalyptus in breastfeeding women. Ingestion of significant quantity may cause eucalyptus oil poisoning with depressed central nervous system and can be fatal.[4]

Adult Concerns: Nausea, vomiting, hypersensitivity, contact dermatitis, diarrhea.

Adult Dose:

Pediatric Concerns:

Infant Monitoring:

Alternatives:

References:

1. Takahashi T, Kokubo R, Sakaino M. Antimicrobial activities of eucalyptus leaf extracts and flavonoids from Eucalyptus maculata. Lett Appl Microbiol. 2004;39(1):60-64.
2. Gray AM, Flatt PR. Antihyperglycemic actions of Eucalyptus globulus(Eucalyptus) are associated with pancreatic and extra-pancreatic effects in mice. J Nutr. 1998 Dec;128(12):2319-2323.
3. Silva J, Abebe W, Sousa SM, Duarte VG, Machado MI, Matos FJ. Analgesic andanti-inflammatory effects of essential oils of Eucalyptus. J Ethnopharmacol. 2003 Dec;89(2-3):277-283.
4. TRC Healthcare. Eucalyptus. In: Natural Medicines Comprehensive Database [Internet Database]. Stockton, CA: Therapeutic Research Faculty. Updated May 23, 2011. Accessed May 24, 2011.

EVEROLIMUS

Trade: Afinitor, Zortress

Category: Antineoplastic

LRC: L5 - No Data-Hazardous

Everolimus is a macrolide immunosuppressant intended for acute rejection prophylaxis after kidney transplantation. Everolimus blocks growth factor-driven transduction signals in the T-cell response to alloantigen. It is currently used as an immunosuppressant to prevent organ transplant rejections. It has a large molecular weight and is unlikely to enter the milk compartment at high levels. However, it is very fetotoxic in pregnant women and its use in breastfeeding mothers should be avoided.

It is not known if everolimus is transferred into human milk. Everolimus and/or its metabolites passed to the milk of lactating rats at a concentration 3.5 times higher than in maternal serum. We recommend that the mother withhold breastfeeding for a minimum of 150 hours.

T 1/2	30 h	MW	958.22 Da	PB	74%
Tmax	1-2 h	RID		Vd	1.57 L/kg
Oral	30%	M/P		pKa	9.96

Adult Concerns: Fatigue, headache, fever, stomatitis, hypertension, diarrhea, anorexia, changes in liver and renal function, hematuria, hyperglycemia, changes in electrolytes, hypercholesterolemia, peripheral edema, skin reactions.

Adult Dose: Initial dose: 0.75 mg twice daily.

Pediatric Concerns:

Infant Monitoring: Withhold breastfeeding for a minimum of 150 hours.

Alternatives:

References:

1. Pharmaceutical manufacturers prescribing information.

EVOLOCUMAB

Trade: Repatha

Category: Monoclonal Antibody

LRC: L3 - No Data-Probably Compatible

Evolocumab is a monoclonal antibody used in combination with a statin medication to treat hyperlipidemia.[1] At this time there are no data regarding the transfer of this medication to human milk. Based on this medication's large molecular weight, it is unlikely to enter milk in clinically relevant concentrations. The low oral bioavailability of this protein also suggests little absorption in the infant's gut. In addition, the manufacturer reports that although human IgG is present in milk, IgG antibodies do not appear to enter the infant's circulation in clinically relevant amounts.

Despite the fact that the molecular weight of this medication is very large and the amount in breast milk is expected to be exceptionally low, there are no long-term data concerning the safety of using immune modulating medications in breastfeeding mothers. Further there are current data that suggest that other IgG drugs do transfer to milk, although minimally, and perhaps the breastfed infant. Therefore, some caution is recommended, especially in the colostral phase. Each woman should understand the benefits and risk of using this type of medication in lactation.

T 1/2	11-17 days	MW	144,000 Da	PB	
Tmax	3-4 days	RID		Vd	0.05 L/kg
Oral	Low to nil	M/P		pKa	

Adult Concerns: Dizziness, fatigue, hypertension, nausea, diarrhea, myalgia, influenza, bruising, infusion reactions, immunogenicity, hypersensitivity reactions.

Adult Dose: 140 mg subcutaneously once every 2 weeks.

Pediatric Concerns:

Infant Monitoring: Diarrhea, poor feeding/poor weight gain.

Alternatives:

References:

1. Pharmaceutical manufacturer product monograph, 2017.

EXEMESTANE

Trade: Aromasin

Category: Antineoplastic

LRC: L5 - No Data-Hazardous

Exemestane is an irreversible, steroidal aromatase inactivator. It acts as a false substrate for the aromatase enzyme, causing its inactivation. Exemestane significantly lowers circulating estrogen concentrations in women, and it is useful in the treatment of estrogen receptor-positive breast cancer.[1] After maximum plasma concentrations are reached, levels decline polyexponentially with a mean terminal half-life of about 24 hours. It is 90% bound to plasma proteins. No data are available on its transfer into human milk. Steroids in general do not transfer significantly, so exemestane levels in milk are probably low. However, this product works irreversibly. Any present in milk could potentially suppress estrogen levels in a breastfed infant. It is not advisable to breastfeed an infant while consuming this product. A withholding period of 5-7 days is recommended should the mother opt to discontinue taking this product and restart breastfeeding.

T 1/2	24 h	MW	296.4 Da	PB	90%
Tmax	1.2 h	RID		Vd	
Oral		M/P		pKa	

Adult Concerns: Anxiety, dizziness, trouble sleeping, nausea, vomiting, abdominal or stomach pain, constipation, diarrhea, loss of appetite, general feeling of discomfort or illness, general feeling of tiredness or weakness, hot flashes, increased sweating.

Adult Dose: 25 mg once daily.

Pediatric Concerns:

Infant Monitoring: Withhold breastfeeding for 5-7 days after use of this product.

Alternatives:

References:
1. Pharmaceutical manufacturers prescribing information.

EXENATIDE

Trade: Byetta, Bydureon

Category: Antidiabetic, other

LRC: L3 - No Data-Probably Compatible

Exenatide improves glycemic control in people with type-2 diabetes mellitus.[1] It enhances glucose-dependent insulin secretion by the pancreatic beta cell, suppresses glucagon secretion, and slows gastric emptying. Exenatide leads to an increase in both glucose-dependent synthesis of insulin, and in vivo secretion of insulin from pancreatic beta cells. Exenatide therefore promotes insulin release from beta cells in the presence of elevated glucose concentrations.

Exenatide is a 39-amino acid peptide and has a molecular weight of 4,186 Da which is far too large to enter milk in clinically relevant amounts. While it is reported to enter rodent milk at extremely low levels, we do not have human studies. The plasma levels of this product are extraordinarily low (picograms), and we would imagine the transfer to human milk is much lower. It would be unlikely that this product would enter milk in clinically relevant amounts, nor would it be orally bioavailable in infants. But as yet, we have no data in breastfeeding mothers and caution is recommended if this product is used.

T 1/2	2.4 h	MW	4186 Da	PB	
Tmax	2.1 h	RID		Vd	0.4 L/kg
Oral	Nil	M/P		pKa	

Adult Concerns: Dizziness, headache, dyspepsia, nausea, vomiting, diarrhea, feeling jittery.

Adult Dose: Highly variable, consult prescribing information.

Pediatric Concerns: None reported.

Infant Monitoring: Vomiting, diarrhea or constipation and signs of hypoglycemia- drowsiness, lethargy, pallor, sweating, tremor.

Alternatives:

References:
1. Pharmaceutical manufacturers prescribing information.

EZETIMIBE

Trade: Zetia

Category: Antihyperlipidemic

LRC: L3 - No Data-Probably Compatible

Ezetimibe reduces blood cholesterol by inhibiting the absorption of cholesterol from the small intestine.[1] It appears to act at the brush border of the small intestine and inhibits the absorption of cholesterol leading to a direct reduction in delivery of cholesterol to the liver. No data are available on the transfer of this agent to milk. Although this medication has a long half-life and is very lipophilic, it has high protein binding and a reasonably poor oral bioavailability so it is unlikely to produce significant levels in the milk or infant. However, it is not clear at all if it would be safe for use in a breastfed infant who needs high levels of cholesterol. Some caution is recommended until more data are available.

T 1/2	22 h	MW	409 Da	PB	>90%
Tmax	4-12 h	RID		Vd	
Oral	35-60%	M/P		pKa	9.48

Adult Concerns: Viral infection, headache, fatigue, and gastrointestinal symptoms such as diarrhea and abdominal pain have been reported but these symptoms are rather low in incidence.

Adult Dose: 10 mg daily.

Pediatric Concerns: No data available on transfer to human milk. Some caution is recommended.

Infant Monitoring: Weight gain, growth.

Alternatives: Cholestyramine salts.

References:
1. Pharmaceutical manufacturers prescribing information.

FAMCICLOVIR

Trade: Famvir

Category: Antiviral

LRC: L3 - No Data-Probably Compatible

Famciclovir is an antiviral agent used in the treatment of uncomplicated herpes zoster infection (shingles) and genital herpes. It is rapidly metabolized to the active metabolite, penciclovir. Although similar to acyclovir, no data are available on levels in human milk. Oral bioavailability of famciclovir (77%) is much better than acyclovir (15-30%). Studies with rodents suggest that the milk/plasma ratio is greater than 1.[1] Because famciclovir provides few advantages over acyclovir, at this point acyclovir would probably be preferred in a nursing mother although the side-effect profile is still minimal with this product.

T 1/2	2-4 h	MW	321 Da	PB	<20%
Tmax	1 h	RID		Vd	0.91-1.25 L/kg
Oral	69-85%	M/P	>1	pKa	3.84

Adult Concerns: Headache, dizziness, fever, anorexia, nausea, diarrhea.

Adult Dose: 500 mg two to three times daily.

Pediatric Concerns: None reported via milk.

Infant Monitoring: Vomiting, diarrhea, weight gain.

Alternatives: Acyclovir(L2)

References:
1. Pharmaceutical manufacturers prescribing information.

FAMOTIDINE

Trade: Pepcid, Pepcid AC

Category: Gastric Acid Secretion Inhibitor

LRC: L1 - Limited Data-Compatible

Famotidine is a typical histamine-2 receptor antagonist that reduces stomach acid secretion. In one study of eight lactating women receiving 40 mg/day, the peak concentration in breast milk was 72 µg/L and occurred at 6 hours postdose.[1] The milk/plasma ratios were 0.41, 1.78, and 1.33 at 2, 6, and 24 hours, respectively.

T 1/2	2.5-3.5 h	MW	337 Da	PB	15-20%
Tmax	1-3 h	RID	1.9%	Vd	0.94-1.33 L/kg
Oral	40-45%	M/P	0.41-1.78	pKa	9.29

Adult Concerns: Headache, dizziness, diarrhea or constipation.

Adult Dose: 20-40 mg twice daily.

Pediatric Concerns: None reported. Pediatric indications are available.

Infant Monitoring:

Alternatives: Ranitidine(L2)

References:
1. Courtney TP, Shaw RW, Cedar E, et al. Excretion of famotidine in breast milk. Br J Clin Pharmacol. 1988;26:639.

FEBUXOSTAT

Trade: Adenuric, Uloric

Category: Antigout

LRC: L3 - No Data-Probably Compatible

Febuxostat is a xanthine oxidase (XO) inhibitor indicated for the chronic management of hyperuricemia in patients with gout. It is not known whether this drug is excreted in human milk. Due to its high protein binding and somewhat low oral bioavailability, minimal amounts are expected to enter breast milk. Febuxostat is transferred in the milk of rats.[1] Until more is known, caution is recommended while administering this drug in lactating women. Initially, in adults, febuxostat may increase plasma concentrations of urate and uric acid, and treatment should not be started until an acute attack of gout has completely subsided; an NSAID or colchicine should be given for at least 6 months after starting febuxostat.[1]

T 1/2	5-8 h	MW	316.4 Da	PB	99%
Tmax	1 h	RID		Vd	
Oral	49%	M/P		pKa	

Adult Concerns: Nausea, changes in liver function, arthralgias.

Adult Dose: 40-80 mg per day.

Pediatric Concerns:

Infant Monitoring:

Alternatives:

References:
1. Pharmaceutical manufacturers prescribing information.

FELBAMATE

Trade: Felbatol

Category: Anticonvulsant

LRC: L4 - No Data-Possibly Hazardous

Felbamate is an oral antiepileptic agent for partial seizures and Lennox-Gastaut syndrome. Due to serious side effects, the FDA recommends that felbamate be given only to patients with serious seizures refractory to all other medications. Felbamate is known to be secreted in rodent milk and was detrimental to their offspring.[1] No data are available on the transfer of this drug to human milk. Due to the incidence of severe side effects, extreme caution is recommended with this medication in breastfeeding mothers.

T 1/2	20-23 h	MW	238 Da	PB	25%
Tmax	1-4 h	RID		Vd	0.7-1 L/kg
Oral	90%	M/P		pKa	14.98

Adult Concerns: Aplastic anemia, weight gain, flu-like symptoms, tachycardia, nausea, vomiting, headache, insomnia.

Adult Dose: 1200 mg per day in 3-4 divided doses.

Pediatric Concerns: None reported, but caution is urged.

Infant Monitoring: Sedation or irritability, not waking to feed/poor feeding and weight gain, nausea, vomiting, insomnia.

Alternatives:

References:
1. Pharmaceutical manufacturers prescribing information.

FELODIPINE

Trade: Agon SR, Plendil, Plendil ER, Renedil

Category: Calcium Channel Blocker

LRC: L3 - No Data-Probably Compatible

Felodipine is a calcium channel antagonist structurally related to nifedipine.[1] No data are available on the transfer of this drug into human milk. Because we have numerous studies on others in this family, it is advisable to use nifedipine or others that have breastfeeding studies available.

T 1/2	11-16 h	MW	384 Da	PB	>99%
Tmax	2.5-5 h	RID		Vd	
Oral	20%	M/P		pKa	<1

Adult Concerns: Headache, fatigue, dizziness, hypotension, arrhythmias, flushing, edema, constipation.

Adult Dose: 2.5-10 mg daily.

Pediatric Concerns: None reported via milk at this time.

Infant Monitoring: Drowsiness, lethargy, pallor, poor feeding, and weight gain.

Alternatives: Nifedipine(L2), Nimodipine(L2), Verapamil(L2)

References:
1. Pharmaceutical manufacturers prescribing information.

FENOFIBRATE

Trade: Tricor

Category: Antihyperlipidemic

LRC: L3 - No Data-Probably Compatible

Fenofibrate reduces total cholesterol, LDL cholesterol, and triglycerides.[1] No data are available on its transfer into human milk; however, agents that reduce plasma cholesterol are not usually considered suitable for use in breastfeeding mothers. Milk levels of cholesterol are higher because the newborns need high levels of cholesterol for neurodevelopment. Some caution is recommended at this time.

T 1/2	20 h	MW	361 Da	PB	99%
Tmax		RID		Vd	
Oral	85%	M/P		pKa	

Adult Concerns: Headache, abdominal pain, constipation, back pain, elevated liver function tests, changes in renal function, elevated CPK, urticaria.

Adult Dose: 160 mg per day.

Pediatric Concerns: None reported via milk, but this agent should be used with care in breastfeeding mothers due to the infants need for cholesterol.

Infant Monitoring: Weight gain, growth.

Alternatives:

References:
1. Pharmaceutical manufacturers prescribing information.

FENOLDOPAM

Trade: Corlopam

Category: Antihypertensive

LRC: L3 - No Data-Probably Compatible

Fenoldopam is a dopamine agonist used to treat severe hypertension in both adults and children.[1] It is not known whether this drug transfers into milk. Further, dopamine agonists are known to suppress prolactin release from the pituitary, so some concern exists for the use of this product in breastfeeding mothers as prolactin suppression could cause a decrease in milk production. However, its brief half-life would preclude large quantities from entering the milk compartment.

T 1/2	5 min	MW	305 Da	PB	
Tmax		RID		Vd	0.6 L/kg
Oral		M/P		pKa	9.71

Adult Concerns: Headache, dizziness, flushing hypotension, arrhythmias, nausea, changes in liver function and renal, hyperglycemia, hypokalemia.

Adult Dose: Do not exceed 1.6 µg/kg/minute.

Pediatric Concerns: In children, the most common adverse effects were hypotension and tachycardia. This medication is used in children aged <1 month to age 12 at doses of up to 0.8 µg/kg/minute for severe hypertension.

Infant Monitoring: Drowsiness, lethargy, pallor, poor feeding, and weight gain.

Alternatives:

References:
1. Pharmaceutical manufacturers prescribing information.

FENTANYL

Trade: Duragesic, Lazanda, Onsolis, Sublimaze, Subsys

Category: Analgesic

LRC: L2 - Limited Data-Probably Compatible

Fentanyl is a potent narcotic analgesic used (IV, IM, transdermally) during labor and delivery. When used parenterally, its half-life is exceedingly short.[1] The transfer of fentanyl into human milk has been documented but is low.

In a group of 10 women receiving a total dose of 50 to 400 µg fentanyl IV during labor, the concentration of fentanyl in milk was generally below the level of detection (<0.05 ng/mL).[2] In a few samples, the levels were between 0.05 and 0.15 ng/mL. Using this data, an infant would ingest less than 3% of the weight-adjusted maternal dose per day.

In another study of 13 women who received 2 µg/kg IV after delivery and cord clamping, fentanyl concentration in colostrum was extremely low.[3] Peak colostrum concentrations occurred at 45 minutes following intravenous administration and averaged 0.4 µg/L. Colostrum levels dropped rapidly and were undetectable after 10 hours. The authors conclude that with these small concentrations and fentanyl's low oral bioavailability, intravenous fentanyl analgesia may be used safely in breastfeeding women. The relatively low level of fentanyl found in human milk is presumably a result of the short maternal half-life, and the rather rapid redistribution out of the maternal plasma compartment. It is apparent that fentanyl transfer to milk under most clinical conditions is poor and is probably clinically unimportant.

In a study of 5 women undergoing surgery with midazolam premedication and induction with propofol and fentanyl, milk samples were obtained at 5, 7, 9, 11, and 24 hours post fentanyl administration.[4] These women were on average 11 weeks postpartum and produced about 325 mL/day of milk. The median amount of fentanyl recovered in milk within 24 hours post-dose was 0.024 µg or 0.024% of the maternal dose (100 µg). The weight-normalized infant dose was 0.005 µg/kg. None of the infants were given their mothers' milk during this study.

In addition, there is one case report of a woman receiving a transdermal fentanyl patch, 100 µg/hour, for chronic pain throughout pregnancy and lactation.[5] Within 24 hours of birth her infant was started on morphine for treatment of opioid withdrawal, this infant's morphine treatment continued for 29 days in the NICU. Breast milk was given to the infant starting two weeks postpartum when the mother's postpartum pain medication regimen returned to baseline (fentanyl patch alone at 100 µg/hour). On day 27 of life, the infant's blood and maternal milk was sampled;

the infant's blood was undetectable for both fentanyl and its metabolite norfentanyl (sensitivity 0.1 ng/mL). The mother's milk had 6.4 µg/L of fentanyl and 6.2 µg/L of norfentanyl. The author of this case report estimated that the average 1-month-old, ingesting 200 mL/kg of milk/day, would receive about 1.3 µg/kg/day of fentanyl in milk.

T 1/2	2-4 h (IV)	MW	336 Da	PB	80-85%
Tmax		RID	2.9% - 5%	Vd	4-6 L/kg
Oral	50-75%	M/P		pKa	8.4

Adult Concerns: Sedation, respiratory depression/apnea, hypotension, bradycardia, nausea, vomiting, constipation.

Adult Dose: 25-35 µg IV every 30-60 min as needed.

Pediatric Concerns: None reported via milk at this time.

Infant Monitoring: Sedation, slowed breathing rate, pallor, constipation, and appropriate weight gain.

Alternatives: Sufentanil.

References:

1. Madej TH, Strunin L. Comparison of epidural fentanyl with sufentanil. Analgesia and side effects after a single bolus dose during elective caesarean section. Anaesthesia. 1987;42(11):1156-1161.
2. Leuschen MP, Wolf LJ, Rayburn WF. Fentanyl excretion in breast milk. Clin Pharm. 1990;9(5):336-337.
3. Steer PL, Biddle CJ, Marley WS, Lantz RK, Sulik PL. Concentration of fentanyl in colostrum after an analgesic dose. Can J Anaesth. March 1992;39(3):231-235.
4. Nitsun M, Szokol JW, Saleh HJ, et al. Pharmacokinetics of midazolam, propofol, and fentanyl transfer to human breast milk. Clin Pharmacol Ther. 2006;79(6):549-557.
5. Cohen RS. Fentanyl transdermal analgesia during pregnancy and lactation. J Hum Lact. August 2009;25(3):359-361.

FENUGREEK

Trade:

Category: Herb

LRC: L3 - Limited Data-Probably Compatible

Fenugreek is commonly sold as the dried, ripe seed and extracts are used as an artificial flavor for maple syrup.[1] The seeds contain from 0.1 to 0.9% diosgenin.[2] Several coumarin compounds have been noted in the seed as well as a number of alkaloids such as trigonelline, gentianin, and carpaine. The seeds also contain approximately 8% of a foul-smelling oil. Fenugreek has been noted to reduce plasma cholesterol in animals when 50% of their diet contained fenugreek seeds.[3] The high fiber content may have accounted for this change although it may be due to the steroid saponins. A hypoglycemic effect has also been noted. When added to the diet of diabetic dogs, a decrease in insulin dose and hyperglycemia was noted.[4] It is not known if these changes are due to the fiber content of the seeds or a chemical component. Fenugreek has been reported to increase the anticoagulant effect of warfarin.[5]

In a group of 10 women (non-placebo controlled) with infants born between 24 to 38 weeks gestation (mean=29 weeks) who ingested 3 fenugreek capsules 3 times daily (Nature's Way) for a week, the average milk production during the week increased significantly from a mean of 207 mL/day (range 57-1057 mL) to 464 mL/day (range 63-1140 mL).[6] No untoward effects were reported.

In a study of 26 mothers of preterm infants (less than 31 weeks gestation) compared the use of fenugreek, 1725 mg (3 tablets) 3 times daily for 21 days to a placebo. Mothers initiated pumping within 12 hours of delivery and kept a daily record. Prolactin levels were drawn weekly and were not significantly changed. Data analysis revealed no statistical difference between the mothers receiving fenugreek or those receiving placebo in terms of milk volume. No adverse effects were noted in mothers or infants.[7] This study suggests that fenugreek is probably ineffective.

When dosed in moderation, fenugreek has limited toxicity and is listed in the US as a GRAS herbal (Generally Regarded As Safe). A maple syrup odor via urine and sweat is commonly reported. Higher doses may produce hypoglycemia although this is largely unsubstantiated. Fenugreek's reputation as a galactagogue is widespread but undocumented. The transfer of fenugreek into milk is unknown, untoward effects have only rarely been reported.

Allergic reactions have been reported in patients sensitive to chickpeas and peanuts.[8]

Adult Concerns: Maple syrup odor in urine and sweat. Diarrhea, hypoglycemia.

Adult Dose: 6 grams per day.

Pediatric Concerns: Maple syrup odor of infant urine; one case of suspected gastrointestinal bleeding in a premature infant has been reported.

Infant Monitoring: Maple syrup odor in urine.

Alternatives: Metoclopramide(L2), Domperidone(L3)

References:
1. DerMarderosian A, Beutler JA. The Review of Natural Products (Facts and Comparisons). St Louis, MO: Wolters Kluwer Health; 2014.
2. Sauvaire Y, Baccou JC. Extraction of diosgenin, (25R)-spirost-5-ene-3beta-ol; problems of the hydrolysis of the saponins. Lloydia. 1978;41:247.
3. Valette G, Sauvaire Y, Baccou JC, Ribes G. Hypocholesterolaemic effect of fenugreek seeds in dogs. Atherosclerosis. 1984;50(1):105-111.
4. Ribes G, Sauvaire Y, Baccou JC, et al. Effects of fenugreek seeds on endocrine pancreatic secretions in dogs. Ann Nutr Metab. 1984;28(1):37-43.
5. Lambert JP, Cormier A. Potential interaction between warfarin and boldo-fenugreek. Pharmacotherapy. 2001;21(4):509-512.
6. Swafford S, Berens P. Effect of fenugreek on breast milk production. Abstract 5th International Meeting of the Academy of Breastfeeding Medicine; September 11-13, 2000; Tucson, Ariz: Academy of Breastfeeding Medicine News and Views; 2000;6(3).
7. Reeder C, Legrand A, O'Conner-Von S. The effect of fenugreek on milk production and prolactin levels in mothers of premature infants. J Human Lact. 2011:27:74. Abstract.
8. Patil SP, Niphadkar PV, Bapat MM. Allergy to fenugreek (Trigonella foenum graecum). Ann Allergy Asthma Immunol. 1997;78(3):297-300.

FERRIC OXIDE

Trade:

Category: Antipruritic

LRC: L1 - No Data-Compatible

Ferric oxide is an iron salt used topically as an astringent/antipruritic agent. Absorption topically is negligible. Commonly found in Calamine lotion along with zinc oxide, it used as an antipruritic and astringent agent to treat various conditions such as sunburn, eczema, poison ivy, insect stings, and other skin irritations.

T 1/2	6 h	MW	159 Da	PB	
Tmax	2 h	RID		Vd	
Oral	10-35%	M/P		pKa	

Adult Concerns: Topically applied, observe for irritation and pain.

Adult Dose:

Pediatric Concerns:

Infant Monitoring:

Alternatives:

References:

FERROUS FUMARATE

Trade: PalaFeR, Iron

Category: Metals

LRC:

Ferrous fumarate is a form of iron salt that is commonly found in over-the-counter dietary supplements, both alone and in combination with other vitamins. It is used to treat iron deficiency anemia. The secretion of iron salts in breast milk appears to be very low, although the bioavailability of iron present in milk is high. According to the American Academy of Pediatrics the average intake of iron in a healthy term breastfed infant is about 0.27 mg/day through 6 months of age.[1] This was determined by the average concentration of iron in breast milk (0.35 mg/L) and the average milk intake of a healthy term infant (0.78 L/day).[1] Furthermore, most infants do not require iron supplementation before 6 months of age and at this time iron-rich complementary foods can be slowly introduced.[2] There are some infants that may be at higher risk of iron deficiency and require supplementation earlier, these infants are often premature, small for gestational age, have inadequate iron stores at birth, or are suffering from a hematologic disorder.

The American Food and Nutrition Board recommends that breastfeeding women have a dietary intake of 9-10 mg of elemental iron per day.[3] The use of relatively high doses in iron deficient, breastfeeding mothers is probably suitable. Iron transports very poorly into the milk compartment and thus supplementation is unlikely to increase milk iron levels. Iron supplements are generally regarded as safe by the U.S. Food and Drug Administration and are commonly used by postpartum women.[4]

*Note that the dosage of commercially available iron salts (e.g. ferrous gluconate, ferrous sulfate, etc.) is expressed both in terms of the parent compound and the quantity of elemental iron delivered.

T 1/2		MW	170 Da	PB	
Tmax		RID		Vd	
Oral	10-90%	M/P		pKa	

Adult Concerns: Nausea, vomiting, abdominal pain, diarrhea, constipation.

Adult Dose: 35-200 mg of elemental iron per day.

Pediatric Concerns: None reported via milk.

Infant Monitoring: Constipation, diarrhea.

Alternatives:

References:
1. Baker RD, Greer FR, The Committee on Nutrition. Diagnosis and prevention of iron deficiency and iron deficiency anemia in infants and young children (0-3 years of age). Pediatrics. 2010;126:1040-1050.
2. American Academy of Pediatrics. Breastfeeding and the use of human milk. Pediatrics. 2005;115(2):496-506.
3. Food and Nutrition Board, Institute of Medicine, National Academies. Dietary Reference Intakes for Vitamin A, Vitamin K, Arsenic, Boron, Chromium, Copper, Iodine, Iron, Manganese, Molybdenum, Nickel, Silicon, Vanadium, and Zinc. Washington, DC: National Academies Press; 2001. www.nap.edu.
4. SCOGS Report #35. Select Committee on GRAS Substances: U.S. Food and Drug Administration; 1980.

FERROUS GLUCONATE

Trade: Ferate, Fergon, Iron

Category: Metals

LRC:

Ferrous gluconate is a form of iron salt that is commonly found in over-the-counter dietary supplements, both alone and in combination with other vitamins. It is used to treat iron deficiency anemia. The secretion of iron salts in breast milk appears to be very low, although the bioavailability of iron present in milk is high. According to the American Academy of Pediatrics the average intake of iron in a healthy term breastfed infant is about 0.27 mg/day through 6 months of age.[1] This was determined by the average concentration of iron in breast milk (0.35 mg/L) and the average milk intake of a healthy term infant (0.78 L/day).[1] Furthermore, most infants do not require iron supplementation before 6 months of age and at this time iron-rich complementary foods can be slowly introduced.[2] There are some infants that may be at higher risk of iron deficiency and require supplementation earlier, these infants are often premature, small for gestational age, have inadequate iron stores at birth, or are suffering from a hematologic disorder.

The American Food and Nutrition Board recommends that breastfeeding women have a dietary intake of 9-10 mg of elemental iron per day.[3] The use of relatively high doses in iron deficient, breastfeeding mothers is probably suitable. Iron transports very poorly into the milk compartment and thus supplementation is unlikely to increase milk iron levels. Iron supplements are generally regarded as safe by the U.S. Food and Drug Administration and are commonly used by postpartum women.[4]

*Note that the dosage of commercially available iron salts (e.g. ferrous gluconate, ferrous sulfate, etc.) is expressed both in terms of the parent compound and the quantity of elemental iron delivered.

T 1/2		MW	448 Da	PB	
Tmax		RID		Vd	
Oral	10-90%	M/P		pKa	

Adult Concerns: Nausea, vomiting, abdominal pain, diarrhea, constipation.

Adult Dose: 35-200 mg of elemental iron per day.

Pediatric Concerns: None reported via milk.

Infant Monitoring: Constipation, diarrhea.

Alternatives:

References:
1. Baker RD, Greer FR, The Committee on Nutrition. Diagnosis and prevention of iron deficiency and iron deficiency anemia in infants and young children (0-3 years of age). Pediatrics. 2010;126:1040-1050.
2. American Academy of Pediatrics. Breastfeeding and the use of human milk. Pediatrics. 2005;115(2):496-506.

3. Food and Nutrition Board, Institute of Medicine, National Academies. Dietary Reference Intakes for Vitamin A, Vitamin K, Arsenic, Boron, Chromium, Copper, Iodine, Iron, Manganese, Molybdenum, Nickel, Silicon, Vanadium, and Zinc. Washington, DC: National Academies Press; 2001. www.nap.edu.
4. SCOGS Report #35. Select Committee on GRAS Substances: U.S. Food and Drug Administration; 1980.

FERROUS SULFATE

Trade: Feosol, Fer-In-Sol, Feratab, Slow-Fe, Iron

Category: Metals

LRC:

Ferrous sulfate is a form of iron salt that is commonly found in over-the-counter dietary supplements, both alone and in combination with other vitamins. It is used to treat iron deficiency anemia. The secretion of iron salts in breast milk appears to be very low, although the bioavailability of iron present in milk is high. According to the American Academy of Pediatrics the average intake of iron in a healthy term breastfed infant is about 0.27 mg/day through 6 months of age.[1] This was determined by the average concentration of iron in breast milk (0.35 mg/L) and the average milk intake of a healthy term infant (0.78 L/day).[1] Furthermore, most infants do not require iron supplementation before 6 months of age and at this time iron-rich complementary foods can be slowly introduced.[2] There are some infants that may be at higher risk of iron deficiency and require supplementation earlier, these infants are often premature, small for gestational age, have inadequate iron stores at birth, or are suffering from a hematologic disorder.

The American Food and Nutrition Board recommends that breastfeeding women have a dietary intake of 9-10 mg of elemental iron per day.[3] The use of relatively high doses in iron deficient, breastfeeding mothers is probably suitable. Iron transports very poorly into the milk compartment and thus supplementation is unlikely to increase milk iron levels. Iron supplements are generally regarded as safe by the U.S. Food and Drug Administration and are commonly used by postpartum women.[4]

*Note that the dosage of commercially available iron salts (e.g. ferrous gluconate, ferrous sulfate, etc.) is expressed both in terms of the parent compound and the quantity of elemental iron delivered.

T 1/2		MW	152 Da	PB	
Tmax		RID		Vd	
Oral	10-90%	M/P		pKa	

Adult Concerns: Nausea, vomiting, abdominal pain, diarrhea, constipation.

Adult Dose: 35-200 mg of elemental iron per day.

Pediatric Concerns: None reported via milk.

Infant Monitoring: Constipation, diarrhea.

Alternatives:

References:
1. Baker RD, Greer FR, The Committee on Nutrition. Diagnosis and prevention of iron deficiency and iron deficiency anemia in infants and young children (0-3 years of age). Pediatrics. 2010;126:1040-1050.
2. American Academy of Pediatrics. Breastfeeding and the use of human milk. Pediatrics. 2005;115(2):496-506.
3. Food and Nutrition Board, Institute of Medicine, National Academies. Dietary Reference Intakes for Vitamin A, Vitamin K, Arsenic, Boron, Chromium, Copper, Iodine, Iron, Manganese, Molybdenum, Nickel, Silicon, Vanadium, and Zinc. Washington, DC: National Academies Press; 2001. www.nap.edu.
4. SCOGS Report #35. Select Committee on GRAS Substances: U.S. Food and Drug Administration; 1980.

FERUMOXYTOL

Trade: Feraheme

Category: Mineral Supplement

LRC: L3 - No Data-Probably Compatible

Ferumoxytol is a uniquely formulated injectable iron replacement product. It consists of iron oxide within a carbohydrate shell.[1] This distinctive formulation allows the drug to pass through the extracellular compartment undeterred and enter the macrophages of the liver, spleen, and bone marrow where eventually iron oxide is released to become a part of the storage iron pool. Iron may also be transferred from here into the plasma to be incorporated into hemoglobin. This unique design makes it effective for the treatment of iron deficiency anemia due to chronic kidney disease.

There are currently no studies on its transfer to human milk. Ferumoxytol is an iron-carbohydrate complex. It is polar and non lipid-soluble. Following intravenous injection, it is primarily confined to the intravascular space. It is highly unlikely that ferumoxytol would enter breast milk or be orally bioavailable in the infant.

T 1/2	9.3-15 h	MW	750,000 Da	PB	
Tmax	0.32 h	RID		Vd	0.045 L/kg
Oral		M/P		pKa	

Adult Concerns: Dizziness, hypotension, nausea, diarrhea, constipation, peripheral edema, rash, serious hypersensitivity reactions.

Adult Dose: 2 doses of 510 mg IV, 3-8 days apart.

Pediatric Concerns: No known adverse reactions via milk at this time. Product has been used in the pediatric population.[2]

Infant Monitoring:

Alternatives: Iron sucrose(L2)

References:
1. Pharmaceutical manufacturers prescribing information.
2. Hassan N, Cahill J, Rajasekaran S, Kovey K. Ferumoxytol infusion in pediatric patients with gastrointestinal disorders: first case series. Ann Pharmacother. December 2011;45(12):e63. Epub November 24, 2011.

FESOTERODINE

Trade: Toviaz

Category: Anticholinergic

LRC: L3 - No Data-Probably Compatible

Fesoterodine is an antimuscarinic agent used in the treatment of overactive bladder dysfunction.[1] It is rapidly metabolized in vivo to produce its active metabolite tolterodine. Tolterodine is a muscarinic anticholinergic agent similar in effect to atropine but is more selective for the bladder. Tolterodine levels in milk have been reported in mice; offspring exposed to extremely high levels had slightly reduced body weight gain, but no other untoward effects. While it is more selective for the bladder, adverse effects including blurred vision, constipation, and dry mouth have still occurred in adults. While we have no data on human milk, it is unlikely concentrations will be high enough to produce untoward effects in infants.

T 1/2	7 h	MW	527.66 Da	PB	50%
Tmax	5 h	RID		Vd	2.41 L/kg
Oral	52%	M/P		pKa	

Adult Concerns: Insomnia, dry eyes, dry mouth, constipation, changes in liver enzymes, urinary retention.

Adult Dose: 4-8 mg once daily.

Pediatric Concerns: No data at this time.

Infant Monitoring: Insomnia, dry mouth, constipation, urinary retention, weight gain.

Alternatives:

References:
1. Pharmaceutical manufacturers prescribing information.

FEXOFENADINE

Trade: Allegra, Allegra Allergy 12 Hour, Allegra Allergy 24 Hour, Allegra ODT

Category: Antihistamine

LRC: L2 - Limited Data-Probably Compatible

Fexofenadine is a non-sedating histamine-1 receptor antagonist and is the active metabolite of terfenadine. It is indicated for symptoms of allergic rhinitis and other allergies. Unlike terfenadine, no cardiotoxicity has been reported with this product. In a study of four women receiving 60 mg/day terfenadine, no terfenadine was found in milk.[1]

However, the metabolite (fexofenadine) was present in small amounts. The average milk level of fexofenadine was 41 µg/L while the maternal plasma averaged 309 ng/mL. The time to peak for milk was 4.3 hours and the half-life in milk was 14.2 hours. The AUC0-12 was 320 ng/hr/mL for milk and 1,590 ng/hr/mL for plasma. The authors estimate that only 0.45% of the weight-adjusted maternal dose would be ingested by the infant.

T 1/2	14.4 h	MW	538 Da	PB	60-70%
Tmax	2.6 h	RID	0.5% - 0.7%	Vd	
Oral	Complete	M/P	0.21	pKa	4.04

Adult Concerns: Drowsiness, fatigue, headache, dry mouth, throat irritation, dyspepsia, nausea.

Adult Dose: 60 mg twice daily.

Pediatric Concerns: None reported.

Infant Monitoring: Drowsiness, fatigue.

Alternatives:

References:
1. Lucas BD Jr, Purdy CY, Scarim SK, Benjamin S, Abel SR, Hilleman DE. Terfenadine pharmacokinetics in breast milk in lactating women. Clin Pharmacol Ther. 1995;57(4):398-402.

FIDAXOMICIN

Trade: Dificid

Category: Antibiotic, Macrolide

LRC: L3 - No Data-Probably Compatible

Fidaxomicin is a macrolide antibiotic used for the treatment of Clostridium difficile infection.[1] Following oral ingestion, this antibiotic acts locally in the gastrointestinal tract against C. difficile, with minimal systemic absorption. There are currently no studies on the transfer of this drug or its active metabolite into human milk. But a review of its pharmacokinetic properties suggests that transfer to breast milk would be minimal, if any transfer does occur, absorption from the infant's gut should be minimal due to low oral bioavailability. However, until more established data is available, it is advisable to use this drug with caution in breastfeeding women.

T 1/2	11.7 h (11.2 h for metabolite)	MW	1,058 Da	PB	
Tmax	1-5 h	RID		Vd	
Oral	Minimal	M/P		pKa	

Adult Concerns: Nausea, vomiting, abdominal pain, anemia. Bowel obstruction and gastrointestinal hemorrhage are rare side effects.

Adult Dose: 200 mg twice daily for 10 days.

Pediatric Concerns:

Infant Monitoring: Vomiting, diarrhea, changes in gastrointestinal flora, and rash.

Alternatives: Metronidazole(L2), Vancomycin(L1)

References:
1. Pharmaceutical manufacturers prescribing information.

FILGRASTIM

Trade: Granix, Neupogen, Nivestim, Ratiograstim, Zarzio, Neulasta

Category: Hematopoietic

LRC: L4 - No Data-Possibly Hazardous

Filgrastim is a Granulocyte Colony Stimulating Factor (GCSF) that can be used for numerous indications; however, one of its main indications is to decrease the risk of infection and duration of neutropenia in those with non-myeloid malignancies receiving myelosuppressive chemotherapy.[1]

At this time, there are no data regarding the transfer of filgrastim to human milk; however, there is one case report of lenograstim (exogenous GCSF product) used in lactation. A 30-year-old breastfeeding mother (4 months post-partum) was a peripheral blood stem cell transplant donor for her sister; this woman was given lenograstim 300 µg/day sc on day 1 and then 600 µg/day sc on days 2-4 after she stopped breastfeeding.[2] On day 4 the WBC increased rapidly so her dose was decreased back to 300 µg/day for days 5 and 6. The GCSF was measured in this patient's milk before and after she was given lenograstim. Before administration the level of GCSF was <5 pg/mL; the peak level after administration occurred at 6 days and was 85.7 pg/mL.

One breastfeeding mother received subcutaneous injections of filgrastim at 600 µg on day 1, 300 µg twice daily on days 2-5, and 300 µg once on day 6. G-CSF levels were determined in her 25-day-old infant.[3] G-CSF levels were measured once daily just before the first dose of each day. G-CSF levels were detectable (>10 ng/L) in milk 12 hours post injection. Milk levels peaked at 188 ng/L at 22 hours after the initial injection, and slowly declined after 43 hours to undetectable levels at 79 hours.

The oral absorption of filgrastim is unlikely. In one case of oral administration of filgrastim at 100 µg daily for 5 days, filgrastim was not absorbed.[4]

T 1/2	3.5 h sc; 3.85 h IV	MW	18,800 Da	PB	
Tmax	2-8 h sc	RID		Vd	0.15 L/kg
Oral	Nil	M/P		pKa	

Adult Concerns: Headache, fever, cough, shortness of breath, Adults Respiratory Distress Syndrome (ARDS), changes in liver function, bone pain, malaise, injection site reactions.

Adult Dose: 5-10 µg/kg once daily subcutaneously or IV.

Pediatric Concerns: No reports of infants exposed to filgrastim in lactation are available at this time. Pediatric data exists for children greater than 7 months of age.

Infant Monitoring: Irritability, unexplained fever, difficulty breathing; if clinical suspicion of adverse effects a CBC or LFTs could be drawn.

Alternatives:

References:

1. Pharmaceutical manufacturers prescribing information.
2. Shibata H, Yamane T, Aoyama Y, et al. Excretion of granulocyte colony stimulating factor into human breast milk. Acta Haematol. 2003;110:200-201.
3. Kaida K, Ikegame K, Fujioka T, et al. Kinetics of granulocyte colony-stimulating factor in the human milk of a nursing donor receiving treatment for mobilization of the peripheral blood stem cells. Acta Haematol. 2007;118(3):176-177. Epub October 3, 2007.
4. Calhoun DA, Maheshwari A, Christensen RD. Recombinant granulocyte colony-stimulating factor administered enterally to neonates is not absorbed. Pediatrics. August 2003;112(2):421-423.

FINGOLIMOD

Trade: Gilenya

Category: Immune Modulator

LRC: L5 - No Data-Hazardous

Fingolimod is an immune modulator and prodrug that binds to the surface of lymphocytes and redirects them from the blood and graft sites to the lymph nodes, thus reducing the immune response in patients with Multiple Sclerosis (MS).[1] It reportedly assists in the repair of brain glial and precursor cells following injury in this syndrome. Fingolimod reportedly slows the progression of disability and reduces the frequency and severity of symptoms in patients with MS. While it decreases the heart rate, it increases the risk of infection and raises liver enzymes. Asthmatic patients may have an increase in the use of their rescue inhalers. The most common side effects include headache, flu, diarrhea, back pain, abnormal liver enzymes, and cough. It is unknown if fingolimod passes into human breast milk, but it is excreted in rat milk.[2] Due to its high volume of distribution and high protein binding, levels in human milk are expected to be be low.

However, several deaths have been reported, and the FDA has recommended that all patients starting fingolimod treatment be monitored for signs of bradycardia for at least 6 hours after the first dose. The FDA is now recommending hourly pulse and blood pressure monitoring for all patients starting treatment, with electrocardiogram monitoring prior to dosing and at the end of the observation period; monitoring should continue until any symptoms resolve. The period should extend past 6 hours in patients at higher risk, in some cases overnight. This product is hazardous and breastfeeding is not recommended.

T 1/2	6-9 days	MW	307.5 Da	PB	99.7%
Tmax	12-16 h	RID		Vd	17.4 L/kg
Oral	93%	M/P		pKa	

Adult Concerns: Headache, flu, diarrhea, back pain, abnormal liver enzymes, cough, macular edema, weakness, dizziness, bradycardia, hypertension.

Adult Dose: 0.5 mg daily.

Pediatric Concerns:

Infant Monitoring: Breastfeeding is not recommended.

Alternatives:

References:

1. Kappos L, Comi AJ, Montalban X, et al. Oral fingolimod (FTY720) for relapsing multiple sclerosis. N Engl J Med. September 14, 2006;355(11):1124-1140.
2. Pharmaceutical manufacturers prescribing information.

FLAVOXATE

Trade: Urispas

Category: Renal-Urologic Agent

LRC: L3 - No Data-Probably Compatible

Flavoxate is used as an antispasmodic to provide relief of painful urination, urgency, nocturia, urinary frequency, or incontinence.[1] It exerts a direct smooth muscle relaxation on the bladder wall and has been used in children for enuresis. No data are available on its transfer to human milk.

T 1/2	<10 h	MW	391 Da	PB	
Tmax	2 h	RID		Vd	
Oral	Complete	M/P		pKa	7.3

Adult Concerns: Drowsiness, dry mouth and throat, nervousness, headache, confusion, nausea, vomiting, blurred vision. Do not use with pyloric or duodenal obstruction, gastrointestinal hemorrhage, or obstructive uropathies.

Adult Dose: 100-200 mg three to four times daily.

Pediatric Concerns: None reported via milk.

Infant Monitoring: Drowsiness, dry mouth, vomiting.

Alternatives:

References:

1. Pharmaceutical manufacturers prescribing information.

FLECAINIDE ACETATE

Trade: Tambocor

Category: Antiarrhythmic

LRC: L3 - Limited Data-Probably Compatible

Flecainide is a potent antiarrhythmic used to suppress dangerous ventricular arrhythmias. In a group of 11 breast-feeding mothers receiving 100 mg oral flecainide (mean 3.2 mg/kg/day) every 12 hours for 5.5 days beginning 1 day postpartum, apparent steady-state levels of flecainide in both milk and plasma were achieved in most cases by day 4 of the study.[1] Highest daily average concentration of flecainide in milk ranged from 270 to 1,529 µg/L (mean 953 µg/L) for the 11 subjects. Mean milk/plasma ratios were 3.7, 3.2, 3.5, and 2.6 on study days 2, 3, 4, and 5 respectively. After the last dose of flecainide, peak milk levels of the drug occurred at 3 to 6 hours and then declined mono-exponentially. The half-life for elimination of flecainide from milk was 14.7 hours and is very similar to the plasma elimination half-life of flecainide in healthy human subjects.

Based on the pharmacokinetics of flecainide in infants, the expected average steady-state plasma concentration of flecainide in a newborn infant consuming all of the milk production of its mother (approximately 700 mL/day at the highest flecainide level of 1,529 µg/L), the average daily intake by the infant would be 1.07 mg. In a normal 4-kg infant, the average plasma concentration in a breastfed infant would not be expected to exceed about 62 ng/mL. The average plasma level in infants treated with therapeutic doses is 360 ng/mL. In another study of one patient receiving 100 mg every 12 hours, milk levels of flecainide averaged 0.99 mg/L on day 4 and 5 postpartum.[2]

Levels of flecainide in milk are moderate to very low. Some caution is recommended.

T 1/2	12-22 h	MW	414 Da	PB	50%
Tmax	4.5 h	RID	4.9% - 5.2%	Vd	
Oral	90%	M/P	2.6-3.7	pKa	9.3

Adult Concerns: Dizziness, blurred vision, dyspnea, arrhythmias, heart failure, nausea, vomiting. Flecainide should be reserved for patients with life-threatening arrhythmias. Withdrawal from flecainide therapy should be gradual due to the possibility of fatal cardiac arrest.

Adult Dose: 50-100 mg twice daily.

Pediatric Concerns: No adverse effects yet reported via milk.

Infant Monitoring: Drowsiness, lethargy, changes in sleep, changes in vision, pallor, poor feeding, weight gain.

Alternatives:

References:
1. McQuinn RL, Pisani A, Wafa S, et al. Flecainide excretion in human breast milk. Clin Pharmacol Ther. 1990;48(3):262-267.
2. Wagner X, Jouglard J, Moulin M, Miller AM, Petitjean J, Pisapia A. Coadministration of flecainide acetate and sotalol during pregnancy: lack of teratogenic effects, passage across the placenta, and excretion in human breast milk. Am Heart J. 1990;119(3 pt 1):700-702.

FLIBANSERIN

Trade: Addyi

Category: Hypoactive sexual desire disorder

LRC: L4 - No Data-Possibly Hazardous

Flibanserin is indicated for the treatment of premenopausal women with acquired, generalized hypoactive sexual desire disorder (HSDD) as characterized by low sexual desire.[1] Its exact mechanism of action is currently unknown; however, it is known to be a 5-HT1A agonist, 5HT2A antagonist and moderate antagonist at 5-HT2B, 5-HT2C and dopamine D4 receptors. There are no data regarding the transfer of this medication to human milk or its safety in lactation. The manufacturer does report that it enters rodent milk. Based on this medication's moderate molecular weight, high protein binding and poor oral bioavailability high concentrations in milk are not anticipated. Until lactation data is available, caution is recommended with the use of this product.

T 1/2	11 h	MW	390.4 Da	PB	98%
Tmax	0.75 - 4 h	RID		Vd	
Oral	33%	M/P		pKa	

Adult Concerns: Dizziness, drowsiness, fatigue, insomnia, anxiety, dry mouth, nausea, abdominal pain, constipation. Major drug reaction with alcohol with severe low blood pressure resulting. DO NOT USE ALCOHOL WITH THIS DRUG.

Adult Dose: 100 mg once daily at bedtime.

Pediatric Concerns: No data in lactation at this time.

Infant Monitoring: Drowsiness, insomnia, irritability, vomiting, constipation, poor weight gain. Severe hypotension in mother if consumed with alcohol.

Alternatives:

References:
1. Pharmaceutical manufacturer prescribing information.

FLUCELVAX

Trade:

Category: Vaccine

LRC: L3 - No Data-Probably Compatible

Flucelvax is the only egg-free influenza vaccine approved by the FDA. The 0.5 ml intramuscular inactivated vaccine is made by Novartis and is administered to adults 18 and older to prevent infection of influenza A and B virus subtypes.

The manufacturer advises caution to those that have displayed Guillain-Barre syndrome within 6 weeks of a previous influenza vaccine as well as those with a latex allergy as the tip of the prefilled syringe contains rubber latex. It is contraindicated in individuals with an allergy to any component of the vaccine.

The vaccine has a 55% efficacy in all culture-confirmed influenza cases as compared to placebo.[1]

Adult Concerns: Pain and redness at injection site, headache, fatigue, myalgia, and malaise. Adverse reactions include; pain (28%) and redness (13%) at the injection site, headache (13%), fatigue, myalgia (11%), and malaise (10%).[1]

Adult Dose:

Pediatric Concerns:

Infant Monitoring:

Alternatives:

References:
1. http://www.novartisvaccinesdirect.com/pdf/Flucelvax_PI.pdf
2. http://www.fda.gov/downloads/BiologicsBloodVaccines/Vaccines/ApprovedProducts/UCM332069.pdf

FLUCLOXACILLIN

Trade: Flopen, Floxapen, Flu-Amp, Flu-Clomix, Flucil, Fluclox, Flucloxacillin, Magnapen, Staphylex

Category: Antibiotic, Penicillin

LRC: L1 - Limited Data-Compatible

Flucloxacillin, is a penicillinase-resistant penicillin frequently used for resistant staphylococcal infections. Only trace amounts are secreted in human milk.[1] Its congener, cloxacillin, is commonly used to treat mastitis in breastfeeding mothers and has been used in thousands of breastfeeding patients without problem. Changes in gut flora are possible but unlikely.

T 1/2	1.5 h	MW	454 Da	PB	94%
Tmax	1 h	RID		Vd	0.11 L/kg
Oral	50%	M/P		pKa	2.7

Adult Concerns: Nausea, vomiting, diarrhea, constipation, skin rashes; hemolytic anemia and interstitial nephritis have been reported rarely.

Adult Dose: 250-500 mg four times daily.

Pediatric Concerns: None reported via milk.

Infant Monitoring: Vomiting, diarrhea, changes in gastrointestinal flora, and rash.

Alternatives: Cloxacillin(L2), Dicloxacillin(L2)

References:
1. Pharmaceutical manufacturers prescribing information.

FLUCONAZOLE

Trade: Diflucan

Category: Antifungal

LRC: L2 - Limited Data-Probably Compatible

Fluconazole is a synthetic triazole antifungal agent and is frequently used for vaginal, oropharyngeal, and esophageal candidiasis. Many of the triazole antifungals (itraconazole, terconazole) have similar mechanisms of action and are considered fungistatic in action. In vivo studies have found fluconazole to have fungistatic activity against a variety of fungal strains including *Candida albicans*, *C. tropicalis*, *C. glabrata*, and *C. neoformans*. The pharmacokinetics are similar following both oral and IV administration. The drug is almost completely absorbed orally (>90%). Peak plasma levels occur in 1-2 hours after oral administration.

Fluconazole is transferred to human milk with a milk/plasma ratio of approximately 0.85.[1] Following a single 150 mg dose, milk levels at 2, 5, 24 and 48 hours were reported to be 2.93, 2.66, 1.76, and 0.98 µg/mL respectively.

Maternal plasma levels at 2, 5, 24, and 48 hours were 6.4, 2.79, 2.52, and 1.19 μg/mL respectively.[1] The plasma half-life of fluconazole is 35 hours and its breast milk half-life is 30 hours. From these data, and assuming an average milk level of 2.3 mg/L, an infant consuming 150 mL/kg/day of milk would receive an average of 0.34 mg/kg/d of fluconazole or 16% of the weight-adjusted maternal dose, and less than 5.8% of the pediatric dose (6 mg/kg/day).

In another study of one patient receiving 200 mg daily (1.5 times the above dose) for 18 days, the peak milk concentration was 4.1 mg/L at 2 hours following the dose.[2] However, the mean concentration of fluconazole in milk was not reported. Taken together, these two studies suggest a relative infant dose of 16 - 22% of the maternal dose.

T 1/2	30 h	MW	306 Da	PB	11-12%
Tmax	1-2 h	RID	16.4% - 21.5%	Vd	0.6 L/kg
Oral	>90%	M/P	0.46-0.85	pKa	1.76

Adult Concerns: Headache, dizziness, QTc prolongation, nausea, vomiting, diarrhea, abdominal pain, changes in liver function, hypokalemia, skin rashes.

Adult Dose: 50-200 mg daily.

Pediatric Concerns: No complications from exposure to breast milk have been reported.

Infant Monitoring: Vomiting, diarrhea.

Alternatives:

References:
1. Force RW. Fluconazole concentrations in breast milk. Pediatr Infect Dis J. 1995;14(3):235-236.
2. Schilling CG, Seay RE, Larson TA, et al. Excretion of fluconazole in human breast milk (abstract # 130). Pharmacotherapy. 1993;13:287.

FLUCYTOSINE

Trade: Ancobon

Category: Antifungal

LRC: L4 - No Data-Possibly Hazardous

Flucytosine is an antifungal medication used in the treatment of Candida and Cryptococcus UTI's, meningitis, pulmonary infections, and systemic infections. Flucytosine is often combined with amphotericin B in systemic infections due to emergence of resistant strains to flucytosine alone. There are no studies on transfer of flucytosine to breast milk. Due to the low protein binding (2-4%), small molecular weight (129.1 Da), and high oral bioavailability (78-89%), a moderate amount of the drug will be expected to be transferred to milk. A small amount of flucytosine (4%) may be metabolized to 5-fluorouracil. Due to the side effects of flucytosine, breastfeeding is not recommended with this drug. The half-life increases with decreasing renal function. The oral dose in neonates is 25-100 mg/kg/day; adult dose 50-150 mg/kg/day divided q 6 hours. Target trough levels are 25-50 mg/L and peak levels 50-100 mg/L. This product is probably too hazardous to use in breastfeeding women.[1-3]

T 1/2	3-8 h	MW	129.1 Da	PB	2-4 %
Tmax	2 h (PO) faster if IV	RID		Vd	0.6 L/kg
Oral	78-89 %	M/P		pKa	2.9

Adult Concerns: Hepatotoxicity, bone marrow suppression, fatigue, hypoglycemia, hypokalemia, vomiting, diarrhea, abdominal pain, chest pain, rash.

Adult Dose: 50-150 mg/kg/day.

Pediatric Concerns:

Infant Monitoring: Not recommended in lactation; if used in lactation, infant plasma drug levels should be monitored along with renal function, hepatic function, and bone marrow function.

Alternatives:

References:
1. Pharmaceutical manufacturers prescribing information.
2. Daneshmend TK, Warnock DW. Clinical pharmacokinetics of systemic antifungaldrugs. Clin Pharmacokinet. January-February 1983;8(1):17-42.
3. Vermes A, Guchelaar HJ, Dankert J. Flucytosine: a review of its pharmacology, clinical indications, pharmacokinetics, toxicity and drug interactions. J Antimicrob Chemother. August 2000;46(2):171-179.

FLUDEOXYGLUCOSE F 18

Trade: Fludeoxyglucose F 18, F18, Sodium Fluoride-18

Category: Diagnostic Agent, Radiopharmaceutical Imaging

LRC: L4 - Limited Data-Possibly Hazardous

Fludeoxyglucose F 18 (FDG) is a positron-emitting radiopharmaceutical used in conjunction with positron emission tomography (PET Scanning) to detect alterations in tissue glucose metabolism and is useful in detecting brain tumors, certain malignancies, chronic coronary artery disease, partial epilepsy, and Alzheimer's disease.[1-3] FDG, as a glucose analog, is taken up by high-glucose-metabolizing cells throughout the body. About 75% is sequestered within the cell until metabolized or decayed. The radioactive Fluorine-18 decays rapidly within the cell with a half-life of 110 minutes. About 20% of the dose is rapidly cleared renally by 2 hours. The urine is therefore radioactive for several hours after administration of this isotope. Thus, about 20% of the dose is rapidly cleared from the body. Only 80% remains to decay. By 24 hours (13 half-lives) only 1 part in 8200 parts of the initial radiation remains.[4] In five half-lives, about 98.5% would be decayed away. Fludeoxyglucose F 18 is rapidly distributed to all parts of the body that have significant glucose metabolism, including the breast.

In a group of six lactating women, who received between 50-160 MBq FDG, amounts reported in milk were very low.[5] Decay-corrected activity measurable in breast milk ranged from 5.54 to 19.3 Bq/mL/MBq injected. Interestingly, the levels in breast tissue were quite high, but this product seems to be sequestered in lactocytes in breast tissue without penetrating into milk. The calculated maximum cumulative dose to the infant, 0.085 mSv with no interruption of breastfeeding, is well below the recommended limit of 1 mSv. Indeed, a higher radiation dose is received by the infant from close contact with the breast than from ingestion of radioactive milk. The authors suggest pumping of the milk and feeding in bottles by another individual to reduce direct exposure to radiation.

International Commission of Radiological Protection (ICRP) recommends no breastfeeding interruption; however, close contact restriction of a few hours is recommended (see radiopharmaceutical breastfeeding and close contact restriction table).[6,7] The half-life of the F-18 is short, only 110 minutes. Due to concentration in some tissues such as the bladder, radiation exposure could be a problem and emptying of the breast at routine intervals "might" help reduce radiation exposure to breast tissue. The USPDI (1994) recommends interruption of breastfeeding for 12-24 hours. At 9 hours, 98.5% of the radioisotope remaining in the tissues would be decayed away.[8] It is likely that after 9 hours, almost all radioisotope would be decayed to almost background levels.

In another recent study of a woman who received 222 MBq of F-18 FDG, and who was breastfeeding only on one side, the uptake of F-18 was clearly evident but only on the side from which the mother breastfed. No estimates of dose in milk were reported.[9]

Recommend pumping and dumping of breast milk after the procedure for at least 4-9 hours to minimize radiation.[6] Because the infant receives more radiation from close contact with the breast, close contact should probably be avoided for about 4 hours and minimized close contact for the next 10 hours, due to release of gamma radiation from the mother.

T 1/2	110 min	MW	181.3 Da	PB	
Tmax		RID		Vd	
Oral	Complete	M/P		pKa	

Adult Concerns: Hypersensitivity reactions- itching, edema and rash.

Adult Dose: 185 to 370 MBq IV.

Pediatric Concerns: None reported, but possible radiation exposure if breastfed prior to 9 hours after dose. Avoid direct contact with mothers' skin before 9 hours.

Infant Monitoring:

Alternatives:

References:

1. Jamieson D, Alavi A, Jolles P, Chawluk J, Reivich M. Positron emission tomography in the investigation of central nervous system disorders. Radiol Clin North Am. 1988;26(5):1075-1088.
2. Jones SC, Alavi A, Christman D, Montanez I, Wolf AP, Reivich M. The radiation dosimetry of 2 [F-18] fluoro-2-deoxy-D-glucose in man. J Nucl Med. 1982;23(7):613-617.
3. Som P, Atkins HL, Bandoypadhyay D, et al. A fluorinated glucose analog, 2-fluoro-2-deoxy-D-glucose (F-18): nontoxic tracer for rapid tumor detection. J Nucl Med. 1980;21(7):670-675.
4. Fludeoxyglucose F-18, http://en.wikipedia.org/wiki/Fludeoxyglucose_(18F).
5. Hicks RJ, Binns D, Stabin MG. Pattern of uptake and excretion of (18)F-FDG in the lactating breast. J Nucl Med. August 2001;42(8):1238-1242.

6. Leide-Svegborn S. Radiation exposure of patients and personnel from a PET/CT procedure with 18F-FDG. Radiat Prot Dosimetry. April-May 2010;139(1-3):208-213. Epub February 18, 2010.

7. ICRP. Radiation dose to patients from radiopharmaceuticals - addendum 3 to ICRP publication 53. ICRP publication 106. Ann ICRP. 2008;38(1-2):1-197.

8. Gupta RK, Tripathi M, Sahoo MK, et al. Asymmetrical F-18 flurorodeoxyglucose uptake in the breasts: a dilemma solved by patient history. Indian J Nucl Med. January-March 2016;31(1):83-84. doi:10.4103/0972-3919.172377.

FLUDROCORTISONE

Trade: Florinef, Myconef

Category: Corticosteroid

LRC: L3 - No Data-Probably Compatible

Fludrocortisone is a halogenated derivative of hydrocortisone with very potent mineralocorticoid activity and is generally used to treat Addison's disease.[1,2] Although its glucocorticoid effect is 15 times more potent than hydrocortisone, it is primarily used for its powerful ability to retain sodium in the vascular compartment (mineralocorticoid activity). It is not known if fludrocortisone penetrates into milk but if it is similar to other corticosteroids, it is very unlikely that the amount in milk would be clinically relevant until extremely high doses are used; caution is recommended.

T 1/2	3.5 h	MW	380 Da	PB	42%
Tmax	1.7 h	RID		Vd	
Oral	Complete	M/P		pKa	12.55

Adult Concerns: Hypertension, sodium retention, cardiac hypertrophy, congestive heart failure, and headache.

Adult Dose: 0.1-0.4 mg daily.

Pediatric Concerns: None via milk.

Infant Monitoring: Feeding, growth, and weight gain.

Alternatives:

References:
1. Pharmaceutical manufacturers prescribing information.
2. DrugBank, 2019.

FLUMAZENIL

Trade: Anexate, Romazicon, Antabenz

Category: Antidote

LRC: L3 - No Data-Probably Compatible

Flumazenil is a benzodiazepine receptor antagonist that blocks the effect of benzodiazepines on the CNS. Flumazenil may be considered suitable for use in lactation as this medication has a very short half-life. When administering this medication to a breastfeeding client for a benzodiazepine overdose, breastfeeding may need to be withheld due to the amount of benzodiazepine in milk, and the potential risk of adverse effects in the breastfeeding infant (respiratory depression, sedation). This may require 12-24 hours interruption to allow maternal levels of benzodiazepine to decline. Flumazenil would be minimally absorbed (16%) orally by a breastfed infant.

T 1/2	4-11 min	MW	303 Da	PB	50%
Tmax	6-10 min	RID		Vd	0.5 L/kg
Oral	16%	M/P		pKa	1.7

Adult Concerns: Dizziness, agitation, anxiety, flushing/sweating, palpitations, shortness of breath, vasodilation, dry mouth, vomiting.

Adult Dose: 0.2 mg IV, with repeated doses as needed.

Pediatric Concerns: None reported at this time.

Infant Monitoring: In infants tolerant to benzodiazepines, may cause acute hyperreactivity reactions to this benzodiazepine blocker. This could include seizures.

Alternatives:

References:

1. Pharmaceutical manufacturer prescribing information.

FLUNARIZINE

Trade: Sibelium

Category: Calcium Channel Blocker

LRC: L4 - No Data-Possibly Hazardous

Flunarizine is a calcium channel blocker primarily indicated for use in migraine headache prophylaxis and peripheral vascular disease. It has a very long half-life and a huge volume of distribution, which contributes to the long half-life.[1] No data are available on the transfer of this product to human milk. However, due to its incredibly long half-life and high volume of distribution, it is possible that this product, over time, could build up and concentrate in a breastfed infant. Other calcium channel blockers may be preferred. Use with extreme caution.

T 1/2	19 days	MW	404 Da	PB	99%
Tmax	2-4 h	RID		Vd	43.2 L/kg
Oral	Complete	M/P		pKa	7.7

Adult Concerns: Extrapyramidal symptoms in elderly patients, depression, porphyria, thrombophlebitis, drowsiness, headache, dizziness.

Adult Dose: 10 mg daily.

Pediatric Concerns: None reported via milk, but caution is advised.

Infant Monitoring: Drowsiness, lethargy, pallor, poor feeding, and weight gain.

Alternatives: Nifedipine(L2), Nimodipine(L2), Verapamil(L2)

References:

1. Pharmaceutical manufacturers prescribing information.

FLUNISOLIDE

Trade: Aerobid, Bronalide, Nasalide, Rhinalar, Syntaris

Category: Corticosteroid

LRC: L3 - No Data-Probably Compatible

Flunisolide is a potent corticosteroid used to reduce airway hyperreactivity in asthmatics. It is also available for intranasal use for allergic rhinitis. Generally, only small levels of flunisolide are absorbed systemically (about 40%) thereby reducing systemic effects and presumably breast milk levels as well.[1] After inhalation of 1 mg, systemic availability was only 40% and plasma level was 0.4-1 ng/mL. Adrenal suppression in children has not been documented even after therapy of 2 months with 1,600 μg/day. Once absorbed, flunisolide is rapidly removed from the plasma compartment by first-pass uptake in the liver. Although no data on breast milk levels are yet available, it is unlikely that the level secreted in milk is clinically relevant.

T 1/2	1.8 h	MW	435 Da	PB	
Tmax	30 min	RID		Vd	1.8 L/kg
Oral	21% (oral)	M/P		pKa	13.73

Adult Concerns: Irritation due to vehicle, not drug itself. Loss of taste, nasal irritation, flu-like symptoms, sore throat, headache.

Adult Dose: 1 mg daily.

Pediatric Concerns: None reported. Can be used in children down to age 6.

Infant Monitoring: Feeding, growth, and weight gain.

Alternatives:

References:

1. Pharmaceutical manufacturers prescribing information.

FLUNITRAZEPAM

Trade: Rohypnol

Category: Sedative-Hypnotic

LRC: L4 - No Data-Possibly Hazardous

Flunitrazepam is a prototypic benzodiazepine. Frequently called the "Date Rape Pill," it induces rapid sedation and significant amnesia, particularly when mixed with alcohol.[1,2] Effects last about 8 hours. It is recommended for adult insomnia and for pediatric preanesthetic sedation. Due to its long half-life of 20 to 30 hours and being highly orally bioavailable, flunitrazepam should not be used routinely during lactation.

T 1/2	20-30 h	MW	313 Da	PB	80%
Tmax	2 h	RID		Vd	3.6 L/kg
Oral	80-90%	M/P		pKa	1.8

Adult Concerns: Drowsiness, amnesia, sedation, ataxia, headache, memory impairment, tremors.

Adult Dose: 2 mg daily.

Pediatric Concerns: None reported via milk.

Infant Monitoring: Sedation, slowed breathing rate, not waking to feed/poor feeding, and weight gain (see other benzodiazepine alternatives).

Alternatives:

References:
1. Kanto J, Erkkola R, Kangas L, Pitkanen Y. Placental transfer of flunitrazepam following intramuscular administration during labour. Br J Clin Pharmacol. 1987;23(4):491-494.
2. Kanto J, Kangas L, Leppanen T. A comparative study of the clinical effects of oral flunitrazepam, medazepam, and placebo. Int J Clin Pharmacol Ther Toxicol. 1982;20(9):431-433.

FLUOCINOLONE

Trade: Capex Shampoo, Dermotic, Flucort-N, Retisert, Synalar

Category: Corticosteroid

LRC: L3 - No Data-Probably Compatible

Fluocinolone acetonide is a corticosteroid primarily used topically to reduce skin inflammation and relieve itching.[1] It is a synthetic hydrocortisone derivative. Typical dosage strength is 0.01 - 0.025%. Fluocinolone is a corticosteroid primarily intended for topical use. It is considered a medium-potency steroid. Following topical application to the skin, only a small amount is systemically absorbed. No data are currently available of its use in breastfeeding women. It is unlikely fluocinolone would be excreted into human milk in clinically relevant levels following topical administration.

T 1/2		MW		PB	>90%
Tmax		RID		Vd	
Oral		M/P		pKa	13.35

Adult Concerns: Contact dermatitis, dry skin, pruritus, erythema, atrophy of skin, shiny skin, papules, hypopigmentation. May cause systemic adverse effects if used on large area, under occlusive dressing, and broken skin. Systemic side effects: HPA axis suppression, secondary infections.

Adult Dose: Apply on affected areas 2-4 times daily.

Pediatric Concerns:

Infant Monitoring: Feeding, growth and weight gain.

Alternatives:

References:
1. Pharmaceutical manufacturers prescribing information.

FLUOCINOLONE + HYDROQUINONE + TRETINOIN

Trade: Tri-Luma

Category: Dermatologic Agents

LRC: L3 - No Data-Probably Compatible

This combination drug product is indicated for the short-term intermittent treatment of moderate to severe melasma of the face. It is a combination drug product containing corticosteroid (fluocinolone), retinoid (tretinoin), and bleaching agent (hydroquinone).

Percutaneous absorption of unchanged tretinoin, hydroquinone, and fluocinolone acetonide into the systemic circulation of two groups of healthy volunteers (total n=59) was found to be minimal following 8 weeks of daily topical application of 1 g (Group I, n=45) or 6 g (Group II, n=14) of fluocinolone + hydroquinone + tretinoin. For tretinoin, quantifiable plasma concentrations were obtained in 57.78% (26 out of 45) of Group I and 57.14% (8 out of 14) of Group II subjects. The exposure to tretinoin as reflected by the C_{max} values ranged from 2.01 to 5.34 ng/mL (Group I) and 2.0 to 4.99 ng/mL (Group II). Thus, daily topical application of this combination drug product resulted in a minimal increase of normal endogenous levels of tretinoin. The circulating tretinoin levels represent only a portion of total tretinoin-associated retinoids, which would include metabolites of tretinoin and that sequestered into peripheral tissues. For hydroquinone, quantifiable plasma concentrations were obtained in 18% (8 out of 44) of Group I subjects. The exposure to hydroquinone as reflected by the C_{max} values ranged from 25.55 to 86.52 ng/mL. All Group II subjects (6 g dose) had postdose plasma hydroquinone concentrations below the quantifiable limit. For fluocinolone acetonide, Groups I and II subjects had all postdose plasma concentrations below quantifiable limits.

We do not have specific data on this combination product, but levels of the individual products are not high and milk levels will be much lower. However, caution is still recommended and a risk:benefit analysis must justify its use in breastfeeding mothers.

T ½	Fluo/hydro/tret: / /2 h	MW	Fluo/hydro/tret: 452.49/110.11/300 Da	PB	Fluo/hydro/tret: >90%/
Tmax		RID		Vd	Fluo/hydro/tret:/ /0.44 L/kg
Oral		M/P		pKa	Fluo/hydro/tret: 13.35/9.96/4.79

Adult Concerns: Erythema, desquamation, burning, dryness, and pruritus at the site of topical application. The hydroquinone content may occasionally cause a blue-black pigmentation of skin at the site of application known as ochronosis.

Adult Dose:

Pediatric Concerns: No reports in the literature. Risks are moderate to low.

Infant Monitoring:

Alternatives:

References:
1. Pharmaceutical manufacturers prescribing information.

FLUORESCEIN

Trade: Fluor-I-Strip, Fluorescein sodium, Fluorescite, Fluorets, Ful-Glo, Funduscein-10, Ophthifluor

Category: Disclosing Agent

LRC: L4 - Limited Data-Possibly Hazardous

Sodium fluorescein is a yellow, water-soluble dye. A 2% fluorescein ophthalmic solution or an impregnated fluorescein strip is used topically to detect corneal abrasions, for fitting of hard contact lenses, and intravenously for fluorescein angiography.

Fluorescein is used in two ways. One, in which a small amount is added directly to the eye generally by ophthalmologists and optometrists, and secondly, when much larger quantities are administered intravenously (5 mL of 10% solution). In a study of one patient who received an intravenous dose of fluorescein (5 mL of 10% fluorescein=500 mg), breast milk levels were monitored for over 76 hours.[1] Concentrations of 372 μg/L at 6 hours and 170 μg/L at 76 hours after the dose were reported. In this patient, the half-life of fluorescein in breast milk appeared quite long, approximating 62 hours. While the authors conclude that this is a high dose via milk, in another patient who received slightly more (910 mg IV), the patient's plasma levels of fluorescein monoglucuronide were 37,000 μg/L.[2]

Using this data, it would appear that an approximation of the milk/plasma ratio would be about 0.018, which suggests that very little of the absolute maternal dose enters milk. Nevertheless, fluorescein-induced phototoxicity remains a possibility in an infant fed breast milk containing sodium fluorescein. One case of severe fluorescein phototoxicity has been reported in an infant receiving fluorescein intravenously.[2] If the infant is not undergoing phototherapy, it would appear that there is little risk to a breastfeeding infant.

The ophthalmic use of fluorescein is probably quite safe in breastfeeding women, as plasma levels are insignificant. The intravenous use of high doses of fluorescein is of concern. Patients who receive IV doses should be warned to pump and discard milk for up to 7 days to allow for clearance of rather prolonged levels of fluorescein in the plasma compartment and milk of the mother.

T 1/2	62 h (IV)	MW	376 Da	PB	70-85%
Tmax	1 h	RID	0.8%	Vd	0.5 L/kg
Oral	50%	M/P		pKa	9.32

Adult Concerns: Fluorescein-induced phototoxicity following IV fluorescein. Nausea, vomiting, dizziness, syncope, pruritus, seizures, following IV therapy. Severe reactions are rare. Oral fluorescein appears to elicit very few adverse reactions.

Adult Dose: 500 mg IV.

Pediatric Concerns: None reported via milk, but avoid phototherapy if used.

Infant Monitoring: Observe for phototoxicity if extensively exposed to light, particularly phototherapy for hyperbilirubinemia.

Alternatives:

References:
1. Maquire AM, Bennett J. Fluorescein elimination in human breast milk. Arch Ophthalmol. 1988;106(6):718-719.
2. Kearns GL, Williams BJ, Timmons OD. Fluorescein phototoxicity in a premature infant. J Pediatr. 1985;107(5):796-798.

FLUORIDE

Trade:

Category: Cariostatic

LRC: L2 - Limited Data-Probably Compatible

Fluoride is an essential element required for bone and teeth development. It is available as salts of sodium and stannic (tin). Excessive levels are known to stain teeth irreversibly. One study shows breast milk levels of 0.024-0.172 ppm in milk (mean=0.077 ppm) of a population exposed to fluoridated water (0.7 ppm).[1]

In another study of breastfeeding women from areas low and rich in fluoride, milk fluoride levels were similar.[2] The mean fluoride concentration was 0.36 µmol/L for colostrum and 0.37 µmol/L for mature milk in the region with 1 ppm fluoride enriched water. In the region with 0.2 ppm fluoride, the mean fluoride concentration of colostrum was 0.28 µmol/L. There was no statistical difference in any of these milk fluoride levels.

One randomized controlled trial compared a group of women (n=85) who took a food supplement containing fluoride 1,500 µg/L per dose to a control group (n=83) given a placebo dose.[3] The area in which the women were recruited from was known to have a low fluoride content in the water. After 6 weeks the fluoride group had a statistically significantly higher amount of fluoride in milk compared to the placebo group (515 µg/L vs 476 µg/L). The fluoride group also had a statistically significant increase in their own milk concentration of fluoride (468 µg/l to 515 µg/L). The authors of this study believe their results confirm that there may be a plasma-milk barrier that regulates excessive amounts of fluoride from entering milk.

T 1/2	6 h	MW	19 Da	PB	
Tmax		RID		Vd	0.5-0.7 L/kg
Oral	90% (Na)	M/P		pKa	3.15

Adult Concerns: Stained enamel, nausea, allergic rash.

Adult Dose: 0.7 mg/L in drinking water.

Pediatric Concerns: No known adverse effects in breastfed infants at this time.

Infant Monitoring:

Alternatives:

References:
1. Latifah R, Razak IA. Fluoride levels in mother's milk. J Pedod. 1989;13(2):149-154.
2. Spak CJ, Hardell LI, De Chateau P. Fluoride in human milk. Acta Paediatr Scand. 1983;72(5):699-701.
3. Campus G, Congiu G, Cocco F, et al. Fluoride content in breast milk after the use of fluoridated food supplement. A randomized clinical trial. Am J Dent. 2014;27:199-202.

FLUOROURACIL

Trade: 5FU, Adrucil, Carac, Cytosafe, Effluderm, Efudex, Fluoroplex

Category: Antineoplastic, Dermatological

LRC: L4 - Limited Data-Possibly Hazardous

Fluorouracil (5-FU) is a uracil analog used to treat a number of cancers.[1] It is used topically for actinic keratosis, breast cancer, colorectal cancer, condyloma acuminatum, and many other cancers. Oral absorption is highly variable but averages less than 50-80%. Topical absorption through intact skin is less than 6-10%. Ninety percent of the dose is accounted for during the first 24 hours, following intravenous administration. Those receiving topical therapy would not need to discontinue breastfeeding, if the surface area is minimal. If large body areas were exposed to this therapy, significant absorption could occur.

With intravenous administration of fluorouracil, the mean half-life of elimination from plasma is approximately 16 minutes, with a range of 8-20 minutes, and is dose dependent. No intact drug can be detected in the plasma three hours after an intravenous injection.

A breastfeeding mother diagnosed with rectal cancer was treated with 5-flourouracil based chemoradiotherapy.[2] During treatment with 5-FU 200 mg/m^2/day the mother pumped and dumped her breast milk twice a day as she desired to continue breastfeeding her 9-month-old after treatment was completed. The four maternal 5-FU plasma samples ranged from 11.14 to 114.95 μmol. All 33 breast milk samples taken from before therapy initiation, throughout drug administration, and up to 10 days after treatment were undetectable. Based on the pharmacokinetics of this drug the authors were not surprised by this finding; however, they do suggest that this should be confirmed in additional breastfeeding women. In this case, the infant did not resume breastfeeding after maternal treatment was finished as the infant refused the breast.

Mothers receiving injected 5-FU (IV, IM, IP) should be advised to withhold breastfeeding for a minimum of 24 hours after exposure. 5-FU is also sometimes used intraocularly following retinal surgery. Animal studies suggest that retention in the vitreous humor is long lasting, thus the drug would be slowly released into the plasma compartment over several days. The doses here are small (5 mg) and are unlikely to produce significant plasma levels or milk levels of this drug.

T 1/2	16 min	MW	130 Da	PB	8-12%
Tmax	Immediate (IV)	RID		Vd	15.5 L/kg
Oral	0-80%	M/P		pKa	7.76

Adult Concerns: Nausea, vomiting, anorexia, blood dyscrasia, bone marrow suppression, myocardial toxicity, dyspnea, cardiogenic shock, rashes.

Adult Dose: 6-12 mg/kg injection (IV) daily.

Pediatric Concerns: None reported but caution is recommended.

Infant Monitoring: Wait 24 hours or more to largely reduce any risk.

Alternatives:

References:
1. Pharmaceutical manufacturers prescribing information.
2. Peccatori FA, Giovannetti E, Pistilli B, et al. "The only thing I know is that I know nothing": 5-fluorouracil in human milk. Ann Oncol. February 2012;23(2):543-544.

FLUOXETINE

Trade: Lovan, Prozac, Zactin

Category: Antidepressant, SSRI

LRC: L2 - Limited Data-Probably Compatible

Fluoxetine is a very popular serotonin reuptake inhibitor (SSRI) currently used for depression and a host of other syndromes. Fluoxetine absorption is rapid and complete, and the parent compound is rapidly metabolized to nor-fluoxetine, which is an active metabolite with a long half-life (360 hours).[1]

Both fluoxetine and norfluoxetine appear to permeate breast milk with a highly variable milk/plasma ratio (0.2-0.9). In one patient taking 20 mg/day, plasma levels of fluoxetine and norfluoxetine were 100.5 μg/L and 194.5 μg/L, respectively while levels in milk were 28.8 μg/L and 41.6 μg/L, respectively.[2] In another patient receiving 20 mg daily at bedtime, the milk concentration of fluoxetine was 67 μg/L and norfluoxetine 52 μg/L at 4 hours.[3] At 8 hours post-dose, the concentrations fell to 17 μg/L and 13 μg/L, respectively. Using this information, the authors estimated that the total daily dose to the infant was only 15-20 μg/kg per day. In another study of 10 breastfeeding women receiving 0.39 mg/kg/day of fluoxetine, the average breast milk levels for fluoxetine and norfluoxetine ranged from 24.4-181.1 μg/L and 37.4-199.1 μg/L, respectively.[4] Peak milk concentrations occurred within 6 hours. The milk/plasma ratios for fluoxetine and norfluoxetine were 0.88 and 0.72 respectively. Fluoxetine plasma levels in one infant were undetectable (<1 ng/mL). Based on these findings, an infant consuming 150 mL/kg/day of milk would be exposed to approximately 9.3-57 μg/kg/day total fluoxetine (and metabolite), which represents 5-9% of the maternal dose. No adverse effects were noted in the infants in this study.

In another case, severe colic, fussiness, and crying was reported.[5] The mother was receiving a dose of 20 mg fluoxetine per day. Concentrations of fluoxetine and norfluoxetine in breastmilk were 69 μg/L and 90 μg/L, respectively. The plasma levels in the infant for fluoxetine and norfluoxetine were 340 ng/mL and 208 ng/mL, respectively, which is almost twice that of normal maternal ranges. The author does not report the maternal plasma levels but suggests they were similar to Isenberg's adult levels (100.5 ng/mL and 194.5 ng/mL for fluoxetine and norfluoxetine). In this infant, the plasma levels would approach those of a mother receiving twice the above 20 mg dose per day (40 mg/day). The symptoms resolved upon discontinuation of fluoxetine by the mother.[5]

In another case, an infant exposed in utero and postpartum via milk to fluoxetine, carbamazepine, and buspirone had moderate plasma fluoxetine levels that continued to increased in the 3 weeks postpartum.[6] The infant's plasma levels of fluoxetine went from undetectable on day 13 to 61 ng/mL on day 21. The mean adult therapeutic range was 145 ng/mL. The infant in this study reportedly exhibited seizure-like activity at 3 weeks, 4 months, and 5 months of age. This activity was never witnessed by a healthcare provider or confirmed with diagnostic testing (including multiple EEGs and MRI). However, the mother reported three 60-90 second episodes in 1 hour at 3 weeks of life where the infant's "eyes rolled back, her upper limbs stretched out, and she became limp." At 4 months of age the mother reported 10-12 episodes a week where the infant became limp and unresponsive for a few seconds and then at 5.5 months of age the baby had peripheral cyanosis lasting 10-15 minutes. This study cautions that seizure-like activity and toxicity may occur in infants exposed to fluoxetine; however, the exact cause of the seizure-like episodes remains unknown and could be attributed to in utero medication exposure, one of the other medication exposures via breast milk or an underlying medical condition of the infant. In this case, the authors reported that the infant had normal development and no further episodes at 1 year of age.

Ilett reports that in a group of 14 women receiving 0.51 mg/kg/day fluoxetine, the mean M/P ratio was 0.67 (range 0.35 to 0.13) and 0.56 for norfluoxetine.[7] Mean total infant dose in fluoxetine equivalents was 6.8% of the weight-adjusted maternal dose. The reported infant fluoxetine and norfluoxetine plasma levels ranged from 20-252 μg/L and 17-187 μg/L, respectively.

Neonatal withdrawal syndrome was reported in one infant exposed in utero.[8] The mother was taking 20 mg/day and delivered at 27 weeks. The baby was treated with nasal CPAP and phenobarbital at a dose of 5 mg/kg/day because the symptoms were interpreted as convulsions. The clinical picture was interpreted as neonatal withdrawal syndrome.[8] In a similar case, the infant became comatose at 11 days postpartum with high plasma levels of norfluoxetine.[9] It is not known if these reported side effects (seizures, colic, fussiness, crying) are common, although this author has received numerous other personal communications similar to this.

Another case report of a preterm infant, born at 35 weeks, demonstrated toxicity from in utero exposure of maternal fluoxetine 40 mg daily.[10] At 4 hours of age, the infant was tachypneic and had signs of respiratory distress (grunting, nasal flaring, retractions). Antibiotics where initiated and a sepsis work-up was completed. The tachypnea resolved within 24 hours but the infant was found to be jittery and agitated. The infant was also noted to have seizure-like activity, with 3-4 episodes occurring by 36 hours of life. The infant exhibited an erythematous rash on both cheeks, petechiae on the abdomen, chest, and extremities, and scleral icterus. Although the seizure-like activity peaked at 5-8 episodes per day the skin changes resolved within 48-72 hours and the jitteriness and tremors decreased over time and resolved by 144 hours. The infant was discharged from hospital by 172 hours. Plasma levels of fluoxetine and norfluoxetine at 96 hours of age were 92 and 34 ng/mL, respectively, which is within the adult therapeutic range. This infant at 4 months of age had normal neurodevelopment. This case report describes fluoxetine toxicity from a neonatal adaptation perspective and is more likely to be due to in utero exposure than excessive drug exposure via breast milk.

The risk to newborns may be reduced by reducing or eliminating the use of SSRIs just prior to delivery, or switching to an alternate antidepressant while breastfeeding (sertraline, paroxetine, etc.). While we do not know the real risk of side effects, they are apparently low for the population. If the patient cannot tolerate switching to another antidepressant, then fluoxetine should be continued. Age at initiation of therapy is of importance. Use in older infants (4-6 months or older) is virtually without complications because they can metabolize and excrete the medication more rapidly. Data published in 1999 also suggest that weight gain in infants breastfed from mothers who were taking fluoxetine demonstrated a growth curve significantly below that of infants who were breastfed by mothers who did not take the drug. The average deficit in measurements taken between 2 and 6 months of age was 392 grams body weight. None of these infants were noted to have unusual behavior.[11]

An investigation was undertaken to study the effects of fluoxetine on the platelet 5-HT levels of the infant following lactational exposure to the drug.[12] Eleven mothers on 20-40 mg fluoxetine daily, along with their infants with ages ranging between 1 week to 6.5 months of age, were included in this study. 5-HT levels of maternal and infant plasma were assessed before taking the first fluoxetine dose, and then again at 4-12 weeks after initiation of fluoxetine therapy. It was found that although the 5-HT levels in the maternal plasma decreased by 9-28% after initiation of therapy while no such difference was noted in 10 of the infants' plasma studied. However, post-exposure 5-HT levels in one infant decreased by 40%, but these levels normalized 4 months later. No untoward effects were reported in any of the infants. The authors of this study concluded that while lactational exposure to fluoxetine 20-40 mg/day causes minimal changes in platelet 5-HT levels of most infants, some caution is still recommended with its use until more studies are done on this subject.

Current data on sertraline and escitalopram suggest these medications have difficulty entering milk, and more importantly, the infant. Therefore, they are preferred agents over fluoxetine for therapy of depression in breastfeeding mothers.[13] Women who can only take fluoxetine should be advised to continue breastfeeding and observe the infant for side effects. Fluoxetine therapy during breastfeeding is by no means contraindicated and has been used by many women.

T 1/2	2-3 days (fluoxetine)	MW	345 Da	PB	94.5%
Tmax	1.5 - 12 h	RID	1.6% - 14.6%	Vd	12-43 L/kg
Oral	100%	M/P	0.286-0.67	pKa	8.7

Adult Concerns: Nausea, tachycardia, hypotension, headache, anxiety, nervousness, insomnia, dry mouth, anorexia and visual disturbances.

Adult Dose: 20-60 mg daily.

Pediatric Concerns: Severe colic, fussiness, and crying have been reported in one case study.

Infant Monitoring: Sedation or irritability, not waking to feed/poor feeding, and weight gain.

Alternatives: Sertraline(L2), Escitalopram(L2)

References:

1. Pharmaceutical manufacturer prescribing information.
2. Isenberg KE. Excretion of fluoxetine in human breast milk. J Clin Psychiatry. April 1990;51(4):169.
3. Burch KJ, Wells BG. Fluoxetine/norfluoxetine concentrations in human milk. Pediatrics. April 1992;89(4 pt 1):676-677.
4. Taddio A, Ito S, Koren G. Excretion of fluoxetine and its metabolite, norfluoxetine, in human breast milk. J Clin Pharmacol. January 1996;36(1):42-47.
5. Lester BM, Cucca J, Andreozzi L, Flanagan P, Oh W. Possible association between fluoxetine hydrochloride and colic in an infant. J Am Acad Child Adolesc Psychiatry. November 1993;32(6):1253-1255.
6. Brent NB, Wisner KL. Fluoxetine and carbamazepine concentrations in a nursing mother/infant pair. Clin Pediatr. January 1998;37(1):41-44.
7. Kristensen JH, Ilett KF, Hackett LP, Yapp P, Paech M, Begg EJ. Distribution and excretion of fluoxetine and norfluoxetine in human milk. Br J Clin Pharmacol. October 1999;48(4):521-527.
8. Nordeng H, Lindemann R, Perminov KV, Reikvam A. Neonatal withdrawal syndrome after in utero exposure to selective serotonin reuptake inhibitors. Acta paediatrica (Oslo, Norway : 1992). March 2001;90(3):288-291.
9. Hale TW, Shum S, Grossberg M. Fluoxetine toxicity in a breastfed infant. Clinical Pediatrics. December 2001;40(12):681-684.
10. Mohan CG, Moore JJ. Fluoxetine toxicity in a preterm infant. J Perinatol. October-November 2000;20(7):445-446.
11. Chambers CD, Anderson PO, Thomas RG, et al. Weight gain in infants breastfed by mothers who take fluoxetine. Pediatrics. November 1999;104(5):e61.
12. Epperson CN, Jatlow PI, Czarkowski K, Anderson GM. Maternal fluoxetine treatment in the postpartum period: effects on platelet serotonin and plasma drug levels in breastfeeding mother-infant pairs. Pediatrics. November 2003;112(5):e425.
13. Weissman AM, Levy BT, Hartz AJ, et al. Pooled analysis of antidepressant levels in lactating mothers, breast milk, and nursing infants. Am J Psychiatr. June 2004;161(6):1066-1078.

FLUPENTHIXOL

Trade: Fluanxol, Fluanxol Depot, Pentixol, Depixol

Category: Antipsychotic, Typical

LRC: L3 - Limited Data-Probably Compatible

Flupenthixol (also called flupentixol) is a first-generation antipsychotic that is used for the treatment of chronic schizophrenia.[1] Based on this medication's large size (588 Da), high protein binding (99%) and high volume of distribution it does not readily enter human milk in significant quantities. However, this medication's long half-life (35 hours) should be taken into consideration.

In 1980, a short report was published that quantified maternal milk and blood samples of flupentixol from three of five women who were taking this medication in pregnancy and lactation.[2] The first woman had milk and serum concentrations drawn on day 4 postpartum. This woman was taking 40 mg IM every 2 weeks, and her serum concentration was 1.5 µg/L while her milk concentration was 0.8 µg/L. This same patient had milk samples repeated on day 41 postpartum, a similar serum concentration was found to be 1.3 µg/L while the milk concentration was higher at 1.8 µg/L. The second patient was taking 60 mg IM every 3 weeks, her serum concentration on day 17 postpartum was 1.4 µg/L, and her milk sample was 1.8 µg/L. The third patient who was taking 2 mg a day orally had her levels drawn on day 30 postpartum; she had a serum concentration of 1.5 µg/L and a milk concentration of 1.8 µg/L. The authors of this short report estimated that an infant who ingests about 1 L of breast milk a day would get 2 µg/day of flupentixol. Based on our calculations (using infant intake of 150 mL/kg/day and the maternal 2 mg/day oral dose) we anticipate the relative infant dose to be 1%. The infants were reported to have normal routine clinical examinations and no concerns with growth.

In 1988, a case report was published regarding the use of flupentixol in breast milk.[3] In this case, the woman was taking 1 mg of flupentixol daily with 100 mg of nortriptyline daily starting in the second trimester of her pregnancy. The nortriptyline was stopped 2 weeks prior to delivery; however, medication was restarted at a higher dose (125 mg) along with an increased dose of flupentixol 4 mg on day 1 postpartum. Maternal blood and milk samples and infant blood samples (heel prick taken 2 h post feed) were taken on day 6 and 7 postpartum. The mean maternal milk concentration was 2.8 µg/L. Based on this milk concentration the authors of this report estimated that the infant would receive 0.4 µg/kg/day of flupentixol in breast milk. The relative infant dose they calculated was 0.6% (maternal weight 60 kg, mean concentration 2.8 µg/L), we found very similar results with a relative infant dose of 0.7-1.75% (standard maternal weight 70 kg and mean (2.8 µg/L) and peak milk concentrations (6.8 µg/L)). This infant was exclusively breastfed, and the infant blood levels were <0.3 µg/L on day 7 postpartum. In addition, the authors reported normal motor development and no signs of medication adverse effects at 4 months of age.

Please note: the levels of flupentixol were not at steady-state in this case report; however, based on calculations the authors do not anticipate the findings would vary significantly at steady-state.

T 1/2	35 h (oral); 3 weeks (depot)	MW	507.45 (tablets); 588.82 (depot) Da	PB	99%
Tmax	3-8 h (oral); 4-7 days (depot)	RID	0.7% - 1.75%	Vd	14.1 L/kg
Oral	40%	M/P		pKa	

Adult Concerns: Headache, dizziness, drowsiness, depression, agitation, restlessness, blurred vision, palpitations, QTc prolongation, xerostomia or increased salivation, nausea, constipation, changes in liver function, hematologic changes, extrapyramidal effects.

Adult Dose: 3-6 mg/day in divided doses (oral tablet); 20-40 mg every 2 to 3 weeks (IM depot).

Pediatric Concerns:

Infant Monitoring: Sedation or irritability, apnea, not waking to feed/poor feeding, constipation, weight gain, and extrapyramidal symptoms. Due to long half-life monitor for adverse effects throughout lactation.

Alternatives: Olanzapine(L2), Risperidone(L2)

References:

1. Pharmaceutical manufacturers prescribing information.
2. Kirk L, Jorgensen A. Concentrations of Cis(Z)-flupentixol in maternal serum, amniotic fluid, umbilical cord serum, and milk. Psychopharmacology (Berl). 1980;72(1):107-108.
3. Matheson I, Skjaeraasen J. Milk concentrations of flupenthixol, nortriptyline and zuclopenthixol and between-breast differences in two patients. Eur J Clin Pharmacol. 1988;35(2):217-220.

FLUPHENAZINE

Trade: Anatensol, Modecate, Moditen, Permitil, Prolixin

Category: Antipsychotic, Typical

LRC: L3 - No Data-Probably Compatible

Fluphenazine is a phenothiazine tranquilizer and presently has the highest milligram potency of this family. Fluphenazine decanoate injections (IM) provide extremely long plasma levels with half-lives approaching 14.3 days at steady state. Members of this family generally have milk/plasma ratios ranging from 0.5 to 0.7.[1] No specific reports on fluphenazine breast milk levels have been located; use with caution.

T 1/2	ora/inj: 14-16 h/ 14 days	MW	591 Da	PB	91-99%
Tmax	oral/inj: 2 h/ 8-10 h	RID		Vd	3.14 L/kg
Oral	Complete	M/P		pKa	3.9, 8.1

Adult Concerns: Depression, seizures, appetite stimulation, blood dyscrasias, weight gain, hepatic toxicity, sedation.

Adult Dose: 1-5 mg daily.

Pediatric Concerns: None reported, but observe for sedation.

Infant Monitoring: Sedation or irritability, apnea, not waking to feed/poor feeding, weight gain.

Alternatives: Risperidone (L2), olanzapine(L2)

References:
1. Ayd FJ. Excretion of psychotropic drugs in breast milk. Int Drug Ther Newslett. 1973;8:33-40.

FLURAZEPAM

Trade: Dalmane

Category: Sedative-Hypnotic

LRC: L4 - No Data-Possibly Hazardous

Flurazepam is a sedative, hypnotic generally used as an aid for sleep. It belongs to the benzodiazepine (Valium) family. It is rapidly and completely metabolized to several long half-life active metabolites. Because most benzodiazepines are secreted into human milk, flurazepam entry into milk should be expected.[1] However, no specific data on flurazepam breastmilk levels are available. Shorter-acting benzodiazepines with no active metabolites, such as lorazepam, are preferred during lactation provided their use is short-term or intermittent and the lowest effective dose is used.[2]

T 1/2	Flurazepam: 2.3 h. Active Metabolites: 47 to 100 h	MW	388 Da	PB	97%
Tmax		RID		Vd	3.4 L/kg
Oral	Complete	M/P		pKa	1.9, 8.2

Adult Concerns: Sedation, dizziness, confusion, apnea, ataxia, and changes in liver enzymes.

Adult Dose: 15-30 mg daily.

Pediatric Concerns: None reported via milk at this time.

Infant Monitoring: Sedation, slowed breathing rate, not waking to feed/poor feeding, and weight gain.

Alternatives: Lorazepam(L3)

References:
1. Drug Facts and Comparisons 2017.
2. Maitra R, Menkes DB. Psychotropic drugs and lactation. N Z Med J. 1996;109(1024):217-218.

FLURBIPROFEN

Trade: Ansaid, Froben, Ocufen

Category: NSAID

LRC: L2 - Limited Data-Probably Compatible

Flurbiprofen is a nonsteroidal analgesic similar in structure to ibuprofen but used both as an ophthalmic preparation (in eyes) and an oral medication. In one study of 12 women given nine oral doses (50 mg/dose, 3-5 days postpartum) the milk levels of flurbiprofen in two women ranged from 0.05 to 0.07 mg/L but was <0.05 mg/L in 10 of the 12 women.[1] Concentrations in breast milk and plasma of nursing mothers suggest that a nursing infant would receive less than 0.1 mg flurbiprofen per day, a level considered exceedingly low. In another study of 10 nursing mothers following a single 100-mg dose, the average peak concentration of flurbiprofen in breast milk was 0.09 mg/L.[2] Both of these studies suggest that the amount of flurbiprofen transferred to human milk would be clinically insignificant to the infant.

T 1/2	3.8-5.7 h	MW	244 Da	PB	99%
Tmax	1.5 h	RID	0.7% - 1.4%	Vd	0.1 L/kg
Oral	Complete	M/P	0.008 - 0.013	pKa	4.2

Adult Concerns: Headache, dizziness, amnesia, nervousness, depression, insomnia, tinnitus, dyspepsia, nausea, vomiting, abdominal pain, diarrhea, gastrointestinal bleeding, changes in liver and renal function, edema, weakness.

Adult Dose: 200-300 mg daily.

Pediatric Concerns: None reported.

Infant Monitoring: Vomiting, diarrhea.

Alternatives: Ibuprofen(L1)

References:
1. Smith IJ, Hinson JL, Johnson VA, et al. Flurbiprofen in post-partum women: plasma and breast milk disposition. J Clin Pharmacol. 1989;29(2):174-184.
2. Cox SR, Forbes KK. Excretion of flurbiprofen into breast milk. Pharmacotherapy. 1987;7(6):211-215.

FLUTAMIDE

Trade: Chimax, Eulexin, Flucinom, Flutamin

Category: Anticancer

LRC: L4 - No Data-Possibly Hazardous

Flutamide is an oral nonsteroidal antiandrogen, that is used in the treatment of prostatic carcinoma. It works by inhibiting the uptake and binding of androgen in target tissues. Flutamide may also be used in women to lower high androgen levels in the treatment of polycystic ovarian syndrome. The transfer of flutamide to human milk is unknown, but the use of an antiandrogen drug in a breastfeeding woman with a male infant is potentially dangerous.[1]

T 1/2	6 h	MW	276.2 Da	PB	92-94%
Tmax	2 h	RID		Vd	
Oral	Complete	M/P		pKa	

Adult Concerns: Drowsiness or insomnia, changes in mood, anxiety, hot flashes, hypertension, nausea, vomiting, anorexia, changes in liver function, gynecomastia, galactorrhea.

Adult Dose: 250 mg 1-3 times daily.

Pediatric Concerns: No data are available for breastfed infants at this time.

Infant Monitoring: This product would be highly risky for a male infant.

Alternatives:

References:
1. Pharmaceutical manufacturers prescribing information.

FLUTICASONE

Trade: Cutivate, Flixonase, Flixotide, Flonase, Flovent, Veramyst

Category: Corticosteroid

LRC: L3 - No Data-Probably Compatible

Fluticasone is a typical steroid primarily used intranasally for allergic rhinitis and via inhalation for asthma. When instilled intranasally, the absolute bioavailability is less than 2%, so virtually none of the dose is absorbed systemically.[1] Oral absorption following inhaled fluticasone is approximately 30%, although almost instant first-pass absorption virtually eliminates plasma levels of fluticasone.[2] Peak plasma levels following inhalation of 880 μg is only 0.1 to 1 ng/mL. Adrenocortical suppression following oral or even systemic absorption at normal doses is extremely rare due to limited plasma levels.[3] Plasma levels are not detectable when using suggested doses. Although fluticasone is secreted into milk of rodents, the dose used was many times higher than found under normal conditions. With the above limited oral and systemic bioavailability, and rapid first-pass uptake by the liver, it is not likely that milk levels will be clinically relevant, even with rather high doses.

T 1/2	7.8 h	MW	500 Da	PB	91%
Tmax	15-60 min	RID		Vd	4.2 L/kg
Oral	Oral (1%), Inhaled (18%)	M/P		pKa	13.56

Adult Concerns: Intranasal: pruritus, headache (1-3%), burning (3-6%), epistaxis. Adverse effects associated with inhaled fluticasone include headache, nasal congestion, and oral candidiasis.

Adult Dose: 50-110 µg inhalation daily.

Pediatric Concerns: No effects have been reported in breastfeeding infants. When used topically on large surface areas, some adrenal suppression has been noted. In children receiving up to 5 times the normal inhaled dose (1000 µg/day), some growth suppression was noted.

Infant Monitoring: Feeding, growth, and weight gain.

Alternatives:

References:
1. Pharmaceutical manufacturers prescribing information.
2. Harding SM. The human pharmacology of fluticasone propionate. Respir Med. 1990;84(suppl A):25-29.
3. Todd G, Dunlop K, McNaboe J, Ryan MF, Carson D, Shields MD. Growth and adrenal suppression in asthmatic children treated with high-dose fluticasone propionate. Lancet. 1996;348(9019):27-29.

FLUVASTATIN

Trade: Lescol, Lescol XL, Vastin

Category: Antihyperlipidemic

LRC: L3 - No Data-Probably Compatible

Fluvastatin is an inhibitor of cholesterol synthesis in the liver. Fluvastatin levels in human milk are reported to be twice that of serum levels, although no exact data could be found.[1] The effect on the infant is unknown, statins could reduce cholesterol synthesis. Cholesterol and other products of cholesterol biosynthesis are essential components for neonatal development; therefore, it is not clear if it would be safe for use in a breastfed infant who needs high levels of cholesterol. Caution is recommended until more data are available.

T 1/2	1.2 h	MW	411 Da	PB	>98%
Tmax	<1 h	RID		Vd	
Oral	20-30%	M/P	2	pKa	4.56

Adult Concerns: Headache, dizziness, nausea, abdominal pain, diarrhea, changes in liver function, weakness, myalgia.

Adult Dose: 20-40 mg daily.

Pediatric Concerns: None reported, but reduced plasma cholesterol levels could occur.

Infant Monitoring: Weight gain, growth.

Alternatives:

References:
1. Pharmaceutical manufacturers prescribing information.

FLUVOXAMINE

Trade: Alti-Fluvoxamine, Faverin, Floxyfral, Luvox, Myroxim

Category: Antidepressant, SSRI

LRC: L2 - Limited Data-Probably Compatible

Fluvoxamine is a serotonin reuptake inhibitor with antidepressant action. Although structurally dissimilar to the other serotonin reuptake inhibitors, fluvoxamine provides increased synaptic serotonin levels in the brain. It has several hepatic metabolites which are not active. Its primary indications are for the treatment of obsessive-compulsive disorders (OCD) although it also functions as an antidepressant. There are a number of significant drug-drug interactions with this product.

In a case report of one 23-year-old mother and following a dose of 100 mg twice daily for 2 weeks, the maternal plasma level of fluvoxamine base was 0.31 mg/L and the milk concentration was 0.09 mg/L.[1] The authors reported a theoretical dose to the infant of 0.0104 mg/kg/day of fluvoxamine, which is only 0.5% of the maternal dose. According to the authors, the infant suffered no unwanted effects as a result of this intake and this dose poses little risk to a nursing infant. In a study of one patient receiving 100 mg twice daily, the AUC milk/serum ratio averaged 1.32. The absolute daily dose of fluvoxamine ingested by the newborn was calculated to be 48 µg/kg/day and the relative dose was calculated to be 1.58% of the weight-adjusted maternal dose.[2] In another study of two breastfeeding women, the AUC average concentration of fluvoxamine in milk was 36 and 256 µg/L respectively.[3] The absolute infant dose was estimated at 5.4 and 38.4 µg/kg/day with a relative infant dose (% of maternal dose) of 0.8% and 1.38%. A Denver assessment on one infant indicated normal development. Fluvoxamine was not detected in the plasma of either infant (limit of detection=2 µg/L). In a case report of a single mother receiving 25 mg three times daily, the highest milk concentration was 40 µg/L.[4] Using this data, an infant would ingest approximately 6 µg/kg/day, which is 0.62% of the maternal weight-adjusted dose. Interestingly, the maternal serum concentration at 10 hours was 20 ng/mL while the infant plasma level was 9 ng/mL. Considering the clinical dose to the infant is low, this plasma level in the infant appears high. The authors suggest this may be an atypical case, or that this infant's clearance of fluvoxamine is poor. The infant showed no symptoms of adverse effects. Yoshida reported a case of a mother receiving 100 mg/day, and an infant 15 weeks postpartum.[5] In this case the concentration of fluvoxamine in maternal serum and milk was 170 µg/L and 50 µg/L respectively and a milk/plasma ratio of 0.29. The authors estimated the dose to the infant at 7.5 µg/kg/day. Developmental assessments of the infant at 4 months and 21 months suggested normal development. In a report of two breastfeeding women receiving 300 mg/day, Piontek was unable to detect any fluvoxamine in the plasma of two breastfed infants.[6]

In summary, the data from these all the mentioned cases suggests that only minuscule amounts of fluvoxamine are transferred to infants, that plasma levels in infants are too low to be detected, and no adverse effects have been noted.

T 1/2	15.6 h	MW	318 Da	PB	80%
Tmax	3-8 h	RID	0.3% - 1.4%	Vd	
Oral	53%	M/P	1.34	pKa	9.4

Adult Concerns: Somnolence, insomnia, nervousness, nausea.

Adult Dose: 50-300 mg daily.

Pediatric Concerns: None reported via milk at this time.

Infant Monitoring: Sedation or irritability, not waking to feed/poor feeding, and weight gain.

Alternatives: Sertraline(L2), Escitalopram(L2)

References:

1. Wright S, Dawling S, Ashford JJ. Excretion of fluvoxamine in breast milk. Br J Clin Pharmacol. 1991;31(2):209.
2. Hagg S, Granberg K, Carleborg L. Excretion of fluvoxamine into breast milk. Br J Clin Pharmacol. 2000;49(3):286-288.
3. Kristensen JH, Hackett LP, Kohan R, Paech M, Ilett KF. The amount of fluvoxamine in milk is unlikely to be a cause of adverse effects in breastfed infants. J Hum Lact. 2002;18(2):139-143.
4. Arnold LM, Suckow RF, Lichtenstein PK. Fluvoxamine concentrations in breast milk and in maternal and infant sera. J Clin Psychopharmacol. 2000;20(4):491-493.
5. Yoshida K, Smith B, Kumar RC. Fluvoxamine in breast-milk and infant development. Br J Clin Pharmacol. 1997;44(2):210-211.
6. Piontek CM, Wisner KL, Perel JM, Peindl KS. Serum fluvoxamine levels in breastfed infants. J Clin Psychiatry. 2001;62(2):111-113.

FOLIC ACID

Trade: Bioglan Daily, Folacin, Folvite, Megafol, Wellcovorin

Category: Vitamin

LRC: L1 - Limited Data-Compatible

Folic acid is an essential vitamin Individuals most susceptible to folic acid deficiency are pregnant women, and those receiving anticonvulsants or birth control medications. Folic acid supplementation is now strongly recommended in women prior to becoming pregnancy due to a documented reduction of spinal cord malformations. Folic acid is actively secreted in breast milk even if mother is deficient.[1] If maternal diet is adequate, folic acid is not generally required. The infant receives all required from a normal milk supply. Cooperman determined milk folic acid content to be 15.2 ng/mL in colostrum, 16.3 ng/mL in transitional, and 33.4 ng/mL in mature milk.[2] In one study of 11 breastfeeding mothers receiving 0.8-1 mg/day of folic acid, the folic acid secreted into human milk averaged 45.6 µg/L.[3] Excessive doses (>1 mg/day) during or before pregnancy are not generally recommended. Patients on anticonvulsants often use 4 mg/day. These doses are not generally hazardous.

T 1/2		MW	441 Da	PB	
Tmax	30-60 min	RID		Vd	
Oral	76-93%	M/P		pKa	4.17

Adult Concerns: Allergies, rash, nausea, anorexia, bitter taste.

Adult Dose: 0.4-0.8 mg daily.

Pediatric Concerns: None reported.

Infant Monitoring:

Alternatives:

References:
1. Cooperman JM, Dweck HS, Newman LJ, Garbarino C, Lopez R. The folate in human milk. Am J Clin Nutr. 1982;36(4):576-580.
2. Tamura T, Yoshimura Y, Arakawa T. Human milk folate and folate status in lactating mothers and their infants. Am J Clin Nutr. 1980;33(2):193-197.
3. Smith AM, Picciano MF, Deering RH. Folate supplementation during lactation: maternal folate status, human milk folate content, and their relationship to infant folate status. J Pediatr Gastroenterol Nutr. 1983;2(4):622-628.

FOLLICLE STIMULATING HORMONES

Trade: Bravelle (Urofollitropin), FSH, Fertinex (Urofollitropin), Fertinorm HP, Follistim (Follitropin Beta), Follitropin Alpha, Follitropin Beta, Gonal-F (Follitropin Alpha), Metrodin, Metrodin (Urofollitropin), Urofollitropin, Fostimon

Category: Pituitary Hormone

LRC: L3 - No Data-Probably Compatible

Follicle-stimulating hormone (FSH) is a glycoprotein gonadotropin secreted by the anterior pituitary in response to gonadotropin-releasing hormone (GnRH) from the hypothalamus.[1-3] FSH and luteinizing hormone bind to receptors in the testis and ovary and regulate gonadal function by promoting sex steroid production and gametogenesis. In the female, FSH induces growth of the Graafian follicle in the ovary preparatory to the release of the ovum. Approximately 15 µg is secreted daily by the pituitary in normal individuals. Numerous forms of FSH are available and are listed below, but all work similarly. FSH is a large molecular weight peptide (34,000 Da) and is very unlikely to enter milk or be orally bioavailable to an infant. However, it is not known if the administration of FSH, and the subsequent maternal changes in estrogen and progesterone, would alter the production of milk. It is however likely, since the onset of pregnancy is commonly followed by a decrease in milk production in most mothers.

Urofollitropin is a preparation of gonadotropin (FSH) extracted from the urine of postmenopausal women. Follitropin alpha and follitropin beta are human FSH preparations of recombinant DNA origin. Menotropins are combination products containing both FSH and luteinizing hormone (LH).

T 1/2	3.9 and 70.4 h	MW	34,000 Da	PB	
Tmax	6-18 h	RID		Vd	0.06, 1.08 L/kg
Oral	None	M/P		pKa	

Adult Concerns: Pulmonary and vascular complications, ovarian hyperstimulation, abdominal pain, fever and chills, abdominal pain, nausea, vomiting, diarrhea, pain at injection site, bruising. Ovarian hyperstimulation.

Adult Dose: 75 units daily.

Pediatric Concerns: None reported via milk. FSH is very unlikely to penetrate milk, and it would not be orally bioavailable. However, observe closely for reduced milk production.

Infant Monitoring:

Alternatives:

References:
1. Sharma V, Riddle A, Mason, et al. Studies on folliculogenesis and in vitro fertilization outcome after the administration of follicle-stimulating hormone at different times during the menstrual cycle. Fertil Steril. 1989;51:298-303.
2. Kjeld JM, Harsoulis P, Kuku SF, et al. Infusions of hFSH and hLH in normal men: kinetics of human follicle stimulating hormone. Acta Endocrinologica. 1976;81:225-233.
3. Yen SSC, Llerena LA, Pearson OH, et al. Disappearance rates of endogenous follicle-stimulating hormone in serum following surgical hypophysectomy in man. J Clin Endocrinol. 1970;30:325-329.

FONDAPARINUX SODIUM

Trade: Arixtra

Category: Anticoagulant

LRC: L3 - No Data-Probably Compatible

Fondaparinux sodium is a synthetic pentasaccharide used to treat and prevent deep vein thrombosis. Fondaparinux sodium causes antithrombin III-mediated inhibition of factor Xa, which inhibits the coagulation cascade and thrombus development.[1] As a pentasaccharide, it would neither be likely to enter the milk compartment due to its large molecular weight, or be orally bioavailable in an infant if any drug managed to reach the milk compartment. No data are available on the transmission of fondaparinux sodium to a nursing infant, but based on the kinetic profile it is highly unlikely that it would be passed to the infant.

T 1/2	17-21 h	MW	1,728 Da	PB	94%
Tmax	2-3 h	RID		Vd	0.1-0.16 L/kg
Oral	Nil	M/P		pKa	

Adult Concerns: Bleeding (e.g. bruising on the skin, blood in urine or stool), changes in liver function, anemia, thrombocytopenia, and rash.

Adult Dose: 2.5-10 mg daily.

Pediatric Concerns: None reported via milk at this time.

Infant Monitoring: Rare- bruising on the skin, blood in urine, vomit, or stool.

Alternatives:

References:
1. Pharmaceutical manufacturers prescribing information.

FORMOTEROL

Trade: Foradil Aerolizer, Symbicort

Category: Antiasthma

LRC: L3 - No Data-Probably Compatible

Formoterol fumarate is a long-acting selective beta-2 adrenoceptor agonist used for asthma and COPD. Following inhalation of a 120 μg dose, the maximum plasma concentration of 92 pg/mL occurred within 5 minutes.[1] No data are available on its transfer to human milk, but the extremely low plasma levels would suggest that milk levels would be incredibly low, if even measurable. Studies of oral absorption in adults suggests that while absorption is good, plasma levels are still below detectable levels and may require large oral doses prior to attaining measurable plasma levels.[2] It is not likely the amount present in human milk would be clinically relevant to a breastfed infant.

T 1/2	10 h	MW	840 Da	PB	64%
Tmax	5 min	RID		Vd	
Oral	Good	M/P		pKa	

Adult Concerns: Tremor, headache, dizziness, restlessness, palpitations, nausea, dry mouth, muscle cramps, and cough. Low serum potassium and elevated blood glucose levels can occur with high doses. Blood pressure and heart rate are minimally affected.

Adult Dose: 12 μg every 12 hours.

Pediatric Concerns: None reported via milk.

Infant Monitoring: Irritability, insomnia, arrhythmias, weight loss, tremor.

Alternatives: Salmeterol, Albuterol(L1)

References:
1. Pharmaceutical manufacturers prescribing information.
2. Tattersfield AE. Long-acting beta 2-agonists. Clin Exp Allergy. 1992;22(6):600-605.
3. Maesen FP, Smeets JJ, Gubbelmans HL, Zweers PG. Bronchodilator effect of inhaled formoterol vs salbutamol over 12 hours. Chest. 1990;97(3):590-594.

FOSCARNET SODIUM

Trade: Foscavir

Category: Antiviral

LRC: L5 - No Data-Hazardous

Foscarnet is an antiviral used to treat mucocutaneous herpes simplex manifestations and cytomegalovirus infections in patients with cancer or AIDS. It is not known if foscarnet is secreted in human milk, but studies in animals indicate levels in milk were three times higher than serum levels (suggesting a milk/plasma ratio of 3).[1,2] Foscarnet is a potent and potentially dangerous drug that could cause significant renal toxicity, seizures, and deposition in bone and teeth. Use of this drug in breastfeeding women should be with extreme caution.

Please note: The Centers for Disease Control and Prevention recommend that HIV-1 infected mothers do not breastfeed their infants to avoid postnatal transmission of HIV-1.

T 1/2	3-4 h	MW	192 Da	PB	14-17%
Tmax	Immediate (IV)	RID		Vd	0.5 L/kg
Oral	12-21%	M/P	3	pKa	7.27

Adult Concerns: Headache, fever, seizures, confusion, anxiety, hyper or hypotension, arrhythmias, nausea, vomiting, diarrhea, changes in renal function and electrolytes, anemia, edema, tremor.

Adult Dose: 34-51 mg/kg injection (IV) daily.

Pediatric Concerns: None reported but caution is urged.

Infant Monitoring: Not recommended in breastfeeding.

Alternatives:

References:
1. Pharmaceutical manufacturers prescribing information.
2. Sjovall J, Karlsson A, Ogenstad S, Sandstrom E, Saarimaki M. Pharmacokinetics and absorption of foscarnet after intravenous and oral administration to patients with human immunodeficiency virus. Clin Pharmacol Ther. 1988;44(1):65-73.

FOSFOMYCIN TROMETAMOL

Trade: Monuril, Monurol

Category: Antibiotic, Other

LRC: L3 - Limited Data-Probably Compatible

Fosfomycin trometamol is a broad-spectrum antibiotic used primarily for uncomplicated urinary tract infections. It is believed safe for use in pregnancy and has been used in children less than 1 year of age. Fosfomycin absorption is largely dependent on the salt form; trometamol salts are modestly absorbed (34-58%) and calcium salts are poorly absorbed (<12%). Fosfomycin secreted into human milk would likely be in the calcium form and is unlikely to be absorbed as secreted in human milk. Foods and the acidic milieu of the stomach both significantly reduce oral absorption.[1-3] Levels secreted into human milk have been reported to be about 10% of the maternal plasma level.[4] Generally, a single 3-g oral dose is effective treatment for many urinary tract infections in women. It is not likely that the levels present in breast milk would produce untoward effects in a breastfeeding infant.

T 1/2	4-8 h	MW	138 Da	PB	<3%
Tmax	1.5-3 h	RID		Vd	0.22 L/kg
Oral	34-58%	M/P	0.1	pKa	7.82

Adult Concerns: Nausea, vomiting, diarrhea, epigastric discomfort, anorexia. Skin rashes and pruritus have been reported.

Adult Dose: 3 g single dose.

Pediatric Concerns: None reported via milk.

Infant Monitoring: Vomiting, diarrhea, changes in gastrointestinal flora and rash.

Alternatives:

References:
1. Bergan T. Degree of absorption, pharmacokinetics of fosfomycin trometamol and duration of urinary antibacterial activity. Infection. 1990;18(suppl 2):S65-S69.
2. Bergan T. Pharmacokinetic comparison between fosfomycin and other phosphonic acid derivatives. Chemotherapy. 1990;36(suppl 1):10-18.
3. Segre G, Bianchi E, Cataldi A, Zannini G. Pharmacokinetic profile of fosfomycin trometamol (Monuril). Eur Urol. 1987;13(suppl 1):56-63.
4. Kirby WM. Pharmacokinetics of fosfomycin. Chemotherapy. 1977;23(suppl 1):141-151.

FOSINOPRIL

Trade: Monopril, Staril

Category: ACE Inhibitor

LRC: L3 - Limited Data-Probably Compatible

Fosinopril is a prodrug that is metabolized by the gut and liver upon absorption to fosinoprilat, which is an ACE inhibitor used as an antihypertensive. The manufacturer reports that the ingestion of 20 mg daily for three days resulted in detectable levels in human milk, although no values were provided.[1] Consider ramipril, enalapril, or captopril as alternatives. While fosinopril is not considered incompatible with breastfeeding, the lack of detail regarding the available data warrants caution when using this drug, particularly during the neonatal period.

Both the ACE inhibitor family and the specific Angiotensin II receptor blockers are contraindicated in pregnancy and thus should be used with caution in women who are planning a subsequent pregnancy in the near future.

T 1/2	11-35 h	MW	564 Da	PB	95%
Tmax	3 h	RID		Vd	
Oral	30-36%	M/P		pKa	3.78

Adult Concerns: Headache, dizziness, fatigue, hypotension, abnormal taste, cough, nausea, diarrhea, constipation, changes in renal function/urine output, hyperkalemia, rash.

Adult Dose: 20-40 mg daily.

Pediatric Concerns: None reported via milk at this time.

Infant Monitoring: Drowsiness, lethargy, pallor, poor feeding, and weight gain.

Alternatives: Ramipril(L3), Enalapril(L2), Captopril(L2)

References:
1. Pharmaceutical manufacturers prescribing information.

FOSPHENYTOIN

Trade: Cerebyx

Category: Anticonvulsant

LRC: L2 - Limited Data-Probably Compatible

Fosphenytoin is a prodrug of phenytoin. Following the parenteral injection of fosphenytoin, it is rapidly converted to the anticonvulsant phenytoin with a brief half-life of 15 minutes.[1] Thus, the active drug is phenytoin.

Phenytoin is an old and efficient anticonvulsant. It is secreted in small amounts in breast milk. The effect on infant is generally considered minimal if the levels in the maternal circulation are kept in low-normal range (10 µg/mL). Phenytoin levels peak in milk at 3.5 hours. In one study of six women receiving 200-400 mg/day, plasma concentrations varied from 12.8 to 78.5 µmol/L, while their milk levels ranged from 1.61 to 2.95 mg/L.[2] The milk/plasma ratios were low, ranging from 0.06 to 0.18. In only two of these infants were plasma concentrations of phenytoin detectable (0.46 and 0.72 µmol/L). No untoward effects were noted in any of these infants. Others have reported milk levels of 6 µg/mL[3], or 0.8 µg/mL.[4] Although the actual concentration in milk varies significantly between studies, the milk/plasma ratio appears relatively similar at 0.13 to 0.45. Breast milk concentrations varied from 0.26 to 1.5 mg/L depending on the maternal dose. In a mother receiving 250 mg twice daily, milk levels were 0.26 and the milk/plasma ratio was 0.45.[5] The maternal plasma level of phenytoin was 0.58. In another study of two patients receiving 300-600 mg/d, the average milk level was 1.9 mg/L.[6] The maximum observed milk level was 2.6 mg/L. The neonatal half-life of phenytoin is highly variable for the first week of life. Monitoring of the infants' plasma may be useful although it is not definitely required. All of the current studies indicate rather low levels of phenytoin in breast milk and minimal plasma levels in breastfeeding infants.

T 1/2	15 min	MW	406 Da	PB	99%
Tmax	0.5 h	RID		Vd	0.06-0.15 L/kg
Oral		M/P		pKa	6.06

Adult Concerns: Headache, nausea, ecchymosis, nystagmus, tremor.

Adult Dose: 4-6 mg phenytoin equivalents/kg/day.

Pediatric Concerns: Only one case of methemoglobinemia, drowsiness, and poor sucking has been reported with phenytoin. Most other studies suggest no problems.

Infant Monitoring: Sedation or irritability, not waking to feed/poor feeding, and weight gain. Based on clinical symptoms some infants may require monitoring of liver enzymes.

Alternatives: Phenytoin(L2)

References:

1. Pharmaceutical manufacturers prescribing information.
2. Steen B, Rane A, Lonnerholm G, Falk O, Elwin CE, Sjoqvist F. Phenytoin excretion in human breast milk and plasma levels in nursed infants. Ther Drug Monit. 1982;4(4):331-334.
3. Svensmark O, Schiller PJ, Buchthal F. 5, 5-Diphenylhydantoin (dilantin) blood levels after oral or intravenous dosage in man. Acta Pharmacol Toxicol (Copenh). 1960;16:331-346.
4. Kaneko S, Sato T, Suzuki K. The levels of anticonvulsants in breast milk. Br J Clin Pharmacol. 1979;7(6):624-627.
5. Rane A, Garle M, Borga O, Sjoqvist F. Plasma disappearance of transplacentally transferred diphenylhydantoin in the newborn studied by mass fragmentography. Clin Pharmacol Ther. 1974;15(1):39-45.
6. Mirkin BL. Diphenylhydantoin: placental transport, fetal localization, neonatal metabolism, and possible teratogenic effects. J Pediatr. 1971;78(2):329-337.

FROVATRIPTAN SUCCINATE

Trade: Frova

Category: Antimigraine

LRC: L3 - No Data-Probably Compatible

Frovatriptan is a 5-HT1B/1D (serotonin) receptor agonist used to treat migraine headaches. Activating these receptors is believed to constrict cranial blood vessels and block the release of pro-inflammatory neuropeptides from the trigeminal nerve. Although the oral bioavailability of frovatriptan is low (30%), it is still about twice that of sumatriptan (14%).

No studies examining frovatriptan secretion into human milk or adverse effects in infants have been published. Some transfer is likely based on this medication's size and low protein binding; however, the clinical significance of this is unknown. Consider sumatriptan as the preferred alternative as the half-life of frovatriptan is significantly longer (26 hours vs. 2-3 hours).

T 1/2	26 h	MW	379 Da	PB	15%
Tmax	2-4 h	RID		Vd	3 L/kg
Oral	30%	M/P		pKa	10.6

Adult Concerns: Dizziness, drowsiness, tinnitus, flushing, hot tingling sensations, dry mouth, chest pain, arrhythmias, hypertension, nausea, vomiting, diarrhea, abdominal pain, weakness, paresthesia.

Adult Dose: 2.5 mg orally, may repeat in 2 hours if needed.

Pediatric Concerns: None reported via milk at this time.

Infant Monitoring: Drowsiness, vomiting, poor feeding.

Alternatives: Sumatriptan(L3), NSAIDs, Acetaminophen(L1)

References:

1. Pharmaceutical manufacturers prescribing information.

FUROSEMIDE

Trade: Frusemide, Frusid, Lasix, Uremide

Category: Diuretic

LRC: L3 - Limited Data-Probably Compatible

Furosemide is a potent loop diuretic with a rather short duration of action. Furosemide has been found in breast milk although the levels are unreported. Furosemide is frequently used in neonates in pediatric units, so pediatric use is common. The oral bioavailability of furosemide in newborns is exceedingly poor and very high oral doses are required (1-4mg/kg BID).[1] It is very unlikely the amount transferred into human milk would produce any effects in a nursing infant although its maternal use could suppress lactation.

T 1/2	92 min	MW	331 Da	PB	>98%
Tmax	1-2 h	RID		Vd	
Oral	60-70%	M/P		pKa	9.83

Adult Concerns: Headache, dizziness, hypotension, ototoxicity, hyperglycemia, hyponatremia, hypokalemia, hyperuricemia, changes in renal function.

Adult Dose: 40-80 mg twice daily.

Pediatric Concerns: None reported via milk at this time.

Infant Monitoring: Observe for fluid loss, dehydration, lethargy; monitor maternal milk supply.

Alternatives:

References:
1. Pharmaceutical manufacturers prescribing information.

GABAPENTIN

Trade: Horizant, Neurontin

Category: Anticonvulsant

LRC: L2 - Limited Data-Probably Compatible

Gabapentin is an older anticonvulsant used primarily for partial (focal) seizures with or without secondary generalization. It is also used for postherpetic neuralgia or neuropathic pain. Unlike many anticonvulsants, gabapentin is almost completely excreted renally without metabolism, it does not induce hepatic enzymes and is remarkably well tolerated.[1-3]

In a study of one breastfeeding mother who was receiving 1800 mg/day, milk levels were 11.1, 11.3, and 11 mg/L at 2, 4, and 8 hours respectively, following a dose of 600 mg. The milk/plasma ratio was calculated to be 0.86 and the relative infant dose was 2.3%. No adverse effects from gabapentin were noted in the infant.[4,5] In another patient receiving 2400 mg/day milk levels were 9.8, 9, and 7.2 mg/L at 2, 4, and 8 hours respectively, after a dose of 800 mg. Using these data, an infant would consume approximately 3.7% to 6.5% of the weight-adjusted maternal dose per day. No adverse events were noted in these two infants. In another study of five mother-infant pairs receiving 900-3200 mg gabapentin per day, the mean milk/plasma ratio ranged from 0.7 to 1.3 from 2 weeks to 3 months postpartum.[6] At 2-3 weeks, two of the five infants had detectable concentrations of gabapentin (1.3 and 1.5 µmol) and one was undetectable. These levels were far below the normal plasma levels in the mothers (11-45 µmol). Assuming a daily milk intake of 150 mL/kg/day, the infant dose of gabapentin was estimated to be 0.2-1.3 mg/kg/day, which is equivalent to 1.3-3.8% of the weight-normalized dose received by the mother. The plasma levels of gabapentin collected after 3 months of breastfeeding in another infant was 1.9 µmol. The authors concluded that the plasma levels measured were low if at all detectable in the infants, and no adverse effects were reported in these infants.

In summary, published data reveals that the infant plasma levels following lactational exposure to gabapentin are probably too low to cause untoward effects in the breastfed infant. However, new data suggests that withdrawal in infants exposed in utero to gabapentin increases the risk of neonatal withdrawal.[7]

T 1/2	5-7 h	MW	171 Da	PB	<3%
Tmax	1-3 h	RID	6.6%	Vd	0.8 L/kg
Oral	50%-60%	M/P	0.7-1.3	pKa	3.68, 10.70

Adult Concerns: Dizziness, somnolence, weight gain, vomiting, tremor, and CNS depression. Abrupt withdrawal may induce severe seizures.

Adult Dose: 300-600 mg three times daily.

Pediatric Concerns: None reported via breastmilk at this time.

Infant Monitoring: Sedation or irritability, not waking to feed/poor feeding, vomiting, tremor.

Alternatives:

References:
1. Goa KL, Sorkin EM. Gabapentin: A review of its pharmacological properties and clinical potential in epilepsy. Drugs. 1993;46(3):409-427.
2. Ramsay RE. Clinical efficacy and safety of gabapentin. Neurology. 1994;44(6 Suppl 5):S23-S30.
3. Dichter MA, Brodie MJ. New antiepileptic drugs. N Engl J Med. 1996;334(24):1583-1590.
4. Hale TW, Ilett KF, Hackett P. Personal communication, 2002.

5. Kristensen JH, Ilett KF, Hackett LP, Kohan R. Gabapentin and breastfeeding: A case report. J Hum Lact. 2006;22(4):426-428.
6. Ohman I, Vitols S, Tomson T. Pharmacokinetics of gabapentin during delivery, in the neonatal period, and lactation: does a fetal accumulation occur during pregnancy? Epilepsia. 2005 Oct;46(10):1621-1624.
7. Huybrechts KF, Bateman BT, Desai RJ, et al. Risk of neonatal drug withdrawal after intrauterine co-exposure to opioids and psychotropic medications: cohort study. BMJ. 2017 Aug;358:j3326. doi:10.1136/bmj.j3326. PubMed PMID: 28768628.

GADOBENATE

Trade: MultiHance

Category: Diagnostic Agent, Radiological Contrast Media

LRC: L3 - Limited Data-Probably Compatible

Gadobenate is a gadolinium-containing radiocontrast agent used in MRIs. Although free gadolinium is neurotoxic, it is safe when bound to the parent molecule in the contrast medium. There have been limited studies on its transfer to human milk; it is unlikely to accumulate in therapeutic levels in milk.[1] The American College of Radiology concludes that it is safe for a mother-infant dyad to continue breastfeeding after the administration of a gadolinium-containing contrast medium.[2] In another review, only tiny amounts of gadolinium contrast agents reach the milk compartment and virtually none of this is absorbed orally by the infant.[3]

T 1/2	1.17-2.02 h	MW	1,058.15 Da	PB	Low
Tmax		RID		Vd	
Oral	Poor	M/P		pKa	2.39

Adult Concerns: Dizziness, nausea, vomiting, headache, taste alteration, dry mouth.

Adult Dose:

Pediatric Concerns: None reported via breast milk.

Infant Monitoring:

Alternatives:

References:

1. Pharmaceutical manufacturers prescribing information.
2. ACR Committee on Drugs and Contrast Media. Administration of contrast medium to breastfeeding mothers. ACR Bull. 2004:42-43.
3. Webb JA, Thomsen HS, Morcos SK, Members of Contrast Media Safety Committee of European Society of Urogenital Radiology (ESUR). The use of iodinated and gadolinium contrast media during pregnancy and lactation. Eur Radiol. 2005 Jun;15(6):1234-1240. Epub 2004 Dec 18.

GADOBUTROL

Trade: Gadavist

Category: Diagnostic Agent, Radiological Contrast Media

LRC: L3 - Limited Data-Probably Compatible

This is a non-radioactive gadolinium-containing contrast agent used in MRI scans. Limited data from the manufacturer reports that levels of similar compounds in milk are only 0.01% to 0.04% of the maternal dose; clinically it is thought that less than 0.1% of the maternal dose enters milk.[1] This agent is also expected to have limited oral absorption. In a rodent study, less than 0.01% of the total administered dose was transferred to the neonatal pup via milk, mostly within 3 hours of administration.

The base gadolinium molecule is toxic in "free" form and is always chelated to various compounds. High Risk gadolinium molecules include gadodiamide and gadoversetamide in which gadolinium is prone to be released from chelation. Medium risk forms include Gadofosveset trisodium (Vasovist), gadoxetic acid disodium (Primovist), and gadobenate dimeglumine (MultiHance). Low risk forms include: Gadoterate meglumine (Dotarem), gadoteridol (ProHance) and gadobutrol (Gadovist).[2]

T 1/2	1.81 h	MW	604 Da	PB	
Tmax	2 min	RID		Vd	
Oral	Nil	M/P		pKa	

Adult Concerns: Headache, nausea, dysgeusia.

Adult Dose:

Pediatric Concerns: Limited oral absorption.

Infant Monitoring:

Alternatives:

References:
1. Pharmaceutical manufacturers prescribing information.
2. Puac P, Rodríguez A, Vallejo C, Zamora CA, Castillo M. Safety of contrast material use during pregnancy and lactation. Magn Reson Imaging Clin N Am. 2017 Nov;25(4):787-797. PubMed PMID: 28964468.

GADODIAMIDE

Trade: Omniscan

Category: Diagnostic Agent, Radiological Contrast Media

LRC: L3 - No Data-Probably Compatible

Gadodiamide is a gadolinium-containing nonionic, non-iodinated water soluble contrast medium commonly used in Magnetic Resonance Imaging (MRI) scans.[1] It is quite similar to Magnevist, another gadolinium-containing agent. These agents penetrate peripheral compartments poorly. As such, they are extremely unlikely to enter milk. Data for gadopentetate (Magnevist) support this, as its transfer to milk is negligible (<0.04%). Neither of these compounds is well absorbed orally, and neither is metabolized to any degree. It is likely that gadodiamide will penetrate milk only minimally. The American College of Radiology concludes that it is safe for a mother-infant to continue breastfeeding after the administration of a gadolinium-containing contrast medium. In another review, only tiny amounts of gadolinium contrast agents reach the milk compartment and virtually none of this is absorbed orally by the infant.[2] Recent data suggest that gadodiamide is one of the gadolinium chelates that is of highest risk of becoming unchelated, and being absorbed in the mother or via milk.[3] Low risk forms include: Gadoterate meglumine (Dotarem), gadoteridol (ProHance), and gadobutrol (Gadovist).

T 1/2	77 min	MW	591.67 Da	PB	
Tmax		RID		Vd	
Oral		M/P		pKa	2.77

Adult Concerns: Nausea, headache, dizziness, fatigue, abdominal pain, diarrhea, hot flashes, myocardial infraction, nephrogenic systemic fibrosis.

Adult Dose:

Pediatric Concerns:

Infant Monitoring:

Alternatives:

References:
1. Pharmaceutical manufacturers prescribing information.
2. Webb JA, Thomsen HS, Morcos SK; Members of Contrast Media Safety Committee of European Society of Urogenital Radiology (ESUR). The use of iodinated andgadolinium contrast media during pregnancy and lactation. Eur Radiol. 2005 Jun;15(6):1234-1240. Epub 2004 Dec 18.
3. Puac P, Rodríguez A, Vallejo C, Zamora CA, Castillo M. Safety of contrast material use during pregnancy and lactation. Magn Reson Imaging Clin N Am. 2017 Nov;25(4):787-797. PubMed PMID: 28964468.

GADOPENTETATE DIMEGLUMINE

Trade: Gadolinium, Magnevist, Magnevistan, Magnograf, Viewgam

Category: Diagnostic Agent, Radiological Contrast Media

LRC: L2 - Limited Data-Probably Compatible

Gadopentetate is a radiopaque agent used in magnetic resonance imaging of the kidney. It is non-ionic, non-iodinated, has low osmolarity, and contains a gadolinium ion as the radiopaque entity. Following a dose of 7 mmol (6.5 g), the amount of gadopentetate secreted in breast milk was 3.09, 2.8, 1.08, and 0.5 μmol/L at 2, 11, 17, and 24 hours respectively.[1] The cumulative amount excreted from both breasts in 24 hours was only 0.023% of the administered dose. Oral absorption is minimal, only 0.8% of gadopentetate is absorbed. These authors suggest that only 0.013

micromole of a gadolinium-containing compound would be absorbed by the infant in 24 hours, which is incredibly low. They further suggest that 24 hours of pumping would eliminate risk, although this seems rather extreme in view of the short (1.6 hours) half-life, poor oral bioavailability, and limited milk levels.

In another study of 19 lactating women who received 0.1 mmol/kg and one additional woman who received 0.2 mmol/kg, the cumulative amount of gadolinium excreted in breastmilk during 24 hours was 0.57 µmol/L.[2] This resulted in an excreted dose of <0.04% of the IV administered maternal dose. A similar amount was noted in the patient receiving a double dose (0.2 mmol/kg). As a result, for any neonate weighing more than 1000 gm, the maximal orally ingested dose would be less than 1% of the permitted intravenous dose of 0.2 mmol/kg. According to the authors, the very small amount of gadopentetate dimeglumine transferred to a nursing infant does not warrant a potentially traumatic 24-hour suspension of breastfeeding for lactating women.

Presently the use of gadolinium radiocontrast agents in infants is controversial. Gadolinium metal ions apparently bind to brain tissue in humans and is concerning for long-term development.

T 1/2	1.5-1.7 h	MW		PB	
Tmax		RID	0.02%-0.04%	Vd	
Oral	0.8%	M/P		pKa	

Adult Concerns: Headache, dizziness, nausea, vomiting, pain at injection site, hypersensitivity.

Adult Dose:

Pediatric Concerns: None reported in three studies.

Infant Monitoring:

Alternatives:

References:
1. Rofsky NM, Weinreb JC, Litt AW. Quantitative analysis of gadopentetate dimeglumine excreted in breast milk. J Magn Reson Imaging. 1993;3(1):131-132.
2. Kubik-Huch RA, Gottstein-Aalame NM, Frenzel T, et al. Gadopentetate dimeglumine excretion into human breast milk during lactation. Radiology. 2000;216(2):555-558.

GADOTERATE

Trade: Dotarem

Category: Diagnostic Agent, Radiological Contrast Media

LRC: L3 - No Data-Probably Compatible

Gadoterate is a gadolinium-based contrast agent indicated for intravenous use with Magnetic Resonance Imaging (MRI), in adult and pediatric patients above 2 years of age.[1] Limited data from the manufacturer reports that levels of gadolinium-based contrast agents are low in human milk; 0.01% to 0.04% of the maternal dose. The American College of Radiology and the Contrast Media Safety Committee of European Society of Urogenital Radiology conclude that it is safe for a mother to continue breastfeeding her infant after the administration of a gadolinium-containing contrast medium.[2,3]

The base gadolinium molecule is toxic in "free" form and is always chelated to various compounds. High Risk gadolinium molecules include gadodiamide and gadoversetamide in which gadolinium is prone to be released from chelation. Medium risk forms include Gadofosveset trisodium (Vasovist), gadoxetic acid disodium (Primovist), and gadobenate dimeglumine (MultiHance). Low risk forms include: Gadoterate meglumine (Dotarem), gadoteridol (ProHance) and gadobutrol (Gadovist).[4]

T 1/2	1.6 h	MW	754 Da	PB	None
Tmax		RID		Vd	0.25 L/kg
Oral		M/P		pKa	

Adult Concerns: Headache, bradycardia, abnormal taste, nausea, feeling of pain, burning or warmth, coldness at injection site.

Adult Dose: 0.2 mL/kg.

Pediatric Concerns: No known data in lactation.

Infant Monitoring:

Alternatives:

References:
1. Pharmaceutical manufacturers prescribing information.
2. American College of Radiology, Committee on Drugs and Contrast Media. ACR manual on contrast media version8. 2012:79.
3. Webb JA, Thomsen HS, Morcos SK; Members of Contrast Media Safety Committee of European Society of Urogenital Radiology (ESUR). The use of iodinated and gadolinium contrast media during pregnancy and lactation. Eur Radiol. 2005 Jun;15(6):1234-1240. Epub 2004 Dec 18.
4. Puac P, Rodríguez A, Vallejo C, Zamora CA, Castillo M. Safety of contrast material use during pregnancy and lactation. Magn Reson Imaging Clin N Am. 2017 Nov;25(4):787-797. PubMed PMID: 28964468.

GADOTERIDOL

Trade: Prohance

Category: Diagnostic Agent, Radiological Contrast Media

LRC: L3 - No Data-Probably Compatible

Gadoteridol is a non-ionic, non-iodinated gadolinium chelate complex used as a radiocontrast agent in MRI scans. The metabolism of gadoteridol is unknown, but a similar gadolinium salt (gadopentetate) is not metabolized at all. The half-life is brief (1.6 hours), and the volume of distribution is very small. This suggests that gadoteridol does not penetrate tissues well and is unlikely to penetrate milk in significant quantities. A similar compound, gadopentetate, is barely detectable in breast milk. Although not reported, the oral bioavailability is probably similar to gadopentetate, which is minimal to none. No data are available on the transfer of gadoteridol to human milk, although it is probably minimal.[1] The American College of Radiology concludes that it is safe for a mother-infant dyad to continue breastfeeding after the administration of a gadolinium-containing contrast medium. In another review, only tiny amounts of gadolinium contrast agents reach the milk compartment and virtually none of this is absorbed orally by the infant.[2]

T 1/2	1.57 h	MW		PB	
Tmax		RID		Vd	
Oral	Poor	M/P		pKa	

Adult Concerns: Hypersensitivity, nausea, urticaria, taste alteration, rash, abdominal cramp, nephrogenic systemic fibrosis.

Adult Dose: 0.1 mmol/kg (0.2 mL/kg)

Pediatric Concerns:

Infant Monitoring:

Alternatives:

References:
1. Pharmaceutical manufacturers prescribing information.
2. Webb JA, Thomsen HS, Morcos SK; Members of Contrast Media Safety Committee of European Society of Urogenital Radiology (ESUR). The use of iodinated andgadolinium contrast media during pregnancy and lactation. Eur Radiol. 2005 Jun;15(6):1234-1240. Epub 2004 Dec 18.

GADOVERSETAMIDE

Trade: Optimark

Category: Diagnostic Agent, Other

LRC: L3 - No Data-Probably Compatible

Gadoversetamide is a paramagnetic agent used as a contrast agent in magnetic resonance imaging (MRI). It does not enter most compartments and is confined to extracellular water with a low volume of distribution.[1] As with gadopentetate, this agent is very unlikely to penetrate milk or be orally bioavailable. However, no human data are available. Rat studies show some penetration of gadoversetamide into rat milk but rodent lactation studies do not correlate with humans. The American College of Radiology concludes that it is safe for a mother-infant dyad to continue breastfeeding after the administration of a gadolinium-containing contrast medium. In another review, only tiny amounts of gadolinium contrast agents reach the milk compartment and virtually none of this is absorbed orally by the infant.[2]

Recent data suggest that gadoversetamide is one of the gadolinium chelates that is of highest risk of becoming unchelated, and being absorbed in the mother or via milk.[3] Low risk forms include: Gadoterate meglumine (Dotarem), gadoteridol (ProHance) and gadobutrol (Gadovist).

T 1/2	1.7 h	MW	661 Da	PB	
Tmax		RID		Vd	0.162 L/kg
Oral		M/P		pKa	

Adult Concerns: Headache, vasodilatation, taste perversion, dizziness, nausea, and paresthesia are most commonly observed.

Adult Dose:

Pediatric Concerns:

Infant Monitoring:

Alternatives:

References:

1. Pharmaceutical manufacturers prescribing information.
2. Webb JA, Thomsen HS, Morcos SK; Members of Contrast Media Safety Committee of European Society of Urogenital Radiology (ESUR). The use of iodinated and gadolinium contrast media during pregnancy and lactation. Eur Radiol. 2005 Jun;15(6):1234-1240. Epub 2004 Dec 18.
3. Puac P, Rodríguez A, Vallejo C, Zamora CA, Castillo M. Safety of contrast material use during pregnancy and lactation. Magn Reson Imaging Clin N Am. 2017 Nov;25(4):787-797. PubMed PMID: 28964468.

GADOXETATE DISODIUM

Trade: Eovist, Primovist

Category: Diagnostic Agent, Radiological Contrast Media

LRC: L3 - No Data-Probably Compatible

Gadoxetate disodium is a gadolinium contrast agent that is given intravenously for magnetic resonance imaging of the liver.[1] The transfer of Gadoxetate to human milk is unknown; according to the manufacturer, breastfeeding should be withheld for at least 10 hours after the IV administration of this agent (in mothers with normal renal function). Due to the molecular weight and kinetics of gadoxetate, virtually none of this contrast agent is expected to be transferred to human milk or absorbed by the infant's gastrointestinal tract; therefore, there is no need to withhold breastfeeding.

T 1/2	0.95 h	MW	725.7 Da	PB	<10%
Tmax		RID		Vd	0.21 L/kg
Oral	Nil	M/P		pKa	

Adult Concerns: Headache, dizziness, feeling of warmth, hypertension, nausea, back pain.

Adult Dose: 0.025 mmol/kg (0.1 mL/kg).

Pediatric Concerns: No data are available in breastfeeding mothers.

Infant Monitoring:

Alternatives:

References:

1. Pharmaceutical manufacturing prescribing information.

GAMMA HYDROXYBUTYRIC ACID

Trade: GBH, GHB, Gamma-OH, Liquid Ecstasy, Oxybutyrate, Somsanit

Category: Sedative-Hypnotic

LRC: L5 - No Data-Hazardous

Gamma hydroxybutyrate (GHB) is a powerful, rapidly acting central nervous system depressant. GHB is indicated for the treatment of cataplexy in patients with narcolepsy, and in other countries, is sometimes used an anesthetic-hypnotic agent for general anesthesia. A natural component in the body, its function remains unknown. It is presently banned in the United States and many other countries. It is used for its ability to produce euphoric and hallucinogenic state, and for its alleged ability to release growth hormone that stimulates muscle growth. Ingestion leads to loss of muscle tone, relaxation, bradycardia to tachycardia, slowed respiration, and loss of inhibitions. Other side effects include delusions, depression, vomiting, nausea, hallucinations, seizures, delirium, agitation, amnesia, and coma. It can be used as a date-rape drug.[1]

It has a rather brief half-life (20-60 minutes) and <5% remains in the plasma compartment following 10 hours, and virtually none is detected in the urine after 12 hours. While these levels would depend on the dose, if the patient has returned to normal, milk levels after 12 hours would probably be low to undetectable. Although we do not have milk levels reported, but they would probably be significant during peak exposure. In patients that have dosed repeatedly for hours, a 24 hour pump and discard would be advisable. This product is strongly additive with alcohol as it is metabolized by alcohol dehydrogenase. This is a dangerous product that should never be used in breastfeeding mothers. Mothers exposed to this agent should pump and discard their milk for a minimum of 12-24 hours depending on the dose before returning the infant to the breast.

T 1/2	20-60 min	MW	126 Da	PB	
Tmax	45 min	RID		Vd	0.4 L/kg
Oral	Good	M/P		pKa	

Adult Concerns: Ingestion leads to loss of muscle tone, relaxation, bradycardia to tachycardia, slowed respiration, and loss of inhibitions. Other side effects include delusions, depression, vomiting, nausea, hallucinations, seizures, delirium, agitation, amnesia, and coma.

Adult Dose: Varies by indication.

Pediatric Concerns: No reported levels in milk, but due to its chemistry, it is likely to enter the milk compartment. Dangerous to infants.

Infant Monitoring: Sedation, slowed breathing rate, not waking to feed/poor feeding, loss of muscle tone, seizures, and weight gain.

Alternatives:

References:
1. Baselt RC. Disposition of Toxic Drugs and Chemicals in Man. 6th ed. Foster City, CA: Chemical Toxicology Institute; 2002:472-475.

GANCICLOVIR

Trade: Cytovene, Valcyte, Vitracert, Zirgan

Category: Antiviral

LRC: L3 - No Data-Probably Compatible

Ganciclovir is a guanosine derivative that, upon phosphorylation, inhibits DNA replication by herpes simplex viruses (HSV). It is provided as an ophthalmic gel, insert, oral tablet, or intravenous liquid. Ganciclovir ophthalmic gel is indicated for the treatment of acute herpetic keratitis (dendritic ulcers). The estimated maximum daily dose of ganciclovir administered as one drop, five times per day is 0.375 mg. Compared to maintenance doses of systemically administered ganciclovir of 900 mg (oral valganciclovir) and 5 mg/kg (IV ganciclovir), the ophthalmically administered daily dose is approximately 0.04% and 0.1% of the oral dose and IV doses, respectively, thus minimal systemic exposure is expected. It is not known whether topical ophthalmic ganciclovir administration would result in sufficient systemic absorption to produce detectable quantities in breast milk, but it is unlikely. Be aware that the oral and intravenous doses may produce much higher plasma and maternal milk levels than the ophthalmic product. Caution should be exercised when oral or intravenous products are administered to nursing mothers.[1]

T 1/2	1.7-5.8 h	MW	255 Da	PB	1%-2 %
Tmax	1.8 h	RID		Vd	0.2 L/kg
Oral	5%	M/P		pKa	

Adult Concerns: Fever, vomiting, diarrhea, anorexia, changes in renal function, leukopenia, neutropenia, thrombocytopenia, anemia, pruritis.

Adult Dose: 900 mg orally once or twice daily.

Pediatric Concerns: None reported via milk at this time.

Infant Monitoring: Vomiting, diarrhea, weight gain. Caution if IV or oral dosage form is used maternally.

Alternatives:

References:
1. Pharmaceutical manufacturers prescribing information.

GANIRELIX ACETATE

Trade: Antagon (ganirelix), Cetrorelix, Cetrotide (cetrorelix)

Category: Female Reproductive Agent

LRC: L3 - No Data-Probably Compatible

Ganirelix is a leutinizing hormone releasing hormone antagonist (LHRH antagonist) use in management of female infertility. Ganirelix acts by competitively inducing a rapid, reversible suppression of gonadotropin secretion.[1] This subsequently inhibits release of luteinizing hormone. The midcycle LH surge initiates several physiologic actions including ovulation, resumption of meiosis in the oocyte, and luteinization. This product is used to prevent the premature LH surge found in some infertile women. No data are available on the transfer of this decapeptide to human milk but it is unlikely due to its peptide structure and its larger molecular weight. In addition, it is very unlikely this decapeptide would be stable in the infants' gastrointestinal tract or orally bioavailable.

Cetrorelix acetate is also an LHRH antagonist similar in action to ganirelix.

T 1/2	12.8-16.2 h	MW	1570 Da	PB	82
Tmax	1.1 h	RID		Vd	0.62 L/kg
Oral	Nil	M/P		pKa	4.2, 9.8

Adult Concerns: Adverse events include abdominal pain, fetal death, headache, ovarian hyperstimulation syndrome, and vaginal bleeding.

Adult Dose: 250 μg subcutaneously daily.

Pediatric Concerns: None reported via milk, but no studies are available.

Infant Monitoring:

Alternatives:

References:
1. Pharmaceutical manufacturers prescribing information.

GATIFLOXACIN

Trade: Tequin, Zymar, Zymaxid

Category: Antibiotic, Quinolone

LRC: L3 - No Data-Probably Compatible

Gatifloxacin is a fluoroquinolone antibiotic similar to ofloxacin, levofloxacin, and ciprofloxacin.[1,2] While the manufacturer reports that gatifloxacin is secreted into animal milk, no data are available in humans. There are other fluoroquinolones with data regarding drug entry into human milk (e.g., ciprofloxacin, ofloxacin). The most likely risk to an infant is a change in gut flora.

Gatifloxacin ophthalmic solution: No data on its transfer to human milk is available, but the maximum plasma levels reported in one set of users was only 2.7 ng/mL. The mean C_{max} and estimated daily exposure values were 1600 and 1000 times lower than the C_{max} and AUC reported after therapeutic 400 mg oral dose of moxifloxacin.[1] Thus ophthalmic exposure is extremely unlikely to produce clinically relevant levels in milk. Following the administration of a gatifloxacin ophthalmic solution (0.3% or 0.5%) to one eye of six healthy male subjects each in an escalated dosing regimen starting with a single two-drop dose, then two drops four times daily for 7 days and finally two drops eight times daily for 3 days, serum gatifloxacin levels were below the lower limit of quantification (5 ng/mL) in all subjects.[2] Due to the very low plasma gatifloxacin levels achieved after ophthalmic use, it is highly unlikely that infant plasma levels following breast milk exposure would be significant enough to cause clinical effects.

Because fluoroquinolones have limited safety data in pediatric and breastfeeding patients, use in lactation is not recommended if alternative therapies exist.[2]

T 1/2	7.1 h	MW	402 Da	PB	20%
Tmax	1-2 h	RID		Vd	1.5 L/kg
Oral	96%	M/P		pKa	5.94, 9.21

Adult Concerns: Diarrhea, nausea, vaginitis, headache, dizziness, allergic reaction, chills, fever, palpitations, abdominal pain and other symptoms have been reported. CNS agitation, nervousness, insomnia, and paranoia have been reported.

Adult Dose: 400 mg daily.

Pediatric Concerns: None reported via milk, no published data available yet.

Infant Monitoring: Vomiting, diarrhea, changes in gastrointestinal flora, and rash.

Alternatives: Ofloxacin(L2), Levofloxacin(L2)

References:
1. Giamarellou H, Kolokythas E, Petrikkos G, Gazis J, Aravantinos D, Sfikakis P. Pharmacokinetics of three newer quinolones in pregnant and lactating women. Am J Med. 1989;87(5A):49S-51S.
2. Pharmaceutical manufacturers prescribing information.

GEMCITABINE

Trade: Gemzar

Category: Antineoplastic

LRC: L4 - No Data-Possibly Hazardous

Gemcitabine is a nucleoside analog used for the treatment of metastatic breast cancer, non-small cell lung cancer, and pancreatic cancer. Gemcitabine elimination follows a two-phase elimination curve. The terminal elimination half-life is reported to be 49 minutes in females but can range to as high as 638 minutes following long infusions.[1] The volume of distribution following short infusions (<70 min) was 50 L/m^2 (1.24 L/kg), indicating that gemcitabine, after short infusions, is not extensively distributed in tissues. For long infusions, the volume of distribution rose to 370 L/m^2 (9.14 L/kg), reflecting slow equilibration of gemcitabine within the tissue compartment. Gemcitabine is metabolized to an active metabolite, gemcitabine triphosphate, which can be extracted from peripheral blood mononuclear cells. The half-life of the terminal phase for gemcitabine triphosphate from mononuclear cells ranges from 1.7 to 19.4 hours. Within 1 week, 92%-98% of the dose was recovered, almost entirely in the urine. No data are available on its transfer to milk. Women should be advised to withhold breastfeeding for a minimum of 7 days.

T 1/2	49 min short infusions; long infusions 245-638 min; active metabolite 1.7-19.4 h	MW	299.7 Da	PB	Negligible
Tmax	30 min (IV)	RID		Vd	1.24-9.14 L/kg
Oral		M/P		pKa	3.6

Adult Concerns: Drowsiness, stomatitis, vomiting, changes in liver and renal function, hematuria, proteinuria, leukopenia, neutropenia, thrombocytopenia, anemia, edema, rash.

Adult Dose: Varies by protocol.

Pediatric Concerns:

Infant Monitoring: Withhold breastfeeding for at least 7 days.

Alternatives:

References:
1. Pharmaceutical manufacturers prescribing information.

GEMFIBROZIL

Trade: Ausgem, Gemcor, Gemhexal, Lopid

Category: Antihyperlipidemic

LRC: L3 - No Data-Probably Compatible

Gemfibrozil is a hypolipidemic agent primarily used to lower triglyceride levels by decreasing serum very low density lipoproteins.[1] A slight reduction in serum cholesterol may likewise occur. Following a dose of 800 mg, mean peak maternal plasma levels were 33 μg/mL. There are no data on its transfer to human milk. Cholesterol and other products of cholesterol biosynthesis are essential components for fetal and neonatal development; therefore, it is not clear if it would be safe for use in a breastfed infant who needs high levels of cholesterol. Some caution is recommended until more data are available.

T 1/2	1.5 h	MW	250 Da	PB	99%
Tmax	1-2 h	RID		Vd	
Oral	97%	M/P		pKa	4.7

Adult Concerns: Dry mouth, epigastric pain, changes in liver function, constipation, diarrhea, flatulence. Changes in blood chemistry including hematocrit, white blood cells, hemoglobin.

Adult Dose: 600 mg twice daily.

Pediatric Concerns: None reported via milk, but risk versus benefit evaluation is recommended.

Infant Monitoring: Weight gain, growth.

Alternatives:

References:
1. DrugBank, 2019.

GEMIFLOXACIN MESYLATE

Trade: Factive

Category: Antibiotic, Quinolone

LRC: L3 - No Data-Probably Compatible

A member of the fluoroquinolone family, gemifloxacin is used to treat a wide range of infections caused by gram-positive and gram-negative bacteria. It acts by inhibiting bacterial DNA synthesis.[1] No data are available on the transfer of gemifloxacin to human milk. Some fluoroquinolones are excreted into breast milk (e.g., ciprofloxacin, ofloxacin). Because fluoroquinolones have limited safety data in pediatric and breastfeeding patients, use in lactation is not recommended if alternative therapies exist.

T 1/2	7 h	MW	485 Da	PB	60%-70%
Tmax	0.5-2 h	RID		Vd	4.2 L/kg
Oral	71%	M/P		pKa	

Adult Concerns: Headache, nausea, vomiting, diarrhea, changes in liver and renal function, neutropenia, thrombocytopenia, rash.

Adult Dose: 320 mg daily.

Pediatric Concerns: No data are available.

Infant Monitoring: Vomiting, diarrhea, changes in gastrointestinal flora, and rash.

Alternatives:

References:
1. Pharmaceutical manufacturers prescribing information.

GENTAMICIN

Trade: Alocomicin, Cidomycin, Garamycin, Garatec, Palacos, Septopal

Category: Antibiotic, Aminoglycoside

LRC: L2 - Limited Data-Probably Compatible

Gentamicin is a narrow spectrum antibiotic generally used for gram-negative infections. The oral absorption of gentamicin (<1%) is generally nil with the exception of premature neonates, where small amounts may be absorbed.[1] In one study of 10 women given 80 mg three times daily IM for 5 days postpartum, milk levels were measured on day 4.[2] Gentamicin levels in milk were 0.42, 0.48, 0.49, and 0.41 mg/L at 1, 3, 5, and 7 hours respectively. The milk/plasma ratios were 0.11 at 1 hour and 0.44 at 7 hours. Plasma gentamicin levels in neonates were small, found in only 5 of the 10 neonates, and averaged 0.41 µg/mL. The authors estimate that daily ingestion via breast milk would be 307 µg for a 3.6 kg neonate (normal neonatal dose= 2.5 mg/kg every 12 hours). These amounts would be clinically irrelevant in most infants.

There has been one case report of an infant with "two grossly bloody stools" on day 5 of maternal antibiotic therapy (antibiotic therapy ended hours before infants symptoms occurred).[3] The mother was receiving Clindamycin 600mg IV q6h and Gentamicin 80mg IV q8h for endometritis; however, it should be noted that the infant was also on 48 hours of ampicillin and gentamicin, while neonatal sepsis was ruled out, at the same time the mother was receiving her treatment. The infant temporarily stopped breastfeeding for 12 hours and symptoms resolved (8 month follow-up - no further concerns).

T 1/2	2-3 h	MW	477 Da	PB	<10%-30%
Tmax	30-90 min (IM)	RID	2.1%	Vd	0.28 L/kg
Oral	<1%	M/P	0.11-0.44	pKa	8.2

Adult Concerns: Headache, ototoxicity, nausea, vomiting, diarrhea, changes in liver and renal function, hematologic changes.

Adult Dose: 1.5-2.5 mg/kg every 8 hours.

Pediatric Concerns: None reported.

Infant Monitoring: Vomiting, diarrhea, changes in gastrointestinal flora, and rash.

Alternatives:

References:
1. Nelson JD, McCracken GH, Jr. The current status of gentamicin for tne neonate and young infant. Am J Dis Child. 1972;124(1):13-14.
2. Celiloglu M, Celiker S, Guven H, Tuncok Y, Demir N, Erten O. Gentamicin excretion and uptake from breast milk by nursing infants. Obstet Gynecol. 1994;84(2):263-265.
3. Mann CF. Clindamycin and breast-feeding. Pediatrics. 1980;66(6):1030-1031.

GENTIAN VIOLET

Trade: Crystal Violet, Gentian Violet, Methylrosaniline chloride

Category: Antifungal

LRC: L2 - No Data-Probably Compatible

Gentian violet (GV) is an older product that, when used topically and orally, is an exceptionally effective antifungal and antimicrobial.[1] It is a strong purple dye that is difficult to remove. Gentian violet has been found to be equivalent to ketoconazole and far superior to nystatin in treating oral (not esophageal) candidiasis in patients with advanced AIDS. It is also useful in treating purulent infections of the ear infected with methicillin-resistant *Staphylococcus aureus*.[3] Gentian violet (GV) solutions generally come as 1%-2% solutions dissolved in a 10% solution of alcohol. For use with infants, the solution should be diluted with distilled water to 0.25% to 0.5% gentian violet. This reduces the irritant properties of GV and reduces the alcohol content as well. While the alcohol is irritating to the nipple, it is not detrimental to the infant.[2] Higher concentrations of GV are known to be very irritating, leading to oral ulceration and necrotic skin reactions in children. If used, a small swab should be soaked in the solution, and then swabbed in the infant's gingivae. Apply it directly to the affected areas in the mouth no more than once or twice daily for no more than 3-7 days. Direct application to the nipple has been reported.

T 1/2		MW	408 Da	PB	
Tmax		RID		Vd	
Oral		M/P		pKa	

Adult Concerns: Oral ulceration, stomatitis, nausea, vomiting, diarrhea, staining of skin and clothing.

Adult Dose: Apply no more than 3-5 consecutive days.

Pediatric Concerns: Irritation leading to buccal ulcerations and necrotic skin reactions if used excessively and in higher concentrations. Nausea, vomiting, diarrhea.

Infant Monitoring: Mucosal ulcerations, vomiting, diarrhea.

Alternatives:

References:
1. DrugBank, 2019.
2. Newman J. Personal communication, 1997.
3. Kayama C, Goto Y, Shimoya S, et al. Effects of gentian violet on refractory discharging ears infected with methicillin-resistant *staphylococcus aureus*. J Otolaryngol. 2006;35(6):384-386.

GLATIRAMER

Trade: Copaxone

Category: Immune Suppressant

LRC: L3 - No Data-Probably Compatible

Glatiramer is a synthetic polypeptide indicated for the treatment of relapsing, remitting multiple sclerosis.[1] It is primarily indicated for those who do not respond to interferons. Glatiramer is a mixture of random polymers of four amino acids: L-alanine, L-glutamic acid, L-lysine, and L-tyrosine.[1,2] Its molecular weight ranges from 4,700 to 13,000 Da, which would reduce its ability to enter milk. It is antigenically similar to myelin basic protein, a natural component of the myelin sheath of neurons. This medication is known to have high polarity and is very hydrophilic and cannot cross the blood-brain barrier, thus this medication is thought to exert most of its effect in the periphery.[2] After this medication is absorbed subcutaneously it is degraded into free amino acids and small oligopeptides, thus it cannot be measured in the plasma. No data are available on its transfer to human milk, but it is very unlikely. If ingested orally, it would also most likely be depolymerized into individual amino acids, so toxicity is unlikely.

T 1/2		MW	4700+ Da	PB	
Tmax		RID		Vd	
Oral	Minimal	M/P		pKa	

Adult Concerns: Dizziness, anxiety, abnormal dreams, fever, chest pain, palpitations, dyspnea, sweating, nausea, urinary urgency, weakness, tremor, infection.

Adult Dose: 20 mg subcutaneously once daily.

Pediatric Concerns: None via milk.

Infant Monitoring:

Alternatives:

References:
1. Pharmaceutical manufacturers prescribing information.
2. Neuhaus O, Kieseier BC, hartung HP. Pharmacokinetics and pharmacodynamics of the interferon-betas, glatiramer acetate, and mitoxantrone in multiple sclerosis. J Neurol Sci. 2007;259:27-37.

GLIPIZIDE

Trade: Glibenese, Glucotrol, Glucotrol XL, Melizide, Minidiab

Category: Antidiabetic, Sulfonylurea

LRC: L2 - Limited Data-Probably Compatible

Glipizide is a potent hypoglycemic agent that belongs to sulfonylurea family.[1] It is formulated in regular and extended release formulations, and it is used for the treatment of non insulin-dependent (type II) diabetes. It reduces glucose levels by stimulating insulin secretion from the pancreas.

A 2005 publication reported the results of two independent studies that included women with type II diabetes starting glyburide or glipizide postpartum.[2] In the second study, two mothers received daily doses of glipizide 5 mg.[1] Maternal serum and milk samples were drawn 1-2 weeks postpartum just prior to the dose (trough) and 4 hours postdose (peak). All four milk samples were below the limit of detection (0.08 µg/mL). The maximum theoretical infant dose and relative infant dose were calculated using the limit of detection. The mean theoretical infant dose was less than 12 µg/kg/day. The relative infant dose in this study was high (~27%); however, this is reflective of the assay's sensitivity, not what was detected in milk (levels undetectable). In addition, the infants had blood glucose levels monitored and both were normal.

T 1/2	2-5 h	MW	446 Da	PB	98%-99%
Tmax	1-3 h	RID		Vd	0.15 L/kg
Oral	90%-100%	M/P		pKa	5.9

Adult Concerns: Hypoglycemia, jaundice, nausea, vomiting, diarrhea, constipation.

Adult Dose: 15-40 mg daily.

Pediatric Concerns: None reported via milk at this time.

Infant Monitoring: Vomiting, diarrhea and signs of hypoglycemia- drowsiness, lethargy, pallor, sweating, tremor.

Alternatives: Insulin(L2), Metformin(L1), Glyburide(L2)

References:
1. Pharmaceutical manufacturers prescribing information.
2. Feig DS, Briggs GG, Kraemer JM, et al. Transfer of glyburide and glipizide into breast milk. Diabetes Care. 2005;28:1851-1855.

GLUCOSAMINE

Trade:

Category: Antiarthritic

LRC: L3 - No Data-Probably Compatible

Glucosamine is an endogenous amino monosaccharide that has been reported to be effective in resolving symptoms of osteoarthritis. It is one of the salt forms of the amino sugar glucosamine, which is a constituent of cartilage proteoglycans. Administered in large doses, most is sequestered in the liver with only minimal amounts reaching other tissues, thus oral bioavailability is low. Most of the oral dose is hepatically metabolized and subsequently incorporated into other plasma proteins.[1] No data are available on transfer to human milk. Because glucosamine is primarily sequestered and metabolized in the liver, and because the plasma levels are almost undetectable, it is unlikely that any would enter human milk. Further, the fact that it is so poorly bioavailable, it is unlikely that an infant would absorb clinically relevant amounts.

T 1/2	0.3 h	MW	179 Da	PB	0%
Tmax		RID		Vd	0.035 L/kg
Oral	<26%	M/P		pKa	8.23, 11.73

Adult Concerns: Headache, nausea, dyspepsia, vomiting, drowsiness, and skin rash. Peripheral edema and tachycardia have been reported. Some reports of exacerbation of asthma by glucosamine.

Adult Dose: 500 mg three times daily.

Pediatric Concerns: None reported via milk.

Infant Monitoring:

Alternatives:

References:

1. Setnikar I, Palumbo R, Canali S, Zanolo G. Pharmacokinetics of glucosamine in man. Arzneimittelforschung. 1993;43(10):1109-1113.

GLYBURIDE

Trade: Daonil, Diabeta, Diaformin, Euglucon, Gen-Glybe, Micronase

Category: Antidiabetic, Sulfonylurea

LRC: L2 - Limited Data-Probably Compatible

Glyburide is a second generation sulfonylurea agent useful in the treatment of non-insulin-dependent (type II) diabetes mellitus.[1] It belongs to the sulfonylurea family (tolbutamide, glipizide) of hypoglycemic agents of which glyburide is one of the most potent. Glyburide apparently stimulates insulin secretion, thus reducing plasma glucose.

A 2005 publication reported the results of two independent studies that included women with type II diabetes starting glyburide or glipizide postpartum.[2] In the first study, women were given single doses of glyburide postpartum and breast milk samples were taken at 2, 4, 6, and 8 hours postdose. Six of these mothers received a single 5 mg dose of glyburide, and two of these mothers received a single 10 mg dose; all breast milk samples were below the limit of detection (0.005 μg/mL). The maximum theoretical infant dose and relative infant dose were calculated using the limit of detection. The mean theoretical infant dose was less than 0.75 μg/kg/day. The mean relative infant dose for the 5 mg and 10 mg doses were both less than 1.05% and 0.7%, respectively.

In the second study, three mothers received daily doses of glyburide 5 mg.[2] Maternal serum and milk samples were drawn on day 5-8 postpartum just prior to the dose (trough) and 4 hours post dose (peak). All milk samples were below the limit of detection (0.08 μg/mL). The maximum theoretical infant dose and relative infant dose were calculated using the limit of detection. The mean theoretical infant dose was less than 12 μg/kg/day. The relative infant dose in this study was high (~28%); however, this is reflective of the assays sensitivity, not what was detected in milk (levels undetectable). In addition, two of the three infants had blood glucose levels monitored and both were normal.

T 1/2	4-13.7 h	MW	494 Da	PB	99%
Tmax	2-4 h	RID	0.53%-1.05%	Vd	0.73 L/kg
Oral	Complete	M/P		pKa	5.3

Adult Concerns: Headache, dizziness, diarrhea or constipation, anorexia, changes in liver enzymes, hypoglycemia, skin rashes.

Adult Dose: 1.25-20 mg daily.

Pediatric Concerns: None reported via milk at this time.

Infant Monitoring: Vomiting, diarrhea, weight gain and signs of hypoglycemia- drowsiness, lethargy, pallor, sweating, tremor.

Alternatives: Insulin(L2), Metformin(L1)

References:
1. Pharmaceutical manufacturers prescribing information.
2. Feig DS, Briggs GG, Kraemer JM, et al. Transfer of glyburide and glipizide into breast milk. Diabetes Care. 2005;28:1851-1855.

GOSERELIN ACETATE IMPLANT

Trade: Histrelin, Supprelin (Histrelin), Trelstar (Triptorelin), Triptorelin, Vantas (Histrelin), Zoladex

Category: Luteinizing Hormone Releasing Hormone Antagonist

LRC: L3 - No Data-Probably Compatible

Goserelin acetate is a synthetic decapeptide analog of luteinizing hormone releasing hormone (LHRH) and it acts as a potent inhibitor of pituitary gonadotropin secretion.[1] Following initial administration in males, goserelin causes an initial increase in serum luteinizing hormone (LH) and follicle stimulating hormone (FSH) levels. Chronic administration of goserelin leads to sustained suppression of these pituitary gonadotropins, and serum levels of testosterone in males. In females, a down-regulation of the pituitary gland following chronic exposure leads to suppression of gonadotropin secretion, a decrease in serum estradiol to levels consistent with the menopausal state. Serum LH and FSH are suppressed to follicular phase levels within 4 weeks. No data are available on its transfer to human milk but due to its structure and molecular weight it is very unlikely to enter milk, or to be orally bioavailable in the infant.

Histrelin acetate and Triptorelin pamoate are also luteinizing hormone releasing hormone (gonadotropin releasing hormone) agonists, similar to goserelin.

T 1/2	2.3 h	MW	1269 Da	PB	Low
Tmax	12-15 days	RID		Vd	0.28 L/kg
Oral		M/P		pKa	6.2

Adult Concerns: Headache, changes in mood, insomnia, hot flashes, sweating, nausea, abdominal pain, sexual dysfunction, vaginitis, pelvic pain, decreased bone mineral density, edema, acne.

Adult Dose: 3.6 mg subcutaneously every 28 days.

Pediatric Concerns: None reported via milk.

Infant Monitoring: It is not known how it may affect milk production, some caution is recommended concerning loss of milk supply.

Alternatives:

References:
1. Pharmaceutical manufacturers prescribing information.

GRAMICIDIN

Trade:

Category: Antibiotic, Other

LRC: L3 - No Data-Probably Compatible

Gramicidin is a mixture of three antibiotic compounds (Gramicidin A, B and C) that are bactericidal against gram-positive bacteria.[1] It is used in combination with neomycin and polymyxin B for treatment of superficial infections of the eye (e.g., conjunctivitis). Currently, there is no information about its entry into human milk.

Adult Concerns: Itching, swelling, eye redness.

Adult Dose:

Pediatric Concerns:

Infant Monitoring:

Alternatives:

References:
1. Pharmaceutical manufacturers prescribing information.

GRANISETRON

Trade: Kytril

Category: Antiemetic

LRC: L3 - No Data-Probably Compatible

Granisetron is an antinauseant and antiemetic agent commonly used with chemotherapy. Following a 1 mg IV dose, the peak plasma concentration was 3.63 ng/mL.[1] No data are available on its transfer to human milk, but its levels are likely to be low. Further, other medications within this antiemetic family (see ondansetron) are used in children (> 1 month of age). It is unlikely that this product will be overtly toxic to a breastfed infant. However, when used with chemotherapeutic agents, long waiting periods should be used for elimination of the chemotherapeutic agents anyway.

T 1/2	3-14 h	MW	349 Da	PB	65%
Tmax	1 h	RID		Vd	2-4 L/kg
Oral	60%	M/P		pKa	9

Adult Concerns: Headache, asthenia, somnolence, insomnia, fever, QTc prolongation, dyspepsia, abdominal pain, diarrhea or constipation, changes in liver enzymes, oliguria.

Adult Dose: 2 mg orally.

Pediatric Concerns: None reported via milk at this time.

Infant Monitoring: Sedation or insomnia, diarrhea.

Alternatives: Ondansetron(L2)

References:
1. Pharmaceutical manufacturers prescribing information.

GRISEOFULVIN

Trade: Fulcin, Fulvicin, Gris-PEG, Griseostatin, Grisovin, Grisovin-FP

Category: Antifungal

LRC: L3 - Limited Data-Probably Compatible

Griseofulvin is an older class antifungal. Enhanced safety profiles with the newer families of antifungals have reduced the use of griseofulvin. The drug is primarily effective against tinea species and not *Candida albicans*.[1,2] There are no data available for humans. In one study in cows following a dose of 10 mg/kg/day for 5 days (human dose =5 mg/kg/day) milk concentrations were 0.16 mg/L. Although these data cannot be directly extrapolated to humans, they indicate transfer to milk in some species. Oral use in adults is associated with low risk of hepatic cancer. Griseofulvin is still commonly used in pediatric tinea capitis (ringworm), where it is a preferred medication.

T 1/2	9-24 h	MW	353 Da	PB	
Tmax	4-8 h	RID		Vd	
Oral	27%-72%	M/P		pKa	

Adult Concerns: Headache, dizziness, fatigue, insomnia, confusion, nausea, vomiting, diarrhea, changes in liver and renal function, jaundice, leukopenia, skin rashes.

Adult Dose: 500-1000 mg daily (micro) or 330-375 mg daily (ultra).

Pediatric Concerns: None reported from breast milk.

Infant Monitoring: Insomnia, lethargy, vomiting, diarrhea. If clinical symptoms of jaundice check liver function and bilirubin.

Alternatives: Fluconazole(L2)

References:
1. Pharmaceutical manufacturers prescribing information.
2. Huddleston WA. Antifungal activity of penicillium griseofulvin mycelium. Vet Rec. 1970;86(3):75-76.

GUAIFENESIN

Trade: Iophen, Mucinex

Category: Expectorant

LRC: L3 - No Data-Probably Compatible

Guaifenesin is an expectorant that thins bronchial secretions and loosens phlegm (mucus) to make a more productive cough.[1] It does not suppress coughing and should not be used in persistent coughs. No data are available on transfer to human milk. In general, clinical studies documenting the efficacy of guaifenesin are lacking, and the usefulness of this product as an expectorant is highly questionable.

Poor efficacy of these drugs (expectorants in general) would suggest that they do not provide enough justification for use in lactating mothers. But untoward effects have not been reported.

Note: Guaifenesin is often found in combination products, suitability of other ingredients in the product also need to be considered.

T 1/2	1 h	MW	198 Da	PB	
Tmax		RID		Vd	1 L/kg
Oral	Complete	M/P		pKa	13.62

Adult Concerns: Sedation, nausea, dyspepsia, vomiting, diarrhea, sedation, skin rash.

Adult Dose: 200-400 mg every 4 hours.

Pediatric Concerns: None reported via milk at this time.

Infant Monitoring: Sedation.

Alternatives:

References:
1. Pharmaceutical manufacturers prescribing information.

HALOPERIDOL

Trade: Haldol, Peridol, Serenace

Category: Antipsychotic, Typical

LRC: L3 - Limited Data-Probably Compatible

Haloperidol is a potent antipsychotic agent that is reported to increase prolactin levels in some patients. In one study of a woman treated for puerperal hypomania and receiving 5 mg twice daily, the concentration of haloperidol in milk was 0, 23.5, 18, and 3.25 µg/L on day 1, 6, 7, and 21 respectively.[1] The corresponding maternal plasma levels were 0, 40, 26, and 4 µg/L on day 1, 6, 7, and 21 respectively. The milk/plasma ratios were 0.58, 0.69, and 0.81 on days 6, 7, and 21 respectively. After 4 weeks of therapy the infant showed no symptoms of sedation and was feeding well. In another study after a mean daily dose of 29.2 mg, the concentration of haloperidol in breast milk was 5 µg/L at 11 hours postdose.[2]

In a study of three women on chronic haloperidol therapy receiving 3, 4, and 6 mg daily, milk levels were reported to be 32, 17, and 4.7 µg/L.[3] The latter levels (4.7) were taken from a patient believed to be noncompliant. Since the levels in milk are significant, some caution is recommended in breastfeeding mothers. In another study of nine mothers receiving 1 to 40 mg/day haloperidol, breast milk samples were randomly collected 12-15 hours after the dose. Levels in milk ranged from undetectable to 24.9 µg/L and were interestingly, not correlated with the dose.[4] In four of these infants, serum concentrations ranged from 0.8 to 2.1 µg/L.

T 1/2	12-38 h	MW	376 Da	PB	92%
Tmax	2-6 h	RID	0.2%-12%	Vd	18-30 L/kg
Oral	60%	M/P	0.58-0.81	pKa	8.3

Adult Concerns: Sedation, tachycardia, hypotension, anemia, extrapyramidal symptoms, hypersomnia, poor feeding, and slowing in motor movements in the infant.

Adult Dose: 0.5-5 mg two to three times daily.

Pediatric Concerns: None reported via milk.

Infant Monitoring: Sedation or irritability, apnea, not waking to feed/poor feeding, constipation, weight gain, and extrapyramidal symptoms.

Alternatives: Risperidone(L2), Olanzapine(L2), Aripiprazole(L3)

References:

1. Whalley LJ, Blain PG, Prime JK. Haloperidol secreted in breast milk. Br Med J (Clin Res Ed). 1981;282(6278):1746-1747.
2. Stewart RB, Karas B, Springer PK. Haloperidol excretion in human milk. Am J Psychiatry. 1980;137(7):849-850.
3. Ohkubo T, Shimoyama R, Sugawara K. Measurement of haloperidol in human breast milk by high-performance liquid chromatography. J Pharm Sci. 1992;81(9):947-949.
4. Yoshida K, Smith B, Craggs M, Kumar R. Neuroleptic drugs in breast-milk: a study of pharmacokinetics and of possible adverse effects in breast-fed infants. Psychol Med. 1998 Jan;28(1):81-91.

HEPARIN

Trade: Canusal, Hepalean, Heparin, Heplok, Pularin

Category: Anticoagulant

LRC: L2 - No Data-Probably Compatible

Heparin is an anticoagulant. It is a large molecule that is used subcutaneously and intravenously. Due to its high molecular weight (12,000-15,000 Da), it is unlikely any would transfer into breast milk.[1] Any present in milk would be rapidly destroyed in the gastric contents of the infant.

T 1/2	1-2 h	MW	12,000-15,000 Da	PB	
Tmax	20 min	RID		Vd	
Oral		M/P		pKa	3.5-4

Adult Concerns: Bruising on the skin, hemorrhage, blood in urine or stool, thrombocytopenia and pain/bruising at injection site.

Adult Dose: 5,000 units sc every 8-12 hours (prophylaxis dose).

Pediatric Concerns: None reported via milk at this time.

Infant Monitoring: Rare bruising on the skin, blood in urine, vomit or stool.

Alternatives: Dalteparin(L2)

References:

1. McEvoy GK, ed. Heparin Sodium. Bethesda, MD: AHFS Drug Information, American Society of Health-System Pharmacists, Inc.; 2012.

HEPATITIS A + HEPATITIS B VACCINE

Trade: Twinrix

Category: Vaccine

LRC: L3 - No Data-Probably Compatible

Hepatitis A + hepatitis B vaccine combination is used for the prevention of hepatitis A and hepatitis B infection.[1] It contains the hepatitis A vaccine as well as the recombinant hepatitis B vaccine. It is used in those 18 years of age and older. It is administered in a three-dose vaccine series at 0, 1, and 6 months. Hepatitis A vaccine is prepared from inactivated hepatitis A virus. There is no contraindication for receiving the vaccine during breastfeeding. Hepatitis B vaccine is an inactivated non-infectious hepatitis B surface antigen vaccine. No data are available on its use in breastfeeding mothers, but it is unlikely to produce untoward effects on a breastfeeding infant since it is an inactivated virus. Hepatitis A + hepatitis B bivalent vaccine is probably compatible with breastfeeding.

Adult Concerns: Headache, fatigue, seizures (rare), diarrhea, redness, swelling tenderness, pain at the site of injection, hypersensitivity reactions.

Adult Dose: 1 mL intramuscular.

Pediatric Concerns:

Infant Monitoring:

Alternatives:

References:
1. Pharmaceutical manufacturers prescribing information.

HEPATITIS A INFECTION

Trade:

Category: Infectious Disease

LRC: L3 - No Data-Probably Compatible

The hepatitis A virus (HAV) belongs to the family of picornaviruses.[1] The most common mode of transmission is feco-oral. It is therefore more common in underdeveloped countries where hygiene is a regular source of concern. Other modes include transmission through contaminated food, transfusion of infected blood products, transplacental transmission,[2] and perinatal transmission.[3] In the United States, some of the most common risk factors include ingestion of contaminated food, close contact with a child/children at a day care center, international travel and use of intravenous drugs. Hepatitis A infection is an acute, self-limiting illness characterized by malaise, fever, anorexia and jaundice. It should also be noted that hepatitis A infection in children less than 6 years of age is asymptomatic 70% of the time.[1]

A majority of the adult population is immune to hepatitis A due to prior exposure. Fulminant hepatitis A infection is rare in infants and young children; chronic infection does not occur and a carrier state is unknown. Once infection occurs, viral shedding continues from onset up to 3 weeks. No reports were found in the literature of direct transmission of hepatitis A virus in breast milk. Therefore, in view of the potential benefits of breastfeeding, it is recommended that a lactating mother with acute hepatitis A infection may continue to breastfeed. However, it is of prime importance to ensure that she take all necessary sanitary precautions to minimize feco-oral transmission to the infant. Measures such as regular handwashing before holding the baby or coming in contact with items or clothing belonging to the infant should be undertaken. Unless the mother is jaundiced and acutely ill, breastfeeding can continue without interruption. Note that in infected children or infants, viral shedding can occur in their stools, despite being asymptomatic. Therefore, care givers of infected children at home and at day care centers should be cautious and maintain all hygienic and sanitary precautions to avoid exposure.

Hepatitis A vaccine and lactation: Since the hepatitis A vaccine is an inactivated vaccine, it is considered suitable in lactating women. Therefore, lactating women traveling to endemic areas are recommended to receive the vaccine as per the general travel immunization guidelines.

Adult Concerns: Jaundice, fever, malaise.

Adult Dose:

Pediatric Concerns: None reported. Protect with immune globulin injection.

Infant Monitoring: Jaundice, fever, malaise.

Alternatives:

References:
1. AAP CoID. Hepatitis A. In: Pickering LKBC, Kimberlin DW, Long SS, eds. Red book: 2009 Report of the Committee on Infectious Diseases. 29th ed. Elk Grove Village, IL: American Academy of Pediatrics; 2009:329-337.
2. Leikin E, Lysikiewicz A, Garry D, Tejani N. Intrauterine transmission of hepatitis A virus. Obstet Gynecol. 1996;88(4 Pt 2):690-691.
3. Motte A, Blanc J, Minodier P, Colson P. Acute hepatitis A in a pregnant woman at delivery. Int J Infect Dis. 2009;13(2):e49-e51.

HEPATITIS A VACCINE

Trade: Havrix, Vaqta

Category: Vaccine

LRC: L3 - No Data-Probably Compatible

Hepatitis A vaccine is indicated for protection against hepatitis A infection. There are two hepatitis A vaccines approved by the FDA for use in the United States, Vaqta and Havrix.[1,2] Both vaccines are made from inactivated hepatitis A virus. Both vaccine doses for adults are 1 mL initially, then a booster dose of 1 mL between 6 and 12 months after the first dose. For children, Vaqta recommends an initial dose of 0.5mL for children 2 to 17 years of age and a booster of 0.5 mL between 6 to 18 months after the initial dose. Havrix also recommends 0.5 mL for both doses but the booster should be given between 6 and 12 months of age. Seroconversion occurs within 1 month in 99% of cases and is expected to provide protective immunity for 20 years. Children should receive prophylaxis with the vaccine starting at 2 years of age for prevention of disease. The only contraindications to use of hepatitis

A vaccine are hypersensitivity to the components. The vaccine is not approved for children under 2 years of age. Hepatitis A vaccine should not be administered with live vaccines. Travelers should be vaccinated at least 1 month prior to departure. For post exposure prophylaxis, the CDC recommends the patient be tested for IgM antibody to confirm hepatitis A infection before treating any contacts of the patient. If positive, household and sexual contacts should receive immune globulin 0.02 mL/kg within 2 weeks of exposure. If the person received the vaccine at least 1 month before exposure, then they do not need the immune globulin. The vaccine should be administered the same day as the immune globulin. There is no contraindication for receiving the vaccine during breastfeeding.

According to the CDC, the inactivated virus is unlikely to cause harmful effects to infants that are breastfed. However, the administration of immune globulin should be considered instead of the vaccine.

Adult Concerns: Headache, fever, malaise, loss of appetite, nausea, vomiting, rash, pain at injection site, hypersensitivity reactions.

Adult Dose:

Pediatric Concerns:

Infant Monitoring:

Alternatives:

References:
1. Duff B, Duff P. Hepatitis A vaccine: ready for prime time. Obstet Gynecol. 1998 Mar;91(3):468-471. Review.
2. Pharmaceutical manufacturers prescribing information.
3. www.cdc.gov/breastfeeding/recommendations/vaccinations.htm

HEPATITIS B IMMUNE GLOBULIN

Trade: H-BIG, HEP-B-Gammagee, Hyperhep

Category: Immune Serum

LRC: L2 - Limited Data-Probably Compatible

Hepatitis B immune globulin (HBIG) is a sterile solution of immunoglobulin (10%-18% protein) containing a high titer of antibodies to hepatitis B surface antigen.[1] It is most commonly used as prophylaxis therapy for infants born to hepatitis B surface antigen positive mothers. The carrier state can be prevented in about 75% of such infections in newborns given HBIG immediately after birth. HBIG is generally administered to infants born to HBsAg positive mothers who wish to breastfeed. The prophylactic dose for newborns is 0.5 mL IM (thigh) as soon after birth as possible, preferably within 12 hours.[2] The infant should also be immunized with hepatitis B vaccine (0.5 mL IM) within 12 hours of birth, and then follow up with their healthcare provider to receive subsequent doses. Its use in a breastfeeding mother would not harm a breastfeeding infant.

T 1/2		MW		PB	
Tmax	1-6 days	RID		Vd	
Oral	None	M/P		pKa	

Adult Concerns: Pain at injection site, erythema, rash, dizziness, malaise.

Adult Dose: 0.06 mL/kg post-exposure.

Pediatric Concerns: Pain at injection site, erythema, rash.

Infant Monitoring:

Alternatives:

References:
1. Pharmaceutical manufacturers prescribing information.
2. Centers for Disease Control and Prevention [Online]. Epidemiology and prevention of vaccine-preventable diseases, August 2015 . http://www.cdc.gov/vaccines/pubs/pinkbook/hepb.html. Accessed July 26, 2016.

HEPATITIS B INFECTION

Trade: Hepatitis B Infection

Category: Infectious Disease

LRC: L4 - Limited Data-Possibly Hazardous

Hepatitis B virus (HBV) is a DNA virus belonging to the family hepadnaviridae.[1] Its antigenic structure is unique and is of prime diagnostic significance. Mode of transmission is mainly through blood and tissue fluids. The virus has been found to exist in human milk, serum, semen, and saliva. Accordingly, various modes of transmission have been reported such as via transfusion of infected blood and blood products, use of contaminated needles, sharing of contaminated needles by illicit intravenous drug abusers, sexual contact, both heterosexual and homosexual, as well as perinatal transmission. Interestingly, transmission by sharing of razors and toothbrushes is also known.[1] HBV is one among the many carcinogenic viruses known to man, feared for its potential to cause hepatocellular carcinoma (liver cancer).[1] Hepatitis B virus (HBV) causes a wide spectrum of infections, ranging from a mild asymptomatic form to a fulminant fatal hepatitis. Chronic infection and carrier status is also known to occur.

Infants of mothers who are HBV positive (HBsAg) should be given hepatitis B immune globulin (HBIG) (preferably within 12 hours of birth) and a Hepatitis B vaccination at birth, which is believed to effectively reduce the risk of post-natal transmission, particularly via blood or body fluids from the mother.[4] While present in milk, it is not clear if HBV is infectious. These injections should be followed by the complete hepatitis B vaccine series.

Hepatitis B antigen has been detected in breast milk.[2-4] Thus far, several older studies have indicated that breastfeeding poses no additional risk of transmission if these immunizations are completed, and thus far no cases of vertical transmission (maternal to child) of hepatitis B via breast milk have been reported.[5-7] According to the World Health Organization, "The risk of transmission associated with breast milk is negligible compared to the high risk of exposure to maternal blood and body fluids at birth, and hepatitis B vaccination will substantially reduce perinatal transmission and virtually eliminate any risk of transmission through breastfeeding or breast milk feeding." In summary, without evidence of cracked, bleeding nipples, or lesions, breastfeeding did not contribute to maternal child transmission of HBV after proper immunoprophylaxis in infants and should be recommended.[7]

Adult Concerns: Hepatitis, increased risk of liver cancer.

Adult Dose:

Pediatric Concerns: None reported if immunized with HBIG and HB vaccination.

Infant Monitoring:

Alternatives:

References:

1. AAP CoID. Hepatitis B. In: Pickering LKBC, Kimberlin DW, Long SS, eds. Red Book: 2009 Report of the Committee on Infectious Diseases. 28th ed. Elk Grove Village, IL: American Academy of Pediatrics; 2009:337-356.
2. Boxall EH, Flewett TH, Dane DS, Cameron CH, MacCallum FO, Lee TW. Letter: Hepatitis-B surface antigen in breast milk. Lancet. 1974;2(7887):1007-1008.
3. Beasley RP, Stevens CE, Shiao IS, Meng HC. Evidence against breast-feeding as a mechanism for vertical transmission of hepatitis B. Lancet. 1975;2(7938):740-741.
4. Woo D, Cummins M, Davies PA, Harvey DR, Hurley R, Waterson AP. Vertical transmission of hepatitis B surface antigen in carrier mothers in two west London hospitals. Arch Dis Child. 1979;54(9):670-675.
5. Hill JB, Sheffield JS, Kim MJ, Alexander JM, Sercely B, Wendel GD. Risk of hepatitis B transmission in breast-fed infants of chronic hepatitis B carriers. Obstet Gynecol. 2002;99(6):1049-1052.
6. Qiu L, Binns CW, Zhao Y, Zhang K, Xie X. Hepatitis B and breastfeeding in Hangzhou, Zhejiang Province, People's Republic of China. Breastfeed Med. 2010;5(3):109-112.
7. Shi Z, Yang Y, Wang H, et al. Breastfeeding of newborns by mothers carrying hepatitis B virus: a meta-analysis and systematic review. Arch Pediatr Adolesc Med. 2011;165(9):837-846.

HEPATITIS B VACCINE

Trade: Energix-B, Heptavax-B, Recombivax HB

Category: Vaccine

LRC: L2 - Limited Data-Probably Compatible

Hepatitis B vaccine is an inactivated non-infectious hepatitis B surface antigen vaccine. It can be used in pediatric patients at birth. No data are available on its use in breastfeeding mothers, but it is unlikely to produce untoward effects on a breastfeeding infant since it is an inactivated virus. Hepatitis B vaccination is approximately 80%-95% effective in preventing acute hepatitis B infections.[1,2] It requires at least 3 immunizations and the immunity lasts about 5-7 years. In infants born of HB surface antigen positive mothers, the American Academy of Pediatrics recommends that hepatitis B vaccine (along with HBIG) should be administered to the infant within 1-12 hours of birth (0.5 mL IM) and then follow up with their health care provider to receive subsequent doses. If so administered, breastfeeding poses no additional risk for acquisition of HBV by the infant.

Adult Concerns: Pain at injection site, swelling, erythema, fever.

Adult Dose: Three injections over 6 months.

Pediatric Concerns: Fever, malaise, fatigue when directly injected. None reported via breast milk.

Infant Monitoring:

Alternatives:

References:
1. Pharmaceutical manufacturers prescribing information.
2. American Academy of Pediatrics. Committee on Infectious Diseases. Red Book, Elk Grove Village, IL: American Academy of Pediatrics; 1997.

HEPATITIS C INFECTION

Trade: HCV, Hepatitis C Infection

Category: Infectious Disease

LRC: L3 - Limited Data-Probably Compatible

Hepatitis C virus (HCV) is an RNA virus belonging to the flaviviridae family.[1] The primary mode of spread is by parenteral route through exposure to HCV-contaminated blood or blood products. Besides this, sexual transmission of HCV has also been described, although rare. Infected individuals usually include illicit intravenous drug users and those who maintain sexual relations with multiple partners. In fact, 75% of those chronically infected with HCV are illicit drug users.[1] A small proportion of those infected also include health care professionals, hemophiliacs, and those requiring hemodialysis. In addition, those who received blood and/or its products before 1992 are also at higher risk for acquiring the disease. Although perinatal transmission can occur, its incidence is known to be low (5%-6%).[1-3] Symptoms of acute infection are anorexia, nausea, fatigue, and jaundice. The majority of those infected become chronic asymptomatic carriers.

In one study of 17 HCV positive mothers, 11 of the 17 had HCV antibodies present in milk, but zero of the 17 had HCV-RNA in milk after birth, suggesting that the virus itself was not detected in milk.[4] However, in later studies, although HCV RNA and anti-HCV antibody have been detected in colostrum and breast milk, no greater risk of HCV transmission has been found in breastfed infants as compared to bottle-fed infants.[1,5-10] Currently a number of other studies have yet to document transmission of HCV by breast milk.[11,12] Mothers infected with HCV should be advised that transmission of HCV by breastfeeding is possible but has not been documented. Available data seem to suggest an elevated risk of vertical transmission of HCV occurs in those co-infected with HIV and in women with elevated titers of HCV RNA. The risk of transmission of HCV via breast milk in such cases is unknown at this time. In one study, while transmission of HCV was significantly higher (21%) in HIV infected individuals, perinatal transmission of HCV was not associated with breastfeeding.[13] HCV-infected women should be counseled that transmission of HCV by breastfeeding is theoretically possible but has not yet been documented.[1,14]

The Centers for Disease Control and Prevention (CDC) does not consider chronic hepatitis C infection in the mother as a contraindication to breastfeeding. The decision to breastfeed should be based largely on informed discussion between the mother and her health care provider. In view of the potential benefits of breastfeeding, a mother with HCV infection may continue to breastfeed. It may be prudent however, for mothers who are seropositive for HCV to abstain from breastfeeding if their nipples are cracked and bleeding.[1,15]

Adult Concerns: Cirrhosis and liver cancer.

Adult Dose:

Pediatric Concerns:

Infant Monitoring:

Alternatives:

References:
1. AAP CoID. Hepatitis C. In: Pickering LK BC, Kimberlin DW, Long SS, eds. Red Book: 2009 Report of the Committee on Infectious Diseases. 28th ed. Elk Grove Village, IL: American Academy of Pediatrics; 2009:362.
2. Nagata I, Shiraki K, Tanimoto K, Harada Y, Tanaka Y, Okada T. Mother to infant transmission of hepatitis C virus. J Pediatrics. 1992;120:432-434.
3. Shiraki K, Ohto H, Inaba N, et al. Guidelines for care of pregnant women carrying hepatitis C virus and their infants. Pediatr Int. 2008;50(1):138-140.
4. Grayson ML, Braniff KM, Bowden DS, Turnidge JD. Breastfeeding and the risk of vertical transmission of hepatitis C virus. Med J Aust. 1995;163(2):107.
5. Airoldi J, Berghella V. Hepatitis C and pregnancy. Obstet Gynecol Surv. 2006;61(10):666-672.
6. Powell M, Bailey J, Maggio LA. Clinical inquiries. How should you manage children born to hepatitis C-positive women? J Fam Pract. 2010;59(5):289-290.
7. Bhola K, McGuire W. Does avoidance of breast feeding reduce mother-to-infant transmission of hepatitis C virus infection? Arch Dis Child. 2007;92(4):365-366.
8. Polywka S, Schroter M, Feucht HH, Zollner B, Laufs R. Low risk of vertical transmission of hepatitis C virus by breast milk. Clin Infect Dis. 1999;29(5):1327-1329.
9. Ruiz-Extremera A, Salmeron J, Torres C, et al. Follow-up of transmission of hepatitis C to babies of human immunodeficiency virus-negative women: the role of breast-feeding in transmission. Pediatr Infect Dis J. 2000;19(6):511-516.

10. Kumar RM, Shahul S. Role of breast-feeding in transmission of hepatitis C virus to infants of HCV-infected mothers. J Hepatol. 1998 Aug;29(2):191-197.

11. Lin HH, Kao JH, Hsu HY, et al. Absence of infection in breast-fed infants born to hepatitis C virus-infected mothers. J Pediatr. 1995;126(4):589-591.

12. Zanetti AR, Tanzi E, Paccagnini S, et al. Mother to infant transmission of hepatitis C virus. Lancet. 1995;345(8945):289-291.

13. Paccagnini S, Principi N, Massironi E, et al. Perinatal transmission and manifestation of hepatitis C virus infection in a high risk population. Pediatr Infect Dis J. 1995;14(3):195-199.

14. Lawrence RA. Breastfeeding: A Guide for the Medical Profession. St. Louis: Mosby Publishers; 1994.

15. Mast EE. Mother-to-infant hepatitis C virus transmission and breastfeeding. Adv Exp Med Biol. 2004;554:211-216.

HEPATITIS E INFECTION

Trade: Hepatitis E

Category: Infectious Disease

LRC: L4 - Limited Data-Possibly Hazardous

Hepatitis E virus (HEV) is an RNA virus belonging to the family hepeviridae.[1] Mode of transmission is mainly by feco-oral route. Therefore, this infection is largely prevalent in developing countries where maintaining food and water hygiene is an everyday challenge. However, other modes of spread such as parenteral and vertical have also been reported.[2-5] In the United States, the only reported cases are those seen in travelers returning from countries endemic for HEV. A small proportion of the cases also include those infected with the hepatitis E virus of swine origin.[1,2] Hepatitis E infection is a self-limiting illness of acute onset associated with fever, malaise, anorexia, abdominal pain, jaundice, and tea-colored urine.[6]

A study was conducted to investigate the transmission of HEV through breast milk.[7] The colostrum samples from 93 mothers who were HEV infected were studied. All 93 samples revealed the presence of anti-HEV antibody and/or HEV RNA. However, the titers in the colostrum samples were much lower as compared to the maternal serum titers. Eighty-six of these women, who were anti-HEV positive but clinically asymptomatic at the time of delivery exclusively breast-fed their infants. Although anti-HEV antibody and/or HEV RNA was found in the colostrum of these women, their infants remained healthy until 3 months of age. The infants of the remaining six women with acute HEV illness at the time of delivery, developed symptomatic HEV illness and became anti-HEV antibody positive within 6-8 weeks of delivery. Also, the anti-HEV antibody titers in the breast milk samples of these women also correspondingly increased. However, none of these six infants were breastfed, suggesting close contact and feco-oral transmission being the most probable route of spread. Therefore, the authors of this study suggest that asymptomatic women with low anti-HEV titers may safely breastfeed their infants. However, in view of possible feco-oral spread due to close contact between mother and child, mothers should be counseled to maintain all sanitary and hygienic conditions while caring for their infants. Women who are clinically ill with high anti-HEV titers or high viral RNA load are suggested to refrain from breastfeeding in view of possible transmission by either feco-oral route or via contaminated breast milk.

In conclusion, the hepatitis E virus has been isolated in breast milk, but the extent of its infectivity to the infant is still unknown. Feco-oral transmission still appears to be the primary mode of transmission, therefore, mothers with hepatitis E infection are encouraged to take all sanitary precautions while caring for their infants. Measures such as regular hand washing before holding the baby or coming in contact with items or clothing belonging to the infant are recommended. It is advisable that mothers with active, symptomatic HEV infection temporarily refrain from breastfeeding until the symptoms subside. HEV infection is a self-limiting illness, and unlike hepatitis B and C, is not known for chronicity and does not exist in carrier state.[1] Therefore, mothers may safely continue breastfeeding once the acute illness subsides.

Adult Concerns: Self-limiting illness of acute onset associated with fever, malaise, anorexia, abdominal pain, jaundice and tea-colored urine.

Adult Dose:

Pediatric Concerns:

Infant Monitoring:

Alternatives:

References:

1. AAP CoID. Hepatitis E. In: Pickering LKBC, Kimberlin DW, Long SS, eds. Red Book: 2009 Report of the Committee on Infectious Diseases. 28th ed. Elk Grove Village, IL: American Academy of Pediatrics; 2009:362.

2. Aggarwal R, Naik S. Epidemiology of hepatitis E: current status. J Gastroenterol Hepatol. 2009;24(9):1484-1493.

3. Acharya SK, Panda SK. Hepatitis E: water, water everywhere - now a global disease. J Hepatol. 2011;54(1):9-11.

4. Fiore S, Savasi V. Treatment of viral hepatitis in pregnancy. Expert Opin Pharmacother. 2009;10(17):2801-2809.

5. Khuroo MS, Kamili S, Jameel S. Vertical transmission of hepatitis E virus. Lancet. 1995;345(8956):1025-1026.

6. Bazaco MC, Albrecht SA, Malek AM. Preventing foodborne infection in pregnant women and infants. Nurs Womens Health. 2008;12(1):46-55.

7. Chibber RM, Usmani MA, Al-Sibai MH. Should HEV infected mothers breast feed? Arch Gynecol Obstet. 2004;270(1):15-20.

HEROIN

Trade: Heroin

Category: Analgesic

LRC: L5 - Limited Data-Hazardous

Heroin is diacetylmorphine (diamorphine), a prodrug that is rapidly converted to 6-monoacetylmorphine and then to morphine (both are active metabolites).[1] With oral use, rapid and complete first-pass metabolism occurs in the liver; morphine levels peak about 30 minutes after the oral dose. When smoked or snorted the onset of heroin can be within seconds and peak in minutes. When injected the onset of heroin is within seconds; this route completely avoids first-pass metabolism. The half-life of diamorphine is only 3 minutes, with the large majority of the prodrug converted to morphine; the duration of effect is anticipated to be about 3-5 hours. It is also well known that with repeated use tolerance can develop.

At this time, there are no data regarding the transfer of heroin to human milk; however, we do know that morphine can enter human milk in significant quantities.[2-5] The relative infant dose for morphine ranges from 9%-35%.[2-5] Morphine is considered suitable for short term use in breastfeeding mothers when non-opioid pain therapy is inadequate (e.g., given as needed for postoperative pain).

Unfortunately, we are unable to quantify the dose of heroin used recreationally and the amount of morphine that enters milk, thus use in lactation is likely to be dangerous for the breastfed infant. While it could be argued that recreational users could continue to breastfeed if they avoid doing so while under the influence of heroin or prior to its use, this is not advisable as it requires some understanding of the dose used and the kinetics of morphine. Additional concerns with heroin use in lactation also need to be assessed prior to initiating breastfeeding, in a woman with a history of heroin use, such as risk factors for HIV and the potential for subsequent use. Heroin use should be avoided in lactation.[6]

T 1/2	2-6 mins heroin; 2 h morphine	MW	369 Da	PB	35%
Tmax	0.5-1 h	RID		Vd	1-6 L/kg
Oral	< 35%	M/P	2.45	pKa	7.6

Adult Concerns: Sedation, euphoria, wakeful then drowsy, respiratory depression, flushing, hypotension, dry mouth, nausea, vomiting, abdominal cramps, constipation.

Adult Dose:

Pediatric Concerns: No data available at this time.

Infant Monitoring: Sedation, slowed breathing rate, pallor, poor feeding, constipation, and appropriate weight gain. Avoid in lactation.

Alternatives: Methadone(L2)

References:

1. National Institute of Health. National Institute on Drug Abuse DrugFacts: Heroin 2014. https://www.drugabuse.gov/publications/drugfacts/heroin. Online Accessed Mar 25, 2016.
2. Feilberg VL, Rosenborg D, Broen CC, Mogensen JV. Excretion of morphine in human breast milk. Acta Anaesthesiol Scand. 1989;33(5):426-428.
3. Wittels B, Scott DT, Sinatra RS. Exogenous opioids in human breast milk and acute neonatal neurobehavior: a preliminary study. Anesthesiology. 1990;73(5):864-869.
4. Baka NE, Bayoumeu F, Boutroy MJ, et al. Colostrum morphine concentrations during postcesarean intravenous patient-controlled analgesia. Anesth Analg. 2002;94:184-187.
5. Robieux I, Koren G, Vandenbergh H, Schneiderman J. Morphine excretion in breast milk and resultant exposure of a nursing infant. J Toxicol Clin Toxicol. 1990;28(3):365-370.
6. American Academy of Pediatrics, Committee on Drugs. Transfer of drugs and other chemicals into human milk. Pediatrics. 2001;108(3):776-789.

HERPES SIMPLEX VIRUS

Trade:

Category: Infectious Disease

LRC: L4 - Limited Data-Possibly Hazardous

The Herpes Simplex virus (HSV) belongs to the family of herpes viruses and consists of two distinct species - HSV-1 and HSV-2. HSV-1 is transmitted by direct contact with either the infected lesions or infected oral secretions. HSV-2 is sexually transmitted and occurs as a result of direct contact with either the infected genital lesions or infected genital secretions.

A number of cases of herpes simplex transmission via breast milk have been reported.[1-6] In one such report, breast milk samples obtained from 34 lactating women were investigated for the presence of HSV DNA by in situ hybridization technique. Sixteen out of the 34 milk samples were found to be positive for HSV DNA. DNA of both HSV-1 and HSV-2 were found. This study implies that transmission of the herpes simplex virus through breast milk is a possibility and this may play a role in causing HSV infections in infants.[3] HSV-1 and HSV-2 have also been isolated from human milk, even in the absence of vesicular lesions or drainage.[4,5] In one case, a breastfed infant who was born healthy developed disseminated HSV illness postnatally.[1] It is believed that the infection was acquired via breast milk since HSV-1 was detected in the mother's milk sample. The mother, however, did not give any history of herpes infection. Therefore, it is advisable that due caution be exercised in breastfeeding women with active herpes lesions of any kind, oral or genital. Lactating mothers, especially those with perioral herpetic lesions, should be counseled about the modes of transmission of herpes and should be warned against any direct contact between the infant and the oral lesions, such as the kind that occurs while kissing or nuzzling the infant. While holding the infant close, any active lesions anywhere should be appropriately covered to avoid direct contact with the infant.

In general, breast milk does not appear to be a common mode of transmission of the herpes simplex virus. However, women with active lesions on one breast should avoid breastfeeding from the affected breast until the lesions completely dry up, and may continue to breastfeed from the opposite breast. Other active lesions on the body should be adequately covered to avoid contact with the infant.

Adult Concerns: Skin eruptions, CNS changes, gingivostomatitis, skin lesions, fever.

Adult Dose:

Pediatric Concerns: Transfer of virus to infants has been reported, but may be from exposure to lesions. Cover lesions on breast.

Infant Monitoring: Fever, skin lesions.

Alternatives:

References:

1. Dunkle LM, Schmidt RR, O'Connor DM. Neonatal herpes simplex infection possibly acquired via maternal breast milk. Pediatrics. 1979;63(2):250-251.
2. Quinn PT, Lofberg JV. Maternal herpetic breast infection: another hazard of neonatal herpes simplex. Med J Aust. 1978;2(9):411-412.
3. Kotronias D, Kapranos N. Detection of herpes simplex virus DNA in maternal breast milk by in situ hybridization with tyramide signal amplification. In Vivo. 1999;13(6):463-466.
4. Light IJ. Postnatal acquisition of herpes simplex virus by the newborn infant: a review of the literature. Pediatrics. 1979;63(3):480-482.
5. Sullivan-Bolyai JZ, Fife KH, Jacobs RF, Miller Z, Corey L. Disseminated neonatal herpes simplex virus type 1 from a maternal breast lesion. Pediatrics. 1983;71(3):455-457.
6. Whitley RJ, Nahmias AJ, Visintine AM, Fleming CL, Alford CA. The natural history of herpes simplex virus infection of mother and newborn. Pediatrics. 1980;66(4):489-494.

HEXACHLOROPHENE

Trade: Dermalex, Phisohex, Sapoderm, Septi-Soft, Septisol

Category: Antiseptic

LRC: L4 - No Data-Possibly Hazardous

Hexachlorophene is an antibacterial that is an effective inhibitor of gram-positive organisms.[1] It is generally used topically as a surgical scrub and sometimes vaginally in mothers. Due to its lipophilic structure, it is well absorbed through intact and denuded skin producing significant levels in plasma, brain, fat, and other tissues in both adults and infants. It has been implicated in causing brain lesions (spongiform myelinopathy), blindness, and respiratory failure in both animals and humans.[2] Although there are no studies reporting concentrations of this compound in breast milk, it is probably transferred to some degree. Transfer into breast milk is known to occur in rodents. Topical use in infants is absolutely discouraged due to the high absorption of hexachlorophene through an infant's skin and proven toxicity.

T 1/2		MW	407 Da	PB	
Tmax		RID		Vd	
Oral	Complete	M/P		pKa	8.79

Adult Concerns: Seizures, respiratory failure, hypotension, brain lesions, blindness in overdose.

Adult Dose:

Pediatric Concerns: Following direct application- CNS injury, seizures, irritability have been reported in neonates. Toxicity via breast milk has not been reported.

Infant Monitoring: AVOID in lactation.

Alternatives:

References:
1. Pharmaceutical manufacturers prescribing information.
2. Tyrala EE, Hillman LS, Hillman RE, Dodson WE. Clinical pharmacology of hexachlorophene in newborn infants. J Pediatr. 1977;91(3):481-486.

HISTAMINE

Trade:

Category: Diagnostic Agent, Other

LRC: L3 - No Data-Probably Compatible

Histamine is a normal substance found in the mast cells and plays a major role in the allergic response, neurotransmission, gastric acid secretion, and bronchial constriction.[1] Physiologically, it interacts at any of three different cellular receptors - H1, H2, and H3. These receptors are in high concentrations in bronchi (H1), gastric, and other tissues (H2, H3). Histamine is primarily stored in the mast cells, which when destabilized by allergens, etc., releases histamine into the tissues and initiates the normal response to histamine. Histamine is primarily used pharmacologically as a diagnostic agent, to induce gastric acid release, or more often, stimulate bronchoconstriction in the diagnosis of asthma. Histamine is rapidly metabolized with a plasma half-life less than 3 minutes. No data are available on its transfer to human milk, but it is probably minimal. Waiting as little as 2 hours following exposure would largely eliminate all risks associated with the use of histamine in a breastfeeding mother.

T 1/2	<3 min	MW	307 Da	PB	
Tmax		RID		Vd	
Oral	Minimal	M/P		pKa	6.9, 10.4

Adult Concerns: Headache, dizziness, blurred vision, flushing, vasodilation, hyper or hypotension, tachycardia, bronchoconstriction, asthma symptoms, hyperacidity, vomiting, diarrhea.

Adult Dose: Highly variable.

Pediatric Concerns: None reported in breastfeeding infants.

Infant Monitoring: A 1-2 hour waiting period after the procedure is recommended.

Alternatives:

References:
1. Pharmaceutical manufacturers prescribing information.

HIV INFECTION

Trade: AIDS

Category: Infectious Disease

LRC: L5 in developed countries

The AIDS (HIV) virus has been isolated from human milk. In addition, recent reports from throughout the world have documented the transmission of HIV through human milk.[1-3] There are more than nine cases in the literature currently suggesting that HIV-1 is secreted and can be transmitted horizontally to the infant via breast milk.[4,5] Women who develop a primary HIV infection while breastfeeding may shed especially high concentrations of HIV viruses and pose a high risk of transmission to their infants. In some studies, the risk of transmission during primary infection was 29%. In various African populations, recent reports suggest the incremental risk of transmitting HIV via breastfeeding ranges from 3% to 12%.[6] Because the risk is now well documented, mothers infected with HIV in the United States and other countries with safe alternative sources of feeding should be advised not to breastfeed their infants.[7] Mothers at risk for HIV should be screened and counseled prior to initiating breastfeeding. A new study outlining Nevirapine infant dosing early postnatally to prevent HIV transmission via milk has been published.[8]

Adult Concerns:

Adult Dose:

Pediatric Concerns:

Infant Monitoring: Potential infection via milk; breastfeeding is not recommended.

Alternatives:

References:

1. Commitee on Pediatric AIDS. Human milk, breastfeeding, and transmission of human immunodeficiency virus in the United States. Pediatrics. 1995;96:977-979.
2. Oxtoby MJ. Human immunodeficiency virus and other viruses in human milk: placing the issues in broader perspective. Pediatr Infect Dis J. 1988;7(12):825-835.
3. Goldfarb J. Breastfeeding. AIDS and other infectious diseases. Clin Perinatol. 1993;20(1):225-243.
4. Van de PP, Simonon A, Hitimana DG, et al. Infective and anti-infective properties of breastmilk from HIV-1-infected women. Lancet. 1993;341(8850):914-918.
5. Dunn DT, Newell ML, Ades AE, Peckham CS. Risk of human immunodeficiency virus type 1 transmission through breastfeeding. Lancet. 1992;340(8819):585-588.
6. St. Louis ME, et al. The timing of HIV-1 transmission in an African setting. Presented at the First National Conference on Human Retroviruses and Related Infections; December 12-16; Washington DC, 1993.
7. AAP CoID. Report of the committee on Infectious Diseases. Elk Grove Village, IL: American Academy of Pediatrics; 1994.
8. Cressey TR, Punyawudho B, Le Coeur S, et al. Assessment of nevirapine prophylactic and therapeutic dosing regimens for neonates. J Acquir Immune Defic Syndr. 2017 Aug;75(5):554-560.

HOMATROPINE

Trade: Acidobyl, Arkitropin, Homatromide, Homatropaire, Isopto Homatropine, Novatropine

Category: Anticholinergic

LRC: L3 - No Data-Probably Compatible

Homatropine belongs to the antimuscarinic family of drugs, which are similar to atropine. Homatropine is rarely used today to treat duodenal or stomach ulcers or intestine problems. In rare instances, it may also be used to prevent nausea, vomiting, and motion sickness. There are no adequate and well-controlled studies or case reports of its use in breastfeeding women. However, the use of this product could produce significant drying, such as constipation, dry eyes, urinary retention, and other typical anticholinergic symptoms. The infrequent ophthalmic use of this product in breastfeeding mothers is probably not a contraindication to its use in breastfeeding women.

T 1/2		MW	370 Da	PB	
Tmax		RID		Vd	
Oral		M/P		pKa	9.65

Adult Concerns: Blurred vision, photophobia, eye irritation, increased ocular pressure, photophobia, dry mouth.

Adult Dose: Instill one or two drops of 2% or 5% solution two to three times a day.

Pediatric Concerns: None reported via milk.

Infant Monitoring: Dry mouth, constipation, urinary retention.

Alternatives:

References:

HONEY, MANUKA

Trade: Honey, Manuka, Manuka Honey

Category: Herb

LRC: L3 - No Data-Probably Compatible

Manuka honey is a monofloral honey produced in New Zealand and Australia from nectar of the manuka tree. It is believed to have antibacterial properties due to the presence of a unique manuka factor. Manuka honey is commonly used in wound healing centers for its antimicrobial effect.[1] Since food-grade honey is frequently contaminated with botulism spores, we should assume the same for manuka honey. Hence, infants should not be given oral manuka honey for at least 12 months, unless it is heat-sterilized.

Adult Concerns: Allergic reaction, stinging or burning because of its natural acidity, digestive problems from incomplete fructose metabolism causing bloating, abdominal pain, and diarrhea.

Adult Dose:

Pediatric Concerns: Do not administer directly to an infant less than 12 months of age.

Infant Monitoring:

Alternatives:

References:
1. Song JJ, Salcido R. Use of honey in wound care: an update. Adv Skin Wound Care. 2011 Jan;24(1):40-44; quiz 45-6. doi: 10.1097/01. ASW.0000392731.34723.06. PubMed PMID: 21150765.

HTLV-1

Trade: Human T-lymphotropic virus

Category: HTLV viral disease

LRC: L5 - Limited Data-Hazardous

Human T-lymphotropic virus Type 1 (HTLV-1), also called the adult T-cell lymphoma virus type 1, is a retrovirus that causes several diseases such as neurological disease (HTLV-1 associated myelopathy/tropical spastic paraparesis), adult T-cell leukemia/lymphoma (ATL), opportunistic infections such as strongyloides stercoralis hyperinfection, uveitis, rheumatic syndromes and other autoimmune conditions as Sjogren's syndrome, polymyositis, thyroiditis, and predisposition to helminthic and bacterial infections scabies, disseminated molluscum contagiosum, and extrapulmonary histoplasmosis.

Transmission of HTLV-1 is believed to occur by sexual contact, from mother to child via breastfeeding, through exposure to contaminated blood, either through blood transfusion or sharing of contaminated needles.

It may be transmitted during pregnancy. In a study, it has been reported that out of the 216 children born from 81 HTLV-1 infected mothers, only 21 were found to be HTLV-1 seropositive, giving a crude HTLV-1 transmission rate of 9.7% .[1] In another study, mother-to-child transmission during the intrauterine period or peripartum has been reported to occur in less than 5% of cases.[2] Testing of newborns born to HTLV-seropositive mothers with an adequate close medical follow-up should also be done.

Several studies have documented that it is transmitted through breastfeeding, therefore breastfeeding may not be recommended. HTLV-1 infection is more prevalent among breastfed children than bottle-fed children.[2] In one study, fresh human milk from HTLV-1 carrier mothers was inoculated orally to common marmoset, which led to HTLV-1 infection.[1] The source of HTLV-1 in breast milk is thought to be T lymphocytes the majority of cells in breast milk are CD14+ macrophages.[3] However, a study has reported that basal mammary epithelial cells are also susceptible to HTLV infection and are capable of transferring HTLV infection by contributing to the seeding of milk with HTLV.[3]

Mothers should be advised to stop breastfeeding, which seems to be the best and easiest way to prevent mother-to-child transmission of HTLV-1. Testing maternal anti-HTLV antibody titer and proviral load before delivery would be an optimal preventive strategy. If screening test is positive, restriction of breastfeeding in HTLV-1 seropositive mothers should be recommended.[4] Early weaning and bottle feeding are the primary options for reducing the risk of HTLV-1 transmission by infected mothers.[5]

Adult Concerns: Neurological disease (HTLV-1 associated myelopathy/tropical spastic paraparesis), adult T-cell leukemia/lymphoma (ATL), opportunistic infections such as *strongyloides stercoralis* hyper-infection, uveitis, rheumatic syndromes, and other autoimmune conditions as Sjogren's syndrome, polymyositis, thyroiditis, and predisposition to helminthic, and bacterial infections scabies, disseminated molluscum contagiosum, and extrapulmonary histoplasmosis.

Adult Dose:

Pediatric Concerns: Transmission via breast milk has been documented.

Infant Monitoring: Breastfeeding is not recommended.

Alternatives:

References:
1. Kinoshita K, Yamanouchi K, Ikeda S, et al. Oral infection of a common marmoset with human T-cell leukemia virus type I (HTLV-I) by inoculating fresh human milk of HTLV-I carrier mothers. Jpn J Cancer Res. 1985;76:1147-1153.
2. Ando Y, Nakano S, Saito K, et al. Hinuma transmission of adult T-cell leukemia retrovirus (HTLV-I) from mother to child: comparison of bottle- with breast-fed babies. Jpn J Cancer Res. 1987;78:322-324.
3. LeVasseur RJ, Southern SO, Southern PJ. Southern Mammary epithelial cells support and transfer productive human T-cell lymphotropic virus infections. J Hum Virol. 1998;1:214-223.

4. Carneiro-Proietti AB, Catalan-Soares B, Proietti FA. Human T-cell lymphotropic viruses (HTLV-I/II) in South America: should it be a public health concern? J Biomed Sci. 2002;9:587-595.
5. Hisada M, Maloney EM, Sawada T, et al. Virus markers associated with vertical transmission of human T lymphotropic virus type 1 in Jamaica. Clin Infect Dis. 2002;34(12):1551-1557.

HUMAN IMMUNE GLOBULIN

Trade: Carimune, Flebogamma, Gammagard, Gammaked, Gammaplex, Hizentra, Octagam, Privigen, Vivaglobin

Category: Immune Serum

LRC: L2 - No Data-Probably Compatible

Intravenous Immunoglobulin (IVIG) is a human blood product containing primarily IgG1 that is used in the treatment of immune deficiencies, inflammatory illnesses, immune thrombocytopenic purpura (ITP) and acute infections.[1] The dose and route of administration varies depending on the clinical indication. The amount of IVIG available in maternal systemic circulation depends on the route of administration, when given IV and IM about 100% and 40% is available in maternal serum, respectively.

Although there are only limited data on the transfer of immunoglobulins to human milk, we believe that the molecule is too large to enter into the milk compartment in clinically relevant amounts. Therefore, milk levels are relatively low[2] and only minimally bioavailable orally.

T 1/2	21 days	MW	150,000 Da	PB	
Tmax	Immediate (IV), 2-5 days (SQ)	RID		Vd	
Oral	Nil	M/P		pKa	

Adult Concerns: Headache, fever, chills, dizziness, anxiety, chest tightness, flushing, hypertension, dyspepsia, nausea, vomiting, changes in liver and renal function, autoimmune hemolytic anemia, thrombocytopenia, hemorrhage, thrombosis, arthralgia, myalgia, infusion, and local injection site reactions.

Adult Dose:

Pediatric Concerns: None reported via milk at this time. IVIG is used in the pediatric population; however, long-term data is limited.

Infant Monitoring:

Alternatives:

References:
1. Pharmaceutical manufacturer drug information, 2013.
2. Jensen, RG. Handbook of Milk Composition. San Diego, CA: Academic Press; 1995:161.

HUMAN PAPILLOMAVIRUS INFECTION

Trade: HPV infection

Category: Infectious Disease

LRC: L3 - Limited Data-Probably Compatible

Human papillomaviruses (HPV) are DNA viruses and some of the most common sexually communicable diseases in the world. They are responsible not only for the presence of anogenital warts, but are also the contributing virus to the formation of flat warts, respiratory papillomatosis, and common skin warts. In addition, certain forms of papillomavirus are leading causes of cancer and dysplasia. Out of more than 100 types of this virus, more than 18 are classified as high risk, with types 16, 18, 31, and 45 being most commonly implicated in the development of cervical cancer. Types 16 and 18 are also linked to the development of oropharyngeal cancer. Types 6 and 11 are also of concern, as they most commonly result in anogenital warts, respiratory papillomatosis, and conjunctival papillomas and carcinomas.[1] Papillomaviruses are spread widely throughout the population and can reach prevalence rates of as high as 50% in school children, where cutaneous warts are common.

As a rule, close contact is required for transmission of these viruses from one individual to the next. This is evidenced by the high incidence of cutaneous warts in school children, as well as the link between public pools and plantar warts. Due to the viral nature of warts, they are often seen in immunocompromised patients. Anogenital warts most often are transferred through sexual contact and often resolve spontaneously without causing clinical effects. In the event that anogenital warts occur frequently or for prolonged periods of time, the risk for cervical cancer increases greatly.[1] It is possible to transfer HPV to an infant through the birth canal or from non-genital sites. The incubation period is varied, ranging from a few months to several years in length. It is possible that a neonate who is exposed to HPV virus will never develop clinical symptoms or may only show presence of the virus over the course of many years.[1]

HPV has been found to enter the breast milk in one study.[2] During this study, approximately 4% of women were found to have HPV-16 DNA in breast milk samples. However, it was not established if the presence of DNA stemmed from virus in the milk or somewhere else. Another study addressed the findings of the previous one, again evaluating if HPV DNA was present within the breast milk. This study did not find any evidence of high risk HPV within milk. At the current time, the authors of the study do not believe that evidence exists that suggests maternal to infant transfer of the virus, which would require discontinuation of breastfeeding while the mother is infected with this disease.[3]

References:
1. American Academy of Pediatrics. Human Papillomaviruses. In: Pickering LK, Baker CJ, Kimberlin DW, Long SS, eds. Red Book: 2009 Report of the Committee on Infectious Diseases. 28th ed. Elk Grove Village, IL: American Academy of Pediatrics; 2009:477-479.
2. Sarkola M, Rintala M, Grénman S, Syrjänen S. Human Papillomavirus DNA detected in breast milk. Pediatr Infect Dis J. 2010;27(6):557-558.
3. Mammas IN, Zaravinos A, Sourvinos G, Myriokefalitakis N, Theodoridou M, Spandidos DA. Can "high-risk" human papillomaviruses (HPVs) be detected in human breast milk? Acta Paediatr. 2011 May;100(5):705-707.

HUMAN PAPILLOMAVIRUS VACCINE

Trade: Cervarix (HPV2), Gardasil (HPV4)

Category: Vaccine

LRC: L3 - No Data-Probably Compatible

There are three versions of the HPV vaccine currently on the market that vary in the number of HPV types they are active against. The active agent in all three products is a set of purified protein derivatives produced via a recombinant mutant of *Saccharomyces cerevisiae* or *Trichoplusia ni*. The proteins in the vaccine do not constitute an intact virus particle, nor do they have the potential to be infectious. It is not known whether vaccine antigens or antibodies are excreted in human milk.[1] Both the Centers for Disease Control and Prevention and the American College of Obstetricians and Gynecologists advise proceeding with vaccination in an exclusively breastfeeding patient.[2,3]

Adult Concerns: Headache, dizziness, fever, nausea, myalgia and injection site pain, swelling, and redness.

Adult Dose: 0.5 mL IM per dose.

Pediatric Concerns: No data available.

Infant Monitoring:

Alternatives:

References:
1. Pharmaceutical manufacturer prescribing information.
2. ACOG Committee opinion no. 588: human papillomavirus vaccination. 2014 Mar.
3. Centers for Disease Control and Prevention (CDC). FDA licensure of bivalent human papillomavirus vaccine (HPV2, Cervarix) for use in females and updated HPV vaccination recommendations from the Advisory Committee on Immunization Practices (ACIP). MMWR Morb Mortal Wkly Rep. 2010 May;59(20):626-629.

HYALURONIC ACID

Trade: Cystistat, Durolane, Euflexxa, Eyestil, Healon, Hyalgan, Hylaform, Juvederm, OrthoVisc, Orthovisc, Provisc, Restylane, Suplasyn, Synvisc

Category: Cartilaginous Defect Repair Agent

LRC: L3 - No Data-Probably Compatible

Hyaluronic acid forms a viscoelastic solution in water, thus functioning as a joint lubricant, vitreous humor during ophthalmic surgery, and even decreasing the depth of wrinkles when injected intradermally. Sodium hyaluronate is a polysaccharide commonly found in humans in the extracellular matrix of connective tissues.[1] There are no data available on the transfer of hyaluronic acid into breast milk, but it would be minimal to nil. The repeating chains can be quite large, and therefore size would prohibit any drug that did get absorbed from transferring to the milk compartment. A similar product is Hyalgan, which is sodium hyaluronate.

T 1/2		MW	Large Da	PB	
Tmax		RID		Vd	
Oral		M/P		pKa	

Adult Concerns: Pain at injection site. Arthralgia, bursitis, etc.

Adult Dose:

Pediatric Concerns: None reported via milk at this time.

Infant Monitoring:

Alternatives:

References:
1. Pharmaceutical manufacturers prescribing information.

HYDRALAZINE

Trade: Alphapress, Apresoline

Category: Antihypertensive

LRC: L2 - Limited Data-Probably Compatible

Hydralazine is a popular antihypertensive used for severe pre-eclampsia and gestational and postpartum hypertension. In a study of one breastfeeding mother receiving 50 mg three times daily, the concentrations of hydralazine in breastmilk at 0.5 and 2 hours after administration was 762, and 792 nmol/L respectively.[1] The respective maternal serum levels were 1525, and 580 nmol/L at the aforementioned times. From these data, an infant consuming 1000 mL of milk would consume only 0.17 mg of hydralazine, an amount too small to be clinically relevant. The published pediatric dose for hydralazine is 0.75 to 1 mg/kg/day. Since the levels in milk are far less than the clinical pediatric doses, hydralazine is probably compatible with breastfeeding.

T 1/2	1.5-8 h	MW	160 Da	PB	87%
Tmax	2 h	RID	1.2%	Vd	1.6 L/kg
Oral	30%-50%	M/P	0.49-1.36	pKa	7.1

Adult Concerns: Headache, flushing, hypotension, tachycardia, anorexia, paresthesias, peripheral edema, agranulocytosis.

Adult Dose: 10-25 mg four times daily.

Pediatric Concerns: None reported via breast milk at this time.

Infant Monitoring: Drowsiness, lethargy, pallor, poor feeding and weight gain.

Alternatives:

References:
1. Liedholm H, Wahlin-Boll E, Hanson A, Ingemarsson I, Melander A. Transplacental passage and breast milk concentrations of hydralazine. Eur J Clin Pharmacol. 1982;21(5):417-419.

HYDROCHLOROTHIAZIDE

Trade: Direma, Diuchlor H, Esidrex, Esidrix, Hydrodiuril, Modizide, Oretic, Tekturna HCT

Category: Diuretic

LRC: L2 - Limited Data-Probably Compatible

Hydrochlorothiazide (HCTZ) is a typical thiazide diuretic.[1] There is one published case report of a woman taking 50 mg of hydrochlorothiazide every morning. On day 28 postpartum, both maternal and infant blood and maternal milk were sampled multiple times over a 24 hour period. Maternal blood and milk samples peaked at 7 hours postdose and were about 425 μg/L and 120 μg/L, respectively. The mean concentration in milk was about 80 μg/L, this corresponded with an infant dose of 0.05 mg/day and a relative infant dose of 1.6%. The infants blood samples were undetectable (less than 20 ng/mL), laboratory parameters were normal (electrolytes, blood sugar, BUN) and no adverse effects were reported.

Some authors suggest that HCTZ can produce thrombocytopenia in nursing infants, although this is remote and unsubstantiated. Thiazide diuretics could potentially reduce milk production by depleting maternal blood volume although it is seldom observed.

T 1/2	5.6-14.8 h	MW	297 Da	PB	58%
Tmax	2 h	RID	1.68%	Vd	3 L/kg
Oral	72%	M/P	0.25	pKa	7.9, 9.2

Adult Concerns: Headache, dizziness, hypotension, hyperglycemia, hypokalemia, changes in renal function, and rash.

Adult Dose: 25-100 mg daily.

Pediatric Concerns: None reported via milk at this time.

Infant Monitoring: Observe for fluid loss, dehydration, lethargy, weight gain; monitor maternal milk supply.

Alternatives: Labetalol(L2), Nifedipine(L2)

References:
1. Miller ME, Cohn RD, Burghart PH. Hydrochlorothiazide disposition in a mother and her breast-fed infant. J Pediatr. 1982;101(5):789-791.

HYDROCODONE

Trade: Hysingla ER, Zohydro ER

Category: Analgesic

LRC: L3 - Limited Data-Probably Compatible

Hydrocodone is a narcotic analgesic and antitussive structurally related to codeine although somewhat more potent. Its active metabolite is hydromorphone. Its use has been found to be very effective in the relief of postpartum and post-operative pain. It has also been found to be effective for the alleviation of pain associated with mastitis.[1]

Hydrocodone is commonly used in breastfeeding mothers throughout the world. In a study of two breastfeeding women taking hydrocodone for various periods, patient one received a total of 63,525 μg (998.8 μg/kg) over 86.5 hours.[2] Patient two, received 9,075 μg (123.5 μg/kg) over 36 hours. In patient one, the AUC of the drug concentration in milk was 4,946.1 μg/L.hr and an average milk concentration of 57.2 μg/L. The authors estimate the relative infant dose at 3.1%. In patient two, the AUC of the drug concentration in milk was 735.6 μg/L. hr and an average milk concentration of 20.4 μg/L. The authors estimate the relative infant dose at 3.7%. This paper concluded that high doses of hydrocodone in mothers who are nursing newborn or premature infants can be concerning.

In another, more recent study, hydrocodone and hydromorphone levels were measured in 125 breast milk samples obtained from 30 women who were receiving 0.14-0.21 mg/kg/day (10-15 mg/day) of hydrocodone for the alleviation of postpartum pain.[3] It was found that fully breastfed infants receive on an average of 2.4% (range: 0.2%-9%) of the maternal hydrocodone dose. When considering total opiate exposure to both hydrocodone and hydromorphone combined, it was found that the total opiate dosage in the infants amounted to 0.7% of the therapeutic dosage commonly used in older infants. This is reassuring and suggests that when used in standard clinical dosages, the total opiate exposure to the infant is minimal and possibly clinically irrelevant. However, when calculating the hydromorphone to hydrocodone ratios in the breast milk samples of these women, it was found that breast milk samples from two of the women had a high hydromorphone to hydrocodone ratio of 2.8 and 3.1. These women were possibly rapid metabolizers. Although the total opiate exposure to the infants of these two women was still well below the regular pediatric therapeutic dosages, this finding raises concerns of possible untoward effects in the infants when hydrocodone is used in high doses, especially in those women who are rapid metabolizers. In conclusion, this study suggests that when used in standard postpartum dosages, hydrocodone appears to be probably safe in breastfeeding mothers of newborn infants. However, the authors advise against the use of high doses for prolonged periods of time, due to possible neonatal sedation and respiratory depression.

It is recommended that for treatment of postpartum pain, hydrocodone dosages should be limited to no more than 30 mg/day. If higher doses are required, then the infant should be closely monitored for possible untoward effects such as sedation and apnea. Doses more than 40 mg/day should be avoided.[3]

T 1/2	3.8 h	MW	299 Da	PB	19%-45%
Tmax	1.3 h	RID	2.21%-3.7%	Vd	3.3-4.7 L/kg
Oral	Complete	M/P		pKa	8.9

Adult Concerns: Sedation, dizziness, respiratory depression/apnea, bradycardia, nausea, constipation.

Adult Dose: 5-10 mg every 6 h as needed.

Pediatric Concerns: Sedation observed in one infant whose mother consumed 20 mg hydrocodone + 1300 mg acetaminophen every 4 hours.[2] Neonatal sedation and apnea are possible, especially with doses more than 30 mg/day.

Infant Monitoring: Sedation, slowed breathing rate, pallor, constipation, and appropriate weight gain.

Alternatives: Hydromorphone(L3)

References:
1. Bodley V, Powers D. Long-term treatment of a breastfeeding mother with fluconazole-resolved nipple pain caused by yeast: a case study. J Hum Lact. 1997 Dec;13(4):307-311.3.
2. Anderson PO, Sauberan JB, Lane JR, Rossi SS. Hydrocodone excretion into breast milk: the first two reported cases. Breastfeed Med. 2007;2(1):10-14.
3. Sauberan JB, Anderson PO, Lane JR, et al. Breast milk hydrocodone and hydromorphone levels in mothers using hydrocodone for-postpartum pain. Obstet Gynecol. 2011 Mar;117(3):611-617.

HYDROCORTISONE ENEMA

Trade: Anucort, Colocort, Cortenema, Hycort Enema, Proctosol, Rectoid

Category: Corticosteroid

LRC: L3 - No Data-Probably Compatible

Hydrocortisone is a typical corticosteroid with weak glucocorticoid and mineralocorticoid activity.[1] The amount transferred to human milk has not been reported, but as with most steroids, is believed minimal. Hydrocortisone rectal suspension is absorbed from the colon, it acts both topically and systemically. Although rectal hydrocortisone has a low incidence of reported adverse reactions, prolonged use presumably may cause typical steroid systemic reactions.

Hydrocortisone administered rectally is probably okay if used short-term. Transfer of hydrocortisone into milk is probably low, although we have no data. No adverse effects have been reported in breastfed infants.

T 1/2	1-2 h	MW	362 Da	PB	90%
Tmax		RID		Vd	0.48 L/kg
Oral	96%	M/P		pKa	12.58

Adult Concerns: Burning, pain rectal bleeding; headache, changes in mood, insomnia, nervousness, seizure, hypertension, arrhythmias, heart failure, edema, vomiting, peptic ulcers, weight gain, changes in liver function, hyperglycemia, changes in electrolytes, leukocytosis, muscle weakness, osteoporosis.

Adult Dose: 100 mg nightly (60 ml) rectally.

Pediatric Concerns: None via breastfeeding have been reported.

Infant Monitoring: Feeding, growth, and weight gain.

Alternatives:

References:
1. Pharmaceutical manufacturers prescribing information.

HYDROCORTISONE SODIUM SUCCINATE

Trade: A-hydrocort, Cortisol, Solu-cortef

Category: Anti-Inflammatory

LRC: L3 - No Data-Probably Compatible

It is an anti-inflammatory glucocorticoid, which contains hydrocortisone sodium succinate as the active ingredient. Hydrocortisone sodium succinate has the same metabolic and anti-inflammatory actions as hydrocortisone, which is naturally occurring glucocorticoid. Sodium succinate ester of hydrocortisone is highly water-soluble which permits the immediate intravenous administration of high doses of hydrocortisone in a small volume and high blood levels of hydrocortisone are achieved rapidly. It is used in allergic states like asthma, dermatitis, endocrine disorders, hematologic disorders, rheumatic disorders, etc.

Systemically administered corticosteroids appear in human milk and can suppress growth and interfere with endogenous corticosteroid production in infants only if it is taken in large doses for many days. In small doses, most steroids are certainly not contraindicated in nursing mothers. Following administration, wait at least 4 hours if possible prior to feeding infant to reduce exposure. With high doses (>200 mg/day), particularly for long periods, hydrocortisone could potentially produce problems in infant growth and development. Brief applications of high dose steroids are probably not contraindicated as the overall exposure is low. With prolonged high dose therapy, the infant should be closely monitored.

T 1/2	8-12 h	MW	484.52 Da	PB	>90%
Tmax	1-2 h	RID		Vd	34 L/kg
Oral	96%	M/P		pKa	12.58

Adult Concerns: Headache, changes in mood, insomnia, nervousness, seizure, hypertension, arrhythmias, heart failure, edema, vomiting, weight gain, changes in liver function, hyperglycemia, changes in electrolytes, leukocytosis, muscle weakness, osteoporosis.

Adult Dose: Oral 20-50 mg daily; IV 100-500 mg daily.

Pediatric Concerns: No reported via milk at this time.

Infant Monitoring: Vomiting, diarrhea, feeding, growth, and weight gain.

Alternatives:

References:
1. Pharmaceutical manufacturers prescribing information.

HYDROCORTISONE TOPICAL

Trade: Aquacort, Cortate, Cortef, Cortone, Dermacort, Dermaid, Egocort, Emo-Cort, Hycor, Westcort

Category: Corticosteroid

LRC: L2 - No Data-Probably Compatible

Hydrocortisone is a typical corticosteroid with glucocorticoid and mineralocorticoid activity. When applied topically it suppresses inflammation and enhances healing. Initial onset of activity when applied topically is slow and may require several days for response. Absorption topically is dependent on placement; percutaneous absorption is 1% from the forearm, 2% from rectum, 4% from the scalp, 7% from the forehead, and 36% from the scrotal area.[1] The amount transferred into human milk has not been reported, but as with most steroids, is believed minimal. Applied to the nipple, only small amounts should be applied and then only after feeding; larger quantities should be removed prior to breastfeeding. 0.5% to 1% ointments, rather than creams, are generally preferred.

T 1/2	1-2 h	MW	362 Da	PB	90%
Tmax		RID		Vd	0.48 L/kg
Oral	96%	M/P		pKa	12.58

Adult Concerns: Local irritation - burning, dryness, skin atrophy, striae.

Adult Dose: Apply topically four times daily.

Pediatric Concerns: None reported via milk.

Infant Monitoring: Feeding, growth, and weight gain.

Alternatives:

References:
1. Derendorf H, Mollmann H, Barth J, Mollmann C, Tunn S, Krieg M. Pharmacokinetics and oral bioavailability of hydrocortisone. J Clin Pharmacol. 1991;31(5):473-476.

HYDROMORPHONE

Trade: Dilaudid, Exalgo, Hydromorph Contin

Category: Analgesic

LRC: L3 - Limited Data-Probably Compatible

Hydromorphone is a potent semisynthetic narcotic analgesic used to alleviate moderate to severe pain.[1] It is approximately 7-10 times more potent than morphine, but is used in equivalently lower doses. Further, it is not subject to rapid metabolism like many other opioids.

In a group of eight women who received 2 mg of intranasal hydromorphone, the milk levels ranged from about 6 µg/L at 1-1.5 hours to 0.2 µg/L at 24 hours (estimated from graph).[2] The observed milk/plasma ratio averaged 2.56 and the half-life of hydromorphone in breast milk was 10.5 hours. The infants in this study were not nursed during the 24 hour study period.

The authors of this study estimated a relative infant dose of 0.67% and reported that based on their calculations, if a women was given 4 mg of hydromorphone every 6 hours, her infant would ingest about 0.002 mg/kg/day or 2.2 µg of the 4 mg taken by the mother.[2] This is significantly less than the clinical oral dose recommended for infants and children with pain (0.03-0.06 mg/kg/dose every 4 hours prn).

A recent report suggests that repeated use of rather high doses of hydromorphone (4 mg every 4 hours) lead to respiratory difficulties in a full-term infant at 6 days postpartum.[3] After a dose of naloxone, the infant recovered rapidly.

T 1/2	2.6 h IV & oral immediate release; 11 h oral extended release	MW	321.8 Da	PB	8%-19%
Tmax	< 1 h oral immediate release	RID	0.67%	Vd	4 L/kg
Oral	60%	M/P	2.56	pKa	10.11

Adult Concerns: Sedation, respiratory depression/apnea, hypotension, nausea, vomiting, constipation, urinary retention, weakness.

Adult Dose: 2-4 mg orally every 4-6 hours as needed or 0.2-1 mg IV every 2-3 hours as needed.

Pediatric Concerns: None reported via milk at this time.

Infant Monitoring: Sedation, slowed breathing rate, pallor, constipation, and appropriate weight gain.

Alternatives: Acetaminophen(L1), NSAIDs, Oxycodone(L3)

References:
1. Pharmaceutical manufacturers prescribing information.
2. Edwards JE, Rudy AC, Wermeling DP, Desai N, McNamara PJ. Hydromorphone transfer into breast milk after intranasal administration. Pharmacotherapy. 2003 Feb;23(2):153-158.
3. Schultz ML, Kostic M, Kharasch S. A case of toxic breast-feeding? Pediatr Emerg Care. 2017 Jan.35(1):e9-e10. doi: 10.1097/PEC.0000000000001009.

HYDROQUINONE

Trade:

Category: Dermatologic Agents

LRC: L3 - No Data-Probably Compatible

Hydroquinone is used for depigmentation of skin due to conditions such as freckles, melasma, senile lentigo, and inactive chloasma.[1] Hydroquinone is rapidly and extensively absorbed from the gut of animals. Absorption via the skin is slower but may be more rapid with vehicles such as alcohols. The transcutaneous absorption is reported to be about 35%, which is relatively high for topical preparations. Hydroquinone distributes rapidly and widely and is metabolized to p-benzoquinone and other products. The excretion of hydroquinone and its metabolites is rapid and occurs primarily via the urine. No data are available on its transfer to human milk. Although it is quite polar and water soluble, it also has a rather high pKa (9.96), which could lead to some trapping in human milk. While it does not seem to be very toxic, its chronic use in breastfeeding mothers is probably not warranted for such benign syndromes that could wait until the mother has weaned the infant off the breast.

T 1/2		MW	110 Da	PB	
Tmax		RID		Vd	
Oral		M/P		pKa	9.96

Adult Concerns: Mild skin irritation and sensitivity, dryness, and fissuring of paranasal and infraorbital areas. Cases of intoxication and death have been reported from the oral ingestion of photographic developing agents. Dermal applications of hydroquinone at concentration levels below 3% in different bases caused negligible effects in male volunteers. However, there are case reports suggesting that skin lightening creams containing 2% hydroquinone have produced leucoderma, as well as ochronosis.

Adult Dose: Apply 2%-4% solutions twice daily. Limit areas treated.

Pediatric Concerns: No reports of its use in breastfeeding mothers.

Infant Monitoring: While not highly risky, its use in breastfeeding mothers may not be justified.

Alternatives: Azelaic acid(L3)

References:
1. Pharmaceutical manufacturers prescribing information.

HYDROXYAMPHETAMINE + TROPICAMIDE

Trade: Paremyd

Category: Mydriatic-Cycloplegic

LRC: L3 - No Data-Probably Compatible

An ophthalmic solution that is a combination of hydroxyamphetamine hydrobromide and tropicamide is currently marketed under the name of Paremyd.[1] It is indicated for use in routine diagnostic ophthalmic procedures and is recommended for topical administration in the form of eye drops. Hydroxyamphetamine is an adrenergic agent and tropicamide has anticholinergic effects. Together, they produce an additive mydriatic effect that facilitates better visualization during ophthalmic procedures. Clinically relevant mydriasis occurs within 30-60 minutes and lasts for 3 hours. The doses used are too low to produce significant systemic levels, and therefore, the amount that enters the milk should likely be too low to produce any untoward effects in the infants. Nevertheless, it is advisable to observe the infant for possible side-effects; a brief withholding period of 3-4 hours could eliminate most risk.

T 1/2		MW		PB	
Tmax	30-60 min	RID		Vd	
Oral		M/P		pKa	

Adult Concerns: Dryness of eyes, blurring of vision, photophobia. Rare adverse effects are myocardial infarction, ventricular arrhythmias, precipitation of glaucoma.

Adult Dose: 1-2 drops.

Pediatric Concerns:

Infant Monitoring: Dry mouth, restlessness, constipation.

Alternatives:

References:
1. Pharmaceutical manufacturers prescribing information.

HYDROXYCHLOROQUINE

Trade: Plaquenil

Category: Antimalarial

LRC: L2 - Limited Data-Probably Compatible

Hydroxychloroquine (HCQ) is effective in the treatment of malaria but is also used in immune syndromes such as rheumatoid arthritis and systemic lupus erythematous (SLE). HCQ is known to produce significant retinal damage and blindness if used over a prolonged period, and this could occur (theoretically but unlikely) in breastfed infants. Patients on this product should see an ophthalmologist routinely. It has a huge volume of distribution (Vd) that suggests milk levels will be quite low.

In one study of a mother receiving 400 mg HCQ daily, the concentrations of HCQ in breast milk were 1.46, 1.09, and 1.09 mg/L at 2.0, 9.5, and 14 hours after the dose.[1] The average milk concentration was 1.1 mg/L. The milk/plasma ratio was approximately 5.5. On a body-weight basis, the infant's dose would be 2.9% of the maternal dose. In another study of one mother receiving 200 mg twice daily, milk levels were much lower than the previous study. Only a total of 3.2 µg of hydroxychloroquine was detected in her milk over 48 hours.[2]

Two breastfeeding mothers taking hydroxychloroquine were tested to determine the concentration in their breast milk 1 week after delivery. The concentrations were 344 and 1424 ng/mL, which corresponded to an infant dose of 0.06 and 0.2 mg/kg/day respectively.[3] Hydroxychloroquine is mostly metabolized to chloroquine and has an incredibly long half-life. The pediatric dose for malaria prophylaxis is 5 mg/kg/week, far larger than the dose received via milk. Due to its huge volume of distribution, milk levels are generally quite low, and therefore this drug may be considered compatible with breastfeeding.

T 1/2	>40 days	MW	336 Da	PB	63%
Tmax	1-2 h	RID	2.9%	Vd	8.3-11.6 L/kg
Oral	74%	M/P	5.5	pKa	8.3, 9.7

Adult Concerns: Headache, arrhythmias, ataxia, dizziness, nervousness, nightmares, seizures, alopecia, hearing and ocular changes including deafness and blindness, vomiting, diarrhea, anorexia, changes in liver enzymes, leukopenia, aplastic anemia, thrombocytopenia, myopathies, skin reactions.

Adult Dose: 400 mg daily (varies by indication).

Pediatric Concerns: None reported via milk at this time.

Infant Monitoring: Irritability, insomnia, vomiting, diarrhea, weight gain. With prolonged exposure monitor vision.

Alternatives:

References:
1. Nation RL, Hackett LP, Dusci LJ, Ilett KF. Excretion of hydroxychloroquine in human milk. Br J Clin Pharmacol. 1984;17(3):368-369.
2. Ostensen M, Brown ND, Chiang PK, Aarbakke J. Hydroxychloroquine in human breast milk. Eur J Clin Pharmacol. 1985;28(3):357.
3. Costedoat-Chalumeau N, Amoura Z, Aymard G, et al. Evidence of transplacental passage of hydroxychloroquine in humans. Arthritis Rheum. 2002;46(4):1123-1124.

HYDROXYPROPYL METHYLCELLULOSE

Trade:

Category: Other

LRC: L3 - No Data-Probably Compatible

Hydroxypropyl methylcellulose, or hypromellose, is an inert polymer most often used as an excipient in other pharmaceutical preparations, as well as a lubricant in the treatment of dry eye. Studies conducted in rats have shown that very little of hypromellose is absorbed orally, with as much as 96.9% being excreted in the feces in less than 48 hours of administration.[1] It is likely that the kinetics are similar in humans, as other substances in the same class have shown similar behavior.[2] Though it lacks data regarding its safety in lactation, due to its inert nature and low oral bioavailability, it is likely that hypromellose is compatible with breastfeeding.

T 1/2	4 h	MW	748.8 Da	PB	
Tmax		RID		Vd	
Oral	3.1%	M/P		pKa	

Adult Concerns: Blurred vision, cataract, conjunctival hyperemia, dry eye, iritis, macular retinal edema, pain in eye, posterior capsule opacification, raised intraocular pressure, retinal hemorrhage.

Adult Dose: Ophthalmic: one to two drops in each eye.

Pediatric Concerns:

Infant Monitoring:

Alternatives:

References:
1. Kitagawa H, Satoh T, Yokoshima T, Nanbo T. Absorption, distribution and excretion of hydroxypropyl-methylcellulose phthalate in the rat. Pharmacometrics. 1971;5:1-4.
2. Cappon GD, Fleeman TL, Rocca MS, Cook JC, Hurtt ME. Embryo/fetal development studies with hydroxypropyl methylcellulose acetate succinate (HPMCAS) in rats and rabbits. Birth Defects Res B Dev Reprod Toxicol. 2003;68:421- 427. doi: 10.1002/bdrb.10039

HYDROXYQUINOLINE

Trade:

Category: Antibiotic, Other

LRC: L3 - No Data-Probably Compatible

Hydroxyquinoline, also referred to as oxyquinoline, is used as an antibacterial and antifungal in individuals requiring the use of a pessary. Its derivatives have also seen use in many industries, specifically by pesticide, nylon, and dye industries. It is currently not known if this substance is present in breast milk or if it would cause untoward effects in a breastfed child. Animal experiments indicate that small doses of ingested hydroxyquinoline may be detrimental to health. This agent was able to cause death in animal subjects with an LD50 of 1200 mg/kg in rats.[1] Absorption may occur through the skin, potentially causing headache, nausea, nervousness, and sleeplessness. It is unlikely that this drug would cause a large number of adverse effects when used to disinfect a pessary.

T 1/2		MW	145.16 Da	PB	
Tmax		RID		Vd	
Oral		M/P		pKa	~8.5

Adult Concerns: Headache, nausea, nervousness, sleeplessness, eye irritation, dermal irritation.

Adult Dose:

Pediatric Concerns:

Infant Monitoring:

Alternatives:

References:
1. 8-Hydroxyquinoline Material Safety Data Sheet. Santa Cruz, CA: Santa Cruz Biotechnology, Inc. Issued May 17, 2008. Accessed July 26, 2011.

HYDROXYTRYPTOPHAN

Trade: 5-HTP, 5-Hydroxytryptophan, L-Tryptophan

Category: Amino Acid Supplement

LRC: L4 - No Data-Possibly Hazardous

5-Hydroxytryptophan (5-HTP) is a natural aromatic amino acid that is the immediate precursor of the neurotransmitter serotonin. L-Tryptophan is another amino acid formerly used to treat depression.

L-Tryptophan: L-tryptophan (LTP), once absorbed, is rapidly transported to the liver where some of it is incorporated into proteins, and some passes unchanged into the general circulation. It is a precursor of serotonin. One of the major problems with the use of LTP is that when used at higher doses, metabolism to kynurenine is highly induced, and the majority of LTP is subsequently metabolized rather than converted into serotonin. Even under the best of circumstances, less than 3% of the LTP is likely to be converted to serotonin in the brain. L-Tryptophan crosses the blood-brain barrier only poorly. As the doses increase, the creation of the metabolite kynurenine tends to block entry of LTP into the brain. As the doses of LTP used are extraordinarily high, 2000-6000 mg/day cost and adverse effects are significant.[1] Older formulations created with contaminants were responsible for the eosinophilia-myalgia syndrome.

5-HTP: 5-HTP is rapidly absorbed, and approximately 70% of the dose is bioavailable. The remaining 30% is converted to serotonin by intestinal cells which may lead to some nausea. 5-HTP readily crosses the blood-brain barrier (24% in CSF) and is one step closer to serotonin production. The dose of 5-HTP is much lower, averaging 100-300 mg/day, and some studies have found it equivalent to tricyclic antidepressants[2] and fluvoxamine (an SSRI) in treating depression.[3] Although several cases of eosinophilia-myalgia syndrome have been reported with the use of 5-HTP[4,5], both of these patients had defective metabolic mechanisms for converting 5-HTP.

Unfortunately, there are no data on the transfer of exogenously supplied LTP or 5-HTP to human milk. For instance, it is not apparently known if high maternal plasma levels would produce elevated milk levels. While it is true human milk contains higher levels of LTP, presumably to stimulate serotonin levels in the infant's CNS, it is not known if high maternal doses would likewise produce high milk levels. Because the infant's neurologic development is incredibly sensitive to serotonin levels, and because we do not know if supplementation with LTP or 5-HTP could produce high milk levels leading to overdose in the infant, we do not recommend the use of L-tryptophan or 5-HTP supplementation in breastfeeding mothers until we know more about corresponding milk levels.

T 1/2	4.3 h	MW	393 Da	PB	19%
Tmax	3-6 h	RID		Vd	0.6 L/kg
Oral	<70%	M/P		pKa	6.96

Adult Concerns: Anorexia, diarrhea, nausea, and vomiting have been reported.

Adult Dose:

Pediatric Concerns: None reported via milk.

Infant Monitoring: Observe for vomiting, diarrhea, and weight gain.

Alternatives: Selective serotonin reuptake inhibitors, tricyclic antidepressants.

References:
1. Murray MT, Pizzorno JE. 5-Hydroxytryptophan. In: Murray MT, Pizzorno JE, eds. Textbook of Natural Medicine. Philadelphia: Churchill Livingstone; 1999:783-796.
2. van Praag HM. Management of depression with serotonin precursors. Biol Psychiatry. 1981;16(3):291-310.
3. Poldinger W, Calanchini B, Schwarz W. A functional-dimensional approach to depression: serotonin deficiency as a target syndrome in a comparison of 5-hydroxytryptophan and fluvoxamine. Psychopathology. 1991;24(2):53-81.
4. Sternberg EM, Van Woert MH, Young SN, et al. Development of a scleroderma-like illness during therapy with L-5-hydroxytryptophan and carbidopa. N Engl J Med. 1980;303(14):782-787.
5. Michelson D, Page SW, Casey R, et al. An eosinophilia-myalgia syndrome related disorder associated with exposure to L-5-hydroxytryptophan. J Rheumatol. 1994;21(12):2261-2265.

HYDROXYUREA

Trade: Hydrea

Category: Antimetabolite

LRC: L4 - Limited Data-Possibly Hazardous

Hydroxyurea is an antineoplastic agent used to treat melanoma, leukemias, and other neoplasms. It is well absorbed orally and rapidly metabolized to urea by the liver. In one study following a dose of 500 mg three times daily for 7 days, milk samples were collected 2 hours after the last dose.[1] The concentration of hydroxyurea in breast milk averaged 6.1 mg/L (range 3.8 to 8.4 mg/L). This is about 4.3% of the maternal dose, which is probably too low to bother a breastfeeding infant. Approximately 80% of the dose is excreted renally within 12 hours in adults. As this product is potentially toxic, mothers receiving hydroxyurea should probably withhold breastfeeding for a minimum of 12-24 hours after the dose.

T 1/2	3-4 h	MW	76 Da	PB	
Tmax	2 h	RID	4.3%	Vd	0.48-1.62 L/kg
Oral	Complete	M/P		pKa	10.14

Adult Concerns: Headache, dizziness, fever, malaise, alopecia, mucositis, vomiting, constipation or diarrhea, anorexia, changes in liver and renal function, leukopenia, neutropenia, anemia.

Adult Dose: 80 mg/kg every 3 days.

Pediatric Concerns: None reported via milk at this time.

Infant Monitoring: Withhold breastfeeding for a minimum of 12-24 hours after the dose.

Alternatives:

References:

1. Sylvester RK, Lobell M, Teresi ME, Brundage D, Dubowy R. Excretion of hydroxyurea into milk. Cancer. 1987;60(9):2177-2178.

HYDROXYZINE

Trade: Atarax, Vistaril

Category: Antihistamine

LRC: L2 - Limited Data-Probably Compatible

Hydroxyzine is an antihistamine structurally similar to cyclizine and meclizine. It produces significant CNS depression and anticholinergic side effects (e.g., dry mouth).[1] Hydroxyzine is largely metabolized to cetirizine. No data are available on its secretion into breast milk, but since it is largely metabolized to cetirizine, its pharmacological behavior should be similar to cetirizine. Cetirizine is one of the preferred antihistamines during breastfeeding since it is non-sedating.

T 1/2	3-7 h in children, 20 h in adults.	MW	375 Da	PB	
Tmax	2 h	RID		Vd	13-31 L/kg
Oral	Complete	M/P		pKa	2.1, 7.1

Adult Concerns: Sedation, hypotension, dry mouth, constipation, urinary retention.

Adult Dose: 50-100 mg four times daily.

Pediatric Concerns: None reported via milk.

Infant Monitoring: Sedation, dry mouth, constipation, urinary retention.

Alternatives: Cetirizine(L2), Loratadine(L1)

References:

1. Paton DM, Webster DR. Clinical pharmacokinetics of H1-receptor antagonists (the antihistamines). Clin Pharmacokinet. 1985;10(6):477-497.

HYOSCYAMINE

Trade: Anaspaz, ED-Spaz, Hyoscine, Levsin, NuLev

Category: Cholinergic Antagonist

LRC: L3 - Limited Data-Probably Compatible

Hyoscyamine is an anticholinergic, antisecretory agent that belongs to the belladonna alkaloid family. It is the levo-isomer of atropine. Its typical effects are to dry secretions, produce constipation, dilate pupils, blur vision, and cause urinary retention.[1] Hyoscyamine is used to provide symptomatic relief to various gastrointestinal disorders including spasms, peptic ulcers, irritable bowel syndrome, pancreatitis, colic, and cystitis.[2] Although no exact amounts are listed, hyoscyamine is thought to be secreted into breast milk in trace amounts.[1] Thus far, no untoward effects from breastfeeding while using hyoscyamine have been found. Hyoscyamine drops have in the past been used directly in infants for colic although it is no longer recommended for this use. As with atropine, infants and children are especially sensitive to anticholinergics and their use is discouraged. Use with caution in breastfeeding mothers.

T 1/2	2-3.5 h	MW	289 Da	PB	50%
Tmax	40-90 min (oral)	RID		Vd	
Oral	81%	M/P		pKa	9.7

Adult Concerns: Drowsiness, confusion, blurred vision, dry mouth, hypotension, bradycardia, constipation, urinary retention, dermatitis, memory loss, hallucinations.

Adult Dose: 0.125-0.25 mg four times daily.

Pediatric Concerns: Decreased heart rate and anticholinergic effects from direct use, but none reported from breast milk ingestion.

Infant Monitoring: Sedation or irritability, drying of oral and ophthalmic secretions, urinary retention, constipation.

Alternatives:

References:
1. Pharmaceutical manufacturers prescribing information.
2. DrugBank, 2019.

IBANDRONATE

Trade: Boniva

Category: Calcium Regulator

LRC: L3 - No Data-Probably Compatible

Ibandronate is a bisphosphonate, which acts by inhibiting osteoclast-mediated bone resorption. It is therefore used in the treatment and prevention of postmenopausal osteoporosis.[1] Following oral or intravenous administration, 40% to 50% of the drug is rapidly removed from the circulation and binds to bone. This reduces plasma concentrations to 10% of peak plasma within 3 hours of an intravenous dose, or within 8 hours of an oral dose. It is currently not known if ibandronate is transferred to human milk. When administered in lactating rats, the concentration of ibandronate that appeared in the milk was 1.5 times the plasma concentrations. A review of the pharmacokinetic profile suggests that due to its relatively high protein binding and low oral bioavailability, this drug will probably not attain clinically significant plasma levels in the infant. However, until more established data is available on the transfer of ibandronate to human milk, some caution is recommended when considering administration in a breast-feeding mother.

T 1/2	4.6 - 25.5 h	MW	359.24 Da	PB	85.7%-99.5%
Tmax	0.5-2 h	RID		Vd	1.23 L/kg
Oral	0.6%	M/P		pKa	

Adult Concerns: Headache, dizziness, insomnia, hypertension, abdominal pain, dyspepsia, vomiting, constipation, hypercholesterolemia, osteonecrosis of the jaw, back pain.

Adult Dose: 3 mg IV every 3 months or 150 mg orally once a month.

Pediatric Concerns:

Infant Monitoring: Changes in sleep, vomiting, diarrhea or constipation.

Alternatives: Alendronate, Pamidronate(L3)

References:
1. Pharmaceutical manufacturers prescribing information.

IBUPROFEN

Trade: Advil, Motrin, NeoProfen
Category: NSAID
LRC: L1 - Extensive Data-Compatible

Ibuprofen is a nonsteroidal anti-inflammatory analgesic (NSAID). It is frequently used for fever in infants and children. Ibuprofen enters milk only in very low levels (less than 0.6% of maternal dose). Even large doses produce very small milk levels. In one patient receiving 400 mg twice daily, milk levels were less than 0.5 mg/L.[1] In another study of 12 women who received 400 mg doses every 6 hours for a total of five doses, all breast milk levels of ibuprofen were less than 1 mg/L, the lower limit of the assay.[2]

In another study of a single mother following the use of six 400 mg doses over 42.5 hours, ibuprofen levels at 30 minutes following the first dose were 13 mg/L.[3] The highest reported level in milk (180 µg/L) was after the third 400 mg dose at 20.5 hours. The authors suggested that an infant would receive approximately 17 µg/kg/day following maternal doses of 1.2 grams daily.

Thirteen breastfeeding mothers who had taken a minimum of three 200 mg tablets of ibuprofen, at least 7 days after delivery were included in a study to determine ibuprofen concentration in mature milk (n = 20, 7 excluded).[4] Breast milk samples were taken from milk that was pumped 1.5 to 8 hours after the third dose of ibuprofen. In addition, two maternal blood samples were taken 30 minutes to 2 hours and 4 to 6 hours post third ibuprofen dose. On average, the women in this study were 34 years-old, 60.4 kg, took 1046 mg/day of ibuprofen and had been breastfeeding for 263 days. The mean concentration of ibuprofen was 361 µg/L and 15.5 mg/L for milk and serum, respectively. The milk plasma ratio was 0.025. The infants received a mean dose of 68 µg/kg/day (range 8-262 µg/kg/day) of ibuprofen from breast milk. The typical infant dose of ibuprofen is 10 mg/kg/dose every 6-8 hours (max 40 mg/kg/day); therefore, the amount of drug received in breast milk was well below the recommended dose used in infants.[5] In addition, the relative infant dose was estimated to be 0.38% (range 0.04%-1.15%). This study also confirmed the hypothesis that the amount of drug in mature milk would decrease as the duration of lactation increased, as the amount of protein in milk decreases over time (ibuprofen is highly protein bound).[4]

Based on years of clinical experience with ibuprofen for postpartum pain and its use in lactation, it is one of the analgesics of choice in breastfeeding women.

T 1/2	1.8-2.5 h	MW	206 Da	PB	>99%
Tmax	1-2 h	RID	0.12%-0.66%	Vd	0.14 L/kg
Oral	80%	M/P		pKa	4.4

Adult Concerns: Headache, dizziness, nervousness, tinnitus, dyspepsia, nausea, vomiting, abdominal pain, constipation, diarrhea, gastrointestinal bleeding, changes in renal function, edema.

Adult Dose: 400 mg every 4-6 hours.

Pediatric Concerns: None reported from breastfeeding.

Infant Monitoring: Vomiting, diarrhea.

Alternatives: Acetaminophen(L1)

References:
1. Weibert RT, Townsend RJ, Kaiser DG, Naylor AJ. Lack of ibuprofen secretion into human milk. Clin Pharm. 1982;1(5):457-458.
2. Townsend RJ, Benedetti TJ, Erickson SH, et al. Excretion of ibuprofen into breast milk. Am J Obstet Gynecol. 1984;149(2):184-186.
3. Walter K, Dilger C. Ibuprofen in human milk. Br J Clin Pharmacol. 1997;44:211-212.
4. Rigourd V, de Villepin B, Amirouche A, et al. Ibuprofen concentrations in human mature milk-first data about pharamcokinetics study in breast milk with AOR-10127 "Antalait" study. Ther Drug Monit. 2014;7:1-7.
5. Pharmaceutical manufacturers prescribing information.

IFOSFAMIDE

Trade: Holoxan, Holoxane, Ifex, Ifolem
Category: Alkylating Agent
LRC: L4 - No Data-Possibly Hazardous

Ifosfamide is structurally similar to cyclophosphamide and is used in breast cancer. This family of drugs requires activation (metabolism) by the liver to produce the active cytotoxic agents. The oral bioavailability of ifosfamide is near 100% and reaches a peak at 1-2 hours.[1] The elimination half-life varies by dose and frequency and ranges from 4.6-15 hours. Transport of ifosfamide and its metabolites into the CNS is exceedingly low (approximately 1/6th of the plasma compartment). This would suggest milk levels will probably be low when they are ultimately determined. The kinetics of this agent are highly variable depending on the renal function, creatinine clearance, liver function, etc. Waiting periods before returning to breastfeeding should be adjusted for this factor. Withhold breastfeeding for at least 72 hours.

T 1/2	4.6-15 h	MW	261 Da	PB	20%
Tmax	1 h	RID		Vd	0.72 L/kg
Oral	92%-100%	M/P		pKa	

Adult Concerns: Agitation, confusion, hallucinations, fever, alopecia, vomiting, anorexia, changes in liver and renal function, hematuria, metabolic acidosis, leukopenia, anemia, thrombocytopenia.

Adult Dose: Varies by protocol.

Pediatric Concerns:

Infant Monitoring: Hazardous, withhold breastfeeding for at least 72 hours.

Alternatives:

References:
1. Pharmaceutical manufacturer information, 2014.

ILOPERIDONE

Trade: Fanapt

Category: Antipsychotic, Atypical

LRC: L3 - No Data-Probably Compatible

Iloperidone is an atypical antipsychotic used in the treatment of schizophrenia.[1] The dose of iloperidone must be increased slowly and administered twice daily to decrease the orthostatic hypotensive effects of the drug. Iloperidone also prolongs the QT interval and has the potential to cause leukopenia, neutropenia and agranulocytosis; therefore, ECG monitoring and monitoring of blood parameters are often done during initial therapy. There are no studies regarding the use of iloperidone in lactation; however, it is known to be excreted in rat milk. Based on its large volume of distribution and high protein binding it may have difficulty entering breast milk. It should be noted that this medication does have a long half-life and very little information is available on its use in breastfeeding women, so other alternatives with more lactation data need to be considered (e.g., risperidone, quetiapine).[2]

T 1/2	18-33 h	MW	426.5 Da	PB	95%
Tmax	2-4 h	RID		Vd	19-40 L/kg
Oral	96%	M/P		pKa	

Adult Concerns: Dizziness, somnolence, orthostatic hypotension, tachycardia, dry mouth, nausea, weight gain, extrapyramidal symptoms.

Adult Dose: 6-12 mg orally twice daily.

Pediatric Concerns:

Infant Monitoring: Sedation or irritability, apnea, dry mouth, not waking to feed/poor feeding, extrapyramidal symptoms, and weight gain.

Alternatives: Risperidone(L2), Quetiapine(L2), Aripiprazole(L3)

References:
1. Pharmaceutical manufacturers prescribing information.
2. Howland RH. Update on newer antipsychotic drugs. J Psychosoc Nurs Ment Health Serv. 2011 Apr;49(4):13-15. doi: 10.3928/02793695-20110311-99.

ILOPROST

Trade: Ventavis

Category: Antihypertensive

LRC: L3 - No Data-Probably Compatible

Iloprost is a prostacylin that is used to treat pulmonary arterial hypertension.[1] This medication dilates the systemic and pulmonary arterial vasculature; with long-term use iloprost can modify pulmonary vascular resistance and suppress vascular smooth muscle proliferation. This drug can also affect platelet aggregation when aerosolized.

Currently there are no data regarding iloprost in human milk. When lactating rats were given 1 mg/kg/day IV, their pups were found to have a higher risk of mortality. When rats were given 250 mg/kg/day orally of iloprost (maternally toxic dose - 13% iloprost) their pups were also found to be at a greater risk of death. Less than 1% of the iloprost IV dose and its metabolites were found in rodent milk. No postnatal development or reproductive complications were reported in breastfed rodents.

T 1/2	20-30 min	MW	360.49 Da	PB	60%
Tmax	5 min	RID		Vd	0.7-0.8 L/kg
Oral		M/P		pKa	

Adult Concerns: Headache, insomnia, flushing, syncope, hypotension, palpitations, jaw pain, vomiting, changes in liver and renal failure, flu like symptoms.

Adult Dose: 5 µg dose inhaled six to nine times daily.

Pediatric Concerns: No data in breastmilk at this time.

Infant Monitoring: Drowsiness, lethargy or insomnia, pallor, poor feeding, vomiting, and weight gain.

Alternatives:

References:
1. Pharmaceutical manufacturers prescribing information.

IMATINIB MESYLATE

Trade: Gleevec

Category: Antineoplastic

LRC: L4 - Limited Data-Possibly Hazardous

Imatinib mesylate is a tyrosine kinase inhibitor used to treat several different types of tumors and leukemias. The parent drug has a half-life of about 18 hours, while the active metabolite the N-desmethyl derivative has a half-life of about 40 hours.[1]

There are now four case reports of women who have taken imatinib during lactation; however, only one of the infants was breastfed. The first case report is of a 40-year-old female with Chronic Myeoloid Leukemia (CML), who was taking imatinib 400 mg once daily. Plasma and breast milk samples were taken 4 weeks postpartum just prior to the dose and then at 1, 2, 3, 4, and 9 hours after.[2] The samples were tested for both imatinib and the main active metabolite (N-desmethyl derivative). The steady state plasma concentrations of the drug and its metabolite were 3 to 3.2 µg/mL and 0.8 to 1.1 µg/mL respectively. The steady state breast milk concentrations of the drug and its metabolite were 1.1 to 1.4 µg/mL and 0.8 µg/mL, respectively. According to the authors the samples were repeated at 2 months postpartum and the results were similar. The milk/plasma ratio was 0.5 for imatinib and 0.9 for the metabolite and the daily infant dose was about 3 mg or 10% of the maternal dose. Although the infant in this case report was breastfed, no information was provided in regards to the infants monitoring or health outcomes.

In the second case, the woman was also receiving 400 mg of imatinib daily for CML.[3] This time breast milk levels were collected 15 hours after the dose taken on postpartum day 7. The concentration of imatinib was 596 ng/mL and the active metabolite was 1,513 ng/mL. This study also estimated the average infant daily dose to be fairly small at 1.2 to 2 mg. The infant in this case report was not breastfed.

In the third report, a 34-year-old female with CML was receiving 400 mg of imatinib daily. The woman did not breastfeed her infant, but did supply breast milk samples for up to 171 hours postpartum.[4] Steady-state was achieved in the breast milk by about day two. By 51 hours, the plasma concentration of imatinib was 2010 ng/mL and the active metabolite was 284 ng/mL. The concentrations of drug and active metabolite in breast milk at 51 hours were 1153 ng/mL and 1024 ng/mL respectively. By 171 hours, the imatinib levels decreased to 797 ng/mL and the metabolite concentration remained steady at 1052 ng/mL.

The fourth case involved a 27-year-old female with CML who also took imatinib 400 mg daily; this woman did not breastfeed her infant but did supply breast milk samples, which were taken on days 7, 14, 15, and 16 postpartum.[5] The imatinib maternal blood concentration 12 hours after the dose on the second day postpartum was 2385 ng/mL. The breast milk samples ranged from as low as 1430 ng/mL 14 hours after the dose on day 7 to as high as 2623 ng/mL 10 hours after the dose on day 14.

Although the daily infant dose is estimated to be low in comparison to the typical maternal dose, the effect of chronic exposure to low doses of imatinib are unknown, and due to the potential for serious sequelae (infection, changes in liver function, etc.) the benefits of breast milk versus risks of imatinib exposure should be seriously considered. Withhold breastfeeding for at least 10 days after treatment.

T 1/2	18 h parent; 40 h metabolite	MW	590 Da	PB	95%
Tmax	2-4 h	RID	5.54%-6.89%	Vd	
Oral	98%	M/P	0.5/0.9 (metabolite)	pKa	12.45

Adult Concerns: Headache, fatigue, insomnia, dizziness, alopecia, hypotension, mucositis, dyspepsia, nausea, vomiting, constipation, changes in liver and renal function, changes in electrolytes, leukopenia, neutropenia, thrombocytopenia, anemia, pruritus, edema.

Adult Dose: 400-800 mg/day.

Pediatric Concerns: No known adverse effects via milk at this time.

Infant Monitoring: Fever, frequent infections, changes in sleep, feeding, or weight gain. Based on clinical symptoms, some infants may require monitoring of their hematology or liver function. Withhold breastfeeding for at least 10 days after treatment.

Alternatives:

References:
1. Pharmaceutical manufacturers prescribing information.
2. Gambacorti-Passerini CB, Tornaghi L, Marangon E, et al. Imatinib concentrations in human milk. Blood. 2007;109(4):1790.
3. Russell MA, Carpenter MW, Akhtar MS, Lagattuta TF, Egorin MJ. Imatinib mesylate and metabolite concentrations in maternal blood, umbilical cord blood, placenta and breast milk. J Perinatology. 2007;27:241-243.
4. Kronenberger R, Schleyer E, Bornhauser M, Ehninger G, Gattermann N, Blum S. Imatinib in breast milk. Ann Hematol. 2009;88:1265-1266.
5. Ali R, Ozkalemkas F, Kimya Y, et al. Imatinib use during pregnancy and breast feeding: a case report and review of the literature. Arch Gynecol Obstet. 2009;280:169-175.

IMIPENEM + CILASTATIN

Trade: Primaxin IV

Category: Antibiotic, Carbapenem

LRC: L3 - No Data-Probably Compatible

Imipenem/cilastatin is a combination drug product that is indicated for use in a variety of infections including infections of the bone or joint, skin and subcutaneous tissues, lower respiratory tract infections, and systemic bacterial infections.[1] Experience with this drug in breastfeeding women is limited; however, there is no evidence that the use of this drug will have adverse effects in the breastfed infant. Cilastatin is added to extend the half-life of an antibiotic called imipenem, structurally similar to penicillins. Both imipenem and cilastatin are poorly absorbed orally and must be administered IM or IV. Transfer to breast milk is probably minimal but no data are available at this time. At this time, meropenem (another carbapenem) would be recommended if appropriate for treatment of the maternal condition as concentrations in milk are known to be very low.

T 1/2	60 min	MW	Imip/cila: 317/380 Da	PB	Imip/cila: 20%/40%
Tmax	Immediate (IV)	RID		Vd	Widely distributed
Oral	Poor	M/P		pKa	

Adult Concerns: Seizures, fever, dizziness, somnolence, hypotension, nausea, diarrhea, vomiting, abdominal pain, changes in liver function, pancytopenia.

Adult Dose: 500 mg IV q 6 h.

Pediatric Concerns: None reported via milk at this time; pediatric safety has been established in the neonatal and pediatric population.

Infant Monitoring: Vomiting, diarrhea, changes in gastrointestinal flora, and rash.

Alternatives: Meropenem(L3)

References:
1. Pharmaceutical manufacturers prescribing information.

IMIPRAMINE

Trade: Impril, Melipramin, Tofranil

Category: Antidepressant, Tricyclic

LRC: L2 - Limited Data-Probably Compatible

Imipramine is a classic tricyclic antidepressant. Imipramine is metabolized to desipramine, the active metabolite. Milk levels approximate those of maternal serum. In a patient receiving 200 mg daily at bedtime, the milk levels at 1, 9, 10, and 23 hours were 29, 24, 12, and 18 µg/L respectively.[1] However, in this study the mother was not in a therapeutic range. In another study of four women receiving 75-150 mg/day imipramine, levels of imipramine plus desipramine in fore milk ranged from 34-408 µg/L and in hind milk ranged from 48 to 622 µg/L.[2] In several breastfed infants, levels of imipramine plus desipramine ranged from 0.6 µg/L in one individual (maternal dose = 75 mg/day) to 5.5 µg/L (maternal dose = 100 mg/day).[3] Therapeutic plasma levels in older children 6-12 years typically range 200-225 µg/L.

One small study that followed four groups of women prescribed TCAs throughout different stages of reproduction found no adverse events in the group of infants whose mothers were prescribed these medications in lactation.[4] This study included 21 women (14 on imipramine) that initiated tricyclic antidepressant therapy at a mean of 10.3 weeks postpartum and breastfed on treatment for a mean of 12 weeks.

T 1/2	8-16 h	MW	280 Da	PB	90%
Tmax	1-2 h	RID	0.1%-4.4%	Vd	20-40 L/kg
Oral	90%	M/P	0.5-1.5	pKa	9.5

Adult Concerns: Sedation, agitation, confusion, insomnia, hypotension, arrhythmias, dry mouth, vomiting, diarrhea or constipation, anorexia, changes in liver function, urinary retention.

Adult Dose: 75-100 mg daily.

Pediatric Concerns: None reported.

Infant Monitoring: Sedation or irritability, dry mouth, not waking to feed/poor feeding, constipation, urinary retention, weight gain.

Alternatives: Amoxapine(L2)

References:
1. Sovner R, Orsulak PJ. Excretion of imipramine and desipramine in human breast milk. Am J Psychiatry. 1979;136(4A):451-452.
2. Yoshida K, Smith B, Kumar R. Psychotropic drugs in mothers' milk: a comprehensive review of assay methods, pharmacokinetics and of safety of breast-feeding. J Psychopharmacol. 1999;13(1):64-80. Review.
3. Yoshida K, Smith B, Craggs M, et al. Investigation of pharmacokinetics and possible adverse effects in infants exposed to tricyclic antidepressants in breast-milk. J Affect Disord. 1997;43:225-237.
4. Misri S, Sivertz K. Tricyclic drugs in pregnancy and lactation: a preliminary report. Int J Psychiatry Med. 1991;21:157-171.

IMIQUIMOD

Trade: Aldara, Beselna, Imimor, Zyclara

Category: Immune Modulator

LRC: L3 - No Data-Probably Compatible

Imiquimod is a toll-like receptor 7 agonist that activates immune cells to produce cytokines and helps regulate co-stimulatory molecule expression. The drug also improves the function of antigens in acquired immune cells. Imiquimod is used for the treatment of plantar warts and actinic keratoses. After topical administration of the 5% cream, serum levels of metabolites were generally found to be low and in one study, only quantifiable in three subjects at the end of a 21 day application.[1] The adult use of imiquimod 3.75% cream in the treatment of actinic keratoses produced similarly low serum levels when applied for 3 weeks. The amount given in this study was 18.75 mg each day for 21 days, applied to 200 square cm of skin. At the end of the study, mean steady state serum concentrations measured 0.323 ng/mL.[1] This concentration is much lower than the 500 ng/mL needed to elicit systemic induction of interferon alpha or interleukin 1 receptor antagonists.[2]

Imiquimod has been used in young children. In a study determining the pharmacokinetics of imiquimod in children, serum levels of this drug were shown to be extremely low. After administration of 12.5-37.5 mg imiquimod each day to children aged 2-12, it was found that the median maximum concentration in serum was ≤ 0.5 ng/mL for single doses and ≤1 ng/mL for multiple doses. One outlier was reported with concentrations as high as 9.7 ng/mL. Children in this study were all treated for molluscum contagiosum with 5% imiquimod cream. Amounts given to each child varied based on the weight of the subject and extent of disease.[3]

While there are no data on the excretion of imiquimod into human milk, milk levels will likely be far lower than 323 ng/L, which would be far too low to produce clinical effects in an infant. The manufacturer recommends that caution be used when administering imiquimod to nursing women.

T 1/2	20 h topical; 2 h subcutaneous	MW	240.3 Da	PB	
Tmax	9-12 h	RID		Vd	
Oral	47%	M/P		pKa	

Adult Concerns: Headache, fever, fatigue, dyspepsia, vomiting, diarrhea, anorexia, myalgia, edema, local site reactions (most common).

Adult Dose: Variable topically.

Pediatric Concerns:

Infant Monitoring: Vomiting and poor feeding.

Alternatives:

References:
1. Kulp J, Levy S, Fein MC, Adams M, Furst J, Meng TC. Pharmacokinetics ofimiquimod 3.75% cream applied daily for 3 weeks to actinic keratoses on the face and/or balding scalp. Arch Dermatol Res. 2010 Sep;302(7):539-544.
2. Miller RL, Gerster JF, Owens ML, Slade HB, Tomai MA. Imiquimod applied topically:a novel immune response modifier and new class of drug. Int J Immunopharmacol. 1999;21:1-14.K.
3. Myhre PE, Levy ML, Eichenfield LF, Kolb VB, Fielder SL, Meng TC. Pharmacokinetics and safety of imiquimod 5% cream in the treatment of molluscum contagiosum in children. Pediatr Dermatol. 2008;25(1);88-95.

INDAPAMIDE

Trade: Dapa-Tabs, Lozide, Lozol, Nadide, Napamide, Natrilix

Category: Diuretic

LRC: L3 - No Data-Probably Compatible

Indapamide is the first of a new class of indoline diuretics used to treat hypertension. No data are available on transfer of this diuretic to human milk.[1] Numerous other diuretics are available and have been studied in breastfeeding mothers. See hydrochlorothiazide, or furosemide as an alternatives.

T 1/2	14 h	MW	366 Da	PB	71%
Tmax	0.5-2 h	RID		Vd	
Oral	Complete	M/P		pKa	8.8

Adult Concerns: Dizziness, irritability, lethargy, hypotension, nausea, vomiting, constipation, changes in electrolytes, muscle cramps, rash.

Adult Dose: 2.5-5 mg daily.

Pediatric Concerns: None reported at this time.

Infant Monitoring: Observe for fluid loss, dehydration, lethargy; monitor maternal milk supply.

Alternatives: Hydrochlorothiazide(L2), Furosemide(L3)

References:
1. Pharmaceutical manufacturers prescribing information.

INDINAVIR

Trade: Crixivan

Category: Antiviral

LRC: L5 - Limited Data-Hazardous if Maternal HIV Infection

Indinavir binds to the protease active site and inhibits the activity of the enzyme in HIV virus.[1] This inhibition prevents cleavage of the viral polyproteins resulting in the formation of immature non-infectious viral particles. In a rodent study, indinavir milk levels were quite high, although usually this does not correlate closely with human milk.

In a study of a single female patient who was receiving 600 mg twice daily during the first 5 days postpartum, levels of indinavir in colostrum were 90%-540% of the maternal plasma levels.[2] This should have been expected, as the milk compartment was virtually open to all plasma components the first few days postpartum. Levels of indinavir after the first week postpartum will likely be much less than above. Viral titers in milk were equivalent to those in the HAART-treated mothers, and were very low (<400 copies/mL).

Note: This medication is an L5 to highlight the contraindication of breastfeeding when the mother is known to be infected with HIV, this medication is not an L5 based on its risk to the infant in breast milk. The Centers for Disease Control and Prevention recommend that HIV-1 infected mothers do not breastfeed their infants to avoid postnatal transmission of HIV-1.

T 1/2	1.4-2.2 h	MW	711.88 Da	PB	60%
Tmax	0.8 h	RID		Vd	
Oral	30%	M/P		pKa	13.19

Adult Concerns: Headache, dizziness, fatigue, fever, abdominal pain, anorexia, changes in liver function, hyperbilirubinemia, kidney stones, hematuria, hyperglycemia, neutropenia, thrombocytopenia.

Adult Dose: 800 mg every 8 hours.

Pediatric Concerns:

Infant Monitoring: Breastfeeding is not recommended in mothers who have HIV.

Alternatives:

References:
1. Lewis JS, 2nd, Terriff CM, Coulston DR, Garrison MW. Protease inhibitors: a therapeutic breakthrough for the treatment of patients with human immunodeficiency virus. Clin Ther. 1997 Mar-Apr;19(2):187-214.
2. Colebunders R, Hodossy B, Burger D, et al. The effect of highly active antiretroviral treatment on viral load and antiretroviral drug levels in breast milk. AIDS. 2005 Nov;19(16):1912-1915.

INDOCYANINE GREEN

Trade: IC-Green, Indocyanine Green

Category: Diagnostic Agent, Other

LRC: L3 - No Data-Probably Compatible

Indocyanine green is a cyanine fluorescent dye used in various medical procedures, including liver blood flow, ophthalmic angiography, and hepatic function.[1] Biologically, it has a plasma half-life of 150-180 seconds and is rapidly transferred into the gall bladder and the intestine for elimination. Due to its large molecular weight, it would most likely have limited entry into breast milk; however, should it enter milk its short half-life would reduce any potential risk to the infant. By 30 minutes, almost all of the dye should be eliminated from the maternal plasma compartment.

T 1/2	2-3 min	MW	774 Da	PB	
Tmax		RID		Vd	
Oral	Nil	M/P		pKa	

Adult Concerns: Possible anaphylactic or urticarial reactions have been reported in patients with or without history of allergy to iodides.

Adult Dose: 5 mg.

Pediatric Concerns: None reported in breastfeeding infants.

Infant Monitoring:

Alternatives:

References:

1. Pharmaceutical manufacturers prescribing information.

INDOMETHACIN

Trade: Arthrexin, Hicin, Indocid, Indocin, Indoptol

Category: NSAID

LRC: L3 - Limited Data-Probably Compatible

Indomethacin is a potent, nonsteroidal anti-inflammatory agent (NSAID) frequently used in arthritis. It is also used in newborns in neonatal units to close a patent ductus arteriosus. There is one case report of convulsions in an infant of a breastfeeding mother who received indomethacin early postpartum (day 7).[1] In another report of 16 women who received 75 mg to 300 mg daily (rectally), 20 milk samples were analyzed and 12 were less than 20 μg/L (limit of detection) and the median milk/plasma ratio was 0.37.[2] The eight measurable samples ranged from 23 to 115 μg/L. The authors suggest the total infant dose, assuming daily milk intake of 150 mL/kg, would range from 0.07% to 0.98% of the weight adjusted maternal dose. Plasma samples derived from six of the seven infants were below the sensitivity of the assay (<20 μg/L) and 47 μg/L in only one infant. Dose calculations for all 16 infants showed that absolute doses ranged from <0.003 to 0.017 mg/kg/day. No adverse effects were noted in this study.

Based on the reported studies, indomethacin levels in breast milk are probably too low to cause any significant adverse effects in the breastfed infant. Therefore, indomethacin use is probably compatible with breastfeeding. But since one case of convulsions has been reported with its early postpartum use, it is advisable to exercise caution in premature and newborn infants. Other NSAIDs with more data in lactation should be considered (e.g., ibuprofen).

T 1/2	4.5 h	MW	357 Da	PB	>90%
Tmax	1-2 :2-4 (SR) h	RID	1.2%	Vd	0.33-0.40 L/kg
Oral	90%	M/P	0.37	pKa	4.5

Adult Concerns: Headache, dizziness, malaise, depression, tinnitus, dyspepsia, epigastric pain, nausea, vomiting, diarrhea, changes in renal function, anemia, bleeding, hyperhidrosis, hot flashes, edema.

Adult Dose: 25-50 mg two to three times daily.

Pediatric Concerns: One case of seizures in a breastfed neonate. Additional report suggests no untoward effects.

Infant Monitoring: Vomiting, diarrhea.

Alternatives: Ibuprofen(L1)

References:

1. Eeg-Olofsson O, Malmros I, Elwin CE, Steen B. Convulsions in a breast-fed infant after maternal indomethacin. Lancet. 1978;2(8082):215.
2. Lebedevs TH, Wojnar-Horton RE, Yapp P, et al. Excretion of indomethacin in breast milk. Br J Clin Pharmacol. 1991;32(6):751-754.

INFLIXIMAB

Trade: Remicade

Category: Monoclonal Antibody

LRC: L3 - Limited Data-Probably Compatible

Infliximab is a monoclonal antibody to tumor necrosis factor-alpha (TNF-alpha) used to treat Crohn's disease and rheumatoid arthritis. Infliximab is a very large molecular weight IgG antibody and is largely retained in the vascular system.

A woman initiated on infliximab 4 months after delivery because of a rheumatoid arthritis flare collected milk samples starting on day 10 post first infusion (160 mg) until day 2 post second infusion (165 mg).[1] The concentration of drug in milk increased from day 10 to 20 post first infusion and peaked 1 day after the second infusion at 473 ng/mL. Although an overestimate, we used the peak level to calculate a relative infant dose of 3%. In this case, the infant was not given maternal milk.

In a study of one breastfeeding patient who received 5 mg/kg IV, infliximab levels were determined in milk at 0, 2, 4, 8, 24, 48, 72 hours, and 4, 5, and 7 days.[2] Infliximab was not detectable in milk at any of the sample times (detection limit <0.1 μg/mL).

In another study of a breastfeeding mother who received 5 infusions of infliximab 10 mg/kg during her pregnancy, infliximab was again undetectable in milk.[3] The baby's serum level after delivery was 39.5 µg/mL, likely due to placental transfer. The half-life of the drug appeared to be prolonged in the newborn.[2]

Another breastfeeding mother's milk was tested 24 hours and 1 week following her first infusion of a 5 mg/kg dose. The milk levels were also below the limit of quantification.[4]

In 2008, another case reported was published of a 22-year-old female receiving 10 mg/kg of infliximab throughout pregnancy and lactation. In this case, no infliximab was detected in breast milk for 30 days following her infusion. The infant was followed up to 27 months of age and no developmental concerns were identified.[5]

In a report of three patients who took infliximab until around 30 weeks gestational age and then restarted during lactation, infliximab levels were undetectable in breast milk.[6] The first participant was a 29-year-old woman who took 5 mg/kg of infliximab every 8 weeks until week 31 of pregnancy. The woman delivered her infant at 38 weeks and restarted infliximab 3 days after delivery. On postpartum day 9, a serum sample was drawn at 74.27 µg/mL and on postpartum day 10 breast milk samples were taken and found to be undetectable (< 10 µg/mL). The second participant was a 32-year-old woman who took 5 mg/kg of infliximab every 8 weeks until week 32 of pregnancy. The woman delivered her infant at 39 weeks and restarted infliximab 10 days after delivery. On postpartum day 15 serum samples were drawn from the mother and infant and were found to be 62.62 µg/mL and < 10 µg/mL, respectively. The breast milk levels were also < 10 µg/mL. The third participant was a 24-year-old woman who started infliximab therapy during her pregnancy at 19 weeks, doses were given at 19, 21, and 25 weeks. Her infant was delivered at 36 weeks, and she restarted infliximab therapy 2 weeks postpartum. The doses were then given every 8 weeks. On day 57, postpartum serum samples were drawn from the mother and infant and were found to be 59.97 µg/mL and < 10 µg/mL. The breast milk level was also undetectable in this case. During follow-up of the three infants no adverse events or increased rates of infection were reported. In addition, all three infants were found to have normal immunity from childhood immunizations given during this time.

In another study of three patients who were at least 5 days postpartum and receiving 5 mg/kg doses, infliximab levels in milk were detectable within 12 hours of injection and peaked at 90-105 ng/mL on day 2-3 after infusion. Corresponding blood levels ranged from 18-64 µg/mL.[7] Please note, levels in milk are still only 0.5% of the levels in maternal serum. In addition, these mothers were studied early postnatally when the milk compartment is still able to leak large molecular weight proteins (i.e., IgG) into milk.

The infants of two women taking 300 mg of infliximab during lactation were followed for 18 and 22 months after birth.[8] In the first report, the maternal milk samples were 1/20th of her serum concentration (200 ng/mL milk; 4700 ng/mL serum) and the infant was found to have undetectable serum levels. These samples were drawn 34 weeks postpartum and 3 weeks after the last infliximab infusion. In the second report, the mother's milk samples were drawn on day 1 and 4 post infliximab infusions and were found to be 94.6 ng/mL and 119.7 ng/mL. Serum samples were drawn 4 weeks later in the mother and infant 5 days after an infliximab infusion and were found to be 78,300 ng/mL and 1700 ng/mL. This infant was exclusively breastfed for the first 3 months of life (prior to initiation of maternal infliximab), and was then partially breastfed until serum levels were drawn. After maternal and infant serum levels were obtained the mother decided to discontinue breastfeeding. In both of these cases, the infants reached their developmental milestones as expected and no adverse events were reported. The authors of this study postulated that immunoglobulins such as infliximab might be absorbed via the immunoglobulin G-transporting neonatal Fc receptor (FcRn) that is expressed in intestinal cells of adults and fetuses.

Although the molecular weight of this medication is very large and the amount in breast milk is very low, there are no long-term data concerning the safety of using immune modulating medications in breastfeeding mothers. Further there are current data that suggest that other IgG drugs also transfer to milk, and perhaps the breastfed infant. Therefore, some caution is recommended and each woman should understand the benefits and risk of using this type of medication in lactation.

T 1/2	8-9.5 days	MW	149,100 Da	PB	
Tmax		RID	0.32%-3.01%	Vd	3 L/kg
Oral		M/P		pKa	

Adult Concerns: Headache, fatigue, hypertension, dyspnea, dyspepsia, nausea, diarrhea, changes in liver enzymes, development of antinuclear antibodies, anemia, arthralgia, infusion reactions, and increased susceptibility to infection.

Adult Dose: 5 mg/kg IV at 0, 2, and 6 weeks, then maintenance doses every 4-8 weeks.

Pediatric Concerns: None reported via milk at this time.

Infant Monitoring: Fever, frequent infections, poor feeding/poor weight gain.

Alternatives:

References:

1. Hale TW, Fasanmade A. Personal communication, 2002.
2. Forger F, Matthias T, Oppermann M, et al. Infliximab in breast milk. ABSTRACT. Lupus. 2004;13:753.

3. Vasiliauskas EA, Church JA, Silverman N, Barry M, Targan SR, Dubinsky MC. Case report: evidence for transplacental trasfer of maternally administered infliximab to the newborn. Clin Gastroenterol Hepatol. 2006;4:1255-1258.

4. Peltier M, James D, Ford J, Wagner C, Davis H, Hanauer S. Infliximab levels in breast-milk of a nursing Crohn's patient. Am J Gastroenterol. 2001;96(9):S312.

5. Stengel JZ, Arnold HL. Is infliximab safe to use while breastfeeding? World Gastroenterol. 2008 May;14(19):3085-3087.

6. Kane S, Ford J, Cohen R, Wagner C. Absence of infliximab in infants and breast milk from nursing mothers receiving therapy for Crohn's disease before and after delivery. J Clin Gastroenterol. 2009 Aug;43(7):613-616.

7. Ben-Horin S, Yavzori M, Kopylov U, et al. Detection of infliximab in breast milk of nursing mothers with inflammatory bowel disease. J Crohns Colitis. 2011 Dec;5(6):555-558.

8. Fritzsche J, Pilch A, Mury D, Schaefer C, Weber-Schoendorfer C. Infliximab and adalimumab use during breastfeeding. J Clin Gastroenterol. 2012;46(8):718-719.

INFLUENZA

Trade:

Category: Infectious Disease

LRC: L2 - No Data-Probably Compatible

The influenza virus is an orthomyxovirus and consists of 3 types - influenza type A, type B, and type C. Most influenza epidemics are caused by type A and type B. The influenza A virus is further classified into several subtypes, some of the most commonly known are H1N1, H1N2, and H3N2.

The influenza virus is highly contagious and is transmitted from person to person through infected respiratory droplets present in the air or on surfaces. Therefore, wearing a mask to avoid inhalation of contaminated aerosol droplets and regular hand washing after contact with potentially contaminated surfaces has been recommended to decrease the risk of exposure to the virus. The incubation period is 1 to 4 days. The patient is infectious for 24 hours before the onset of symptoms. Once infected, a patient remains infectious for 3 to 7 days.[1] Influenza is characterized by moderate to high degree fever, chills, rigors, malaise, myalgia and is associated with upper respiratory tract symptoms such as cough, nasal congestion, and rhinitis.

The protective benefits of breast milk in fighting respiratory illnesses in the infant has been well established. It was found that breast milk mediates an increased production of type 1 interferons in the respiratory tract of infants with influenza. Therefore, infants with influenza illness are encouraged to breastfeed.[2] In view of its potential benefits and since no established data on transfer of the influenza virus into breast milk exists, mothers with influenza are encouraged to continue breastfeeding. It should be noted that exposure of infant to maternal illness is inevitable since the mother is contagious 24 hours prior to onset of symptoms, therefore when symptoms develop baby might already be infected, at that moment maternal antibodies, which are transferred by milk to the infant, will protect him against virus. Lactating women with influenza can be safely treated with either oseltamivir, zanamivir, or baloxavir since as they are considered compatible with breastfeeding.[3] The infant should be closely monitored for any signs of respiratory illness and be treated accordingly.

If H1N1 is the virus implicated, and you are breastfeeding, a cautious approach may include protecting your baby from exposure to flu virus by washing your hands thoroughly prior to handling the infant, and using a face mask while breastfeeding.

Adult Concerns: Fever, sore throat, malaise, arthralgias, nausea, vomiting, diarrhea.

Adult Dose:

Pediatric Concerns:

Infant Monitoring: Fever, lethargy, vomiting, diarrhea.

Alternatives: Oseltamivir(L2), baloxavir(L3)

References:

1. AAP CoID. Influenza. In: Pickering LKBC, Kimberlin DW, Long SS, eds. Red Book: 2009 Report of the Committee on Infectious Diseases. 28th ed. Elk Grove Village, IL: American Academy of Pediatrics; 2009:400-412.

2. Melendi GA, Coviello S, Bhat N, Zea-Hernandez J, Ferolla FM, Polack FP. Breastfeeding is associated with the production of type I interferon in infants infected with influenza virus. Acta Paediatr. 2010;99(10):1517-1521.

3. Tanaka T, Nakajima K, Murashima A, Garcia-Bournissen F, Koren G, Ito S. Safety of neuraminidase inhibitors against novel influenza A (H1N1) in pregnant and breastfeeding women. CMAJ. 2009;181(1-2):55-58.

INFLUENZA VIRUS VACCINES

Trade: Afluria, Agriflu, Flu Vaccine, Flu-Imune, FluLaval, FluMist, Fluarix, Fluogen, Fluviral, Fluvirin, Fluzone, Vaccine- Influenza

Category: Vaccine

LRC: L1 - Limited Data-Compatible

Influenza virus vaccines come in two forms. One that is non-viable and requires injection, and the second, a live but attenuated vaccine for application in the nasal passages.

Injectable (Flu-Immune, Fluogen, Fluzone, Flucelvax, etc.): This influenza vaccine is prepared from inactivated, non-viable influenza viruses and infection of the neonate via milk would not be expected. There are no reported side effects, nor published contraindications for using influenza virus vaccine during lactation.[1,2] Influenza vaccine is now indicated for breastfeeding mothers and their infants by the American Academy of Pediatrics.

Intranasal Live Influenza Virus Vaccine (FluMist): This vaccine consists of a live but attenuated and heat unstable form of influenza virus. Virus instilled in the nasal mucosa replicate, thus producing immunity in the host. Viruses that escape the nasal mucosa are unstable and die quickly. It is not known if this virus reaches the human milk compartment, but it is highly unlikely the virus could survive at this temperature in the plasma nor the milk compartment of the mother.

The CDC and the FDA recommend that all breastfeeding women be immunized. This will further protect the breastfed infant as these antibodies will pass into milk, and help protect the newborn breastfed infant from infection. Contents of influenza vaccines change from year to year. Presently, some multi-dose vials contain a small amount of mercury, but there is no evidence that this would even pass to a breastfeeding infant. Single dose vials typically do not contain mercury. The live attenuated vaccine, FluMist, is not recommended for breastfeeding women, although we know the risks are low.

The CDC encourages the inactivated influenza vaccine for children 6-23 months and their close contacts and caregivers.

Adult Concerns: Fever, myalgia.

Adult Dose: 0.5 mL injection once.

Pediatric Concerns: None reported in breastfeeding mothers.

Infant Monitoring:

Alternatives:

References:
1. Kilbourne ED. Questions and answers. Artificial influenza immunization of nursing mothers not harmful. JAMA. 1973;226:87.
2. Pharmaceutical manufacturers prescribing information.
3. www.cdc.gov/breastfeeding/recommendations/vaccinations.htm

INSULIN

Trade: Humalog, Humulin, Iletin, Mixtard, Monotard, Novolin, Protaphane

Category: Antidiabetic, other

LRC: L2 - No Data-Probably Compatible

Insulin is an anti-diabetic agent used in the management of Type I and II diabetes and gestational diabetes.[1] Insulin is a large peptide that is not known to be transported into milk in clinically significant amounts. A small pilot study demonstrated that insulin is transported into breastmilk; however, no difference in insulin breastmilk levels were found in non-diabetics, type II diabetics not on insulin therapy and type I diabetics on insulin therapy.[2] At this time, it is thought that even if insulin is found in breastmilk, it would not lead to hypoglycemia in the infant. I would not be orally bioavailable.

T 1/2	4-6 min	MW	~6,000 varies depending on type of insulin	PB	
Tmax		RID		Vd	0.37 L/kg
Oral	Nil	M/P		pKa	Varies depending on type of insulin

Adult Concerns: Hypoglycemia, hypokalemia, atrophy or hypertrophy of subcutaneous fat tissue, pain at injection site.

Adult Dose: Highly Variable.

Pediatric Concerns: None reported via milk.

Infant Monitoring: Signs of hypoglycemia- drowsiness, lethargy, pallor, sweating, tremor.

Alternatives:

References:
1. Pharmaceutical manufacturers prescribing information.
2. Whitmore TJ, Trengove NJ, Graham DF, Hartmann PE. Analysis of insulin in human breast milk in mothers with type 1 and type 2 diabetes mellitus. Int J Endocrinol. 2012;2012:1-9.

INSULIN GLARGINE

Trade: Lantus

Category: Antidiabetic, other

LRC: L1 - No Data-Compatible

Insulin glargine (rDNA origin) is a recombinant human insulin analog that is long-acting (up to 24 hours).[1] Insulin glargine differs from human insulin in that the amino acid asparagine at position A-21 is replaced by glycine and two arginines are added to the C-terminus of the B-chain. This product when administered subcutaneously precipitates and forms crystals that are slow absorbing, thus producing a sustained release formulation with a half-life of about 198 minutes. Insulin is a large peptide that is not known to be transported into milk in clinically significant amounts. A small pilot study demonstrated that insulin is transported into breastmilk; however, no difference in insulin breastmilk levels were found in non-diabetics, type II diabetics not on insulin therapy and type I diabetics on insulin therapy.[2] At this time, it is thought that even if insulin is found in breastmilk, it would not lead to hypoglycemia in the infant.

T 1/2	5-15 min	MW	6,063 Da	PB	5%
Tmax	6 h	RID		Vd	0.15 L/kg
Oral	Nil	M/P		pKa	

Adult Concerns: Hypoglycemia, hypokalemia, atrophy or hypertrophy of subcutaneous fat tissue, pain at injection site.

Adult Dose: Highly variable.

Pediatric Concerns: None reported in breastfeeding infants.

Infant Monitoring: Signs of hypoglycemia- drowsiness, lethargy, pallor, sweating, tremor.

Alternatives:

References:
1. Pharmaceutical manufacturers prescribing information.
2. Whitmore TJ, Trengove NJ, Graham DF, Hartmann PE. Analysis of insulin in human breast milk in mothers with type 1 and type 2 diabetes mellitus. Int J Endocrinol. 2012;2012:1-9.

INTERFERON ALFA-2B

Trade: Intron A

Category: Antineoplastic

LRC: L3 - No Data-Probably Compatible

Interferon alfa-2b is indicated for the treatment of hepatitis B and C.[1] While we have no data on its use in breastfeeding mothers, other data on interferons (alfa and beta) suggest they do not readily enter the milk, and milk levels will be exceedingly low.

Following an intravenous dose of 30 million IU, the amount of interferon transferred into human milk was only slightly elevated (1551 IU/mL) when compared to control milk (1249 IU/mL). These data suggest that even following enormous doses, interferon is probably too large in molecular weight to transfer into human milk in clinically relevant amounts.

When combined with ribavirin for Hepatitis C, breastfeeding is not recommended (due to ribavirin content). There is also a pegylated form of this medication (PegIntron), pegylation confers protection against enzymatic degradation systemically. The pegylated form has a much longer half-life of 40 hours.

T 1/2	2-3 h	MW	19,271 Da	PB	
Tmax	3-12 h (IM, SC)	RID	0.05%	Vd	0.44 L/kg
Oral	83% (IM); 90% (SC)	M/P		pKa	

Adult Concerns: Alopecia, fever, chills, headache, fatigue, cough, dry mouth, hypertension, nausea, vomiting, diarrhea, anorexia, changes in liver function, neutropenia, anemia, myalgia, flu-like symptoms, weakness, rash.

Adult Dose: 3-10 million units SC or IM three times a week (varies by indication).

Pediatric Concerns: None reported via milk at this time.

Infant Monitoring: Drowsiness, dry mouth, vomiting, diarrhea, weight gain.

Alternatives:

References:
1. Kumar AR, Hale TW, Mock RE. Transfer of interferon alfa into human breast milk. J Hum Lact. 2000;16(3):226-228.

INTERFERON ALFA-2B + RIBAVIRIN

Trade: Rebetron

Category: Antiviral

LRC: L4 - No Data-Possibly Hazardous

This is a combination product containing the antiviral ribavirin and the immunomodulator drug called interferon alfa-2b. This new combination product is indicated for the long-term treatment of hepatitis C.

Ribavirin is a synthetic nucleoside used as an antiviral agent and is effective in a wide variety of viral infections. It has been used acutely in respiratory syncytial virus infections in infants without major complications. However, its current use in breastfeeding patients, for treatment of Hepatitis C infections, when combined with interferon alfa (Rebetron) for periods up to one year may be more problematic as high concentrations of ribavirin could accumulate in the breastfed infant over time. No data are available on its transfer to human milk, but it is probably low and its oral bioavailability is low as well. However, ribavirin concentrates in peripheral tissues and in the red blood cells in high concentrations over time (Vd= 40 L/kg).[1] Its elimination half-life at steady state averages 298 hours, which reflects slow elimination from non-plasma compartments. Red cell concentrations on average are 60 fold higher than plasma levels and may account for the occasional hemolytic anemia. It is likely the acute exposure of a breastfed infant would produce minimal side effects. However, chronic exposure over 12 months may be more risky, so caution is recommended.

Interferon alfa-2b is indicated for the treatment of hepatitis B and C.[1] While we have no data on its use in breastfeeding mothers, other data on interferons (alfa and beta) suggest they do not readily enter the milk, and milk levels will be exceedingly low. Some interferons are known to be secreted into human milk normally and may contribute to the antiviral properties of human milk. However, interferons are large in molecular weight (16-28,000 Da) which would limit their transfer into human milk. Following treatment with a massive dose of 30 million units IV of interferon alpha in a breastfeeding patient, the amount of interferon alpha transferred into human milk was 894, 1004, 1551, 1507, 788, 721 IU at 0 (baseline), 2, 4, 8, 12, and 24 hours respectively.[2] In a more recent study of the transfer of Interferon Beta-1a, average milk concentrations were 46.7, 97.4, 66.4, 77.5, 103.1, 108.3, 124, and 87.9 pg/mL at 0, 1, 4, 8, 12, 24, 48, and 72 hours, respectively, after dosing. Using the highest value measured (179 pg/mL), the estimated relative infant dose would be 0.006% of the maternal dose.[3] Thus interferon levels in milk are probably exceedingly low.

T 1/2	INF/rib: 2-3 h/298 h	MW	INF/rib: 19,271/244 Da	PB	INF/rib: /none
Tmax	INF/rib: 3-12 h/1.5 h	RID		Vd	INF/rib: 0.44/40.8 L/kg
Oral	INF/rib: 90%/64%	M/P		pKa	

Adult Concerns: Alopecia, fever, chills, headache, fatigue, cough, dry mouth, hypertension, nausea, vomiting, diarrhea, anorexia, changes in liver function, leukopenia, neutropenia, anemia, myalgia, flu-like symptoms, weakness, rash.

Adult Dose: INF 3 million units SC or IM three times a week + ribavirin 400 mg in the morning and 600 mg at night.

Pediatric Concerns: None reported via breast milk at this time.

Infant Monitoring: Not recommended for chronic exposure via breastmilk.

Alternatives:

References:
1. Lertora JJ, Rege AB, Lacour JT, et al. Pharmacokinetics and long-term tolerance to ribavirin in asymptomatic patients infected with human immunodeficiency virus. Clin Pharmacol Ther. 1991;50(4):442-449.
2. Kumar AR, Hale TW, Mock RE. Transfer of interferon alfa into human breast milk. J Hum Lact. 2000;16(3):226-228.
3. Hale TW, Siddiqui AA, Baker TE. Transfer of Interferon beta-1a into Human Breastmilk. Breastfeed Med. 2012 Apr;7(2):123-125.

INTERFERON ALPHA-N3

Trade: Alferon N

Category: Immune Modulator

LRC: L2 - Limited Data-Probably Compatible

Interferon alpha is a pure clone of a single interferon subspecies with antiviral, antiproliferative, and immunomodulatory activity. The alpha-interferons are active against various malignancies and viral syndromes such as hairy cell leukemia, melanoma, AIDS-related Kaposi's sarcoma, condyloma acuminata, and chronic hepatitis B and C infections.[1] Other forms of interferons such as the Alfa-2b (Intron A or PegIntron) are also available. Very little is known about the secretion of interferons in human milk although some interferons are known to be secreted normally and may contribute to the antiviral properties of human milk. However, interferons are large in molecular weight (16,000-27,000 Da), which would limit their transfer into human milk. Following treatment with a massive dose of 30 million units IV in one breastfeeding patient, the amount of interferon alpha transferred into human milk was 894, 1004, 1551, 1507, 788, 721 units at 0 (baseline), 2, 4, 8, 12, and 24 hours respectively.[2] Hence, even following a massive dose, no change in breastmilk levels were noted from baseline. One thousand international units is roughly equivalent to 500 nanograms of interferon.

The oral absorption of interferons is controversial and is believed to be minimal. Interferons are relatively nontoxic unless extraordinarily large doses are administered parenterally. Interferons are sometimes used in infants and children to treat idiopathic thrombocytopenia (ITP).

T 1/2		MW	16,000 - 27,000 Da	PB	
Tmax		RID		Vd	
Oral		M/P		pKa	

Adult Concerns: Insomnia, depression, headache, fatigue, fever, chills, changes in vision, changes in taste, dyspepsia, nausea, vomiting, diarrhea, leukopenia, myalgia, flu-like symptoms, weakness.

Adult Dose: 0.05-0.5 mL per wart twice weekly.

Pediatric Concerns: None reported via milk.

Infant Monitoring: Changes in sleep, vomiting, diarrhea, weight gain.

Alternatives:

References:
1. Pharmaceutical manufacturers prescribing information.
2. Kumar AR, Hale TW, Mock RE. Transfer of interferon alfa into human breast milk. J Hum Lact. 2000;16(3):226-228.

INTERFERON BETA-1A

Trade: Avonex, Betaferon, Rebif

Category: Immune Modulator

LRC: L2 - Limited Data-Probably Compatible

Interferon Beta-1A is a moderately large glycoprotein (166 amino acids) with antiviral, antiproliferative, and immunomodulator activity presently used for reducing the severity and frequency of exacerbations of relapsing-remitting multiple sclerosis.[1] Interferons are large in molecular weight, generally containing 166 amino acids, which would limit their transfer into human milk. Their oral absorption is controversial but is believed to be minimal. In addition, most researchers find that plasma levels of interferons following IM injection are detectable for only a few hours, generally less than 15 hours following the dose. Thus the transfer of interferons into the plasma compartment are thought to be minimal and brief.

In a recent study of the transfer of Interferon Beta-1a in six mothers receiving 30 μg per week, average milk concentrations were 46.7, 97.4, 66.4, 77.5, 103.1, 108.3, 124, and 87.9 pg/mL at 0, 1, 4, 8, 12, 24, 48, and 72 hours, respectively, after dosing.[2] Using this data, the RID is 3.6%. Interferons are relatively nontoxic unless extraordinarily large doses are administered parenterally. Interferons are sometimes used in infants and children to treat idiopathic thrombocytopenia (ITP) in huge doses.

T 1/2	10 h	MW	22,500 Da	PB	
Tmax	15 h	RID	3.68%	Vd	Total Body Water L/kg
Oral	Minimal	M/P		pKa	

Adult Concerns: Headache, fatigue, fever, chills, depression, dry mouth, dyspepsia, nausea, diarrhea, changes in liver function, leukopenia, flu-like symptoms.

Adult Dose: 30 μg weekly I.M.

Pediatric Concerns: None reported via milk.

Infant Monitoring: Drowsiness, dry mouth, vomiting, diarrhea, weight gain.

Alternatives:

References:

1. Chofflon M. Recombinant human interferon beta in relapsing-remitting multiple sclerosis: a review of the major clinical trials. Eur J Neurol. 2000;7(4):369-380.
2. Hale TW, Siddiqui AA, Baker TE. Transfer of interferon beta-1a into Human Breastmilk. Breastfeed Med. 2012 Apr;7(2):123-125.

INTERFERON BETA-1B

Trade: Betaseron, Extavia

Category: Immune Modulator

LRC: L2 - Limited Data-Probably Compatible

Interferon Beta-1B is a glycoprotein with antiviral, antiproliferative, and immunomodulatory activity presently used for treatment of multiple sclerosis.[1,2] Very little is known about the secretion of interferons in human milk although some interferons are known to be secreted normally and may contribute to the antiviral properties of human milk. However, interferons are large in molecular weight, generally containing 165 amino acids, which would limit their transfer into human milk. Interferons are relatively nontoxic unless extraordinarily large doses are administered parenterally. Interferons are sometimes used in infants and children to treat idiopathic thrombocytopenia (ITP). The transfer of interferon Beta-1a is essentially nil and it is likely the same for this product, interferon Beta-1b.

T 1/2	8 min - 4.3 h	MW	22, 500 Da	PB	
Tmax		RID		Vd	0.25-2.88 L/kg
Oral	Poor	M/P		pKa	

Adult Concerns: Headache, fatigue, fever, chills, depression, chest pain, dyspepsia, nausea, diarrhea, constipation, changes in liver function, leukopenia, neutropenia, flu-like symptoms.

Adult Dose: 0.25 mg every other day.

Pediatric Concerns: None reported via milk.

Infant Monitoring: Drowsiness, vomiting, diarrhea, constipation, weight gain.

Alternatives:

References:

1. Hale TW, Siddiqui AA, Baker TE. Transfer of interferon beta-1a into Human Breastmilk. Breastfeed Med. 2012 Apr;7(2):123-125.

INULIN

Trade:

Category: Diagnostic Agent, Other

LRC: L3 - No Data-Probably Compatible

Inulin is an insoluble oligosaccharide that is used as both a fiber supplement and a diagnostic agent for renal function.[1] This agent is not metabolized and is eliminated rapidly through urine when administered intravenously. When administered orally, inulin is not broken down and is instead used as a prebiotic in the gut to promote the growth of bifidobacteria. In the event of hydrolysis, the primary product of inulin is fructose. It is unlikely that this agent will be excreted into breast milk. Inulin has been suspected of altering the absorption of several other nutrients such as calcium and glucose.

T 1/2		MW	6179.36 Da	PB	
Tmax		RID		Vd	
Oral	0%	M/P		pKa	11.63

Adult Concerns: Bloating, flatulence, abdominal discomfort.

Adult Dose:

Pediatric Concerns:

Infant Monitoring:

Alternatives:

References:
1. Kaur N, Gupta AK. Applications of inulin and oligofructose in health and nutrition. J Biosci. 2002 Dec;27(7):703-714.

IODINATED GLYCEROL

Trade: Organidin, R-GEN

Category: Expectorant

LRC: L4 - Limited Data-Possibly Hazardous

Iodinated glycerol is a mucolytic-expectorant. This product contains 50% organically bound iodine. High levels of iodine are known to be secreted in milk.[1] Milk/plasma ratios as high as 26 have been reported. Following absorption by the infant, high levels of iodine could lead to severe thyroid depression in infants. Normal iodine levels in breast milk are already four times higher than the RDA for infants. Expectorants, including iodine, work very poorly. Recently, many iodine containing products have been replaced with guaifenesin, which is considered safer. High levels of iodine-containing drugs should not be used in lactating mothers.

T 1/2		MW	258 Da	PB	
Tmax		RID		Vd	
Oral	Complete	M/P		pKa	

Adult Concerns: Depressed thyroid function, metallic taste, nausea, vomiting, diarrhea, acne, dermatitis.

Adult Dose:

Pediatric Concerns: Iodine concentrates in milk and should not be administered to breastfeeding mothers. Infantile thyroid suppression is likely.

Infant Monitoring: Reduced thyroid function.

Alternatives:

References:
1. Postellon DC, Aronow R. Iodine in mother's milk. JAMA. 1982;247(4):463.

IODINE

Trade: Iodex, Iodoflex, Iodosorb, Potassium Iodide

Category: Antiseptic

LRC: L4 - Limited Data-Possibly Hazardous

Iodine is an essential dietary element that can be commonly found in many foods. It is most commonly used as the potassium or sodium salt. Iodine is also used as a topical antiseptic, although its use impairs wound healing and it is no longer recommended. Another use of iodine (potassium iodide) is for treatment of thyrotoxicosis, as large doses suppress thyroxine production by the thyroid gland. Foods such as seaweed, kelp, yogurt, milk, iodinated salt, and fish contain higher levels of iodine.

Seaweed and kelp may contain up to 20 times the recommended daily intake. Recommended dietary allowance for iodine by the US Institute for Medicine in breastfeeding women is 290 µg/day. Excessive iodine exposure may cause hypothyroidism in infants. High levels of iodine are known to be pumped into human milk.[1] Milk/plasma ratios as high as 26 have been reported.

Following absorption by the infant, high levels of iodine could lead to severe thyroid depression in infants. Normal iodine levels in breast milk are already four times higher than the RDA for infants. In one study, infant subclinical hypothyroidism has been associated with excessive iodine in breast milk (198-8484 µg/L) probably due to seaweed consumption (more than 2000 µg/day of iodine).[2] Iodine odor from a breastfed infant has been reported from a mother who used povidone-iodine vaginal gel for 6 days; however, no thyroid abnormalities were observed.[3] High levels of iodine-containing drugs should not be used in lactating mothers. Limit doses to ranges close to the RDA (290 µg/day).

Two case reports have been published regarding infant hypothyroidism after exposure to iodine in breast milk.[4,5] In the first case report, the mother was applying iodine soaked gauze to her C-section scar after the birth of her 31 week preterm infant.[4] On day 4 of life the infants thyroid function was found to be normal; however, upon repeat 2 weeks later the infant had an elevated TSH and borderline T4. The results were thus repeated again one week later and the TSH was even higher and the T4 and fT4 were low. On learning of the maternal history, the infant's urine was tested for iodine, it was above normal at 684 µg/L (normal 42-350 µg/L) and the maternal milk concentration was tested, 1911 µg/L (normal 5-185 µg/L). The infant was treated with L-thyroxine and the mother pumped and dumped her milk for 1 week after stopping iodine therapy. The infant was eventually discharged from NICU on L-thyroxine, and had no long-term complications.

In the second case report, a 15-day-old infant was found to have a high TSH, low fT4, and high urine iodine concentration 410 µg/L.[5] The mother reported using iodine antiseptic for her episiotomy and her milk concentration was 300 µg/L. This infant was also treated with L-thyroxine, and the authors reported no long-term complications.

Mothers who are exposed to radioactive iodine, such as from nuclear accidents, should take potassium iodide once or twice to reduce exposure of their thyroid glands to the radioactive iodine. Breastfeeding women should only take potassium iodide if they are contaminated with radioactive iodine and advised to do so by their governmental agencies. Non-radioactive iodine transfers into the thyroid gland avidly and prevents radioactive iodine transfer. Radioactive iodine transfers into breast milk at high levels and therefore can transfer to the breastfed baby.

The Endocrine Society, the American Thyroid Association, the Teratology Society, and the American Academy of Pediatrics recommend that women receive prenatal vitamins containing no more than 150 µg of iodine daily during preconception, pregnancy, and lactation. Taking a higher dose or more frequent doses can result in adverse health effects and can even be fatal. Finally, ONLY use potassium iodide if you are advised to by your physician or government health care agency, and ONLY if you are exposed to high levels of radioactive iodine. Do not exceed a maximum daily dose of 290 µg if you are breastfeeding.

T 1/2		MW	127 Da	PB	
Tmax		RID		Vd	
Oral	High	M/P	up to 26	pKa	Completely ionized

Adult Concerns: Topical: Eczema, irritation, increase TSH, edema. Iodine intoxication: Fever, headache, hypothyroidism, metallic taste, arthralgia, pulmonary edema, rash, urticaria, lymp node enlargement.

Adult Dose: 150 µg/day, Pregnant: 220 µg/day, Lactation: 290 µg/day.

Pediatric Concerns: Hypothyroidism.[4,5]

Infant Monitoring: May consider monitoring for hypothyroidism if exposure in milk occurred (TSH, fT4).

Alternatives:

References:

1. Postellon DC, Aronow R. Iodine in mother's milk. JAMA. 1982;247(4):463.
2. Chung HR, Shin CH, Yang SW, Choi CW, Kim BI. Subclinical hypothyroidism in Korean preterm infants associated with high levels of iodine in breast milk. J Clin Endocrinol Metab. 2009 Nov;94(11):4444-4447. Epub 2009 Oct 6.
3. Iodine. In: REPROTOX® Database [Internet database]. Greenwood Village, Colo: Thomson Reuters (Healthcare) Inc. Updated periodically. Accessed July 13, 2011.
4. Smith VC, Svoren BM, Wolfsdorf JI. Hypothyroidism in a breast-fed preterm infant resulting from maternal topical iodine exposure. J Pediatr. 2006;149:566-567.
5. Kurtoglu S, Akin L, Akin MA, Coban D. Iodine overload and severe hypothyroidism in two neonates. J Clin Res Pediatr Endocrinol. 2009;1(6):275-277.

IODIPAMIDE

Trade: Cholografin, Sinografin

Category: Diagnostic Agent, Radiological Contrast Media

LRC: L3 - No Data-Probably Compatible

Iodipamide is an ionic radiopaque contrast agent used to view the gallbladder and biliary tract. It is used in both adults and pediatric patients.[1] No data are available on the transfer of iodipamide to human milk; however, it is unlikely when compared to other similar agents. It has a very short half-life, and it is highly protein bound. Based on kinetic data, the American College of Radiology suggests that it is safe for a mother to continue breastfeeding after receiving iodinated X-ray contrast media.[2]

T 1/2	30 min	MW		PB	Very High
Tmax		RID		Vd	
Oral	10%	M/P		pKa	2.63

Adult Concerns: Hypotension, flushing, nausea, vomiting, changes in renal function, hypersensitivity reaction. With rapid administration: warmth sensation, fever, chills, dizziness, restlessness.

Adult Dose:

Pediatric Concerns: None reported via breast milk.

Infant Monitoring:

Alternatives:

References:

1. Pharmaceutical manufacturers prescribing information.
2. ACR Committee on Drugs and Contrast Media. Administration of contrast medium to breastfeeding mothers. Reston, VA: American College of Radiology; 2004:42-43.

IODIXANOL

Trade: Visipaque

Category: Diagnostic Agent, Radiological Contrast Media

LRC: L3 - No Data-Probably Compatible

Iodixanol is an intravenous, nonionic, water soluble radiocontrast medium with iodine concentrations of 270 and 320 mg/mL.[1] It has been studied and approved in children 1 year of age and older, as well as in adults. There are no studies on the transfer of iodixanol to human milk; however, it is unlikely that iodixanol would transfer to milk in any therapeutic level. Its poor oral bioavailability would further reduce any risk to an infant. Based on kinetic data, the American College of Radiology suggests that it is safe for a mother to continue breastfeeding after receiving iodinated X-ray contrast media.[2]

T 1/2	123 min	MW	1550.2 Da	PB	None
Tmax		RID		Vd	
Oral	Poor	M/P		pKa	11.43

Adult Concerns: Anaphylaxis, local injection site reactions, taste perversion, headache, pruritus, nausea, rash, paresthesia, renal failure, myocardial infarction.

Adult Dose:

Pediatric Concerns:

Infant Monitoring:

Alternatives:

References:

1. Pharmaceutical manufacturers prescribing information
2. ACR Committee on Drugs and Contrast Media. Administration of contrast medium to breastfeeding mothers. Reston, VA: American College of Radiology; 2004:42-43.

IOHEXOL

Trade: Accupaque, Myelo-Kit, Omnigraf, Omnipaque, Omnitrast

Category: Diagnostic Agent, Radiological Contrast Media

LRC: L2 - Limited Data-Probably Compatible

Iohexol is a nonionic radiocontrast agent. Radiopaque agents (except barium) are iodinated compounds used to visualize various organs during X-ray, CAT scans, and other radiological procedures. These compounds are highly iodinated, benzoic acid derivatives. Although under usual circumstances iodine products are contraindicated in nursing mothers (due to ion trapping in milk), these products are unique, in that they are extremely inert and are largely cleared without metabolism. The iodine is organically bound to the structure and is not biologically active.

In a study of four women who received 0.755 gm/kg (350 mg iodine/mL) of iohexol IV, the mean peak level of iohexol in milk was 35 mg/L at 3 hours post-injection.[1] The average concentration in milk was only 24.6 mg/L over 24 hours. Assuming a daily milk intake of 150 mL/kg body weight, the amount of iohexol transferred to an infant during the first 24 hours would be 3.7 mg/kg (or 1.7 mg iodine/kg) which corresponds to 0.5% of the maternal dose.

As a group, radiocontrast agents are virtually unabsorbed after oral administration (<0.1%).[2] Iohexol has a brief half-life of just two hours, and the estimated dose ingested by the infant is only 0.5% of the radiocontrast dose used clinically for various scanning procedures in infants. Although most company package inserts suggest that an infant be removed from the breast for 24 hours, no untoward effects have been reported with these products in breastfed infants. Because the amount of iohexol transferred to milk is so small, the authors conclude that breastfeeding is acceptable after intravenously administered iohexol. Based on kinetic data, the American College of Radiology suggests that it is safe for a mother to continue breastfeeding after receiving iodinated X-ray contrast media.[3]

T 1/2	2-3.4 h	MW	821.14 Da	PB	None
Tmax		RID	0.49%-0.59%	Vd	
Oral	Poor	M/P		pKa	11.73

Adult Concerns: Dizziness, headache, anxiety, arrhythmias, heart failure, nausea, vomiting, diarrhea, renal dysfunction, injection site reactions, allergic reactions - bronchospasm, anaphylaxis.

Adult Dose:

Pediatric Concerns: None reported in one study.

Infant Monitoring:

Alternatives:

References:
1. Nielsen ST, Matheson I, Rasmussen JN, Skinnemoen K, Andrew E, Hafsahl G. Excretion of iohexol and metrizoate in human breast milk. Acta Radiol. 1987;28(5):523-526.
2. Pharmaceutical manufacturers prescribing information.
3. ACR Committee on Drugs and Contrast Media. Administration of contrast medium to breastfeeding mothers. Reston, VA: American College of Radiology; 2004:42-43.

IOPAMIDOL

Trade: Gastromiro, Iopamiro, Iopamiron, Isovue, Niopam, Pamitra, Radiomiron, Scanlux, Solutrast

Category: Diagnostic Agent, Radiological Contrast Media

LRC: L3 - No Data-Probably Compatible

Iopamidol is a nonionic radiocontrast agent used for numerous radiological procedures. Although it contains significant iodine content (20%-37%), the iodine is covalently bound to the parent molecule, and the bioavailability of the iodine molecule is miniscule. As with other ionic and nonionic radiocontrast agents, it is primarily extracellular and intravascular, it does not pass the blood-brain barrier, and it would be extremely unlikely that it would penetrate into human milk. However, no data are available on its transfer to human milk. As with most of these products, it is poorly absorbed from the gastrointestinal tract and rapidly excreted from the maternal circulation, due to an extremely short half-life.[1] Based on kinetic data, the American College of Radiology suggests that it is probably safe for a mother to continue breastfeeding after receiving iodinated X-ray contrast media.[2]

T 1/2	2 h	MW		PB	Very Low
Tmax		RID		Vd	
Oral	None	M/P		pKa	

Adult Concerns: Headache, seizure, pain, hot flashes, chest pain, dyspnea, nausea, vomiting, abdominal pain, diarrhea, nephropathy, rash, hives.

Adult Dose:

Pediatric Concerns:

Infant Monitoring:

Alternatives:

References:
1. Pharmaceutical manufacturers prescribing information.
2. ACR Committee on Drugs and Contrast Media. Administration of contrast medium to breastfeeding mothers. Reston, VA: American College of Radiology; 2004:42-43.

IOPANOIC ACID

Trade: Biliopaco, Cistobil, Colegraf, Colepak, Neocontrast, Telepaque

Category: Diagnostic Agent, Radiological Contrast Media

LRC: L2 - Limited Data-Probably Compatible

Iopanoic acid is a radiopaque organic iodine compound similar to dozens of other radiocontrast agents. It contains 66.7% by weight of iodine. As with all of these compounds, the iodine is organically bound to the parent molecule, and only minimal amounts are free in solution or metabolized by the body. In a group of five breastfeeding mothers who received an average of 2.77 g of iodine (as iopanoic acid), the amount of iopanoic acid excreted into human milk during the following 19-29 hours was 20.8 mg or about 0.08% of the maternal dose.[1] No untoward effects were noted in the infants. Since the amounts that enter breastmilk are too minimal to cause any significant adverse effects in an infant, iopanoic acid is probably compatible with breastfeeding. Based on kinetic data, the American College of Radiology suggests that it is probably safe for a mother to continue breastfeeding after receiving iodinated x-ray contrast media.[2]

T 1/2	33 % eliminated in 24 h	MW	570.93 Da	PB	High
Tmax		RID		Vd	
Oral	Well absorbed	M/P		pKa	4.8

Adult Concerns: Nausea, vomiting, diarrhea, renal failure.

Adult Dose:

Pediatric Concerns:

Infant Monitoring:

Alternatives:

References:
1. Holmdahl KH. Cholecystography during lactation. Acta Radiol. 1956;45(4):305-307.
2. ACR Committee on Drugs and Contrast Media. Administration of contrast medium to breastfeeding mothers. Reston, VA: American College of Radiology; 2004:42-43.

IOPENTOL

Trade: Imagopaque, Ivepaque

Category: Diagnostic Agent, Radiological Contrast Media

LRC: L3 - No Data-Probably Compatible

Iopentol is a new non-ionic contrast medium that is not yet available in the United States. There are no studies on the transfer of iopentol to human milk; however, as with virtually all of the radio contrast agents, it is unlikely that iopentol would transfer to milk in any therapeutic level. The poor oral bioavailability further reduces risk to an infant.[1]

T 1/2	2 h	MW	835.2 Da	PB	3%
Tmax		RID		Vd	
Oral	Poor	M/P		pKa	

Adult Concerns: Heat sensation, nausea.

Adult Dose:

Pediatric Concerns:

Infant Monitoring:

Alternatives:

References:
1. Pharmaceutical manufacturers prescribing information.

IOPROMIDE

Trade: Clarograf, Proscope, Ultravist

Category: Diagnostic Agent, Radiological Contrast Media

LRC: L3 - No Data-Probably Compatible

Iopromide is a nonionic, water soluble X-ray contrast agent. Its iodine content is 48.12%, and it is available in 150, 240, 300, and 370 mg iodine/mL.[1] No data are available on the transfer of iopromide into human milk, but others in this family transfer at extraordinarily low levels, and none are orally bioavailable. Therefore, iopromide use is not likely to pose a threat to an infant and should not be a contraindication for breastfeeding. Based on kinetic data, the American College of Radiology suggests that it is probably safe for a mother to continue breastfeeding after receiving iodinated X-ray contrast media.[2]

T 1/2	2 h	MW	791.1 Da	PB	1%
Tmax		RID		Vd	
Oral	Poor	M/P		pKa	

Adult Concerns: Headache, nausea, vomiting, vasodilation, angina pectoris, back pain, urinary urgency, nephropathy, anaphylaxis.

Adult Dose:

Pediatric Concerns:

Infant Monitoring:

Alternatives:

References:
1. Pharmaceutical manufacturers prescribing information.
2. ACR Committee on Drugs and Contrast Media. Administration of contrast medium to breastfeeding mothers. Reston, VA: American College of Radiology; 2004:42-43.

IOTHALAMATE

Trade: Angio-Conray, Conray 325, Conray 400, Conray-30, Conray-43, Conray-60, Cysto-Conray, Cysto-Conray II, Vascoray

Category: Diagnostic Agent, Radiological Contrast Media

LRC: L3 - No Data-Probably Compatible

Iothalamate is an iodinated contrast medium, available in iodine concentrations ranging from 81 mg iodine/mL to 400 mg iodine/mL.[1] No data are available on the transfer to human milk; however, levels in milk are expected to be low to undetectable, and oral bioavailability is low. Therefore, risk to the infant would be minimal. Based on kinetic data, the American College of Radiology suggests that it is safe for a mother to continue breastfeeding after receiving iodinated X-ray contrast media.[2,3]

T 1/2	90-92 min	MW		PB	Low
Tmax		RID		Vd	
Oral		M/P		pKa	

Adult Concerns: Hypersensitivity, local injection site reactions, venous thrombosis, skin necrosis.

Adult Dose:

Pediatric Concerns:

Infant Monitoring:

Alternatives:

References:
1. Pharmaceutical manufacturers prescribing information.
2. ACR Committee on Drugs and Contrast Media. Administration of contrast medium to breastfeeding mothers. Reston, VA: American College of Radiology; 2004:42-43.
3. Webb JA, Thomsen HS, Morcos SK, Members of Contrast Media Safety Committee of European Society of Urogenital R. The use of iodinated and gadolinium contrast media during pregnancy and lactation. Eur Radiol. 2005 Jun;15(6):1234-1240.

IOVERSOL

Trade: Optiject, Optiray

Category: Diagnostic Agent, Radiological Contrast Media

LRC: L3 - No Data-Probably Compatible

Ioversol is a typical iodinated radiocontrast agent used in computed tomographic imaging (CAT scans). The concentration of iodine varies from 16% organically bound iodine (160) to 35% iodine (350).[1] Ioversol is not metabolized, but it is excreted largely unchanged. Iodine is only minimally released; therefore, thyroid function tests remain unchanged with exception of iodine uptake studies (PBI, radioactive iodine uptake). The vascular half-life is brief, only 20 minutes. No data are available on its transfer into milk, but many others in this family have been studied and transfer to milk occurs at extraordinarily low levels. Further, none of these agents are orally bioavailable. Therefore, ioversol is probably compatible with breastfeeding. Based on kinetic data, the American College of Radiology suggests that it is probably safe for a mother to continue breastfeeding after receiving iodinated X-ray contrast media.[2]

T 1/2	1.5 h	MW	807.12 Da	PB	Very low
Tmax		RID		Vd	
Oral	Nil	M/P		pKa	11.34

Adult Concerns: Headache, chest pain, hot flashes, nausea, vomiting, back pain, rash, hives, burning sensation, nephropathy, hypersensitivity.

Adult Dose:

Pediatric Concerns:

Infant Monitoring:

Alternatives:

References:
1. Pharmaceutical manufacturers prescribing information.
2. ACR Committee on Drugs and Contrast Media. Administration of contrast medium to breastfeeding mothers. Reston, VA: American College of Radiology; 2004:42-43.

IOXAGLATE

Trade: Hexabrix, Hexabrix 160, Hexabrix 200, Hexabrix 320

Category: Diagnostic Agent, Radiological Contrast Media

LRC: L3 - No Data-Probably Compatible

Ioxaglate is an ionic dimer that offers a lower osmolarity and consequently less pain upon injection. It contains 32% iodine and is approved for both children and adults. No data are available on the transfer to human milk; however, levels are expected to be low as its molecular weight is high and its oral bioavailability is low. Based on kinetic data, the American College of Radiology suggests that it is safe for a mother to continue breastfeeding after receiving iodinated X-ray contrast media.[1]

T 1/2	60-140 min	MW	1268 Da	PB	Low
Tmax		RID		Vd	
Oral	Nil	M/P		pKa	

Adult Concerns: Nausea, vomiting, warmth sensation, thromboembolic events, nephropathy, hypersensitivity.

Adult Dose:

Pediatric Concerns:

Infant Monitoring:

Alternatives:

References:
1. ACR Committee on Drugs and Contrast Media. Administration of contrast medium to breastfeeding mothers. Reston, VA: American College of Radiology; 2004:42-43.

IOXILAN

Trade: Oxilan

Category: Diagnostic Agent, Radiological Contrast Media

LRC: L3 - No Data-Probably Compatible

Ioxilan is an iodinated radio-opaque contrast agent used for diagnostic purposes. Ioxilan contains 48.1% by weight of iodine. As with all of these compounds, the iodine is organically bound to the parent molecule, and only minimal amounts are free in solution or metabolized by the body. In the case of ioxilan, 93.7% of the original amount injected is excreted unchanged in the urine within 24 hours of administration. This suggests that very little free iodine is actually available systemically. As with other iodinated radiocontrast agents, ioxilan is excreted unchanged and little or no iodine is secreted into human milk.[1] Therefore, a brief interruption of breastfeeding for a few hours would virtually eliminate all risks. Based on kinetic data, the American College of Radiology suggests that it is probably safe for a mother to continue breastfeeding after receiving iodinated X-ray contrast media.[2]

T 1/2	137 min	MW	791.12 Da	PB	Negligible
Tmax	Immediately	RID		Vd	0.1 L/kg
Oral		M/P		pKa	6.8

Adult Concerns: Hypersensitivity to iodine may cause severe, sometimes life-threatening reactions. The risk of reaction increases with history of previous reactions to radiocontrast agents.

Adult Dose: 86 grams IV.

Pediatric Concerns: No untoward effects reported.

Infant Monitoring:

Alternatives:

References:
1. Holmdahl KH. Cholecystography during lactation. Acta Radiol. 1956;45(4):305-307.
2. ACR Committee on Drugs and Contrast Media. Administration of contrast medium to breastfeeding mothers. Reston, VA: American College of Radiology; 2004;42-43.

IOXITALAMIC ACID

Trade: Telebrix

Category: Diagnostic Agent, Radiological Contrast Media

LRC: L3 - No Data-Probably Compatible

Ioxitalamic acid is available in both an oral solution and an injectable solution, in concentrations ranging from 12% to 38% iodine.[1] It is used in both adults and children. There are no data available on the transfer of ioxitalamic acid to breast milk, although levels are likely to be low and oral bioavailability is extremely low. As a result, any small amount ingested would pose little threat to a breastfeeding infant. Based on kinetic data, the American College of Radiology suggests that it is safe for a mother to continue breastfeeding after receiving iodinated X-ray contrast media.[2]

T 1/2		MW		PB	
Tmax		RID		Vd	
Oral	None	M/P		pKa	

Adult Concerns: Dizziness, change in taste, nausea, vomiting, warmth sensation.

Adult Dose:

Pediatric Concerns:

Infant Monitoring:

Alternatives:

References:
1. Pharmaceutical manufacturers prescribing information.
2. ACR Committee on Drugs and Contrast Media. Administration of contrast medium to breastfeeding mothers. Reston, VA: American College of Radiology; 2004:42-43.

IPILIMUMAB

Trade: Yervoy

Category: Monoclonal Antibody

LRC: L4 - Limited Data-Possibly Hazardous

Ipilimumab is an IgG1 monoclonal antibody that binds to human cytotoxic T-lymphocyte antigen 4.[1] This interaction promotes antitumor immune responses. Ipilimumab is indicated for the treatment of unresectable or metastatic melanoma.

Thus far there is only one case report of a woman given ipilimumab 3 mg/kg IV every 3 weeks for four doses postpartum.[2] The milk levels increased about 5 days after the infusion and continued to increase with subsequent doses. The peak and trough concentrations in milk were 147 ng/mL and 41 ng/mL, respectively. The average level of ipilimumab in milk was 75.36 ng/mL, this corresponds with an average infant dose of 53,481 ng/day. The authors further quantified the amount of drug an infant would receive over the 84-day course of maternal therapy as 4.5 mg. In this case the woman was asked not to breastfed until 3 weeks after her last infusion, thus the safety of this medication in lactation remains unknown.

Although the molecular weight of this medication is very large and the amount in breast milk appears to be low, there are no long-term data concerning the safety of using immune modulating medications in breastfeeding mothers. Further there are current data that suggest that other IgG drugs do transfer to milk, and perhaps the breastfed infant. Therefore, some caution is recommended and each woman should understand the benefits and risk of using this type of medication in lactation.

T 1/2	15.4 days	MW	148,000 Da	PB	
Tmax		RID	0.38%	Vd	0.1 L/kg
Oral	Low	M/P		pKa	

Adult Concerns: Headache, fatigue, fever, shortness of breath, hypothyroidism, hypophysitis, anorexia, nausea, vomiting, diarrhea or constipation, abdominal pain, changes in liver function, anemia, pruritus, severe rash.

Adult Dose: 3 mg/kg IV over 90 minutes every 3 weeks.

Pediatric Concerns: No known reports of exposure via milk at this time.

Infant Monitoring: Fever, frequent infections, poor feeding/poor weight gain. Based on clinical symptoms some infants may require monitoring of their hematology, thyroid, or liver function.

Alternatives:

References:
1. Pharmaceutical manufacturers prescribing information.
2. Ross E, Robinson SE, Amato C, et al. Therapeutic monoclonal antibodies in human breast milk: a case study. Melanoma Res. 2014;24:177-180.

IPODATE

Trade: Bilivist, Biloptin, Gastrographin, Oragrafin, Solu-Biloptin, Solubiloptine

Category: Diagnostic Agent, Radiological Contrast Media

LRC: L3 - No Data-Probably Compatible

Not available in the United States, Ipodate is an iodine-containing oral contrast agent used for examining the gallbladder and bile ducts when gallstones are suspected. There are no studies on the transfer of ipodate to human breast milk. However, this product releases some of its iodine content and could increase iodine levels in human milk. While it is likely that minimal drug would transfer to the milk compartment, released iodine may increase levels in milk significantly. A brief 24 hour interruption of breastfeeding is suggested. Caution should be used.[1]

T 1/2	45% gone in 24 h	MW	619 Da	PB	High
Tmax		RID		Vd	
Oral	High	M/P		pKa	

Adult Concerns: Nausea, vomiting, hypersensitivity.

Adult Dose:

Pediatric Concerns:

Infant Monitoring:

Alternatives:

References:
1. Pharmaceutical manufacturers prescribing information.

IPRATROPIUM BROMIDE

Trade: Atrovent

Category: Antiasthma

LRC: L2 - No Data-Probably Compatible

Ipratropium is an anticholinergic drug that is used via inhalation for dilating the bronchi of asthmatics.[1] Ipratropium is a quaternary ammonium compound, and although no data exists, it probably penetrates into breast milk in exceedingly small levels due to its structure. It is unlikely that the infant would absorb any, due to the poor tissue distribution and oral absorption of this family of drugs.

T 1/2	1.6 h	MW	412 Da	PB	0%-9%
Tmax	1-2 h	RID		Vd	
Oral	7 %	M/P		pKa	

Adult Concerns: Nervousness, dizziness, dry mouth, bitter taste, nausea, gastrointestinal distress.

Adult Dose: 36 µg four times daily.

Pediatric Concerns: None reported. Used in pediatric patients.

Infant Monitoring: Irritability, insomnia, arrhythmias, weight loss, tremor.

Alternatives:

References:
1. Pharmaceutical manufacturers prescribing information.

IRBESARTAN

Trade: Avapro

Category: Angiotensin II Receptor Antagonist

LRC: L3 - No Data-Probably Compatible

Irbesartan is an angiotensin-II receptor antagonist used as an antihypertensive. Low concentrations are known to be secreted into rodent milk, but human studies are lacking.[1] No data are available on its use in lactating mothers, thus other medications should be used if suitable for the maternal medical condition (e.g., ramipril, labetalol, nifedipine). In addition, its use early postpartum in lactating mothers should be approached with caution, particularly in mothers with premature infants.

Both the ACE inhibitor family and the specific angiotensin-II receptor blockers are contraindicated in pregnancy and thus should be used with caution in women who are planning a subsequent pregnancy in the near future.

T 1/2	11-15 h	MW	428 Da	PB	90%
Tmax	1.5-2 h	RID		Vd	1.3 L/kg
Oral	60%-80%	M/P		pKa	4.24

Adult Concerns: Headache, dizziness, fatigue, hypotension, nausea, diarrhea, constipation, changes in renal function/urine output, hyperkalemia.

Adult Dose: 150-300 mg daily.

Pediatric Concerns: None reported via milk at this time.

Infant Monitoring: Drowsiness, lethargy, pallor, poor feeding, and weight gain.

Alternatives: Captopril(L2), Enalapril(L2), Ramipril(L3)

References:
1. Pharmaceutical manufacturers prescribing information.

IRON DEXTRAN

Trade: Dexferrum, Infed, Iron

Category: Metals

LRC: L2 - No Data-Probably Compatible

Iron dextran is a colloidal solution of ferric hydroxide in a complex with partially hydrolyzed low molecular weight dextran.[1,2] It is used for severe iron deficiency anemia. Its molecular weight is approximately 180,000 Da. Approximately 99% of the iron in iron dextran is present as a stable ferric-dextran complex. Following intramuscular (IM) injection, iron dextran is absorbed from the site principally through the lymphatic system and subsequently transferred to the reticuloendothelial system in the liver for metabolism. The initial phase of absorption lasts 3 days, which accounts for 60% of an IM dose. The other 40% requires a few weeks to several months for complete absorption.

While there are no data available on the transfer of iron dextran to human milk, there has been one study that reported no change in the milk iron concentrations of women given IV iron sucrose postpartum.[3] Based on the large molecular weight of iron dextran, it too is unlikely to enter breast milk in significant concentrations. Further, iron is transferred to human milk by a tightly controlled pumping system that first chelates the iron to a high molecular weight protein and then transfers it into the milk compartment. It is generally well known that oral dietary supplements of iron in breastfeeding mothers do not change milk levels of iron significantly.[1] In breastfeeding mothers, supplementing with high doses is probably not contraindicated due to the poor passage of iron to milk.

Adult Concerns: Headache, dizziness, syncope, fever, chills, flushing, chest pain, hypotension, changes in taste, nausea, vomiting, abdominal pain, diarrhea, leukocytosis, arthralgia, myalgia, anaphylaxis.

Adult Dose: Doses vary based on iron deficiency, can be given IM or IV.

Pediatric Concerns: None via breast milk.

Infant Monitoring:

Alternatives:

References:
1. Lawrence RA. Breastfeeding: A Guide for the Medical Profession. St. Louis: Mosby Publishers; 1994.
2. Pharmaceutical manufacturers prescribing information.
3. Breymann C, von Seefried Bettina, Stahel M, et al. Milk iron content in breast-feeding mothers after administration of intravenous iron sucrose complex. J Perinat Med. 2007;35:115-118.

IRON SUCROSE

Trade: Venofer, Iron

Category: Metals

LRC: L2 - Limited Data-Probably Compatible

Iron sucrose is used in the treatment of iron-deficiency anemia.[1] When given intravenously, it is sequestered in the liver where it is metabolized, and free iron is released into the circulation and incorporated into hemoglobin. At this time, there has been one study that compared the transfer of iron to milk in 10 women with iron deficiency given IV iron to five women with iron deficiency not given treatment.[2] These women were given 100 mg of IV iron sucrose 2-3 days after delivery; milk samples were taken before treatment and for 4 days after. When the milk samples were compared to those of the five women not given IV iron, there was no difference in the mean baseline concentrations or the levels measured over the 4 day observation period.

T 1/2	6 h	MW	34,000-60,000 Da	PB	
Tmax		RID		Vd	0.11 L/kg
Oral	Poor	M/P		pKa	

Adult Concerns: Headache, dizziness, syncope, fever, chills, flushing, chest pain, hypotension, changes in taste, nausea, vomiting, abdominal pain, diarrhea, leucocytosis, arthralgia, myalgia, anaphylaxis.

Adult Dose: Doses vary based on iron deficiency, typically 1000 mg elemental IV iron in divided doses.

Pediatric Concerns: No data available.

Infant Monitoring:

Alternatives:

References:
1. Pharmaceutical manufacturers prescribing information.
2. Breymann C, von Seefried Bettina, Stahel M, et al. Milk iron content in breast-feeding mothers after administration of intravenous iron sucrose complex. J Perinat Med. 2007;35:115-118.

ISOMETHEPTENE MUCATE + CAFFEINE + ACETAMINOPHEN

Trade: Prodrin

Category: Antimigraine

LRC: L3 - No Data-Probably Compatible

Isometheptene is a mild stimulant (sympathomimetic) that apparently acts by constricting dilated cranial and cerebral arterioles, thus reducing vascular headaches. It is commonly combined with caffeine and acetaminophen for migraine headaches. caffeine, also a cranial vasoconstrictor, is added to further enhance the vasoconstrictor effect. It is also used as a central stimulant for relief of headache. Acetaminophen, an effective non-narcotic analgesic, reduces the perception of pain impulses originating from dilated cerebral vessels; no hyperacidity of stomach and less allergies than aspirin.

Nothing is known about the transfer of isometheptene to human milk. Due to its size and molecular composition, it is likely to attain low to moderate levels in breast milk. Because better drugs exist for migraine therapy, this product is probably not a good choice for breastfeeding mothers. Consider sumatriptan, rizatriptan, amitriptyline, or propranolol as alternatives.

T 1/2	ISO/Caf/Acet: / 4.9 h/2 h	MW	ISO/Caf/Acet: 493/191 /151 Da	PB	ISO/Caf/Acet: /36%/25%
Tmax		RID		Vd	
Oral	Complete	M/P		pKa	

Adult Concerns: Dizziness, skin rash, hypertension. Isometheptene Mucate, Caffeine, and Acetaminophen is contraindicated in Glaucoma and/or severe cases of renal disease, hypertension, organic heart disease, hepatic disease, and in those patients who are on monoamine oxidase inhibitor (MAOI) therapy.

Adult Dose: One to two caplets STAT, followed by one caplet every hour until relieved. No more than five caplets within 12 hours

Pediatric Concerns: None reported via milk at this time.

Infant Monitoring: Not recommended in lactation.

Alternatives: Sumatriptan(L3), rizatriptan(L3), amitriptyline(L2), or propranolol(L2) as alternatives.

References:
1. Pharmaceutical manufacturers prescribing information.

ISONIAZID

Trade: INH, Isotamine, Pycazide, Rimifon

Category: Antitubercular

LRC: L3 - Limited Data-Probably Compatible

Isoniazid (INH) is an antimicrobial agent primarily used to treat tuberculosis. Following doses of 5 and 10 mg/kg, one report measured peak milk levels at 6 mg/L and 9 mg/L, respectively.[1] Isoniazid was not measurable in the infant's serum but was detected in the urine of several infants. In another study, following a maternal dose of 300 mg of isoniazid, the concentration of isoniazid in milk peaked at 3 hours at 16.6 mg/L while the acetyl derivative (AcINH) was 3.76 mg/L.[2] The 24-hour excretion of INH in milk was estimated at 7 mg. The authors felt this dose was potentially hazardous to a breastfed infant.

In a well-done study in seven exclusively lactating women (at 33 days or steady state) who were receiving 300 mg isoniazid daily in a single dose (and rifampin and ethambutol), the mean (AUC) of isoniazid in plasma and milk was 18.4 µg/mL/24 hours and 14.4 µg/mL/24 hours respectively.[3] The mean milk/plasma ratio (AUC) was 0.89 and the calculated relative infant dose was 1.2%. In this nicely done study, peak levels are clearly evident at 1 hour and fall rapidly at 4 hours. Suggest the mom avoid breastfeeding for 2 hours following administration of INH to avoid the peak plasma concentrations at 2 hours.

T 1/2	1.1-3.1 h	MW	137 Da	PB	10%-15%
Tmax	1-2 h (oral)	RID	1.2%-18%	Vd	0.6 L/kg
Oral	Complete	M/P		pKa	1.9, 3.5

Adult Concerns: Dizziness, depression, lethargy, fever, blurred vision, vomiting, anorexia, changes in liver function, agranulocytosis, anemia, peripheral neuropathy, arthralgia, rash. Pyridoxine (vitamin B6) 25-50 mg/day is recommended for those at risk of neuropathy (e.g., pregnant women, breastfeeding women, those with malnutrition) and 100 mg/day is recommended for those with neuropathy.[4]

Adult Dose: 5 mg/kg daily.

Pediatric Concerns: None reported via milk at this time.

Infant Monitoring: Drowsiness, lethargy, vomiting, and weight gain. If clinical symptoms arise (e.g., yellowing of the skin or eyes) check liver function tests.

Alternatives:

References:

1. Snider DE Jr, Powell KE. Should women taking antituberculosis drugs breast-feed? Arch Intern Med. 1984;144(3):589-590.
2. Berlin CM, Lee C. Isoniazid and acetylisoniazid disposition in human milk, saliva and plasma. Fed Proc. 1979;38:426.
3. Singh N, Golani A, Patel Z, Maitra A. Transfer of isoniazid from circulation to breast milk in lactating women on chronic therapy for tuberculosis. BJCP. 2008;65(3):418-422.
4. Nahid P, Doman SE, Alipanah N, et al. Official american thoracic society/centers for disease control and prevention/infectious diseases society of america clinical practice guidelines: treatment of drug-susceptible tuberculosis. CID. 2016;63:e147-e195.

ISOPROTERENOL

Trade: Isoprenaline, Isuprel, Medihaler-Iso

Category: Antiarrhythmic

LRC: L3 - No Data-Probably Compatible

Isoproterenol is a non-selective beta agonist that is used for both bronchospasm during anesthesia and the treatment of certain arrhythmias.[1] This medication is available in both inhaled and injectable forms. At this time, there are no data regarding the amount of isoproterenol that enters milk. Based on this medication's short half-life, significant levels are not expected in milk.

T 1/2	4 min (IV); 5 min (inh)	MW	247.7 Da	PB	
Tmax		RID		Vd	
Oral		M/P		pKa	9.81

Adult Concerns: Dizziness, headache, restlessness, insomnia, angina, hyper or hypotension, arrhythmias, shortness of breath, nausea, vomiting, tremor, weakness.

Adult Dose: Varies by indication.

Pediatric Concerns: No known adverse events at this time.

Infant Monitoring: Irritability, insomnia, weight loss, tremor, lethargy.

Alternatives:

References:

1. Pharmaceutical manufacturer prescribing monograph, 2006.

ISOSORBIDE DINITRATE

Trade: Carvasin, Cedocard, Coronex, Dilatrate, Isordil

Category: Vasodilator

LRC: L3 - No Data-Probably Compatible

Isosorbide dinitrate and its mononitrate cousin are vasodilating agents used in the treatment of angina and congestive heart failure, and many other syndromes. The treatment of anal fissures with isosorbide dinitrate early postpartum may impact breastfeeding. Absorption is highly variable but once absorbed it is metabolized to a 2-mononitrate and 5-mononitrate derivatives. The 5-mononitrate has a half-life of approximately 5 hours. No data are available on the transfer of isosorbide dinitrate into human milk although small amounts may enter milk.

T 1/2	5 h (metabolite)	MW		PB	Low
Tmax	1 h	RID		Vd	2-4 L/kg
Oral	10%-90%	M/P		pKa	

Adult Concerns: Headache, nervousness, dizziness, heart palpitations, low blood pressure, weakness, itching, and rash.

Adult Dose: 5-20 mg orally two to three times a day, varies by indication.

Pediatric Concerns: No data are available on the transfer of isosorbide dinitrate to human milk. Methemoglobinemia has been reported in pure nitrite poisoning from drinking water, but this is highly unlikely to occur with the use of this drug. Use with some caution.

Infant Monitoring: Drowsiness, lethargy, pallor, poor feeding, and weight gain.

Alternatives:

References:
1. Pharmaceutical manufacturers prescribing information.

ISOSORBIDE MONONITRATE

Trade: Corangin, Dynamin, Elantan, Imdex, Imdur

Category: Vasodilator

LRC: L3 - No Data-Probably Compatible

Isosorbide mononitrate and its dinitrate cousin are vasodilating agents used in the treatment of angina and congestive heart failure, and many other syndromes. While we have no data on the transfer of isosorbide mononitrate to human milk, we know that the transfer of nitrates to human milk in general is quite poor from maternal diet and water (see nitroglycerin).

T 1/2	6.2 h	MW	191 Da	PB	<5%
Tmax	30-60 min	RID		Vd	0.6 L/kg
Oral	93%	M/P		pKa	

Adult Concerns: Headache, arrhythmias, hypotension, edema, flushing, methemoglobinemia.

Adult Dose: Highly variable.

Pediatric Concerns: None reported. Use with some caution.

Infant Monitoring: Drowsiness, lethargy, pallor, poor feeding, and weight gain.

Alternatives:

References:
1. Pharmaceutical manufacturers prescribing information.

ISOSULFAN BLUE

Trade: Lymphazurin

Category: Diagnostic Agent, Radiological Contrast Media

LRC: L4 - No Data-Possibly Hazardous

Isosulfan blue is a contrast agent used for visualization of the lymphatic system drainage. Each mL of solution contains 10 mg isosulfan blue, 6.6 mg sodium monohydrogen phosphate, and 2.7 mg potassium dihydrogen phosphate.[1] Isosulfan blue has a higher rate of success in detecting sentinel lymph nodes than does Technetium-99m sulfur colloid (TSC).[2] Severe anaphylactic reactions have been reported with this product.[3] Methylene blue dye has been shown to be equally effective without the same chance of severe adverse effects, and thus its use is increasing.[4] No data are available on the transfer of isosulfan blue to breast milk, and therefore caution should be used in breastfeeding mothers. Urine is blue for at least 24 hours. Suggest a waiting period of approximately 48 hours.

T 1/2		MW	566.7 Da	PB	50%
Tmax		RID		Vd	
Oral		M/P		pKa	

Adult Concerns: Localized swelling and itching.

Adult Dose: 0.5 mL into 3 interdigital spaces.

Pediatric Concerns: No data were available.

Infant Monitoring:

Alternatives:

References:
1. Pharmaceutical manufacturers prescribing information.
2. Saha S, Dan AG, Berman B, et al. Lymphazurin 1% versus 99mTc sulfur colloid for lymphatic mapping in colorectal tumors: a comparative analysis. Ann Surg Oncol. 2003;11(1):21-26.
3. Stefanutto TB, Shapiro WA, Wright PMC. Anaphylactic reaction to isosulphan blue. Br J Anesth. 2002;89(3):527-528.
4. Thevarajah S, Huston TL, Simmons RM. A comparison of the adverse reactions associated with isosulfan blue versus methylene blue dye in sentinel lymph node biopsy for breast cancer. Am J Surg. 2005;189(2):236-239.

ISOTRETINOIN

Trade: Roaccutane, Isotrex, Absorica, Amnesteem, Claravis, Myorisan, Epuris

Category: Antiacne

LRC: L5 - No Data-Hazardous

Isotretinoin is a synthetic derivative of the vitamin A family called retinoids. Isotretinoin is known to be incredibly teratogenic producing profound birth defects in exposed fetuses.[1] It is primarily used for cystic acne, where it is extremely effective if used by skilled physicians. While only 25% reaches the plasma, the remaining is either metabolized in the gastrointestinal tract or removed during first pass by the liver. It is distributed to the liver, adrenals, ovaries, and lacrimal glands. Unlike vitamin A, isotretinoin is not stored in the liver. Secretion into milk is unknown but is likely as with other retinoids. Isotretinoin is extremely lipid soluble, and concentrations in milk may be significant. The manufacturer strongly recommends against using isotretinoin in a breastfeeding mother.

T 1/2	>20 h	MW	300 Da	PB	99.9%
Tmax	3.2 h	RID		Vd	
Oral	25%	M/P		pKa	4

Adult Concerns: Headache, fatigue, changes in sleep, elevated serum triglycerides, hyperglycemia, colitis, weight loss, elevations in liver enzymes, agranulocytosis (rare), anemia, arthralgias, myalgias, bruising, abnormal wound healing, changes in skin pigmentation, erythema, dry skin, pruritus, rash.

Adult Dose: 0.5-2 mg/kg daily.

Pediatric Concerns: None reported at this time.

Infant Monitoring: Not recommended in lactation.

Alternatives:

References:
1. Pharmaceutical manufacturers prescribing information.

ISRADIPINE

Trade: DynaCirc, Vascal

Category: Calcium Channel Blocker

LRC: L3 - No Data-Probably Compatible

Isradipine is a calcium channel blocker used in the management of hypertension.[1] It is not known if isradipine is secreted into human milk. Although this medication is highly protein bound, it has a high volume of distribution and a large first-pass effect (low bioavailability) other calcium channel blockers are preferred as they transfer to milk minimally (see nifedipine).

T 1/2	8 h	MW	371 Da	PB	95%
Tmax	1.5 h	RID		Vd	3 L/kg
Oral	15-24%	M/P		pKa	

Adult Concerns: Headache, dizziness, fatigue, hypotension, palpitations, dyspnea, nausea, vomiting ,diarrhea, edema.

Adult Dose: 2.5-10 mg twice daily.

Pediatric Concerns: None reported at this time.

Infant Monitoring: Drowsiness, lethargy, pallor, poor feeding, and weight gain.

Alternatives: Nifedipine(L2), Verapamil(L2), Nimodipine(L2)

References:
1. Pharmaceutical manufacturers prescribing information.

ITRACONAZOLE

Trade: Sporanox, Onmel

Category: Antifungal

LRC: L3 - Limited Data-Probably Compatible

Itraconazole is an antifungal agent active against a variety of fungal strains. It is extensively metabolized to hydroxy-itraconazole, an active metabolite.[1] Itraconazole has an enormous volume of distribution, and large quantities (20-fold compared to plasma) concentrate in fatty tissues, liver, kidney, and skin. In a study of two women who received two oral doses of 200 mg itraconazole 12 hours apart, the average milk concentrations at 4, 24, and 48 hours after the second dose were 70, 28, and 16 µg/L, respectively.[2] After 72 hours, itraconazole levels in one mother were 20 µg/L and undetectable in the other. Reported milk/plasma ratios at 4, 24, and 48 hours were 0.51, 1.61, and 1.77 respectively. However, itraconazole oral absorption in an infant is somewhat unlikely as it requires an acidic milieu for absorption, which may be unlikely in a diet high in milk. Itraconazole has also been reported to induce significant bone defects in newborn animals, and it is not cleared for pediatric use. Until further studies are done, fluconazole is probably a preferred choice in breastfeeding mothers.

T 1/2	64 h	MW	706 Da	PB	99.8%
Tmax	2-5 h	RID	0.2%	Vd	10 L/kg
Oral	55%	M/P	0.51-1.77	pKa	

Adult Concerns: Dizziness, hypertension, nausea, vomiting, diarrhea, epigastric pain, abnormal liver enzymes, rash.

Adult Dose: 200-400 mg daily.

Pediatric Concerns: None reported via breastmilk. Absorption via milk is unlikely.

Infant Monitoring: Vomiting, diarrhea.

Alternatives: Fluconazole(L2)

References:
1. Pharmaceutical manufacturers prescribing information.
2. Janssen Pharmaceuticals, personal communication, 1996.

IVACAFTOR

Trade: Kalydeco

Category: Other

LRC: L3 - No Data-Probably Compatible

Ivacaftor is a transmembrane conductance regulator (CFTR) potentiator, indicated specifically for the treatment of cystic fibrosis due to the G551D mutation in the CFTR gene.[1] Currently there are no data available on the transfer of ivacaftor in human milk. Due to its high protein binding and high volume of distribution, it is unlikely that it would enter into milk in significant quantities. However, since so little is known about this drug, caution is urged.

T 1/2	12 h	MW	392.49 Da	PB	99%
Tmax	4 h	RID		Vd	5 L/kg
Oral		M/P		pKa	

Adult Concerns: Headache, dizziness, nasal congestion, nausea, abdominal pain, changes in liver function, hyperglycemia, diarrhea, myalgia, rash.

Adult Dose: 150 mg every 12 hours.

Pediatric Concerns:

Infant Monitoring: Vomiting, diarrhea, nasal congestion.

Alternatives:

References:

1. Pharmaceutical manufacturers prescribing information.

IVERMECTIN

Trade: Mectizan, Stromectol, Sklice Lotion

Category: Anthelmintic

LRC: L3 - Limited Data-Probably Compatible

Ivermectin is now widely used to treat human onchocerciasis, lymphatic filariasis, and other worms and parasites such as head lice. In a study of four women given 150 µg/kg orally, the maximum breast milk concentration averaged 14.13 µg/L.[1] Milk/plasma ratios ranged from 0.39 to 0.57 with a mean of 0.51. Highest breast milk concentration was at 4-6 hours. Average daily ingestion of ivermectin was calculated at 2.1 µg/kg, which is 10-fold less than the adult dose. No adverse effects were reported in the breastfed infant. Ivermectin is probably compatible with breastfeeding.

A new topical formulation of ivermectin (Sklice) has just been introduced for head lice in infants (6 months and older).

T 1/2	18 h	MW		PB	93%
Tmax	4 h	RID	1.3%	Vd	3-3.5 L/kg
Oral	Variable	M/P	0.39-0.57	pKa	12.47

Adult Concerns: Headache, transient hypotension, pruritus.

Adult Dose: 150-200 µg/kg once.

Pediatric Concerns: None reported via milk.

Infant Monitoring:

Alternatives:

References:

1. Ogbuokiri JE, Ozumba BC, Okonkwo PO. Ivermectin levels in human breast milk. Eur J Clin Pharmacol. 1994;46(1):89-90.
2. Pharmaceutical manufacturers prescribing information.

KETAMINE

Trade: Anesject, Brevinaze, Calypsol, Ketalar, Ketamax, Ketanest, Spravato

Category: Anesthetic

LRC: L3 - No Data-Probably Compatible

Ketamine is a rapid acting general anesthetic agent with analgesia and anesthetic effects. It is increasingly more popular, as it has fewer hemodynamic problems, and reduced postoperative sedation.[1,2] One major benefit of ketamine is the production of excellent analgesia with minimal respiratory depression. No data are available on the transfer of ketamine into human milk. It has a short half-life of 2.5 hours but its redistribution half-life out of the plasma (to muscle and tissues) is brief (10-15 min), thus milk levels are likely to be low.[3]

Recently a new intranasal preparation was released for treatment of depression. No data on breastmilk levels are available at this dose or route of administration.

T 1/2	2.5 h	MW	274 Da	PB	47%
Tmax	1 minute IV	RID		Vd	2.4 L/kg
Oral	20-30%	M/P		pKa	7.5

Adult Concerns: Sedation, hallucinations, diplopia, nystagmus, hypertension and tachycardia or hypotension and bradycardia, arrhythmias, increase in respiratory rate or less commonly respiratory depression, nausea, vomiting, increased muscle tone.

Adult Dose: Varies 1-2 mg/kg IV. Intranasal dose: 56 or 84 mg twice weekly

Pediatric Concerns: None reported via milk. Rapid redistribution from the plasma would probably reduce levels in milk.

Infant Monitoring: Observe for sedation, irritability, poor feeding.

Alternatives: Propofol(L2), Fentanyl(L2)

References:

1. Bergman SA. Ketamine: review of its pharmacology and its use in pediatric anesthesia. Anesth Prog. 1999;46(1):10-20.
2. White M, de GP, Renshof B, van KE, Dzoljic M. Pharmacokinetics of S(+) ketamine derived from target controlled infusion. Br J Anaesth. 2006 Mar;96(3):330-334.
3. Pharmaceutical manufacturers prescribing information.

KETOCONAZOLE

Trade: Extina, Nizoral, Nizoral A-D, Xolegel

Category: Antifungal

LRC: L2 - Limited Data-Probably Compatible

Ketoconazole is an antifungal similar in structure to miconazole and clotrimazole. It is used orally, topically, and via shampoo.[1] Ketoconazole is not detected in plasma after chronic shampooing. In a study of one patient (82 kg) receiving 200 mg daily for 10 days, milk samples were taken at 1.75, 3.25, 6, 8, and 24 hours after the tenth dose.[2] The average concentration of ketoconazole over the 24 hours was 68 μg/L while the C_{max} at 3.25 hours was 0.22 mg/L. The absorption of ketoconazole is highly variable, and could be reduced in infants due to the alkaline condition induced by milk ingestion.[3] Regardless, ketoconazole is probably safe in breastfeeding infants.

T 1/2	2-8 h	MW	531 Da	PB	99%
Tmax	1-2 h	RID	0.3%	Vd	
Oral	Variable (75%)	M/P		pKa	2.94, 6.51

Adult Concerns: Dizziness, fever, chills, nausea, vomiting, diarrhea, abdominal pain, changes in liver function, itching.

Adult Dose: 200-400 mg daily.

Pediatric Concerns: None reported in one case.

Infant Monitoring: Vomiting, diarrhea.

Alternatives: Fluconazole(L2)

References:

1. Pharmaceutical manufacturers prescribing information.
2. Moretti ME, Ito S, Koren G. Disposition of maternal ketoconazole in breast milk. Am J Obstet Gynecol. 1995;173(5):1625-1626.
3. Force RW, Nahata MC. Salivary concentrations of ketoconazole and fluconazole: implications for drug efficacy in oropharyngeal and esophageal candidiasis. Ann Pharmacother. 1995;29(1):10-15.

KETOROLAC

Trade: Acular, Toradol

Category: NSAID

LRC: L2 - Limited Data-Probably Compatible

Ketorolac is a popular, nonsteroidal analgesic. In a study of 10 lactating women who received 10 mg orally four times daily, milk levels of ketorolac were not detectable in four of the subjects.[1] In the six remaining patients, the concentration of ketorolac in milk 2 hours after a dose ranged from 5.2 to 7.3 μg/L on day 1 and 5.9 to 7.9 μg/L on day two. In most patients, the breast milk level was never above 5 μg/L. The maximum daily dose an infant could absorb (maternal dose= 40 mg/day) would range from 3.16 to 7.9 μg/day assuming a milk volume of 400 mL or 1000 mL. An infant would therefore receive less than 0.2% of the daily maternal dose (Please note, the original paper contained a misprint on the daily intake of ketorolac, mg instead of μg).

Ketorolac has been extensively studied in neonates, infants, and children.[2,3] The half-life is brief and in some cases is undetectable in the infant plasma after 4 hours.[2] For a complete review of the pediatric use of ketorolac see Buck.[3]

T 1/2	2.5 h	MW	255 Da	PB	99%
Tmax	0.5 - 1 h,	RID	0.14% - 0.2%	Vd	0.18-0.21 L/kg
Oral	>81%	M/P	0.015-0.037	pKa	3.5

Adult Concerns: Headache, dizziness, drowsiness, tinnitus, hypertension, dyspepsia, nausea, vomiting, abdominal pain, constipation, diarrhea, gastrointestinal bleeding, anorexia, changes in liver and renal function, anemia, edema.

Adult Dose: 10 mg every 6 hours.

Pediatric Concerns: None reported in one study.

Infant Monitoring: Vomiting, diarrhea.

Alternatives: Ibuprofen(L1), celecoxib(L2)

References:
1. Wischnik A, Manth SM, Lloyd J, Bullingham R, Thompson JS. The excretion of ketorolac tromethamine into breast milk after multiple oral dosing. Eur J Clin Pharmacol. 1989;36(5):521-524.
2. Cohen MN, Christians U, Henthorn T, et al. Pharmacokinetics of single-dose intravenous ketorolac in infants aged 2-11 months. Anesth Analg. 2011 Mar;112(3):655-660.
3. Buck ML. Use of intravenous ketorolac for postoperative analgesia in infants. Pediatr Pharmacother Newsl. 2011 Aug;17(8).

KETOROLAC TROMETHAMINE

Trade: Acuvail, Sprix

Category: NSAID

LRC: L2 - Limited Data-Probably Compatible

Ketorolac is a popular, nonsteroidal analgesic used in eye drops. While oral or IV ketorolac produce low levels in breast milk, it is exceedingly unlikely that the ophthalmic product will produce high enough levels systemically in the mother to ever produce measurable levels in breast milk.

Milk levels of ketorolac are low with the usual oral dosage,[1] but have not been measured after higher injectable dosages. Maternal use of ketorolac eye drops would not be expected to cause any adverse effects in breastfed infants. To substantially diminish the amount of drug that reaches the breast milk after using eye drops, place pressure over the tear duct by the corner of the eye for 1 minute or more, then remove the excess solution with an absorbent tissue.

T 1/2	4-6 h	MW	376.41 Da	PB	99%
Tmax	30-60 min	RID		Vd	
Oral	99%	M/P		pKa	3.5

Adult Concerns: Headache, dizziness, drowsiness, tinnitus, hypertension, dyspepsia, nausea, vomiting, abdominal pain, constipation, diarrhea, gastrointestinal bleeding, anorexia, changes in liver and renal function, anemia, edema.

Adult Dose: One drop (0.25 mg) four times daily.

Pediatric Concerns:

Infant Monitoring: Vomiting, diarrhea.

Alternatives:

References:
1. Wischnik A, Manth SM, Lloyd J, Bullingham R, Thompson JS. The excretion of ketorolac tromethamine into breast milk after multiple oral dosing. Eur J Clin Pharmacol. 1989;36(5):521-524.

KETOTIFEN

Trade: Alaway, Claritin Eye, Zaditen, Zaditor, Zyrtec Itchy-Eye Drops

Category: Antihistamine

LRC: L3 - No Data-Probably Compatible

Ketotifen is a second-generation H1 antihistamine. It is used ophthalmically to treat red eye and allergic conjunctivitis.[1] Ketotifen has been shown to enter breast milk in animal studies, however it is unknown if it is excreted in human breast milk.[1] It is unknown if enough drug enters systemic circulation after topical administration to produce significant quantities in breast milk. This drug has a molecular weight of 425.5, an oral bioavailability of 50%, and is distributed widely throughout the body. Based on these kinetics, it is unlikely that this drug would pose a significant risk to breastfed infants.

T 1/2	21 h	MW	425.5 Da	PB	75%
Tmax	2-4 h	RID		Vd	56 L/kg
Oral	50%	M/P		pKa	8.43

Adult Concerns: Syncope, rash, contact dermatitis, hyperglycemia, weight gain, xerostomia, dizziness, headache, somnolence, dyspnea, pharyngitis, rhinitis.

Adult Dose: 1 drop in each eye twice daily; 1-2mg oral twice daily.

Pediatric Concerns:

Infant Monitoring: Sedation or insomnia, dry mouth.

Alternatives:

References:
1. Product Information: Zaditor(TM), Ketotifen Ophthalmic Solution 0.025%. Duluth, GA: Novartis Ophthalmics; 2012.

L-METHYLFOLATE

Trade: Deplin, Metafolin

Category: Vitamin

LRC: L3 - No Data-Probably Compatible

L-Methylfolate, also called Metafolin, is the active biological isomer of folate and the form of circulating folate. Approximately 10% of the population lacks the enzymes necessary to metabolize folic acid to L-methylfolate. L-Methylfolate is the form transported across cell membranes, and is bioactive. No data are available on the transport of this form of folate into human milk. However, several studies of folic acid supplementation in breastfeeding mothers clearly suggest that folate is actively transported into human milk, but most importantly, supplementing of the mother only marginally if at all, increases milk folate levels.[1,2] This suggests that even following supplementation, milk levels would be unlikely to increase, unless the mother is deficient. Thus, this product is probably not hazardous to use in a breastfeeding mother.

T 1/2		MW	455 Da	PB	
Tmax		RID		Vd	
Oral	Complete	M/P		pKa	

Adult Concerns:

Adult Dose: 7.5 mg daily.

Pediatric Concerns: None reported via milk.

Infant Monitoring:

Alternatives: Folic acid(L1)

References:
1. Tamura T, Yoshimura Y, Arakawa T. Human milk folate and folate status in lactating mothers and their infants. Am J Clin Nutr. 1980;33:193-197.
2. Smith AM, Picciano MF, Deering RH. Folate supplementation during lactation: maternal folate status, human milk folate content, and their relationship to infant folate status. J Pediatr Gastroenterol Nutr. 1983;2:622-628.

LABETALOL

Trade: Normodyne, Presolol, Trandate

Category: Beta Adrenergic Blocker

LRC: L2 - Limited Data-Probably Compatible

Labetalol is a selective beta-blocker with moderate lipid solubility that is used as an antihypertensive and for treating angina. In one study of 3 women receiving 600-1200 mg/day, the peak concentrations of labetalol in breast milk were 129, 223, and 662 µg/L respectively.[1] In only one infant were measurable plasma levels found (18 µg/L) following a maternal dose of 600 mg. Therefore, only small amounts are secreted in human milk.

T 1/2	6-8 h	MW	328 Da	PB	50%
Tmax	1-2 h (oral)	RID	0.2% - 0.6%	Vd	5.1-9.4 L/kg
Oral	30-40%	M/P	0.8-2.6	pKa	8.05

Adult Concerns: Headache, dizziness, insomnia, depression, fatigue, chest pain, bradycardia, ventricular arrhythmia, hypotension, heart failure, wheezing, taste disturbances, vomiting, heartburn, myalgia, infusion reactions.

Adult Dose: 200-400 mg twice daily.

Pediatric Concerns: None reported via milk at this time.

Infant Monitoring: Drowsiness, lethargy, pallor, poor feeding, and weight gain.

Alternatives: Nifedipine(L2), Metoprolol(L2)

References:
1. Lunell NO, Kulas J, Rane A. transfer of labetalol into amniotic fluid and breast milk in lactating women. Eur J Clin Pharmacol. 1985;28(5):597-599.

LACOSAMIDE

Trade: Vimpat

Category: Anticonvulsant

LRC: L3 - No Data-Probably Compatible

Lacosamide is an anticonvulsant used as adjunctive therapy in the treatment of partial-onset seizures in adults with epilepsy.[1] Lacosamide selectively enhances slow inactivation of voltage-gated sodium channels, thus stabilizing hyperexcitable neuronal membranes and blocking repetitive firing. Due to its small molecular weight (250 Da), poor protein binding and low Vd (0.6 L/kg) levels in milk may be significant. No data are available on its transfer to human milk, but caution is recommended until we have more data.

T 1/2	12.48 h	MW	250 Da	PB	15%
Tmax	1-4 h	RID		Vd	0.6 L/kg
Oral	100%	M/P		pKa	

Adult Concerns: Fatigue, headache, depression, insomnia, agitation, memory impairment, vertigo, diplopia, blurred vision, nystagmus, dyspepsia, nausea, vomiting, diarrhea, weakness, ataxia, tremor, pruritus.

Adult Dose: 200-400 mg daily in two divided doses.

Pediatric Concerns: None reported via milk, but caution is recommended. In pediatric patients it can cause drowsiness, irritability, GI upset and motor instability.[2]

Infant Monitoring: Sedation or irritability, not waking to feed/poor feeding, weight gain, vomiting, diarrhea, tremor.

Alternatives: Lamotrigine(L2), Carbamazepine(L2)

References:
1. Pharmaceutical manufacturers prescribing information.
2. Grosso S, Parisi P, Spalice A, Verrotti A, Balestri P. Efficacy and safety of lacosamide in infants and young children with refractory focal epilepsy. Eur J Paediatr Neurol. 2014;18(1):55-59.

LACTASE

Trade: Lactaid, SureLac

Category: Dietary Supplement

LRC: L3 - No Data-Probably Compatible

Lactase is an enzyme that metabolizes lactose (milk sugar) in the small intestine to glucose and galactose. This enzyme is naturally produced in 77% of U.S. adult populations and 100% of human infants.[1] There are no adequate and well-controlled studies or case reports in breastfeeding women, however used orally, this product is probably safe for breastfeeding women.

Adult Concerns: None reported.

Adult Dose: 1-2 capsules with milk.

Pediatric Concerns:

Infant Monitoring:

Alternatives:

References:
1.   Bersaglieri T, Sabeti PC, Patterson N, et al. Genetic signatures of strong recent positive selection at the lactase gene. Am J Hum Genet. 2004 Jun;74(6):1111-1120. Epub 2004 Apr 26.

LACTULOSE

Trade: Bifiteral, Cephulac, Chronulac, Constilac, Constulose, Duphalac, Enulose, Evalose, Generlac

Category: Laxative

LRC: L3 - No Data-Probably Compatible

Lactulose is an osmotic laxative used for the treatment of constipation, it increases the number of bowel movements per day, and the number of days on which bowel movements occur.[1] Lactulose is also used in the treatment and prevention of portal systemic encephalopathy. Lactulose works by reducing the concentration levels of ammonia in the blood. The transfer of lactulose to human milk is unlikely as lactulose is poorly absorbed.

T 1/2		MW	342.2 Da	PB	
Tmax		RID		Vd	
Oral	Minimal	M/P		pKa	

Adult Concerns: Flatulence, intestinal cramps, diarrhea, nausea, and vomiting.

Adult Dose: 15 to 60 mL daily.

Pediatric Concerns: None observed in breastfeeding mothers. Commonly used in infants.

Infant Monitoring:

Alternatives: Polyethylene glycol (PEG).

References:
1.   Pharmaceutical manufacturers prescribing information.

LAMIVUDINE

Trade: 3TC, Epivir-HBV

Category: Antiviral

LRC: L5 - Limited Data-Hazardous if Maternal HIV Infection

Lamivudine is a synthetic nucleoside analog antiviral used for the treatment of Hepatitis B or HIV infections. It is presently in numerous other combination products (Combivir, Ziagen, etc.). In a study of 20 women receiving either 300 mg once daily or 150 mg twice daily one week postpartum, the mean breast milk concentration was 1.22 mg/L (range = 0.5-6.09) or 0.183 mg/kg/day.[1] This is significantly less than the clinical dose normally administered to infants (4-8 mg/kg/day). The authors suggested that the amount ingested via breast milk was negligible relative to therapeutic dosing and would not provide adequate antiretroviral drug concentrations for a neonate.

In another study of 18 women receiving antiretroviral treatment for HIV infections (150 mg BID lamivudine and 200 mg BID nevirapine), median lamivudine concentrations in maternal serum, breast milk, and the infant's serum were 678 ng/mL, 1828 ng/mL, and 28 ng/mL, respectively.[2] The median milk/serum ratio was 3.34 for lamivudine. The median infant concentration of lamivudine (28 ng/mL) was 5% of the inhibitory concentration (50%), which is 550 ng/mL. This data suggests that the serum levels of lamivudine attained in the infant are probably too low to produce side effects in the infant, and certainly too low to treat HIV effectively in the infant.

In 2007, 40 women were given zidovudine, lamivudine, and nevirapine from 28 weeks gestational age to 1 month postpartum to evaluate the potential efficacy of using these medications to prevent the transmission of perinatal HIV.[3] All women in this study were instructed not to breastfeed their infants. Milk samples were collected five times a day from delivery to day 7 postpartum, and blood samples were collected on day 3 (time 0) and day 7 (time 7); the samples were used to quantify the amount of HIV RNA and DNA in milk and the concentrations of each medication in maternal plasma and milk. The mean concentrations of lamivudine at times 0 and 7 in maternal plasma were 200 μg/L and 400 μg/L. The mean concentrations of lamivudine at times 0 and 7 in milk were 400 μg/L and 400 μg/L. The milk/plasma ratios were 3.3 and 2.9 at times 0 and 7, respectively. We used the milk levels from times 0 and 7 to estimate the relative infant dose for lamivudine to be 1.4%.

In 2009, a study was published that assessed 67 women taking combination antiretroviral therapy from 34 to 36 weeks through 6 months postpartum.[4] These women took one Combivir tablet twice daily (lamivudine 150 mg + zidovudine 300 mg/tab) with nevirapine 200 mg x 14 days then 200 mg twice a day. Lamivudine milk samples were taken within 24 hours of delivery, then at weeks 2, 6, 14, and 24 postpartum. The median values for each parameter were estimated across all study visits; the maternal concentration was 508 ng/mL (290-800 ng/mL), the milk concentration was 1,214 ng/mL (862 to 1651 ng/mL), and the milk/plasma ratio was 2.56. The authors of this study estimated that an infant would receive about 182 µg/kg/day of lamivudine (2% of the infant dose 4 mg/kg twice a day) if they consumed about 150 mL/kg/day of breast milk. We calculated the relative infant dose to be 4.2%, which is equivalent to the infant dose estimated by the authors of this study. The authors also noted that the median infants lamivudine plasma concentration from weeks 2-24 was 23 ng/mL, this was just above the upper limit of the IC50 for HIV (0.6-21 ng/mL). The long-term effects and risk of resistance from these levels in infants who become infected with HIV are unknown at this time.

Another study that evaluated the safety of maternal antiretrovirals for prophylaxis against HIV transmission to the infant during lactation also reported the milk levels of lamivudine (n=206 samples).[5] This study tested maternal serum and breast milk on the day of delivery and at months 1, 3, and 6 postpartum. Infant levels were also taken at months 1, 3, and 6 of age. The median drug concentrations of lamivudine in maternal serum, breast milk, and the infant were 844 ng/mL (430-1,350 ng/mL), 446 ng/mL (269-683 ng/mL), and 18 ng/mL (7-35 ng/mL), respectively. The milk/plasma ratio was 0.59. The relative infant dose that we calculated using the maternal dose of 150 mg twice a day and median milk level was 1.56%. This study reported infant adverse events (e.g. pneumonia, diarrhea, changes in liver function, neutropenia, thrombocytopenia), but was unable to determine which medication caused the effects based on drug levels; please see study for adverse event details.

A publication in 2013 followed women taking antivirals in pregnancy and breastfeeding and studied maternal milk samples 30 days postpartum.[6] Forty-five breast milk samples were available, and the median milk concentration was 0.14 µg/mL. In addition, the median milk to plasma ratio was 0.74. The relative infant dose calculated using this median milk sample and a maternal dose of lamivudine 150 mg bid was 0.5%.

In a 2014 study of HIV RNA in milk and the pharmacokinetics of maternal medications, 30 women were given one Combivir tablet twice a day (zidovudine 300 mg + lamivudine 150 mg/tab) with two tablets of Aluvia twice a day (lopinavir 200 mg + ritonavir 50 mg) starting post delivery until breastfeeding was stopped or 28 weeks.[7] Samples were taken pre-dose (time 0) and then at 2, 4, and 6 hours postdose when the women were enrolled at either 6, 12, or 24 weeks postpartum. The median drug concentrations of lamivudine in maternal serum, breast milk, and the infant were 717 ng/mL (588-945 ng/mL), 944 ng/mL (682-1112 ng/mL), and 18 ng/mL (10-28 ng/mL), respectively. The milk to plasma ratio was 1.21. The RID that we calculated using the maternal dose of 150 mg twice a day and median milk level was 3.3%.

Another study that evaluated lamivudine use in pregnancy to prevent vertical transmission of Hepatitis B reported that 40 infants were breastfed in this study while their mothers took this medication for 4 weeks postpartum; no adverse events were reported that were attributed to medication exposure in breast milk.[8]

Note: This medication is an L5 to highlight the contraindication of breastfeeding when the mother is known to be infected with HIV; this medication is not an L5 based on its risk to the infant in breast milk. The Centers for Disease Control and Prevention recommend that HIV-1 infected mothers do not breastfeed their infants to avoid postnatal transmission of HIV-1.

T 1/2	5-7 h	MW	229 Da	PB	<36%
Tmax	1-1.5 h	RID	0.49% - 6.4%	Vd	0.9-1.7 L/kg
Oral	82%	M/P	3.34	pKa	

Adult Concerns: Headache, fatigue, malaise, lactic acidosis, severe hepatomegaly, pancreatitis, nausea, vomiting, and myalgia.

Adult Dose: 100 mg daily for hepatitis B infections.

Pediatric Concerns: None reported via milk at this time.

Infant Monitoring: Somnolence, vomiting, diarrhea, weakness. Breastfeeding is not recommended in mothers who have HIV.

Alternatives:

References:

1. Moodley J, Moodley D, Pillay K, et al. Pharmacokinetics and antiretroviral activity of lamivudine alone or when coadministered with zidovudine in human immunodeficiency virus type 1-infected pregnant women and their offspring. J Infect Dis. 1998;178(5):1327-1333.
2. Shapiro RL, Holland DT, Capparelli E, et al. Antiretroviral concentrations in breast-feeding infants of women in Botswana receiving antiretroviral treatment. J Infect Dis. 2005 Sep;192(5):720-727.
3. Giuliano M, Guidotti G, Andreotti M, et al. Triple antiviral prophylaxis administered during pregnancy and after delivery significantly reduces breast milk viral load. J Acquir Immune Defic Syndr. 2007;44:286-291.

4. Mirochnick M, Thomas T, Capparelli E, et al. Antiretroviral concentrations in breast-feeding infants of mothers receiving highly active antiretroviral therapy. Antimicrob Agents Chemother. 2009;53(3);1170-1176.
5. Palombi L, Pirillo MF, Andreotti M, et al. Antiretroviral prophylaxis for breastfeeding transmission in Malawi: drug concentrations, virological efficacy and safety. Antivir Ther. 2012;17:1511-1519.
6. Shapiro RL, Rossi S, Ogwu A, et al. Therapeutic levels of lopinavir in late pregnancy and abacavir passage into breast milk in the Mma Bana Study, Botswana. Antivir Ther. 2013;18(4):585-590.
7. Corbett AH, Kayira D, White NR, et al. Antiretroviral pharmacokinetics in mothers and breastfeeding infants from 6 to 24 weeks postpartum: results of the BAN study. Antivir Ther. 2014;19(6):587-595.
8. Greenup AJ, Tan PK, Nguyen V, et al. Efficacy and safety of tenofovir disoproxil fumarate in pregnancy to prevent perinatal transmission of hepatitis B virus. J Hepatol. 2014;61:501-507.

LAMOTRIGINE

Trade: Lamictal, Lamictal XR

Category: Anticonvulsant

LRC: L2 - Significant Data-Compatible

Lamotrigine is a newer anticonvulsant primarily indicated for treatment of simple and complex partial seizures and treatment of manic disorders. In a study of a 24-year-old female receiving 300 mg/day of lamotrigine during pregnancy, the maternal serum and cord levels of lamotrigine at birth were 3.88 µg/mL in the mother and 3.26 µg/mL in the cord blood.[1] By day 22, the maternal serum level was 9.61 µg/mL, the milk concentration was 6.51 mg/L, and the infant's serum level was 2.25 µg/mL. Following a reduction in dose, the prior levels decreased significantly over the next few weeks. The milk/plasma ratio at the highest maternal serum level was 0.562. The estimated infant dose was approximately 2-5 mg per day assuming a maternal dose of 200-300 mg per day. The infant was reported to have developed normally.

In another study of a single mother receiving 200 mg/day lamotrigine, milk levels of lamotrigine immediately prior to the next dose (trough) at steady state were 3.48 mg/L (13.6 µmole).[2] The authors estimated the daily infant dose to be 0.5 mg/kg/day. The above authors suggest that infants, while developing normally, should probably be monitored periodically for plasma levels of lamotrigine.

The manufacturer reports that in a group of five women (no dose listed), breast milk concentrations of lamotrigine ranged from 0.07-5.03 mg/L.[3] Breast milk levels averaged 40-45% of maternal plasma levels. No untoward effects were noted in the infants.

In a study by Ohman of nine breastfeeding women at 3 weeks postpartum, the median milk/plasma ratio was 0.61, and the breastfed infants maintained lamotrigine concentrations of approximately 30% of their mother's plasma levels.[4] The authors estimated the dose to the infant to be 0.2-1 mg/kg/day. No adverse effects were noted in the infants.

One further study of six breastfeeding women taking 175-800 mg/day (mean 400 mg) resulted in average infant doses of 0.45 mg/kg/day, and an average infant plasma concentration of 0.6 mg/L. No adverse effects in the infants were noted.[5]

In a study of four mothers with partial epilepsy on lamotrigine monotherapy, serum levels of lamotrigine in nursing newborns ranged from <1 to 2 µg/mL on day 10 of life.[6] Three babies had lamotrigine levels >1 µg/mL. Lamotrigine levels in newborns were on average 30% (range 20-43%) of the maternal drug level. Unfortunately, no decline was noted in two children with repeat levels at 2 months. The authors suggested significant genetic variability in the infants' ability to metabolize this drug. Close monitoring of the infant plasma levels was recommended.

In a well-done study of 30 women taking lamotrigine for seizures, the average milk/plasma ratio was 0.413.[7] Infant plasma levels were 18.3% of maternal plasma levels. The theoretical daily infant dose was 0.51 mg/kg/day and the relative infant dose was 9.2% (range=3.1-21.1%). Most importantly, this study indicates that there is wide variability in milk levels that seem to be more related to the pharmacogenetic makeup of the individual than the dose. It is important to remember that although the theoretic infant dose in these studies ranges from 0.51 mg/kg/day to perhaps as high as 1 mg/kg/day, this is still significantly less than the therapeutic dose (4.4 mg/kg/day) administered to a 17-day-old infant with neonatal seizures.[8]

One case of severe apnea has been reported in a 16-day-old breastfed infant.[9] In this case, the mother was receiving 850 mg/day (dose increased throughout pregnancy), and had a plasma level of 14.93 µg/mL. The plasma level of the infant was 4.87 µg/mL. Interestingly, the milk/plasma ratio was higher, 0.79 to 0.96, suggesting higher transfer to milk than in the above studies.

In a study of nine women during pregnancy, delivery, and lactation, the median umbilical cord blood to maternal serum was 1.01 (range:0.56-1.42) while the median lamotrigine ratio of breast milk to maternal serum concentration was 0.59 (range 0.35-0.86). It was noted that the concentration in breast milk was found to decrease with time after delivery.[10]

The use of lamotrigine in breastfeeding mothers produces significant plasma levels in some breastfed infants, although they are apparently not high enough to produce side effects in most cases. Exposure in utero is considerably higher, and levels will probably drop postnatally in newborn infants who are breastfed. Nevertheless, it is advisable to monitor the infant's plasma levels closely to ensure safety. In two recent studies by Meador et al, no untoward effects on IQ level were noted in children at age 3 years when exposed to lamotrigine during pregnancy and breastfeeding.[11,12]

A Norwegian study published in 2013 assessed the adverse effects of antiepileptic medications via breast milk in infants who were also exposed in utero.[13] The study evaluated mothers' reports of their children's behavior, motor, social, and language skills at 6, 18, and 36 months using validated screening tools. At age 6 months, infants of mothers using antiepileptic drugs in utero had a significantly higher risk of impaired fine motor skills when compared to control group infants. In addition, infants exposed to multiple antiepileptics also had a greater risk of fine motor and social impairment when compared to control group infants. However, it was noted that continuous breastfeeding in the first 6 months did demonstrate a trend toward improvement in all of the developmental domains. In addition, The study demonstrated that continuous breastfeeding (daily for more than 6 months) in children of women using antiepileptic drugs in utero reduced the impairment in development at 6 and 18 months when compared with those with no breastfeeding or breastfeeding for less than 6 months. At 18 months, children in the drug-exposed group had an increased risk of impaired development compared with the reference group; the risks were highest in children who stopped breastfeeding early. Within the drug-exposed group, this impairment was statistically significant for autistic traits; 22.4% with discontinued breastfeeding were affected compared with 8.7% with prolonged breastfeeding. By 36 months, prenatal antiepileptic drug exposure was associated with impaired development such as autistic traits, reduced sentence completeness, and aggressive symptoms, regardless of breastfeeding during the first year of life. The authors concluded that women with epilepsy should be encouraged to breastfeed regardless of their antiepileptic medication.

In 2014 a prospective observational study looked at long-term neurodevelopment of infants exposed to antiepileptic drugs in utero and lactation.[14] This study included women taking carbamazepine, lamotrigine, phenytoin, or valproate as monotherapy for epilepsy. In this study, 42.9% of the infants were breastfed for a mean of 7.2 months. The IQ of these children at 6 years of age was statistically significantly lower in children who were exposed to valproate in utero (7-13 IQ points lower). It was also noted that higher doses of medication (primarily with valproate) were associated with lower IQ scores. The children's IQ scores were found to be higher if the maternal IQ was higher, the mother took folic acid near the time of conception and if the child was breastfed (4 points higher). In addition, verbal abilities were also found to be significantly higher in children that were breastfed. Although this study has many limitations (e.g. small sample size, difficulties with patient follow-up) it does provide data up to age 6 that suggest benefits of breastfeeding are not outweighed by risks of maternal drug therapy in milk.

Lamotrigine clearance increases during pregnancy and with drug interactions such as concurrent use of hormonal contraceptive drugs. One study recommends to taper the lamotrigine dose on postpartum days 3 and 7 so that by day 10 the woman can be back to her pre-pregnancy dose (or dose + 50 mg/d); this is thought to reduce maternal toxicity (e.g. dizziness, blurred vision, double vision, or imbalance) as maternal clearance returns to the pre-pregnancy state. According to another study, the pre-pregnancy dose can be achieved over 2-3 weeks postpartum. It is recommended to monitor the patient's clinical status and check therapeutic drug levels prior to pregnancy, during each trimester of pregnancy, postpartum, and with the addition or changes to other medications such as hormonal contraceptive regimens.[15,16]

Recently, we were informed of an unpublished case of a breastfed infant presenting early postpartum with a rash and elevated liver enzymes. The rash persisted until the infant discontinued breastfeeding. As a rash is prognostic of lamotrigine toxicity, infants exposed to lamotrigine while breastfeeding who present with a rash, should discontinue breastfeeding until the cause of the rash is determined.

T 1/2	29 h	MW	256 Da	PB	55%
Tmax	1-4 h	RID	9.2% - 18.27%	Vd	0.9-1.3 L/kg
Oral	98%	M/P	0.562	pKa	5.7

Adult Concerns: Headache, faintness, dizziness, drowsiness, fatigue, ataxia, dyspepsia, nausea, vomiting, tremor, and rash.

Adult Dose: 100-400 mg/day.

Pediatric Concerns: There has been one reported case of severe neonatal apnea in an infant.[12] Mild thrombocytosis has also been reported in one study in seven of eight infants (range 329,000-652,000).[7] Breast milk levels are relatively high and reported infant plasma levels are 15-30% of maternal levels.

Infant Monitoring: Sedation or irritability, not waking to feed/poor feeding, weight gain, and rash. Based on clinical symptoms some infants may require monitoring of liver enzymes or CBC.

Alternatives:

References:
1. Rambeck B, Kurlemann G, Stodieck SR, May TW, Jurgens U. Concentrations of lamotrigine in a mother on lamotrigine treatment and her newborn child. Eur J Clin Pharmacol. 1997;51(6):481-484.
2. Tomson T, Ohman I, Vitols S. Lamotrigine in pregnancy and lactation: a case report. Epilepsia. 1997;38(9):1039-1041.

3. Biddlecombe RA. Analysis of breast milk samples for lamotrigine. Internal document BDCR/93/0011. Glaxo-Wellcome 2004.
4. Ohman I, Vitols S, Tomson T. Lamotrigine in pregnancy: pharmacokinetics during delivery, in the neonate, and during lactation. Epilepsia. 2000;41(6):709-713.
5. Page-Sharp M, Kristensen JH, Hackett LP, et al. Transfer of lamotrigine into breast milk. Ann Pharmacother. 2006;40:1470-1471.
6. Liporace J, Kao A, D'Abreu A. Concerns regarding lamotrigine and breast-feeding. Epilepsy Behav. 2004;5(1):102-105.
7. Newport DJ, Pennell PB, Calamaras MR, et al. Lamotrigine in breast milk and nursing infants: determination of exposure. Pediatrics. 2008;122(1):e223-e231.
8. Barr PA, Buettiker VE, Antony JH. Efficacy of lamotrigine in refractory neonatal seizures. Pediatr Neurol. 1999 Feb;20(2):161-163.
9. Nordmo E, Aronsen L, Wasland K, Smabrekke L, Vorren S. Severe apnea in an infant exposed to lamotrigine in breast milk. Ann Pharmacother. 2009 Nov;43(11):1893-1897.
10. Fotopoulou C, Kretz R, Bauer S, et al. Prospectively assessed changes in lamotrigine-concentration in women with epilepsy during pregnancy, lactation and the neonatal period. Epilepsy Res. 2009 Jul;85(1):60-64.
11. Meador KJ, Baker GA, Browning N, et al. Effects of breastfeeding in children of women taking antiepileptic drugs. Neurology. 2010 Nov;75(22):1954-1960.
12. Meador KJ, Baker GA, Browning N, et al. Cognitive function at 3 years of age after fetal exposure to antiepileptic drugs. N Eng J Med. 2009 Apr;360(16):1597-1605.
13. Veiby G, Engelsen BA, Gilhus NE. Early child development and exposure to antiepileptic drugs prenatally and through breastfeeding: a prospective cohort study on children of women with epilepsy. JAMA Neurol. 2013;70(11):1367-1374.
14. Meador KJ, Baker GA, Browning N, et al. Breastfeeding in children of women taking antiepileptic drugs cognitive outcomes at age 6. JAMA Pediatr. 2014;168(8):729-736.
15. Pennell PB, Peng L, Newport DJ, et al. Lamotrigine in pregnancy: clearance, therapeutic drug monitoring, and seizure frequency. Neurology. 2008 May;70(22 Pt 2):2130-2136.
16. Gentile S. Lamotrigine in pregnancy and lactation. Arch Womens Ment Health. 2005 May;8(1):57-58.

LANSOPRAZOLE

Trade: Prevacid, Prevacid NapraPak, Prevpac, Zoton

Category: Gastric Acid Secretion Inhibitor

LRC: L2 - No Data-Probably Compatible

Lansoprazole is a new proton pump inhibitor that suppresses the release of acid protons from the parietal cells in the stomach, effectively raising the pH of the stomach.[1] Lansoprazole is secreted in animal milk; however, there are no human data at this time. Lansoprazole is structurally similar to omeprazole and it is very unstable in stomach acid and to a large degree is denatured by acidity of the infant's stomach. A new study shows milk levels of omeprazole are minimal, it is likely milk levels of lansoprazole would be similar.

T 1/2	1.5 h	MW	369 Da	PB	97%
Tmax	1.7 h	RID		Vd	0.5 L/kg
Oral	80% (Enteric only)	M/P		pKa	8.85

Adult Concerns: Headache, dizziness, nausea, diarrhea, constipation, abdominal pain, changes in liver and renal function, anemia.

Adult Dose: 15-30 mg once daily (varies by indication).

Pediatric Concerns: None reported via milk at this time.

Infant Monitoring: Unlikely to be absorbed while dissolved in milk due to instability in acid.

Alternatives: Omeprazole(L2), Ranitidine(L2), Famotidine(L1)

References:
1. Pharmaceutical manufacturers prescribing information.

LAPATINIB

Trade: Tykerb

Category: Antineoplastic

LRC: L4 - No Data-Possibly Hazardous

Lapatinib is an orally active drug for the treatment of breast cancer (naive, ER+/EGFR+/HER2+ breast cancer patients) (triple positive) and other solid tumors. It is a dual tyrosine kinase inhibitor.[1,2] There are no data available on its use in breastfeeding mothers. Due to its large molecular weight, high volume of distribution, and high protein binding, milk levels will probably be exceedingly low once determined. Withhold breastfeeding for at least 48 to 120 hours.

T 1/2	24 h		MW	943 Da		PB	>99%
Tmax	4 h		RID			Vd	31.4 L/kg
Oral	Poor		M/P			pKa	

Adult Concerns: Alopecia, headache, fatigue, insomnia, shortness of breath, dyspepsia, mucositis, dyspepsia, nausea, vomiting, diarrhea, abdominal pain, anorexia, changes in liver function, weakness, dry skin, skin rashes.

Adult Dose: Varies according to cancer type/treatment.

Pediatric Concerns:

Infant Monitoring: Withhold breastfeeding for at least 48 to 120 hours.

Alternatives:

References:
1. Pharmaceutical manufacturers prescribing information.
2. Medina PJ, Goodin S. Lapatinib: a dual inhibitor of human epidermal growth factor receptor tyrosine kinases. Clin Ther. 2008 Aug;30(8):1426-1447. Review.

LATANOPROST

Trade: Optimol, Xalatan

Category: Antiglaucoma

LRC: L3 - No Data-Probably Compatible

Latanoprost is a prostaglandin F2-alpha analog used ophthalmically for the treatment of ocular hypertension and glaucoma. One drop used daily is usually effective.[1] No data are available on the transfer of this product to human milk, but it is unlikely. Prostaglandins are, by nature, rapidly metabolized. Plasma levels are barely detectable and then only for 1 hour after use. Combined with the short half-life, minimal plasma levels, and poor oral bioavailability, its transfer to milk is extremely unlikely.

T 1/2	<30 min		MW	432.59 Da		PB	
Tmax	<1 h		RID			Vd	0.16 L/kg
Oral	Nil		M/P			pKa	14.47

Adult Concerns: Ocular irritation, headache, rash, muscle aches, joint pain.

Adult Dose: 1 drop in affected eye daily.

Pediatric Concerns: None reported via milk.

Infant Monitoring:

Alternatives:

References:
1. Pharmaceutical manufacturers prescribing information.

LEAD

Trade:

Category: Metals

LRC: L5 - Limited Data-Hazardous

Lead is an environmental pollutant. It serves no useful purpose in the body and tends to accumulate in the body's bony structures based on their exposure. Due to the rapid development of the nervous system, children are particularly sensitive to elevated levels. Lead apparently transfers to human milk at a rate proportional to maternal blood levels, but the absolute degree of transfer is controversial. Studies of milk lead levels vary enormously and probably reflect the enormous difficulty in accurately measuring lead in milk. In mothers who have previously been exposed to high-lead environments, the greatest chance of lead toxicity will be with her first pregnancy. Her blood levels will be highest postpartum because blood lead levels increase during lactation, and her baby's greatest chance of toxicity will be prenatal, because intestinal absorption of lead from milk is low.[1] One study evaluated lead transfer to human milk in a population of women with an average blood lead level of 45 µg/dL (considered very high).[2] The average lead level in milk was 2.47 µg/dL. Using these parameters, the average intake in an infant would be 8.1 µg/kg/day.

The daily permissible level by WHO is 5 µg/kg/day. Using these parameters, mothers contaminated with lead should not breastfeed their infants.

However, in another study of two lactating women whose blood lead levels were 29 and 33 µg/dL, the breast milk levels were <0.005 µg/mL and <0.010 µg/mL respectively.[3] Although both infants had high lead levels (38 µg/dL and 44 µg/dL), it was probably derived from the environment or in utero. Using this data, breastfeeding would appear to be safe. In a larger study of Shanghai mothers (n=165), the transfer of lead to the fetus was highly correlated with maternal blood lead levels (maternal blood vs. cord= 13.2 µg/dL and 6.9 µg/dL).[4] Lead levels in the cord blood and breast milk increased with the lead levels in the maternal blood, with coefficients of correlation of 0.714 and 0.353 respectively. The average concentration of lead in breast milk for 12 occupationally exposed women (lead-exposed jobs) was 52.7 µg/L, which was almost 12 times higher than that for the occupationally non-exposed population (4.43 µg/dL). These results suggest that lead levels in milk could pose a potential health hazard to the breastfed infant but only in those mothers with high plasma lead levels.

In another rather elegant study of milk lead levels, Gulson et.al. collected samples from 21 mothers and 24 infants over a 6-month period.[5] They reported lead concentrations in milk ranging from 0.09-3.1 µg Pb/kg or ppb (mean 0.73 µg/kg) while the blood lead levels were all less than 5 µg/dL with exception of one mother. The major source of lead to the infant during this period was from maternal bone and diet. Nashashibi reports on the transfer of lead from the mother to fetus and into her breast milk.[6] In a group of 47 women, the mean maternal blood lead concentration was 14.9 µg/dL, while in milk the mean lead level was 2 µg/dL. Mean lead level in cord blood was 13.1 µg/dL. These data suggest a close correlation between maternal blood and cord blood lead levels, and maternal blood and milk levels. Lead exposure to military personnel on firing ranges has been questioned. Lead levels in frequent target shooters are known to be elevated as a result of exposure to lead from unjacketed bullets and lead in primers. Breastfeeding mothers should avoid confined, unventilated ranges, but brief exposure to military firing in well-ventilated areas with jacketed bullets is probably safe. Individuals should avoid dust in such areas, sweeping, or cleaning of fire ranges.[7]

In the last decade, the permissible blood level (according to CDC) in children has dropped from 25 to less than 10 µg/dL. Lead poisoning is known to significantly alter IQ and neurobehavioral development, particularly in infants. Therefore, infants receiving breast milk from mothers with high lead levels should be closely monitored, and both mother and infant may require chelation and the infant transferred to formula. Depending on the choice of chelator, mothers undergoing chelation therapy to remove lead may mobilize significant quantities of lead and should not breastfeed during the treatment period unless the chelator is Succimer. For treatment, see entries on Penicillamine and Succimer.

T 1/2	20-30 years (bone)	MW	207 Da	PB	
Tmax		RID		Vd	
Oral	5-10%	M/P		pKa	

Adult Concerns: Constipation, abdominal pain, anemia, anorexia, vomiting, lethargy.

Adult Dose:

Pediatric Concerns: Pediatric lead poisoning, but appears unlikely via milk. More likely environmental.

Infant Monitoring: Constipation, anemia, vomiting, lethargy.

Alternatives:

References:

1. Manton WI, Angle CR, Stanek KL, Kuntzelman D, Reese YR, Kuehnemann TJ. Release of lead from bone in pregnancy and lactation. Environ Res. 2003;92:139-151.
2. Namihira D, Saldivar L, Pustilnik N, Carreon GJ, Salinas ME. Lead in human blood and milk from nursing women living near a smelter in Mexico City. J Toxicol Environ Health. 1993;38(3):225-232.
3. Baum C, Shannon M. Lead-Poisoned lactating women have insignificant lead in breast milk. J Clin Toxicol. 1995;33(5):540-541.
4. Li PJ, Sheng YZ, Wang QY, Gu LY, Wang YL. Transfer of lead via placenta and breast milk in human. Biomed Environ Sci. 2000;13(2):85-89.
5. Gulson BL, Jameson CW, Mahaffey KR, et al. Relationships of lead in breast milk to lead in blood, urine, and diet of the infant and mother. Environ Health Perspect. 1998;106(10):667-674.
6. Nashashibi N, Cardamakis E, Bolbos G, Tzingounis V. Investigation of kinetic of lead during pregnancy and lactation. Gynecol Obstet Invest. 1999;48(3):158-162.
7. Gelberg KH, Depersis R. Lead exposure among target shooters. Arch Environ Occup Health. 2009 Summer;64(2):115-120.

LEDIPASVIR + SOFOSBUVIR

Trade: Harvoni

Category: Antiviral

LRC: L3 - No Data-Probably Compatible

Ledipasvir + sofosbuvir are a combination medication that are part of the new second-generation direct-acting antivirals used to treat chronic hepatitis C (HCV).[1,2] This combination drug can be used on its own or in combination with ribavirin to treat HCV.[2] At present no data are available on the transfer of ledipasvir or sofosbuvir to human milk. The manufacturer reports that ledipasvir and the main inactive metabolite of sofosbuvir (GS-331007; half-life 27 hours) enter rat milk.[1] Based on the pharmacokinetics of both of these medications, we anticipate they will enter human milk to some degree.

Ledipasvir + sofosbuvir in combination with ribavirin is not recommended for use in breastfeeding patients at this time. Ribavirin lacks lactation data but has the potential to accumulate in breast milk because of its long half-life (298 hours at steady-state). See ribavirin monograph for more details.

T 1/2	led: 47 h; Sof: 0.4 h, 27 h (inactive metabolite)	MW	led: 889; sof: 529 Da	PB	led: 99.8%; sof: 61-65%
Tmax	led: 4-4.5 h; sof: 0.5-2 h, 2-4 h (inactive metabolite)	RID		Vd	
Oral		M/P		pKa	

Adult Concerns: Headache, fatigue, insomnia, nausea, diarrhea, changes in liver function, and increased bilirubin.

Adult Dose: One tablet once daily (led: 90 mg + sof: 400 mg).

Pediatric Concerns: No data in lactation at this time.

Infant Monitoring: Changes in sleep or feeding, diarrhea, weight gain; if clinical symptoms arise consider checking liver function and bilirubin.

Alternatives:

References:
1. Pharmaceutical manufacturers prescribing information.
2. Spera AM, Eldin TK, Tosone G, et al. Antiviral therapy for hepatitis C: has anything changed for pregnant/lactation women? World J Hepatol. 2016;8(12):557-565.

LEFLUNOMIDE

Trade: Arava

Category: Anti-Inflammatory

LRC: L5 - No Data-Hazardous

Leflunomide is an anti-inflammatory and immunosuppressant agent used for the treatment of rheumatoid arthritis.[1] Leflunomide is metabolized to an active metabolite teriflunomide, which has a long half-life and slow elimination. This product is a potent immunosuppressant with a potential elevated risk of malignancy, liver injury, hematologic changes, and infection. At this time there are no data regarding its transfer to human milk; use of this product while breastfeeding would not be recommended.

T 1/2	18-19 days	MW	270 Da	PB	99%
Tmax	6-12 h	RID		Vd	0.16 L/kg
Oral	80%	M/P		pKa	10.41

Adult Concerns: Alopecia, headache, dizziness, changes in sleep, hypertension, chest pain, respiratory tract infections, nausea, vomiting, abdominal pain, diarrhea, changes in liver function, hypokalemia, hyperglycemia, pancytopenia, severe skin rashes.

Adult Dose: 20 mg daily.

Pediatric Concerns: None reported via milk at this time.

Infant Monitoring: Not recommended in lactation.

Alternatives:

References:
1. Pharmaceutical manufacturers prescribing information.

LENOGRASTIM

Trade: Granocyte, Neutrogin

Category: Hematopoietic

LRC: L4 - No Data-Possibly Hazardous

Lenograstim is a Granulocyte Colony Stimulating Factor (GCSF) that is identical to native GCSF. Lenograstim can be used for numerous indications; one of the main indications is to decrease the risk of infection and duration of neutropenia in those with non-myeloid malignancies receiving myelosuppressive chemotherapy.[1] Lenograstim enters the milk of both rats and humans.[1,2]

A 30-year-old breastfeeding mother (4 months postpartum) was a peripheral blood stem cell transplant donor for her sister. This woman was given lenograstim 300 µg/day sc on day 1 and then 600 µg/day sc on days 2-4 after she stopped breastfeeding.[2] On day 4 the WBC increased so rapidly that her dose was decreased to 300 µg/day for days 5 and 6. The GCSF was measured in this woman's milk before and after she was given lenograstim. Before administration the level of GCSF was <5 pg/mL; the peak milk level after administration occurred on days 6 and was 85.7 pg/mL.

Endogenous GCSF in human milk is apparently protected from degradation and is absorbed from specific GCSF receptors expressed on the villous enterocytes of the infant.[2] Until the safety of exogenously administered GCSF is assessed and the absorption in the neonates gut is quantified, use in lactation is not recommended unless the infant's white blood cell count is also monitored.

T 1/2	2.3-7.5 h sc; 0.8- 4 h IV	MW	20,000 Da	PB	
Tmax	6 h sc	RID		Vd	0.052 L/kg
Oral		M/P		pKa	

Adult Concerns: Headache, fever, cough, shortness of breath, Adults Respiratory Distress Syndrome (ARDS), changes in liver function, bone pain, malaise, injection site reactions.

Adult Dose: 5-10 µg/kg once daily subcutaneously or IV.

Pediatric Concerns: No reports of infants exposed to lenograstim in lactation are available at this time. Pediatric data exists for children greater than 4.5 months of age.

Infant Monitoring: Irritability, unexplained fever, difficulty breathing; if clinical suspicion of adverse effects a CBC or LFTs could be drawn.

Alternatives:

References:
1. Pharmaceutical manufacturers prescribing information.
2. Shibata H, Yamane T, Aoyama Y, et al. Excretion of granulocyte colony stimulating factor into human breast milk. Acta Haematol. 2003;110:200-201.

LETROZOLE

Trade: Femara

Category: Aromatase Inhibitor

LRC: L5 - No Data-Hazardous

Letrozole is a non-competitive inhibitor of estrogen synthesis, and it is used for the treatment of estrogen-dependent tumors, particularly breast cancer and sometimes for the inducing of ovulation in infertile women. Letrozole's terminal elimination half-life is about 2 days and steady-state plasma concentration after daily 2.5 mg dosing is reached in 2-6 weeks.[1] It has a high volume of distribution and is generally used for long periods. It is well absorbed orally. No data are available on its transfer to human milk but one should expect the levels are low.

However, this product works irreversibly and any present in milk could potentially suppress estrogen levels in a breastfed infant. The transfer of small amounts of this agent to an infant could seriously impair bone growth or sexual development of an infant and for this reason it is probably somewhat hazardous to use in a breastfeeding mother. It has a very long half-life, which is concerning in a breastfed infant and could lead to higher plasma levels over time. It is not advisable to breastfeed an infant while consuming this product. Discontinue breastfeeding while taking this product or for a period of 10 days following its discontinuation.

T 1/2	48 h	MW	285 Da	PB	Weak
Tmax		RID		Vd	1.9 L/kg
Oral	90%	M/P		pKa	

Adult Concerns: Fatigue, chest pain, edema, hot flushes, hypertension, nausea, constipation, diarrhea, vomiting, bone pain, back pain, arthralgia, limb pain, dyspnea, cough, and chest wall pain.

Adult Dose: 2.5 mg daily.

Pediatric Concerns: None reported via milk, but this agent is probably too hazardous to use in a breastfeeding woman.

Infant Monitoring: AVOID in lactation.

Alternatives:

References:
1. Pharmaceutical manufacturers prescribing information.

LEUCOVORIN CALCIUM

Trade: Fusilev

Category: Vitamin

LRC: L3 - No Data-Probably Compatible

Leucovorin is an active form of folic acid, also known as the methotrexate rescue drug. Its active component is folinic acid and its active metabolite is 5-methyltetrahydrofolate. The oral administration of leucovorin causes a significant increase in plasma folate activity. This property has been employed in the management of methotrexate toxicity as well as toxicities due to other anti-folates such as pyrimethamine and trimethoprim. Leucovorin is also used for the management of folate-deficient megaloblastic anemia, and in advanced colorectal cancer.[1] Currently there are no studies available on the transfer of leucovorin to human milk. However, considering that leucovorin is basically an active form of folic acid, which is a physiological nutrient, it is highly unlikely that leucovorin should cause any significant harm to the breastfed infant.

When using this medication in lactation, consider the indication. If treating an adverse effect of another drug, consider its suitability in lactation.

T 1/2	3.5-5.7 h (oral), 6.2 h (IV or IM)	MW	511.51 Da	PB	
Tmax	1.72-2.3 h (oral), 52 min (IM), 10 min (IV)	RID		Vd	
Oral	97%	M/P		pKa	

Adult Concerns: Diarrhea, nausea, vomiting, stomatitis, fatigue, and hypersensitivity reaction.

Adult Dose: Do not exceed 25 mg oral dose.

Pediatric Concerns:

Infant Monitoring: Vomiting, diarrhea.

Alternatives:

References:
1. Pharmaceutical manufacturers prescribing information.

LEUPROLIDE ACETATE

Trade: Eligard, Lupron, Prostap, Viadur

Category: Gonadotropin Releasing Hormone Agonist

LRC: L5 - No Data-Hazardous

Leuprolide is a synthetic nonapeptide analog of naturally occurring gonadotropin-releasing hormone with greater potency than the naturally occurring hormone. After initial stimulation, it inhibits gonadotropin release from the pituitary and after sustained use, suppresses ovarian and testicular hormone synthesis (2-4 weeks).[1] Almost complete suppression of estrogen, progesterone, and testosterone occurs.[2] It is not known whether leuprolide transfers to human milk, but due to its nonapeptide structure, it is not likely that its transfer would be extensive. In addition, animal studies have found that it has zero oral bioavailability; therefore, it is unlikely it would be orally bioavailable in the human infant if ingested via milk. Its effect on lactation is unknown, but it could suppress lactation particularly early postpartum. Leuprolide would reduce estrogen and progestin levels to menopausal ranges, which could potentially suppress lactation. Interestingly, several studies show no change in prolactin levels although these were not in lactating women. One study of a hyperprolactinemic patient showed significant suppression of prolactin which is the reason for the L5 risk categorization. It is of little risk to the breastfed infant, only to milk production.

T 1/2	3.6 h	MW	1400 Da	PB	43-49%
Tmax	4-6 h	RID		Vd	0.52 L/kg
Oral	None	M/P		pKa	9.6

Adult Concerns: Vasomotor hot flashes, gynecomastia, edema, bone pain, thrombosis, and gastrointestinal disturbances, body odor, fever, headache.

Adult Dose: 3.75 mg every month.

Pediatric Concerns: May suppress lactation, particularly early in lactation.

Infant Monitoring:

Alternatives:

References:
1. Sennello LT, Finley RA, Chu SY, et al. Single-dose pharmacokinetics of leuprolide in humans following intravenous and subcutaneous administration. J Pharm Sci. 1986;75(2):158-160.
2. Chantilis SJ, Barnett-Hamm C, Byrd WE, Carr BR. The effect of gonadotropin-releasing hormone agonist on thyroid-stimulating hormone and prolactin secretion in adult premenopausal women. Fertil Steril. 1995;64(4):698-702.

LEVALBUTEROL

Trade: Xopenex

Category: Antiasthma

LRC: L2 - No Data-Probably Compatible

Levalbuterol is the active (R)-enantiomer of the drug substance racemic albuterol. It is a popular and new bronchodilator used in asthmatics.[1] No data are available on breast milk levels. After inhalation, plasma levels are incredibly low averaging 1.1 ng/mL. It is very unlikely that enough would enter milk to produce clinical effects in an infant. This product is used in children for asthma and other causes of bronchospasm.

T 1/2	3.3 h	MW	275 Da	PB	
Tmax	0.5 (inhalation)	RID		Vd	27.14 L/kg
Oral	100%	M/P		pKa	9.621

Adult Concerns: Tachycardia, tremors, dizziness, dyspepsia.

Adult Dose: 90 µg every 4-6 h as needed.

Pediatric Concerns: None reported via milk.

Infant Monitoring: Irritability, insomnia, arrhythmias, weight loss, tremor.

Alternatives:

References:
1. Pharmaceutical manufacturers prescribing information.

LEVETIRACETAM

Trade: Keppra

Category: Anticonvulsant

LRC: L2 - Limited Data-Probably Compatible

Levetiracetam is a popular broad-spectrum antiepileptic agent. In a study of a single patient who received levetiracetam at 7 days postpartum (dose unreported), the breast milk concentrations of levetiracetam were 99 µmol three hours after administration. The corresponding plasma levels were 32 µmol (milk/plasma ratio= 3.09). The mother was also ingesting phenytoin (3 x 100 mg/day) as well as valproic acid (4 x 500 mg/day). The infant was preterm (36 weeks) and unstable at birth. After the addition of levetiracetam at day 7, the infant became increasingly hypotonic and fed poorly. The infant was removed from the breast and 96 hours later the infant's plasma levetiracetam levels were 6 µmol. The authors strongly advise avoidance of levetiracetam and close monitoring of the infant in breastfeeding mothers.[1] In this case, the infant was exposed to three anticonvulsants, and it is difficult to suggest that levetiracetam was solely responsible for the hypnotic condition. This is further supported by the study below.

In another study of eight women receiving 1500 to 3500 mg/day who were studied at birth (seven patients) and one at 10 months, the mean umbilical cord serum/maternal serum ratio was 1.14 (n=4) at birth suggesting extensive transport of levetiracetam to the fetus.[2] The mean milk/maternal serum concentration ratio was 1 (range, 0.7-1.33) at 3 to 5 days after delivery (n= 7). Maternal milk levels ranged from 28 to 153 µmol(4.8-26 µg/mL) but averaged 74 µmol(12.6 mg/L). At 3 to 5 days after delivery, the infants had very low levetiracetam serum concentrations <10-15 µmol(1.7-2.5 µg/mL), a finding that persisted during continued breastfeeding. One infant had a levetiracetam level of 77 µmol(13 µg/mL) at day 1, but <10 µmol at day 4, suggesting infants clear this product rapidly, and that breastfeeding contributes only a minimal dose. No adverse effects were noted in any of the breastfeeding infants. The authors conclude that levetiracetam passes to the infant, but breastfed infants have very low serum concentrations, suggesting a rapid elimination of levetiracetam.

Another study of 14 women receiving 1000 to 3000 mg per day had a milk/plasma ratio of 1.05, with an infant dose of 2.4 mg/kg/day, or 7.9% of the maternal dose. Plasma concentrations in the infants were 13% of those in the mother's plasma, ranging from 4 to 20 µmol/L. There was no evidence of accumulation of levetiracetam in this study. The authors suggest that this study should be reassuring for breastfeeding mothers taking levetiracetam.[3]

T 1/2	6-8 h	MW	170 Da	PB	<10%
Tmax	1 h	RID	3.4% - 7.8%	Vd	0.7 L/kg
Oral	100%	M/P	1	pKa	

Adult Concerns: Headache, dizziness, somnolence, irritability, hypertension, anorexia, nausea, vomiting, constipation, abdominal pain, ataxia, weakness.

Adult Dose: 1000 - 3000 mg daily.

Pediatric Concerns: No adverse effects reported in one study of eight patients and in another with 14 patients. One case report of an infant that became increasingly hypotonic and fed poorly after addition of levetiracetam; however, it should be noted that this infant was exposed to multiple seizure medications in milk.[1]

Infant Monitoring: Sedation or irritability, not waking to feed/poor feeding, and weight gain.

Alternatives: Gabapentin(L2), Lamotrigine(L2)

References:
1. Kramer G, Hosli I, Glanzmann R, et al. Levetiracetam accumulation in human breast milk. Epilepsia. 2002;43(supplement 7):105.
2. Johannessen SI, Helde G, Brodtkorb E. Levetiracetam concentrations in serum and in breast milk at birth and during lactation. Epilepsia. 2005;46:775-777.
3. Tomson T, Palm R, Källén K, et al. Pharmacokinetics of levetiracetam during pregnancy, delivery, in the neonatal period, and lactation. Epilepsia. 2007;48(6):1111-1116.

LEVMETAMFETAMINE

Trade: Vicks Vapor Inhaler

Category: Decongestant

LRC: L3 - No Data-Probably Compatible

Levmetamfetamine is the levorotary (R-enantiomer) of methamphetamine and is used topically as a nasal decongestant.[1] Levmetamfetamine is used as a nasal decongestant for the temporary relief of nasal congestion due to a cold, hay fever, or other upper respiratory allergies. While it produces local vasoconstriction, it has few CNS effects in humans. There are no data on the use of this product in breastfeeding women. Some will probably transfer to human milk, although its oral absorption is probably low and the clinical side effects in an infant are probably minimal.

T 1/2	9-20 h	MW	149.2 Da	PB	
Tmax		RID		Vd	
Oral	Low	M/P		pKa	

Adult Concerns: Dizziness, hypertension, tachycardia, temporary burning, stinging, sneezing, and increased nasal discharge. Increased nasal congestion with prolonged use.

Adult Dose:

Pediatric Concerns: Observe for tachycardia, and symptoms of sympathetic stimulation.

Infant Monitoring: Irritability, poor sleep, poor feeding, tremor, weight loss.

Alternatives:

References:
1. Pharmaceutical manufacturers prescribing information.

LEVOBUNOLOL

Trade: Betegan, Ophtho-Bunolol

Category: Antiglaucoma

LRC: L3 - No Data-Probably Compatible

Levobunolol is an ophthalmic beta-blocker used to treat glaucoma.[1] Some systemic absorption has been reported, with resultant bradycardia in patients. No data on transfer to human milk are available. Use with caution.

T 1/2	6.1 h	MW	291 Da	PB	
Tmax	3 h	RID		Vd	5.5 L/kg
Oral	Complete	M/P		pKa	14.09

Adult Concerns: Headache, dizziness, fatigue, lethargy, bradycardia, hypotension.

Adult Dose: 1-2 drops twice daily.

Pediatric Concerns: None reported via milk, but transfer of other beta-blockers is reported.

Infant Monitoring: Lethargy, apnea, bradycardia, hypotension.

Alternatives:

References:
1. Pharmaceutical manufacturers prescribing information.

LEVOCABASTINE

Trade: Livostin

Category: Antihistamine

LRC: L3 - No Data-Probably Compatible

Levocabastine is an antihistamine primarily used via nasal spray and eye drops.[1] It is used for allergic rhinitis and ophthalmic allergies.[1] After application to eye or nose, very low levels are attained in the systemic circulation (<1 ng/mL). In one nursing mother, it was calculated that the daily dose of levocabastine in the infant was about 0.5 µg, far too low to be clinically relevant.

T 1/2	33-40 h	MW	420.52 Da	PB	
Tmax	1-2 h	RID		Vd	
Oral	100%	M/P		pKa	

Adult Concerns: Sedation, dry mouth, fatigue, eye and nasal irritation.

Adult Dose: 1 drop in each eye four times daily or 2 sprays in each nostril bid.

Pediatric Concerns: None reported via milk.

Infant Monitoring: Sedation, dry mouth.

Alternatives:

References:
1. Pharmaceutical manufacturers prescribing information.

LEVOCARNITINE

Trade: Carnitor, Carnitor SF

Category: Dietary Supplement

LRC: L3 - No Data-Probably Compatible

Levocarnitine supplements carnitine, a natural metabolic compound that facilitates the transfer of fatty acids into the mitochondria, thus ensuring energy production. A deficiency can be associated with excess acyl CoA esters and disruption of intermediary metabolism.[1] Supplementation has not been studied in nursing mothers but it is not likely hazardous.

T 1/2	17.4 h	MW	161 Da	PB	Low
Tmax	3.3 h	RID		Vd	
Oral	10-20%	M/P		pKa	4.2

Adult Concerns: Injection site pain, hypotension, diarrhea, hypervolemia, and pharyngitis.

Adult Dose: 990 mg two to three times/day.

Pediatric Concerns: No data available.

Infant Monitoring:

Alternatives:

References:
1. Pharmaceutical manufacturers prescribing information.

LEVOCETIRIZINE

Trade: Xyzal

Category: Antihistamine

LRC: L2 - No Data-Probably Compatible

Levocetirizine is a third-generation non-sedating antihistamine. It is the active metabolite (L-enantiomer) of cetirizine.[1] It has twice the binding affinity at the H1-receptor compared to cetirizine. No data on the transfer to human milk are available at this time. Just as with cetirizine, it is probably compatible with breastfeeding.

T 1/2	8 h	MW	389 Da	PB	92%
Tmax	1 h	RID		Vd	0.4 L/kg
Oral	Complete	M/P		pKa	

Adult Concerns: Sedation, fatigue, dry mouth.

Adult Dose: 5 mg daily.

Pediatric Concerns: None reported via milk.

Infant Monitoring: Sedation, dry mouth.

Alternatives:

References:
1. Pharmaceutical manufacturers prescribing information.

LEVOFLOXACIN

Trade: Levaquin, Quixin

Category: Antibiotic, Quinolone

LRC: L2 - Limited Data-Probably Compatible

Levofloxacin is a pure (S) enantiomer of the racemic fluoroquinolone ofloxacin.[1] In one case report of a mother receiving 500 mg/day, the 24-hour average milk level was reported to be approximately 5 µg/mL.[2] A peak level of 8.2 µg/mL was reported, and occurred at 5 hours after the dose. The half-life of levofloxacin in milk was estimated to be

7 hours, which would result in undetectable amounts in milk after 48 hours. The authors report the absolute infant dose would be 1.23 mg/kg/day, although this was calculated from the highest milk level of eight samples. While the peak levels were reported to be 8.2 μg/mL, the average milk level reported was 5 μg/mL. Using this data, the relative infant dose would range from 10.5% to 17%. However, the time-to-peak interval reported in this case was 5 hours, rather than 1-1.8 hours reported following both oral and IV doses in the prescribing information. Of the 10 reported levels in this study, only one was above 5 μg/mL. Thus, the reported average level of 5 μg/mL is probably consistent with other data. This suggests a milk/plasma ratio of approximately 0.95, which is probably correct. Thus, levofloxacin concentrations in milk peak around 1-1.8 hours and at levels close to maternal plasma levels.

Because fluoroquinolones have limited safety data in pediatric and breastfeeding patients, use during lactation is not recommended if alternative therapies exist.[1]

T 1/2	6-8 h	MW	370 Da	PB	24-38%
Tmax	1-1.8 h	RID	10.5% - 17.2%	Vd	1.27 L/kg
Oral	99%	M/P	0.95	pKa	6.05, 8.22

Adult Concerns: Nausea, vomiting, diarrhea, abdominal cramps, gastrointestinal bleeding.

Adult Dose: 500 mg daily.

Pediatric Concerns: None reported in one case report.

Infant Monitoring: Vomiting, diarrhea, changes in gastrointestinal flora and rash.

Alternatives:

References:
1. Pharmaceutical manufacturers prescribing information.
2. Cahill JB, Bailey EM, Chien S, Johnson GM. Levofloxacin secretion in breast milk: a case report. Pharmacother. 2005;25(1):116-118.

LEVOMILNACIPRAN

Trade: Fetzima

Category: Antidepressant, other

LRC: L3 - No Data-Probably Compatible

Levomilnacipran is a selective serotonin and norepinephrine reuptake inhibitor (SNRI) that is used in the treatment of depression.[1] At this time there is no data regarding the transfer of levomilnacipran to human milk; the manufacturer states that this drug is secreted in rat milk. Based on this medication's half-life, low protein binding, and small molecular weight, we anticipate it will enter milk.

In addition, there is some lactation data regarding the use of a similar medication, milnacipran, which is used to treat fibromyalgia. According to a single study where eight lactating women received a single dose of 50 mg of milnacipran hydrochloride, it was found that milnacipran transfers to human milk. Based on peak plasma concentrations, the maximum estimated daily infant dose was 5% of the maternal dose. It should be noted that the kinetics of levomilnacipran and milnacipran are slightly different.

T 1/2	12 h	MW	282.8 Da	PB	22%
Tmax	6-8 h	RID		Vd	5.5-6.8 L/kg
Oral	92%	M/P		pKa	

Adult Concerns: Agitation, aggressive behavior, anxiety, dry eyes, tachycardia, palpitations, orthostatic hypotension, nausea, vomiting, constipation, urinary hesitancy, changes in liver function, extrapyramidal symptoms, dry skin.

Adult Dose: 40 to 120 mg once daily.

Pediatric Concerns:

Infant Monitoring: Sedation or irritability, not waking to feed/poor feeding, constipation, decreased wet diapers, weight gain.

Alternatives: Sertraline(L2), Citalopram(L2), Escitalopram(L2), Duloxetine(L3)

References:
1. Pharmaceutical manufacturers prescribing information.

LEVOTHYROXINE

Trade: Eltroxin, Levothroid, Levoxyl, Oroxine, Synthroid, Thyroid, Thyroxine, Tirosint, Unithroid

Category: Thyroid Supplement

LRC: L1 - Limited Data-Compatible

Levothyroxine is also called T4. Most studies indicate that minimal levels of maternal thyroid are transferred to human milk, and further, that the amount secreted is extremely low and insufficient to protect a hypothyroid infant even while nursing.[1-3] The amount secreted after supplementing a breastfeeding mother is highly controversial and numerous reports conflict. Anderson[4] indicates that levothyroxine is not detectable in breast milk although others using sophisticated assay methods have shown extremely low levels (4 ng/mL). It is generally recognized that some thyroxine will transfer but the amount will be extremely low. It is important to remember that supplementation with levothyroxine is designed to bring the mother to a euthyroid state, which is equivalent to the normal breastfeeding female. Hence, the risk of using exogenous thyroxine is no different than in a normal euthyroid mother. Liothyronine (T3) appears to transfer to milk in higher concentrations than levothyroxine (T4), but liothyronine is seldom used in clinical medicine due to its short half-life (2.5 days).

T 1/2	6-7 days	MW	798 Da	PB	99%
Tmax	2-4 h	RID		Vd	
Oral	50-80%	M/P		pKa	7.43

Adult Concerns: Nervousness, tremor, agitation, weight loss.

Adult Dose: 75-125 µg daily.

Pediatric Concerns: None reported via milk.

Infant Monitoring:

Alternatives:

References:
1. Mizuta H, Amino N, Ichihara K, et al. Thyroid hormones in human milk and their influence on thyroid function of breast-fed babies. Pediatr Res. 1983;17(6):468-471.
2. Oberkotter LV. Thyroid function and human breast milk. Am J Dis Child. 1983;137(11):1131.
3. Sack J, Amado O, Lunenfeld B. Thyroxine concentration in human milk. J Clin Endocrinol Metab. 1977;45(1):171-173.

LIDOCAINE

Trade: Burn-O-Jel, Burnamycin, Lidoderm, Topicaine, Xylocaine

Category: Anesthetic, Local

LRC: L2 - Limited Data-Probably Compatible

Lidocaine is an antiarrhythmic and a local anesthetic. It is used intravenously, orally, and topically. In one study of a breastfeeding mother who received IV lidocaine for ventricular arrhythmias, the mother received approximately 965 mg over 7 hours including the bolus starting doses.[1] At 7 hours, breast milk samples were drawn and the concentration of lidocaine was 0.8 mg/L or 40% of the maternal plasma level (2 mg/L). Assuming that the mother's plasma was maintained at 5 µg/mL (therapeutic= 1.5-5 µg/mL), an infant consuming 1 L per day of milk would ingest approximately 2 mg/day. This amount is exceedingly low in view of the fact that the oral bioavailability of lidocaine is very poor (35%). The lidocaine dose recommended for pediatric arrhythmias is 1 mg/kg given as a bolus. Once absorbed by the liver, lidocaine is rapidly metabolized. These authors suggest that a mother could continue to breastfeed while on parenteral lidocaine. Dryden and Lo have reported the transfer of lidocaine following tumescent liposuction in a 80-kg patient.[2] The areas undergoing liposuction were infiltrated with a 52.5 mg/kg dose of lidocaine dissolved in 8400 mL of solution (total= 4200 mg). Milk samples were drawn 17 hours, and plasma levels were drawn 18 hours following the procedure because other studies show lidocaine peaks in the plasma compartment at this time postoperatively. Milk levels of lidocaine were 0.55 mg/L while plasma levels were 1.2 mg/L. Breast milk levels were 46% of the serum level. The authors conclude that it is unlikely that toxic levels would be reached in a nursing infant.

In a study of 27 parturients who received an average of 82.1 mg bupivacaine and 183.3 mg lidocaine via an epidural catheter, lidocaine milk levels at 2, 6, and 12 hours post administration were 0.86, 0.46, and 0.22 mg/L respectively.[3] Levels of bupivacaine in milk at 2, 6, and 12 hours were 0.09, 0.06, and 0.04 mg/L respectively. The milk/serum ratio bases upon area under the curve values (AUC) were 1.07 and 0.34 for lidocaine and bupivacaine respectively. Based on AUC data of lidocaine and bupivacaine milk levels, the average milk concentration of these agents over 12 hours was 0.5 and 0.07 mg/L. Most of the infants had a maximal APGAR score. In a study of seven nursing mothers who received 3.6-7.2 mL of 2% lidocaine without adrenaline, the concentration of lidocaine in milk 3 and 6 hours after injection averaged 97.5 µg/L and 52.7 µg/L respectively.[4] These authors suggest that mothers who receive local injections of lidocaine can safely breastfeed.

When administered as a local anesthetic for dental and other surgical procedures, only small quantities are used, generally less than 40 mg. However, following liposuction, the amount used via instillation in the tissues is quite high. Nevertheless, maternal plasma and milk levels do not seem to approach high concentrations and the oral bioavailability in the infant would be quite low (<35%). The topical application of lidocaine preparations to the nipple is not recommended. Oral doses as low as 100 mg have produced seizures in toddlers. Doses in infants would be much less. Two toddlers developed seizures following a dose of 15 mg/kg of 1% dibucaine ointment. For viscous lidocaine (2%) in infants and children less than 3 years of age, no more than 1.25 mL (equivalent to 25 mg) should be applied topically to the skin every 3 hours. Thus topical use to a mother's nipple is potentially hazardous.

Lidocaine patches (Lidoderm) transfer minimal levels to the plasma compartment. Following exposure to three patches on the back over a 36-hour period, plasma levels at 12 hours after application of each patch were only 130 ng/mL (Cmax=11 hours). Levels in milk would likely be insignificant.

Following the use of tumescent lidocaine for liposuction, doses of lidocaine are quite high and with added epinephrine, the elimination half-life is greatly extended requiring up to 24 hours or longer for complete elimination. Following doses of 19.4 to 52 mg/kg with liposuction, elevated plasma levels peaked at 12 hours and were sustained beyond 24 hours.[5] Mothers undergoing liposuction or other procedures using these high doses should avoid breastfeed for at least 48 hours.

T 1/2	1.8 h	MW	234 Da	PB	70%
Tmax	Immediate (IM, IV)	RID	0.5% - 3.1%	Vd	1.3 L/kg
Oral	<35%	M/P	0.4	pKa	7.9

Adult Concerns: Bradycardia, confusion, cardiac arrest, drowsiness, seizures, bronchospasm.

Adult Dose: Varies by indication.

Pediatric Concerns: None reported via milk. However, oral doses as low as 100 mg have produced seizures in toddlers. Doses via milk would be much less. Two toddlers developed seizures following a dose of 15 mg/kg of 1% dibucaine ointment.

Infant Monitoring:

Alternatives:

References:

1. Zeisler JA, Gaarder TD, De Mesquita SA. Lidocaine excretion in breast milk. Drug Intell Clin Pharm. 1986;20(9):691-693.
2. Dryden RM, Lo MW. Breast milk lidocaine levels in tumescent liposuction. Plast Reconstr Surg. 2000;105(6):2267-2268.
3. Ortega D, Viviand X, Lorec AM, Gamerre M, Martin C, Bruguerolle B. Excretion of lidocaine and bupivacaine in breast milk following epidural anesthesia for cesarean delivery. Acta Anaesthesiol Scand. 1999;43(4):394-397.
4. Giuliani M, Grossi GB, Pileri M, Lajolo C, Casparrini G. Could local anesthesia while breast-feeding be harmful to infants? J Pediatr Gastroenterol Nutr. 2001;32(2):142-144.
5. Klein JA, Jeske DR. Estimated maximal safe dosages of tumescent lidocaine. Anesth Analg. 2016 May;122(5):1350-1359.

LINACLOTIDE

Trade: Linzess

Category: Gastrointestinal Agent

LRC: L3 - No Data-Probably Compatible

Linaclotide is a guanylate cyclase-C (GC-C) enzyme agonist used to treat irritable bowel syndrome with constipation and chronic idiopathic constipation.[1] Both the parent drug and its active metabolite bind to the GC-C enzyme and act on the luminal surface of the intestine. This results in an increase in secretion of chloride and bicarbonate into the intestinal lumen, resulting in increased intestinal fluid and quicker gastrointestinal transit. Both linaclotide and its active metabolite are degraded in the intestinal lumen to smaller peptides and natural amino acids that are excreted in the stool. Linaclotide is minimally absorbed with negligible systemic availability following oral administration.

It is not known if linaclotide is excreted in human milk.[1] However, its ability to transfer into human milk is probably low because neither the parent drug or its active metabolite is measurable in plasma following the recommended oral dose.

T 1/2		MW	1526.8 Da	PB	
Tmax		RID		Vd	
Oral		M/P		pKa	

Adult Concerns: Gastroesophageal reflux disease (GERD), vomiting, diarrhea, abdominal pain, flatulence.

Adult Dose: Irritable bowel syndrome: 290 μg once daily; Chronic idiopathic constipation: 145 μg once daily.

Pediatric Concerns: Contraindicated in pediatric patients less than 6 years of age due to deaths in juvenile mice after 1-2 daily doses.

Infant Monitoring: Diarrhea, dehydration.

Alternatives:

References:
1. Pharmaceutical manufacturers prescribing information.

LINAGLIPTIN

Trade: Tradjenta

Category: Antidiabetic, other

LRC: L3 - No Data-Probably Compatible

Linagliptin is a dipeptidyl peptidase IV (DPP-4) inhibitor. Inhibition of this enzyme prolongs active incretin levels, which increases insulin release and decreases glucagon secretion in the presence of elevated plasma glucose.[1] This medication does not appear to increase the risk of hypoglycemia in healthy subjects. There are no data available on the transfer of linagliptin to human milk. Levels will probably be quite low due to its size and kinetics. The infant's growth should be monitored carefully until data support the safe use of this drug in breastfeeding women.

T 1/2	12 h	MW	472.54 Da	PB	70-80%
Tmax	1.5 h	RID		Vd	15.9 L/kg
Oral	30%	M/P	4:1 in animals	pKa	8.6

Adult Concerns: Nasopharyngitis, cough, diarrhea, hypersensitivity, myalgia, pancreatitis.

Adult Dose: 5 mg daily.

Pediatric Concerns:

Infant Monitoring: Signs of hypoglycemia- drowsiness, lethargy, pallor, sweating, tremor.

Alternatives:

References:
1. Pharmaceutical manufacturer prescribing information.

LINDANE

Trade: Desintan, Hexit, Kwell, Kwellada, Quellada, Scabene

Category: Pediculicide

LRC: L4 - Limited Data-Possibly Hazardous

Lindane is an older pesticide also called gamma benzene hexachloride. It is primarily indicated for treatment of pediculus capitis (head lice) and less so for scabies (crab lice).[1] Lindane has been banned in California, the United Kingdom, and many western countries due to concerns about neurotoxicity and adverse effects on the environment. Because of its lipophilic nature, it is significantly absorbed through the skin of neonates (up to 13%) and has produced elevated liver enzymes, seizures, and hypersensitivity. Lindane is transferred into human milk although the exact amounts are unpublished. Estimates by the manufacturer indicate that the total daily dose of an infant ingesting 1 L of milk daily (30 ng/mL) would be approximately 30 μg/day, an amount that would probably be clinically insignificant. Although there are reports of some resistance, head lice and scabies should generally be treated with permethrin and other products (NIX, Elimite), which are much safer in pediatric patients.

T 1/2	18-21 h	MW	290 Da	PB	
Tmax	6 h	RID		Vd	
Oral		M/P		pKa	

Adult Concerns: Dermatitis, seizures (excess dose), nervousness, irritability, anxiety, insomnia, dizziness, aplastic anemia, thrombocytopenia, neutropenia.

Adult Dose: Topical.

Pediatric Concerns: Potential CNS toxicity includes lethargy, disorientation, restlessness, and tonic-clonic seizures.

Infant Monitoring: Seizures, irritability, insomnia.

Alternatives: Malathion(L3), Permethrin(L2)

References:
1. Pharmaceutical manufacturers prescribing information.

LINEZOLID

Trade: Zyvox, Zyvoxam, Zyvoxid

Category: Antibiotic, Other

LRC: L3 - Limited Data-Probably Compatible

Linezolid is an oxazolidinone antibiotic primarily used for Gram-positive infections.[1] It is active against many strains, including methicillin-resistant *Staphylococcus aureus* (MRSA), vancomycin-resistant *Enterococcus faecium* (VREF), and others. Linezolid was found in the milk of lactating rats at concentrations similar to plasma levels although the dose administered, and milk concentrations were not reported in the product monograph.

In 2009, a 32-year-old healthy breastfeeding volunteer took a single 600-mg oral dose of linezolid; this study quantified the amount of linezolid in breast milk and determined that the AUC0-24 was 100.79 µg.h/mL (C_{avg} = 4.2 µg/mL and the C_{max} in milk was 12.36 µg/mL).[2] The relative infant doses were calculated based on both the C_{avg} and C_{max} (over estimate) and were found to be 3.67% and 10.81%, respectively.

There is currently one case report with steady-state breast milk data in a breastfeeding mother who took linezolid 600 mg orally every 12 hours to treat her MRSA mastitis.[3] This patient took breast milk samples on day 1 of therapy (single dose data) and day 14 (steady state data). The Cavg of linezolid on day 1 and day 14 were 6.16 µg/mL and 12.24 µg/mL, respectively. The C_{max} milk levels were 9.75 µg/mL on day 1 and 18.73 µg/mL on day 14.

The relative infant dose (maternal weight of 102 kg) was 7.85% and 15.61% on days 1 and 14, respectively.[3] The estimated infant exposure based on this RID would be 0.924 mg/kg/day on day 1, and 1.836 mg/kg/day on day 14, which is significantly less than the recommended 10 mg/kg/dose administered every 8-12 hours in neonates requiring linezolid drug therapy.[1,3] Note that even when we calculated the relative infant dose using the C_{max} on day 14 (RID=23.88%) the anticipated infant dose was 2.81 mg/kg/day, still well below the typical infant treatment dose. In this case-report the infant was not breastfed, thus the adverse effects of exposure to linezolid in breast milk are still unknown.[3]

In another case report of a woman receiving 600 mg linezolid twice daily, breast milk levels ranged from 3.5 to 12.2 µg/mL with an average of 8.1 µg/mL.[4] In this case, the infant's plasma levels of linezolid, after 44 hours, were undetectable.

T 1/2	5.2 h	MW	337 Da	PB	31%
Tmax	1.5-2.2 h	RID	1.07% - 15.61%	Vd	0.71 L/kg
Oral	100%	M/P		pKa	1.7

Adult Concerns: Headache, insomnia, dizziness, changes in hearing or vision, tongue discoloration, taste perversion, nausea, vomiting, diarrhea, constipation, changes in liver or renal function, anemia, thrombocytopenia, leukopenia, neutropenia. Serotonin syndrome when used with other pro-serotonergic medications (e.g. SSRIs, SNRIs).

Adult Dose: 600 mg every 12 hours.

Pediatric Concerns: None reported via milk at this time, pediatric data is also limited.

Infant Monitoring: Vomiting, diarrhea, changes in gastrointestinal flora and rash; if clinical symptoms arise a CBC or liver function tests may be warranted.

Alternatives: Vancomycin(L1), Clindamycin(L2)

References:
1. Pharmaceutical manufacturers prescribing information.
2. Sagirli O, Onal A, Toker S, Oztunc A. Determination of linezolid in human breast milk by high-performance liquid chromatography with ultraviolet detection. J AOAC Int. 2009;92(6):1658-1662.
3. Rowe HE, Felkins K, Cooper SD, Hale TW. Transfer of linezolid into breast milk. J Hum Lact. 2014;30(4):410-412. doi: 10.1177/0890334414546045.
4. Lim FH, Lovering AM, Currie A, Jenkins DR. Linezolid and lactation: measurement of drug levels in breast milk and the nursing infant. J Antimicrob Chemother. 2017 Sep;72(9):2677-2678. doi: 10.1093/jac/dkx159. PubMed PMID: 28541475.

LIOTHYRONINE

Trade: Cytomel, Tertroxin

Category: Thyroid Supplement

LRC: L2 - No Data-Probably Compatible

Liothyronine is also called T3. It is seldom used for thyroid replacement therapy due to its short half-life. It is generally recognized that only minimal levels of thyroid hormones are secreted in human milk although several studies have shown that hypothyroid conditions only became apparent when breastfeeding was discontinued.[1,2] Although some studies indicate that breastfeeding may briefly protect hypothyroid infants, it is apparent that the levels of T4 and T3 are too low to provide long-term protection from hypothyroid disease.[3-6] Levels of T3 reported in milk vary but, in general, are around 238 ng/dL and considerably higher than T4 levels. The maximum amount of T3 ingested daily by an infant would be 357 ng/kg/day, or approximately 1/10 the minimum requirement. From these studies, it is apparent that only exceedingly low levels of T3 are secreted in human milk and are insufficient to protect an infant from hypothyroidism.

T 1/2	2.5 days	MW	651 Da	PB	Low
Tmax	1-2 h	RID		Vd	
Oral	95%	M/P		pKa	8.49

Adult Concerns: Tachycardia, tremor, agitation, hyperthyroidism.

Adult Dose: 25-75 µg daily.

Pediatric Concerns: None reported via milk.

Infant Monitoring:

Alternatives:

References:

1. Bode HH, Vanjonack WJ, Crawford JD. Mitigation of cretinism by breast-feeding. Pediatrics. 1978;62(1):13-16.
2. Rovet JF. Does breast-feeding protect the hypothyroid infant whose condition is diagnosed by newborn screening? Am J Dis Child. 1990;144(3):319-323.
3. Varma SK, Collins M, Row A, Haller WS, Varma K. Thyroxine, tri-iodothyronine, and reverse tri-iodothyronine concentrations in human milk. J Pediatr. 1978;93(5):803-806.
4. Hahn HB Jr, Spiekerman AM, Otto WR, Hossalla DE. Thyroid function tests in neonates fed human milk. Am J Dis Child. 1983;137(3):220-222.
5. Letarte J, Guyda H, Dussault JH, Glorieux J. Lack of protective effect of breast-feeding in congenital hypothyroidism: report of 12 cases. Pediatrics. 1980;65(4):703-705.
6. Franklin R, O'Grady C, Carpenter L. Neonatal thyroid function: comparison between breast-fed and bottle-fed infants. J Pediatr. 1985;106(1):124-126.

LIRAGLUTIDE

Trade: Victoza

Category: Antidiabetic, other

LRC: L3 - No Data-Probably Compatible

Liraglutide is a medication that is used with diet and exercise to improve glycemic control in Type II diabetes.[1] Liraglutide is a glucagon-like peptide-1 (GLP-1) receptor agonist that increases the release of insulin when blood glucose is high, delays gastric emptying, and reduces the secretion of glucagon.

It is currently not known if liraglutide is excreted in human milk; however, in rats, this drug is excreted in concentrations of approximately 50% of maternal plasma. The molecular weight of this medication is about 3750 Da; this size of molecule would have great difficulty entering breast milk. In addition, this medication is given subcutaneously for therapeutic effect; thus very little of this medication would be absorbed by the infant orally if found in breast milk. There is reportedly a slightly increased risk of thyroid C-cell tumors/malignancy in rodent and human studies. The risk of this in a breastfed infant would be expected to be very low. The benefits and risks of this medication should be discussed with each individual as there are numerous medication alternatives for this indication with more data in breastfeeding.

T 1/2	13 h	MW	3751.2 Da	PB	>98%
Tmax	8-12 h	RID		Vd	0.07 L/kg
Oral		M/P		pKa	

Adult Concerns: Headache, nausea, vomiting ,diarrhea, constipation, hypoglycemia, malignancy, injection site reactions.

Adult Dose: 1.2 mg subcutaneously once daily (increase to 1.8 mg daily for glycemic control).

Pediatric Concerns:

Infant Monitoring: Vomiting, diarrhea and signs of hypoglycemia- drowsiness, lethargy, pallor, sweating, tremor

Alternatives: Metformin(L1), Glyburide(L2), Insulin(L2)

References:
1. Pharmaceutical manufacturers prescribing information.

LISDEXAMFETAMINE

Trade: Vyvanse

Category: CNS Stimulant

LRC: L3 - Limited Data-Probably Compatible

Lisdexamfetamine dimesylate is a prodrug and is rapidly metabolized to dextroamphetamine in the gastrointestinal tract.[1] Dextroamphetamine is a potent and long-acting amphetamine. Following a 20-mg daily dose of racemic amphetamine administered at 10:00, 12:00, 14:00, and 16:00 hours each day (total= 80 mg/day) to a breastfeeding mother, amphetamine concentrations were determined in milk at 10 days and 42 days postpartum. Samples were taken at 20 minutes prior to the 10:00 hour dose and immediately prior to the 14:00 hour dose. Milk levels were 55 and 118 µg/L respectively.[2] Corresponding maternal plasma levels were 20 and 40 ng/mL at the same times. Milk/plasma ratios at these times were 2.8 and 3 respectively. At 42 days, breast milk levels of amphetamine were 68 and 138 µg/L while maternal plasma levels were 9 and 21 ng/mL respectively. Milk/plasma ratios in the 42-day samples were 7.5 and 6.6 respectively. Although the milk/plasma ratios appear high, using a daily milk intake of 150 mL/kg/day, the relative infant dose would be only 1.8% of the weight-normalized maternal dose, which probably accounts for the fact that the infant in this study was unaffected. In another study of four mothers who received 15-45 mg/day dextroamphetamine, the average absolute infant dose was 21 (11-39) µg/kg/day.[3] The authors suggest the relative infant dose was 5.7% (4-10.6). Plasma levels in the infants ranged from undetectable to 18 µg/L. No untoward effects were noted in any of the four infants.

The above data suggest that with normal therapeutic doses, the dose of dextroamphetamine in milk is probably subclinical. However, abuse of this medication is common, and doses can be extraordinarily high. Thus mothers should be strongly advised to withhold breastfeeding for 24 hours following the non-clinical use of dextroamphetamine.

T 1/2	6.8 h	MW	455 Da	PB	16-20%
Tmax	3.5 h	RID	1.8% - 6.2%	Vd	3.2 - 5.6 L/kg
Oral	96%	M/P	2-5.2	pKa	

Adult Concerns: Nervousness, insomnia, anorexia, hyperexcitability.

Adult Dose: 30-70 mg daily.

Pediatric Concerns: Possible insomnia, irritability, anorexia, reduced weight gain, or poor sleeping patterns in infants. However in these studies, none of the infants were affected.

Infant Monitoring: Agitation, irritability, poor sleeping patterns, poor weight gain.

Alternatives: Methylphenidate(L2)

References:
1. Pharmaceutical manufacturers prescribing information.
2. Steiner E, Villen T, Hallberg M, Rane A. Amphetamine secretion in breast milk. Eur J Clin Pharmacol. 1984;27(1):123-124.
3. Ilett KF, Hackett LP, Kristensen JH, Kohan R. Transfer of dexamphetamine into breast milk during treatment for attention deficit hyperactivity disorder. Br J Clin Pharmacol. 2006;63(3): 371-375.

LISINOPRIL

Trade: Carace, Lisoril, Prinil, Prinivil, Zestril

Category: ACE Inhibitor

LRC: L3 - No Data-Probably Compatible

Lisinopril is a long-acting ACE inhibitor used as an antihypertensive.[1] No breastfeeding data are available on this product. ACE inhibitors in general do not transfer to human milk significantly. They should be used with caution in extremely premature infants due to renal toxicity. Consider enalapril, benazepril, or captopril as alternatives.

Both the ACE inhibitor family and the specific Angiotensin II receptor blockers are contraindicated in pregnancy and thus should be used with caution in women who are planning a subsequent pregnancy in the near future.

T 1/2	12 h	MW	442 Da	PB	Low
Tmax	7 h	RID		Vd	
Oral	25%	M/P		pKa	3.85

Adult Concerns: Headache, dizziness, fatigue, hypotension, abnormal taste, cough, nausea, diarrhea, constipation, changes in renal function/urine output, hyperkalemia, rash.

Adult Dose: 20-40 mg daily.

Pediatric Concerns: None reported via milk at this time.

Infant Monitoring: Drowsiness, lethargy, pallor, poor feeding, and weight gain.

Alternatives: Captopril(L2), Enalapril(L2), Ramipril(L3)

References:
1. Pharmaceutical manufacturers prescribing information.

LITHIUM CARBONATE

Trade: Camcolit, Carbolit, Duralith, Eskalith, Liskonum, Lithane, Lithicarb, Lithobid

Category: Antipsychotic, other

LRC: L4 - Limited Data-Possibly Hazardous

Lithium is a potent antimanic drug used in bipolar disorder. Its use in the first trimester of pregnancy may be associated with a number of birth anomalies, particularly cardiovascular.[1] If used during pregnancy, the dose required is generally elevated due to the increased renal clearance during pregnancy. Soon after delivery, maternal lithium levels should be closely monitored as the mother's renal clearance drops to normal in the next several days to weeks. Several cases of lithium toxicity have been reported in newborns.

A woman who received lithium 1000 mg/day throughout pregnancy and lactation had both her and her infant's serum level drawn near birth and in lactation.[2] Fifteen minutes after delivery the maternal lithium concentration was 0.33 mEq/L and the newborn's level at the same time was 0.35 mEq/L. On day 17 postpartum, the maternal level was 0.84 mEq/L and the newborn's level had decreased to 0.04 mEq/L. The maternal milk level was sampled on day 70 after birth and was 0.12 mEq/L; the corresponding maternal serum level that day was 0.5 mEq/L. The authors also reported no adverse effects or concerns with this newborns development.

In a study of a 36-year-old mother who received lithium during and after pregnancy, the infant's serum lithium level was similar to the mother's at birth (maternal dose = 400 mg) but dropped to 0.03 mmol/L by the sixth day.[3] While the mother's dose increased to 800 mg/day postpartum, the infant's serum level did not rise above 10% of the maternal serum levels. At 42 days postpartum, the maternal and infant serum levels were 1.1 and 0.1 mmol/L, respectively. The maternal milk concentration peaked near day 28 at 0.7 mmol/L and stabilized at about 0.3 mmol/L thereafter. Using this data, the RID ranged from 2.7% to 6.3%. Although the infant was reported to have low tone for the first 48 hours of life, all labs/diagnostic tests and development were normal up to 10 weeks of life when breastfeeding stopped.

Some toxic effects have been reported; however, these adverse effects appear to be more attributable to in utero exposure.[4] A mother receiving 600-1200 mg lithium daily during pregnancy gave birth to a full-term baby girl. Within hours of birth the infant was floppy, unresponsive, and found to have a heart murmur. These symptoms resolved by Day 3; however, the infant was readmitted to hospital on Day 5 of life with lethargy and an elevated lithium level. The maternal and infant plasma levels on Day 5 were 1.5 mEq/L and 0.6 mEq/L, respectively. The concentration of lithium in breast milk was 0.6 mEq/L, and a recommendation was made to stop breastfeeding on Day 5. On Day 7, the infant exhibited inverted T waves on ECG and the lithium level was rechecked at 0.21 mEq/L. In this case, all symptoms resolved by Day 8.

In another case report, lithium milk levels were drawn 7 days postpartum.[5] In this case the woman was taking lithium 900 mg/day, and her plasma lithium level was 0.9 mEq/L both immediately before and after delivery. Her milk and infant's plasma levels were both 0.3 mEq/L on Day 7.

In a case report of a mother receiving 300 mg three times daily and breastfeeding her infant at 2 weeks postpartum, the mother and infant's lithium levels were 0.62 and 0.31 mmol/L, respectively.[6] The infant had a subsequent level drawn at 4 weeks which was stable at 0.29 mmol/L. The infant's neurobehavioral development and thyroid function were reported as normal.

In a group of 11 breastfeeding mothers who received 600 to 1500 mg/day of lithium, the authors found wide interpatient variability in lithium dose offered to the infant through breast milk.[7] The authors reported that the relative infant doses ranged from 0 to 30% (mean 12.2%). In addition, one infant had serum levels 17-20% of maternal levels at 4 weeks of life, and a second infant had serum concentrations 50% of maternal levels at Day 25 of life. In both cases no adverse effects were reported, but breastfeeding was discontinued in the second case due to concern of the high infant level.

In a group of 10 breastfeeding women who received 600 to 1200 mg/day of lithium (average 850 mg/day), the authors sampled maternal serum and milk 8 to 27 weeks postpartum.[8] The average maternal serum trough concentration was 0.76 mEq/L (range 0.41-1.31 mEq/L). The average breast milk concentration was 0.35 mEq/L (range 0.19-0.48 mEq/L), and the average infant concentration was 0.16 mEq/L (range 0.09-0.25 mEq/L). In this study the infants were breastfed for an average of 4 months and no infants had serious adverse effects; changes in thyroid and kidney function were observed in three infants but were considered minimal and transient. However, in one case an infant had a slightly elevated TSH after a normal TSH at newborn screening. In this case the mother was asked to stop breastfeeding. She chose to discontinue her medication and breastfeed and the infant's TSH normalized.

One mother consuming 1200 mg of lithium carbonate daily produced toxic lithium levels of 4.19 mmol/L at 20 hours post dose.[10] Lithium levels at 4 days after discontinuing breastfeeding were 0.11 mmol/L (day 4) and undetectable on day 6.[9]

From these studies it is apparent that lithium can permeate milk and is absorbed by the breastfed infant. If the infant continues to breastfeed, it is strongly suggested that the infant be closely monitored for serum lithium levels, and BUN/creatinine after 6 weeks or so, and cardiac defects such as Ebstein's anomaly. Levels drawn too early (7 days) may only reflect in utero exposure. Lithium does not reach steady state levels for approximately 10 or more days, postpartum. Clinicians may wish to wait at least this long prior to evaluating the infant's serum lithium level, unless symptoms occur. In addition, lithium is known to reduce thyroxine production, and periodic thyroid evaluation should be considered. Because hydration status of the infant can alter lithium levels dramatically, the clinician should observe changes in hydration carefully. A number of studies of lithium suggest that lithium administration is not an absolute contraindication to breastfeeding, if the physician monitors the infant closely for plasma lithium levels.[8] Current studies, as well as unpublished experience, suggest that the infant's plasma levels rise to about 20-50% of the maternal level, most often without untoward effects in the infant.[7,8] Recent evidence suggests that certain anticonvulsants and atypical antipsychotics may be suitable to treat some patients with bipolar disorder. Because these medications are probably safer to use in breastfeeding mothers, the clinician may wish to explore the use of these medications in certain breastfeeding mothers suffering from bipolar symptoms.

The decision to breastfeed while taking lithium depends upon a case-by-case evaluation of the mother's illness course, risk factors, and personal preference, as well as the future health of and potential risk to the infant.

T 1/2	18-36 h	MW	6.941 Da	PB	0%
Tmax	2-4 h	RID	0.87% - 7.29%	Vd	0.7-1 L/kg
Oral	80-100%	M/P	0.24-0.66	pKa	

Adult Concerns: Dizziness, confusion, lethargy, restlessness, alopecia, nystagmus, blurred vision, excessive salivation, arrhythmias, hypotension, nausea, vomiting, diarrhea, anorexia, frequent urination, leukocytosis, tremor.

Adult Dose: 900-2400 mg/day in 3-4 divided doses.

Pediatric Concerns: Some toxic effects have been reported; however, these adverse effects appear to be more attributable to in utero exposure.[3,4]

Infant Monitoring: Neurobehavioral development, drowsiness, irritability, dry mouth or excessive salivation, thyroid function, vomiting, constipation, hydration, renal function, urination, tremor.

Alternatives: Carbamazepine(L2), Lamotrigine(L2)

References:
1. Schou M. Lithium treatment during pregnancy, delivery, and lactation: an update. J Clin Psychiatry. 1990;51(10):410-413.
2. Weinstein MR, Goldfield M. Lithium carbonate treatment during pregnancy (report of a case). Dis Nerv Syst. 1969;30(12):828-832.
3. Sykes PA, Quarrie J, Alexander FW. Lithium carbonate and breast-feeding. Br Med J. 1976;2(6047):1299.
4. Tunnessen WW Jr, Hertz CG. Toxic effects of lithium in newborn infants: a commentary. J Pediatr. 1972;81(4):804-807.
5. Fries H. Lithium in pregnancy. Lancet. 1970;1(7658):1233.
6. Montgomery A. Use of lithium for treatment of bipolar disorder during pregnancy and lactation. Acad Breastfeed Med News Views. 1997;3(1):4-5.
7. Moretti ME, Koren G, Verjee Z, Ito S. Monitoring lithium in breast milk: an individualized approach for breast-feeding mothers. Ther Drug Monit. 2003 Jun;25(3):364-366. Review.
8. Viguera AC, Newport, DJ, Ritchie J, et al. Lithium in breast milk and nursing infants: clinical implications. Am J Psychiatry. 2007;164(2):342-345.
9. Tanaka T, Moretti ME, Verjee ZH, Shupak M, Ivanyi KE, Ito S. A pitfall of measuring lithium levels in neonates. Ther Drug Monit. 2008 Dec;30(6):752-754. doi: 10.1097/FTD.0b013e3181898978. Erratum in: Ther Drug Monit. 2009 Feb;31(1):137. PMID: 19057375.
10. Armstrong C. ACOG guidelines on psychiatric medication use during pregnancy and lactation. Am Fam Physician. 2008;78(6):772-778.

LOMEFLOXACIN

Trade: Maxaquin, Okacin

Category: Antibiotic, Quinolone

LRC: L3 - No Data-Probably Compatible

Lomefloxacin belongs to the fluoroquinolone family of antibiotics.[1] It is reported that lomefloxacin is excreted in the milk of lactating animals; however, no human data is available at this time. There are other fluoroquinolones with lactation data (e.g. ciprofloxacin, ofloxacin). Because fluoroquinolones have limited safety data in pediatric and breastfeeding patients, use in lactation is not recommended if alternative therapies exist.[1]

T 1/2	8 h	MW	351 Da	PB	20.6%
Tmax	0.7-2 h	RID		Vd	2 L/kg
Oral	92%	M/P		pKa	6.75

Adult Concerns: Gastrointestinal distress, diarrhea, colitis, headaches, phototoxicity.

Adult Dose: 400 mg daily.

Pediatric Concerns: None reported with this drug.

Infant Monitoring: Vomiting, diarrhea, changes in gastrointestinal flora, and rash.

Alternatives: Norfloxacin, Ofloxacin(L2), trovafloxacin.

References:
1. Pharmaceutical manufacturers prescribing information.

LOPERAMIDE

Trade: Imodium

Category: Antidiarrheal

LRC: L2 - Limited Data-Probably Compatible

Loperamide is an antidiarrheal drug. Because it is minimally absorbed orally (0.3%), only extremely small amounts are secreted in breast milk. Following a 4-mg oral dose twice daily in six women (early postpartum), milk levels 12 hours postdose averaged 0.18 µg/L, and 6 hours after the second dose were 0.27 µg/L.[1] A breastfeeding infant consuming 165 mL/kg/day of milk would ingest 2000 times less than the recommended daily dose. It is very unlikely these reported levels in milk (Relative infant dose= 0.03%) would ever produce clinical effects in a breastfed infant.

T 1/2	10.8 h	MW	477 Da	PB	
Tmax	4-5 h	RID	0.03%	Vd	
Oral	0.3%	M/P	0.5-0.36	pKa	8.6

Adult Concerns: Fatigue, dizziness, dry mouth, vomiting, abdominal pain, constipation, hyperglycemia.

Adult Dose: 4 mg at onset of diarrhea, then 2 mg after each loose bowel movement (max 16 mg/day).

Pediatric Concerns: One case of mild delirium has been reported in a 4-year-old.

Infant Monitoring: Drowsiness, dry mouth, vomiting, constipation.

Alternatives:

References:
1. Nikodem VC, Hofmeyr GJ. Secretion of the antidiarrhoeal agent loperamide oxide in breast milk. Eur J Clin Pharmacol. 1992;42(6):695-696.

LOPINAVIR + RITONAVIR

Trade: Kaletra

Category: Antiviral

LRC: L5 - Limited Data-Hazardous if Maternal HIV Infection

Lopinavir + Ritonavir is a combined drug product used for treatment of HIV infection in combination with other antiretroviral agents.[1]

Lopinavir: A study which evaluated the safety of maternal antiretrovirals for prophylaxis against HIV transmission to the infant during lactation also reported the milk levels of lopinavir (n=23 samples).[2] This study tested maternal serum and breast milk on the day of delivery and at months 1, 3, and 6 postpartum. Infant levels were also taken at months 1, 3, and 6 of age. The median drug concentrations of lopinavir in maternal serum, breast milk and the infant were 5392 ng/mL (2330-10,084 ng/mL), 1,834 ng/mL (557-3950 ng/mL), and 105 ng/mL (12-518 ng/mL), respectively. The milk/plasma ratio was 0.38. The relative infant dose that we calculated using the maternal dose of 400 mg twice a day and median milk level was 2.4%. This study also reported other infant adverse events (e.g. pneumonia, diarrhea, changes in liver function, neutropenia, thrombocytopenia), but was unable to determine which medication caused the effects based on drug levels; please see study for adverse event details. A publication in 2013 followed women taking antivirals in pregnancy and breastfeeding, and studied maternal milk samples 30 days postpartum.[3] Fourteen breast milk samples were available; the median milk concentration of lopinavir was 0.06 µg/mL. In addition, the median milk/plasma ratio was 0.007.

In 2014, a study was published which looked at HIV RNA in milk and the pharmacokinetics of maternal medications in milk to prevent transmission of HIV to the infant during lactation.[4] In this study 30 women were given one Combivir tablet twice a day (zidovudine 300 mg + lamivudine 150 mg/tab) with 2 tablets of Aluvia twice a day (lopinavir 200 mg + ritonavir 50 mg) starting after delivery until breastfeeding was stopped or 28 weeks. Samples were taken pre-dose (time 0) and then at 2, 4, and 6 hours postdose when the women were enrolled at either 6, 12, or 24 weeks postpartum. The median drug concentrations of lopinavir in maternal serum, breast milk, and the infant were 7790 ng/mL (4510-10,130 ng/mL), 1430 ng/mL (750-2070 ng/mL) and undetectable, respectively. The milk/plasma ratio was 0.194. The RID that we calculated using the maternal dose of 400 mg twice a day and median milk level was 1.88%.

Ritonavir: A study that evaluated the safety of maternal antiretrovirals for prophylaxis against HIV transmission to the infant during lactation also reported the milk levels of ritonavir (n=23 samples).[2] This study tested maternal serum and breast milk on the day of delivery and at months 1, 3, and 6 postpartum. Infant levels were also taken at months 1, 3, and 6 of age. The median drug concentrations of ritonavir in maternal serum, breast milk, and the infant were 422 ng/mL (160-982 ng/mL), 79 ng/mL (31-193 ng/mL) and 7 ng/mL (0-138 ng/mL), respectively. The milk/plasma ratio was 0.2. The relative infant dose that we calculated using the maternal dose of 100 mg twice a day and median milk level was 0.42%. This study also reported other infant adverse events (e.g. pneumonia, diarrhea, changes in liver function, neutropenia, thrombocytopenia), but was unable to determine which medication caused the effects based on drug levels; please see study for adverse event details.

In 2014, a study was published which looked at HIV RNA in milk and the pharmacokinetics of maternal medications in milk to prevent transmission of HIV to the infant during lactation.[4] In this study 30 women were given one Combivir tablet twice a day (zidovudine 300 mg + lamivudine 150 mg/tab) with 2 tablets of Aluvia twice a day (lopinavir 200 mg + ritonavir 50 mg) starting after delivery until breastfeeding was stopped or 28 weeks. Samples were taken pre-dose (time 0) and then at 2, 4, and 6 hours postdose when the women were enrolled at either 6, 12, or 24 weeks postpartum. The median drug concentrations of ritonavir in maternal serum, breast milk, and the infant were 364 ng/mL (280-489 ng/mL), 79 ng/mL (47-112 ng/mL) and undetectable, respectively. The milk to plasma ratio was 0.195. The RID that we calculated using the maternal dose of 100 mg twice a day and median milk level was 0.42%.

Note: This medication combination is an L5 to highlight the contraindication of breastfeeding when the mother is known to be infected with HIV; this medication combination is not an L5 based on its risk to the infant in breast milk. The Centers for Disease Control and Prevention recommend that HIV infected mothers do not breastfeed their infants to avoid postnatal transmission of HIV.[5]

T 1/2	3-5 h	MW	Lop/rit: 629/721 Da	PB	98%-99%
Tmax	Lop/rit: 2-6 h /2-4 h	RID	Lop: 0.08% - 0.24%; rit: 0.42%	Vd	Lop/rit: 0.92-1.86/0.16-0.56 L/kg
Oral	Lop/rit: Low/80%	M/P		pKa	Lop/rit: 13.39/13.68

Adult Concerns: Headache, fatigue, insomnia, anxiety, vomiting, abdominal pain, diarrhea, changes in liver function, elevated cholesterol and triglycerides, elevated blood sugar, neutropenia, thrombocytopenia, skin rash.

Adult Dose: Lopinavir/ritonavir: 400/100 mg (two 200/50 mg tablets or 5 mL oral solution) twice daily.

Pediatric Concerns: No known adverse events in breastfed infants at this time.

Infant Monitoring: Breastfeeding is not recommended in mothers who have HIV.

Alternatives:

References:
1. Pharmaceutical manufacturers prescribing information.
2. Palombi L, Pirillo MF, Andreotti M, et al. Antiretroviral prophylaxis for breastfeeding transmission in Malawi: drug concentrations, virological efficacy and safety. Antivir Ther. 2012;17:1511-1519.

3. Shapiro RL, Rossi S, Ogwu A, et al. Therapeutic levels of lopinavir in late pregnancy and abacavir passage into breast milk in the Mma Bana Study, Botswana. Antivir Ther. 2013;18(4):585-590.

4. Corbett AH, Kayira D, White NR, et al. Antiretroviral pharmacokinetics in mothers and breastfeeding infants from 6 to 24 weeks postpartum: results of the BAN study. Antivir Ther. 2014;19(6):587-595.

5. World Health Organization. Global Programme on AIDS. Consensus Statement from the WHO/UNICEF Consultation on HIV Transmission and Breast-Feeding. Geneva: WHO; 1992.

LORATADINE

Trade: Alavert, Claritin, Clear-Atadine

Category: Antihistamine

LRC: L1 - Limited Data-Compatible

Loratadine is a long-acting antihistamine with minimal sedative properties. Six women 1-12 months postpartum were given a single 40-mg dose of loratadine and instructed not to breastfeed their infant post dose.[1] Maternal blood and milk samples were drawn at multiple time points from 0-48 hours post dose. The peak maternal plasma concentrations of loratadine and its active metabolite descarboethoxyloratadine were 30.5 ng/mL and 18.6 ng/mL, respectively. This produced peak milk concentrations of 29.2 ng/mL and 16 ng/mL of loratadine and its metabolite, respectively. Therefore the total peak milk concentrations of loratadine and its metabolite following a 40-mg maternal dose is 45.2 ng/mL. Over 48 hours, the amount of loratadine transferred via milk was 4.2 µg, which was 0.01% of the maternal dose. Through 48 hours, only 6 µg of descarboethoxyloratadine (7.5 µg loratadine equivalents) was excreted in breast milk, which was 0.019% of the maternal dose. This amounts to a total of 11.7 µg or 0.029% of the administered dose of loratadine and its active metabolite transferred to milk over 48 hours. According to the authors, a 4-kg infant would receive only 2.9 µg/kg of loratadine. It is very unlikely this dose would present a hazard to breastfed infants. The half-life in neonates is not known although it is likely quite long. Pediatric formulations are available.

T 1/2	8.4 h (range 3-20 h)	MW	383 Da	PB	97%
Tmax	1.3 h	RID	0.77% - 1.19%	Vd	
Oral	Complete	M/P	1.2	pKa	4.33

Adult Concerns: Sedation, dry mouth, fatigue, nausea, tachycardia, palpitations.

Adult Dose: 10 mg daily.

Pediatric Concerns: None reported via milk at this time.

Infant Monitoring: Sedation, dry mouth.

Alternatives: Cetirizine(L2)

References:

1. Hilbert J, Radwanski E, Affrime MB, Perentesis G, Symchowicz S, Zampaglione N. Excretion of loratadine in human breast milk. J Clin Pharmacol. 1988;28(3):234-239.

LORAZEPAM

Trade: Almazine, Ativan

Category: Antianxiety

LRC: L3 - Limited Data-Probably Compatible

Lorazepam is one of the benzodiazepines with a shorter half-life and no active metabolite.[1] It is frequently used for relief of anxiety symptoms (short-term) and pre-surgically for sedation. Although this medication has a shorter half-life than other benzodiazepines, and is preferred in lactation because of this, it should be noted that the infant half-life (~30 hours) appears to be much longer than the adult half-life (12 hours).[2]

In one breastfeeding patient receiving 2.5 mg twice daily for 5 days postpartum, the breast milk levels were 12 µg/L.[3] In another patient 4 hours after an oral dose of 3.5 mg, milk levels averaged 8.5 µg/L which is an RID of only 2.6%.[4] Summerfield reports an average milk/plasma ratio of 0.22. It would appear from these studies that the amount of lorazepam secreted in milk would be clinically insignificant under most conditions.

In another study that included 124 breastfeeding women and their infants (aged 2-24 months), two infants (1.6%) were reported as having CNS depression.[5] The three most commonly taken benzodiazepines were lorazepam (52%), clonazepam (18%), and midazolam (15%). There was no correlation between infant sedation and maternal benzodiazepine dose or duration of use. The two mothers who reported infants with sedation were taking more medications that also cause similar CNS adverse effects than those without infant concerns (mean of 3.5 versus 1.7 medications).

The benzodiazepine family, as a rule, is not ideal for breastfeeding mothers due to relatively long half-lives and the development of dependence. However, it is apparent that the shorter-acting benzodiazepines are safer during lactation provided their use is short-term or intermittent and the lowest effective maternal dose is used.[6]

T 1/2	12 h	MW	321 Da	PB	85-93%
Tmax	2 h	RID	2.6% - 2.9%	Vd	1.3 L/kg
Oral	90%	M/P	0.15-0.26	pKa	10.61

Adult Concerns: Sedation, agitation, respiratory depression, withdrawal syndrome.

Adult Dose: 1 mg two-three times a day as needed.

Pediatric Concerns: None reported via milk at this time.

Infant Monitoring: Sedation, slowed breathing rate, not waking to feed/poor feeding, and weight gain.

Alternatives: Oxazepam(L2), Midazolam(L2)

References:
1. Pharmaceutical manufacturers prescribing information.
2. Young, TE, Mangum, B., eds. NeoFax 2010. 23rd ed. Montvale, NJ: Thomson Reuters; 2010.
3. Whitelaw AG, Cummings AJ, McFadyen IR. Effect of maternal lorazepam on the neonate. Br Med J (Clin Res Ed). 1981;282(6270):1106-1108.
4. Summerfield RJ, Nielsen MS. Excretion of lorazepam into breast milk. Br J Anaesth. 1985; 57(10):1042-1043.
5. Kelly LE, Poon S, Madadi P, Koren G. Neonatal benzodiazepines exposure during breastfeeding. J Pediatr. 2012;161(3):448-451.
6. Maitra R, Menkes DB. Psychotropic drugs and lactation. N Z Med J. 1996;109(1024):217-218.

LOSARTAN

Trade: Cozaar

Category: Angiotensin II Receptor Antagonist

LRC: L3 - No Data-Probably Compatible

Losartan is an angiotensin II receptor blocker (ARB) used in the management of hypertension.[1] No data are available on its transfer to human milk. Although it penetrates the CNS significantly, its high protein binding would probably reduce its ability to enter milk significantly. However, no data are available on levels in milk.

Both the ACE inhibitor family and the specific Angiotensin II receptor blockers are contraindicated in pregnancy and thus should be used with caution in women who pregnant.

T 1/2	Los/metabolite: 2.1 h / 7.4 h	MW	422.9 Da	PB	99.8%
Tmax	1 h	RID		Vd	0.17-0.49 L/kg
Oral	33%	M/P		pKa	5.5

Adult Concerns: Headache, dizziness, fatigue, hypotension, nausea, diarrhea, constipation, changes in renal function/urine output, hyperkalemia.

Adult Dose: 25-50 mg one - two times daily.

Pediatric Concerns: None reported via milk at this time.

Infant Monitoring: Drowsiness, lethargy, pallor, poor feeding, and weight gain.

Alternatives: Captopril(L2), Enalapril(L2), Ramipril(L3)

References:
1. Pharmaceutical manufacturers prescribing information.

LOTEPREDNOL

Trade: Alrex, Lotemax

Category: Corticosteroid

LRC: L3 - No Data-Probably Compatible

Loteprednol is a corticosteroid used ophthalmically to decrease inflammation due to allergy or other inflammatory conditions. The preparation comes in 0.2% and 0.5% concentrations. The drug is mainly metabolized in the cornea.

Renal excretion is nil. No reports have been located on use during lactation.[1,2] In general, steroids, particularly oph-thalmic steroids, would virtually never enter milk in clinically relevant amounts.

T 1/2	2.8 h	MW	467 Da	PB	95%
Tmax		RID		Vd	
Oral	Minimal	M/P		pKa	

Adult Concerns: Dry eyes, blurred vision, itching, eye irritation, cataracts, headache, rhinitis, increase in intraocular pressure.

Adult Dose: One drop in affected eye four times daily.

Pediatric Concerns:

Infant Monitoring: Feeding, growth, and weight gain.

Alternatives:

References:
1. Pharmaceutical manufacturer prescribing information.
2. Howes J, Novack GD. Failure to detect systemic levels, and effects of loteprednol etabonate and its metabolite, PJ-91, following chronic ocular adminstration. J Ocul Pharmacol Ther. 1998;14:153-158.

LOVASTATIN

Trade: Mevacor

Category: Antihyperlipidemic

LRC: L3 - No Data-Probably Compatible

Lovastatin is an effective inhibitor of hepatic cholesterol synthesis. It is primarily used for hypercholesterolemia. Small but unpublished levels are known to be secreted in human breast milk.[1] The effect on the infant is unknown and statins could reduce cholesterol synthesis. Cholesterol and other products of cholesterol biosynthesis are essential components for neonatal development; therefore, it is not clear if it would be safe for use in a breastfed infant who needs high levels of cholesterol. Caution is recommended until more data are available.

T 1/2	1.1-1.7 h	MW	405 Da	PB	>95%
Tmax	2-4 h	RID		Vd	
Oral	5-30%	M/P		pKa	14.91

Adult Concerns: Headache, abdominal pain, dyspepsia, diarrhea, flatulence, constipation, changes in liver function, weakness, myalgia.

Adult Dose: 20-80 mg daily.

Pediatric Concerns: None reported but its use is not recommended.

Infant Monitoring: Weight gain, growth.

Alternatives:

References:
1. Pharmaceutical manufacturers prescribing information.

LOXAPINE

Trade: Loxapac, Loxitane

Category: Antipsychotic, Typical

LRC: L4 - No Data-Possibly Hazardous

Loxapine is a typical antipsychotic similar to clozapine that produces pharmacologic effects similar to the phenothi-azines and haloperidol family.[1] The drug does not appear to have antidepressant effects and may lower the seizure threshold. It is a powerful tranquilizer and has been found to be secreted in the milk of animals, but no data are available for human milk. This is a potent tranquilizer that could produce significant sequelae in breastfeeding infants. Numerous well studied alternatives exist, such as olanzapine, risperidone, and aripiprazole. Caution is urged.

T 1/2	19 h	MW	328 Da	PB	
Tmax	1-2 h	RID		Vd	
Oral	33%	M/P		pKa	6.6

Adult Concerns: Drowsiness, tremor, rigidity, extrapyramidal symptoms.

Adult Dose: 10-50 mg two-four times daily.

Pediatric Concerns: None reported, but extreme caution is recommended.

Infant Monitoring: Sedation or irritability, apnea, not waking to feed/poor feeding, constipation, weight gain, and extrapyramidal symptoms.

Alternatives: Olanzapine(L2), Risperidone(L2), Aripiprazole(L3)

References:
1. Pharmaceutical manufacturers prescribing information.

LUBIPROSTONE

Trade: Amitiza

Category: Gastrointestinal Agent

LRC: L3 - No Data-Probably Compatible

Lubiprostone is used for treating chronic idiopathic constipation. It is a local-acting chloride channel activator, which in turn increases chloride-rich intestinal fluid secretion without altering other serum electrolyte concentrations. Increasing the intestinal fluid secretion results in an increased motility in the intestine, and increased passage of stool.[1] No data are available on its transfer to human milk, but given that the oral absorption is nil, plasma levels in the adult are undetectable, and lubiprostone is 94% protein-bound, the amount delivered to a breastfeeding infant through milk would likely be nil. Monitor baby for signs of diarrhea but this is unlikely.

T 1/2	0.9-1.4 h	MW	390.46 Da	PB	94%
Tmax	1.14 h	RID		Vd	
Oral	Nil	M/P		pKa	9.68

Adult Concerns: Headache, nausea, diarrhea.

Adult Dose: 24 µg twice daily.

Pediatric Concerns: No data are available.

Infant Monitoring: Diarrhea.

Alternatives:

References:
1. Pharmaceutical manufacturers prescribing information.

LURASIDONE

Trade: Latuda

Category: Antipsychotic, Atypical

LRC: L3 - No Data-Probably Compatible

Lurasidone hydrochloride is an atypical antipsychotic agent used in the treatment of schizophrenia.[1] The efficacy of lurasidone in schizophrenia is thought to be mediated through a combination of central dopamine type 2 (D2) and serotonin type 2 (5-HT 2A) receptor antagonism. Lurasidone is present in rat milk, but there are no studies in humans. Due to its high protein binding and low oral bioavailability, lurasidone is not likely to enter breast milk in clinically relevant amounts. Until more data are available in humans, caution is recommended. Well studied alternatives include quetiapine, risperidone, and aripiprazole.

T 1/2	18 h	MW	529.14 Da	PB	99%
Tmax	1-3 h	RID		Vd	88.2 L/kg
Oral	9 to 19%	M/P		pKa	

Adult Concerns: Drowsiness, dizziness, insomnia, anxiety, agitation, orthostatic hypotension, dry mouth, dyspepsia, nausea, vomiting, abdominal pain, decreased appetite, hyperglycemia, increased triglycerides, increased prolactin, changes in renal function, weight gain, extrapyramidal symptoms.

Adult Dose: 40-80 mg daily.

Pediatric Concerns: No data in lactation at this time.

Infant Monitoring: Sedation or irritability, apnea, not waking to feed/poor feeding, extrapyramidal symptoms, and weight gain.

Alternatives: Quetiapine(L2), Risperidone(L2), Aripiprazole(L3)

References:
1. Pharmaceutical manufacturing prescribing information, 2011.

LUTEIN

Trade: Carotenoids

Category: Dietary Supplement

LRC: L3 - No Data-Probably Compatible

Lutein is a xanthophyll carotenoid that is the main carotenoid in the retina and eye lens. Breast milk is the main source of lutein for a breastfed infant. In one study, lutein concentration in breast milk was 159 µg/L at day 3 and 62.6 µg/L at day 30 while breastfeeding women were ingesting 1209-1258 µg of lutein daily.[1] There are no controlled studies in breastfeeding women; however, the risk of side effects to infant is probably minimal. Lutein should be given only if the potential benefit justifies the potential risk to the infant.

T 1/2		MW	569 Da	PB	
Tmax		RID	52.2% - 138.2%	Vd	
Oral		M/P		pKa	18.22

Adult Concerns: None reported.

Adult Dose: 2-6 mg/day.

Pediatric Concerns:

Infant Monitoring:

Alternatives:

References:
1. Cena H, Castellazzi AM, Pietri A, Roggi C, Turconi G. Lutein concentration in human milk during early lactation and its relationship with dietary lutein intake. Public Health Nutr. 2009 Oct;12(10):1878-1884. Epub 2009 Feb 16.

LUTROPIN ALFA

Trade: Luveris

Category: Female Reproductive Agent

LRC: L3 - No Data-Probably Compatible

Lutropin Alfa is a human luteinizing hormone (LH) of DNA recombinant origin used in the treatment of female infertility due to LH deficiency.[1] Endogenous LH promotes ovulation as well as the growth and development of the ovarian follicle. There are no studies currently on the transfer of lutropin alfa to breast milk. However, due to its high molecular weight, transfer is unlikely. Nonetheless, some caution is recommended. It is not known if the administration of LH, and the subsequent maternal changes in estrogen and progesterone, would alter the production of milk. It is however likely, since the onset of pregnancy is commonly followed by a decrease in milk production in most mothers. Use in lactating women only if potential benefits to mother outweighs potential risks to infant.

T 1/2	11-18 h	MW	23,390 Da	PB	
Tmax	4-16 h	RID		Vd	0.14-0.2 L/kg
Oral	56% (subcutaneous)	M/P		pKa	

Adult Concerns: Nausea, diarrhea, constipation, abdominal pain, headache. Cystic ovaries, ovarian hypertrophy, and hyperstimulation.

Adult Dose: 75 international units given subcutaneously.

Pediatric Concerns:

Infant Monitoring:

Alternatives:

References:
1. Pharmaceutical manufacturers prescribing information.

LYME DISEASE

Trade: Borrelia burgdorferi infection

Category: Infectious Disease

LRC: L4 - Limited Data-Possibly Hazardous

Lyme disease is caused by infection with the spirochete, *Borrelia burgdorferi*. It is a vector-borne illness transmitted by the hard Ixodes scapularis tick that generally inhabits wooded, forested areas. Lyme disease is prevalent in regions of central and eastern Europe and in eastern Asia.[1] In the United States, it is prevalent in three major geographical zones that include southern New England, eastern mid-Atlantic and upper Midwest.[2] People of all ages may be affected. Transmission of infection is most effective 48 to 72 hours after the attachment of the infected tick.[1]

This spirochete is transferred in utero to the fetus.[3] The only evidence of possible transmission of Borrelia burgdorferi to human milk was when urine and breast milk samples from patients with skin manifestations of LD were studied using nested PCR for detection of Borrelia burgdorferi DNA. Borrelia burgdorferi DNA was detected in breast milk samples of two lactating women who presented with erythema migrans, a characteristic rash associated with Lyme disease. The 6-month-old infant of one mother had to be hospitalized after developing fever and vomiting of unknown etiology, but the infant recovered subsequently. Therefore, although transmission of B. burgdorferi to human milk may occur, it is not known if transmission occurs via milk.[4]

If diagnosed postpartum or in a breastfeeding mother, the mother should be treated immediately. In adults, preferred oral therapy is doxycycline (100 mg orally twice daily for 10-21 days), amoxicillin (500 mg three times daily for 14-21 days), or cefuroxime axetil (500 mg orally twice daily for 14-21 days).[5] In breastfeeding patients, doxycycline, amoxicillin, or cefuroxime are preferred and doxycycline can be used up to 3 weeks. Alternative therapy for adults with contraindications to first-line therapies include macrolide antibiotics (clarithromycin, azithromycin), both of which are suitable for use in lactation.

It is not known if Lyme disease is infectious via milk. However, because the spirochete antigen has been found in breast milk, initiation of maternal treatment with an appropriate antibiotic should be instituted rapidly.

Adult Concerns: Acute Lyme disease: rash and influenza-like symptoms.

Adult Dose:

Pediatric Concerns:

Infant Monitoring: Lyme rash, flu-like symptoms.

Alternatives:

References:
1. Bhate C, Schwartz RA. Lyme disease: Part I. Advances and perspectives. J Am Acad Dermatol. 2011 Apr;64(4):619-636; quiz 637-8. doi:10.1016/j.jaad.2010.03.046.
2. AAP CoID. Lyme Disease (Lyme Borreliosis, Borrelia burgdorferi Infection). In: Pickering LK BC, Kimberlin DW, Long SS, eds. Red Book: 2009 Report of the Committee on Infectious Diseases. 28th ed. Elk Grove Village, IL: American Academy of Pediatrics; 2009:430-435.
3. Stiernstedt G. Lyme borreliosis during pregnancy. Scand J Infect Dis Suppl 1990; 71:99-100
4. Schmidt BL, Aberer E, Stockenhuber C, Klade H, Breier F, Luger A. Detection of Borrelia burgdorferi DNA by polymerase chain reaction in the urine and breast milk of patients with Lyme borreliosis. Diagn Microbiol Infect Dis. 1995;21(3):121-128.
5. Wormser GP, Dattwyler RJ, Shapiro ED, et al. The clinical assessment, treatment, and prevention of Lyme disease, human granulocytic anaplasmosis and babesiosis: clinical practice guidelines by the Infectious Diseases Society of America. Clin Infect Dis. 2006;43(9):1089-1034.

LYSERGIC ACID DIETHYLAMIDE (LSD)

Trade: LSD

Category: Drugs of Abuse

LRC: L5 - No Data-Hazardous

Lysergic acid diethylamide (LSD) is a powerful hallucinogenic drug.[1] No data are available on transfer to breast milk. However, due to its extreme potency and its ability to pass through the blood-brain barrier, LSD is likely to penetrate milk and produce hallucinogenic effects in the infant. This drug is definitely CONTRAINDICATED. Maternal urine may be positive for LSD for 34-120 hours post ingestion.

T 1/2	3 h	MW	268 Da	PB	
Tmax	30-60 min (oral)	RID		Vd	
Oral	Complete	M/P		pKa	7.8

Adult Concerns: Hallucinations, dilated pupils, salivation, nausea.

Adult Dose:

Pediatric Concerns: None reported via milk, but due to potency, hallucinations are likely. Contraindicated.

Infant Monitoring: Avoid breastfeeding.

Alternatives:

References:
1. Ellenhorn MJ, Barceloux DG. Medical Toxicology. New York, NY: Elsevier; 1988.

MACITENTAN

Trade: Opsumit

Category: Antihypertensive

LRC: L4 - No Data-Possibly Hazardous

Macitentan is an endothelin receptor antagonist used for the treatment of pulmonary arterial hypertension.[1] Currently, there are no data regarding the transfer of macitentan into breast milk as this is a new medication. Animal data has demonstrated that macitentan and its active metabolite enter rat milk. Based on this medication's properties it may enter human milk. This medication has a high molecular weight (588 Da), and high protein binding (>99%), which favor poor drug entry into human milk; however, this medication's active metabolites' long half-life (48 hours) and small volume of distribution (0.7 L/kg) favor entry into human milk.

This medication is used to delay disease progression, improve symptoms, and reduce hospitalization. The benefits of this medication were seen when taken for an average of 2 years; consider delaying treatment until after lactation has ceased. At this time, this medication is not recommended for use in breastfeeding mothers.

T 1/2	16 h (drug); 48 h (active metabolite)	MW	588.27 Da	PB	>99%
Tmax	8 h	RID		Vd	0.7 L/kg
Oral		M/P		pKa	7.76

Adult Concerns: Headache, nasopharyngitis, bronchitis, influenza, urinary tract infection, changes in liver function, anemia. This medication may effect male fertility.

Adult Dose: 10 mg once daily.

Pediatric Concerns: Safety has not been established in the pediatric population at this time.

Infant Monitoring: Lab work could be drawn if clinical signs of liver dysfunction, anemia, or frequent infections.

Alternatives:

References:
1. Pharmaceutical manufacturers prescribing information.

MAGNESIUM HYDROXIDE

Trade: Magnolax

Category: Laxative

LRC: L1 - Limited Data-Compatible

Magnesium hydroxide is used as an antacid and laxative. Magnesium hydroxide is poorly absorbed from maternal gastrointestinal tract. Only about 15-30% of an orally ingested magnesium product is absorbed. Magnesium rapidly deposits in bone (>50%) and is significantly distributed to tissue sites. In a comparative report of the laxative efficacy of senna vs mineral oil or magnesium hydroxide, 50 postpartum women were administered senna, while the other 50 received either mineral oil or magnesium hydroxide. Doses were administered on first postpartum day, with additional doses administered on the following days. No alterations in bowel habits or abnormal stools were noted in any of the breastfed infants, indicating that magnesium hydroxide exposure through breast milk is clinically insignificant in an infant.[1]

T 1/2		MW	58 Da	PB	33%
Tmax		RID		Vd	
Oral	15-30%	M/P		pKa	

Adult Concerns: Hypotension, nausea, diarrhea.

Adult Dose: 5-30 mL PRN.

Pediatric Concerns: None reported.

Infant Monitoring:

Alternatives:

References:
1. Baldwin WF. Clinical study of senna administration to nursing mothers. Can Med Assoc J. 1963;89:566-568.

MAGNESIUM SALICYLATE

Trade: Doan's Extra Strength, Doan's Regular, Keygesic-10, Momentum, Novasal

Category: Salicylate, Non-Aspirin

LRC: L3 - No Data-Probably Compatible

Magnesium salicylate is a topical analgesic most often used to treat back pain. Studies concerning the passage of magnesium salicylate into breast milk have not been conducted, though it has been documented that salicylic acid is transferred to breast milk.[1] As with other topical preparations, this drug does not enter the systemic circulation to the degree that an oral dosage form would. The American Academy of Pediatrics generally deems topical preparations of salicylate derivatives to be compatible with breastfeeding.[2]

T 1/2	2-3 h; 12 h at high doses	MW	138.12 Da	PB	50-80%
Tmax	5 h topical	RID		Vd	0.17 L/kg
Oral		M/P		pKa	

Adult Concerns: Burning, itching, hypermagnesemia, bleeding (less risk than aspirin), hypersensitivity reaction.

Adult Dose: 650 mg every 4 hours; use topically PRN.

Pediatric Concerns:

Infant Monitoring: Vomiting, diarrhea.

Alternatives:

References:
1. Gilman AG, Rall TW, Nies AS, et al. In: Gilman AG, Rall TW, Nies AS, et al., eds. Goodman and Gilman's The Pharmacological Basis of Therapeutics. 8th ed. New York, NY: Pergamon Press; 1990.
2. Anon: American academy of pediatrics committee on drugs: transfer of drugs and other chemicals into human milk. Pediatrics. 2001;108(3):776-789.

MAGNESIUM SULFATE

Trade:

Category: Laxative

LRC: L1 - Limited Data-Compatible

Magnesium is a normal plasma electrolyte. It is used pre- and postnatally in women with preeclampsia to both prevent and treat eclamptic seizures. In one study of 10 preeclamptic patients who received a 4-g IV loading dose followed by 1 g per hour IV for more than 24 hours, the average milk magnesium levels in treated subjects were 6.4 mg/

dL, only slightly higher than controls (untreated) which were 4.77 mg/dL.[1] On day 2, the average milk magnesium levels in treated groups were 3.83 mg/dL, which was not significantly different from untreated controls, 3.19 mg/dL. By day 3, the treated and control groups' breast milk levels were identical (3.54 vs. 3.52 mg/dL).

The mean maternal serum magnesium level on day 1 in treated groups was 3.55 mg/dL, which was significantly higher than control untreated, 1.82 mg/dL. In both treated and control subjects, levels of milk magnesium were approximately twice those of maternal serum magnesium levels, with the milk-to-serum ratio being 1.9 in treated subjects and 2.1 in control subjects. This study clearly indicates a normal concentrating mechanism for magnesium in human milk. It is well known that oral magnesium absorption is very poor, averaging only 4%.[2] Further, this study indicates that in treated groups, infants would only receive about 1.5 mg of oral magnesium more than the untreated controls. It is very unlikely that the amount of magnesium in breast milk would be clinically relevant.

T 1/2	<3 h	MW	120 Da	PB	30%
Tmax	Immediate (IV)	RID	0.2%	Vd	
Oral	4%	M/P	1.9	pKa	

Adult Concerns: IV-sedation, decreased respiratory rate, hypotension, muscle weakness, systemic flushing/warmth during infusion.

Adult Dose: 4 g IV load, then 1 g/hour infusion for 24 hours.

Pediatric Concerns: None reported via milk.

Infant Monitoring: Diarrhea.

Alternatives:

References:

1. Cruikshank DP, Varner MW, Pitkin RM. Breast milk magnesium and calcium concentrations following magnesium sulfate treatment. Am J Obstet Gynecol. 1982;143(6):685-688.
2. Morris ME, LeRoy S, Sutton SC. Absorption of magnesium from orally administered magnesium sulfate in man. J Toxicol Clin Toxicol. 1987;25:371-382.

MALATHION

Trade: A-Lices, Ovide, Prioderm, Quellada M

Category: Pediculicide

LRC: L3 - No Data-Probably Compatible

Malathion is a common pesticide. It is used in lotions (0.5%) for the treatment of resistant lice and scabies.[1] It should not be used in neonates, although one case report of its use in a 7-month-old infant suggests it is relatively safe. Less than 10% of malathion is absorbed transcutaneously and is rapidly metabolized and excreted. While it belongs to the organophosphate family of insecticides, it is so rapidly metabolized and eliminated by humans that it is relatively non-toxic under normal conditions. Since so little is absorbed systemically after its topical use, maternal levels attained will not be sufficiently high to produce significant levels in breast milk or in the infant. Therefore, no significant clinical effects are expected in the infant following its use in breastfeeding mothers.[2,3]

T 1/2	7.6 h	MW		PB	
Tmax		RID		Vd	
Oral	Complete	M/P		pKa	

Adult Concerns: Skin irritation, stinging.

Adult Dose:

Pediatric Concerns: None observed via breastfeeding.

Infant Monitoring:

Alternatives: Permethrin(L2)

References:

1. Pharmaceutical manufacturers prescribing information.
2. Ostrea EM Jr, Bielawski DM, Posecion NC Jr, et al. A comparison of infant hair, cord blood, and meconium analysis to detect fetal exposure to environmental pesticides. Environ Res. 2008 Feb;106(2): 277-283.
3. Lebwohl M, Clark L, Levitt J. Therapy for head lice based on life cycle, resistance, and safety consideration. Pediatrics. 207;119:965-974. Online access: http://pediatrics.aapublications.org/content/119/5/965.full.html

MANNITOL

Trade: Osmitrol

Category: Diuretic

LRC: L3 - No Data-Probably Compatible

Mannitol is a hexahydroxy alcohol chemically related to mannose and is used as an osmotic diuretic.[1] As such, it does not readily enter the cellular compartment and remains in the extracellular compartment, thus it would not enter lactocytes. Hepatic metabolism is minimal and the drug is primarily excreted unchanged in the urine by glomerular filtration. The elimination half-life is 71-100 minutes. Mannitol does not normally enter the CNS or the eye. It is freely filtered by the kidneys with less than 10% tubular reabsorption, which is the basis for its use as a diuretic. It is not known if it enters the milk compartment, but it is likely only during the first few days postpartum when the tight junctions in the alveolar system are immature. After 48-72 hours the entry of mannitol into human milk is probably minimal. Oral absorption in infants would be minimal except early postpartum when their gastrointestinal tract is relatively porous.

T 1/2	71-100 min	MW	182 Da	PB	0%
Tmax		RID		Vd	Low L/kg
Oral	17%	M/P		pKa	13.5

Adult Concerns: Hypernatremia, hyponatremia, elevated potassium, diarrhea, kidney failure, pulmonary edema, and congestive heart failure.

Adult Dose: Highly variable.

Pediatric Concerns: None reported via milk. Due to its osmotic diuresis, it is possible that it could briefly reduce the production of milk.

Infant Monitoring: Observe for fluid loss, dehydration, lethargy.

Alternatives:

References:
1. Pharmaceutical manufacturers prescribing information

MAPROTILINE

Trade: Ludiomil

Category: Antidepressant, Tricyclic

LRC: L3 - No Data-Probably Compatible

Maprotiline is a unique structured (tetracyclic) antidepressant dissimilar to others but has clinical effects similar to the tricyclic antidepressants. While it has fewer anticholinergic side effects than the tricyclics, it is more sedating and has similar toxicities in overdose. In one study following an oral dose of 50 mg three times daily, milk and maternal blood levels were greater than 200 µg/L.[1] Milk/plasma ratios varied from 1.3 to 1.5. While these levels are quite low, it is not known if they are hazardous to a breastfed infant; caution is recommended.

T 1/2	27-58 h	MW	277 Da	PB	88%
Tmax	12 h	RID	1.4%	Vd	22.6 L/kg
Oral	100%	M/P	1.5	pKa	10.5

Adult Concerns: Drowsiness, sedation, vertigo, blurred vision, dry mouth, and urinary retention. Skin rashes, seizures, myoclonus, mania, and hallucinations have been reported.

Adult Dose: 25-75 mg daily.

Pediatric Concerns: None reported via milk, but caution is recommended.

Infant Monitoring: Sedation or irritability, dry mouth, not waking to feed/poor feeding, constipation, urinary retention, weight gain.

Alternatives: Sertraline(L2), Escitalopram(L2), Venlafaxine(L2)

References:
1. Riess W. The relevance of blood level determinations during the evaluation of maprotiline in man. In: Murphy, ed. Research and Clinical Investigations in Depression. Northhampton: Cambridge Medical Publications; 1976:19-37.

MEASLES + MUMPS + RUBELLA + VARICELLA VACCINE

Trade: MMRV, ProQuad

Category: Vaccine

LRC: L2 - No Data-Probably Compatible

The measles + mumps + rubella + varicella (MMRV) vaccine is a combined vaccine, recommended for prevention of measles, mumps, rubella, and varicella infection.[1]

MMR vaccine is a mixture of live, attenuated viruses from measles, mumps, and rubella strains. It is usually administered to children at 12-15 months of age. Rubella, and perhaps measles and mumps virus, are undoubtedly transferred via breast milk and have been detected in throat swabs of 56% of breastfeeding infants.[2-5] Infants exposed to the attenuated viruses via breast milk had only mild symptoms. If medically required, MMR vaccine can be administered early postpartum.[6] A live attenuated varicella vaccine (Varivax - Merck) was recently approved for marketing by the US Food and Drug Administration. It is not known if the vaccine-acquired VZV is secreted in human milk, nor its infectiousness to infants. Interestingly, in two women with varicella zoster infections, the virus was not cultured from milk. The antibody from the varicella zoster vaccine has been isolated in breast milk along with the DNA.[7,8] Both the AAP[9] and the Centers for Disease Control and Prevention approve the use of varicella zoster vaccines in breastfeeding mothers, if the risk of infection is high.

The ACIP has stated that breastfeeding women may be administered both the live and killed vaccines.[10] As a general rule, vaccines are often safe to use during breastfeeding.[11]

Adult Concerns: Redness, pain, swelling, tenderness at site of injection, fever, skin reactions, hypersensitivity reaction. Seizures, Guillain-Barre syndrome, meningitis have rarely occurred. Not to be given in pregnancy.

Adult Dose: 0.5 mL subcutaneous.

Pediatric Concerns: Mild symptoms of rubella have been reported in one newborn infant via milk after maternal rubella vaccination.[5] Consult pediatrician prior to maternal vaccination for risks/benefits discussion if infant is known to be immunocompromised; caution is recommended.

Infant Monitoring:

Alternatives:

References:

1. Product Information: PROQUAD(R) powder for solution subcutaneous injection, measles, mumps, rubella, varicella virus vaccine live solution subcutaneous injection. Merck, Whitehouse Station, NJ, 2009.
2. Buimovici-Klein E, Hite RL, Byrne T, Cooper LZ. Isolation of rubella virus in milk after postpartum immunization. J Pediatr. 1977;91(6):939-941.
3. Losonsky GA, Fishaut JM, Strussenberg J, Ogra PL. Effect of immunization against rubella on lactation products. I. Development and characterization of specific immunologic reactivity in breast milk. J Infect Dis. 1982;145(5):654-660.
4. Losonsky GA, Fishaut JM, Strussenberg J, Ogra PL. Effect of immunization against rubella on lactation products. II. Maternal-neonatal interactions. J Infect Dis. 1982;145(5):661-666.
5. Landes RD, Bass JW, Millunchick EW, Oetgen WJ. Neonatal rubella following postpartum maternal immunization. J Pediatr. 1980;97(3):465-467.
6. Lawrence RA. Breastfeeding: A Guide for the Medical Profession. St. Louis: Mosby Publishers; 1994.
7. Frederick IB, White RJ, Braddock SW. Excretion of varicella-herpes zoster virus in breast milk. Am J Obstet Gynecol. 1986;154(5):1116-1117.
8. Yoshida M, Yamagami N, Tezuka T, Hondo R. Case report: detection of varicella-zoster virus DNA in maternal breast milk. J Med Virol. 1992 Oct;38(2):108-110.
9. American Academy of Pediatrics. 1997 Red Book: Report of the Committee on Infectious Diseases. 24th ed. Elk Grove Village, IL: American Academy of Pediatrics; 1997.
10. Anon. General recommendations on immunization; recommendations of the advisory committee on immunization practices (AICP) and the American academy of family physicians (AAFP). MMWR. 2002;51(RR02):1-36.
11. Schaefer C. Drugs During Pregnancy and Lactation. Amsterdam, The Netherlands: Elsevier Science B.V.; 2001.

MEASLES + MUMPS + RUBELLA VACCINE (MMR VACCINE)

Trade: MMR, Priorix

Category: Vaccine

LRC: L2 - Limited Data-Probably Compatible

MMR vaccine is a mixture of live, attenuated viruses from measles, mumps, and rubella strains. It is usually administered to children at 12-15 months of age. Rubella, and perhaps measles and mumps virus, are undoubtedly transferred via breast milk and have been detected in throat swabs of 56% of breastfeeding infants.[1-4] Infants exposed to the attenuated viruses via breast milk had only mild symptoms. If medically required, MMR vaccine can be administered early postpartum.[5] The Advisory Committee on Immunization Practices has stated that breastfeeding women may be administered both the live and killed vaccines.[6] As a general rule, vaccines are often safe to use during breastfeeding.[7]

Adult Concerns: Mild symptoms, fever, flu-like symptoms.

Adult Dose: 0.5 mL subcutaneous injection in outer aspect of upper arm.

Pediatric Concerns: Mild symptoms of rubella have been reported in one newborn infant via milk after maternal rubella vaccination.[4]

Infant Monitoring:

Alternatives:

References:
1. Buimovici-Klein E, Hite RL, Byrne T, Cooper LZ. Isolation of rubella virus in milk after postpartum immunization. J Pediatr. 1977;91(6):939-941.
2. Losonsky GA, Fishaut JM, Strussenberg J, Ogra PL. Effect of immunization against rubella on lactation products. I. Development and characterization of specific immunologic reactivity in breast milk. J Infect Dis. 1982;145(5):654-660.
3. Losonsky GA, Fishaut JM, Strussenberg J, Ogra PL. Effect of immunization against rubella on lactation products. II. Maternal-neonatal interactions. J Infect Dis. 1982;145(5):661-666.
4. Landes RD, Bass JW, Millunchick EW, Oetgen WJ. Neonatal rubella following postpartum maternal immunization. J Pediatr. 1980;97(3):465-467.
5. Lawrence RA. Breastfeeding: A Guide for the Medical Profession. St. Louis: Mosby Publishers; 1994.
6. Guidelines for Vaccinating Pregnant Women. Centers for Disease Control and Prevention, March 2014. http://www.cdc.gov/vaccines/pubs/preg-guide.htm, 2014.
7. Schaefer C, Schaefer C. Drugs During Pregnancy and Lactation. Amsterdam, The Netherlands: Elsevier Science B.V.; 2001.

MEASLES VIRUS VACCINE, LIVE

Trade: Attenuvax

Category: Vaccine

LRC: L2 - Limited Data-Probably Compatible

Measles vaccine is a live, attenuated vaccine indicated for the prevention of measles illness. It is administered at 12-15 months of age, as part of the routine childhood immunization schedule. It is usually administered along with the mumps and rubella vaccine, in the form of the MMR vaccine. There are currently no reports of transfer of the live measles virus vaccine to breast milk. The American Advisory Committee on Immunization Practices has stated that breastfeeding women may be administered both the live and killed vaccines.[1] As a general rule, vaccines are often safe to use during breastfeeding.[2] The WHO considers measles vaccine compatible with breastfeeding. Therefore, a lactating mother vaccinated with the measles vaccine may continue to breastfeed her child.

Further, breastfeeding provides an additional benefit toward protection against measles in the infant. Protective measles antibodies have been detected in breast milk and are transferred to the infant via breastfeeding.[3] It has been found that breastfeeding for more than 3 months is associated with a 30% decreased risk of clinical measles, and can provide protection up to the age of 10 years.[4] However, this protection is not equally as efficacious as that following measles vaccination. Therefore, while a lactating mother who has received the measles vaccine may continue to breastfeed, this does not preclude the importance of measles vaccination in the infant.

Adult Concerns: Headache, dizziness, rash, fever, diarrhea. Serious side effects: Anaphylaxis, encephalitis, thrombocytopenia, Steven-Johnson syndrome.

Adult Dose: 0.5 mL subcutaneous injection.

Pediatric Concerns: Mothers of immunodeficient infants should not breastfeed following use of this vaccine.

Infant Monitoring:

Alternatives:

References:
1. Anon. General recommendations on immunization; recommendations of the advisory committee on immunization practices (AICP) and the American academy of family physicians (AAFP). MMWR. 2002;51(RR02):1-36.
2. Schaefer C, Schaefer C. Drugs During Pregnancy and Lactation. Amsterdam, The Netherlands: Elsevier Science B.V.; 2001.
3. Adu FD, Adeniji JA. Measles antibodies in the breast milk of nursing mothers. Afr J Med Med Sci. 1995 Dec;24(4):385-388.
4. Silfverdal SA, Ehlin A, Montgomery SM. Breast-feeding and a subsequent diagnosis of measles. Acta Paediatr. 2009 Apr;98(4):715-719. Epub 2008 Dec 24.

MEBENDAZOLE

Trade: Sqworm, Vermox

Category: Anthelmintic

LRC: L3 - No Data-Probably Compatible

Mebendazole is an anthelmintic used primarily for pinworms although it is active against roundworms, hookworms, and a number of other nematodes. Mebendazole is poorly absorbed orally. In one patient who received 100 mg twice daily for three days, milk production was drastically reduced.[1] However in another report of four postpartum breast-feeding mothers who received 100 mg twice daily for 3 days, milk levels of mebendazole were undetectable in one patient sample. No change in milk production was noted in the latter study.[2] Considering the poor oral absorption and high protein binding, it is unlikely that mebendazole would be transmitted to the infant in clinically relevant concentrations.

T 1/2	2.8-9 h	MW	295 Da	PB	High
Tmax	0.5-7 h	RID		Vd	
Oral	2-10%	M/P		pKa	8.44

Adult Concerns: Diarrhea, abdominal pain, nausea, vomiting, headache. Observe mother for reduced production of breast milk.

Adult Dose: 100 mg twice daily.

Pediatric Concerns: None reported via milk. May inhibit milk production.

Infant Monitoring:

Alternatives: Pyrantel(L3)

References:
1. Rao TS. Does mebendazole inhibit lactation? N Z Med J. 1983;96(736):589-590.
2. Kurzel RB, Toot PJ, Lambert LV, Mihelcic AS. Mebendazole and postpartum lactation. N Z Med J. 1994; 107(988):439.

MECLIZINE

Trade: Antivert

Category: Antiemetic

LRC: L3 - No Data-Probably Compatible

Meclizine is an antihistamine frequently used for nausea, vertigo, and motion sickness although it is inferior to scopolamine. Meclizine was previously used for nausea and vomiting of pregnancy in the USA, and still is in many countries.[1] No data are available on its secretion in breast milk. There are no pediatric indications for this product. The use of meclizine while breastfeeding is probably safe; however, monitoring for sedation in the infant is advised.

T 1/2	6 h	MW	391 Da	PB	
Tmax	3 h	RID		Vd	7 L/kg
Oral	Complete	M/P		pKa	

Adult Concerns: Drowsiness, sedation, dry mouth, blurred vision.

Adult Dose: 25-100 mg daily.

Pediatric Concerns: None reported.

Infant Monitoring: Sedation, dry mouth.

Alternatives: Dimenhydrinate(L2), Diphenhydramine(L2), Scopolamine(L3)

References:
1. Pharmaceutical manufacturers prescribing information.

MECLOFENAMATE

Trade: Meclomen

Category: NSAID

LRC: L3 - Limited Data-Probably Compatible

Meclofenamate is a nonsteroidal anti-inflammatory agent (NSAID) used in the treatment of mild to moderate pain and dysmenorrhea. NSAIDs, as a class, are secreted minimally in breast milk. Data from the manufacturer of meclofenamate reports the drug has been found in trace amounts in breast milk.[1] Trace amounts of meclofenamate are not expected to cause clinical effects in the breastfeeding infant.

T 1/2	0.8 to 2.1 h	MW	336.15 Da	PB	99%
Tmax	0.5-2 h	RID		Vd	23 L/kg
Oral	Complete	M/P		pKa	

Adult Concerns: Headache, dizziness, nervousness, tinnitus, dyspepsia, nausea, vomiting, abdominal cramps, gastrointestinal bleeding, changes in liver and renal function, edema.

Adult Dose: 50 mg every 4-6 hours.

Pediatric Concerns:

Infant Monitoring: Vomiting, diarrhea.

Alternatives: Ibuprofen(L1)

References:

1. Pharmaceutical manufacturers prescribing information.

MEDROXYPROGESTERONE

Trade: Cycrin, DMPA, Depo-Provera, Divina, Farlutal, Provelle, Provera, Ralovera, Sayana

Category: Female Reproductive Agent

LRC: L4 - Limited Data-Possibly Hazardous

Medroxyprogesterone is a synthetic progestin compound. It is used orally for amenorrhea, dysmenorrhea, uterine bleeding, and infertility. It is used intramuscularly for contraception. Due to its poor oral bioavailability, it is seldom used orally. Saxena has reported that the average concentration in milk is 1.03 µg/L.[1] Koetswang reported average milk levels of 0.97 µg/L.[2]

In a series of studies, the World Health Organization reviewed the developmental skills of children and their weight gain following exposure to progestin-only contraceptives during lactation.[3,4] These studies documented that no adverse effects on overall development, or rate of growth, were notable. Further, they suggested there is no apparent reason to deny lactating women the use of progestin-only contraceptives, preferably after 6 weeks postpartum. There have been consistent and controversial studies suggesting that males exposed to early postnatal progestins have higher feminine scores. However, Ehrhardt's studies have provided convincing data that males exposed to early progestins were no different than controls.[5]

A number of other short- and long-term studies available on development of children have found no differences with control groups.[6,7] Interestingly, an excellent study of the transfer of DMPA into breastfed infants has been published.[8] In this study of 13 breastfeeding women who received 150-mg injections of DMPA on day 43 and again on day 127 postpartum, urine and plasma collections in infants (n=22) from day 38 to day 137 were collected. Urinary follicle stimulating hormone (FSH), luteinizing hormone (LH), unconjugated testosterone, unconjugated cortisol, medroxyprogesterone, and metabolites were measured. No differences (from untreated controls) were found in LH, FSH, or unconjugated testosterone urine levels in the infants. Urine cortisol levels were not altered from those of control infants. Medroxyprogesterone or its metabolites were at no time detected in any of the infant urine samples. This data concludes that only small trace amounts of medroxyprogesterone acetate (MPA) are transferred to breastfeeding infants and that these amounts are not expected to have any influence on breastfeeding infants. In support of this, using calculations based on MPA levels in the blood of DMPA users and a plasma-to-milk MPA ratio, Benagiano and Fraser suggest that the actual amounts of MPA in the infant's system is probably at or below trace levels.[9] Koetsewant states that the small amount of MPA present in milk is unlikely to have any significant clinical adverse effects on the infant.[2] A long-term follow-up study by Jimenez found no changes in growth, development, and health status in 128 breastfed infants at 4.5 years of age.[10] DMPA mothers lactated significantly longer than controls in this study.

The use of DMPA in breastfeeding women is common and somewhat controversial. DMPA has been documented to significantly elevate prolactin levels in breastfeeding mothers (administered 6 weeks postpartum)[11] and increase milk production in some mothers.[12] With progestins, clinical experience has found that some women may experience a decline in milk production or arrested early production, following an injection of DMPA, particularly when the progestin is used early postpartum (12-48 hours).[13] At present there are no published data to support this, nor is the relative incidence of this untoward effect known.

Therefore, in some instances, it might be advisable to recommend treatment with oral progestin-only contraceptives postpartum rather than DMPA, so that women who experience reduced milk supply could easily withdraw from the medication without significant loss of breast milk supply. Progestins should be avoided early postnatally if possible.[13] See Contraception - Hormonal Monograph for further details.

T 1/2	14.5 h	MW	344 Da	PB	
Tmax		RID		Vd	
Oral	0.6-10%	M/P		pKa	17.82

Adult Concerns: Fluid retention, gastrointestinal distress, menstrual disorders, breakthrough bleeding, weight gain.

Adult Dose: 5-10 mg daily.

Pediatric Concerns: None reported via milk, although unsubstantiated reports of reduced milk supply have been made.

Infant Monitoring: Small amounts are present in human milk. Possible suppression of milk production early postpartum is reported.

Alternatives:

References:

1. Saxena BN, Shrimanker K, Grudzinskas JG. Level of contraceptive steroids in breast milk and plasma of lactating women. Contraception. 1977;16:605-613.
2. Koetsawang S, Nukulkarn P, Fotherby K, Shrimanker K, Mangalam M, Towobola K. Transfer of contraceptive steroids in milk of women using long-acting gestagens. Contraception. 1982;25(4):321-331.
3. Progestogen-only contraceptives during lactation: I. Infant growth. World Health Organization task force for epidemiological research on reproductive health; special programme of research, development and research training in human reproduction. Contraception. 1994;50(1):35-53.
4. Progestogen-only contraceptives during lactation: II. Infant development. World Health Organization, task force for epidemiological research on reproductive health; special programme of research, development, and research training in human reproduction. Contraception. 1994;50(1):55-68.
5. Ehrhardt AA, Grisanti GC, Meyer-Bahlburg HF. Prenatal exposure to medroxyprogesterone acetate (MPA) in girls. Psychoneuroendocrinology. 1977;2(4):391-398.
6. Schwallie PC. The effect of depot-medroxyprogesterone acetate on the fetus and nursing infant: a review. Contraception. 1981;23(4):375-386.
7. Pardthaisong T, Yenchit C, Gray R. The long-term growth and development of children exposed to Depo-Provera during pregnancy or lactation. Contraception. 1992;45(4):313-324.3.
8. Virutamasen P, Leepipatpaiboon S, Kriengsinyot R, et al. Pharmacodynamic effects of depot-medroxyprogesterone acetate (DMPA) administered to lactating women on their male infants. Contraception. 1996; 54(3):153-157.
9. Benagiano G, Fraser I. The Depo-Provera debate. Commentary on the article "Depo-Provera, a critical analysis". Contraception. 1981;24(5):493-528.
10. Jimenez J, Ochoa M, Soler MP, Portales P. Long-term follow-up of children breast-fed by mothers receiving depot-medroxyprogesterone acetate. Contraception. 1984;30(6):523-533.
11. Ratchanon S, Taneepanichskul S. Depot medroxyprogesterone acetate and basal serum prolactin levels in lactating women. Obstet Gynecol. 2000;96(6):926-928.
12. Fraser IS. Long acting injectable hormonal contraceptives. Clin Reprod Fertil. 1982;1(1):67-88.
13. Kennedy KI, Short RV, Tully MR. Premature introduction of progestin-only contraceptive methods during lactation. Contraception. 1997;55(6):347-350.

MEFLOQUINE

Trade: Lariam

Category: Antimalarial

LRC: L2 - Limited Data-Probably Compatible

Mefloquine is an antimalarial and a structural analog of quinine. It is concentrated in red cells and therefore has a long half-life.[1] Following a single 250-mg dose in two women, the milk/plasma ratio was only 0.13 to 0.16 the first 4 days of therapy.[2] The concentration of mefloquine in milk ranged from 32 to 53 μg/L. Unfortunately, these studies were not carried out after steady-state conditions, which would probably increase to some degree the amount transferred to the infant. According to the manufacturer, mefloquine is secreted in small concentrations approximating 3% of the maternal dose. Assuming a milk level of 53 μg/L and a daily milk intake of 150 mL/kg/day, an infant would ingest approximately 8 μg/kg/day of mefloquine, which is not sufficient to protect the infant from malaria. The dose for malaria prophylaxis is 5 mg/kg once weekly in an infant. Thus far, no untoward effects have been reported.

T 1/2	10-21 days	MW	414 Da	PB	98%
Tmax	1-2 h	RID	0.1% - 0.2%	Vd	19 L/kg
Oral	85%	M/P	0.13-0.27	pKa	<2, 8.6

Adult Concerns: Headache, fever, fatigue, abnormal dreams, irritability, tinnitus, visual disturbances, vomiting, diarrhea, anorexia, myalgias.

Adult Dose: 250 mg every week.

Pediatric Concerns: None reported via milk at this time.

Infant Monitoring: Irritability, insomnia, vomiting, diarrhea, weight gain.

Alternatives:

References:
1. Pharmaceutical manufacturers prescribing information.
2. Edstein MD, Veenendaal JR, Hyslop R. Excretion of mefloquine in human breast milk. Chemotherapy. 1988;34(3):165-169.

MEGESTROL

Trade: Megace, Megace ES

Category: Progestin

LRC: L4 - No Data-Possibly Hazardous

Megestrol is a progesterone derivative indicated in the management of advanced breast and endometrial cancer, and also used in the management of cachexia associated with AIDS.[1] Currently there are no data available of its use in breastfeeding women, or of its transfer to breast milk. However, being a progesterone derivative, its effects are probably similar to other progestins, in that its use during lactation may suppress milk production. Thus it is advisable to wait as long as possible postpartum (at least 6-8 weeks) prior to instituting therapy with progesterone to avoid reducing the milk supply.

The direct effects of progesterone therapy on the nursing infant is generally unknown, but it is believed minimal to none as natural progesterone is poorly bioavailable to the infant via milk. Several cases of gynecomastia in infants have been reported but are extremely rare.

T 1/2	34 h	MW	384.51 Da	PB	
Tmax	1-5 h	RID		Vd	
Oral		M/P		pKa	

Adult Concerns: Headache, mood swings, insomnia, hypertension, hot flashes, nausea, vomiting, diarrhea, impotence, amenorrhea, hyperglycemia, anemia, leukopenia, thromboembolism, edema, weight gain.

Adult Dose: 400-800 mg per day.

Pediatric Concerns:

Infant Monitoring: Small amounts are present in human milk. Possible suppression of milk production early postpartum is reported.

Alternatives:

References:
1. Pharmaceutical manufacturers prescribing information.

MELATONIN

Trade:

Category: Pineal Gland Hormone

LRC: L3 - No Data-Probably Compatible

Melatonin (N-acetyl-5-methoxytryptamine) is a normal hormone secreted by the pineal gland in the human brain. It is circadian in rhythm, with nighttime values considerably higher than daytime levels. It is postulated to induce a sleep-like pattern in humans. It is known to be passed into human milk and is believed responsible for entraining the newborn brain to phase shift its circadian clock to that of the mother by communicating time-of-day information to the newborn.

On average, the amount of melatonin in human milk is about 35% of the maternal plasma level but can range to as high as 80%.[1] Post-feeding milk levels appear to more closely reflect the maternal plasma level than pre-feeding values, suggesting that melatonin may be transported into milk at night, during the feeding, rather than being stored in fore-milk. In neonates, melatonin levels are low and progressively increase up to the age of 3 months when the characteristic diurnal rhythm is detectable.[2] Nighttime melatonin levels reach a maximum at the age of 1-3 years and thereafter decline to adult values.[3-5] While nighttime maternal serum levels average 280 pmol/L, milk levels averaged 99 pmol/L in a group of 10 breastfeeding mothers.[1] The effect of orally administered melatonin in newborns is unknown.

T 1/2	30-50 min	MW	232 Da	PB	
Tmax	0.5-2 h	RID		Vd	
Oral	Complete	M/P	0.35-0.8	pKa	

Adult Concerns: Headache and confusion, drowsiness, fatigue, hypothermia, and dysphoria in depressed patients.

Adult Dose:

Pediatric Concerns: None reported.

Infant Monitoring: Drowsiness, fatigue.

Alternatives:

References:
1. Illnerova H, Buresova M, Presl J. Melatonin rhythm in human milk. J Clin Endocrinol Metab. 1993;77(3):838-841.
2. Hartmann L, Roger M, Lemaitre BJ, Massias JF, Chaussain JL. Plasma and urinary melatonin in male infants during the first 12 months of life. Clin Chim Acta. 1982;121(1):37-42.
3. Aldhous M, Franey C, Wright J, Arendt J. Plasma concentrations of melatonin in man following oral absorption of different preparations. Br J Clin Pharmacol. 1985;19(4):517-521.
4. Attanasio A, Rager K, Gupta D. Ontogeny of circadian rhythmicity for melatonin, serotonin, and N-acetylserotonin in humans. J Pineal Res. 1986;3(3):251-256.
5. Dollins AB, Lynch HJ, Wurtman RJ, et al. Effect of pharmacological daytime doses of melatonin on human mood and performance. Psychopharmacology (Berl). 1993;112(4):490-496.

MELOXICAM

Trade: Mobic

Category: NSAID

LRC: L3 - No Data-Probably Compatible

Meloxicam is a nonsteroidal anti-inflammatory drug that appears more closely for the COX-2 receptors.[1] No data are available for transfer to human milk although it does transfer to rodent milk. Due to its long half-life and good bioavailability, another NSAID would probably be preferred.

T 1/2	20.1 h	MW	351 Da	PB	99.4
Tmax	4.9 h	RID		Vd	0.14 L/kg
Oral	89%	M/P		pKa	4.2

Adult Concerns: Headache, dizziness, insomnia, tinnitus, dyspepsia, nausea, vomiting, abdominal pain, diarrhea, gastrointestinal bleeding, changes in renal function, edema, arthralgia.

Adult Dose: 7.5 mg/day.

Pediatric Concerns: None reported via milk.

Infant Monitoring: Vomiting, diarrhea.

Alternatives: Ibuprofen(L1), Naproxen(L3)

References:
1. Pharmaceutical manufacturers prescribing information.

MELPHALAN

Trade: Alkeran

Category: Antineoplastic

LRC: L5 - No Data-Hazardous

Melphalan is an alkylating agent used in the treatment of multiple myeloma and ovarian carcinoma. Oral bioavailability in adults is highly variable and ranges from 56-93%.[1] Due to the wide variability, it is most commonly used intravenously at higher doses. The terminal elimination half-life is 1.5 hours but can vary to as high as 3 hours. Penetration into CNS fluid is low. No data are available on its transfer to human milk, but levels are expected to be quite low. Mothers should be advised to withhold breastfeeding for at least 24 hours following treatment.

T 1/2	1.5 h	MW	305.2 Da	PB	60%-90%
Tmax	1-2 h	RID		Vd	0.5 L/kg
Oral	56-93%	M/P		pKa	2.5

Adult Concerns: Nausea, vomiting, myelosuppression, secondary malignancy, hypersensitivity, thrombocytopenia, leukopenia.

Adult Dose: Varies by protocol.

Pediatric Concerns: No lactation data at this time.

Infant Monitoring: Withhold breastfeeding for at least 24 hours after treatment.

Alternatives:

References:
1. Pharmaceutical manufacturers prescribing information.

MEMANTINE

Trade: Ebixa, Namenda

Category: NMDA Receptor Antagonist

LRC: L3 - No Data-Probably Compatible

Memantine is used to treat moderate to severe dementia associated with Alzheimer's disease.[1] It blocks NMDA receptors, blocking glutamate from exciting the neuronal cells. The over-excitation of NMDA receptors is postulated to contribute to the disease. It binds to the magnesium binding site for longer periods of time than magnesium, causing receptor blockade under excessive stimulation. There are no data available on the transfer of memantine into human milk.

T 1/2	60-80 h	MW	216 Da	PB	45%
Tmax	3-7 h	RID		Vd	9-11 L/kg
Oral	Complete	M/P		pKa	10.7

Adult Concerns: Headache, dizziness, confusion, cough, hypertension, vomiting, constipation.

Adult Dose: 20 mg/day.

Pediatric Concerns: No data are available.

Infant Monitoring: Constipation, vomiting and cough.

Alternatives:

References:
1. Pharmaceutical manufacturers prescribing information.

MENINGOCOCCAL VACCINE

Trade: Menactra (MCV4), Menomune (MPSV4), Menveo (MODC)

Category: Vaccine

LRC: L1 - No Data-Compatible

Meningococcal polysaccharide vaccine is a freeze-dried preparation of group-specific antigens from Neisseria meningitidis.[1] This vaccine is not infectious and is useful in preventing endemic and epidemic meningitis and meningococcemia in children and young adults. There are no contraindications for using this in breastfeeding mothers other than allergic hypersensitivity to some of the ingredients.

Adult Concerns: Pain, erythema, induration at injection site. Headaches, malaise, chills and elevated temperature have been reported.

Adult Dose: 0.5 mL subcutaneously.

Pediatric Concerns: None via milk.

Infant Monitoring:

Alternatives:

References:
1. Pharmaceutical manufacturers prescribing information.

MENOTROPINS

Trade: Humegon, Menopur, Pergonal, Repronex

Category: Gonadotropin

LRC: L3 - No Data-Probably Compatible

Menotropins is a purified preparation of gonadotropin hormones extracted from the urine of postmenopausal women. It is a biologically standardized form containing equal activity of follicle stimulating hormone (FSH) and luteinizing hormone (LH).[1-3] Menotropins and human chorionic gonadotropins (see chorionic gonadotropins) are given sequentially to induce ovulation in the anovulatory female. FSH and LH are large molecular weight peptides and would not likely penetrate into human milk. Further, they are unstable in the gastrointestinal tract and their oral bioavailability would be minimal to zero even in an infant.

T 1/2	3.9 and 70.4 h	MW	34,000 Da	PB	
Tmax	6 h	RID		Vd	1.08 L/kg
Oral	0%	M/P		pKa	

Adult Concerns: Ovarian enlargement, cysts, hemoperitoneum, fever, chills, aches, joint pains, nausea, vomiting, abdominal pain, diarrhea, bloating, rash, dizziness.

Adult Dose: Dose and frequency varies by indication, 150-450 units/day.

Pediatric Concerns: None reported via milk. These agents are very unlikely to enter milk. But observe closely for changes in milk production that could occur.

Infant Monitoring:

Alternatives:

References:
1. Sharma V, Riddle A, Mason B, Whitehead M, Collins W. Studies on folliculogenesis and in vitro fertilization outcome after the administration of follicle-stimulating hormone at different times during the menstrual cycle. Fertil Steril. 1989;51(2):298-303.
2. Kjeld JM, Harsoulis P, Kuku SF, Marshall JC, Kaufman B, Fraser TR. Infusions of hFSH and hLH in normal men. I. Kinetics of human follicle stimulating hormone. Acta Endocrinol (Copenh). 1976;81(2):225-233.
3. Yen SC, Llerena LA, Pearson OH, Littell AS. Disappearance rates of endogenous follicle-stimulating hormone in serum following surgical hypophysectomy in man. J Clin Endocrinol Metab. 1970;30(3):325-329.

MENTHOL

Trade:

Category: Anesthetic, Local

LRC: L3 - No Data-Probably Compatible

Menthol is commonly used for topical analgesic and sore throat relief. Only a limited amount of menthol is absorbed systemically from topical application. Application of 300 mg of topical menthol patches produces maximum plasma concentration of 36 ng/mL.[1] Menthol is metabolized rapidly at first-pass metabolism to menthol glucuronide. Only minimal amounts of menthol would be transferred to breast milk. According to one source, only 0.063% of the maternal dose is transferred to breast milk.[2] Adverse effects to infant from breastfeeding are unlikely due to low relative dose and first-pass metabolism. There are no adequate and well-controlled studies in breastfeeding women.[3]

T 1/2	3-6 h (topical)	MW	156 Da	PB	
Tmax	3.4 h (topical)	RID	0.06%	Vd	
Oral		M/P		pKa	

Adult Concerns: Contact dermatitis. If ingested may cause nausea, vomiting, abdominal pain, drowsiness, ataxia.

Adult Dose:

Pediatric Concerns:

Infant Monitoring:

Alternatives:

References:

1. Martin D, Valdez J, Boren J, Mayersohn M. Dermal absorption of camphor, menthol, and methyl salicylate in humans. J Clin Pharmacol. 2004 Oct;44(10):1151-1157.
2. Hausner H, Bredie WL, Mølgaard C, Petersen MA, Møller P. Differential transfer of dietary flavour compounds into human breast milk. Physiol Behav. 2008 Sep 3;95(1-2):118-124. Epub 2008 May 15.
3. Menthol. In: TERIS® Database [Internet database]. Greenwood Village, CO: Thomson Reuters (Healthcare) Inc. Updated periodically. Accessed 06 July, 2011.

MEPERIDINE

Trade: Demerol, Pethidine

Category: Analgesic

LRC: L4 - Limited Data-Possibly Hazardous

Meperidine is a potent opiate analgesic. It is rapidly and completely metabolized by the adult and neonatal liver to an active metabolite, normeperidine. Significant but small amounts of meperidine are secreted in breast milk. In a study of nine nursing mothers 2 hours after a 50-mg IM injection, the average concentration of meperidine in milk was 82 µg/L and the milk/plasma ratio was 1.12.[1] The highest concentration of meperidine in breast milk at 2 hours after the dose was 0.13 mg/L.

In another study of three women, the maximum concentration of meperidine in milk ranged from 134 to 244 µg/L in five patients at 1-2 hours after administration and 76 to 318 µg/L at 2-4 hours after administration of 25 mg intravenously.[2] According to these authors, the maximum infant dose would be approximately 9.5 µg/kg or 1.2% to 3.5% of the weight-adjusted maternal dose.

In a study of two nursing mothers who received varying amounts of meperidine following delivery (up to 1275 mg within 72 hours), the levels in milk of meperidine ranged from 36.2 to 314 µg/L with an average of 225 µg/L. Breast milk levels of normeperidine ranged from zero to 333 µg/L with an average of 142 µg/L.[3] This study clearly shows a much longer half-life for the active metabolite, normeperidine. Normeperidine levels were detected after 56 hours post-administration in human milk (8.1 ng/mL) following a single 50-mg dose. The milk/plasma ratios varied from 0.82 to 1.59 depending on the dose and timing of sampling.

The Sudden Infant Death Syndrome Institute reviewed all cases of infants referred for unexplained apnea, bradycardia, and/or cyanosis in the first week of life (0.5-7 days) over a 1-year period (1984-85).[4] The data demonstrated that opioids could have been a factor as 10 of the 12 infants were exposed to opioids and most of their mothers received more doses than the control group. In this review six mothers were taking codeine, four were taking propoxyphene, and four were also given an intramuscular dose of meperidine.

In the largest study, infant exposure via breast milk after maternal epidural meperidine was assessed in 20 postpartum mother-infant pairs; the women received a mean dose of 670 mg over 41 hours for post-cesarean pain relief.[5] Maternal plasma, infant plasma, and breast milk samples were obtained within 2 hours of cessation of meperidine administration. A second sample was obtained 6 hours later. The combined relative infant dose (RID) for both meperidine and its active metabolite normeperidine at the first sampling time was 1.4%; this decreased to 0.9% within 6 hours. When meperidine and normeperidine concentrations in milk were considered independently, the mean RID for meperidine was 0.5%, while that for normeperidine was 0.65%. Therefore, at all times during the study period, the corresponding RIDs for meperidine and normeperidine remained within acceptable limits. No untoward effects were reported in the breastfed infants. Although the women in this study experienced adequate analgesia, the maternal plasma concentrations of the drug were well below the minimum effective plasma concentration required to provide clinical analgesia. This suggests that the analgesic effect of epidural meperidine is primarily local with little systemic absorption. No untoward effects were noted in the infants during the period of this study.

Published half-lives for meperidine in neonates (13 hours) and normeperidine (63 hours) are long and with time could concentrate in the plasma of a neonate. Wittels' studies clearly indicate that infants from mothers treated with meperidine (post-cesarean) were neurobehaviorally depressed after three days.[6] Infants from similar groups treated with morphine were not affected in the same manner.

T 1/2	2-4 h; active metabolite 15-30 h	MW	247 Da	PB	65-80%
Tmax	30-50 min (IM)	RID	1.1% - 13.3%	Vd	3.7-4.2 L/kg
Oral	<50%	M/P	0.84-1.59	pKa	8.6

Adult Concerns: Sedation, confusion, seizures, hypotension, bradycardia, respiratory depression, nausea, constipation, urinary retention, weakness.

Adult Dose: 50-100 mg every 3-4 h as needed.

Pediatric Concerns: Sedation, poor suckling reflex, neurobehavioral delay. Other narcotics with no active metabolite and a lower relative infant dose are preferred.

Infant Monitoring: Sedation, slowed breathing rate/apnea, pallor, constipation, and not waking to feed/poor feeding.

Alternatives: Fentanyl(L2), Hydrocodone(L3), Hydromorphone(L3)

References:
1. Peiker G, Muller B, Ihn W, Noschel H. Excretion of pethidine in mother's milk (author's transl). Zentralbl Gynakol. 1980;102(10):537-541.
2. Borgatta L, Jenny RW, Gruss L, Ong C, Barad D. Clinical significance of methohexital, meperidine, and diazepam in breast milk. J Clin Pharmacol. 1997;37(3):186-192.
3. Quinn PG, Kuhnert BR, Kaine CJ, Syracuse CD. Measurement of meperidine and normeperidine in human breast milk by selected ion monitoring. Biomed Environ Mass Spectrom. 1986;13(3):133-135.
4. Naumburg EG, Meny RG. Breast milk opioids and neonatal apnea. Pediatr Forum. 1998;142:11-12.
5. Al-Tamimi Y, Ilett KF, Paech MJ, O'Halloran SJ, Hartmann PE. Estimation of infant dose and exposure to pethidine and norpethidine via breast milk following patient-controlled epidural pethidine for analgesia post caesarean delivery. Int J Obstet Anesth. 2011 Apr;20(2):128-134.
6. Wittels B, Scott DT, Sinatra RS. Exogenous opioids in human breast milk and acute neonatal neurobehavior: a preliminary study. Anesthesiology. 1990;73(5):864-869.

MEPIVACAINE

Trade: Carbocaine, Polocaine

Category: Anesthetic, Local

LRC: L3 - No Data-Probably Compatible

Mepivacaine is a long-acting local anesthetic similar to bupivacaine.[1-3] Mepivacaine is used for infiltration, peripheral nerve blocks, and central nerve blocks (epidural or caudal anesthesia). No data are available on the transfer of mepivacaine into human milk; however, its structure is practically identical to bupivacaine and one would expect its entry into human milk is similar and low. Bupivacaine enters milk in exceedingly low levels (see bupivacaine below). Due to higher fetal levels and reported toxicities, mepivacaine is never used antenatally. For use in breastfeeding patients, bupivacaine is preferred.

T 1/2	1.9-3.2 h	MW	246 Da	PB	60-85%
Tmax	30 min	RID		Vd	
Oral		M/P		pKa	7.6

Adult Concerns: Sedation, bradycardia, respiratory sedation, transient burning, anaphylaxis.

Adult Dose: 50-300 mg X 1.

Pediatric Concerns: None reported via milk. Neonatal depression and convulsive seizures occurred in seven neonates 6 hours after delivery.

Infant Monitoring:

Alternatives:

References:
1. Pharmaceutical manufacturers prescribing information.
2. Hillman LS, Hillman RE, Dodson WE. Diagnosis, treatment, and follow-up of neonatal mepivacaine intoxication secondary to paracervical and pudendal blocks during labor. J Pediatr. 1979;95(3):472-477.
3. Teramo K, Rajamaki A. Foetal and maternal plasma levels of mepivacaine and foetal acid-base balance and heart rate after paracervical block during labour. Br J Anaesth. 1971;43(4):300-312.

MERCAPTOPURINE

Trade: 6-MP, Puri-Nethol, Purinethol

Category: Antimetabolite

LRC: L3 - Limited Data-Probably Compatible

Azathioprine is metabolized to 6-mercaptopurine, so both are essentially identical. 6-Mercaptopurine (6-MP) is an anticancer and immunosuppressant drug that acts intracellularly as a purine antagonist, ultimately inhibiting DNA and RNA synthesis.[1] It is commonly used to treat Crohn's disease and ulcerative colitis due to its immunosuppressant effect. Numerous breastfeeding studies are available with respect to azathioprine and 6-MP.

In two mothers receiving 75 mg azathioprine, the concentration of 6-MP in milk varied from 3.5-4.5 µg/L in one mother and 18 µg/L in the second mother.[2] Both levels were peak milk concentrations at 2 hours following the dose. The authors conclude that these levels would be too low to produce clinical effects in a breastfed infant. Using this data for 6-MP, an infant would absorb only 0.1 % of the weight-adjusted maternal dose, which is probably too low to produce adverse effects in a breastfeeding infant. Plasma levels in treated patients is maintained at 50 ng/mL or higher. One infant continued to breastfeed during therapy and displayed no immunosuppressive effects. In another study of two infants who were breastfed by mothers receiving 75-100 mg/day azathioprine, milk levels of 6-MP were not measured. But both infants had normal blood counts, no increase in infections, and above-average growth rate.[3]

Four mothers who were receiving 1.2-2.1 mg/kg/day of azathioprine throughout pregnancy and continued postpartum were studied while breastfeeding. The mothers' blood concentrations of 6-TGN and 6-MMPN (the metabolites of azathioprine) ranged from 234-291 and 284 to 1178 pmol/100 million RBC, respectively. Neither 6-TGN nor 6-MMPN could be detected in the exposed infants. The authors suggest that breastfeeding while taking azathioprine may be safe in mothers with "normal" TPMT enzyme activity (the enzyme responsible for metabolizing 6-TGN).[4]

Four case reports were performed with mothers taking between 50 to 100 mg/day of azathioprine. No adverse events were reported in any of the infants, and milk concentrations in two mothers proved to be undetectable.[5] Ten women at steady state on 75 to 150 mg/day azathioprine provided milk samples on days 3-4, days 7-10, and day 28 after delivery, between 3 and 18 hours after azathioprine administration. 6-MP was detected in only one case, at 1.2 and 7.6 ng/mL at 3 and 6 hours after azathioprine intake on day 28. However, 6-MP and 6-TGN were undetectable in the infants' blood. There were no signs of immunosuppression, even in three preterm neonates. The authors suggest that azathioprine therapy should not deter mothers from breastfeeding.[6] Another study of three mothers taking azathioprine while breastfeeding (doses of 100-175 mg) reported normal blood cell counts in all three infants, and only a low amount of 6-TGN in one infant on day 3. At age 3 weeks, this level decreased below the detectable range.[7] In a group of eight lactating women who received azathioprine (75-200 mg/day), levels in milk ranged from 2-50 µg/L.[8] After 6 hours an average of 10% of the peak values were measured. The authors estimate the infants' dose to be <0.008 mg/kg/24 hours. They suggest that breastfeeding during treatment with azathioprine seems safe and should be recommended. In a 31-year-old mother with Crohn's disease being treated with 100 mg/day azathioprine, peripheral blood levels of 6-MP and 6-TGN in the infant were undetectable at day 8 or after 3 months of therapy.[9] The infant was reported to be normal after 6 months. In a recent study of the long-term follow-up (median 3.3 years) of fetal and breastfeeding exposure to azathioprine (n = 11 infants), there were no differences in rates of infectious disease in azathioprine-treated groups compared to non-treated controls. The authors suggest that breastfeeding following exposure to azathioprine does not increase the risk of infections.[10]

In summary, the transport of 6-mercaptopurine into human milk is apparently quite low. However, this is a strong immunosuppressant and some caution is still recommended if it is used in a breastfeeding mother. Monitor the infant closely for signs of immunosuppression, leukopenia, thrombocytopenia, hepatotoxicity, pancreatitis, and other symptoms of 6-mercaptopurine exposure. The risks to the infant are probably low. Recent long-term data suggest that the rate of infections in treated groups is no different from non-treated controls.

T 1/2	21-90 min	MW	170 Da	PB	19%
Tmax	2 h	RID		Vd	0.9 L/kg
Oral	50%	M/P		pKa	7.6

Adult Concerns: Bone marrow suppression, liver toxicity, nausea, vomiting, diarrhea.

Adult Dose: 1.5-2.5 mg/kg daily.

Pediatric Concerns: No data are available on 6-MP, but data on azathioprine has been published.

Infant Monitoring: If signs of immunosuppression or anemia check CBC; if signs of liver dysfunction (yellowing of skin or whites of eyes), check liver enzymes and bilirubin.

Alternatives: Infliximab(L3)

References:

1. Pharmaceutical manufacturers prescribing information.
2. Coulam CB, Moyer TP, Jiang NS, Zincke H. Breast-feeding after renal transplantation. Transplant Proc. 1982;14(3):605-609.
3. Grekas DM, Vasiliou SS, Lazarides AN. Immunosuppressive therapy and breast-feeding after renal transplantation. Nephron. 1984;37(1):68.
4. Gardiner SJ, Gearry RB, Roberts RL, Zhang M, Barclay ML, Begg EJ. Exposure to thiopurine drugs through breast milk is low based on metabolite concentrations in mother-infant pairs. Br J Clin Pharmacol. 2006;62(4):453-456.
5. Moretti ME, Verjee Z, Ito S, Koren G. Breast-feeding during maternal use of Azathioprine. Ann Pharmacother. 2006;40:2269-2272.
6. Sau A, Clarke S, Bass J, Kaiser A, Marinaki A, Nelson-Piercy C. Azathioprine and breastfeeding- is it safe? BJOG. 2007;114:498-501.

7. Bernard N, Garayt C, Chol F, Vial T, Descotes J. Prospective clinical and biological follow-up of three breastfed babies from azathioprine-treated mothers. Fundam clin Pharmacol. 2007;21 (suppl.1):62-63. Abstract.

8. Christensen LA, Dahlerup JF, Nielsen MJ, Fallingborg JF, Schmiegelow K. Azathioprine treatment during lactation. Aliment Pharmacol Ther. 2008 Nov;28(10):1209-1213. Epub 2008 Aug 30.

9. Zelinkova Z, De Boer IP, Van Dijke MJ, Kuipers EJ, Van Der Woude CJ. Azathioprine treatment during lactation. Aliment Pharmacol Ther. 2009 Jul;30(1):90-91;

10. Angelberger S, Reinisch W, Messerschmidt A, et al. Long-term follow-up of babies exposed to azathioprine in utero and via breastfeeding. J Crohns Colitis. 2011 Apr;5(2):95-100. Epub 2010 Dec 9.

MERCURY

Trade: Mercury

Category: Metals

LRC: L5 - Limited Data-Hazardous

Mercury is an environmental contaminate that is available in multiple salt forms. Elemental mercury, the form found in thermometers, is poorly absorbed orally (0.01%) but completely absorbed via inhalation (>80%).[1] Inorganic mercury causes most forms of mercury poisoning and is available in mercury disk batteries (7-15% orally bioavailable). Organic mercury (methyl mercury fungicides, phenyl mercury) is readily absorbed (90% orally). Mercury poisoning produces encephalopathy, acute renal failure, severe GI necrosis, and numerous other systemic toxicities. Mercury transfers to human milk with a milk/plasma ratio that varies according to the mercury form. Pitkin reports that in the USA that 100 unexposed women had 0.9 µg/L total mercury in their milk.[2] Concentrations of mercury in human milk are generally much higher in populations that ingest large quantities of fish. Mothers known to be contaminated with mercury should not breastfeed.

The transfer of mercury from dental amalgams has been studied to some degree. In mothers with mercury-containing amalgams, the transfer of mercury during gestation to the fetus is generally much higher than from human milk.[3,4] Mercury levels in milk are highest immediately after birth, and these are significantly correlated with the number and size of amalgam fillings present in the mother, although others disagree.[5,6,7] In this study breastmilk levels of mercury dropped significantly after 2 months and are more positively associated with the amount of fish ingested, rather than the number of amalgam fillings. At birth mercury levels in milk averaged 0.9 µg/L (0.25 to 20.3 µg/L) and after 2 months mercury levels averaged 0.25 µg/L (0.25-11.7 µg/L). The authors suggest that the exposure to mercury of breastfed infants from maternal amalgam fillings is of minor importance compared to maternal fish consumption.

Oskarsson suggests, in a study of Swedish women, that the exposure of the infant to mercury from breast milk was less than 0.3 µg/kg/d. This exposure is only approximately one-half the tolerable daily intake for adults recommended by the World Health Organization.[6]

These studies generally conclude that while mercury fillings may increase the transfer of mercury to the infant, it usually occurs in utero. Secondly, the transfer of mercury to human milk is transiently high at birth and then drops significantly at 2 months. Apparently the diet provides the greatest source of maternal mercury to human milk; much less is provided by older amalgam fillings. The removal or replacement of amalgam fillings while pregnant or breastfeeding could potentially increase the transfer of mercury to the infant (this largely depends on the precautions taken by the dentist). This procedure should be postponed if possible.

There are several routine precautions that the dentist could use when removing the old amalgam. Because heat during the grinding process can vaporize the mercury and enhance absorption by the mother, suggest that the dentist use copious amounts of cold water irrigation to minimize heat, use a rubber dam to isolate her mouth from the particles, and use an alternate source of air (oxygen) to minimize mercury vapor inhalation during removal of the amalgam.

While the USA has removed methylmercury from virtually all pediatric immunizations, other countries have not. In infants receiving three doses of hepatitis B vaccine and three DTP vaccines during the first 6 months of life, the exposure to ethylmercury was 25 µg Hg for each vaccine. Infant hair-Hg increased 446% during these six months, while maternal hair-Hg decreased 57%. This provides evidence that the extra mercury exposure is due to the vaccinations rather than maternal milk.[8]

The new compact fluorescent light bulbs commonly in use today contain only 5 mg of mercury. This is 1/100th of the amount used in a single dental amalgam. Exposure to this limited amount would not be hazardous to a breastfeeding infant.

Normal mercury values in blood are <10 ng/mL. Individuals with minimal daily exposure (such as dentists) may routinely have levels around 15 ng/mL. Patients with heavy fish consumption may have levels approaching 20 ng/mL. Levels >50 ng/mL (alkyl Hg) or >200 ng/mL (inorganic Hg2+) constitute significant exposure requiring treatment. For treatment, see entries on Penicillamine and Succimer.

T 1/2	70 days	MW	201 Da	PB	
Tmax		RID		Vd	
Oral	Variable	M/P	0.27 -1.0	pKa	

Adult Concerns: Brain damage, acute renal failure, severe GI necrosis, and numerous other systemic toxicities.

Adult Dose:

Pediatric Concerns: Mercury transfer into milk is significant. Transfer to the infant is a function of levels in the mother. Mercury levels in milk drop significantly after 2 months.

Infant Monitoring: Neurodevelopment.

Alternatives:

References:

1. Wofff MS. Occupationally derived chemicals in breast milk. Am J Ind Med. 1983;4:259-281.
2. Pitkin RM, Bahns JA, Filer LJ, Reynolds WA. Mercury in human maternal and cord blood, placenta, and milk. Proc Soc Exp Med. 1976;151:565-567.
3. Ramirez GB, Cruz MC, Pagulayan O, Ostrea E, Dalisay C. The Tagum study I: analysis and clinical correlates of mercury in maternal and cord blood, breast milk, meconium, and infants' hair. Pediatrics. 2000;106(4):774-781.
4. Yang J, Jiang Z, Wang Y, Qureshi IA, Wu XD. Maternal-fetal transfer of metallic mercury via the placenta and milk. Ann Clin Lab Sci. 1997;27(2):135-141.
5. Drexler H, Schaller KH. The mercury concentration in breast milk resulting from amalgam fillings and dietary habits. Environ Res. 1998;77(2):124-129.
6. Oskarsson A, Schultz A, Skerfving S, Hallen IP, Ohlin B, Lagerkvist BJ. Total and inorganic mercury in breast milk in relation to fish consumption and amalgam in lactating women. Arch Environ Health. 1996;51(3):234-241.
7. Klemann D, Weinhold J, Strubelt O, Pentz R, Jungblut JR, Klink F. Effects of amalgam fillings on the mercury concentrations in amniotic fluid and breast milk. Dtsch Zahnarztl Z. 1990;45(3):142-145.
8. Marques RC, Dórea JG, Fonseca MF, Bastos WR, Malm O. Hair mercury in breast-fed infants exposed to thimerosal-preserved vaccines. Eur J Pediatr. 2007 Sep;166(9):935-941. Epub 2007 Jan 20. PubMed PMID: 17237965.

MEROPENEM

Trade: Meronem, Merrem

Category: Antibiotic, Carbapenem

LRC: L3 - Limited Data-Probably Compatible

Meropenem is a carbapenem antibiotic with similar efficacy to imipenem/cilastatin.[1] This agent is not orally bioavailable to any degree but changes in gastrointestinal flora could occur in a breastfed infant. There is one published case report of meropenem in breastfeeding from 2012. A postpartum female received meropenem 1000 mg IV every 8 hours for 7 days to treat a resistant *E.coli* urinary tract infection.[2] The average and maximum meropenem concentrations in breast milk were found to be 0.48 μg/mL and 0.64 μg/mL. Using the average and maximum milk concentration, the estimated infant doses would be 0.072 mg/kg/day and 0.097 mg/kg/day respectively. The authors of this case report estimated the relative infant doses by using the average and maximum concentrations in breast milk and the maternal weight of 57 kg; they found the RIDs to be 0.13% and 0.18% respectively.

Our estimate of the RIDs using a standard 70-kg maternal weight were 0.17% and 0.23%. There were no adverse effects to the infant during maternal treatment or up to 30 days after completing therapy.[2] This case report demonstrated that meropenem does not readily enter breast milk and that this drug is most likely suitable in lactation.[2]

T 1/2	1.58 - 3.8 h	MW	437 Da	PB	2%
Tmax	Immediate	RID	0.17% - 0.23%	Vd	0.28 L/kg
Oral	Nil	M/P		pKa	3.47

Adult Concerns: Headache, seizures (0.5%), nausea, abdominal pain, diarrhea, and elevated liver function tests have been reported.

Adult Dose: 1 gram IV every 8 hours.

Pediatric Concerns: None reported via breast milk in one case report.

Infant Monitoring: Vomiting, diarrhea, changes in gastrointestinal flora, and rash.

Alternatives: Ertapenem(L2)

References:
1. Pharmaceutical manufacturers prescribing information.
2. Sauberan JB, Bradley JS, Blumer J, Stellwagen LM. Transmission of meropenem in breast milk. Pediatr Infect Dis J. 2012;31:832-834.

MESALAMINE

Trade: Apriso, Asacol, Canasa, Delzicol, Lialda, Mesalazine, Mesasal, Pentasa, Quintasa, Rowasa, Salofalk

Category: Anti-Inflammatory

LRC: L3 - Limited Data-Probably Compatible

Mesalamine, or 5-aminosalicylic acid (5-ASA), is used as an anti-inflammatory, immunosuppressant, and bacteriostatic agent for treatment of ulcerative colitis.[1] This drug comes in a variety of dosages, formulations, and routes of administration, which deliver the drug to particular parts of the GI tract. Absorption and metabolism of mesalamine vary drastically throughout the tract. Rectal suppositories are minimally absorbed, while oral, unformulated (i.e. no enteric coating) suspensions are almost 80% absorbed. Furthermore, the first-pass metabolism of absorbed drug is easily saturable, leading to disproportionately high plasma levels at the higher end of the dosage range.

In one patient receiving 500 mg mesalamine orally three times daily, the concentration of 5-ASA in breast milk was 0.11 mg/L, and the acetyl-5-ASA metabolite was 12.4 mg/L of milk.[2] Using these numbers, the weight-adjusted RID of metabolite and active ingredient would be 8.8%.

In a second case report of a patient receiving 1 g of 5-ASA three times daily, the milk levels for 5-ASA and acetyl-5-ASA were 0.1 µg/mL and 12.3 µg/mL respectively at 11 days postpartum.[3] The authors estimated the infant would receive about 0.015 mg/kg/day of 5-ASA and 2-3 mg/kg/day of acetyl-5-ASA. These results suggest that even with high doses (3 g/day), the amount of 5-ASA transferred is minimal.

In a study of four breastfeeding women, concentrations of 5-ASA in milk were 4-40 µg/L and the N-acetyl-5-ASA were 5-14.9 mg/L. The authors of this study calculated that infants would receive about 0.0006-0.006 mg/kg/day of 5-ASA in milk. [4]

Few adverse effects have been observed in most nursing infants; however, a 3-month-old infant exposed to sulfasalazine in breast milk experienced bloody diarrhea.[5] In this case, the mother was taking 3 g/day of sulfasalazine and the infant was exclusively breastfed. At 2 months of age the infant had its first episode of bloody diarrhea; this recurred 2 weeks later and then persisted until 3 months of age. The diarrhea occurred up to six times per day; all investigations were considered normal, except sulfapyridine was measurable in the infant's blood (5.3 mg/L). When the mother's therapy was stopped, the infant's symptoms resolved 48-72 hours later.

In the second case report, a woman was taking 5-ASA 500 mg rectally twice daily and her infant had multiple episodes of diarrhea.[6] This woman stopped and started her medication multiple times due to her infant's diarrhea and each time the diarrhea started 8-12 hours after she took the medication and resolved 8-12 hours after she stopped. No further episodes occurred after breastfeeding ceased.

Barriuso reports a case of a 4-month-old breastfed infant, with a thrombosis of the superior sagittal sinus secondary to a severe thrombocytosis.[7] The mother, suffering Crohn's disease, had recently discontinued 1 week prior the use of mesalazine throughout her pregnancy and during lactation. The authors hypothesized that the recent discontinuation of mesalamine led to thrombosis.

Be advised that many recent formulations of mesalamine are in colon-delivery systems which probably reduces the overall oral absorption commonly seen in older studies.

T 1/2	0.5-10 h (metabolite)	MW	153 Da	PB	55%
Tmax	4-16 h	RID	0.12% - 8.76%	Vd	0.26 L/kg
Oral	20-40%	M/P	0.27, 5.1	pKa	2.02

Adult Concerns: Headache, dizziness, fever, nausea, vomiting, anorexia, abdominal pain, watery diarrhea, bloody diarrhea, changes in liver function, leukopenia, thrombocytopenia, hemolytic anemia, skin rash, pruritus.

Adult Dose: 800 mg three times daily.

Pediatric Concerns: With 5-ASA and other similar products there has been one reported case of hypersensitivity, as well as multiple case reports of infants with bloody stools and diarrhea. In addition, case reports of pediatric patients taking 5-ASA formulations have also found bloody diarrhea.[6] Caution in infants with G6PD deficiency.

Infant Monitoring: Vomiting, watery diarrhea.

Alternatives:

References:
1. Pharmaceutical manufacturers prescribing information.
2. Jenss H, Weber P, Hartmann F. 5-Aminosalicylic acid and its metabolite in breast milk during lactation. Am J Gastroenterol. 1990 Mar;85(3):331.

3. Klotz U, Harings-Kaim A. Negligible excretion of 5-aminosalicylic acid in breast milk. Lancet. 1993 Sep;342(8871):618-619.
4. Silverman DA, Ford J, Shaw I, Probert CS. Is mesalazine really safe for use in breastfeeding mothers? Gut. 2005 Jan;54(1):170-171.
5. Branski D, Kerem E, Gross-Kieselstein E, Hurvitz H, Litt R, Abrahamov A. Bloody diarrhea--a possible complication of sulfasalazine transferred through human breast milk. J Pediatr Gastroenterol Nutr. 1986 Mar-Apr;5(2):316-317.
6. Nelis GF. Diarrhoea due to 5-aminosalicylic acid in breast milk. Lancet. 1989 Feb;1(8634):383.
7. Esbjorner E, Jarnerot G, Wranne L. Sulphasalazine and sulphapyridine serum levels in children to mothers treated with sulphasalazine during pregnancy and lactation. Acta Paediatr Scand. 1987;76(1):137-142.

MESTRANOL

Trade:

Category: Estrogen

LRC: L3 - No Data-Probably Compatible

Mestranol is a prodrug of ethinyl estradiol. Seventy percent of mestranol is converted in the liver to ethinyl estradiol. Ethinyl estradiol is an estrogenic agent. Although small amounts of estrogens may pass into breast milk, the effects of estrogens on the infant appear minimal. In one study, ethinyl estradiol was not detected in breast milk after administration of 50 μg/day.[1] After administration of 500 μg/day, the level in breast milk was approximately 300 pg/mL.[1] Early postpartum use of estrogens may reduce volume of milk produced and the protein content, but it is variable, controversial, and depends on dose and the individual.[2,3,4,5] Breastfeeding mothers should attempt to wait until lactation is firmly established (6-8 weeks) prior to use of estrogen-containing oral contraceptives. See Contraception monograph for further details.

Adult Concerns: Headache, hypertension, increased breast size, dysmenorrhea, uterine or fibroid growth, bloating, edema, thromboembolism, chloasma.

Adult Dose:

Pediatric Concerns:

Infant Monitoring: Possible suppression of milk production early postpartum is reported.

Alternatives:

References:

1. Nilsson S, Nygren KG, Johansson ED. Ethinyl estradiol in human milk and plasma after oral administration. Contraception. 1978 Feb;17(2):131-139.
2. Booker DE, Pahl IR. Control of postpartum breast engorgement with oral contraceptives. Am J Obstet Gynecol. 1967; 98(8):1099-1101.
3. Kamal I, Hefnawi F, Ghoneim M, Abdallah M, Abdel RS. Clinical, biochemical, and experimental studies on lactation. V. Clinical effects of steroids on the initiation of lactation. Am J Obstet Gynecol. 1970;108(4):655-658.
4. Kora SJ. Effect of oral contraceptives on lactation. Fertil Steril. 1969;20(3):419-423.
5. Koetsawang S, Bhiraleus P, Chiemprajert T. Effects of oral contraceptives on lactation. Fertil Steril. 1972;23(1):24-28.

METAMIZOLE

Trade: Analgin, Dipyrone, Novalgin, Novalgina

Category: Analgesic

LRC: L4 - Limited Data-Possibly Hazardous

Metamizole is an effective analgesic and antipyretic and was removed from the US market due to serious adverse effects including agranulocytosis, aplastic anemia, thrombocytopenic purpura, and hemolytic anemia. However, it is still used in other countries. Recent estimates suggest that the incidence of metamizole-induced agranulocytosis is between 0.2 and 2 cases per million person-days of use. This is lower than many commonly used medications in the United States.

In one patient who took three doses of 500 mg orally over a 16-hour period, metamizole concentrations in the mother's serum and milk and in the infant's serum and urine were 3.3, 4.3 and 3.2, 3.74 μg/mL respectively.[1]

Metamizole was detected in the serum of one breastfed infant and its urine after his mother took 1500 mg of metamizole over a 16-hour period. The infant's metamizole serum concentration was 3.2 mg/L and urine concentration was 3.74 mg/L. Two cyanotic episodes were noted in a 42 day-old infant approximately 30 minutes following the maternal dose of 1500 mg.[1]

In a group of eight women, 3-5 days postpartum, who received 1-g doses of metamizole, milk levels of metamizole metabolites were sampled between 2.5 and 5.5 hours.[2] Four metabolites were measured: 4-methylaminoantipyrine (MAA), 4-aminoantipyrine (AA), 4-formylaminoantipyrine (FAA), and 4-acetylaminoantipyrine (AAA). The sum of the mean concentrations of all four metabolites in milk was 20.37 mg/L. The mean concentration of MAA, the only active metabolite, was 11.2 µg/mL. Using the MAA data, the relative infant dose would be 1.2%. All metabolites were undetectable by 48 hours.

Because of its known complications, such as agranulocytosis and other blood dyscrasias, it is no longer recommended as an analgesic in many countries. Other safer alternatives are available.

T 1/2	2-3 h (4-MAA)	MW	311 Da	PB	58%
Tmax	1 h	RID	1.2% - 3%	Vd	0.57 L/kg
Oral	Complete	M/P	1.37 (MAA)	pKa	

Adult Concerns: Agranulocytosis, aplastic anemia, thrombocytopenic purpura, and hemolytic anemia. Hypotension, skin rash, urticaria, toxic epidermal necrolysis have been reported.

Adult Dose: 500 mg to 1 gram 3-4 times a day.

Pediatric Concerns: Two cyanotic episodes were noted in a 42-day-old infant approximately 30 minutes following the maternal dose of 1500 mg.

Infant Monitoring: Avoid; not recommended in lactation.

Alternatives: Ibuprofen(L1), Acetaminophen(L1)

References:

1. Rizzoni G, Furlanut M. Cyanotic crisis in a breast-fed infant from mother taking dipyrone. Hum Toxicol. 1984;3:505-507.
2. Zylber-Katz E , Linder N, Granit L, Levy M. Excretion of dipyrone metabolites in human breast milk. Eur J Clin Pharmacol. 1986;30:359-361.

METAXALONE

Trade: Skelaxin

Category: Skeletal Muscle Relaxant

LRC: L3 - No Data-Probably Compatible

Metaxalone is a centrally acting sedative used primarily as a muscle relaxant.[1] Its ability to relax skeletal muscle is weak and is probably due to its sedative properties. No data are available on its transfer to breast milk.

T 1/2	11.1 (females) h	MW	221 Da	PB	
Tmax	3.3 h	RID		Vd	11.4 L/kg
Oral		M/P		pKa	13.14

Adult Concerns: Sedation, nausea, vomiting, gastrointestinal upset, hemolytic anemia, abnormal liver function.

Adult Dose: 800 mg 3-4 times daily.

Pediatric Concerns: None reported. No data available.

Infant Monitoring: Sedation, vomiting, gastrointestinal upset.

Alternatives:

References:

1. Pharmaceutical manufacturers prescribing information.

METFORMIN

Trade: Diabex, Diaformin, Diguanil, Glucophage, Glumetza, Glycon, Riomet

Category: Antidiabetic, other

LRC: L1 - Limited Data-Compatible

Metformin belongs to the biguanide family and is used to reduce glucose levels in non-insulin dependent diabetics. It is also used to treat polycystic ovary syndrome. Oral bioavailability is only 50%. In a study of seven women taking metformin (median dose 1500 mg/day), the mean milk/plasma ratio for metformin was 0.35.[1] The average concentration in milk over the dose interval was 0.27 mg/L. The absolute infant dose averaged 0.04 mg/kg/day and the mean relative infant dose was 0.28%. Metformin was present in very low or undetectable concentrations in the plasma of four of the infants who were studied. No health problems were found in the six infants who were evaluated. In another study of five subjects, the median milk/plasma ratio for metformin was 0.47.[2] The median calculated infant dose was 0.2% of the weight-adjusted maternal dose. None of the infants exposed to their mothers' milk had detectable levels of metformin in their plasma, nor were any side effects noted.

In a recent study of five women consuming an average dose of 500 mg twice daily, the mean peak and trough metformin concentrations in breast milk were 0.42 mg/L (range 0.38-0.46 mg/L) and 0.39 mg/L (range 0.31-0.52 mg/L), respectively.[3] The average milk/plasma ratio was 0.63 (range 0.36-1) and the estimated relative infant dose was 0.65% (range 0.43-1.08%). Blood glucose concentrations in three infants were normal, ranging from 47-77 mg/dL. The mothers reported no side effects in the breastfed infants.

In one study of 61 nursing infants whose mothers were taking a median of 2.55 g/day throughout pregnancy and lactation, the growth, motor, and social development of the infants was recorded to be normal. The authors concluded that metformin was safe and effective during breastfeeding in the first 6 months of an infant's life.[4]

T 1/2	6.2 h	MW	165 Da	PB	Minimal
Tmax	2.75 h	RID	0.3% - 0.7%	Vd	9 L/kg
Oral	50%	M/P	0.35-0.63	pKa	12.4

Adult Concerns: Headache, dizziness, nausea, vomiting, abdominal pain, diarrhea, bloating, hypoglycemia, vitamin B12 deficiency, lactic acidosis.

Adult Dose: 500 mg twice daily.

Pediatric Concerns: No side effects noted in three studies. Plasma levels undetectable.

Infant Monitoring: Vomiting, diarrhea and signs of hypoglycemia- drowsiness, lethargy, pallor, sweating, tremor.

Alternatives: Glyburide(L2), Insulin(L2)

References:
1. Hale TW, Kristensen JH, Hackett LP, Kohan R, Ilett KF. Transfer of metformin into human milk. Diabetologia. 2002;45(11):1509-1514.
2. Gardiner SJ, Kirkpatrick CM, Begg EJ, Zhang M, Moore MP, Saville DJ. Transfer of metformin into human milk. Clin Pharmacol Ther. 2003;73(1):71-77.
3. Briggs GG, Ambrose PJ, Nageotte MP, Padilla G, Wan S. Excretion of metformin into breast milk and the effect on nursing infants. Obstet Gynecol. 2005 Jun;105(6):1437-1441.
4. Glueck CJ, Salehi M, Sieve L, Wang P. Growth, motor, and social development in breast-and formula-fed infants of metformin-treated women with polycystic ovary syndrome. J Pediatr. 2006;148:628-632.

METHACHOLINE CHLORIDE

Trade: Arthralgen, Mecholyl, Provocholine

Category: Diagnostic Agent, Bronchial

LRC: L3 - No Data-Probably Compatible

Methacholine is an analog of acetylcholine and is used via inhalation to diagnose asthma. When inhaled in patients prone for asthma, acute bronchoconstriction occurs, confirming the diagnosis of asthma. Although it is unlikely this product would enter milk in clinically relevant amounts, it is also unlikely to survive the gastrointestinal tract. Because this is a one-time test, a brief interruption of breastfeeding for a few hours (about 4 hours) would all but eliminate any risk.

T 1/2	Brief	MW	195 Da	PB	
Tmax	1-4 min	RID		Vd	
Oral	Low to nil	M/P		pKa	

Adult Concerns: Headache, lightheadedness, shortness of breath, wheezing.

Adult Dose: Highly variable.

Pediatric Concerns: None reported via milk.

Infant Monitoring:

Alternatives:

References:
1. Pharmaceutical manufacturers prescribing information.

METHADONE

Trade: Biodone forte, Dolophine, Metadon, Methex, Physeptone

Category: Analgesic

LRC: L2 - Significant Data-Compatible

Methadone is a potent and very long-acting opiate analgesic. It is primarily used to prevent withdrawal in opiate addiction. In one study of 10 women receiving methadone 10-80 mg/day, the average milk/plasma ratio was 0.83.[1] Due to the variable doses used, the milk concentrations ranged from 0.05 mg/L in one patient receiving 10 mg/day, to 0.57 mg/L in a patient receiving 80 mg/day. One infant death has been reported in a breastfeeding mother receiving maintenance methadone therapy, although it is not clear that the only source of methadone to this infant was from breast milk.[2]

In a study of 12 breastfeeding women on methadone maintenance with doses ranging from 20-80 mg/day, the mean concentration of methadone in plasma and milk were 311 (207-416) µg/L and 116 (72-160) µg/L respectively yielding a mean M/P ratio of 0.44 (0.24-0.64).[3] The mean absolute oral dose to the infant was 17.4 (10.8-24) µg/kg/day. This equates to a mean of 2.79% of the maternal dose per day. In this study, 64% of the infants exhibited neonatal abstinence syndrome requiring treatment.

In two women receiving similar doses of methadone, 30 mg twice daily and 73 mg once daily, the average breast milk concentrations were 0.169 mg/L and 0.132 mg/L respectively.[4] The milk/plasma ratios were 1.215 and 0.661 respectively. While the infant of the second mother died at 3 1/2 months of SIDS, it was apparently not due to methadone, as none was present in the infant's plasma and the infant was significantly supplemented with formula.

In an excellent study, eight mother/infant pairs ingesting from 40 to 105 mg/day methadone, the average (AUC) concentration of R-methadone and S-methadone enantiomers varied from 42-259 µg/L and 26-126 µg/L respectively.[5] The relative infant dose was estimated to be 2.8% of the maternal dose. Interestingly, there was little difference in methadone milk levels in immature and mature milk.

Most studies thus far show that only small amounts of methadone pass into breast milk despite doses as high as 105 mg/day. In fact, neonatal abstinence syndromes are well known to occur in breastfeeding infants following delivery. In one study, 58% of infants developed neonatal abstinence syndrome while still breastfeeding.[3] However, some methadone is undoubtedly transferred via milk, and abrupt cessation of breastfeeding during high-dose therapy has resulted in neonatal abstinence in some infants.[6]

In a recent study of eight methadone-maintained lactating women (dose= 50-105 mg/day), the concentration of methadone in milk was low (range: 2-462 ng/mL) and interestingly, was not related to maternal dose.[7] Maternal plasma levels rose over a 4-week period postpartum to reach a high at 30 days. Median milk/plasma ratios ranged from 0.22 to 0.92. The average amount of methadone ingestible by the infant was estimated to be <0.2 mg/day at day 30 postpartum. Infant plasma levels of methadone ranged from 2.2 to 8.1 ng/mL. Again, there was no correlation between maternal dose and infant plasma level. There were no significant neurobehavioral changes noted.

In a study of four methadone-consuming mothers whose doses ranged from 60-110 mg/day, milk levels ranged from as low as 27 ng/mL to as high as 407 ng/mL. While the dose and sampling method was highly variable, the authors estimated that the average daily dose to an infant was about 330 µg/day.[8]

In a group of 20 women consuming 40-200 mg/day (mean 102 mg/day), R-methadone concentrations in milk were 1.3-3 times higher than S-methadone levels in all breast milk samples studied. The average Relative Infant Dose range of R-, S-, and total methadone were 2.7%, 1.6%, and 2.1% respectively.[9]

A 2011 study that verified a method to quantify illicit substances in human milk obtained one milk sample from a woman with a history of heroin use who was put on methadone maintenance therapy. Her milk sample contained 97 µg/L of methadone with 8 µg/L of its metabolite EDDP and a low concentration of morphine 7 µg/L.[10] No details were provided regarding her last heroin use, methadone dose, timing of dose, and milk sample or infant outcomes in this paper.

In summary, the dose of R plus S methadone transferred via milk generally averages less than 2.8% of the maternal dose.[5] This is significantly less than the conventional cut-off value of 10% of the maternal dose corrected for weight. Although the amount in milk is insufficient to prevent neonatal withdrawal syndrome, another new study suggests that it actually reduces the incidence of neonatal abstinence syndrome when infants are breastfed (OR=0.55).[11]

T 1/2	13-55 h	MW	309 Da	PB	89%
Tmax	0.5-1 h	RID	1.9% - 6.5%	Vd	4-5 L/kg
Oral	50%	M/P	0.68 (R)	pKa	8.6

Adult Concerns: Sedation, respiratory depression/apnea, nausea, vomiting, constipation. Withdrawal can occur if not titrated off the medication.

Adult Dose: Usually started at 20 mg daily and titrated to effect.

Pediatric Concerns: Neonatal abstinence syndrome after in utero exposure.

Infant Monitoring: Sedation, slowed breathing rate/apnea, pallor, constipation, and not waking to feed/poor feeding.

Alternatives:

References:

1. Blinick G, Inturrisi CE, Jerez E, Wallach RC. Methadone assays in pregnant women and progeny. Am J Obstet Gynecol. 1975;121(5):617-621.
2. Smialek JE, Monforte JR, Aronow R, Spitz WU. Methadone deaths in children. A continuing problem. JAMA. 1977;238(23):2516-2517.
3. Wojnar-Horton RE, Kristensen JH, Yapp P, Ilett KF, Dusci LJ, Hackett LP. Methadone distribution and excretion into breast milk of clients in a methadone maintenance programme. Br J Clin Pharmacol. 1997;44(6):543-547.
4. Geraghty B, Graham EA, Logan B, Weiss EL. Methadone levels in breast milk. J Hum Lact. 1997;13(3):227-230.
5. Begg EJ, Malpas TJ, Hackett LP, Ilett KF. Distribution of R- and S-methadone into human milk during multiple, medium to high oral dosing. Br J Clin Pharmacol. 2001;52(6):681-685.
6. Malpas TJ, Darlow BA. Neonatal abstinence syndrome following abrupt cessation of breastfeeding. N Z Med J. 1999;112(1080):12-13.
7. Jansson LM, Choo R, Velez ML, et al. Methadone maintenance and breastfeeding in the neonatal period. Pediatrics. 2008;121:106-114.
8. Jansson LM, Choo R, Velez ML, Lowe R, Huestis MA. Methadone maintenance and long-term lactation. Breastfeed Med. 2008 Mar;3(1):34-37.
9. Bogen DL, Perel JM, Helsel JC, Hanusa BH, Thompson M, Wisner KL. Estimated infant exposure to enantiomer-specific methadone levels in breastmilk. Breastfeed Med. 2011 Dec;6:377-384.
10. Marchei E, Escuder D, Pallas CR, et al. Simultaneous analysis of frequently used licit and illicit psychoactive drugs in breast milk by liquid chromatography tandem mass spectrometry. J Pharm Biomed Anal. 2011;55:309–316.
11. Dryden C, Young D, Hepburn M, Mactier H. Maternal methadone use in pregnancy: factors associated with the development of neonatal abstinence syndrome and implications for healthcare resources. BJOG. 2009 Apr;116(5):665-671.

METHAMPHETAMINE

Trade: Anadrex, Desoxyephedrine, Desoxyn, Methedrine, Pervitin

Category: CNS Stimulant

LRC: L5 - Limited Data-Hazardous

Methamphetamine is a potent CNS stimulant; this medication is considered an illicit substance. Methamphetamine is partially metabolized by N-demethylation to amphetamine. In a study of two women who were occasional recreational users of intravenous amphetamines, replicate milk samples were drawn over 24 hours.[1] The IV dose was unknown. In the 24 hours after the dose, average concentrations in milk were 111 ng/mL and 281 ng/mL for methamphetamine and 4 ng/mL and 15 ng/mL for amphetamine in the two subjects. Absolute infant doses for methamphetamine plus amphetamine (as methamphetamine equivalents) were 17.5 µg/kg/day and 44.7 µg/kg/day, respectively, for subjects 1 and 2.

In 2015, a study was published which examined the amount of time required for methamphetamine to be undetectable in maternal urine and breast milk.[2] Thirty-three women were included in the study; 22 of the 33 milk samples were undetectable (average time since last use 72.2 h). Of the remaining 11 samples, only two participants supplied at least four consecutive samples for analysis. The first subject smoked methamphetamine 53 hours prior to delivery; her first milk sample contained 142 ng/mL of methamphetamine. The second subject smoked 68 hours prior to delivery; her first milk sample contained 344.5 ng/mL of methamphetamine. The average infant dose of methamphetamine in the first 24 hours would have been 21.3 µg/kg/day (59.3 µg) and 51.7 µg/kg/day (93 µg) for the infants of these two subjects. In both subjects, the methamphetamine became undetectable around 100 hours after use; however, their urine remained detectable for another 75 and 30 hours, respectively. The excretion half-life in milk was found to be 11.3 hours in subject 1 and 30.3 hours in subject 2; the authors of this study question if there could be a dose-dependent excretion pattern.

Methamphetamine is a potent neurotoxin, known to cause dopaminergic degeneration, with loss of brain dopamine and serotonin neurons. Methamphetamine is a strong CNS stimulant that is strongly addictive. After prolonged use it is known to induce paranoid symptoms. We recommend breastfeeding mothers avoid this drug in lactation. Other strategies to minimize infant exposure include waiting until the urine screen is negative or pumping and discarding milk for at least 100 hours after last maternal use.

T 1/2	4-13.6 h	MW	185.7 Da	PB	
Tmax		RID		Vd	
Oral	64-70%	M/P		pKa	9.87

Adult Concerns: Physical effects may include anorexia, hyperactivity, mydriasis, dry mouth, headache, tachycardia, elevated blood pressure, hyperthermia, diarrhea, arrhythmia, insomnia, stroke and even death. Severe dental decay and acne are common in frequent abusers. Psychological effects include euphoria, increased libido, anxiety, grandiosity, sociability, aggressive behavior, paranoid schizophrenic symptoms, and psychosis.

Adult Dose:

Pediatric Concerns: There is one published case report of an infant death following exposure to methamphetamine in breast milk.[3] According to the authors of this report, the plasma levels in the infant were reportedly too low to induce such symptoms, so the etiology of this death is in question.

Infant Monitoring: AVOID in lactation.

Alternatives:

References:

1. Bartu A, Dusci LJ, Ilett KF. Transfer of methylamphetamine and amphetamine into breast milk following recreational use of methyl-amphetamine. Br J Clin Pharmacol. 2009 Apr;67(4):455-459.
2. Chomchai C, Chomchai S, Kitsommart R. Transfer of methamphetamine (MA) into breast milk and urine of postpartum women who smoked MA tablets during pregnancy: implications for initiation of breastfeeding. J Hum Lact. 2016 May;32(2):333-339.
3. Ariagno R, Karch SB, Middleberg R, Stephens BG, Valdes-Dapena M. Methamphetamine ingestion by a breast-feeding mother and her infant's death: People v Henderson. JAMA. 1995 Jul;274(3):215.

METHENAMINE

Trade: Cystex, Hiprex, Urex

Category: Antibiotic, Other

LRC: L3 - Limited Data-Probably Compatible

Methenamine is a polar heterocyclic organic compound that is converted into formaldehyde in the urinary tract and thus acts as an anti-infective.[1] Methenamine is transferred to breast milk in low amounts. Methenamine was measured at 4.3 mg/L 6-7 hours after a 1 g dose of methenamine hippurate.[2] The relative infant dose was calculated to be 3.62-4.52%. No adverse effects were reported in four neonates that were breastfed while their mothers were taking methenamine.

T 1/2	3-6 h	MW	140 Da	PB	
Tmax		RID	3.6% - 4.5%	Vd	
Oral		M/P	0.88-1.08	pKa	

Adult Concerns: Nausea, rash, vomiting, bladder irritation, pruritus, dyspepsia.

Adult Dose: Hippurate: 1g twice daily, Mandelate 1g four times daily.

Pediatric Concerns:

Infant Monitoring: Vomiting, diarrhea, changes in gastrointestinal flora, and rash.

Alternatives:

References:

1. Lexi-Comp OnlineTM ,Lexi-Drugs OnlineTM. Hudson, Ohio: Lexi-Comp, Inc.; 2011; June 01, 2011.
2. Allgen LG, Holmberg G, Persson B, et al. Biological fate of methenamine in man. Acta Obstet Gynecol Scand. 1979;58:287-293.

METHIMAZOLE

Trade: Tapazole

Category: Antithyroid Agent

LRC: L2 - Limited Data-Probably Compatible

Methimazole, carbimazole, and propylthiouracil (PTU) are used to inhibit the secretion of thyroxine. Carbimazole is a prodrug and is rapidly converted to methimazole.

Levels of methimazole in milk depend on the maternal dose but appear too low to produce clinical effects. In one study of a single patient receiving 2.5 mg methimazole every 12 hours, the milk/serum ratio was 1.16, and we estimate the Cavg to be 40.1 µg/L.[1] This was equivalent to a relative infant dose of approximately 8.4%.

In another study of 35 lactating women receiving 5 to 20 mg/day of methimazole, no changes in the infant thyroid function were noted in any infant, even those at higher doses.[2] Further, studies by Lamberg in 11 women who were treated with the methimazole derivative carbimazole (5-15 mg daily, equal to 3.3 -10 mg methimazole), found all 11 infants had normal thyroid function following maternal treatments.[3] Thus, in small maternal doses, methimazole may also be safe for the nursing mother. In a study of a woman with twins who was receiving up to 30 mg carbimazole daily, the average methimazole concentration in milk was 43 µg/L.[4] The average plasma concentrations in the twin infants were 45 and 52 ng/mL, which is below therapeutic range. Methimazole milk concentrations peaked at 2-4 hours after a carbimazole dose. No changes in thyroid function in these infants were noted.

In a large study of over 134 thyrotoxic lactating mothers and their infants, methimazole therapy was initiated at 10-30 mg/day for 1 month, and reduced to 5-10 mg/day subsequently. Even at methimazole doses of 20 mg/day, no changes in infant TSH, T4, or T3 were noted in over 12 months of study.[5] The authors conclude that both PTU and methimazole can be safely administered during lactation.

T 1/2	6-13 h	MW	114 Da	PB	0%
Tmax	1 h	RID	5.88% - 14.7%	Vd	
Oral	80-95%	M/P	1.16	pKa	10.41

Adult Concerns: Hypothyroidism, hepatic dysfunction, bleeding, drowsiness, skin rash, nausea, vomiting, fever. The treatment of Graves' disease with the antithyroid drug methimazole is associated with a significantly increased risk of acute pancreatitis, and although cases are rare, the risk justifies warnings about this potential adverse event, according to a nationwide controlled study in Denmark spanning more than 20 years.

Adult Dose: 5-30 mg daily.

Pediatric Concerns: None reported in several studies, but propylthiouracil may be a preferred choice in breastfeeding women.

Infant Monitoring: Signs of hypothyroidism; monitor thyroid function if clinical symptoms present.

Alternatives: Propylthiouracil(L2)

References:
1. Tegler L, Lindstrom B. Antithyroid drugs in milk. Lancet. 1980;2(8194):591.
2. Azizi F. Effect of methimazole treatment of maternal thyrotoxicosis on thyroid function in breast-feeding infants. J Pediatr. 1996;128(6):855-858.
3. Lamberg BA, Ikonen E, Osterlund K, et al. Antithyroid treatment of maternal hyperthyroidism during lactation. Clin Endocrinol (Oxf). 1984;21(1):81-87.
4. Rylance GW, Woods CG, Donnelly MC, Oliver JS, Alexander WD. Carbimazole and breastfeeding. Lancet. 1987;1(8538):928.
5. Azizi F, Khoshniat M, Bahrainian M, Hedayati M. Thyroid function and intellectual development of infants nursed by mothers taking methimazole. J Clin Endocrinol Metab. 2000;85(9):3233-3238.

METHOCARBAMOL

Trade: Robaxin, Robaxisal

Category: Skeletal Muscle Relaxant

LRC: L3 - No Data-Probably Compatible

Methocarbamol is a centrally acting sedative and skeletal muscle relaxant.[1] At this time there are no data regarding the transfer of this medication into human milk; minimal amounts have been found in the milk of dogs. Based on this medication's small molecular weight and low protein binding, we do expect it will enter human milk.

T 1/2	1-2 h	MW	241 Da	PB	46-50%
Tmax	1-2 h	RID		Vd	
Oral	Complete	M/P		pKa	13.6

Adult Concerns: Headache, drowsiness, vertigo, blurred vision, seizures, hypotension, metallic taste, dyspepsia, nausea, vomiting, jaundice.

Adult Dose: 1.5 g every 6 hours.

Pediatric Concerns: None reported via milk at this time. Information is limited.

Infant Monitoring: Sedation, vomiting.

Alternatives:

References:
1. Pharmaceutical manufacturers prescribing information.

METHOHEXITAL

Trade: Brevital, Brietal

Category: Anesthetic

LRC: L3 - No Data-Probably Compatible

Methohexital is an ultra-short-acting barbiturate used for induction in anesthesia. The duration of action is approximately half that of thiopental sodium or less than 8 minutes depending on the dose. Although the elimination half-life is 3.9 hours, within 30 minutes there is complete redistribution of methohexital to tissues other than the brain, primarily the liver.[1,2]

In one study of nine women who received 120-150 mg of methohexital for induction of anesthesia, milk levels collected 1-2 hours after surgery ranged from 100 to 407 μg/L in five patients.[3] Levels in the breast milk were found to decline rapidly within the first hour and were undetectable after 24 hours. The maximum level in milk occurred at 63 minutes after administration of anesthesia and was found to be 407 μg/L via breast milk. The authors suggested the infant would receive a maximum of 0.04 mg of methohexital in a typical feeding (100 mL) or between 0.1 to 0.8% of the maternal weight-adjusted dosage. We calculated the relative infant dose to be 2.85-3.56%.

T 1/2	3.9 h	MW	262 Da	PB	73%
Tmax	Instant	RID	2.85% - 3.56%	Vd	
Oral		M/P	1.1	pKa	8.3

Adult Concerns: Hypotension, lethargy, restlessness, confusion, headache, delirium, and excitation.

Adult Dose: 0.75-1.5 mg/kg IV, varies by indication.

Pediatric Concerns: None reported via milk. Levels would be too low.

Infant Monitoring: Observe for sedation, irritability, poor feeding, tremor, muscle rigidity, weight loss.

Alternatives:

References:
1. Pharmaceutical manufacturers prescribing information.
2. McEvoy GE, ed. AHFS Drug Information. Bethesda, MD: American Society of Health-Systems Pharmacists; 2003.
3. Borgatta L, Jenny RW, Gruss L, Ong C, Barad D. Clinical significance of methohexital, meperidine, and diazepam in breast milk. J Clin Pharmacol. 1997;37:186-192.

METHOTREXATE

Trade: Folex, Ledertrexate, Methoblastin, Rheumatrex

Category: Antimetabolite

LRC: L4 - Limited Data-Possibly Hazardous

Methotrexate is a potent and potentially dangerous folic acid antimetabolite used in arthritic and other immunologic syndromes. It is also used as an abortifacient in tubal pregnancies. Methotrexate is secreted in breast milk in small amounts and has been recommended by the American Academy of Pediatrics to be avoided in lactation in a statement published in 2001.[1]

In 1972, a case report was published about a woman who was taking a 22.5 mg/day oral dose of methotrexate to treat a choriocarcinoma. Two hours postdose, the methotrexate concentration in breast milk was 2.6 μg/L with a milk/plasma ratio of 0.08.[2] The cumulative excretion of methotrexate in the first 12 hours after oral administration was only 0.32 μg in milk. These authors concluded that methotrexate therapy in breastfeeding mothers would not pose a contraindication to breastfeeding.

In 2014, a second case report was published about a woman who was taking 25 mg/week of methotrexate subcutaneously to treat rheumatoid arthritis (RA).[3] This woman reinitiated her therapy 151 days postpartum because her disease continued to flare while on sulfasalazine, hydroxychloroquine, and prednisone. The maternal serum concentration was 0.92 μmol 1 hour after her dose was given; breast milk samples taken at 2, 12 and 24 hours after her dose were 0.05 μmol(detectable but below the level of quantification). The authors estimated the average infant dose to be 3.4 μg/kg/day (22.7 μg/L); this was based on the 0.05 μmol concentration remaining steady for the full 24 hours after maternal dose administration. The authors found a relative infant dose of about 1%. This infant continued to breastfeed at 5 months of age when methotrexate was reinitiated in the mother and for another 9 months. No adverse events were reported in the infant.

Following intrathecal administration, plasma levels are highly variable, but generally less than those following a similar dose administered orally or IM. Elimination of methotrexate is by a two-compartment model with a terminal elimination half-life of 8-15 hours in adults (1-6 hours in children).[4] Patients with poor renal function or those given higher doses have prolonged methotrexate half-lives.

In addition, methotrexate is believed to be retained in human tissues (particularly gastrointestinal cells and ovarian cells) for long periods (months).[5] It is apparent that the concentration of methotrexate in human milk is minimal, although due to the toxicity of this agent and the unknown effects on rapidly developing neonatal gastrointestinal cells, it is probably wise to pump and discard the mother's milk for a minimum of 24 hours postdose if given as a single dose (e.g. 50 mg/m² IM for ectopic pregnancy) or administered once weekly (e.g. for RA). The period in which the mother discards her milk may require extending (consider 4 days of interruption) if the dose used is quite high (>75mg) or if the dose is frequently administered (more than once weekly). Being on scheduled doses more than once a week is likely to be a situation where the mother should not breastfeed at all.

In a recent case report of a 29-year-old woman receiving 92 mg IM daily for 3 days, milk levels were collected and assayed for methotrexate.[7] Her child was delivered at 32 weeks weighing 3 pounds. On postpartum day 5, this mother was diagnosed with placenta accreta and treated with intramuscular methotrexate for 3 consecutive days. She received 92 mg methotrexate intramuscularly daily, and was advised not to breastfeed. She collected milk samples on day 2, the zero hour before the second dose and at 1, 2, 4, 8, 12, and 24 hours after taking the dose. Both methotrexate and its metabolite 7-hydroxymethotrexate levels in milk were exceedingly low. On day 2 of therapy, the average milk concentration of methotrexate was 8.6 ng/mL. The maximum concentration (Cmax) of methotrexate occurred at 2 hours and was found to be 16.9 ng/mL. The levels gradually receded and were 4.9 ng/mL at 24 hours. The relative infant dose of methotrexate (RID) was calculated at 0.11%.

Please note: Should the breastfeeding woman wish to have additional children, she should understand that studies have indicated a higher risk of fetal malformations, miscarriage, and fetal death in women on methotrexate months prior to becoming pregnant.[6,7] Therefore, pregnancy should be delayed if either partner is receiving methotrexate for at least 3 months to 1 year following therapy.[8]

T 1/2	8-15 h	MW	454 Da	PB	50%
Tmax	1-2 h (oral); 30-60 min (IM)	RID	0.11% - 0.95%	Vd	0.4-0.8 L/kg
Oral	20-95%	M/P	>0.08	pKa	3.41

Adult Concerns: Dizziness, headache, fatigue, changes in mood, cognitive dysfunction, seizures, alopecia, tinnitus, visual changes, chest pain, hypotension, anorexia, nausea, vomiting, diarrhea, melena, cystitis, changes in liver and renal function, thrombosis, thrombocytopenia, anemia, agranulocytosis, increased risk of infection, skin photosensitivity, serious types of rash.

Adult Dose: 10-25 mg IM or sc once weekly, highly variable.

Pediatric Concerns: None reported via milk, but caution is recommended.

Infant Monitoring: Should patient resume breastfeeding more than 24 hours after the last dose of maternal therapy, monitor the infant for vomiting, diarrhea, blood in the vomit, stool, or urine. Lab work could be drawn if clinical signs of liver or renal dysfunction, anemia, thrombocytopenia, or an inability to fight infection.

Alternatives:

References:

1. American Academy of Pediatrics, Committee on Drugs. Transfer of drugs and other chemicals into human milk. Pediatrics. 2001;108(3):776-789.
2. Johns DG, Rutherford LD, Leighton PC, Vogel CL. Secretion of methotrexate into human milk. Am J Obstet Gynecol. 1972;112(7):978-980.
3. Thorne JC, Nadarajah T, Moretti M, Ito S. Methotrexate use in a breastfeeding patient with rheumatoid arthritis. J Rheumatol. 2014;41(11):2322.
4. Grochow LB, Ames MM. A Clinician's Guide to Chemotherapy Pharmacokinetics and Pharmacodynamics. 1st ed. Baltimore, MD: Williams & Wilkins; 1998.
5. Oliverio VT, Davidson JD. The physiological disposition of dichloromethotrexate-C136 in animals. J Pharmacol Exp Ther. 1962 Jul;137:76-83.
6. Walden PA, Bagshawe KD. Pregnancies after chemotherapy for gestational trophoblastic tumours. Lancet. 1979;2(8154):1241.
7. Baker T, Datta P, Rewers-Felkins K, Hale TW. High-dose methotrexate treatment in a breastfeeding mother with placenta accreta: a case report. Breastfeed Med. 2018 Jul/Aug;13(6):450-452. Epub 2018 Jul 9. PMID: 29985651.
8. Pharmaceutical manufacturers prescribing information.http://mmm.ibreastfeeding.com/drugs/edit/445#tab1

METHSCOPOLAMINE

Trade: Aerohist, Amdry-D, Pamine

Category: Cholinergic Antagonist

LRC: L3 - No Data-Probably Compatible

Methscopolamine is an anticholinergic commonly used for stomach/intestinal spasms, antiemetic, anti-vertigo, urinary antispasmodic, to decrease salivation, to reduce stomach acid secretion and motility, and may be used for other purposes.[1] No data are available on its transfer to milk, but it is probably minimal due to its quaternary ammonium structure. Little is known about its kinetics, but its effect persists for about 4-6 hours. It is rather unlikely that this product would produce clinical levels in infants following ingestion of milk. But infants should be monitored for classic anticholinergic symptoms such as drying of oral and ophthalmic secretions, constipation, and urinary retention.

T 1/2	<4 h	MW	398 Da	PB	
Tmax		RID		Vd	
Oral	10-25%	M/P		pKa	

Adult Concerns: Headache, drowsiness, dizziness, dry mouth, palpitations, urinary retention, constipation.

Adult Dose: 2.5 mg four times a day in adults.

Pediatric Concerns: None reported via milk at this time.

Infant Monitoring: Sedation or irritability, drying of oral and ophthalmic secretions, urinary retention, constipation.

Alternatives:

References:
1. Pharmaceutical manufacturers prescribing information.

METHYL SALICYLATE

Trade:

Category: Salicylate, Non-Aspirin

LRC: L3 - No Data-Probably Compatible

Methyl salicylate is a form of NSAID used to alleviate pain when applied through topical compounds and patches. The American Academy of Pediatrics recommends that salicylates be used with caution in breastfeeding women.[1] The transdermal absorption of methyl salicylate is significant ranging from 15.5% to 22% recovery in the urine.[2] Methyl salicylate is well known to produce acute toxicity and fatalities when ingested by infants and children. While unpublished, the transfer of methyl salicylate to human milk is probably minimal, but mothers should use great caution in using various forms of methyl salicylate while breastfeeding.

T 1/2	2-12 h	MW	152.1 Da	PB	50-80%
Tmax	0.8-2.2 h	RID		Vd	
Oral	15-22%	M/P		pKa	

Adult Concerns: Headache, tinnitus, confusion, nausea, vomiting, stomach pain, gastrointestinal bleed, hypersensitivity reaction, irritation, rash.

Adult Dose: Apply to affected area 3-4 times per day.

Pediatric Concerns:

Infant Monitoring: Rapid breathing, vomiting, diarrhea.

Alternatives:

References:
1. Briggs GG, Freeman RK, Yaffe SJ. Drugs in Pregnancy and Lactation. 5th ed. Baltimore, MD: Williams & Wilkins; 1998.
2. Morra P, Bartle WR, Walker SE, Lee SN, Bowles SK, Reeves RA. Serum concentrations of salicylic acid following topically applied salicylate derivatives. Ann Pharmacother. 1996 Sep;30(9):935-940.

METHYLCELLULOSE

Trade: Citrucel

Category: Laxative

LRC: L1 - No Data-Compatible

Methylcellulose is used as a bulk laxative for the treatment of constipation.[1] There are no data on the excretion of methylcellulose in human milk. However, it stays in the gastrointestinal tract and is totally unabsorbed. It is safe for breastfeeding mothers.

T 1/2		MW	Very large	PB	
Tmax		RID		Vd	
Oral		M/P		pKa	

Adult Concerns: Nausea, vomiting, feeling of fullness, abdominal pain, flatulence, diarrhea.

Adult Dose:

Pediatric Concerns:

Infant Monitoring:

Alternatives:

References:
1. Pharmaceutical manufacturers prescribing information.

METHYLDOPA

Trade: Aldomet, Aldopren, Dopamet, Hydopa, Nova-Medopa, Nudopa

Category: Antihypertensive

LRC: L2 - Limited Data-Probably Compatible

Alpha-methyldopa is a centrally acting antihypertensive. It can be used to treat hypertension during pregnancy. In a study of two lactating women who received a dose of 500 mg, the maximum breast milk concentration of methyldopa ranged from 0.2 to 0.66 mg/L.[1] In another patient who received a 1000-mg dose, the maximum concentration in milk was 1.14 mg/L.[1] The milk/plasma ratios varied from 0.19 to 0.34. The authors indicated that if the infant were to ingest 750 mL of milk daily (with a maternal dose= 1000 mg), the maximum daily ingestion would be less than 855 μg or approximately 0.02% of the maternal dose. In another study of seven women who received 0.75-2 grams/day of methyldopa, the free methyldopa concentrations in breast milk ranged from zero to 0.2 mg/L while the conjugated metabolite had concentrations of 0.1 to 0.9 mg/L.[2] These studies generally indicate that the levels of methyldopa transferred to a breastfeeding infant would be too low to be clinically relevant. However, gynecomastia and galactorrhea has been reported in one full-term 2-week-old female neonate following seven days of maternal therapy with methyldopa, 250 mg three times daily.[3]

T 1/2	105 min	MW	211 Da	PB	Low
Tmax	3-6 h	RID	0.1% - 0.4%	Vd	0.3 L/kg
Oral	25-50%	M/P	0.19-0.34	pKa	2.2

Adult Concerns: Headache, dizziness, depression, hypotension heart failure, bradycardia, dry mouth, gynecomastia, hyperprolactinemia, diarrhea, changes in liver and renal function, weight gain, bone marrow suppression, rash.

Adult Dose: 250-500 mg 3-4 times daily.

Pediatric Concerns: None reported in several studies. Gynecomastia and galactorrhea in one personal communication.

Infant Monitoring: Drowsiness, lethargy, pallor, poor feeding, and weight gain.

Alternatives:

References:
1. White WB, Andreoli JW, Cohn RD. Alpha-methyldopa disposition in mothers with hypertension and in their breast-fed infants. Clin Pharmacol Ther. 1985;37(4):387-390.
2. Jones HM, Cummings AJ. A study of the transfer of alpha-methyldopa to the human foetus and newborn infant. Br J Clin Pharmacol. 1978;6(5):432-434.
3. E.D.M. Personal Communication, 1997.

METHYLENE BLUE

Trade: Atrosept, Dolsed, Prosed, Urimar-T

Category: Diagnostic Agent, Other

LRC: L4 - No Data-Possibly Hazardous

Methylene blue is a blue dye that is used in diagnostic procedures, to treat drug-induced methemoglobinemia, and to prevent ifosfamide-induced encephalopathy in oncology. No data are available on its transfer into human milk, but some should be expected. Oral absorption is variable (53-97%).[1,2] The apparent half-life in humans is approximately 5.25 hours; thus interruption of breastfeeding for 24 hours is probably advisable.

T 1/2	6 h	MW	319 Da	PB	
Tmax		RID		Vd	
Oral		M/P		pKa	3.8

Adult Concerns: Cardiac dysrhythmias and hypertension. Sweating, discoloration of skin, malignant hyperthermia, nausea, vomiting, diarrhea. At high doses or in patients with G6PD-deficiency and infants, methylene blue may catalyze the oxidation of ferrous iron in hemoglobin to ferric iron, causing paradoxical methemoglobinemia and hemolysis. Onset of anemia may be delayed 1o or more days and may require red blood cell transfusions.

Adult Dose: 0.1-0.2 mL/kg IV, varies by indication.

Pediatric Concerns: None reported via milk. Oral absorption is poor.

Infant Monitoring: At high doses or in patients with G6PD-deficiency and infants, methylene blue may catalyze the oxidation of ferrous iron in hemoglobin to ferric iron causing paradoxical methemoglobinemia and hemolysis. Onset of anemia may be delayed 1o or more days and may require red blood cell transfusions.

Alternatives:

References:
1. Peter C, Hongwan D, Kupfer A, Lauterburg BH. Pharmacokinetics and organ distribution of intravenous and oral methylene blue. Eur J Clin Pharmacol. 2000 Jun;56(3):247-250.

METHYLERGONOVINE

Trade: Mergot, Mergotrex, Methergine

Category: Vasopressor

LRC: L2 - Limited Data-Probably Compatible

Methylergonovine is an amine ergot alkaloid used to control postpartum uterine bleeding. This medication is typically given intramuscularly at the time of a postpartum hemorrhage. In a group of eight postpartum women receiving 125 µg three times daily for 5 days, the concentration of methylergonovine in plasma and milk were studied on the morning of day 5 after a 250-µg dose.[1] The milk concentrations ranged from <0.5 µg/L to 1.3 µg/L at one hour postdose and <0.5 µg/L to 1.2 µg/L at 8 hours postdose. In this study, only five of 16 milk samples had detectable methylergonovine levels. Using a dose of 1.3 µg/L of milk, an infant would only consume approximately 0.2 µg/kg/day, which is incredibly low compared to the maternal dose given in this study. The milk/plasma ratio averaged about 0.3.

In a 2004 prospective study following a maternal oral dose of 250 µg in 10 lactating women, the mean time to peak and peak milk concentration of methylergonovine occurred at 1.8 hours and was about 0.657 µg/L (range 410-830 µg/L).[2] The mean milk/plasma ratio was 0.18 at 1 hour and 0.17 at 2 hours postdose. We estimate that the infant would receive about 0.098 µg/kg/day or 2.7% of the maternal dose.

In a 2012 study, 12 lactating women were given methylergonovine 0.125 mg three times a day for 5 days.[3] Milk samples were collected on day one of therapy after the first dose. The peak concentration was 0.437 µg/L at 2 hours and declined to 0.086 µg/L by 5 hours. We used both of these concentrations to estimate an infant would receive between 0.7-3.6% of the maternal dose.

In a study of 10 women given methylergonovine 0.2 mg orally three times a day for 1 week compared to 10 lactating women given no therapy, no difference in maternal prolactin levels or breast milk volume were reported.[4]

However, studies have shown a suppression in prolactin and milk production. One study suggested a 50% decrease in prolactin levels 30 to 75 minutes after a 0.2 mg intramuscular injection of methylergonovine in women 3 days postpartum.[5] Prolactin levels were reported to increase 180 to 240 min after the injection. In a study of 30 lactating women receiving 0.6 mg orally from day 1 to day 7 postpartum, prolactin levels were significantly lower at day 7, while milk production was significantly reduced at days 3 and 7 when compared to untreated women.[6] In a study of 14 postpartum women who received 0.2 mg intramuscularly, plasma prolactin concentrations were lower (141 µg/L) as compared to 15 control subjects (266 µg/L) at 1.5 hours postpartum.[7] The authors did comment that in both groups the mothers were separated from their infants after delivery. No further information regarding breastfeeding status was given.

Short-term use of these agents when clinically indicated does not appear to pose problems in nursing mothers or their infants. The prolonged use of ergot alkaloids should be avoided as they may negatively affect milk production.

T 1/2	3 h (range 1.5 to 12.7 h)	MW	339 Da	PB	36%
Tmax	0.2-0.6 h (IM)	RID	0.72% - 5.46%	Vd	0.55-1 L/kg
Oral	60% (oral)	M/P	0.3	pKa	6.7

Adult Concerns: Dizziness, headache, tinnitus, seizure, chest pain, arrhythmias, myocardial infarction, hypertension, nausea, vomiting, diarrhea, water intoxication, thrombophlebitis.

Adult Dose: 0.2 mg IM, repeat every 2-4 h as needed (max 5 doses).

Pediatric Concerns: None reported at this time.

Infant Monitoring: Vomiting, diarrhea.

Alternatives:

References:
1. Erkkola R, Kanto J, Allonen H, Kleimola T, Mantyla R. Excretion of methylergometrine (methylergonovine) into the human breast milk. Int J Clin Pharmacol Biopharm. 1978;16(12):579-580.
2. Vogel D, Burkhardt T, Rentsch K, et al. Misoprostol versus methylergometrine: pharmacokinetics in human milk. Am J Obstet Gynecol. 2004 Dec;191(6):2168-2173.
3. Nakamichi T, Yawata A, Hojo H, et al. Monitoring of methylergonovine in human breast milk by solid-phase extraction and high-performance liquid chromatography with fluorimetric detection. Pharmazie. 2012;67:482-484.
4. Del Pozo E, Brun DR, Hinselmann M. Lack of effect of methyl-ergonovine on postpartum lactation. Am J Obstet Gynecol. 1975;123(8):845-846.
5. Perez-Lopez FR, Delvoye P, Denayer P, L'Hermite M, Roncero MC, Robyn C. Effectof methylergobasine maleate on serum gonadotrophin and prolactin in humans. Acta Endocrinol (Copenh). 1975;79(4):644-657.
6. Peters F, Lummerich M, Breckwoldt M. Inhibition of prolactin and lactation by methylergometrine hydrogenmaleate. Acta Endocrinol (Copenh). 1979;91(2):213-216.
7. Weiss G, Klein S, Shenkman L, Kataoka K, Hollander CS. Effect of methylergonovine on puerperal prolactin secretion. Obstet Gynecol. 1975;46(2):209-210.

METHYLNALTREXONE BROMIDE

Trade: Relistor

Category: Opioid Antagonist

LRC: L3 - No Data-Probably Compatible

Methylnaltrexone is a peripherally acting, selective antagonist of opioid binding at the mu-opioid receptor.[1] It is a quaternary amine and has limited ability to cross the blood-brain barrier. It is used to decrease the constipating effects of opioids in patients with advanced illness without impacting opioid-mediated analgesic effects on the central nervous system. This medication is typically given to patients who have been resistant to multiple laxatives or combinations of therapies.

According to the manufacturer, methylnaltrexone appears in the milk of lactating rats.[1] At this time, there are no studies in breastfeeding women; however, quaternary amines do not usually enter human milk in clinically relevant amounts. Combined with this drug's poor oral bioavailability, this medication is likely to be compatible with breastfeeding; however, based on this medication's indication, the maternal opioid should also be assessed for suitability in lactation. No adverse effects have been observed in infants exposed to the related drug, naltrexone.[2]

T 1/2	8 h	MW	436.36 Da	PB	11-15.3%
Tmax	0.5 h	RID		Vd	1.1 L/kg
Oral	Poor	M/P		pKa	

Adult Concerns: Dizziness, syncope, nausea, vomiting, flatulence, diarrhea, abdominal pain and cramping, flushing, diaphoresis, opioid withdrawal.

Adult Dose: 8 mg (if 38-62 kg) or 12 mg (if 62-114 kg) subcutaneous every other day.

Pediatric Concerns: None reported via milk at this time.

Infant Monitoring: Irritability, poor feeding, vomiting, diarrhea, weight gain.

Alternatives: Polyethylene glycol 3350.

References:
1. Pharmaceutical manufacturer prescribing information.
2. Chan CF, Page-Sharp M, Kristensen JH, O"Neil G, Ilett KF. Transfer of naltrexone and its metabolite 6, beta-naltrexol into human milk. J Hum Lact. 2004;20(3):322-326.

METHYLPHENIDATE

Trade: Concerta, Daytrana, Metadate CD, Metadate ER, Methylin, Riphenidate, Ritalin, QuilliChew ER, Cotempla, Jornay PM

Category: CNS Stimulant

LRC: L2 - Limited Data-Probably Compatible

The pharmacologic effects of methylphenidate are similar to those of amphetamines and include CNS stimulation.[1] It is presently used for narcolepsy and attention deficit hyperactivity syndrome.

In a study of three women receiving an average of 52 (35-80) mg/day of methylphenidate, the average drug in milk was 19 (13-28) µg/L.[2] The milk/plasma ratio averaged 2.8 (2-3.6). The absolute infant dose averaged 2.9 (2-4.25) µg/kg/day. The average relative infant dose was 0.9% (0.7-1.1). In the one infant studied, plasma levels were <1 µg/L. These levels are probably too low to be clinically relevant. Another case reported a mother taking 15 mg/day with breast milk concentrations averaging 2.5 ng/mL. The daily infant dose was estimated at 0.38 µg/kg, which corresponds to 0.16% of the maternal dose.[3] No drug was detected in breast milk 20-21 hours after the maternal dose.

A mother taking 80 mg/day was determined to have a milk-to-plasma ratio of 2.7, giving an absolute infant dose of 2.3 µg/kg/day, or 0.2% of the maternal dose. Methylphenidate was not detected in the infant's plasma.[4] No adverse effects were noted in any of the infants. These levels are significantly less than for dextroamphetamine.

Dexmethylphenidate hydrochloride is simply the active dextrorotary enantiomer of methylphenidate, and therefore kinetic and breast milk data should be similar to that of methylphenidate.

In another recent case study of a woman who took duloxetine (90 mg QD) and methylphenidate (36 mg daily) during pregnancy and breastfeeding, at 4 weeks postpartum, milk levels of duloxetine were 32.8 ng/mL and of methylphenidate were 7.9 ng/mL.[5] The authors estimated the RID at 0.3 of duloxetine and 0.2% of methylphenidate, respectively.

T 1/2	1.4-4.2 h	MW	233 Da	PB	10-33%
Tmax	1-3 h	RID	0.19% - 0.4%	Vd	1.8-2.65 L/kg
Oral	95%	M/P	2.8	pKa	8.8

Adult Concerns: Nervousness, hyperactivity, insomnia, agitation, and lack of appetite.

Adult Dose: 10 mg 2-3 times daily. Highly variable.

Pediatric Concerns: None reported via milk.

Infant Monitoring: Agitation, irritability, poor sleeping patterns, changes in feeding, poor weight gain.

Alternatives:

References:
1. Pharmaceutical manufacturers prescribing information.
2. Hackett LP, Ilett KF, Kristensen JH, Kohan R, Hale TW. Infant dose and safety of breastfeeding for dexamphetamine and methylphenidate in mothers with attention deficit hyperactivity disorder. Proceedings of the 9th International Congress of Therapeutic Drug Monitoring and Clinical Toxicology, Louisville, USA; April 23-28, 2005, Ther Drug Monit. 2005;27:220. (Abstract # 40).
3. Spigset O, Brede WR, Zahlsen K. Excretion of methylphenidate in Breast Milk. Am J Psychiatry. 2007;164(2):348.
4. Hackett LP, Kristensen JH, Hale TW, Paterson R, Ilett, KF. Methylphenidate and breast-feeding. Ann Pharmacother. 2006;40(10):1890-1891.
5. Collin-Lévesque L, El-Ghaddaf Y, Genest M, et al. Infant exposure to methylphenidate and duloxetine during lactation. Breastfeed Med. 2018 Apr;13(3):221-225. PubMed PMID: 29485905.

METHYLPREDNISOLONE

Trade: Advantan, Depo-Medrol, Medrol, Neo-Medrol, Solu-Medrol

Category: Corticosteroid

LRC: L2 - Limited Data-Probably Compatible

Methylprednisolone (MP) is the methyl derivative of prednisolone. Four milligrams of methylprednisolone is roughly equivalent to 5 mg of prednisone. Multiple dosage forms exist and include the succinate salt which is rapidly active, the methylprednisolone base which is the tablet formulation for oral use, and the methylprednisolone acetate suspension (Depo-Medrol) which is slowly absorbed over many days to weeks. Depo-Medrol is generally used intrasynovially, IM, or epidurally and is slowly absorbed from these sites. They would be very unlikely to affect a breastfed infant, but this depends on dose and duration of exposure.

For a complete description of corticosteroid use in breastfeeding mothers see the Prednisone monograph. In general, the amount of methylprednisolone and other steroids transferred into human milk is minimal as long as the dose does not exceed 80 mg per day.[1] However, relating side effects of steroids administered via breast milk and their maternal doses is rather difficult and each situation should be evaluated individually. Extended use of high doses could predispose the infant to steroid side effects including decreased linear growth rate, but these require rather high doses. Low to moderate doses are believed to have minimal effect on breastfed infants.

High dose pulsed intravenous or oral administrations of methylprednisolone (MP) have become increasingly important as a treatment for acute relapses or progressively worsening of multiple sclerosis (MS).[2-6] Even though prednisolone is approved by the American Academy of Pediatrics for use in breastfeeding women, when MP is used in such high doses in patients with MS, questions concerning when mothers can return to breastfeeding have arisen. There are extensive kinetic data on the plasma levels, metabolism, and clearance of methylprednisolone patients with and without MS.[7,8] In a recent case report of a patient receiving intravenous (1000 mg) doses of MP on three consecutive days, breast milk levels averaged (C_{avg}) 1.094 µg/mL on day 3, 1.290 µg/mL on day two, and 1.382 µg/mL on day 3.[9] The Relative Infant Doses ranged from 1.45%, 1.35%, to 1.15% on days 1, 2, and 3, respectively, based on the C_{avg}. While the infant was not breastfed, these levels in milk are far too low to produce sequelae in a breastfeeding infant. A brief interruption of 12 hours, following IV therapy, would virtually eliminate any risk associated with this therapy in breastfeeding mothers.

In 2015, a case report was published of a 39-year-old woman taking methylprednisolone 1000 mg IV x 3 days for a relapse of MS.[10] Directly after the dose the concentration in milk was 3 mg/L; 4 hours later it was 1.2 mg/L. The authors of this case report found that if an infant were to start feeding 4 hours after the maternal dose the infant would ingest 0.168 mg of methylprednisolone (equivalent to 0.84 mg cortisol or 42% of the daily endogenous production). If the infant waited 8 hours to start feeding the infant would ingest a maximum of 0.048 mg of methylprednisolone (12% of the daily endogenous production; authors noted this could be even lower as concentrations dropped exponentially). We found the relative infant dose to be 3.15% at 4 hours and 1.26% at 8 hours.

Based on the two most recent case reports published, it would seem reasonable to continue breastfeeding while receiving a short course of methylprednisolone; to reduce exposure the mother could wait to feed her infant until 8-12 hours after her dose.[9,10]

T 1/2	2.8 h	MW	374 Da	PB	
Tmax		RID	0.46% - 3.15%	Vd	1.5 L/kg
Oral	Complete	M/P		pKa	2.6, 5

Adult Concerns: Headache, changes in mood, insomnia, nervousness, hypertension, heart failure, arrhythmias, edema, vomiting, peptic ulcers, gastrointestinal bleeding, weight gain, changes in liver function, hyperglycemia, changes in electrolytes, leukocytosis, muscle weakness, osteoporosis.

Adult Dose: 2-60 mg/day in 1-4 divided doses orally.

Pediatric Concerns: None reported via breast milk. High doses and prolonged durations may inhibit epiphyseal bone growth, induce gastric ulcerations, glaucoma, etc.

Infant Monitoring: Feeding, growth, and weight gain. Limit degree and duration of exposure if possible. Short-term use is suitable.

Alternatives: Prednisone(L2)

References:

1. Anderson PO. Corticosteroid use by breast-feeding mothers. Clin Pharm. 1987;6(6):445.
2. Miller DM, Weinstock-Guttman B, Bethoux F, et al. A meta-analysis of methylprednisolone in recovery from multiple sclerosis exacerbations. Mult Scler. 2000;6(4):267-273.
3. Hommes OR, Barkhof F, Jongen PJ, Frequin ST. Methylprednisolone treatment in multiple sclerosis: effect of treatment, pharmacokinetics, future. Mult Scler. 1996;1(6):327-328.
4. Goas JY, Marion JL, Missoum A. High dose intravenous methyl prednisolone in acute exacerbations of multiple sclerosis. J Neurol Neurosurg Psychiatry. 1983;46(1):99.
5. Sellebjerg F, Frederiksen JL, Nielsen PM, Olesen J. Double-blind, randomized, placebo-controlled study of oral, high-dose methylprednisolone in attacks of MS. Neurology. 1998;51(2):529-534.
6. Barnes D, Hughes RA, Morris RW, et al. Randomised trial of oral and intravenous methylprednisolone in acute relapses of multiple sclerosis. Lancet. 1997;349(9056):902-906.
7. Vree TB, Verwey-van Wissen CP, Lagerwerf AJ, et al. Isolation and identification of the C6-hydroxy and C20-hydroxy metabolites and glucuronide conjugate of methylprednisolone by preparative high-performance liquid chromatography from urine of patients receiving high-dose pulse therapy. J Chromatogr B Biomed Sci Appl. 1999; 726(1-2):157-168.
8. Vree TB, Lagerwerf AJ, Verwey-van Wissen CP, Jongen PJ. High-performance liquid chromatography analysis, preliminary pharmacokinetics, metabolism and renal excretion of methylprednisolone with its C6 and C20 hydroxy metabolites in multiple sclerosis patients receiving high-dose pulse therapy. J Chromatogr B Biomed Sci Appl. 1999; 732(2):337-348.

9. Cooper SD, Felkins K, Baker TE, Hale TW. Transfer of methylprednisolone into breast milk in a mother with multiple sclerosis. J Hum Lact. 2015 May;31(2):237-239.

10. Strijbos E, Coenradie S, Touw DJ, Aerden LAM. High-dose methylprednisolone for multiple sclerosis during lactation: concentrations in breast milk. Mult Scler J. 2015;21(6):797-798. doi: 10.1177/1352458514565414.

METHYLSULFONYLMETHANE

Trade: Crystalline DMSO, DMSO2, MSM

Category: Antiarthritic

LRC: L3 - No Data-Probably Compatible

Methylsulfonylmethane (DMSO2, MSM, Crystalline DMSO) is the normal oxidation product of dimethyl sulfoxide (DMSO). It is purportedly used for osteoarthritis and joint inflammations.[1] No data are available on this product, but it is probably distributed and eliminated the same as dimethyl sulfoxide. MSM is well absorbed, and produces significant levels in the CNS, which would suggest it enters milk as well. It is primarily used in osteoarthritis, joint inflammation, bursitis, and allergic rhinitis, although its efficacy is questionable. Its use in pregnant and breastfeeding women is questionable due to the lack of safety data.

T 1/2		MW	94.1 Da	PB	
Tmax		RID		Vd	
Oral		M/P		pKa	

Adult Concerns: Diarrhea, nausea, headache, bloating, fatigue, insomnia, and difficulty with mental acuity.

Adult Dose: <6 grams daily.

Pediatric Concerns:

Infant Monitoring:

Alternatives:

References:
1. Pharmaceutical manufacturers prescribing information.

METHYLTESTOSTERONE

Trade: Android, Methitest, TestRed

Category: Androgen

LRC: L4 - Limited Data-Possibly Hazardous

Methyltestosterone is a synthetic androgen that is metabolized to testosterone. Testosterone is a male sex hormone used to treat testosterone deficiency in males, reverse delayed puberty in males, improve libido, and as part of female-to-male gender reassignment.

Methyltestosterone and testosterone are rarely used in breastfeeding women. It is not known how much testosterone transfers to human milk; however, even small amounts may affect nursing infants. Infants exposed to external androgens may experience accelerated bone maturation without a proportional gain in linear growth, thereby compromising their adult stature. Androgens like testosterone may adversely affect milk supply.[1]

T 1/2	10-100 min	MW	302 Da	PB	98%
Tmax	1-2 h	RID		Vd	
Oral		M/P		pKa	

Adult Concerns: Gynecomastia, polycythemia, hepatitis, hirsutism.

Adult Dose: 10-50 mg daily.

Pediatric Concerns: Aggressive behavior, virilization of genitalia, advanced bone age, hirsuitism.

Infant Monitoring: Virilization of genitalia, advanced bone age, hirsuitism

Alternatives:

References:
1. Pharmaceutical manufacturers prescribing Information, Valeant Pharmaceuticals, 1973.

METOCLOPRAMIDE

Trade: Pramin, Emex, Gastromax, Maxeran, Maxolon, Metozolv ODT, Reglan, Pramin

Category: Stimulant, Gastrointestinal

LRC: L2 - Significant Data-Compatible

Metoclopramide, a dopamine receptor blocker, has multiple functions but is primarily used for increasing the lower esophageal sphincter tone in gastroesophageal reflux in patients with reduced gastric tone. In breastfeeding, it is sometimes used in lactating women to stimulate prolactin release from the pituitary and enhance breast milk production.

Since 1981, a number of publications have documented major increases in breast milk production following the use of metoclopramide, domperidone, or sulpiride. With metoclopramide, the increase in serum prolactin and breast milk production appears dose-related up to a dose of 15 mg three times daily.[1] Many studies show 66 to 100% increases in milk production depending on the degree of breast milk supply in the mother prior to therapy and maybe her initial prolactin levels. Doses of 15 mg/day were found ineffective, whereas doses of 30-45 mg/day were most effective. In most studies, major increases in prolactin were observed such as from 125 ng/mL to 172 ng/mL in one patient.[2] In Kauppila's study[3], the concentration of metoclopramide in milk was consistently higher than the maternal serum levels. The peak occurred at 2-3 hours after administration of the medication. During the late puerperium, the concentration of metoclopramide in the milk varied from 20 to 125 µg/L, which was less than the 28 to 157 µg/L noted during the early puerperium. The authors estimated the daily dose to infant to vary from 6 to 24 µg/kg/day during the early puerperium and from 1 to 13 µg/kg/day during the late phase. These doses are minimal compared to those used for therapy of reflux in pediatric patients (0.1 to 0.5 mg/kg/day). In these studies, only one of five infants studied had detectable blood levels of metoclopramide; hence, no accumulation or side effects were observed.

While plasma prolactin levels in the newborns were comparable to those in the mothers prior to treatment, Kauppila found slight increases in prolactin levels in four of seven newborns following treatment with metoclopramide although a more recent study did not find such changes. However, prolactin levels are highly variable and subject to diurnal rhythm; thus timing is essential in measuring prolactin levels and could account for this inconsistency. In another study of 23 women with premature infants, milk production increased from 93 mL/day to 197 mL/day between the first and 7th days of therapy with 30 mg/day.[4] Prolactin levels, although varied, increased from 18.1 to 121.8 ng/mL. While basal prolactin levels were elevated significantly, metoclopramide seems to blunt the rapid rise of prolactin when milk was expressed. Nevertheless, milk production was still elevated.

Gupta studied 32 mothers with inadequate milk supply.[5] Following a dose of 10 mg three times daily, a 66-100% increase in milk supply was noted. Of 12 cases of complete lactation failure, eight responded to treatment in an average of 3-4 days after starting therapy. In this study, 87.5% of the total 32 cases responded to metoclopramide therapy with greater milk production. No untoward effects were noted in the infants. In a study of five breastfeeding women who were receiving 30 mg/day, daily milk production increased significantly from 150.9 mL/day to 276.4 mL/day in this group.[6] Infant plasma prolactin levels in breastfed infants were determined as well on the fifth postnatal day and no changes were noted; thus, the amount of metoclopramide transferred in milk was not enough to change the infants' prolactin levels. In a study by Lewis in 10 patients who received a single oral dose of 10 mg, the mean maternal plasma and milk levels at 2 hours was 68.5 ng/mL and 125.7 µg/L respectively.[7] Hansen's study showed that 28 women receiving 30 mg/day had no significant increase in milk production as compared to the placebo group.[8] However, this study was initiated with 96 hours of delivery, a time when virtually all mothers would have had exceedingly high plasma prolactin levels anyway. Metoclopramide should not be expected to work as a galactagogue when plasma prolactin levels are high.

It is well recognized that metoclopramide increases a mother's milk supply when her prolactin levels are low, but it is exceedingly dose-dependent, and yet some mothers simply do not respond. In those mothers who do not respond, Kauppila's work suggests that these patients may already have elevated prolactin levels. In his study, three of the five mothers who did not respond with increased milk production, had the highest basal prolactin levels (300-400 ng/mL).[3] Thus it may be advisable to do plasma prolactin levels on under-producing mothers prior to instituting metoclopramide therapy to assess the response prior to treating. Side effects such as gastric cramping and diarrhea limit the compliance of some patients but are rare.

Withdrawing from therapy: It is often found that upon rapid discontinuation of the medication, the supply of milk may in some instances reduce significantly. Tapering of the dose is generally recommended and one possible regimen is to decrease the dose by 10 mg per week. Long-term use of this medication (>4 weeks) may be accompanied by increased side effects such as depression in the mother although some patients have used it successfully for months. The FDA has warned that therapy longer than 3 months may be associated with tardive dyskinesis.

Two recent cases of serotonin-like reactions (agitation, dysarthria, diaphoresis, and extrapyramidal movement disorder) have been reported when metoclopramide was used in patients receiving sertraline or venlafaxine.[9]

Another dopamine antagonist, domperidone, is a preferred choice but is unfortunately not available in the United States. When metoclopramide and domperidone were compared in a 2012 randomized controlled trial, both medications were found to increase milk supply with similar efficacy.[10] Sixty-five women were given 10 mg TID of either domperidone or metoclopramide for 10 days. These women had given birth to preterm infants (average gestation at birth= 28 weeks) and started this medication if they were unable to produce 160 mL/kg/day of milk; most women in this trial started drug therapy about 4 weeks postpartum. Women in the domperidone and metoclopramide groups increased their milk supply by 96.3% and 93.7%, respectively. More women in the metoclopramide group reported adverse effects (7 vs. 3) such as headache, mood swings, dry mouth, change in appetite, and diarrhea.

T 1/2	5-6 h	MW	300 Da	PB	30%
Tmax	1-2 h (oral)	RID	4.7% - 14.3%	Vd	
Oral	30-100%	M/P	0.5-4.06	pKa	14.49

Adult Concerns: Headache, mood swings, depression, arrhythmias, dry mouth, change in appetite, abdominal cramps, diarrhea, extrapyramidal symptoms, itchy skin.

Adult Dose: 10-15 mg three times daily.

Pediatric Concerns: None reported in infants via milk.

Infant Monitoring: Sedation, diarrhea, extrapyramidal symptoms.

Alternatives: Domperidone(L3)

References:

1. Kauppila A, Kivinen S, Ylikorkala O. A dose response relation between improved lactation and metoclopramide. Lancet. 1981;1(8231):1175-1177.
2. Budd SC, Erdman SH, Long DM, Trombley SK, Udall JN Jr. Improved lactation with metoclopramide. A case report. Clin Pediatr (Phila). 1993;32(1):53-57.
3. Kauppila A, Arvela P, Koivisto M, Kivinen S, Ylikorkala O, Pelkonen O. Metoclopramide and breast feeding: transfer into milk and the newborn. Eur J Clin Pharmacol. 1983;25(6):819-823.
4. Ehrenkranz RA, Ackerman BA. Metoclopramide effect on faltering milk production by mothers of premature infants. Pediatrics. 1986;78(4):614-620.
5. Gupta AP, Gupta PK. Metoclopramide as a lactogogue. Clin Pediatr (Phila). 1985;24(5):269-272.
6. Ertl T, Sulyok E, Ezer E, Sarkany I, Thurzo V, Csaba IF. The influence of metoclopramide on the composition of human breast milk. Acta Paediatr Hung. 1991;31(4):415-422.
7. Lewis PJ, Devenish C, Kahn C. Controlled trial of metoclopramide in the initiation of breast feeding. Br J Clin Pharmacol. 1980;9(2):217-219.
8. Hansen WF, McAndrew S, Harris K, Zimmerman MB. Metoclopramide effect on breastfeeding the preterm infant: a randomized trial. Obstet Gynecol. 2005;105(2):383-389.
9. Fisher AA, Davis MW. Serotonin syndrome caused by selective serotonin reuptake-inhibitors-metoclopramide interaction. Ann Pharmacother. 2002;36:67-71.
10. Ingram J, Taylor H, Churchill C, et al. Metoclopramide or domperidone for increasing maternal breast milk output: a randomized controlled trial. Arch Dis Child Fetal Neonatal Ed. 2012;97:F241-F245.

METOPROLOL

Trade: Betaloc, Lopressor, Minax, Toprol-XL

Category: Beta Adrenergic Blocker

LRC: L2 - Limited Data-Probably Compatible

At low doses, metoprolol is a very cardioselective beta-1 blocker, and it is used for hypertension, angina, and tachyarrhythmias. In a study of 3 women 4-6 months postpartum who received 100 mg twice daily for 4 days, the peak concentration of metoprolol ranged from 0.38 to 2.58 µmol/L, whereas the maternal plasma levels ranged from 0.1 to 0.97 µmol/L.[1] The mean milk/plasma ratio was 3. Assuming ingestion of 75 mL of milk at each feeding, and the maximum concentration of 2.58 µmol/L, an infant would ingest approximately 0.05 mg metoprolol at the first feeding and considerably less at subsequent feedings.

In another study of 9 women receiving 50-100 mg twice daily, the maternal plasma and milk concentrations ranged from 4-556 nmol/L and 19-1690 nmol/L respectively.[2] Using this data, the authors calculated an average milk concentration throughout the day as 280 µg/L of milk. This dose is 20-40 times less than a typical clinical dose. The milk/plasma ratio in these studies averaged 3.72. Although the milk/plasma ratios for this drug are in general high, the maternal plasma levels are quite small, so the absolute amount transferred to the infant are quite small. Although these levels are probably too low to be clinically relevant, clinicians should use metoprolol under close supervision.

T 1/2	3-7 h	MW	267 Da	PB	10%
Tmax	2 h	RID	1.4%	Vd	3.2-5.6 L/kg
Oral	40-50%	M/P	3-3.72	pKa	9.7

Adult Concerns: Headache, dizziness, insomnia, depression, fatigue, chest pain, bradycardia, first degree heart block, palpitations, hypotension, heart failure, wheezing, taste disturbances, heartburn, vomiting, constipation, diarrhea, myalgia.

Adult Dose: 100-450 mg daily.

Pediatric Concerns: None reported via milk at this time.

Infant Monitoring: Drowsiness, lethargy, pallor, poor feeding, and weight gain.

Alternatives: Propranolol(L2), Labetalol(L2)

References:

1. Liedholm H, Melander A, Bitzen PO, et al. Accumulation of atenolol and metoprolol in human breast milk. Eur J Clin Pharmacol. 1981;20(3):229-231.
2. Sandstrom B, Regardh CG. Metoprolol excretion into breast milk. Br J Clin Pharmacol. 1980;9(5):518-519.

METRIZAMIDE

Trade: Amipaque

Category: Diagnostic Agent, Radiological Contrast Media

LRC: L2 - Limited Data-Probably Compatible

Metrizamide is a radiographic contrast medium used mainly in myelography. It is water soluble and nonionic. Metrizamide contains 48% bound iodine by molecular weight. The iodine molecule is organically bound and is not available for uptake into breast milk due to minimal metabolism. Following subarachnoid administration of 5.06 g the peak plasma level of 32.9 µg/mL occurred at 6 hours. Cumulative excretion in milk increased with time, but was extremely small with only 1.1 mg or 0.02% of the dose being recovered in milk within 44.3 hours.[1] The drug's high water solubility, nonionic characteristic, and high molecular weight (789) also support minimal excretion into breast milk. This agent is sometimes used as an oral radiocontrast agent.[2] Only minimal oral absorption occurs (<0.4%). The authors suggest that the very small amount of metrizamide secreted in human milk is unlikely to be hazardous to the infant.

T 1/2	>24 h	MW	789 Da	PB	
Tmax	6 h	RID		Vd	
Oral	<0.4 %	M/P		pKa	10.23

Adult Concerns: Headache, irritation of meninges.

Adult Dose:

Pediatric Concerns:

Infant Monitoring:

Alternatives:

References:

1. Ilett KF, Hackett LP, Paterson JW, McCormick CC. Excretion of metrizamide in milk. Br J Radiol. 1981;54(642):537-538.
2. Johansen JG. Assessment of a non-ionic contrast medium (Amipaque) in the gastrointestinal tract. Invest Radiol. 1978;13(6):523-527.

METRIZOATE

Trade: Angiocontrast, Isopaque

Category: Diagnostic Agent, Radiological Contrast Media

LRC: L2 - Limited Data-Probably Compatible

Metrizoate is an ionic radiocontrast agent. Radiopaque agents (except barium) are iodinated compounds used to visualize various organs during X-rays, CAT scans, and other radiological procedures.[1,2] These compounds are highly iodinated benzoic acid derivatives. While iodine products are generally contraindicated in nursing mothers these products are unique, because they are extremely inert and are largely cleared without metabolism. In a study of four women who received metrizoate 0.58 g/kg (350 mg Iodine/mL) IV, the peak level of metrizoate in milk was 14 mg/L at 3 and 6 hours post-injection.[1] The average milk concentration during the first 24 hours was only 11.4 mg/L. During the first 24 hours following injection, it is estimated that a total of 1.7 mg/kg would be transferred to the infant, which is only 0.3% of the maternal dose.

As a group, radiocontrast agents are virtually unabsorbed after oral administration (<0.1%). Metrizoate has a brief half-life of just two hours, and the estimated dose ingested by the infant is only 0.3% of the radiocontrast dose used clinically for various scanning procedures in infants. Although most company package inserts suggest that an infant be removed from the breast for 24 hours, no untoward effects have been reported with these products in breastfed infants. Because the amount of metrizoate transferred into milk is so small, the authors conclude that breastfeeding is acceptable after intravenously administered metrizoate.

T 1/2	60-140 min	MW	627 Da	PB	Very Low
Tmax		RID	0.29%	Vd	
Oral		M/P		pKa	

Adult Concerns: Headache, dizziness, cough, sneezing, tachycardia, hypotension, vomiting, chills, warm sensation, urticaria, allergic reactions- anaphylaxis.

Adult Dose:

Pediatric Concerns:

Infant Monitoring:

Alternatives:

References:

1. Nielsen ST, Matheson I, Rasmussen JN, Skinnemoen K, Andrew E, Hafsahl G. Excretion of iohexol and metrizoate in human breast milk. Acta Radiol.1987;28(5):523-526.
2. Steinberg, Evans JA. Isopaque 440 (metrizoate); a new cardiovascular contrast medium. Experience with 100 consecutive cases. Am J Roentgenol Radium Ther Nucl Med. 1967;101(1):229-233.

METRONIDAZOLE

Trade: Flagyl, Metrocream, Metrolotion, Metrozine, Neo-Metric

Category: Antibiotic, Other

LRC: L2 - Limited Data-Probably Compatible

Metronidazole is indicated in the treatment of vaginitis due to Trichomonas vaginalis and many other types of anaerobic bacterial infections including giardiasis, H. pylori, B. fragilis, and Gardnerella vaginalis.

Metronidazole absorption is time- and dose-dependent and also depends on the route of administration (oral vs. vaginal). Following a 2-g oral dose, milk levels were reported to peak at 50-57 mg/L at 2 hours. Milk levels after 12 hours were approximately 19 mg/L and at 24 hours were approximately 10 mg/L.[1] The average drug concentration reported in milk at 2, 8, 12, and 12-24 hours was 45.8, 27.9, 19.1, and 12.6 mg/L respectively. If breastfeeding were to continue uninterrupted, an infant would consume 21.8 mg via breastmilk. After withholding breastfeeding for 12 hours, an infant would consume only 9.8 mg.

In a group of 12 nursing mothers receiving 400 mg three times daily, the mean milk/plasma ratio was 0.91.[2] The mean milk metronidazole concentration was 15.5 mg/L. Infant plasma metronidazole levels ranged from 1.27 to 2.41 µg/mL. No adverse effects were attributable to metronidazole therapy in these infants. In another study in patients receiving 600 and 1200 mg daily, the average milk metronidazole concentration was 5.7 and 14.4 mg/L respectively.[3] The plasma levels of metronidazole (2 hours) at the 600 mg/day dose were 5 µg/mL (mother) and 0.8 µg/mL (infant). At the 1200 mg/day dose (2 hours), plasma levels were 12.5 µg/mL (mother) and 2.4 µg/mL (infant). The authors estimated the daily metronidazole dose received by the infant at 3 mg/kg with 500 mL milk intake per day, which is well below the typical therapeutic dose for infants of 15-35 mg/kg/day.

For treating trichomoniasis, many physicians now recommend a 2 g single oral dose (stat dose) with an interruption of breastfeeding for 12-24 hours, then reinstitute breastfeeding. Thus far, no reports of untoward effects in breastfed infants have been published with either the 2-g single dose or the 250 mg three times daily for 7-10 days dose regimens. In a study of six women receiving 400 mg three times daily for 3 days, the average milk concentration was 13.5 mg/L with a milk/plasma ratio of 0.9.[4]

It is true that the relative infant dose via milk is moderately high depending on the dose and timing. Infants whose mothers ingest 1.2 g/day will receive approximately 13.5% or less of the maternal dose or approximately 2.3 mg/kg/day. Bennett has calculated the relative infant dose from 11.7% to as high as 24% of the maternal dose.[5] Heisterberg found metronidazole levels in infant plasma to be 16% and 19% of the maternal plasma levels following doses of 600 mg/day and 1200 mg/day.[3] While these levels seem significant, it is still pertinent to remember that metronidazole is a commonly used drug in pregnancy, premature neonates, infants, and children, and 2.3 mg/kg/day is still much less than the therapeutic dose used in infants/children (15-30 mg/kg/day). Thus far, virtually no adverse effects have been reported.

INTRAVENOUS USE: Metronidazole is rapidly and almost completely absorbed orally. In one study of intravenous kinetics, the authors found peak plasma levels of 28.9 µg/mL in adults following a 500-mg TID dose.[6] In another study of oral and intravenous kinetics, the authors used 400 mg orally, and 500 mg intravenously.[7] Following 400 mg orally, the C_{max} at 90 minutes was 17.4 µg/mL. Following 500 mg IV, the C_{max} at 90 minutes was 23.6 µg/mL. Reducing the IV dose to 400 mg would have given a plasma level of approximately 18.8 or an amount similar to the oral plasma level attained in the above group(17.4). From these two sets of data, it is apparent that the peak (C_{max}) following an intravenous dose is only slightly higher than that obtained following oral administration. In an elegant study of plasma kinetics of oral and IV metronidazole (both 500 mg and 2000 mg), Loft found that the AUC (500 mg dose) for oral and IV treatments was virtually identical (101 vs. 100 µg/mL h respectively).[8] The C_{max} (taken from graph) for oral and IV treatments were essentially the same. In another study comparing the plasma kinetics following 800 mg doses orally and IV, Bergan found that plasma levels are virtually identical at 2-3 hours after the dose.[9]

VAGINAL USE: Vaginal absorption of metronidazole is approximately 2% for vaginal gel as compared to oral doses.

Data from older studies with rats and mice have shown that metronidazole is potentially mutagenic/carcinogenic. Thus far, no studies in humans have found it to be mutagenic after man years. In fact, the opposite seems to be the finding.[10,11,12] Roe suggests that metronidazole is "essentially free of cancer risk or other serious toxic side effects."[12] Age-gender stratified analysis did not reveal any association between short-term exposure to metronidazole and cancer in humans.[11]

T 1/2	8.5 h	MW	171 Da	PB	< 20%
Tmax	2-4 h	RID	12.6% - 13.5%	Vd	
Oral	Complete	M/P	1.15	pKa	2.6

Adult Concerns: Dry mouth, bad taste, nausea, vomiting, diarrhea, abdominal discomfort. Drug may turn urine brown.

Adult Dose: 250-500 mg twice daily.

Pediatric Concerns: Numerous studies shown no untoward effects. One letter to the editor suggests an infant developed diarrhea, and a case of lactose intolerance. The link to metronidazole is tenuous.

Infant Monitoring: Dry mouth, vomiting, diarrhea, changes in gastrointestinal flora, urine may turn brown, rash.

Alternatives:

References:

1. Erickson SH, Oppenheim GL, Smith GH. Metronidazole in breast milk. Obstet Gynecol. 1981;57(1):48-50.
2. Passmore CM, McElnay JC, Rainey EA, D'Arcy PF. Metronidazole excretion in human milk and its effect on the suckling neonate. Br J Clin Pharmacol. 1988;26(1):45-51.
3. Heisterberg L, Branebjerg PE. Blood and milk concentrations of metronidazole in mothers and infants. J Perinat Med. 1983;11(2):114-120.
4. Amon I, Amon K. Wirkstoffkonzentrationen von metronidazol bie schwangeren und postpartal. Fortschritte der antimikrobiellen und antineoplastischen. Chemotherapie. 2004;Band 2-4:605-612.
5. Bennett PN. Use of the monographs on drugs: In: Drugs and Human Lactation. Amsterdam: Elsevier; 1996.
6. Ti TY, Lee HS, Khoo YM. Disposition of intravenous metronidazole in Asian surgical patients. Antimicrob Agents Chemother. 1996;40(10):2248-2251.
7. Earl P, Sisson PR, Ingham HR. Twelve-hourly dosage schedule for oral and intravenous metronidazole. J Antimicrob Chemother. 1989;23(4):619-621.
8. Loft S, Dossing M, Poulsen HE, et al. Influence of dose and route of administration on disposition of metronidazole and its major metabolites. Eur J Clin Pharmacol. 1986;30(4):467-473.
9. Bergan T, Leinebo O, Blom-Hagen T, Salvesen B. Pharmacokinetics and bioavailability of metronidazole after tablets, suppositories and intravenous administration. Scand J Gastroenterol Suppl. 1984;91:45-60.
10. Falagas ME, Walker AM, Jick H, Ruthazer R, Griffith J, Snydman DR. Late incidence of cancer after metronidazole use: a matched metronidazole user/nonuser study. Clin Infect Dis. 1998;26(2):384-388.
11. Fahrig R, Engelke M. Reinvestigation of in vivo genotoxicity studies in man. I. No induction of DNA strand breaks in peripheral lymphocytes after metronidazole therapy. Mutat Res. 1997;395(2-3):215-221.
12. Roe FJ. Toxicologic evaluation of metronidazole with particular reference to carcinogenic, mutagenic, and teratogenic potential. Surgery. 1983;93(1 Pt 2):158-164.

METRONIDAZOLE TOPICAL GEL

Trade: Metro-Gel, MetroGel Topical, Metrogel, Metrogyl

Category: Antibiotic, Other

LRC: L2 - No Data-Probably Compatible

Metronidazole topical gel is primarily indicated for rosacea and is a gel formulation containing 0.75% metronidazole. Following topical application of 1 g of metronidazole gel to the face (equivalent to 7.5 mg metronidazole base), the maximum serum concentration was only 66 ng/mL in only one of 10 patients (in three of the 10 patients, levels were undetectable).[1] This concentration is 100 times less than the serum concentrations achieved following the oral ingestion of just one 250-mg tablet. Therefore, the topical application of metronidazole gel provides exceedingly low plasma levels in the mother and minimal to no levels in milk.

T 1/2	8.5 h	MW	171 Da	PB	<20%
Tmax		RID		Vd	
Oral	Complete	M/P	0.4-1.8	pKa	2.6

Adult Concerns: Watery eyes if the gel is applied too close to eyes. Minor skin irritation, redness, burning.

Adult Dose: Apply topically twice daily.

Pediatric Concerns: None reported via milk. Milk levels would be exceedingly low to nil.

Infant Monitoring: Dry mouth, vomiting, diarrhea, changes in gastrointestinal flora, urine may turn brown, rash.

Alternatives:

References:
1.   Pharmaceutical manufacturers prescribing information.

METRONIDAZOLE VAGINAL GEL

Trade: MetroGel Vaginal, Metrogel

Category: Antibiotic, Other

LRC: L2 - No Data-Probably Compatible

Metronidazole is an antibiotic used for the treatment of bacterial vaginosis. Both topical and vaginal preparations of metronidazole contain only 0.75% metronidazole. Plasma levels following administration are exceedingly low.[1] This metronidazole vaginal product produces only 2% of the mean peak serum level concentration of a 500-mg oral metronidazole tablet. The maternal plasma level following use of each dose of vaginal gel averaged 237 µg/L compared to 12,785 µg/L following an oral 500-mg tablet. Milk levels following intravaginal use would probably be exceedingly low. Milk/plasma ratios, although published for oral metronidazole, may be different for this route of administration, primarily due to the low plasma levels attained with this product.

T 1/2	8.5 h	MW	171 Da	PB	10%
Tmax	6-12 h	RID		Vd	
Oral	Complete	M/P		pKa	2.6

Adult Concerns: Mild irritation such as burning to vaginal wall.

Adult Dose: 37.5 mg once daily.

Pediatric Concerns: None reported.

Infant Monitoring: Dry mouth, vomiting, diarrhea, changes in gastrointestinal flora, urine may turn brown, rash.

Alternatives:

References:
1.   Pharmaceutical manufacturers prescribing information.

METYRAPONE

Trade: Metopirone

Category: Diagnostic Agent, Other

LRC: L2 - Limited Data-Probably Compatible

Metyrapone is an inhibitor of endogenous adrenal corticosteroid synthesis and is a diagnostic drug for diagnosis and treatment of adrenocortical hyperfunction. In a case report of a single patient who received 250 mg four times daily for almost 9 weeks, and who was 1 week postpartum, breast milk samples were analyzed for metyrapone and its metabolite. At steady state, the average concentrations in milk and absolute and relative infant doses were 11 µg/L, 1.7 µg/kg/day, and 0.02%, respectively, for metyrapone; and 48.5 µg/L, 7.3 µg/kg/day, and 0.08%, respectively, for its metabolite, rac-metyrapol.[1] The authors suggest that maternal metyrapone use during breastfeeding is unlikely to be a significant risk to an infant.

T 1/2	1.9 h	MW	226 Da	PB	
Tmax	1 h	RID	0.06%	Vd	
Oral	Complete	M/P		pKa	

Adult Concerns: Hypertension, nausea, headache, sedation, rash, acne, alopecia and hirsutism, bone marrow depression, adrenal insufficiency have been reported.

Adult Dose: 30 mg/kg .

Pediatric Concerns: None yet. Levels probably too low.

Infant Monitoring:

Alternatives:

References:
1. Hotham NJ, Ilett KF, Hackett LP, Morton MR, Muller P, Hague WM. Transfer of metyrapone and its metabolite, rac-metyrapol, into breast milk. J Hum Lact. 2009 Nov;25(4):451-454.

MEXILETINE

Trade: Mexitil

Category: Antiarrhythmic

LRC: L2 - Limited Data-Probably Compatible

Mexiletine hydrochloride is an antiarrhythmic agent with activity similar to lidocaine. In a study on one patient who was receiving 600 mg/day in divided doses, the milk level at steady state was 0.8 mg/L, which represented a milk/plasma ratio of 1.1.[1] Mexiletine was not detected in the infant nor were untoward effects noted. In another study on days 2 to 5 postpartum and in a patient receiving 200 mg three times daily, the mean peak concentration of mexiletine in breast milk was 959 μg/L, and the maternal serum was 724 μg/L.[2] In this study the milk/plasma ratio varied from 0.78 to 1.89 with an average of 1.45. It is unlikely this exposure would lead to untoward side effects in a breastfeeding infant.

T 1/2	10-14 h	MW	179 Da	PB	63%
Tmax	2-3 h (oral)	RID	1.4% - 1.6%	Vd	5-7 L/kg
Oral	90%	M/P	1.45	pKa	8.4

Adult Concerns: Arrhythmias, bradycardia, hypotension, tremors, dizziness.

Adult Dose: 200 mg every 8 hours.

Pediatric Concerns: None reported in two studies.

Infant Monitoring: Drowsiness, lethargy, changes in vision, pallor, arrhythmias, poor feeding, weight gain, tremor.

Alternatives:

References:
1. Lewis AM, Patel L, Johnston A, Turner P. Mexiletine in human blood and breast milk. Postgrad Med J. 1981;57(671):546-547.
2. Timmis AD, Jackson G, Holt DW. Mexiletine for control of ventricular dysrhythmias in pregnancy. Lancet. 1980;2(8195 pt 1):647-648.

MICAFUNGIN

Trade: Mycamine

Category: Antifungal

LRC: L3 - No Data-Probably Compatible

Micafungin is an antifungal drug which inhibits the production of a vital component of the fungal cell wall, beta-1,3-D-glucan.[1] It is administered intravenously to treat candida infections such as candidemia, candida peritonitis, abscesses, and esophageal candidiasis, and prevent candida infections in patients undergoing hematopoietic stem cell transplants. It is not known whether micafungin is excreted in human milk; however, based on its physicochemical and pharmacokinetic characteristics it is not likely to enter breast milk in significant amounts. Caution should be exercised when administered to a nursing woman until further information is available.

T 1/2	13-17 h	MW	1292.26 Da	PB	> 99%
Tmax		RID		Vd	0.39 L/kg
Oral		M/P		pKa	9.15

Adult Concerns: Headache, dizziness, insomnia, fever, tachycardia, mucositis, nausea, vomiting, abdominal pain, diarrhea, changes in liver and renal function, hypokalemia, neutropenia, thrombocytopenia, rashes.

Adult Dose: 50-150 mg IV once daily.

Pediatric Concerns: There is safety data available in pediatric patients greater than 4 months of age.

Infant Monitoring: Insomnia, lethargy, vomiting, diarrhea.

Alternatives:

References:
1. Pharmaceutical manufacturers prescribing information.

MICONAZOLE

Trade: Daktarin, Micatin, Monistat 3, Monistat 7, Oravig, Smart Sense Miconazole 1, Topcare Miconazole, Up and Up Miconazole

Category: Antifungal

LRC: L2 - No Data-Probably Compatible

Miconazole is an effective antifungal that is commonly used IV, topically, and intravaginally. After intravaginal application, approximately 1% of the dose is absorbed systemically.[1,2] After topical application, there is little or no absorption (0.1%). It is unlikely that the limited absorption of miconazole from vaginal application would produce significant levels in milk. Milk concentrations following oral and IV miconazole have not been reported. Oral absorption of miconazole is poor, only 25-30%. Miconazole is commonly used in pediatric patients less than 1 year of age.

T 1/2	20-25 h	MW	416 Da	PB	91-93%
Tmax	Immediate (IV)	RID		Vd	
Oral	25-30%	M/P		pKa	6.9

Adult Concerns: Nausea, vomiting, diarrhea, anorexia, itching, rash, local irritation.

Adult Dose: 200-1200 mg three times daily.

Pediatric Concerns: None reported via milk.

Infant Monitoring:

Alternatives:

References:
1. Pharmaceutical manufacturers prescribing information.

MICROFIBRILLAR COLLAGEN HEMOSTAT

Trade: Avitene, Helistat, Hemotene

Category: Hemostatic

LRC: L3 - No Data-Probably Compatible

Microfibrillar collagen hemostat (MCH) is an absorbable topical hemostatic agent of bovine origin. It is used to achieve hemostasis during surgical procedures when conventional methods appear to fail. Chemically it is collagen non-covalently bound to hydrochloric acid.[1,2] Collagen is an inert protein found in skin, ligaments, tendons, and bones. It serves the purpose of providing cytoskeletal stability and inelasticity. Its molecular weight is 300,000 Da. When MCH is applied on a bleeding surface, it attracts platelets to the surface and results in the formation of a platelet plug, which eventually helps control bleeding.[3] MCH is being used increasingly for neurosurgical procedures. This product has been known to excite local and systemic inflammatory reactions. Following its use in neurosurgical procedures, a few cases of seizures, mass occupying granulomas, and encephalomyelitis have been described.[4-7] This product has the potential to pass through the circulatory system from the initial site of application, and deposit in different organs causing organ damage.[8] Its use in breastfeeding women has not been described. However, due to its high molecular weight, its transfer to breast milk is unlikely. Being an inert protein, its systemic absorption following ingestion in milk is unlikely.

T 1/2		MW	300,000 Da	PB	
Tmax		RID		Vd	
Oral		M/P		pKa	

Adult Concerns: Abscess formation, hematoma, alveolitis of jaw when used in dental extraction pockets.

Adult Dose:

Pediatric Concerns:

Infant Monitoring:

Alternatives:

References:

1. Product Information: Avitene(R), microfibrillar collagen hemostat, Avicon, Inc, Ft Worth TX, 1990. Avitene(R), microfibrillar collagen hemostat, Avicon, Inc, Ft Worth TX, 1990.
2. Anon. Avitene(R) - a new topical hemostatic agent. Med Lett Drug Ther. 1977;19:28.
3. Mason RB, Read MS. Some effects of a microcrystalline collagen preparation on blood. Haemostasis. 1974;3:31-45.
4. Apel-Sarid L, Cochrane DD, Steinbok P, Byrne AT, Dunham C. Microfibrillarcollagen hemostat-induced necrotizing granulomatous inflammation developing aftercraniotomy: a pediatric case series. J Neurosurg Pediatr. 2010 Oct;6(4):385-392.
5. Sani S, Boco T, Lewis SL, Cochran E, Patel AJ, Byrne RW. Postoperative acutedisseminated encephalomyelitis after exposure to microfibrillar collagenhemostat. J Neurosurg. 2008 Jul;109(1):149-152.
6. O'Shaughnessy BA, Schafernak KT, DiPatri AJ Jr, Goldman S, Tomita T. Agranulomatous reaction to Avitene mimicking recurrence of a medulloblastoma. Casereport. J Neurosurg. 2006 Jan;104(1 Suppl):33-36.
7. Nakajima M, Kamei T, Tomimatu K, Manabe T. An intraperitoneal tumorous masscaused by granulomas of microfibrillar collagen hemostat (Avitene). Arch Pathol Lab Med. 1995 Dec;119(12):1161-1163.
8. Robicsek F, Duncan GD, Born GV, Wilkinson HA, Masters TN, McClure M. Inherent dangers of simultaneous application of microfibrillar collagen hemostat andblood-saving devices. J Thorac Cardiovasc Surg. 1986 Oct;92(4):766-770.

MIDAZOLAM

Trade: Hypnovel, Versed, Nayzilam Intranasal

Category: Sedative-Hypnotic

LRC: L2 - Limited Data-Probably Compatible

Midazolam is a short-acting benzodiazepine primarily used as an induction or preanesthetic medication. Midazolam has a quick onset of action, rapid elimination, and is more potent than diazepam. With a half-life of only 3 hours, it is preferred for rapid induction and maintenance of anesthesia.

After oral administration of 15 mg for up to 6 days postnatally in 22 women, the mean milk/plasma ratio was 0.15 and the maximum level of midazolam in breast milk was 9 µg/L and occurred 1-2 hours after administration.[1] Midazolam and its hydroxy metabolite were undetectable 4 hours after administration. Therefore, the amount of midazolam transferred to an infant via early milk is minimal, particularly if the baby is breastfed more than 4 hours after administration.

In a study of five women undergoing surgery with IV midazolam premedication and induction with propofol and fentanyl, milk samples were obtained at 5, 7, 9, 11, and 24 hours post midazolam administration.[2] These women were on average 11 weeks postpartum and produced about 325 mL/day of milk. The median amount of midazolam recovered in milk within 24 hours post dose was 0.08 µg or 0.004% of the maternal dose (2 mg). The weight-normalized infant dose was 0.016 µg/kg. None of the infants was given their mother's milk during this study.

In another study that included 124 breastfeeding women and their infants (aged 2-24 months), 2 infants (1.6%) were reported as having CNS depression.[3] The three most commonly taken benzodiazepines were lorazepam (52%), clonazepam (18%), and midazolam (15%). There was no correlation between infant sedation and maternal benzodiazepine dose or duration of use. The two mothers who reported infants with sedation were taking more medications that also cause similar CNS adverse effects than those without infant concerns (mean of 3.5 versus 1.7 medications).

T 1/2	3 h	MW	326 Da	PB	97%
Tmax	0.2-3 h (oral)	RID	0.63%	Vd	1-3.1 L/kg
Oral	40-50%	M/P	0.15	pKa	6.2

Adult Concerns: Sedation, dizziness, confusion, apnea, hypotension.

Adult Dose: 1-2.5 mg IV (varies by indication and route of administration).

Pediatric Concerns: None reported via milk at this time.

Infant Monitoring: Sedation, slowed breathing rate, not waking to feed/poor feeding, and weight gain.

Alternatives: Lorazepam(L3)

References:

1. Matheson I, Lunde PK, Bredesen JE. Midazolam and nitrazepam in the maternity ward: milk concentrations and clinical effects. Br J Clin Pharmacol. 1990;30(6):787-793.
2. Nitsun M, Szokol JW, Saleh HJ, et al. Pharmacokinetics of midazolam, propofol, and fentanyl transfer to human breast milk. Clin Pharmacol Ther. 2006;79(6):549-557.
3. Kelly LE, Poon S, Madadi P, Koren G. Neonatal benzodiazepines exposure during breastfeeding. J Pediatr. 2012;161(3):448-451.

MIDODRINE

Trade: Amatine, Gutron, Midon, ProAmatine

Category: Vasopressor

LRC: L3 - No Data-Probably Compatible

Midodrine is a vasopressor used to increase blood pressure.[1] Midodrine is a prodrug that is metabolized to desglymidodrine. This metabolite is a long-acting alpha-1 agonist. It produces an increase in vascular tone and elevation of blood pressure. Desglymidodrine does not stimulate cardiac beta-1 receptors, nor does it pass the blood-brain barrier. No data are available on its transfer to human milk, but some should be expected. This product is small in molecular weight, belongs to the phenylethylamine family, is lipophilic, and is likely to penetrate milk as do the other members of this family. Some caution is recommended.

T 1/2	3-4 h (metabolite)	MW	290 Da	PB	
Tmax	1-2 h	RID		Vd	
Oral	93%	M/P		pKa	7.8

Adult Concerns: Supine hypertension, pruritus, pilomotor reactions, chills, painful urination retention, and gastrointestinal symptoms have been reported. CNS reactions include headache, insomnia, stimulation, restlessness, dizziness. A vagal reflex may occur following use and produce a reflex bradycardia.

Adult Dose: 10 mg three times daily at 4-hour intervals for orthostatic hypotension.

Pediatric Concerns: None reported via milk, but some caution is recommended. Observe for hypertension, insomnia, and excitement.

Infant Monitoring: Insomnia, excitement, restlessness.

Alternatives:

References:

1. Pharmaceutical manufacturers prescribing information.

MIFEPRISTONE

Trade: Korlym, Mifegyne, Mifeprex, Pencroftonum, RU-486

Category: Antiprogesterone

LRC: L3 - Limited Data-Probably Compatible

Mifepristone is a potent glucocorticoid (GR-II) receptor antagonist when used in higher doses; when used in lower doses it is a selective antagonist of the progesterone receptor. It is used in the treatment of hyperglycemia secondary to hypercortisolism in patients with Cushing syndrome.[1] Because of its antiprogesterone effect, it is used worldwide to terminate pregnancies.[2]

Mifepristone transfers into human milk in low levels, especially when used in low doses. In a study of 12 mothers who received 200 mg or 600 mg of mifepristone orally, the milk levels ranged from undetectable (<0.013 μmol/l) to 0.913 μmol/l. The milk/serum ratio ranged from <0.013:1 to 0.042:1, and the highest calculated RID was 1.5%.[2] Thus, its transfer to human milk is probably negligible.

T 1/2	20-85 h	MW	429.5 Da	PB	99.2%
Tmax	1-4 h	RID		Vd	1.5 L/kg
Oral	69%	M/P		pKa	

Adult Concerns: Nausea, vomiting, fatigue, peripheral edema, headache, dizziness, arthralgia, back pain, hypokalemia, decreased appetite, hypertension, and endometrial hypertrophy.

Adult Dose: 200-1200 mg daily.

Pediatric Concerns: The safety and efficacy in pediatric patients have not been established.

Infant Monitoring:

Alternatives:

References:
1. Pharmaceutical manufacturers prescribing information.
2. Saav I, Fiala C, Hamaleinen JM, Heikinheimo O, Gemzell-Danielsson K. Medical abortion in lactating women – low levels of mifepristone in breast milk. Acta Obstetricia et Gynecologica. 2010;89:618–622.

MIGLITOL

Trade: Diastabol, Glyset

Category: Antidiabetic, Alpha Glucosidase Inhibitor

LRC: L2 - Limited Data-Probably Compatible

Miglitol is an oral alpha-glycosidase inhibitor for use in non-insulin dependent diabetes mellitus.[1] Miglitol delays the digestion of ingested carbohydrates thereby resulting in a small rise in blood glucose concentration following meals. Miglitol does not stimulate insulin release, inhibit lactase, or induce hypoglycemia. The oral absorption of miglitol is saturable in adults in doses higher than 25 mg. A dose of 100 mg is only 50-70% absorbed orally. The manufacturer reports that milk levels are very small. Total excretion in milk accounted for 0.02% of a 100-mg maternal dose. The estimated exposure to a nursing infant is approximately 0.4% of the maternal dose. With such little amounts of transfer into breast milk, it is highly unlikely that miglitol used during lactation will cause significant clinical effects in the breastfed infant. Miglitol is probably compatible with breastfeeding.

T 1/2	2 h	MW	207 Da	PB	<4%
Tmax	2-3 h	RID	0.4%	Vd	0.18 L/kg
Oral	Variable	M/P		pKa	5.9

Adult Concerns: Flatulence, soft stools, diarrhea, abdominal discomfort are the most commonly reported side effects.

Adult Dose: 50 mg three times daily.

Pediatric Concerns: No reports of use in breastfeeding mothers.

Infant Monitoring: Diarrhea and signs of hypoglycemia- drowsiness, lethargy, pallor, sweating, tremor.

Alternatives: Metformin(L1)

References:
1. Pharmaceutical manufacturers prescribing information.

MILK THISTLE

Trade: Holy Thistle, Lady Thistle, Marian Thistle, Silybum, Silymarin

Category: Herb

LRC: L3 - No Data-Probably Compatible

Milk thistle has been used for centuries as a liver protectant.[1] Silymarin, a mixture of three isomeric flavonolignans, consists of silybin, silychristin, and silidianin.[2] Silybin is the most biologically active and is believed to be a potent antioxidant and hepatoprotective agent. Silymarin is poorly soluble in water so aqueous preparations such as teas are ineffective. The oral bioavailability is likewise poor; only 23-47% is absorbed orally. Oral forms are generally concentrated. Silymarin effects are almost exclusively on the liver and kidney and concentrates in liver cells. It is believed to inhibit oxidative damage to cells by increasing glutathione synthesis. It is also believed to stimulate the regenerative capacity of liver cells. While it has been advocated for the stimulation of milk synthesis, little evidence of efficacy exists. No data are available concerning Silymarin transfer to human milk but some probably transfers. It also has rather limited toxicity data with only reports of brief gastrointestinal intolerance and mild allergic reactions.[3,4]

T 1/2		MW	482 Da	PB	
Tmax		RID		Vd	
Oral	23-47%	M/P		pKa	

Adult Concerns: Mild gastrointestinal intolerance and allergic reactions.

Adult Dose: 200-400 mg daily via extracts.

Pediatric Concerns: None reported via milk.

Infant Monitoring: Gastrointestinal intolerance.

Alternatives:

References:

1. Foster S. Milk Thistle-Silybum Marianum. Botanical Series No. 305. Austin, TX : American Botanical Council; 1991:3-7.
2. Leung AY. Encyclopedia of Common Natural Ingredients used in Food, Drugs and Cosmetics. New York, NY: J Wiley and Sons; 1980.
3. Review of Natural Products Facts and Comparisons, 1999.
4. Awang D. Milk thistle. Can Pharm J. 1993 Oct;126:403-404.

MILNACIPRAN

Trade: Savella

Category: Antidepressant, other

LRC: L3 - Limited Data-Probably Compatible

Milnacipran is a selective serotonin and norepinephrine reuptake inhibitor (SNRI) that is used in the treatment of fibromyalgia. It potentiates the serotonergic and noradrenergic activity in the brain. Studies have shown that the drug is secreted in both rat and human milk.[1]

According to a single study where eight lactating women received a single dose of 50 mg of milnacipran hydrochloride, it was found that milnacipran transfers to human milk. Based on peak plasma concentrations, the maximum estimated daily infant dose was 5% of the maternal dose. In most cases, peak concentrations in breast milk were reported 4 hours after maternal dose.[1]

T 1/2	6-8 h	MW	282.8 Da	PB	13%
Tmax	2-4 h	RID		Vd	5.7 L/kg
Oral	85-90%	M/P		pKa	9.6

Adult Concerns: Headache, dizziness, somnolence or insomnia, tachycardia, hypertension, nausea, decreased appetite, constipation, urinary retention, increases in cholesterol.

Adult Dose: 50 mg twice daily.

Pediatric Concerns: No data in lactation at this time.

Infant Monitoring: Sedation or irritability, not waking to feed/poor feeding, constipation, weight gain.

Alternatives: SSRIs, Venlafaxine(L2), Duloxetine(L3)

References:

1. Pharmaceutical manufacturer (Forest) prescribing information, 2014.

MILRINONE

Trade: Corotrop, Primacor

Category: Vasodilator

LRC: L4 - No Data-Possibly Hazardous

Milrinone is a bupyridine inotropic/vasodilator agent. The drug is used in the short-term treatment of heart failure (<48 hours) that is unresponsive to other modalities. There is increased mortality with long-term oral use. Milrinone increases the cardiac output and decreases pulmonary capillary wedge pressure and vascular resistance with mild to moderate increases in heart rate. The drug is well absorbed after oral administration. Blood pressure, heart rate, ECG, fluid and electrolyte balance, and renal function should be monitored during therapy. The half-life is brief, 2.3 hours; therefore waiting 8 hours after last dose prior to restarting breastfeeding should eliminate risk to the infant.[1]

T 1/2	0.8 to 2.3 h	MW	211.2 Da	PB	70%
Tmax		RID		Vd	0.38 L/kg
Oral	80%	M/P		pKa	8.83

Adult Concerns: Headache, supraventricular and ventricular arrhythmias, hypotension, angina, hypokalemia, tremor, thrombocytopenia.

Adult Dose: 50 µg/kg over 10 min, followed by 0.59-1.13 mg/kg infusion over 24 hours.

Pediatric Concerns:

Infant Monitoring: Drowsiness, lethargy, pallor, poor feeding, and weight gain.

Alternatives:

References:

1. Pharmaceutical Manufacturer prescribing information.

MINERAL OIL (PARAFFIN)

Trade:

Category: Laxative

LRC: L3 - No Data-Probably Compatible

Mineral oils are a group of substances derived from petroleum with chain lengths that range in size from 15-40 carbon atoms in length. They are most often used as laxatives and emollients in topical preparations. The size of any given paraffin is indirectly related to its ability to be absorbed. Substances with greater than 34 carbons are unlikely to be absorbed due to size, while smaller molecules of less than 20 carbons are absorbed well but also broken down very quickly in the liver. Mineral hydrocarbons that are of the most concern in human subjects fall within a range of 21-28 carbons.[1,3] Rectal absorption is minimal, due to the greatest degree of absorption occurring in the small intestine.[2] As such, mineral oil is of concern only when ingested or applied topically. Ingested hydrocarbons do distribute widely throughout the body, resulting in concentrations of up to 4.5 mg/g in humans. The present molecules can include cycloalkanes, which are often found in lipogranulomas and are indicative of mineral oil presence.[1,3]

Acceptable daily intakes (ADI) vary between different mineral oils, with differences being based upon composition of any given preparation. In the case of infants less than 3 months of age, it is recommended that mineral oils be no less than 480 Da (approximately 34 carbons), and that at most 5% of the dose consist of molecules with 25 or less carbons. Total intake should not exceed 0-4 mg/kg, and substances less than 25 carbons should not exceed 0.2 mg/kg.[4] Mineral oils do transfer to breast milk, and generally appear in highest concentration toward the start of lactation. Continued breastfeeding has been shown to lower concentrations of paraffins significantly.

In one woman it was shown that n-alkanes deposited in breast milk centered around a length of 23 carbons, with a substantial amount of hydrocarbons of 22-26 carbon lengths, indicating the presence of mineral oils. Direct application of paraffins to the breast results in accumulation of mineral hydrocarbons in the milk fat. Upon administration of Vaseline to the breast for 20 days, mineral hydrocarbons in the milk fat increased to 160 mg/kg.[4] In an infant who ingests 800 mL breast milk containing 3% fat daily, this would amount to a daily intake of 1 mg/kg mineral oils. This clearly exceeds the acceptable daily intake for paraffins less than 25 carbons in length. Application of salves and ointments to the breast is only recommended after feeding, as the infant may ingest up to 40 mg/kg mineral oil from a mother who applies five daily applications of 100 mg to each breast. Based on the compositions of some body creams, this can result in a dose to the infant that measures 40 times the ADI for substances less than 25 carbons in length. Due to the fact that shorter length hydrocarbons are absorbed well by the mother, it is likely that they will also be absorbed by the infant. It should be noted that while longer chain mineral oils are not well absorbed in the gastrointestinal tract; it is possible for them to be absorbed dermally, though the rate of absorption would be very low.[4]

Toxic effects have been shown in rats when exposed to large amounts of paraffin oils, with the most significant endpoint being histiocytosis in lymph nodes.[5] It is recommended that nursing mothers avoid using paraffin containing products for breast care.[4] Mineral oil is commonly used to treat pediatric constipation, although it may prevent the absorption of oil-soluble vitamins.

T 1/2		MW	Varies Da	PB	
Tmax		RID		Vd	
Oral	30-60%, varies based on molecular weight	M/P		pKa	

Adult Concerns: Lipid pneumonitis may occur with aspiration. Nausea, vomiting, cramps, and diarrhea may occur with oral ingestion. Anal seepage may result from rectal application. Impaired absorption of vitamins A, D, E, and K can result.

Adult Dose: Oral: 15-45 mL; Rectal: 118 mL; Topical: Apply as needed.

Pediatric Concerns:

Infant Monitoring:

Alternatives:

References:
1. Rose HG, Liber AF. Accumulation of saturated hydrocarbons in human spleens. J Lab Clin Med. 1966;68:475–483.
2. Curry CE, Butler D. Laxative products. In: Allen LV Jr, Berardi RR, DeSimone EM II, eds. Handbook of Nonprescription Drugs. 12th ed. Washington, DC: American Pharmaceutical Association; 2000.
3. Boitnott JK, Margolis S. Saturated hydrocarbons in human tissues. III. Oil droplets in the liver and spleen. Johns Hopkins Med. J. 1970;127:65–78.
4. Noti A, Grob K, Biedermann M, Deiss U, Brüschweiler BJ. Exposure of babies to C15–C45 mineral paraffins from human milk and breast salves. Regul Toxicol Pharmacol. 2003 Dec;38(3):317-325.
5. Smith JH, Mallett AK, Priston RA, et al. Ninety-day feeding study in Fischer-344 rats of highly refined petroleum-derived food-grade white oils and waxes. Toxicol Pathol. 1996;24:214-230.

MINOCYCLINE

Trade: Akamin, Arestin, Dynacin, Minocin, Minomycin, Amzeeq

Category: Antibiotic, Tetracycline

LRC: L3 - Limited Data-Probably Compatible

Minocycline is a broad-spectrum tetracycline antibiotic with significant side effects in pediatric patients, including dental staining and reduced bone growth.[1] It is probably secreted in breast milk in small but clinically insignificant levels. Because tetracyclines in general bind to milk calcium, they would have reduced absorption in the infant, but minocycline may be absorbed to a greater degree than the older tetracyclines.

In a study of two patients receiving 200 mg orally, the concentration at peak (6 hours) was 0.8 μg/mL.[2] The authors report that the average milk level was 0.5 to 0.8 mg/L for a period of 12 hours postdose, which would transfer approximately 18 μg to the infant. Thus approximately 4.2% of the maternal dose would possibly transfer to the infant via milk. Most of this would be unabsorbed orally by the infant. Due to the risk of dental staining, and epiphyseal problems with tetracyclines in infants and children, prolonged use (more than 3 weeks) of tetracyclines should be avoided.

A new microsomal product (Arestin) used in adults for periodonatal maintenance therapy contains only 1 mg of minocycline per capsule. There would be no risk to the limited use of this product in breastfeeding mothers (< 3-4 weeks).

T 1/2	15-20 h	MW	457 Da	PB	76%
Tmax	3 h	RID	4.2%	Vd	0.14-0.7 L/kg
Oral	90-100%	M/P		pKa	2.8, 5, 7.8, 9.3

Adult Concerns: Headache, fever, dyspepsia, abdominal cramps, vomiting, diarrhea, anorexia, changes in liver and renal function, photosensitivity, agranulocytosis.

Adult Dose: 100 mg twice daily.

Pediatric Concerns: None via breastmilk at this time.

Infant Monitoring: Vomiting, diarrhea, changes in gastrointestinal flora, rash; prolonged exposure may lead to dental staining, and decreased bone growth.

Alternatives:

References:
1. Pharmaceutical manufacturers prescribing information.
2. Mizuno S, Takata M, Sano S, Ueyama T. Minocycline. Jpn J Antibiot. 1969 Dec;22(6):473-479.

MINOXIDIL

Trade: Loniten, Minodyl, Minox

Category: Antihypertensive

LRC: L3 - No Data-Probably Compatible

Minoxidil is a potent vasodilator and antihypertensive. It is also used for hair loss and baldness. When applied topically, only 1.4% of the dose is absorbed systemically. Following an oral dose of 7.5 mg, minoxidil was secreted in human milk in concentrations ranging from trough levels of 0.3 μg/L at 12 hours to peak levels of 41.7-55 μg/L at 1 hour following an oral dose of 7.5 mg.[1] Long-term exposure of breastfeeding infants in women ingesting oral minoxidil may not be advisable. However, in those using topical minoxidil, the limited absorption via skin would minimize systemic levels and significantly reduce risk of transfer to infant via breast milk. It is unlikely that the amount absorbed via topical application would produce clinically relevant concentrations in breast milk.

T 1/2	3.5-4.2 h	MW	209 Da	PB	Low
Tmax	2-8 h	RID	9.1%	Vd	
Oral	90-95%	M/P	0.75-1	pKa	4.6

Adult Concerns: Hypotension, tachycardia, headache, weight gain, skin pigmentation, rash, renal toxicity, leukopenia.

Adult Dose: 10-40 mg daily.

Pediatric Concerns: None reported.

Infant Monitoring: Drowsiness, lethargy, pallor, poor feeding, and weight gain.

Alternatives:

References:
1. Valdivieso A, Valdes G, Spiro TE, Westerman RL. Minoxidil in breast milk. Ann Intern Med. 1985;102(1):135.

MIRABEGRON

Trade: Myrbetriq

Category: Adrenergic Stimulant

LRC: L3 - No Data-Probably Compatible

Mirabegron is a beta-3 adrenergic agonist used to treat overactive bladder (OAB) symptoms.[1] There are no human data regarding the transfer of mirabegron to human milk. Based on this medication's long half-life (50 hours), smaller size (396.5 Da), and moderate protein binding (71%), it is expected that this medication could enter human milk to some degree. However, due to this medication's massive volume of distribution, it is unlikely much will stay in the plasma compartment of the mother or enter the milk compartment. At this time, it is probably compatible for use in a breastfeeding mother; however, there are alternatives that may enter milk to a lesser degree (e.g. oxybutynin).

T 1/2	50 h	MW	396.51 Da	PB	71%
Tmax	3.5 h	RID		Vd	23.9 L/kg
Oral	29-35% (dose dependent)	M/P		pKa	

Adult Concerns: Headache, dizziness, hypertension, tachycardia, nausea, diarrhea, constipation, changes in liver function, urinary retention, urinary tract infections.

Adult Dose: 25 mg or 50 mg extended release tablet once daily.

Pediatric Concerns: None reported via milk at this time. Safety has not been established in pediatric patients.

Infant Monitoring: Vomiting, constipation or diarrhea, urinary retention.

Alternatives: Oxybutynin(L3)

References:
1. Pharmaceutical manufacturer prescribing information.

MIRTAZAPINE

Trade: Avanza, Remeron, Zispin

Category: Antidepressant, other

LRC: L3 - Limited Data-Probably Compatible

Mirtazapine is a unique antidepressant structurally dissimilar to the SSRIs, tricyclic antidepressants, or the monoamine oxidase inhibitors. Mirtazapine has little or no serotonergic-like side effects, fewer anticholinergic side effects than amitriptyline, it produces less sexual dysfunction, and has not demonstrated cardiotoxic or seizure potential in a limited number of overdose cases.[1]

In a study of three women who received 45, 60, and 45 mg/day mirtazapine, the average concentration (AUC) in milk was 77, 75, and 47 µg/L, respectively.[2] The absolute infant dose was 10, 11.3, and 7.1 µg/kg/day, respectively. The relative infant dose was 1.9%, 1.1%, and 1.5% of the weight-normalized maternal dose, respectively. Mirtazapine was below the limit of quantitation in two of the infants and only 1.5 ng/mL in the second infant. The infants were meeting all developmental milestones and were without side effects.

Another study of eight women taking an average of 38 mg/day showed average milk concentrations of 53 µg/L and 13 µg/L of mirtazapine and its metabolite, respectively. The average absolute infant dose was 495 µg/kg/day, indicating a relative infant dose of 1.9%. The authors of this study suggest that breastfeeding is safe during mirtazapine therapy.[3] In another mother who took 22.5 mg/day, milk levels were 130 µg/L 4 hours after dosing and 61 µg/L 10 hours after the dose (foremilk). This suggests the relative infant dose was 3.9-4.4% and 1.8-2.7% respectively of the weight-adjusted maternal dose at these two times. At 12.5 hours postdose, infant plasma levels were undetectable.[4]

T 1/2	20-40 h	MW	265 Da	PB	85%
Tmax	2 h	RID	1.6% - 6.3%	Vd	4.5 L/kg
Oral	50%	M/P	0.76	pKa	7.1

Adult Concerns: Drowsiness (54%), dizziness, dry mouth, constipation, increased appetite (17%), and weight gain (12%) have been reported.

Adult Dose: 15-45 mg daily.

Pediatric Concerns: None reported via milk but observe for sedation.

Infant Monitoring: Sedation or irritability, not waking to feed/poor feeding, and weight gain.

Alternatives: Sertraline(L2), Venlafaxine(L2)

References:

1. Pharmaceutical manufacturers prescribing information.
2. Ilett KF, Hackett LP, Kristensen JH, Rampono J. Distribution and excretion of the novel antidepressant mirtazapine in human milk. International Lactation Consultants Meeting, Sydney; July 31- August 3, 2003.
3. Kristensen JH, Ilett KF, Rampono J, Kohan R, Hackett LP. Transfer of the antidepressant mirtazapine into breast milk. Br J Clin Pharmacol. 2006;63(3):322-327.
4. Klier CM, Mossaheb N, Lee A, Zernig G. Mirtazapine and breastfeeding: maternal and infant plasma levels. Am J Psychiatry. 2007;164(2):348-349.

MISOPROSTOL

Trade: Cytotec

Category: Prostaglandin

LRC: L2 - Limited Data-Probably Compatible

Misoprostol is a prostaglandin E1 compound that is useful in treating multiple conditions such as postpartum hemorrhage and NSAID-induced gastric ulceration.[1] Misoprostol can be administered orally, vaginally, or rectally depending on its indication for use. Intact misoprostol is not detectable in plasma and is rapidly metabolized to misoprostol acid which is biologically active. The peak of misoprostol acid is 6-22 min after oral administration.

In a study of 20 women given a single 600-µg oral dose of misoprostol, the first eight women were sampled immediately postpartum.[2] These eight women had insufficient quantities of colostrum to quantify the concentration of misoprostol in colostrum. From the remaining 12 that were sampled 3-6 days postpartum, misoprostol reached its peak concentration in colostrum about 1 hour after the dose (20.9 pg/mL). The concentrations then declined with each subsequent sample and were less than 1 pg/mL by 5 hours.

In a 2004 prospective study following a maternal oral dose of 200 µg in 10 lactating women, the mean time to peak and peak milk concentration of misoprostol occurred at 1.1 hours and was about 0.0076 µg/L (range 0.0019-0.0307 µg/L).[3] The mean milk/plasma ratio was 0.04 at 0.5 hours and 0.06 at 1 hour postdose. We estimate that the infant would receive less than 0.5% of the maternal dose. Although the authors of this study suggest that misoprostol be taken immediately after a feed and the next feed be given 4 hours postdose, we suggest that this is probably unnecessary as this drug is rapidly eliminated and levels in milk are exceedingly low.

T 1/2	20-40 min	MW	383 Da	PB	80-90%
Tmax	6-22 min (oral)	RID	0.04%	Vd	
Oral	Complete	M/P	0.05	pKa	14.68

Adult Concerns: Headache, fever, chills, nausea, vomiting, diarrhea, abdominal cramps and pain, uterine bleeding, and abortion.

Adult Dose: 100-200 µg four times daily or 600-800 µg as a single dose.

Pediatric Concerns: None reported via milk at this time.

Infant Monitoring: Vomiting, diarrhea.

Alternatives: None.

References:
1. Pharmaceutical manufacturers prescribing information.
2. Abdel-Aleem H, Villar J, Gulmezoglu AM, et al. The pharmacokinetics of the prostaglandin E1 analogue misoprostol in plasma and colostrum after postpartum oral administration. Eur J Obstet Gynecol Reprod Bio. 2003;108:25-28.
3. Vogel D, Burkhardt T, Rentsch K, et al. Misoprostol versus methylergometrine: Pharmacokinetics in human milk. Am J Obstet Gynecol. 2004;191:2168-2173.

MITOMYCIN

Trade: Mitomycin-C, Mutamycin

Category: Antineoplastic

LRC: L5 - No Data-Hazardous

Mitomycin is an alkylating agent used for the treatment of stomach, pancreatic, and numerous other cancers. Oral absorption is erratic due to its instability in aqueous solutions, so it is always used intravenously.[1] It is eliminated via a biexponential curve with a terminal half-life of 23-78 minutes. No data are available on its transfer to human milk. Withhold breastfeeding for a minimum of 24-48 hours.

T 1/2	23-78 min	MW	334 Da	PB	
Tmax		RID		Vd	0.27-1.19 L/kg
Oral		M/P		pKa	3.2, 6.5

Adult Concerns: Loss of appetite, nausea and vomiting, numbness or tingling in fingers and toes, purple-colored bands on nails, skin rash, unusual tiredness or weakness.

Adult Dose: 20 mg/m² IV every 6-8 weeks.

Pediatric Concerns:

Infant Monitoring: Withhold breastfeeding for a minimum of 24-48 hours.

Alternatives:

References:
1. Pharmaceutical manufacturers prescribing information.

MITOXANTRONE

Trade: Formyxan, Genefadrone, Misostol, Mitoxl, Novantrone, Onkotrone, Pralifan

Category: Immune Suppressant

LRC: L5 - Limited Data-Hazardous

Mitoxantrone is an antineoplastic agent used in the treatment of relapsing multiple sclerosis. It is a DNA-reactive agent that intercalates into DNA via hydrogen bonding, causing crosslinks. It inhibits B cell, T cell, and macrophage proliferation. Terminal elimination is described by a three-compartment model. The mean alpha half-life of mitoxantrone is 6-12 minutes, the mean beta half-life is 1.1 to 3.1 hours, and the mean gamma (terminal or elimination) half-life is 23 to 215 hours (median approximately 75 hours).[1]

Distribution to tissues is extensive: steady-state volume of distribution exceeds 1000 L/m². Tissue concentrations of mitoxantrone appear to exceed those in the blood during the terminal elimination phase. In a study of a patient who received three treatments of mitoxantrone (6 mg/m²) on days 1 to 5. Mitoxantrone levels in milk measured 120 ng/mL just after treatment (on the third day of treatment, RID= 12.14%), and dropped to a stable level of 18 ng/mL for the next 28 days (RID=1.8%).[2] This agent has an enormous volume of distribution and is sequestered in at least seven organs including the liver and bone marrow; in another study, 15% of the dose remained 35 days after exposure.[3] Assuming a mother was breastfeeding, these levels would provide about 18 µg/L of milk consumed after the first few days following exposure to the drug. In addition, it would be sequestered for long periods in the infant as well. As this is a DNA-reactive agent, and it has a huge volume of distribution leading to prolonged tissue, plasma, and milk levels, mothers should be strongly advised not to breastfeed following its use.

T 1/2	23-215 h (Median 75 h)	MW	517 Da	PB	78%
Tmax		RID	1.82% - 12.14%	Vd	14-24.7 L/kg
Oral	Poor	M/P		pKa	9.78

Adult Concerns: Headache, fever, fatigue, alopecia, cardiotoxicity, nausea, vomiting, diarrhea, mucositis, anorexia, changes in liver and renal function, leukopenia, neutropenia, thrombocytopenia, pruritus, phlebitis, increased frequency of infection.

Adult Dose: 12 mg/m^2, frequency of administration varies by indication.

Pediatric Concerns: None reported at this time.

Infant Monitoring: Breastfeeding is not recommended.

Alternatives:

References:
1. Pharmaceutical manufacturers prescribing information.
2. Azuno Y, Kaku K, Fujita N, Okubo M, Kaneko T, Matsumoto N. Mitoxantrone and etoposide in breast milk. Am J Hematol. 1995 Feb;48(2):131-132.
3. Alberts DS, Peng YM, Leigh S, Davis TP, Woodward DL. Disposition of mitoxantrone in cancer patients. Cancer Res. 1985 Apr;45(4):1879-1884.

MIVACURIUM

Trade: Mivacrom, Mivacron

Category: Skeletal Muscle Relaxant

LRC: L3 - No Data-Probably Compatible

Mivacurium is a short-acting neuromuscular blocking agent used to relax skeletal muscles during surgery. Its duration is very short (6-9 minutes) and complete recovery generally occurs in 15-30 minutes.[1] No data are available on its transfer to breast milk. However, it has an exceedingly short plasma half-life, a rather large molecular weight, and probably poor to no oral absorption. It is very unlikely that it would be absorbed by a breastfeeding infant.

T 1/2	2 min	MW	1100 Da	PB	
Tmax		RID		Vd	147 L/kg
Oral	Poor	M/P		pKa	

Adult Concerns: Flushing, hypotension, weakness.

Adult Dose: 0.1-0.15 mg/kg every 15 minutes PRN.

Pediatric Concerns: None reported.

Infant Monitoring: Flushing, weakness.

Alternatives:

References:
1. Pharmaceutical manufacturers prescribing information.

MOCLOBEMIDE

Trade: Arima, Aurorix, Manerix

Category: Antidepressant, other

LRC: L4 - Limited Data-Possibly Hazardous

Moclobemide is a monoamine oxidase (MAO) inhibitor. Unlike older MAO inhibitors, moclobemide is a selective and reversible inhibitor of MAO-A isozyme and thus is not plagued with the dangerous side effects of the older MAO inhibitor families. It is an effective treatment for depression.[1]

In a study by Pons in six lactating women who received a single oral dose of 300 mg, the concentration of moclobemide (C$_{max}$) was highest at 3 hours after the dose and averaged 2.7 mg/L.[2] The average (AUC) milk concentration throughout the 12-hour period was 0.97 mg/L hour. The minimal levels of moclobemide found in milk are unlikely to produce untoward effects according to the authors. For adults, serotoninergic syndrome is unlikely, but possible when admixed with SSRI antidepressants, clomipramine, fluoxetine, etc.

T 1/2	1-2.2 h	MW	269 Da	PB	50%
Tmax	2 h	RID	3.4%	Vd	1-2 L/kg
Oral	80%	M/P	0.72	pKa	6.3

Adult Concerns: Dry mouth, headache, dizziness, tremor, sweating, insomnia, and constipation.

Adult Dose: 300-600 mg/day.

Pediatric Concerns: None reported via milk.

Infant Monitoring: Sedation or irritability, insomnia, not waking to feed/poor feeding, constipation, weight gain.

Alternatives:

References:
1. Fulton B, Benfield P. Moclobemide. An update of its pharmacological properties and therapeutic use. Drugs. 1996;52(3):450-474.
2. Pons G, Schoerlin MP, Tam YK, et al. Moclobemide excretion in human breast milk. Br J Clin Pharmacol. 1990;29(1):27-31.

MODAFINIL

Trade: Alertec, Provigil

Category: CNS Stimulant

LRC: L3 - No Data-Probably Compatible

Modafinil is a wakefulness-promoting agent used for the treatment of narcolepsy.[1] Modafinil is a 1:1 mixture of the R- and S-enantiomers. A similar drug, armodafinil, is the R-enantiomer of modafinil, has recently been studied.

In a recent study of armodafinil, a 27-year-old mother who was receiving 250 mg/day armodafinil, delivered an infant at 37 weeks gestational age.[2] Following a dose of 250 mg, the maximum concentration of armodafinil in milk was 2.3 µg/mL and was observed at 2 hours. This level decreased gradually over 24 hours. As the patient was at steady state, the authors observed a milk level of 0.43 µg/mL at zero hour. The calculated area under the curve was 28.96 mg.hr/L. The average infant dose was 0.181 mg/kg/day based on the assumption of the infant's daily intake of 150 mL/kg/day. The relative infant dose (RID) was estimated to be 5.3%. There were no reported complications in the breastfed infant.

T 1/2	15 h	MW	273 Da	PB	60%
Tmax	2-4 h	RID	5.3%	Vd	0.9 L/kg
Oral	Complete	M/P		pKa	8.84

Adult Concerns: May increase incidence of headache, chest pain, palpitations, dyspnea, and transient T-wave changes on ECG. CNS changes include delusions, auditory hallucinations and sleep deprivation. Diarrhea, dry mouth, nausea, and rhinitis have been reported.

Adult Dose: 200-400 mg up to twice daily.

Pediatric Concerns: None reported. Observe for reduced milk supply.

Infant Monitoring: Agitation, irritability, poor sleeping patterns, poor weight gain.

Alternatives:

References:
1. Pharmaceutical manufacturers prescribing information.
2. Aurora S, Aurora N, Datta P, Rewers-Felkins K, Baker T, Hale TW. Evaluating transfer of modafinil into human milk during lactation: a case report. J Clin Sleep Med. 2018 Dec;14(12):2087-2089. PMID: 30518447.

MOMETASONE

Trade: Asmanex, Elocon, Nasonex

Category: Corticosteroid

LRC: L3 - No Data-Probably Compatible

Mometasone is a corticosteroid primarily intended for intranasal and topical use. It is considered a medium-potency steroid, similar to betamethasone and triamcinolone. Following topical application to the skin, less than 0.7% is systemically absorbed over an 8 hour period.[1] It is extremely unlikely mometasone would be excreted in human milk in clinically relevant levels following topical or intranasal administration.

Asmanex is the inhaled version of this steroid for therapy in asthma.

T 1/2	5.8 h	MW	427.36 Da	PB	98-99%
Tmax		RID		Vd	
Oral	Poor	M/P		pKa	

Adult Concerns: Topically: irritation, burning, stinging, and dermal atrophy. Nasally: headache, pharyngitis, epistaxis, and cough.

Adult Dose: Apply topically 2-3 times daily.

Pediatric Concerns: None reported via milk.

Infant Monitoring: Feeding, growth, and weight gain.

Alternatives:

References:
1. Pharmaceutical manufacturers prescribing information.

MONOETHANOLAMINE OLEATE

Trade: Ethamolin

Category: Other

LRC: L3 - No Data-Probably Compatible

Monoethanolamine is a sclerosing agent to treat varicose veins.[1] When injected intravenously, monoethanolamine oleate acts primarily by irritation of the intimal endothelium of the vein and produces an inflammatory response. This results in fibrosis and possible occlusion of the vein. There are no data on its transfer to human milk, but following injection, this product disappears from the plasma within 5 minutes. Hence a brief waiting period of perhaps an hour would significantly reduce any exposure of the milk compartment to this drug. Pump and discard all milk during this hour.

T 1/2	<5 min	MW	344 Da	PB	
Tmax		RID		Vd	
Oral		M/P		pKa	9.4

Adult Concerns: Pulmonary toxicity, allergic reactions, pleural effusion, edema.

Adult Dose:

Pediatric Concerns:

Infant Monitoring:

Alternatives:

References:
1. Pharmaceutical manufacturers prescribing information.

MONTELUKAST SODIUM

Trade: Singulair

Category: Antiasthma

LRC: L4 - Limited Data-Possibly Hazardous

Montelukast is a leukotriene receptor inhibitor used in the treatment of asthma and allergic rhinitis.[1] Montelukast milk levels have been reported in seven exclusively breastfeeding women with infants 1.4-8.2 months of age (mean 4.3 months).[2] Milk levels were determined at 0, 1, 2, 4, 8, and 12 hours postdose. Montelukast levels in milk averaged 5.32 µg/L. The relative infant dose was 0.68% and the absolute infant dose was 0.79 µg/kg/day. There were no adverse events reported in these breastfed infants.

The FDA has just added a Black Box warning over the pediatric use of montelukast, which included side effects such as serious behavior and mood-related change, and suicide in users.

T 1/2	2.7-5.5 h	MW	608 Da	PB	99%
Tmax	2-4 h	RID	0.68%	Vd	0.15 L/kg
Oral	64%	M/P		pKa	

Adult Concerns: Headache, dizziness, fatigue, fever, nasal congestion, dental pain, cough, dyspepsia, gastroenteritis, changes in liver function, weakness. The FDA has just added a Black Box warning over the pediatric use of montelukast, which included side effects such as serious behavior and mood-related change, and suicide in users.

Adult Dose: 10 mg daily.

Pediatric Concerns: None reported via milk.

Infant Monitoring: Irritability, drowsiness, diarrhea. The FDA has just added a Black Box warning over the pediatric use of montelukast, which included side effects such as serious behavior and mood-related change, and suicide in users.

Alternatives: Zafirlukast(L3)

References:

1. Pharmaceutical manufacturers prescribing information.
2. Datta P, Rewers-Felkins K, Baker T, Hale TW. Transfer of montelukast into human milk during lactation. Breastfeed Med. 2017;12(1):54-57.

MORPHINE

Trade: Anamorph, Duramorph, Epimorph, Infumorph, Kapanol, M.O.S., MS Contin, Oramorph, Sevredol, Statex

Category: Analgesic

LRC: L3 - Limited Data-Probably Compatible

Morphine is a potent narcotic analgesic. In a group of five lactating women who required surgery at least 1 month after delivery, different routes of morphine were administered and breast milk samples were analyzed.[1] Two women received epidural morphine, one woman had two 4-mg epidural injections at 0 and 6 hours, and the other had one 4-mg injection at 0 hours. The highest morphine concentration in breast milk was following two 4-mg epidural doses; this concentration was 82 µg/L at 30 minutes post second dose. Three other women were given varying doses of IV/IM morphine; in this case the highest breast milk level was following 15 mg of IV/IM morphine, and this breast milk concentration was 500 µg/L. Although this makes the epidural RID 9.1% and the IV/IM RID 35%, the authors conclude that the maximum amount of morphine given to a nursing child after 4 mg of maternal epidural morphine would be 8 µg/100 mL. The maximum transfer of morphine after IV/IM administration was estimated to be about 50 µg/100mL of breast milk. The oral absorption of morphine is very poor and its first-pass metabolism is high; thus the authors estimate that the amount of drug that would actually reach the infant's systemic circulation would be 2-3 µg/100 mL and 10- 20 µg/100 mL via maternal epidural and IV/IM routes, respectively.

In another study of six women receiving IV morphine via patient-controlled analgesia (PCA) for 20-43 hours post-cesarean section, the concentration of morphine in breast milk ranged from 50-60 µg/L (estimated from graph).[2] The women in this study were given a 0.1-mg/kg IV loading dose of morphine after cord clamping, then PCAs were used with a 1-1.5 mg dose of morphine (6 min lockout period). Once the catheters were discontinued 5-30 mg of oral morphine was available every 2-3 hours as needed for pain. None of the infants in this study was neurobehaviorally delayed when assessed on day 3. Because of the poor oral bioavailability of morphine (26%) it is unlikely these levels would be clinically relevant in a stable breastfeeding infant.

A 2002 study also reviewed the use of IV morphine via patient-controlled analgesia for post-cesarean section pain.[3] In this study seven women were given morphine 4 mg IV followed by 1 mg every 10 min until their visual analog pain score was less than 3. The pump had a 1-mg incremental dose, 10 min lockout, and maximum of 20 mg/4 hours. Maternal blood and milk samples were taken at baseline, 12, 24, 36, and 48 hours. The levels of morphine and morphine-6-glucuronide (M6G) were variable in blood, and ranged from undetectable to 274 µg/L for morphine and undetectable to 559 µg/L for M6G in the first 48 hours. The milk levels of morphine and M6G were also variable, from undetectable to 48 µg/mL for morphine and undetectable to 1084 µg/mL for M6G. The study authors reported that an infant would receive 0.0048 mg/100 mL of milk of morphine and 0.1 mg/100 mL milk for M6G. No infants in this study were breastfed while their mothers received the morphine PCA.

However, data from Robieux suggests the levels transferred to the infant are higher.[4] In this study of a single patient, plasma levels in the breastfed infant were within therapeutic range (4 µg/L) although the infant showed no untoward signs or symptoms. However, this case was somewhat unique in that the mother received daily morphine (50 mg orally every 6 hours) during the third trimester for severe back pain. One week postpartum, the morphine was discontinued and then 5 days later reinstated due to withdrawal effects in the mother. The reported concentrations in foremilk and hindmilk were 100 µg/L and 10 µg/L respectively and the authors suggested that the dose to the infant would be 0.8-12% of the maternal oral dose (0.15 to 2.41 mg/day). Although this study suggests that the amount of morphine transferred in milk could be clinically relevant, the authors calculated the infant dose from the highest milk concentration and a milk intake of 150 mL/kg/day, thus the dose of morphine to the infant would have been substantially lower (53 µg/day). This study seems flawed because the plasma levels and the doses via milk just don't correlate. The reason why this infant showed no untoward effects, may be explained by the fact that it may have exhibited tolerance after in utero exposure, or the plasma levels assayed in this infant were in error.

Infants under 1 month of age have a prolonged elimination half-life and decreased clearance of morphine relative to older infants. The clearance of morphine and its elimination begins to approach adult values by 2 months of age. High doses over prolonged periods could lead to sedation and respiratory problems in newborn infants.

T 1/2	1.5-2 h	MW	285 Da	PB	35%
Tmax	0.5-1 h	RID	9.09% - 35%	Vd	2-5 L/kg
Oral	26%	M/P	1.1-3.6	pKa	8.1

Adult Concerns: Sedation, respiratory depression/apnea, nausea, vomiting, constipation, urinary retention, weakness.

Adult Dose: 10-30 mg oral or 5-15 mg IM or 2.5-5 mg IV every 4 h as needed.

Pediatric Concerns: None reported via milk at this time; sedation and apnea has been reported with codeine use (active metabolite is morphine).

Infant Monitoring: Sedation, slowed breathing rate/apnea, pallor, constipation, and appropriate weight gain.

Alternatives: Acetaminophen(L1), NSAIDs, Hydromorphone(L3), Hydrocodone(L3)

References:
1. Feilberg VL, Rosenborg D, Broen CC, Mogensen JV. Excretion of morphine in human breast milk. Acta Anaesthesiol Scand. 1989;33(5):426-428.
2. Wittels B, Scott DT, Sinatra RS. Exogenous opioids in human breast milk and acute neonatal neurobehavior: a preliminary study. Anesthesiology. 1990;73(5):864-869.
3. Baka NE, Bayoumeu F, Boutroy MJ, et al. Colostrum morphine concentrations during postcesarean intravenous patient-controlled analgesia. Anesth Analog. 2002;94:184-187.
4. Robieux I, Koren G, Vandenbergh H, Schneiderman J. Morphine excretion in breast milk and resultant exposure of a nursing infant. J Toxicol Clin Toxicol. 1990;28(3):365-370.

MOXIFLOXACIN

Trade: Avelox, Moxeza, Vigamox

Category: Antibiotic, Quinolone

LRC: L3 - No Data-Probably Compatible

Moxifloxacin is a quinolone antibiotic for use orally, intravenously, and in the eye.[1] It is a new-generation fluoroquinolone that exhibits improved activity against *Streptococcus pneumoniae* and other species. No data are available on its transfer to human milk so until we have data, one should opt for using ofloxacin or levofloxacin for which published data is available. Moxifloxacin is known to transfer to the milk of goats and sheep, and in studies concerning those two species, the drug entered the milk to a large degree. It was believed that high concentrations in the milk compartment were achieved by way of ion trapping.[2,3] Ophthalmic use of moxifloxacin in the form of eye drops is probably OK due to low systemic levels attained. However, caution is advised with its oral or intravenous use.

Because fluoroquinolones have limited safety data in pediatric and breastfeeding patients, use in lactation is not recommended if alternative therapies exist.[1]

T 1/2	9-16 h	MW	437 Da	PB	50%
Tmax	1-3 h	RID		Vd	1.7-3 L/kg
Oral	90%	M/P		pKa	6.4

Adult Concerns: Headache, dizziness, insomnia, QTc prolongation, nausea, vomiting, diarrhea, changes in bilirubin, hematological changes.

Adult Dose: 400 mg daily.

Pediatric Concerns: No reports available at this time.

Infant Monitoring: Vomiting, diarrhea, changes in gastrointestinal flora and rash.

Alternatives: Ofloxacin(L2), Levofloxacin(L2), norfloxacin, Ciprofloxacin(L3)

References:
1. Pharmaceutical manufacturers prescribing information.
2. Gouda A. Disposition kinetics of moxifloxacin in lactating ewes. Vet J. 2008 Nov;178(2):282-287.
3. Fernandez-Varon E, Villamayor L, Escudero E, Espuny A, Carceles CM. Pharmacokinetics and milk penetration of moxifloxacin after intravenous and subcutaneous administration to lactating goats. Vet J. 2006;172: 302–307.

MULTIVITAMIN

Trade:

Category: Vitamin

LRC: L3 - No Data-Probably Compatible

Basic multivitamins usually contain vitamins A, C, D, E, K, thiamine (B1), riboflavin (B2), niacin (B3), pantothenic acid (B5), pyridoxine (B6), biotin (B7), folic acid (B9), cobalamin (B12), and minerals such as calcium, zinc, potassium iodide, magnesium, manganese, molybdenum, borate(s), cupric, and iron. Other formulations may include other constituents such as lutein, lycopene, gamma-tocopherol, inositol, PABA, choline, trimethylgycine, betaine hydrochloride, lecithin etc.[1] See individual vitamins/minerals for more information. Prenatal vitamins are generally preferred for pregnant and breastfeeding mothers. Prenatal vitamins usually have reduced vitamin A and increased folic acid concentration.

Adult Concerns:

Adult Dose: Typically, one tablet daily.

Pediatric Concerns:

Infant Monitoring:

Alternatives:

References:
1. Dietary Reference Intakes (DRIs). Recommended Dietary Allowances and Adequate Intakes, Vitamins Food and Nutrition Board, Institute of Medicine, National Academies. Updated 2010. Accessed June 23, 2011.

MUMPS VIRUS VACCINE, LIVE

Trade: Mumpsvax

Category: Vaccine

LRC: L3 - No Data-Probably Compatible

Mumps vaccine is a live, attenuated vaccine indicated for the prevention of mumps illness. It is administered at 12-15 months of age, as part of the routine childhood immunization schedule. It is usually administered along with the measles and rubella vaccine, in the form of the MMR vaccine. There are currently no reports of transfer of the live mumps virus vaccine to breast milk. The American Advisory Committee on Immunization Practices has stated that breastfeeding women may be administered both the live and killed vaccines.[1] As a general rule, vaccines are often safe to use during breastfeeding.[2] The WHO considers mumps vaccine compatible with breastfeeding. Therefore, a lactating mother who has received the mumps vaccine may continue to breastfeed her child. Further, the antibodies present in human milk may provide some additional protection against mumps infection in the breastfed child. The breastfed infant should also receive the mumps vaccine as per the routine childhood immunization schedule.

Adult Concerns: Pain at injection site, fever, common cold, lymphadenopathy, rash. Serious side effects: anaphylaxis, encephalitis, thrombocytopenia, Steven-Johnson syndrome, febrile seizure.

Adult Dose: 0.5 mL subcutaneous injection.

Pediatric Concerns:

Infant Monitoring: Avoid in immunocompromised infants.

Alternatives:

References:
1. Anon. General recommendations on immunization; recommendations of the advisory committee on immunization practices (AICP) and the American academy of family physicians (AAFP). MMWR. 2002;51(RR02):1-36.
2. Schaefer C. Drugs During Pregnancy and Lactation. Amsterdam, The Netherlands: Elsevier Science B.V.; 2001.

MUPIROCIN OINTMENT

Trade: Bactroban

Category: Antibiotic, Other

LRC: L1 - No Data-Compatible

Mupirocin is a topical antibiotic used for impetigo, Group A beta-hemolytic streptococcal, staphylococcus, and *Streptococcal pyogenes* infections.[1] Mupirocin is only minimally absorbed following topical application. In one study, less than 0.3% of a topical dose was absorbed after 24 hours. Most remained adsorbed to the corneum layer of the skin. The drug is absorbed orally, but it is so rapidly metabolized that systemic levels are not sustained. It is quite safe for breastfeeding mothers.

T 1/2	17-36 min	MW	501 Da	PB	97%
Tmax		RID		Vd	
Oral	Complete	M/P		pKa	4.78

Adult Concerns: Rash, irritation.

Adult Dose: Apply sparingly.

Pediatric Concerns: None reported. Commonly used in pediatric patients.

Infant Monitoring: Rash.

Alternatives:

References:
1. Pharmaceutical manufacturers prescribing information.

MYCOPHENOLATE

Trade: CellCept

Category: Immune Suppressant

LRC: L5 - No Data-Hazardous

Mycophenolate is an immunosuppressive agent used to prevent rejection of allogenic transplants (kidney, heart, liver, intestine, limb, small bowel, etc.).[1] It is well absorbed and rapidly metabolized to MPA, the active metabolite. MPA glucuronide then subsequently enters the small intestine and is reabsorbed by enterohepatic recirculation. No data are available on its transfer to human milk. The average blood level is about 63.9 µg/mL (AUC) which is relatively high. Until we have data on human breast milk levels, this agent should be considered relatively hazardous.

T 1/2	17.9 h	MW	433 Da	PB	97%
Tmax	1 h	RID		Vd	4 L/kg
Oral	94% (parent)	M/P		pKa	9.76

Adult Concerns: Headache, insomnia, dizziness, hypertension, hypotension, tachycardia, dyspepsia, vomiting, diarrhea, constipation, anorexia, changes in liver and renal function, hyperglycemia, hypercholesterolemia, leukopenia, anemia, thrombocytopenia, edema, tremor, increased frequency of infection.

Adult Dose: 1-1.5 g orally twice daily.

Pediatric Concerns:

Infant Monitoring: Not recommended for use in lactation.

Alternatives: Cyclosporine(L3)

References:
1. Pharmaceutical manufacturers prescribing information.

N-ACETYLCYSTEINE

Trade: Acetadote, Mucomyst, Parvolex, NAC, Acetylcysteine

Category: Antidote

LRC: L3 - No Data-Probably Compatible

N-Acetylcysteine is commonly used in the treatment of acetaminophen overdoses, prevention of contrast-induced nephropathy and in diagnosis and treatment of certain respiratory conditions.[1] It is not known whether acetylcysteine enters human milk. Based on this medications small molecular weight and low volume of distribution, it most likely will enter milk; however, its oral bioavailability is low (10%-30%), thus the amount the infant will be exposed to should be low.

The manufacturer reports that N-acetylcysteine should be completely cleared by 30 hours after the last dose; however, when administering this medication to a breastfeeding woman for an acetaminophen overdose, breastfeeding may need to be withheld due to the amount of acetaminophen in milk, and potential risk of adverse effects to the infant. It may be best to resume breastfeeding once acetaminophen levels are undetectable.

Please note the half-life of N-Acetylcysteine can be increased as much as 80% in patients with severe liver damage.

T 1/2	5.6 h IV	MW	163.2 Da	PB	83%
Tmax	1-2 h Oral	RID		Vd	0.47 L/kg
Oral	10%-30%	M/P		pKa	

Adult Concerns: Anaphylaxis, drowsiness, flushing, tachycardia, cough, bronchospasm, stomatitis, nausea, vomiting, urticaria, rash, edema.

Adult Dose: Acetaminophen Overdose IV: 150 mg/kg loading dose over 1 hour, second dose 50 mg/kg over 4 hours, third dose 100 mg/kg over 16 hours.

Pediatric Concerns: No known adverse reactions from exposure in lactation at this time. In 2015, a small study looking at the benefits of N-acetylcysteine for neonatal neuroprotection in maternal chorioamnionitis reported no adverse events from administering this medication directly to the infant.[2] This medication was given to 12 preterm and term infants at birth (12.5-25 mg/kg/dose IV q12h x five doses).

Infant Monitoring: Drowsiness, vomiting.

Alternatives: None.

References:
1. Pharmaceutical manufacturers prescribing information.
2. Jenkins DD, Wiest DB, Mulvihill DM, et al. Fetal and neonatal effects of N-acetylcysteine when used for neuroprotection in maternal chorioamnionitis. J Pediatr. 2015;212:e1–e9. doi: 10.1016/j.jpeds.2015.09.076.

NABILONE

Trade: Cesamet

Category: Antiemetic

LRC: L3 - No Data-Probably Compatible

Nabilone is a synthetic oral cannabinoid, similar to marijuana. It affects the CNS and has an antiemetic effect due to its interactions with CB1 receptor, in the neural tissues.[1]

Nabilone has potential for abuse due to psychological dependence. Patients have reported changes in mood (euphoria, depression, anxiety, panic, paranoia, psychosis), decrease in cognition and memory, decrease in reality realizations (loss of sense of time and perception of objects, hallucinations), and decrease in drive and impulse. The drug's excretion into breast milk has not been determined. However, this drug is structurally similar to tetrahydrocannabinol, the active ingredient in marijuana, which is known to enter milk. For more information, see cannabis.

T 1/2	2 h (metabolites 35 h)	MW	372.55 Da	PB	Highly bound
Tmax	2 h	RID		Vd	12.5 L/kg
Oral	Complete absorbed by GI	M/P		pKa	

Adult Concerns: Vertigo, headache, drowsiness, dizziness, sleep disturbances, ataxia, dysphoria, visual disturbances, dry mouth, ataxia, hypotension, nausea, anorexia or increased appetite, weakness.

Adult Dose: 1-2 mg daily.

Pediatric Concerns: None reported via milk, but caution recommended.

Infant Monitoring: Sedation, changes in sleep, irritability, dry mouth, weight gain.

Alternatives:

References:
1. Pharmaceutical manufacturers prescribing information.

NABUMETONE

Trade: Relafen, Relifex

Category: NSAID

LRC: L3 - No Data-Probably Compatible

Nabumetone is a nonsteroidal anti-inflammatory agent for arthritic pain.[1] Immediately upon absorption, nabumetone is metabolized to the active metabolite. The parent drug is not detectable in plasma. It is not known if the nabumetone metabolite (6MNA) is secreted in human milk. It is known to be secreted into animal milk and has a very long half-life. Long half-life NSAIDS are not generally recommended in nursing mothers. Ketorolac and ibuprofen are ideal.

T 1/2	22-30 h	MW	228 Da	PB	99%
Tmax	2.5-4 h	RID		Vd	
Oral	38%	M/P		pKa	

Adult Concerns: Headache, dizziness, insomnia, nervousness, tinnitus, dry mouth, stomatitis, dyspepsia, nausea, vomiting, abdominal pain, diarrhea, constipation, gastrointestinal bleeding, changes in liver and renal function, edema.

Adult Dose: 500-1000 mg one to two times daily.

Pediatric Concerns: None reported via milk. Observe for gastrointestinal distress.

Infant Monitoring: Vomiting, diarrhea.

Alternatives: Ibuprofen(L1)

References:
1. Pharmaceutical manufacturers prescribing information.

NADOLOL

Trade: Corgard, Syn-Nadolol

Category: Beta Adrenergic Blocker

LRC: L4 - Limited Data-Possibly Hazardous

Nadolol is a long-acting beta adrenergic blocker used as an antihypertensive. It is secreted into breastmilk in moderately high concentrations. Following a maternal dose of 20 mg/day, breastmilk levels at 38 hours postpartum were 146 μg/L.[1] In another study of 12 women receiving 80 mg daily, the mean steady-state concentrations in milk were 357 μg/L.[2] The time to maximum concentration was 6 hours. The milk/serum ratio was reported to average 4.6. A 5 kg infant would receive 4%-7% of the maternal dose. The authors recommended caution with the use of this beta blocker in breastfeeding patients. Due to its long half-life and high milk/plasma ratio, this would not be a preferred beta blocker.

T 1/2	20-24 h	MW	309 Da	PB	30%
Tmax	2-4 h	RID	4.4% - 6.9%	Vd	1.5-3.6 L/kg
Oral	20-40%	M/P	4.6	pKa	9.7

Adult Concerns: Headache, dizziness, insomnia, depression, fatigue, chest pain, bradycardia, arrhythmias, hypotension, heart failure, wheezing, vomiting, constipation, myalgia.

Adult Dose: 40-80 mg daily.

Pediatric Concerns: None reported, but due to the high M/P ratio of 4.6, this product is not recommended.

Infant Monitoring: Drowsiness, lethargy, pallor, poor feeding, and weight gain.

Alternatives: Propranolol(L2), Metoprolol(L2), Labetalol(L2)

References:
1. Fox RE, Marx C, Stark AR. Neonatal effects of maternal nadolol therapy. Am J Obstet Gynecol. 1985;152(8):1045-1046.
2. Devlin RG, Duchin KL, Fleiss PM. Nadolol in human serum and breast milk. Br J Clin Pharmacol. 1981;12(3):393-396.

NAFCILLIN

Trade: Nafcil, Unipen

Category: Antibiotic, Penicillin

LRC: L1 - No Data-Compatible

Nafcillin is a penicillin antibiotic that is poorly and erratically absorbed orally.[1] The only formulations available are IV and IM. No data are available on concentration in milk, but it is likely small. Oral absorption in the infant would be minimal.

T 1/2	0.5-1.5 h	MW	436 Da	PB	70%-90%
Tmax	30-60 min (IM).	RID		Vd	
Oral	50%	M/P		pKa	

Adult Concerns: Neutropenia, hypokalemia, pseudomembranous colitis, allergic rash.

Adult Dose: 250-1000 mg every 4-6 hours.

Pediatric Concerns: None reported. Nafcillin is frequently used in infants.

Infant Monitoring: Vomiting, diarrhea, changes in gastrointestinal flora, and rash.

Alternatives:

References:
1. Pharmaceutical manufacturers prescribing information.

NAFTIFINE

Trade: Naftin

Category: Antifungal

LRC: L3 - No Data-Probably Compatible

Naftifine hydrochloride is a topical allylamine medication used to treat fungal infections. Naftin is not an imidazole. The drug has anti-inflammatory and antihistaminic effects along with antifungal effects. Some degree of vasoconstriction occurs if an occlusive dressing is used which often occurs with steroid medications. No reported systemic effects have been noted with naftifine, but there have been reports of some local skin irritation. The systemic absorption of naftifine cream is between 2.5% to 6%. It is unknown if naftifine is excreted into breast milk. Theoretically, the estimate of topical absorption between 2.5% to 3.4% could suggest that 0.3 µg/kg of the drug would be excreted into milk.[1-2]

T 1/2	2-3 days	MW	287 Da	PB	
Tmax		RID		Vd	
Oral		M/P		pKa	

Adult Concerns: Stinging, burning, dry skin, skin irritation, pruritus, erythema.

Adult Dose:

Pediatric Concerns:

Infant Monitoring:

Alternatives: Nystatin(L1), Fluconazole(L2)

References:
1. Gupta AK, Ryder JE, Cooper EA. Naftifine: a review. J Cutan Med Surg. 2008 Mar-Apr;12(2):51-58. Review.
2. Briggs G, Freeman R, Yaffe S. A Reference Guide to Fetal and Neonatal Risk: Drugs in Pregnancy and Lactation. 7th ed. vol 1. Philadelphia, PA: Lippincott Williams & WIlkins; 2005.

NALBUPHINE

Trade: Nubain

Category: Analgesic

LRC: L2 - Limited Data-Probably Compatible

Nalbuphine is a potent narcotic analgesic similar in potency to morphine. Nalbuphine is both an antagonist and agonist of opiate receptors and should not be mixed with other opiates due to interference with analgesia. In a group of 20 postpartum mothers who received a single 20 mg IM nalbuphine dose, the total amount of nalbuphine excreted into human milk during a 24 hour period averaged 2.3 μg, which is equivalent to 0.012% of the maternal dosage (not weight adjusted).[1] The mean milk/plasma ratio using the AUC was 1.2. According to the authors, an oral intake of 2.3 μg nalbuphine per day by an infant would not show any measurable plasma concentrations in the neonate.

In another study of 18 mothers who received 0.2 mg/kg every 4 hours over 2-3 days, the average concentration in breast milk was 42 μg/L, with a maximum of 61 μg/L. The reported infant dose was an average of 7 μg/kg/day, with a maximum of 9 μg/kg/day.[2] The authors estimate the RID = 0.59% of the weight-adjusted maternal daily dose and suggest breastfeeding is permissible.

T 1/2	5 h	MW	357 Da	PB	
Tmax	2-15 min (IV, IM)	RID	0.5%-0.8%	Vd	2.4-7.3 L/kg
Oral	16%	M/P	1.2	pKa	

Adult Concerns: Hypotension, sedation, withdrawal syndrome, respiratory depression.

Adult Dose: 10-20 mg every 3-6 hours PRN.

Pediatric Concerns: Levels in milk are low. No complications reported.

Infant Monitoring: Sedation, slowed breathing rate/apnea, pallor, constipation, and appropriate weight gain.

Alternatives:

References:
1. Wischnik A, Wetzelsberger N, Lucker PW. Elimination of nalbuphine in human milk. Arzneimittelforschung. 1988;38(10):1496-1498.
2. Jacqz-Aigrain E, Serreau R, Boissinot C, et al. Excretion of ketoprofen and nalbuphine in human milk during treatment of maternal pain after delivery. Ther Drug Monit. 2007 Dec;29(6):815-818.

NALDEMEDIN

Trade: Symproic

Category: Opioid Antagonist

LRC: L3 - No Data-Probably Compatible

Naldemedin is an opioid antagonist indicated for the treatment of opioid-induced constipation.[1] Naldemedin is an opioid antagonist with binding affinities for mu, delta, and kappa opioid receptors primarily in the periphery and gut. It does not transfer into the CNS, thus it functions as a peripherally-acting mu-opioid receptor antagonist in the GI tract, thus reducing constipation. Infants dependent on opioids may suffer withdrawal.

T 1/2	11 h	MW	742.84 Da	PB	95%
Tmax	0.75 h	RID		Vd	2.2 L/kg
Oral	Good	M/P		pKa	

Adult Concerns: Abdominal pain, diarrhea, nausea, gastroenteritis.

Adult Dose: 0.2 mg orally once daily.

Pediatric Concerns:

Infant Monitoring: Infants addicted to opioid may suffer withdrawal.

Alternatives:

References:
1. Pharmaceutical manufacturers prescribing information.

NALOXONE

Trade: Nalone, Narcan

Category: Opioid Antagonist

LRC: L3 - No Data-Probably Compatible

Naloxone is a narcotic antagonist that when administered occupies the opiate receptor site, or when opiates are present, displaces them from the active site. It is commonly used for the treatment of opiate associated itching, overdose, and now to prevent opiate abuse in patients undergoing withdrawal treatment.[1] Naloxone is poorly absorbed orally and plasma levels in adults are undetectable (<0.05 ng/mL) 2 hours after oral doses. Following intravenous use (0.4 mg), plasma naloxone levels averaged <0.084 µg/mL. Side effects are minimal except in narcotic-addicted patients. Its use in breastfeeding mothers would be unlikely to cause problems as its milk levels would likely be low and its oral absorption is minimal to nil.

When administering this medication to a breastfeeding woman for a narcotic overdose, breastfeeding may need to be withheld for 12-24 hours due to the amount of narcotic in milk, and potential risk of adverse effects (respiratory depression, sedation).

T 1/2	0.5-1.5 h	MW	364 Da	PB	weakly bound
Tmax		RID		Vd	2.6-2.8 L/kg
Oral	Nil	M/P		pKa	7.45, 9.88

Adult Concerns: Withdrawal effects in narcotic-addicted patients. Ventricular tachycardia and fibrillation, hypertension, headache, and rarely seizures have been reported.

Adult Dose: Highly variable but an initial dose of 0.4 to 2 mg intravenously is used for opiate withdrawal.

Pediatric Concerns: No breastfeeding studies are available. This product poses minimal risks to infants of women not addicted to opiates. However, even small amounts present in milk could accelerate slight withdrawal symptoms in infants of narcotic-addicted women.

Infant Monitoring: Tachycardia, withdrawal in chronic opiate-using moms/breastfed infants. When administering this medication to a breastfeeding woman for a narcotic overdose, breastfeeding may need to be withheld due to the amount of narcotic in milk, and potential risk of adverse effects (respiratory depression, sedation).

Alternatives:

References:

1. Pharmaceutical manufacturers prescribing information.

NALTREXONE

Trade: Nalorex, ReVia, Vivitrol

Category: Opioid Antagonist

LRC: L1 - Limited Data-Compatible

Naltrexone is a long acting narcotic antagonist similar in structure to naloxone. Orally absorbed, it has been clinically used in addicts to prevent the action of injected heroin. It occupies and competes with all opioid medications for the opiate receptor. When used in addicts, it can induce rapid and long-lasting withdrawal symptoms. Although the half-life appears brief, the duration of antagonism is long lasting (24-72 hours).[1-5] Naltrexone is quite lipid soluble, has a high pKa, and transfers into the brain easily (brain/plasma ratio = 0.81). It is readily metabolized to 6-beta-naltrexol (active) and two minor metabolites. The activity of naltrexone is believed to be mainly due to parent and 6-beta-naltrexol. The product Vivitrol is a sustained release injectable used once monthly.

In a study of one patient (60 kg) receiving 50 mg/day, the average concentration of naltrexone and 6-beta-naltrexol in milk were 1.7 and 46 µg/L.[6] The milk/plasma ratios of naltrexone and 6-beta-naltrexol were 1.9 and 3.4 respectively. The absolute infant dose was 0.26 and 6.86 µg/kg/day, respectively. The authors suggest the relative infant dose is 0.06 and 1% (range 0.86%-1.06%). The infant was reported to have achieved all expected milestones and showed no drug-related side effects. Naltrexone was undetectable in the infants' plasma and levels of 6-beta-naltrexol were only marginally detectable, at 1.1 µg/L.

T 1/2	4-13 h	MW	341 Da	PB	21%
Tmax	1 h	RID	1.4%	Vd	19 L/kg
Oral	96%	M/P	1.9 (3.4 metabolite)	pKa	7.9

Adult Concerns: Rapid opiate withdrawal symptoms. Dizziness, anorexia, rash, nausea, vomiting, and hepatocellular toxicity. Liver toxicity is common at doses approximately five times normal or less.

Adult Dose: 50-150 mg daily.

Pediatric Concerns: None reported in one case.

Infant Monitoring: Withdrawal in opiate-using moms/breastfed infants.

Alternatives:

References:

1. Bullingham RE, McQuay HJ, Moore RA. Clinical pharmacokinetics of narcotic agonist-antagonist drugs. Clin Pharmacokinet. 1983;8(4):332-343.
2. Crabtree BL. Review of naltrexone, a long-acting opiate antagonist. Clin Pharm. 1984;3(3):273-280.
3. Ludden TM, Malspeis L, Baggot JD, Sokoloski TD, Frank SG, Reuning RH. Tritiated naltrexone binding in plasma from several species and tissue distribution in mice. J Pharm Sci. 1976;65(5):712-716.
4. Verebey K, Volavka J, Mule SJ, Resnick RB. Naltrexone: disposition, metabolism, and effects after acute and chronic dosing. Clin Pharmacol Ther. 1976;20(3):315-328.
5. Wall ME, Brine DR, Perez-Reyes M. Metabolism and disposition of naltrexone in man after oral and intravenous administration. Drug Metab Dispos. 1981;9(4):369-375.
6. Chan CF, Page-Sharp M, Kristensen JH, O"Neil G, Ilett KF. Transfer of naltrexone and its metabolite 6,beta naltrexol into human milk. J Hum Lact. 2004;20(3):322-326.

NAPHAZOLINE

Trade: AK-Con, Albalon, Allersol, Clear Eyes, Naphcon, Ocu-Zoline, Privine, Vasoclear

Category: Decongestant

LRC: L3 - No Data-Probably Compatible

Naphazoline is used for relief of red eyes and as a nasal decongestant (spray). Over the counter products have low naphazoline concentrations (0.05%) such that systemic absorption is probably low, especially from ophthalmic preparations.[1] There are no adequate or well-controlled studies in breastfeeding women; however, the risk of side effects to a breastfed infant is probably minimal.

T 1/2		MW	210 Da	PB	
Tmax		RID		Vd	
Oral		M/P		pKa	

Adult Concerns: Irritation, blurred vision, increased intraocular pressure, dryness, rebound congestion.

Adult Dose: Instill one to two drops every 6 hours.

Pediatric Concerns:

Infant Monitoring:

Alternatives:

References:
1. Pharmaceutical manufacturers prescribing information.

NAPROXEN

Trade: Aleve, Anaprox, Naprosyn

Category: NSAID

LRC: L3 - Limited Data-Probably Compatible

Naproxen is a popular NSAID analgesic. It is known to transfer to breast milk, but not in quantities that would result in untoward effects in a breastfed infant. NSAIDs in general are usually compatible with breastfeeding. In a study done at steady state in one mother consuming 375 mg twice daily, milk levels ranged from 1.76-2.37 mg/L at 4 hours.[1,2] Total naproxen excretion in the infant's urine was only 0.26% of the maternal dose.

One case of prolonged bleeding, hemorrhage, and acute anemia has been reported in a 7-day-old infant.[4] The relative infant dose on a weight-adjusted maternal daily dose would probably be less than 3.3%. Other studies have confirmed naproxen's low transfer into breast milk, showing a 1% concentration compared to the mother's plasma levels.[4,5] Despite very low transfer into milk, there have been some reports of adverse effects in infants whose mothers were administered naproxen. In a study of 20 mothers given this medication, two reported drowsiness in their infants, while one reported vomiting.[6]

Although the amount of naproxen transferred via milk is minimal, one should use this with caution in nursing mothers because of its long half-life. Short term use postpartum or infrequent or occasional use would be compatible with breastfeeding. Ibuprofen levels in milk are exceedingly low, and it is a preferred alternative.

T 1/2	12-15 h	MW	230 Da	PB	99.7%
Tmax	2-4 h	RID	3.3%	Vd	0.09 L/kg
Oral	74%-99%	M/P	0.01	pKa	5

Adult Concerns: Headache, dizziness, hypertension, asthma exacerbations, dyspepsia, peptic ulcer, gastrointestinal bleed, nausea, abdominal pain, diarrhea, changes in liver and renal function, bruising, thrombocytopenia, anemia, edema.

Adult Dose: 250-500 mg twice daily.

Pediatric Concerns: One reported case of prolonged bleeding, hemorrhage, and acute anemia in a 7-day-old infant. Two reported cases of drowsiness in infants, and one case of vomiting.

Infant Monitoring: Vomiting, diarrhea. One reported case of prolonged bleeding, hemorrhage, and acute anemia in a 7-day-old infant. Two reported cases of drowsiness in infants, and one case of vomiting.

Alternatives: Ibuprofen(L1), Celecoxib(L2)

References:
1. Jamali F, Stevens DR. Naproxen excretion in milk and its uptake by the infant. Drug Intell Clin Pharm. 1983;17(12):910-911.
2. Jamali F, Tam YK, Stevens RD. Naproxen excretion in breast milk and its uptake by sucking infant. Drug Intell Clin Pharm. 1982;16:475 (Abstr).
3. Figalgo I. Anemia aguda, rectaorragia y hematuria asociadas a la ingestion de naproxen. Anales Espanoles de Pediatrica. 1989;30:317-319.
4. Pharmaceutical manufacturers prescribing information.
5. Brogden RN. Naproxen: A reveiw of its pharmacological properties and therapeutic efficacy and use. Drugs. 1975;9:326.
6. Ito S, Blajchman A, Stephenson M, et al. Prospective follow-up of adverse reactions in breast-fed infants exposed to maternal medication. Am J Obstet Gynecol. 1993;168(5):1393-1399.

NARATRIPTAN

Trade: Amerge, Naramig, Antimigraine

Category: Antimigraine

LRC: L3 - No Data-Probably Compatible

Naratriptan is a 5-HT1B/1D (serotonin) receptor agonist used to treat migraine headaches.[1] Activating these receptors is believed to constrict cranial blood vessels and block the release of pro-inflammatory neuropeptides from the trigeminal nerve. Although the oral bioavailability of naratriptan (74%) is slower during a migraine, the overall absorption is not affected. In addition, the oral bioavailability of naratriptan is five times greater than sumatriptan (14%).

No studies examining naratriptan secretion into human milk or adverse effects in infants have been published. Some transfer is likely based on this medication's small size and low protein binding; however, the clinical significance of this is unknown. Consider sumatriptan as the preferred alternative.

T 1/2	6-7 h	MW	372 Da	PB	29%
Tmax	2-5 h	RID		Vd	3.73 L/kg
Oral	74%	M/P		pKa	

Adult Concerns: Dizziness, drowsiness, flushing, hot tingling sensations, jaw pain, dry mouth, chest pain, arrhythmias, hypertension, nausea, vomiting, weakness, paresthesia.

Adult Dose: 1-2.5 mg orally, may repeat in 4 hours if needed.

Pediatric Concerns: None reported via milk.

Infant Monitoring: Drowsiness, vomiting, poor feeding.

Alternatives: Sumatriptan(L3), NSAIDs, Acetaminophen(L1)

References:
1. Pharmaceutical manufacturers prescribing information.

NATALIZUMAB

Trade: Tysabri

Category: Monoclonal Antibody

LRC: L3 - Limited Data-Probably Compatible

Natalizumab is a recombinant humanized IgG4k monoclonal antibody used to suppress immunity in patients with multiple sclerosis. In one study of a single 28 year old patient with an infant of 11.5 months, and who received 300 mg IV natalizumab every 4 weeks, levels in milk over a 50 day period were generally low but rising.[1] Following her first injection, levels were below the limit of quantification for the first 13 days, and began to appear in milk slowly. Levels in milk at 14 days were 0.333 µg/mL and rose to a peak of 0.49 µg/mL at day 28.

Following another injection at day 29, levels rose from 0.49 µg/mL to 2.83 µg/mL 20 days later following the second infusion. The relative infant dose at day 50 (assuming a clinical dose of 600 mg total) was 5.3%. This number is quite high and concerning. Using C_{avg}, the RID was 1.74% . However, while the oral absorption of this IgG4 molecule is probably low, we do not know with certainty how much would actually be absorbed in an infant. The infant reportedly was normal in growth and development and had no symptoms of infection.

In another study of two mothers with newborns, natalizumab was detected in the breast milk at a concentration of 1.89 mg/L in one mother. No natalizumab was detected in the milk of the second mother.[2]

Following IV doses of 300 mg natalizumab for the treatment of MS, natalizumab levels in milk ranged from a low of 2 µg/L to 412 µg/L.[3] The authors of this study suggest natalizumab levels in milk are gone 35 days post dose.

Normally, the transfer of native IgG or similar monoclonal antibodies to human milk is low even during the colostral period, and they are easily digested prior to absorption in the GI tract of a mature infant. In the case above, levels in milk apparently tend to rise over time (50 days). The mean average time to steady-state for natalizumab following intravenous injection is reported to be 24 weeks following two injections (every 4 weeks). Assuming this is correct, levels in milk may continue to rise over time and may reach significantly higher levels in milk at steady state. This will require further study.

Although the molecular weight of this medication is very large and the amount in breast milk is low, there are no long-term data concerning the safety of using immune modulating medications in breastfeeding mothers. Further, there are current data that suggest that some monoclonal antibody drugs do transfer to milk, and perhaps the breast-fed infant. Therefore, some caution is recommended, and each woman should understand the benefits and risk of using this type of medication in lactation.

T 1/2	11 days	MW	149,000 Da	PB	
Tmax		RID	5.3%	Vd	0.08 L/kg
Oral	Nil	M/P		pKa	

Adult Concerns: Hypersensitivity reactions have been reported which include urticaria, dizziness, fever, rash, pruritus, nausea, flushing, hypotension, dyspnea, and chest pain.

Adult Dose: 300 mg IV monthly.

Pediatric Concerns: No data are available at this time.

Infant Monitoring: Fever, frequent infections, poor feeding/poor weight gain.

Alternatives:

References:
1. Baker T, Cooper SD, Kessler L, Hale T. Transfer of natalizumab into breast milk in a mother with multiple sclerosis. J Hum Lact. 2015 May;31(2):233-236.
2. Hainke U, Sehr T, Eisele JC, et al. Natalizumab: passage into breast milk and neonatal blood. Mult Scler. 2015;23:690. Abstract EP1324.
3. Proschmann U, Thomas K, Thiel S, Hellwig K, Ziemssen T. Natalizumab during pregnancy and lactation. Mult Scler. 2018 Oct;24(12):1627-1634. PubMed PMID: 28857686.

NATEGLINIDE

Trade: Starlix

Category: Antidiabetic, other

LRC: L3 - No Data-Probably Compatible

Nateglinide is an oral antidiabetic agent used to treat type II diabetes.[1] It lowers blood glucose by stimulating the release of insulin from the pancreas; this medication depends on functioning beta cells for its effect and is glucose dependent (effect diminishes with low blood glucose).

It is not known if nateglinide is excreted in human milk.[1] Studies in rats have shown that nateglinide is excreted in milk although no human data are available. Clinicians should watch infant for hypoglycemia.

T 1/2	1.5 h	MW	317.43 Da	PB	98%
Tmax	1 h	RID		Vd	0.14 L/kg
Oral	73%	M/P		pKa	

Adult Concerns: Hypoglycemia (dizziness, fatigue, palpitations, nausea, increased appetite, sweating, tremor, weakness), diarrhea, changes in liver function.

Adult Dose: 60 mg-120 mg orally TID prior to meals.

Pediatric Concerns: There are no pediatric efficacy or safety data at this time.

Infant Monitoring: Diarrhea and signs of hypoglycemia - drowsiness, lethargy, pallor, sweating, tremor.

Alternatives:

References:
1. Pharmaceutical manufacturers prescribing information.

NEBIVOLOL

Trade: Bystolic

Category: Beta Adrenergic Blocker

LRC: L3 - No Data-Probably Compatible

Nebivolol is a beta-1 selective antagonist used for the treatment of hypertension. No data are available on the transfer of this drug into human milk; however, an overview of the kinetics of this drug suggests that nebivolol will probably produce minimal milk levels. Because of the potential for beta blockers to produce serious adverse reactions in nursing infants, especially bradycardia, nebivolol is not recommended during nursing at this time.

It should be noted that nebivolol is metabolized through the CYP 2D6 pathway; the oral bioavailability is dependent on CYP 2D6 and averages 12% in extensive metabolizers and about 96% in slow metabolizers.[1] When at steady state and taking the same dose, the peak plasma concentrations of unchanged drug was about 23 times higher in the poor metabolizers. In addition, when unchanged drug and active metabolites were considered, the difference in peak plasma concentrations was 1.3 to 1.4 fold. Due to this variation in CYP 2D6 metabolism, the dose of nebivolol should always be adjusted to the individual requirements of the patient (poor metabolizers may require lower doses).

T 1/2	12-19 h	MW	442 Da	PB	98%
Tmax	1.5-4 h	RID		Vd	8-12 L/kg
Oral	12%-96%	M/P		pKa	

Adult Concerns: Headache, dizziness, insomnia, depression, fatigue, chest pain, bradycardia, hypotension, heart failure, wheezing, vomiting, diarrhea, changes in liver and renal function, myalgia.

Adult Dose: 5-40 mg daily.

Pediatric Concerns: Observe infant for sedation, changes in breathing, bradycardia, jitteriness, and hypoglycemia.

Infant Monitoring: Drowsiness, lethargy, pallor, poor feeding and weight gain. Observe infant for sedation, changes in breathing, bradycardia, jitteriness, and hypoglycemia.

Alternatives: Metoprolol(L2), Labetalol(L2)

References:
1. Pharmaceutical manufacturers prescribing information.

NEFAZODONE HCL

Trade: Dutonin, Serzone

Category: Antidepressant, other

LRC: L4 - Limited Data-Possibly Hazardous

Nefazodone is an antidepressant similar to trazodone but structurally dissimilar from the other serotonin reuptake inhibitors. It is rapidly metabolized to three partially active metabolites that have significantly longer half-lives (1.5 to 18 hours).[1]

In a study of one patient receiving 200 mg in the morning and 100 mg at night, the infant at 9 weeks of age (2.1 kg), was admitted for drowsiness, lethargy, failure to thrive, and poor temperature control.[2] The infant was born premature at 27 weeks. The maximum milk concentration of nefazodone was 358 µg/L while the maternal plasma C_{max} was 1270 µg/L. The concentration of the metabolites was reported to be 83 µg/L for triazoledione, 32 µg/L for HO-Nefazodone, and 18 µg/L for m-Chlorophenylpiperazine. The authors estimate the relative infant dose to be 0.45 % of the weight-adjusted maternal dose. The AUC milk/plasma ratio ranged from 0.02 to 0.27.

Unfortunately, no infant plasma samples were taken for analysis. Dodd recently reported a M/P ratio of only 0.1 for nefazodone in a patient receiving 200 mg twice daily.[3] This is approximately one-third of the M/P ratio (0.27) reported by Yapp. However, the Yapp study used AUC data over many points and is probably a more accurate reflection of nefazodone transfer into milk during the day. This medication should probably not be used in breastfeeding mothers with young infants, premature infants, infants subject to apnea, or other weakened infants.

T 1/2	1-4 h	MW	507 Da	PB	>99%
Tmax	1 h	RID	1.2%	Vd	0.9 L/kg
Oral	20%	M/P	0.1-0.27	pKa	6.6

Adult Concerns: Weakness, hypotension, somnolence, dizziness, dry mouth, constipation, nausea, headache.

Adult Dose: 150-300 mg twice daily.

Pediatric Concerns: Drowsiness, lethargy, failure to thrive, and poor temperature control in one infant.

Infant Monitoring: Sedation or irritability, not waking to feed/poor feeding, and weight gain.

Alternatives: SSRIs, Trazodone(L2)

References:

1. Pharmaceutical manufacturers prescribing information.
2. Yapp P, Ilett KF, Kristensen JH, Hackett LP, Paech MJ, Rampono J. Drowsiness and poor feeding in a breast-fed infant: association with nefazodone and its metabolites. Ann Pharmacother. 2000;34(11):1269-1272.
3. Dodd S, Buist A, Burrows GD, Maguire KP, Norman TR. Determination of nefazodone and its pharmacologically active metabolites in human blood plasma and breast milk by high-performance liquid chromatography. J Chromatogr B Biomed Sci Appl. 1999;730(2):249-255.

NEFOPAM

Trade: Acupan

Category: Analgesic

LRC: L3 - Limited Data-Probably Compatible

Nefopam hydrochloride is a non-narcotic analgesic used for postoperative and musculoskeletal pain. The drug also works well for episiotomy pain.[1] The drug has also been used for shivering and intractable hiccoughs. Nefopam is structurally related to diphenhydramine and may be used as an alternative pain control method in patients who are opioid dependent. Nefopam does not appear to cause respiratory depression and is one-third as potent as morphine. Nefopam is well absorbed orally and extensively metabolized by the liver. The drug is excreted largely by the kidney. In a study of five breastfeeding women who were treated with 60 mg nefopam every 4 hours for 48 hours after delivery, levels in milk were similar to plasma (M/P ratio = 1.2). Levels in milk ranged from 5.8 to 298.7 ng/mL with a mean milk level of 90.4 µg/L, and a relative infant dose of 2.6%.[2]

T 1/2	3-8 h	MW	289.8 Da	PB	71%-76 %
Tmax	Oral 1-3 h; IM 1.5 h	RID	2.6%	Vd	
Oral	Well absorbed	M/P	1.2	pKa	9.36

Adult Concerns: Urine retention, headache, insomnia, tachycardia, diaphoresis, lightheadedness, rash, nausea, vomiting, dry mouth, and drowsiness.

Adult Dose: 60 mg every 4 hours.

Pediatric Concerns:

Infant Monitoring: Sedation, urine retention.

Alternatives: Morphine(L3), Hydrocodone(L3), Oxycodone(L3)

References:

1. Bloomfield SS, Barden TP, Mitchell J. Nefopam and propoxyphene in episiotomy pain. Clin Pharmacol Ther. 1980 Apr;27(4):502-507.
2. Liu DT, Savage JM, Donnell D. Nefopam excretion in human milk. Br J Clin Pharmacol. 1987 Jan;23(1):99-101.

NEISSERIA GONORRHEAE

Trade: Gonococcal infection, Gonorrhea

Category: Infectious Disease

LRC: L4 - No Data-Possibly Hazardous

Neisseria gonorrhoeae is a gram negative bacteria, known to cause the sexually transmitted disease gonorrhea. Mode of transmission is mainly through exposure to infected genital secretions during sexual intercourse. Infection in neonates may occur due to exposure to infected secretions during vaginal delivery. Gonorrhea in women may cause infertility. In neonates, gonococcal infection is manifested in the form of an eye infection called gonococcal conjunctivitis or ophthalmia neonatorum. It is characterized by thick purulent conjunctival discharge. As a prophylactic measure, all neonates are routinely administered 1% tetracycline ophthalmic ointment or 0.5% erythromycin ophthalmic ointment in each eye, soon after birth. Neonates who are born to mothers with known gonococcal infection are also administered a single dose of ceftriaxone. Infants who are breastfeeding from an infected mother should be tested for infection and treated accordingly.

There no studies reporting the transfer of *Neisseria gonorrhoeae* to breast milk, although it should be expected. When a lactating mother has been diagnosed with gonorrhea, treatment should be instituted immediately with a single intramuscular dose of ceftriaxone 125 mg. Additionally, the mother should receive a single dose of one-gram azithromycin. Since the mode of transmission is mainly through contact with infected secretions, it is advisable that the mother take all hygienic and sanitary precautions to avoid transmission to the infant.

Adult Concerns: Gonococcal infection in adults or adolescents is usually manifested by thick, purulent discharge from the cervix or urethra. Besides this burning and pain during urination, skin rash, and arthritis are some of the other symptoms. Gonorrhea in women may cause infertility.

Adult Dose:

Pediatric Concerns: In neonates, Gonococcal infection is manifested in the form of an eye infection called gonococcal conjunctivitis or ophthalmia neonatorum. It is characterized by thick purulent conjunctival discharge.

Infant Monitoring: Highly infectious via milk.

Alternatives:

References:

NEOMYCIN

Trade: Neo-Fradin

Category: Antibiotic, Aminoglycoside

LRC: L3 - No Data-Probably Compatible

Neomycin is an antibiotic commonly used for topical treatment of bacterial infections.[1] It is also used in preparation for bowel surgery. There are no adequate and well-controlled studies or case reports in breastfeeding women. However, contact dermatitis is a consistent problem (10% of patients) and this product should probably not be used on breastfeeding mothers, particularly on sore nipples.

T 1/2	2-3 h (12 h at high doses)	MW	614.6 Da	PB	0%-30%
Tmax	1-4 h (oral)	RID		Vd	0.36 L/kg
Oral	0.6%-0.8%	M/P		pKa	12.29

Adult Concerns: Rash, pruritus, nausea, vomiting, nephrotoxicity, ototoxicity, respiratory depression.

Adult Dose:

Pediatric Concerns:

Infant Monitoring: Vomiting, diarrhea, changes in gastrointestinal flora, and rash.

Alternatives:

References:
1. Pharmaceutical manufacturers prescribing information.

NEPAFENAC

Trade: Nevanac

Category: NSAID

LRC: L3 - No Data-Probably Compatible

Nepafenac is a nonsteroidal anti-inflammatory that is used ophthalmically. It is primarily used to treat the inflammation associated with extraction of cataracts and the accompanying pain. Nepafenac has been shown to be excreted in milk during animal studies, however it is not known if it is excreted in human milk.[1] Levels in human plasma are exceedingly low and levels once determined in milk, will be even lower.

T 1/2	0.7-1.1 h	MW	254.28 Da	PB	82.7%-84.3%
Tmax	0.15-0.35 h	RID		Vd	
Oral	6%	M/P		pKa	15.82

Adult Concerns: Vitreous detachment, conjunctival edema, dry eye, foreign body sensation, itching of eye, sticky sensation, photophobia, ocular hyperemia, photophobia, raised intraocular pressure, reduced visual acuity, capsular opacity, headache, hypertension, sinusitis, nausea.

Adult Dose: One drop three times daily.

Pediatric Concerns:

Infant Monitoring: Vomiting, diarrhea.

Alternatives:

References:
1. Pharmaceutical manufacturers prescribing information.

NESIRITIDE

Trade: Natrecor

Category: Natriuretic Peptide

LRC: L3 - No Data-Probably Compatible

Nesiritide is a recombinant form of human B-type natriuretic peptide. It is used to treat acutely decompensated congestive heart failure.[1] No studies have been performed on the concentrations of nesiritide in human milk. However, due to the large molecular weight of this peptide (3464 Da), it is unlikely that it would pass into the milk compartment or be orally bioavailable to a breastfeeding infant.

T 1/2	18 min	MW	3464 Da	PB	
Tmax	1 h	RID		Vd	0.19 L/kg
Oral		M/P		pKa	

Adult Concerns: Hypotension, increased serum creatinine, ventricular tachycardia, nausea, and headache.

Adult Dose: 0.01 μg/kg/minute.

Pediatric Concerns: No data are available. It is unlikely to enter milk.

Infant Monitoring:

Alternatives:

References:
1. Pharmaceutical manufacturers prescribing information.

NETILMICIN

Trade: Netromycin, Nettilin

Category: Antibiotic, Aminoglycoside

LRC: L3 - No Data-Probably Compatible

Netilmicin is a typical aminoglycoside antibiotic. Poor oral absorption limits its use to IM and IV administration although some studies suggest significant oral absorption in infancy.[1,2] Only small levels are believed to be secreted into human milk although no reports exist.

T 1/2	2-2.5 h	MW	476 Da	PB	<10%
Tmax	30-60 min (IM)	RID		Vd	
Oral	Negligible	M/P		pKa	

Adult Concerns: Changes in renal function, hearing loss, changes in gastrointestinal flora.

Adult Dose: 1.3-2.2 mg/kg every 8 hours.

Pediatric Concerns: None reported but observe for gastrointestinal symptoms such as diarrhea.

Infant Monitoring: Vomiting, diarrhea, changes in gastrointestinal flora, and rash.

Alternatives:

References:
1. Pharmaceutical manufacturers prescribing information.
2. McEvoy GE, ed. AFHS Drug Information. New York, NY: McGraw-Hill; 2003.

NEUROMUSCULAR BLOCKING AGENTS

Trade: Anectine, Arduan, Mivacron, Norcuron, Nuromax, Pavulon, Raplon, Tracrium, Zemuron

Category: Neuromuscular Blocker

LRC: L3 - No Data-Probably Compatible

Neuromuscular blocking agents are similar to curare and are primarily used to relax skeletal muscle during surgery.[1,2] They typically have a three phase elimination curve. The first phase elimination is rapid, averaging <5 minutes. The second phase half-life ranges from 7-40 minutes, and a third phase half-life is 2-3 hours. It is not known if any of these agents penetrate into human milk, but it is very unlikely. First they are large in molecular weight, have highly polar structures, and are virtually excluded from most cells. Oral bioavailability is not reported, but it is likely small to nil. A brief waiting period (few hours) after surgery will eliminate most risks associated with the use of these products.

T 1/2	Variable	MW	Large	PB	
Tmax		RID		Vd	
Oral		M/P		pKa	

Adult Concerns: Prolonged apnea, hypotension, arrhythmias, residual muscle weakness, allergic reactions. Histamine-related events include flushing, erythema, pruritus, urticaria, wheezing, and bronchospasm.

Adult Dose: Variable depending on individual agent.

Pediatric Concerns: None reported via milk. They are unlikely to penetrate into milk in significant levels.

Infant Monitoring: Weakness, apnea; a brief waiting period (few hours) after surgery should eliminate most risks.

Alternatives:

References:
1. Pharmaceutical manufacturers prescribing information.
2. Baselt RC. Disposition of Toxic Drugs and Chemicals in Man. Foster City, CA: Chemical Toxicology Institute; 2000.

NEVIRAPINE

Trade: Viramune

Category: Antiviral

LRC: L5 - Limited Data-Hazardous if Maternal HIV Infection

Nevirapine selectively inhibits reverse transcriptase activity and replication of HIV. It is commonly used concomitantly with other antiretroviral drugs to treat HIV.[1] In a study of 20 women receiving 200 mg twice daily at steady state, median nevirapine levels in maternal serum at 4 hours postdose, breast milk, and infant serum were 9534 ng/mL, 6795 ng/mL and 971 ng/mL, respectively.[2] The milk/serum ratio was 0.67. The median infant serum concentration of nevirapine (971 ng/mL) was at least 40 times the 50% inhibitory concentration and similar to peak concentrations after a single 2 mg/kg dose of nevirapine. The authors concluded that HIV-1 inhibitory concentrations of nevirapine are achieved in breastfed infants of mothers receiving nevirapine, exposing infants to the potential for both the beneficial as well as the adverse effects of nevirapine ingestion. Thus far, no untoward effects have been noted in the few infants studied.

In 2007, 40 women were given zidovudine, lamivudine, and nevirapine from 28 weeks gestational age to 1 month postpartum to evaluate the potential efficacy of using these medications to prevent the transmission of perinatal HIV.[3] All women in this study were instructed not to breastfeed their infants. Milk samples were collected five times a day from delivery to day 7 postpartum, blood samples were collected on day 3 (time 0) and day 7 (time 7); the samples were used to quantify the amount of HIV RNA and DNA in milk and the concentrations of each medication in maternal plasma and milk. The mean concentrations of nevirapine at time 0 and 7 in maternal plasma were 3100 µg/L and 3900 µg/L. The mean concentrations of nevirapine at time 0 and 7 in milk were 2300 µg/L and

2200 µg/L. The milk plasma ratios were 0.8 and 0.6 at time 0 and 7, respectively. We used the milk levels from time 0 and 7 to estimate the relative infant dose for nevirapine to range from 5.7%-6.04%.

In 2009, a study was published that assessed 67 women taking combination antiretroviral therapy from 34 to 36 weeks through 6 months postpartum.[4] These women took 1 combivir tablet twice daily (lamivudine 150 mg + zidovudine 300 mg/tab) with nevirapine 200 mg x 14 days then 200 mg twice a day. Nevirapine milk samples were taken within 24 hours of delivery, then at weeks 2, 6, 14, and 24 postpartum. The median values for each parameter were estimated across all study visits, the maternal concentration was 6087 ng/mL (4895 to 7518 ng/mL), the milk concentration was 4546 ng/mL (3480 to 5715 ng/mL) and the milk/plasma ratio was 0.75. The authors of this study estimated that an infant would receive about 682 µg/kg/day of nevirapine (15% of the 4 mg/kg dose used in infants) if they consumed about 150 mL/kg/day of breast milk. We calculated the relative infant dose to be 11.9%, which is equivalent to the infant dose estimated by the authors of this study. The authors also noted that the median infants nevirapine plasma concentration from weeks 2-14 was 896.9 ng/mL, which is above the IC50 for HIV (17 ng/mL) but below the recommended trough plasma concentration of 3000 ng/mL. The long-term effects and risk of resistance from these levels in infants who become infected with HIV are unknown at this time.

Infant nevirapine prophylaxis in the first 6 weeks of life is known to decrease breastfeeding HIV transmission, but the efficacy of continuation of such therapy is not known. Recently, a study was reported of the efficacy and safety of extended administration of nevirapine in a breastfeeding infant of an HIV-infected mother.[5] In this study, 1527 breastfed infants of HIV-infected mothers received 10 mg nevirapine daily for first 6 weeks of life. All the enrolled infants were HIV-negative at the time of initiation of the study. These infants were then randomized into two groups - those receiving nevirapine and those receiving placebo. All the infants were exclusively breastfed during the course of the study. The infants in the nevirapine group were administered age-appropriate increasing doses of nevirapine ranging from 10 mg daily up to 28 mg daily until 6 months of age or until cessation of breastfeeding, whichever occurred earlier. It was found that at 6 months of age, the rate of HIV-1 transmission in the nevirapine group was 1.1% as compared to 2.4% in the control group. This implies a 54% reduction in the rate of mother-to-infant trans-mission of HIV via breast milk. This extended nevirapine regimen was documented to be particularly effective in those mothers with CD4 cell counts of more than 350, who normally do not require antiretroviral therapy for their own health. In such mothers, there was a four-fold reduction in the rate of HIV-1 transmission via breast milk as compared to the control group, making the rate in mothers who are not on antiretroviral therapy equivalent to those who are on antiretroviral therapy. Further, it was revealed that the rate of breastfeeding HIV transmission returns to pretreatment levels once infant nevirapine prophylaxis is stopped. In this studies conclusion, it indicated that infants of mothers who do not require antiretroviral therapy for their own health may continue to exclusively breastfeed for at least 6 months of age, if the infants receive nevirapine prophylaxis during the course of breastfeeding. This could allow the infant to receive the benefits of breast milk while simultaneously avoiding the risks of HIV transmission; however, at this time it is still not recommended that women who have HIV breastfeed.

Another study which evaluated the safety of maternal antiretrovirals for prophylaxis against transmission to the infant during lactation also reported the milk levels of nevirapine (n = 181 samples).[6] This study tested maternal serum and breast milk on the day of delivery and at months 1, 3, and 6 postpartum. Infant levels were also taken at months 1, 3 and 6 of age. The median drug concentrations of nevirapine in maternal serum, breast milk and the infant were 5261 ng/mL (4066-6882 ng/mL), 2901 ng/mL (2097-4684 ng/mL) and 809 ng/mL (535-1061 ng/mL), respectively. The milk to plasma ratio was 0.59. The relative infant dose that we calculated using the maternal dose of 200 mg twice a day and median milk level was 7.6%. In this study, two infants acquired HIV, one at 1 month of age (suggesting in utero transmission) and the other at 3 months of age (from breast milk exposure). Both of these infants acquired NNRTI resistance at 6 months of age and both of these infants were noted to have significant serum levels of nevirapine. This study also reported infant adverse events (e.g., pneumonia, diarrhea, changes in liver function, neutropenia, thrombocytopenia), but was unable to determine which medication caused the effects based on drug levels, please see study for adverse event details.

A publication in 2013, followed women taking antivirals in pregnancy and breastfeeding and studied maternal milk samples 30 days postpartum.[7] Fifteen breast milk samples were available, the median milk concentration was 1.83 µg/mL. In addition, the median milk to plasma ratio was 0.27. The relative infant dose calculated using this median milk sample and a maternal dose of nevirapine 200 mg bid was 4.8%.

In a more recent study, the median(range) of nevirapine in maternal plasma, milk, and infant plasma were 5170 ng/mL (1,320-15,600), 4830 ng/mL (1,360-16,300) and 660 ng/mL (104-3090), respectively.[8] The authors estimated the average and maximum NVP doses from breast milk were 704 µg/kg/day (331-1700) and 888 µg/kg/day (462-2270), respectively. The author estimated the RID dose as 13.8%.

Note: This medication is an L5 to highlight the contraindication of breastfeeding when the mother is known to be infected with HIV, this medication is not an L5 based on its risk to the infant in breast milk. The Centers for Disease Control and Prevention recommend that HIV infected mothers do not breastfeed their infants to avoid postnatal transmission of HIV.

T 1/2	25-30 h	MW	266 Da	PB	60%
Tmax	4 h	RID	4.8%-17.84%	Vd	1.4 L/kg
Oral	90%	M/P	0.67-0.95	pKa	

Adult Concerns: Headache, fatigue, nausea, abdominal pain, diarrhea, changes in liver function, increases in cholesterol, neutropenia, myalgia, rash.

Adult Dose: 200 mg twice daily but highly variable.

Pediatric Concerns: Levels in milk are moderate and levels in infant plasma are supratherapeutic. In one study, two infants acquired HIV, one at 1 month of age (suggesting in utero transmission) and the other at 3 months of age (breast milk exposure).[6] Both of these infants acquired NNRTI resistance at 6 months of age and both of these infants were noted to have significant serum levels of nevirapine. Please see study for adverse event details.

Infant Monitoring: Breastfeeding is not recommended in mothers who have HIV.

Alternatives:

References:

1. Pharmaceutical manufacturer prescribing information.
2. Shapiro RL, Holland DT, Capparelli E, et al. Antiretroviral concentrations in breast-feeding infants of women in Botswana receiving antiretroviral treatment. J Infect Dis. 2005 Sep;192(5):720-727.
3. Giuliano M, Guidotti G, Andreotti M, et al. Triple antiviral prophylaxis administered during pregnancy and after delivery significantly reduces breast milk viral load. J Acquir Immune Defic Syndr. 2007;44:286-291.
4. Mirochnick M, Thomas T, Capparelli E, et al. Antiretroviral concentrations in breast-feeding infants of mothers receiving highly active antiretroviral therapy. Antimicrob Agents Chemother. 2009;53(3):1170-1176.
5. Coovadia HM, Brown ER, Fowler MG, et al. Efficacy and safety of an extended nevirapine regimen in infant children of breastfeeding mothers with HIV-1 infection for prevention of postnatal HIV-1 transmission (HPTN 046): a randomised, double-blind, placebo-controlled trial. Lancet. 2011 Dec;379(9812):221-228.
6. Palombi L, Pirillo MF, Andreotti M, et al. Antiretroviral prophylaxis for breastfeeding transmission in Malawi: drug concentrations, virological efficacy and safety. Antivir Ther. 2012;17:1511-1519.
7. Shapiro RL, Rossi S, Ogwu A, et al. Therapeutic levels of lopinavir in late pregnancy and abacavir passage into breast milk in the Mma Bana Study, Botswana. Antivir Ther. 2013;18(4):585-590.
8. Olagunju A, Khoo S, Owen A. Pharmacogenetics of nevirapine excretion into breast milk and infants' exposure through breast milk versus postexposure prophylaxis. Pharmacogenomics. 2016 Jun;17(8):891-906.

NIACIN

Trade: Niacin-Time, Niacor, Niaspan FCT, Niodan, Slo-Niacin

Category: Vitamin

LRC: L3 - No Data-Probably Compatible

Niacin, also known as vitamin B-3, is an essential dietary substance, and is present in a wide variety of foods and supplements. It is a component of two coenzyme which function in oxidation-reduction reactions essential for tissue respiration. It is also used to reduce cholesterol and other fatty substances in the blood in high doses (2-6 g/day). Pellagra is a disease caused by niacin deficiency, and most often arises due to inadequate dietary intake. The recommended daily allowance for niacin is 14 mg/day for females, with an upper limit of 35 mg/day. In its extended release formulation, niacin has been excreted into human milk.[1] The recommended daily allowance of niacin in lactating women is 18 to 20 mg of the standard release formulation. It is currently unknown if there are clinically significant consequences when breastfeeding an infant while the mother is taking a higher dose of niacin. There is limited data concerning the use of niacin for hypercholesterolemia or hypertriglyceridemia in breastfeeding mothers. Since niacin is known to be hepatotoxic in higher doses, it is recommended that mothers control these conditions with dietary measures while breastfeeding and do not exceed the daily recommended allowance.

T 1/2	45 min	MW	123 Da	PB	
Tmax	45 min	RID		Vd	
Oral	100%	M/P		pKa	4.85

Adult Concerns: Flushing, peripheral dilation, itching, nausea, vomiting, bloating, flatulence, abnormal liver function.

Adult Dose: 10-20 mg/day.

Pediatric Concerns: None reported.

Infant Monitoring: Flushing, vomiting.

Alternatives:

References:

1. Pharmaceutic manufacturers prescribing information, 2014.

NICARDIPINE

Trade: Cardene

Category: Calcium Channel Blocker

LRC: L2 - Limited Data-Probably Compatible

Nicardipine is a typical calcium channel blocker structurally related to nifedipine. In a study of 11 mothers consuming 20-120 mg nicardipine daily in various dosage forms, the milk/plasma ratio at 3 hours postdose averaged 0.25 (range 0.08-0.75), and the milk concentration (Cmax) was 7.3 µg/L (range 1.9-18.8).[1] The mean milk concentration was 4.4 µg/L (range 1.3-13.8). The authors estimate the relative infant dose to be 0.07% (range: 0.3-0.14) of the weight-adjusted maternal dose. Another study of 7 lactating women receiving a dose of 1 to 6.5 mg/hour found 82% of 34 milk samples to have undetectable levels. Six samples contained between 5.1 to 18.5 µg/L. The maximum infant exposure was calculated to be less than 300 ng/day, a level much lower than the dose used in neonates.[2]

T 1/2	6-10 h	MW	480 Da	PB	>95%
Tmax	0.5-2 h	RID	0.07%-0.1%	Vd	0.6-2 L/kg
Oral	35%	M/P	0.25	pKa	

Adult Concerns: Headache, hypotension, arrhythmias, flushing, peripheral edema, constipation.

Adult Dose: 20-50 twice daily.

Pediatric Concerns: None reported via milk at this time.

Infant Monitoring: Drowsiness, lethargy, pallor, poor feeding and weight gain.

Alternatives: Nifedipine(L2), Nimodipine(L2)

References:

1. Jarreau P, Beller CL, Guillonneau M, Jacqz-Aigrain E. Excretion of nicardipine in human milk. Paediatr Perinat Drug Ther. 2000;4(1):28-30.
2. Bartels P, Hanff L, Mathot R, Steegers E, Vulto A, Visser W. Nicardipine in pre-eclamptic patients: placental transfer and disposition in breast milk. BJOG. 2007 Feb;114(2):230-233.

NICOTINE

Trade: Blue Cigs (ENDS), Electronic-cigarettes, Habitrol, NicoDerm, Nicorette, Nicotrol, ProStep

Category: Smoking Cessation Agent

LRC: L3 - Limited Data-Probably Compatible

Nicotine and its metabolite cotinine are both present in milk with a milk/plasma ratio of 2.9. Fifteen lactating women (mean age, 32 years; mean weight, 72 kg) who were smokers (mean of 17 cigarettes per day) participated in a trial of the nicotine patch to assist in smoking cessation.[1] Serial milk samples were collected from the women over sequential 24-hour periods when they were smoking and when they were stabilized on the 21 mg/day, 14 mg/day, and 7 mg/day nicotine patches. Nicotine and cotinine concentrations in milk were not significantly different between smoking (mean of 17 cigarettes per day) and the 21 mg/day patch, but concentrations were significantly lower when patients were using the 14 mg/day and 7 mg/day patches than when smoking. There was also a downward trend in absolute infant dose (nicotine equivalents) from smoking or the 21 mg patch through to the 14 mg and 7 mg patches. Milk intake by the breastfed infants was similar while their mothers were smoking (585 mL/d) and subsequently when their mothers were using the 21 mg (717 mL/d), 14 mg (731 mL/d), and 7 mg (619 mL/d) patches. The authors conclude that the absolute infant dose of nicotine and its metabolite cotinine decreases by about 70% from when subjects were smoking or using the 21 mg patch to when they were using the 7 mg patch. In addition, use of the nicotine patch had no significant influence on the milk intake by the breastfed infant. Undertaking maternal smoking cessation with the nicotine patch is, therefore, a safer option than continued smoking.

With nicotine gum, maternal serum nicotine levels average 30%-60% of those found in cigarette smokers. While patches (transdermal systems) produce a sustained and lower nicotine plasma level, nicotine gum may produce large variations in peak levels when the gum is chewed rapidly, fluctuations similar to smoking itself. Mothers who choose to use nicotine gum and breastfeed should be counseled to refrain from breastfeeding for 2-3 hours after using the gum product. The nicotine inhaler only dispenses about 4 mg of nicotine following 80 inhalations, of which, only 2 mg is actually absorbed. Plasma levels slowly reach levels of about 6 ng/mL in contrast to those of a cigarette, which reach a Cmax of approximately 49 ng/mL in only 5 minutes. These levels (6 ng/mL) are probably too low to affect a breastfeeding infant. Habitual smokeless tobacco users will receive 130-250 mg of nicotine per day compared to 180 mg per day for one pack of cigarettes.

E-cigarettes, also known as electronic nicotine delivery systems (ENDS) are battery-powered devices that look like conventional cigarettes and are designed to mimic and deliver the satisfying effects of a traditional cigarette without exposing the user, or the people around to the harmful compounds of tobacco smoke. E-cigarettes contain mainly 5 FDA-approved ingredients: nicotine, water, propylene glycol, glycerol, and flavoring. While the nicotine content provides the gratifying effects of a regular cigarette, the propylene glycol produces vapor to mimic cigarette smoke. E-cigarettes have therefore become very popular as a safer alternative to cigarette smoking without exposure to tobacco and substances known to cause detrimental effects including lung cancer. However, these products have not been extensively studied and currently are not licensed by the FDA. The amount of nicotine delivered per puff or per cartridge is also obscure. One study compared the peak blood nicotine levels achieved after the use of a 16 mg e-cigarette, a nicotine inhaler, and a conventional cigarette.[2] It was reported that an e-cigarette produced peak blood nicotine levels of 1.3 ng/mL in 19.6 minutes, which is comparable to the levels obtained by a nicotine inhaler (2.1 ng/mL in 32 minutes) and much lower than those obtained by a conventional cigarette (13.4 ng/mL in 14.3 minutes). This study further revealed that the reduction in the desire to smoke is similar to that of a nicotine inhaler but that e-cigarettes are better tolerated by users. Eissenberg later conducted a similar study and reported that the amount of nicotine delivered after 10 puffs of a 16 mg e-cigarette is little to none.[3] Based on these findings, it can be concluded that the amount of nicotine that transfers into breast milk after an acute inhalation of an e-cigarette is probably minimal, and comparable to that of a nicotine inhaler. But it is reported that an average e-cigarette user inhales up to 120 puffs/day.[4] This could possibly amount to significantly higher blood nicotine levels. It is too early to comment on the long-term effects of chronic use of e-cigarettes and more studies are required.

Nicotine has been suggested to cause a decrease in basal prolactin production.[5,6] One study clearly suggests that cigarette smoking significantly reduces breast milk production at 2 weeks postpartum from 514 mL/day in non-smokers to 406 mL/day in smoking mothers.[7] However, Ilett's well-done study above did not detect any change in milk production at all, although the methods of these two studies were not identical. Mothers should be advised to limit smoking as much as possible and to smoke only after they have fed their infant, or to switch to the use of nicotine patches.

T 1/2	2 h (non-patch)	MW	162 Da	PB	4.9%
Tmax	2-4 h	RID		Vd	
Oral	30%	M/P	2.9	pKa	

Adult Concerns: Tachycardia, vomiting, diarrhea, restlessness.

Adult Dose: 7-21 mg daily.

Pediatric Concerns: No untoward effects were noted from nicotine patch study.

Infant Monitoring: Vomiting, diarrhea, rapid heart beat.

Alternatives:

References:
1. Ilett KF, Hale TW, Page-Sharp M, Kristensen JH, Kohan R, Hackett LP. Use of nicotine patches in breast-feeding mothers: transfer of nicotine and cotinine into human milk. Clin Pharmacol Ther. 2003;74(6):516-524.
2. Bullen C, McRobbie H, Thornley S, Glover M, Lin R, Laugesen M. Effect of an electronic nicotine delivery device (e cigarette) on desire to smoke and withdrawal, user preferences and nicotine delivery: randomised cross-over trial. Tob Control. 2010 Apr;19(2):98-103.
3. Eissenberg T. Electronic nicotine delivery devices: ineffective nicotine delivery and craving suppression after acute administration. Tob Control. 2010 Feb;19(1):87-88.
4. Etter JF, Bullen C. Electronic cigarette: users profile, utilization,satisfaction and perceived efficacy. Addiction. 2011 Nov;106(11):2017-2028. doi: 10.1111/j.1360-0443.2011.03505.x. Epub 2011 Jul 27.
5. Benowitz NL. Nicotine replacement therapy during pregnancy. JAMA. 1991;266(22):3174-3177.
6. Matheson I, Rivrud GN. The effect of smoking on lactation and infantile colic. JAMA. 1989;261(1):42-43.
7. Hopkinson JM, Schanler RJ, Fraley JK, Garza C. Milk production by mothers of premature infants: influence of cigarette smoking. Pediatrics. 1992;90(6):934-938.

NICOTINIC ACID

Trade: Niacels, Niacin, Niaspan, Nicobid, Nicolar, Nicotinamide

Category: Vitamin

LRC: L3 - No Data-Probably Compatible

Nicotinic acid, commonly called niacin, is a component of two coenzymes which function in oxidation-reduction reactions essential for tissue respiration. It is converted to nicotinamide in vivo. Although considered a vitamin, large doses (2-6 g/day) are effective in reducing serum LDL cholesterol and triglyceride and increasing serum HDL. From numerous studies, niacin content (even when supplemented with moderately low amounts) seems to vary from about 1.1 to 3.9 mg/L under normal circumstances.[1] Supplementation apparently does increase milk niacin levels. The concentration transferred to milk as a function of dose or following high maternal doses has not been reported, but it is presumed that elevated maternal plasma levels may significantly elevate milk levels of niacin as well. Because niacin is known to be hepatotoxic in higher doses, breastfeeding mothers should not significantly exceed the RDA such as with the 2 g/day doses used to treat hypercholesterolemia.

T 1/2	45 min	MW	123 Da	PB	
Tmax	45 min	RID		Vd	
Oral	Complete	M/P		pKa	4.85

Adult Concerns: Flushing, peripheral dilation, itching, nausea, bloating, flatulence, vomiting. In high doses, some abnormal liver function tests.

Adult Dose: 10-20 mg daily.

Pediatric Concerns: None reported via milk.

Infant Monitoring: Flushing, vomiting.

Alternatives:

References:
1. Pratt jp, Hamil BM, Moyer EZ, et al. Metabolism of women during the reproductive cycle. XVIII. The effect of multivitamin supplements on the secretion of B vitamins in human milk. J Nutr. 1951;44(1):141-157.

NIFEDIPINE

Trade: Adalat, Nefensar XL, Nifecard, Nifedical, Procardia

Category: Calcium Channel Blocker

LRC: L2 - Limited Data-Probably Compatible

Nifedipine is an effective antihypertensive. It belongs to the calcium channel blocker family of drugs. Two studies indicate that nifedipine is transferred to breast milk in varying but generally low levels.

In one study in which the dose was varied from 10-30 mg three times daily, the highest concentration (53.35 µg/L) was measured at 1 hour after a 30 mg dose.[1] Other levels reported were 16.35 µg/L 60 minutes after a 20 mg dose and 12.89 µg/L 30 minutes after a 10 mg dose. The milk levels fell linearly with the milk half-lives estimated to be 1.4 hours for the 10 mg dose, 3.1 hours for the 20 dose, and 2.4 hours for the 30 mg dose. The milk concentration measured 8 hours following a 30 mg dose was 4.93 µg/L. In this study, using the highest concentration found and a daily intake of 150 mL/kg of human milk, the amount of nifedipine intake would only be 8 µg/kg/day (less than 1.8% of the therapeutic pediatric dose). The authors conclude that the amount ingested via breast milk poses little risk to an infant.

In another study, concentrations of nifedipine in human milk 1 to 8 hours after 10 mg doses varied from <1 to 10.3 µg/L (median 3.5 µg/L) in six of 11 patients.[2] In this study, milk levels 3 days after discontinuing medication ranged from <1 to 9.4 µg/L. The authors concluded the exposure to nifedipine through breast milk is not significant. In a study by Penny and Lewis, following a maternal dose of 20 mg nifedipine daily for 10 days, peak breast milk levels at 1 hour were 46 µg/L.[3] The corresponding maternal serum level was 43 µg/L. From this data, the authors suggest a daily intake for an infant would be approximately 6.45 µg/kg/day. Nifedipine has been found clinically useful for nipple vasospasm. Because of the similarity to Raynaud's Phenomenon, sustained release formulations providing 30-60 mg per day are suggested.

T 1/2	1.8-7 h	MW	346 Da	PB	92%-98%
Tmax	45 min-4 h	RID	2.3%-3.4%	Vd	
Oral	50%	M/P	1	pKa	

Adult Concerns: Headache, dizziness, fatigue, hypotension, constipation, peripheral edema.

Adult Dose: 30-60 mg XL/day.

Pediatric Concerns: None reported via milk at this time.

Infant Monitoring: Drowsiness, lethargy, pallor, poor feeding, and weight gain.

Alternatives: Labetalol(L2)

References:
1. Ehrenkranz RA, Ackerman BA, Hulse JD. Nifedipine transfer into human milk. J Pediatr. 1989;114(3):478-480.
2. Manninen AK, Juhakoski A. Nifedipine concentrations in maternal and umbilical serum, amniotic fluid, breast milk and urine of mothers and offspring. Int J Clin Pharmacol Res. 1991;11(5):231-236.
3. Penny WJ, Lewis MJ. Nifedipine is excreted in human milk. Eur J Clin Pharmacol. 1989;36(4):427-428.

NILOTINIB

Trade: Tasigna

Category: Antineoplastic

LRC: L4 - No Data-Possibly Hazardous

Nilotinib is used for the treatment of chronic myelogenous leukemia (CML).[1] Studies suggest it has a relatively favorable safety profile. Nilotinib is an inhibitor of the Bcr-Abl tyrosine kinase. Nilotinib was developed as a second-generation inhibitor of bcr-abl tyrosine kinase that would be effective in patients with imatinib-resistant or -intolerant CML. The drug carries a black box warning for possible heart complications. No data are available on its transfer to human milk. Due to its high protein binding, levels in milk will probably be low. Further, its oral bioavailability is poor, which would reduce oral absorption in infants. This product is significantly toxic and we suggest withholding breastfeeding for 4 days.

T 1/2	17 h	MW	529 Da	PB	98%
Tmax	3 h	RID		Vd	
Oral	30%	M/P		pKa	2.1-5.4

Adult Concerns: Rash, pruritus, nausea, fatigue, headache, prolonged QT interval, gastrointestinal disturbances, increase bilirubin levels, hypophosphatemia, hypokalemia, hyperkalemia, hypocalcemia, hyponatremia, hematologic changes.

Adult Dose: 300-400 mg twice daily.

Pediatric Concerns: Rash, fatigue.

Infant Monitoring: Withhold breastfeeding for 4 days.

Alternatives:

References:
1. Pharmaceutical manufacturers prescribing information.

NIMODIPINE

Trade: Nimotop

Category: Calcium Channel Blocker

LRC: L2 - Limited Data-Probably Compatible

Nimodipine is a calcium channel blocker, although it is primarily used in preventing cerebral artery spasm and improving cerebral blood flow. Nimodipine is effective in reducing neurologic deficits following subarachnoid hemorrhage, acute stroke, and severe head trauma. It is also useful in prophylaxis of migraine.

In one study of a patient 3 days postpartum who received 60 mg every 4 hours for 1 week, breast milk levels paralleled maternal serum levels with a milk/plasma ratio of approximately 0.33.[1] The highest milk concentration reported was approximately 3.5 µg/L, while the maternal plasma was approximately 16 µg/L. In another study [2], a 36-year-old mother received a total dose of 46 mg IV over 24 hours. Nimodipine concentration in milk was much lower than in maternal serum, with a milk/serum ratio of 0.06 to 0.15. During IV infusion, nimodipine concentrations in milk raised initially to 2.2 µg/L and stabilized at concentrations between 0.87 and 1.6 µg/L of milk. Assuming a daily milk intake of 150 mL/kg, the authors estimate an infant would ingest approximately 0.063 to 0.705 µg/kg/day or 0.008% to 0.092% of the weight-adjusted dose administered to the mother. We calculate the RID at 0.001%-0.037%, which is exceedingly low.

T 1/2	9 h	MW	418 Da	PB	95%
Tmax	1 h	RID	0.001%-0.04%	Vd	0.94 L/kg
Oral	13%	M/P	0.06 to 0.33	pKa	

Adult Concerns: Headache, hypotension, diarrhea, nausea, muscle cramps.

Adult Dose: 60 mg every 4 hours.

Pediatric Concerns: None reported via milk at this time.

Infant Monitoring: Drowsiness, lethargy, pallor, poor feeding, and weight gain.

Alternatives: Verapamil(L2), Nifedipine(L2)

References:
1. Tonks AM. Nimodipine levels in breast milk. Aust N Z J Surg. 1995;65(9):693-694.
2. Carcas AJ, Abad-Santos F, de Rosendo JM, Frias J. Nimodipine transfer into human breast milk and cerebrospinal fluid. Ann Pharmacother. 1996;30(2):148-150.

NISOLDIPINE

Trade: Sular, Syscor

Category: Calcium Channel Blocker

LRC: L3 - No Data-Probably Compatible

Nisoldipine is a typical calcium channel blocker antihypertensive.[1] No data are available on its transfer to human milk. For alternatives see nifedipine and verapamil. Due to its poor oral bioavailability, presence of lipids that reduce its absorption and high protein binding, it is unlikely into penetrate milk and be absorbed by the infant.

T 1/2	7-12 h	MW	388 Da	PB	99%
Tmax	6-12 h	RID		Vd	4 L/kg
Oral	5%	M/P		pKa	

Adult Concerns: Hypotension, bradycardia, peripheral edema.

Adult Dose: 20-40 mg daily.

Pediatric Concerns: None reported via milk. Observe for hypotension, sedation although unlikely.

Infant Monitoring: Drowsiness, lethargy, pallor, poor feeding, and weight gain.

Alternatives: Nifedipine(L2), Verapamil(L2), Nimodipine(L2)

References:
1. Pharmaceutical manufacturers prescribing information.

NITAZOXANIDE

Trade: Alinia

Category: Antibiotic, Other

LRC: L3 - No Data-Probably Compatible

Nitazoxanide is a new thiazolide antiprotozoan agent that shows excellent in vitro activity against a wide variety of protozoa and helminths. It is a suitable alternative for metronidazole in many infections including *Giardia lamblia* and *Cryptosporidium parvum*. Once absorbed it is rapidly converted to the active metabolite tizoxanide.[1] No data are available on its transfer to human milk.

T 1/2	1-1.6 h	MW	307 Da	PB	99%
Tmax	4 h	RID		Vd	
Oral	Good	M/P		pKa	

Adult Concerns: Abdominal pain, diarrhea, headache, and nausea have been reported in clinical trials.

Adult Dose: 500 mg every 12 hours with food.

Pediatric Concerns: None reported, but no data are available.

Infant Monitoring: Vomiting, diarrhea, changes in gastrointestinal flora, and rash.

Alternatives: Metronidazole(L2)

References:
1. Pharmaceutical manufacturers prescribing information.

NITRAZEPAM

Trade: Alodorm, Atempol, Mogadon, Nitrazadon, Nitrodos

Category: Sedative-Hypnotic

LRC: L2 - Limited Data-Probably Compatible

Nitrazepam is a benzodiazepine used as a sedative. In a study of nine women who received 5 mg nitrazepam at night, the concentration in milk increased over a period of 5 days from 30 nmol/L to 48 nmol/L.[1] The mean milk/plasma ratio after 7 hours was 0.27 in 32 paired samples and did not vary from day 1 to day 5. The mean concentration of nitrazepam in milk was 13 µg/L and the C_{max} was 0.20 µg/L. Nitrazepam levels in a 6-day-old infant were below the limits of detection. No adverse effects were noted in the infants breastfed for 5 days.

T 1/2	30 h	MW	281 Da	PB	90%
Tmax	0.5-5 h	RID	2.9%	Vd	2-5 L/kg
Oral	53%-94%	M/P	0.27	pKa	11.9

Adult Concerns: Sedation, dizziness, confusion, apnea.

Adult Dose: 5-10 mg daily.

Pediatric Concerns: None reported via milk at this time.

Infant Monitoring: Sedation, slowed breathing rate, not waking to feed/poor feeding, and weight gain.

Alternatives: Lorazepam(L3)

References:

1. Matheson I, Lunde PK, Bredesen JE. Midazolam and nitrazepam in the maternity ward: milk concentrations and clinical effects. Br J Clin Pharmacol. 1990;30(6):787-793.

NITROFURANTOIN

Trade: Furadantin, Furan, Macrobid, Macrodantin

Category: Antibiotic, Other

LRC: L2 - Limited Data-Probably Compatible

Nitrofurantoin is an old urinary tract antimicrobial. It is secreted in breast milk but in very small amounts. In one study of 20 women receiving 100 mg four times daily, none was detected in milk.[1] In another group of nine nursing women who received 100-200 mg every 6 hours, nitrofurantoin was undetectable in the milk of those treated with 100 mg and only trace amounts were found in those treated with 200 mg (0.3-0.5 mg/L milk).[2] In these two patients, the milk/plasma ratio ranged from 0.27 to 0.31.

In a well-done study of four breastfeeding mothers who ingested 100 mg nitrofurantoin with a meal, the milk/serum ratio averaged 6.21 suggesting an active transfer to milk.[3] Regardless of an active transfer, the average milk concentration throughout the day (AUC) was only 1.3 mg/L. According to the authors, the estimated dose an infant would ingest was 0.2 mg/kg/day or 6.8% of the weight-adjusted maternal dose if they consumed 200 mg/day nitrofurantoin. The therapeutic dose administered to infants is 5-7 mg/kg/day.

Use with caution in premature infants and neonates with hyperbilirubinemia. Avoid in infants with G6PD deficiency or in infants less than 1 month of age, due to displacement of bilirubin from albumin binding sites.

T 1/2	20-58 min	MW	238 Da	PB	60%-90%
Tmax		RID	6.8%	Vd	0.8 L/kg
Oral	94%	M/P	0.27-6.2	pKa	7.2

Adult Concerns: Nausea, vomiting, brown urine, hemolytic anemia, hepatotoxicity.

Adult Dose: 50-100 mg four times daily.

Pediatric Concerns: None reported via milk, however, do not use in infants with G6PD deficiency or in infants less than 1 month of age.

Infant Monitoring: Vomiting, diarrhea, changes in gastrointestinal flora and rash; if clinical symptoms of jaundice check bilirubin and CBC if risk of hemolytic anemia.

Alternatives:

References:

1. Hosbach RH, Foster RB. Absence of nitrofurantoin from human milk. JAMA. 1967;202(11):1057.
2. Varsano I, Fischl J, Shochet SB. The excretion of orally ingested nitrofurantoin in human milk. J Pediatr. 1973;82(5):886-887.
3. Gerk PM, Kuhn RJ, Desai NS, McNamara PJ. Active transport of nitrofurantoin into human milk. Pharmacotherapy. 2001;21(6):669-675.

NITROPRUSSIDE

Trade: Nipride, Nitropress

Category: Vasodilator

LRC: L4 - No Data-Possibly Hazardous

Nitroprusside is a rapid acting hypotensive agent of short duration (1-10 minutes). Besides rapid hypotension, nitroprusside is converted metabolically to cyanogen (cyanide radical), which is potentially toxic. Although rare, significant thiocyanate toxicity can occur at higher doses (>2 µg/kg/minute) and longer durations of exposure (>1-2 days).[1] When administered orally, nitroprusside is reported to be inactive, although one report suggests a modest hypotensive effect. No data are available on transfer of nitroprusside nor thiocyanate to human milk. The half-life of the thiocyanate metabolite is approximately 3 days. Because the thiocyanate metabolite is orally bioavailable, some caution is advised if the mother has received nitroprusside for more than 24 hours.[2]

T 1/2	2 min	MW	297.5 Da	PB	
Tmax	less than 2 min	RID		Vd	
Oral		M/P		pKa	

Adult Concerns: Headache, drowsiness, hypotension, nausea, vomiting, methemoglobinemia, cyanide toxicity, hypothyroidism.

Adult Dose: 0.3 µg/kg/minute titrate dose every 5-10 minutes (maximum 10 µg/kg/minute).

Pediatric Concerns: None reported but caution is urged due to thiocyanate metabolite.

Infant Monitoring: Drowsiness, lethargy, pallor, poor feeding, and weight gain.

Alternatives:

References:
1. Page IH, Corcoran AC, Dustan HP, Koppanyi T. Cardiovascular actions of sodium nitroprusside in animals and hypertensive patients. Circulation. 1955;11(2):188-198.
2. Benitz WE, Malachowski N, Cohen RS, Stevenson DK, Ariagno RL, Sunshine P. Use of sodium nitroprusside in neonates: efficacy and safety. J Pediatr. 1985;106(1):102-110.

NITROUS OXIDE

Trade: Entonox

Category: Anesthetic

LRC: L3 - No Data-Probably Compatible

Nitrous oxide is a weak anesthetic gas. It provides good analgesia and weak anesthesia. It is rapidly eliminated from the body due to rapid exchange with nitrogen via the pulmonary alveoli (within minutes).[1,2] A rapid recovery generally occurs in 3-5 minutes. Due to poor lipid solubility, uptake by adipose tissue is relatively poor, and only insignificant traces of nitrous oxide circulate in blood after discontinuing inhalation of the gas. No data exist on the entry of nitrous oxide into human milk. Ingestion of nitrous oxide orally via milk is unlikely.

T 1/2	<3 min	MW	44 Da	PB	
Tmax	15 min	RID		Vd	
Oral	Poor	M/P		pKa	

Adult Concerns: Chronic exposure can produce bone marrow suppression, headaches, hypotension, and bradycardia.

Adult Dose: For inhalation, 50% nitrous oxide with 50% oxygen.

Pediatric Concerns: None reported via milk.

Infant Monitoring: Sedation.

Alternatives:

References:
1. General Anesthetics. In: Drug Evaluations Annual 1995. Chicago, IL: American Medical Association; 1995.
2. Adriani J. General Anesthetics. In: Clinical Management of Poisoning and Drug Overdose. Philadelphia, PA: W.B. Saunders & Co.; 1983.

NIZATIDINE

Trade: Axid, Tazac

Category: Gastric Acid Secretion Inhibitor

LRC: L2 - Limited Data-Probably Compatible

Nizatidine is an antisecretory, histamine-2 antagonist that reduces stomach acid secretion. In one study of five lactating women using a dose of 150 mg daily, milk levels of nizatidine were directly proportional to circulating maternal serum levels, yet were very low.[1] Over a 12 hour period, 96 µg (less than 0.5% of dose) was secreted into milk. No effects on infant have been reported.

T 1/2	1.5 h	MW	331 Da	PB	35%
Tmax	0.5-3 h	RID	0.5%	Vd	
Oral	94%	M/P		pKa	

Adult Concerns: Headache, gastrointestinal distress.

Adult Dose: 150-300 mg daily.

Pediatric Concerns: None reported.

Infant Monitoring:

Alternatives: Famotidine(L1), Ranitidine(L2)

References:

1. Obermeyer BD, Bergstrom RF, Callaghan JT, Knadler MP, Golichowski A, Rubin A. Secretion of nizatidine into human breast milk after single and multiple doses. Clin Pharmacol Ther. 1990;47(6):724-730.

NONOXYNOL 9

Trade: Advantage-S, Aqua Lube Plus, Conceptrol, Delfen Foam, Emko, Encare, Gynol II, Today Sponge

Category: Contraceptive

LRC: L3 - No Data-Probably Compatible

Nonoxynol 9 is a non-ionic surfactant used as a vaginal spermicide. In one rodent study, 0.3% of the nonoxynol 9 maternal dose was present in the breast milk of rats.[1] However, the study could not distinguish between nonoxynol 9 or its metabolite. Studies in rodents are not comparable to those done in humans. There are no controlled studies in breastfeeding women reporting the level of nonoxyl 9 in breast milk. Based on local administration and the high molecular weight, levels in milk are anticipated to be low.

T 1/2		MW	617 Da	PB	
Tmax		RID		Vd	
Oral		M/P		pKa	

Adult Concerns: Vaginal irritation, vaginal discomfort, vaginal pain.

Adult Dose: 1 applicator 1 hour prior intercourse.

Pediatric Concerns:

Infant Monitoring:

Alternatives:

References:

1. Chvapil M, Eskelson CD, Stiffel V, Owen JA, Droegemueller W. Studies on Nonoxynol-9. II. Intravaginal absorption, distribution, metabolism and excretion in rats and rabbits. Contraception. 1980 Sep;22(3):325-339.

NORETHINDRONE

Trade: Aygestin, Brevinor, Camila, Errin, Jolivette, Micronor, NOR-Q.D., Nora-BE, Norethisterone, Norlestrin, Norlutate, Ortho-Micronor

Category: Progestin

LRC: L3 - Limited Data-Probably Compatible

Norethindrone is a typical synthetic progestational agent that is used for oral contraception and other endocrine functions. It is believed to be secreted into breast milk in small amounts. It may reduce lactose content and reduce overall milk volume and nitrogen/protein content, resulting in lower infant weight gain, although these effects are unlikely if doses are kept low.[1-5] Progestin-only mini pills are preferred oral contraceptives in breastfeeding mothers.

However, recent reports claim that norethindrone can be associated with decreased breast milk production. In a report of 13 women taking Micronor (norethindrone) who presented with poor milk production, 10 women experienced an increase in lactation upon withdrawal of Micronor.[6] While norethindrone birth control pills are considered ideal for most breastfeeding mothers, some women retain sensitivity to these products and may suffer from reduced milk production. Each and every breastfeeding mother should be individually counseled about the possible reduction in milk synthesis following the use of this product. It is advisable to wait as long as possible, preferably a minimum of 4 weeks postpartum prior to instituting therapy with progesterone to avoid reducing the milk supply. See contraception, hormonal monograph for more details.

T 1/2	4-13 h	MW	298 Da	PB	97%
Tmax	1-2 h	RID		Vd	
Oral	60%	M/P		pKa	

Adult Concerns: Headache, hypertension, nausea, vomiting, gallbladder disease, changes in liver function, abdominal cramps, bloating, breakthrough bleeding, spotting, amenorrhea, edema, weight gain, thromboembolism (DVT, PE, stroke, MI). Potential suppression of milk supply.

Adult Dose: 0.35-5 mg daily.

Pediatric Concerns: None reported via milk.

Infant Monitoring: Small amounts are present in human milk. Possible suppression of milk production early postpartum is reported.

Alternatives:

References:

1. Kora SJ. Effect of oral contraceptives on lactation. Fertil Steril. 1969;20(3):419-423.
2. Miller GH, Hughes LR. Lactation and genital involution effects of a new low-dose oral contraceptive on breast-feeding mothers and their infants. Obstet Gynecol. 1970;35(1):44-50.
3. Karim M, Ammar R, El Mahgoub S, et al. Injected progestogen and lactation. Br Med J. 1971;1(742):200-203.
4. Lonnerdal B, Forsum E, Hambraeus L. Effect of oral contraceptives on composition and volume of breast milk. Am J Clin Nutr. 1980;33(4):816-824.
5. Laukaran VH. The effects of contraceptive use on the initiation and duration of lactation. Int J Gynaecol Obstet. 1987;25 Suppl:129-142.
6. Norethindrone (Micronor): suspected association with decreased breast milk production. CARN. 2007 July;17(3):4.

NORTRIPTYLINE

Trade: Allegron, Aventyl, Norventyl, Pamelor

Category: Antidepressant, Tricyclic

LRC: L2 - Limited Data-Probably Compatible

Nortriptyline is a tricyclic antidepressant and is the active metabolite of amitriptyline. In 1988, a case report was published regarding the use of nortriptyline in breast milk.[1] In this case, the woman was taking 1 mg of flupentixol daily with 100 mg of nortriptyline daily starting in the second trimester of her pregnancy. The nortriptyline was stopped 2 weeks prior to delivery; however, this medication was restarted at a higher dose (125 mg), along with an increased dose of flupentixol 4 mg on day 1 postpartum. Maternal blood and milk samples and infant blood samples (heel prick taken 2 hours post-feed) were taken on day 6 and 7 postpartum. The woman's milk concentrations of nortriptyline averaged 180 µg/L after 6-7 days of administration.[1] Based on these concentrations, the authors calculated the average daily infant dose was 27 µg/kg/day and the relative infant dose was 1.3% (used maternal weight 60 kg). We found very similar results with a relative infant dose of 1.7% (standard maternal weight 70 kg and mean milk concentration (180 µg/L). In addition, we also calculated the relative infant dose using the peak nortriptyline concentration of 400 µg/L and still only found an RID of 3.4%. This infant was exclusively breastfed, the authors reported normal motor development and no signs of medication adverse effects at 4 months of age.

Please note: the levels of nortriptyline were not at steady-state in this case report; however, based on calculations the authors do not anticipate the findings would vary significantly at steady-state.

Several other authors have been unable to detect nortriptyline in maternal milk and the serum of infants after prolonged exposure.[2,3] A pooled analysis of 35 studies with an average dose of 78 mg/day reported a detectable level of nortriptyline in breast milk in only one patient, with a concentration of 230 ng/mL. The authors suggest that breastfed infants exposed to nortriptyline are unlikely to develop detectable concentrations in plasma, and therefore breastfeeding during nortriptyline therapy is not contraindicated.[4]

In addition, one small study that followed four groups of women prescribed TCAs throughout different stages of reproduction found no adverse events in the group of infants whose mothers were prescribed these medications in lactation.[5] This study included 21 women (two on nortriptyline) that initiated tricyclic antidepressant therapy at a mean of 10.3 weeks postpartum and breastfed on treatment for a mean of 12 weeks.

T 1/2	16-90 h	MW	263 Da	PB	92%
Tmax	7-8.5 h	RID	1.7%-3.36%	Vd	21 L/kg
Oral	51%	M/P	0.87-3.71	pKa	9.7

Adult Concerns: Sedation, blurred vision, dry mouth, constipation, urinary retention.

Adult Dose: 25 mg three to four times daily.

Pediatric Concerns: None reported in several studies.

Infant Monitoring: Sedation or irritability, dry mouth, not waking to feed/poor feeding, constipation, urinary retention, weight gain.

Alternatives: Imipramine(L2), Amitriptyline(L2), SSRIs.

References:

1. Matheson I, Skjaeraasen J. Milk concentrations of flupenthixol, nortriptyline and zuclopenthixol and between-breast differences in two patients. Eur J Clin Pharmacol. 1988;35(2):217-220.
2. Wisner KL, Perel JM. Serum nortriptyline levels in nursing mothers and their infants. Am J Psychiatry. 1991;148(9):1234-1236.
3. Brixen-Rasmussen L, Halgrener J, Jorgensen A. Amitriptyline and nortriptyline excretion in human breast milk. Psychopharmacology (Berl). 1982;76(1):94-95.
4. Weissman AM, Levy BT, Hartz AJ, et al. Pooled analysis of antidepressant levels in lactating mothers, breast milk, and nursing infants. Am J Psychiatry. 2004 June;161(6):1066-1078.
5. Misri S, Sivertz K. Tricyclic drugs in pregnancy and lactation: a preliminary report. Int J Psychiatry Med. 1991;21:157-171.

NYSTATIN

Trade: Candistatin, Mycostatin, Nadostine, Nilstat, Nystan

Category: Antifungal

LRC: L1 - Limited Data-Compatible

Nystatin is an antifungal primarily used for candidiasis topically and orally. The oral absorption of nystatin is extremely poor, and plasma levels are undetectable after oral administration.[1] The likelihood of secretion into milk is remote due to poor maternal absorption. It is frequently administered directly to neonates in neonatal units for candidiasis. In addition, absorption into infant circulation is equally unlikely. Current studies suggest that resistance to nystatin is growing.

T 1/2		MW	926 Da	PB	
Tmax		RID		Vd	
Oral	0%	M/P		pKa	

Adult Concerns: Bad taste, nausea, vomiting, diarrhea.

Adult Dose: Swish and swallow 400,000 to 600,000 units four times a day.

Pediatric Concerns: None reported. Nystatin is commonly used in infants.

Infant Monitoring: Vomiting, diarrhea.

Alternatives: Fluconazole(L2)

References:

1. Rothermel P, Faber M. Drugs in breast milk: a consumer's guide. Birth Family J. 1975;2:76-78.

OCRELIZUMAB

Trade: Ocrevus

Category: Treatment of Multiple Sclerosis

LRC: L4 - No Data-Possibly Hazardous

Ocrelizumab is a recombinant humanized monoclonal antibody directed against CD20-expressing B-cells and is indicated for the treatment of Multiple Sclerosis. It is a glycosylated immunoglobulin G1 (IgG1) and binds to the CD20 cell surface antigen present in B cells involved in multiple sclerosis. While no levels in milk have been published, it is likely they are low, and that present, is probably not orally bioavailable. Other such monoclonal antibodies are virtually unabsorbed orally in humans. There are no published data on the transfer of ocrelizumab into human milk, although it was excreted in the milk of ocrelizumab-treated monkeys. This product could potentially reduce B-cell populations in the gut, and could lead to higher rates of gut infections in infants. Caution is recommended with this antibody.

T 1/2	26 days	MW	145,000 Da	PB	
Tmax		RID		Vd	0.04 L/kg
Oral	Low	M/P		pKa	

Adult Concerns: Upper respiratory tract infections and infusion reactions, skin infections, and lower respiratory tract infections. Pruritus, rash, urticaria, erythema, bronchospasm, throat irritation, oropharyngeal pain, dyspnea, pharyngeal or laryngeal edema, flushing, hypotension, pyrexia, fatigue, headache, dizziness, nausea, and tachycardia have been reported.

Adult Dose: 600 mg every 6 months or 300 mg every 2 weeks times two.

Pediatric Concerns: Observe for GI infections.

Infant Monitoring: Observe for gut, lower and upper respiratory tract infections, herpetic eruptions. If used during pregnancy, observe for pruritus, rash, urticaria, erythema, bronchospasm, throat irritation, oropharyngeal pain, dyspnea, pharyngeal or laryngeal edema, flushing, hypotension, pyrexia, fatigue, dizziness, nausea, and tachycardia.

Alternatives:

References:
1. Pharmaceutical manufacturers prescribing information.

OCTREOTIDE ACETATE

Trade: Octreotide Acetate Injection, Octreotide Acetate Omega, SandoSTATIN, SandoSTATIN LAR

Category: Somatostatin (class)

LRC: L3 - No Data-Probably Compatible

Octreotide is a close analog of and provides activity similar to the natural hormone somatostatin.[1] Octreotide (Sandostatin LAR) is a long acting form consisting of microspheres containing octreotide. Like somatostatin, it also suppresses LH response to GnRH, decreases splanchnic blood flow, and inhibits release of serotonin, gastrin, vasoactive intestinal peptide, secretin, motilin, and pancreatic polypeptide. It is used to treat acromegaly and carcinoid tumors. Due to its molecular weight, transfer to milk is probably minimal. This product, if present in milk, would not likely be absorbed to any degree.

T 1/2	1.9 h	MW	1019 Da	PB	65%
Tmax	SQ: 0.4 h ; IM: 1 h	RID		Vd	0.2 L/kg
Oral		M/P		pKa	

Adult Concerns: Nausea, diarrhea, vomiting, anorexia, abdominal discomfort, flatulence, steatorrhea, hair loss, gallstones.

Adult Dose: IM: 20 mg q4 weeks; SQ: 100-200 µg TID.

Pediatric Concerns:

Infant Monitoring: Vomiting, diarrhea, changes in feeding.

Alternatives:

References:
1. Pharmaceutical manufacturers prescribing information.

OFATUMUMAB

Trade: Arzerra

Category: Antineoplastic

LRC: L4 - No Data-Possibly Hazardous

Ofatumumab is a humanized monoclonal antibody that binds specifically to both the small and large extracellular loops of the CD20 molecule. It is a cytolytic product indicated for the treatment of patients with chronic lymphocytic leukemia (CLL) refractory to fludarabine and alemtuzumab. No data are available on its use in breastfeeding mothers. The major complication is heightened rate of pneumonia or infections due to depletion of B-cells. Due to its large molecular weight and the fact that it is an IgG FAB product, milk levels are likely to be quite low.

Although the molecular weight of this medication is very large and the amount in breast milk is expected to be exceptionally low, there are no long-term data concerning the safety of using immune modulating medications in breastfeeding mothers. Further there are current data that suggest that some IgG drugs do transfer to milk, and perhaps the breastfed infant. Therefore, some caution is recommended, and each woman should understand the benefits and risk of using this type of medication in lactation.

T 1/2	14 days	MW	149,000 Da	PB	
Tmax		RID		Vd	0.07 L/kg
Oral		M/P		pKa	

Adult Concerns: Rash, diarrhea, nausea, neutropenia, anemia, fatigue, pneumonia, cough, dyspnea, upper respiratory tract infection, bronchitis, and fever.

Adult Dose:

Pediatric Concerns: No adverse events have been reported at this time.

Infant Monitoring: Fever, frequent infections, feeding/weight gain.

Alternatives:

References:
1. Pharmaceutical manufacturers prescribing information.

OFLOXACIN

Trade: Floxin, Ocuflox, Tarivid

Category: Antibiotic, Quinolone

LRC: L2 - Limited Data-Probably Compatible

Ofloxacin is a typical fluoroquinolone antimicrobial. Breast milk concentrations are reported equal to maternal plasma levels. In one study in lactating women who received 400 mg oral doses twice daily, drug concentrations in breast milk averaged 0.05-2.41 mg/L in milk (24 hours and 2 hours postdose respectively).[1] The drug was still detectable in milk 24 hours after a dose. Because fluoroquinolones have limited safety data in pediatric and breastfeeding patients, use in lactation is not recommended if alternative therapies exist.[2]

After 10 days of topical ophthalmic dosing, maximum serum ofloxacin concentrations were found to be more than 1000 times lower than those reported after standard oral doses of ofloxacin.[2]

T 1/2	5-7 h	MW	361 Da	PB	32%
Tmax	0.5-2 h	RID	3.1%	Vd	1.4 L/kg
Oral	98%	M/P	0.98-1.66	pKa	

Adult Concerns: Nausea, vomiting, diarrhea, abdominal cramps, gastrointestinal bleeding.

Adult Dose: 200-400 mg twice daily.

Pediatric Concerns: None reported, but caution recommended.

Infant Monitoring: Vomiting, diarrhea, changes in gastrointestinal flora, and rash.

Alternatives: Norfloxacin, Ciprofloxacin(L3)

References:
1. Giamarellou H, Kolokythas E, Petrikkos G, Gazis J, Aravantinos D, Sfikakis P. Pharmacokinetics of three newer quinolones in pregnant and lactating women. Am J Med. 1989;87(5A):49S-51S.
2. Pharmaceutical manufacturer's prescribing information, 2010.

OLANZAPINE

Trade: Zyprexa, Zyprexa Relprevv

Category: Antipsychotic, Atypical

LRC: L2 - Limited Data-Probably Compatible

Olanzapine is an atypical antipsychotic that can be used for treating many disorders such as schizophrenia, bipolar disorder, and augmenting depression.[1] Olanzapine is structurally similar to clozapine and is rather unusual because of its greater affinity for serotonin receptors rather than dopamine receptors.

In a recent and excellent study of seven mother-infant nursing pairs receiving a median dose of olanzapine of 7.5 mg/day (range = 5-20 mg/day), the median infant dose ingested via milk was approximately 1% of the maternal dose.[2] The median milk/plasma AUC ratio was 0.38. Olanzapine was undetected in the plasma of six infants tested. All infants were healthy and experienced no observable side effects. The maximum relative infant dose was approximately 1.2%.

In a case report of a mother taking 20 mg/day, the milk/plasma ratio was 0.35, giving a relative infant dose of about 4% at steady state. This milk was not fed to the infant, so infant plasma levels were not performed.[3]

In a study of five mothers receiving olanzapine at a dose of 2.5-20 mg/day, reported milk/plasma ratios of 0.2 to 0.84, with an average relative infant dose of 1.6%. The authors reported no untoward effects on the infants attributable to olanzapine.[4]

In addition, a study published in 2011 evaluated infants exposed to olanzapine during lactation for early discontinuation of breastfeeding (less than 3 weeks), infant growth and development (speech and motor delays).[5] This study also had a secondary objective, which was to review information available regarding neonatal symptoms of infants exposed in utero. This study included 37 women who took olanzapine in pregnancy and/or lactation and a control group of 51 women; 30 of the 37 women exposed to olanzapine took the medication during pregnancy. Of the participants included, 18 of the 22 breastfed-exposed infants were also exposed in utero, 12 of the 15 non-breastfed infants were exposed in utero and none of the 51 control infants were exposed in utero or lactation. The rate of adverse outcomes in olanzapine-exposed breastfed infants did not differ from those of the non-breastfed and control group. Neonatal symptoms were seen in eight of the 30 olanzapine in utero-exposed infants versus 1 of 51 non-exposed infants. The types of neonatal symptoms recorded included respiratory distress (2), hypotonia (1), poor suck and feeding difficulty (2) and withdrawal syndrome (3); six of the eight symptomatic infants were not breastfed.

In 2013, a retrospective review was published regarding the safety of olanzapine in pregnancy and lactation.[6] This review compiled all pregnancy and breastfeeding data available from the literature and regulatory agencies by accessing the global safety database maintained by Eli Lilly and Company. There were a total of 102 infants exposed to olanzapine in breast milk, the maternal oral olanzapine dose was available for 62 of these cases and ranged from 2.5 to 20 mg a day (average 7.4 mg/day). Thirty women provided the duration of olanzapine exposure via breast milk, this ranged from 2 days to 13 months (average 74 days). The majority of cases reported no adverse effects (82.3%). Of the 15.6% who did report infant concerns, the most common were somnolence (3.9%), irritability (2%), tremor (2%) and insomnia (2%). In 40% of these cases, the adverse events were reported as resolving or resolved, 24% were said not to have resolved and the remaining cases did not provide follow up.

A publication in 2015 described the case of a 33-year-old woman who 2 days after delivering her twins was initiated on sodium valproate for bipolar maintenance therapy.[7] On days 18 to 20 postpartum she developed both psychotic and manic symptoms, thus olanzapine 15 mg and quetiapine 200 mg were added daily at 11 pm. The patient was advised to start breastfeeding 8 hours after her bedtime doses, and to pump and discard her milk accumulated overnight around 7 am each day. Three breast milk samples were collected and saved by the patient at 4 a.m., 8 a.m., and 11 p.m. (before taking her medications) for 27 days within a 48-day period. The median daily concentration of olanzapine was 10.2 ng/mL. The absolute infant dose for olanzapine was 1.29 µg/kg, this corresponded to a relative infant dose of 0.74%. The infants were breastfed using this routine for 15 months, no adverse effects or concerns with development were reported by the pediatrician.

T 1/2	21-54 h	MW	312 Da	PB	93%
Tmax	5-8 h	RID	0.28%-2.24%	Vd	14.3 L/kg
Oral	>57%	M/P	0.38	pKa	5, 7.4

Adult Concerns: Agitation, dizziness, somnolence, constipation, weight gain, elevated liver enzymes.

Adult Dose: 5-10 mg daily.

Pediatric Concerns: Somnolence, irritability, tremor and insomnia have been reported with breast milk exposure.

Infant Monitoring: Sedation or irritability, insomnia, apnea, not waking to feed/poor feeding, extrapyramidal symptoms, tremor, and weight gain.

Alternatives: Risperidone(L2), Quetiapine(L2)

References:

1. Pharmaceutical manufacturers prescribing information.
2. Gardiner SJ, Kristensen JH, Begg EJ, et al. Transfer of olanzapine into breast milk, calculation of infant drug dose, and effect on breast-fed infants. Am J Psychiatry. 2003;160:1428-1431.
3. Ambresin G, Berney P, Schulz P, Bryois C. Olanzapine excretion into breast milk: a case report. J Clin Psychopharmacol. 2004;24(1):93-95.

4. Croke S, Buist A, Hackett LP, Ilett KF, Norman TR, Burrows GD. Olanzapine excretion in human breast milk: estimation of infant exposure. Int J Neuropsychopharmacol. 2002;5:243-247.
5. Gilad O, Merlob P, Stahl B, Klinger G. Outcome of infants exposed to olanzapine during breastfeeding. Breastfeed Med. 2011;6(2):55-58.
6. Brunner E, Falk DM, Jones M, Dey DK, Shatapathy CC. Olanzapine in pregnancy and breatfeeding: a review of data from global safety surveillance. BMC Pharmacol Toxicol. 2013;14:38.
7. Aydin B, Nayir T, Sahin S, Yildiz A. Olanzapine and quetiapine use during breastfeeding excretion into breast milk and safe breastfeeding strategy. J Clin Psychopharmacol. 2015;35(2):206-208.

OLMESARTAN MEDOXOMIL

Trade: Benicar

Category: Angiotensin II Receptor Antagonist

LRC: L3 - No Data-Probably Compatible

Olmesartan is an angiotensin II receptor antagonist used as an antihypertensive. Olmesartan medoxomil is a prodrug and is rapidly metabolized in the gastrointestinal tract to the active olmesartan product. No data are available on its use in lactating mothers, thus other medications should be used if suitable for the maternal medical condition (e.g., ramipril, labetalol, nifedipine). In addition, its use early postpartum in lactating mothers should be approached with caution, particularly in mothers with premature infants.

Both the ACE inhibitor family and the specific Angiotensin II receptor blockers are contraindicated in pregnancy and thus should be used with caution in women who are planning a subsequent pregnancy in the near future.

T 1/2	13 h	MW	558 Da	PB	
Tmax	1-2 h	RID		Vd	0.24 L/kg
Oral	26%	M/P		pKa	

Adult Concerns: Headache, dizziness, fatigue, hypotension, nausea, diarrhea, constipation, changes in renal function/urine output, hyperkalemia.

Adult Dose: 20-40 mg daily.

Pediatric Concerns: None reported via milk at this time.

Infant Monitoring: Drowsiness, lethargy, pallor, poor feeding, and weight gain.

Alternatives: Captopril(L2), Enalapril(L2), Ramipril(L3)

References:
1. Pharmaceutical manufacturers prescribing information.

OLSALAZINE

Trade: Dipentum

Category: Anti-Inflammatory

LRC: L3 - Limited Data-Probably Compatible

Olsalazine is a salicylate which is converted to 5-aminosalicylic acid (active component), olsalazine-sulfate and acetylated-5-ASA in the gastrointestinal tract; 5-ASA is used as an anti-inflammatory, immunosuppressant and bacteriostatic agent for treatment of ulcerative colitis.[1] After oral administration of olsalazine, only 3% is systemically absorbed while the majority is metabolized in the gastrointestinal tract to 5-ASA.

A woman breastfeeding a 4-month-old was given a single 500 mg dose of olsalazine; acetylated-5-ASA achieved concentrations of 0.8, 0.86, and 1.24 µmol/L in her breast milk at 10, 14, and 24 hours respectively.[2] Olsalazine, olsalazine-S, and 5-ASA were undetectable in breast milk. Maternal olsalazine therapy was continued for an additional 2 weeks and the infant had no adverse effects from the medication in milk. While clinically significant levels in milk are remote, infants should be monitored for gastric changes such as diarrhea.

Please see sulfasalazine monograph for further data regarding 5-ASA transfer into breast milk and suitability in lactation.

T 1/2	0.9 h	MW	302 Da	PB	>99%
Tmax	1 h	RID	0.51%	Vd	
Oral	3% (olsalazine)	M/P		pKa	3.53

Adult Concerns: Dizziness, fever, nausea, vomiting, anorexia, abdominal pain, watery diarrhea, bloody diarrhea, changes in liver function, leukopenia, thrombocytopenia, hemolytic anemia, skin rash, pruritus.

Adult Dose: 500 mg twice daily.

Pediatric Concerns: None specifically reported with this product. With other 5-ASA formulations there has been one reported case of hypersensitivity, multiple case reports of infants with bloody stools and diarrhea. In addition, case reports of pediatric patients taking other 5-ASA formulations have also found bloody diarrhea.[3] Caution in infants with G6PD deficiency.[4]

Infant Monitoring: Vomiting, diarrhea.

Alternatives:

References:
1. Pharmaceutical manufacturers prescribing information.
2. Miller LG, Hopkinson JM, Motil KJ, Corboy JE, Andersson S. Disposition of olsalazine and metabolites in breast milk. J Clin Pharmacol. 1993;33(8):703-706.
3. Werlin SL, Grand RJ. Bloody diarrhea-a new complication of sulfasalazine. J Pediatr. 1978 Mar;92(3):450.
4. Esbjorner E, Jarnerot G, Wranne L. Sulphasalazine and sulphapyridine serum levels in children to mothers treated with sulphasalazine during pregnancy and lactation. Acta Paediatr Scand. 1987;76(1):137-142.

OMADACYCLINE

Trade: Nuzyra

Category: Antibiotic, Tetracycline

LRC: L3 - No Data-Probably Compatible

Omadacycline is a modernized tetracycline with broad-spectrum activity that is designed to overcome tetracycline resistance. It is only recommended for treatment of adults with community-acquired bacterial pneumonia and acute skin and skin structure infection. As with all tetracyclines, omadacycline use during pregnancy, infancy, and childhood to the age of 8 years may cause permanent discoloration of the teeth and enamel hypoplasia.

T 1/2	15.5 h	MW	728.9 Da	PB	20%
Tmax	2.5 h	RID		Vd	190 L/kg
Oral	34.5%	M/P		pKa	

Adult Concerns: Alanine aminotransferase increased, hypertension, gamma-glutamyl transferase increased, insomnia, vomiting, constipation, nausea, aspartate aminotransferase increased, headache.

Adult Dose: 100 mg IV daily, or 300 mg daily orally.

Pediatric Concerns: The use of Omadacycline during tooth development (last half of pregnancy, infancy and childhood to the age of 8 years) may cause permanent discoloration of the teeth (yellow-gray-brown) and enamel hypoplasia.

Infant Monitoring: Omadacycline during tooth development (last half of pregnancy, infancy and childhood to the age of 8 years) may cause permanent discoloration of the teeth (yellow-gray-brown) and enamel hypoplasia.

Alternatives:

References:
1. Pharmaceutical manufacturers prescribing information.

OMALIZUMAB

Trade: Xolair

Category: Monoclonal Antibody

LRC: L3 - No Data-Probably Compatible

Omalizumab inhibits the binding of IgE to the high-affinity IgE receptor on the surface of mast cells and basophils. It is a large IgG monoclonal antibody used to treat persistent allergic asthma that cannot be controlled using inhaled corticosteroids. It works by inhibiting IgE binding to the receptor on mast cells and basophils, in turn decreasing the release of mediators in the allergic response.[1] The manufacturer suggests that omalizumab may be secreted into human breast milk based on monkey studies where milk levels were only 0.15% of maternal blood levels, which would be exceedingly low. However, no studies have been performed in humans.

Although the molecular weight of this medication is very large and the amount in breast milk is expected to be exceptionally low, there are no long-term data concerning the safety of using immune modulating medications in breastfeeding mothers. Further there are current data that suggest that some IgG drugs do transfer to milk, and perhaps the breastfed infant. Therefore, some caution is recommended, and each woman should understand the benefits and risk of using this type of medication in lactation.

T 1/2	26 days	MW	149,000 Da	PB	
Tmax	7-8 days	RID		Vd	0.078 L/kg
Oral	62%	M/P		pKa	

Adult Concerns: Headache, dizziness, fatigue, fever, pain, hypotension, thrombocytopenia, injection site reaction.

Adult Dose: Subcutaneous 150-300 mg every 2-4 weeks.

Pediatric Concerns: No data are available.

Infant Monitoring: Fever, frequent infections, poor feeding/poor weight gain.

Alternatives:

References:
1. Pharmaceutical manufacturers prescribing information.

OMEPRAZOLE

Trade: Prilosec

Category: Gastric Acid Secretion Inhibitor

LRC: L2 - Limited Data-Probably Compatible

Omeprazole is a potent inhibitor of gastric acid secretion. In a study of one patient receiving 20 mg omeprazole daily, the maternal serum concentration was negligible until 90 minutes after ingestion and then reached 950 nM at 240 min[1] The breast milk concentration of omeprazole began to rise minimally at 90 minutes after ingestion and peaked after 180 minutes at only 58 nM, or less than 7% of the highest serum level. This would indicate a maximum dose of 3 µg/kg/day in a breastfed infant. Omeprazole milk levels were essentially flat over 4 hours of observation. Omeprazole is extremely acid labile with a half-life of 10 minutes at pH values below 4.[2] Virtually all omeprazole ingested via milk would probably be destroyed in the stomach of the infant prior to absorption.

T 1/2	1 h	MW	345 Da	PB	95%
Tmax	0.5-3.5 h	RID	1.1%	Vd	
Oral	30%-40%	M/P		pKa	

Adult Concerns: Headache, dizziness, nausea, vomiting, diarrhea, constipation, abdominal pain, flatulence, changes in liver and renal function, anemia.

Adult Dose: 20 mg twice daily.

Pediatric Concerns: None reported via milk at this time.

Infant Monitoring: Unlikely to be absorbed while dissolved in milk due to instability in acid.

Alternatives: Ranitidine(L2), Famotidine(L1)

References:
1. Marshall JK, Thompson AB, Armstrong D. Omeprazole for refractory gastroesophageal reflux disease during pregnancy and lactation. Can J Gastroenterol. 1998;12(3):225-227.
2. Pilbrant A, Cederberg C. Development of an oral formulation of omeprazole. Scand J Gastroenterol Suppl. 1985;108:113-120.

ONDANSETRON

Trade: Zofran, Zuplenz

Category: Antiemetic

LRC: L2 - No Data-Probably Compatible

Ondansetron is a selective 5-HT3 receptor antagonist which blocks serotonin both centrally and peripherally.[1] This medication was originally indicated for chemotherapy induced nausea and vomiting but is now being used more frequently for other indications such as postoperative nausea and vomiting. Ondansetron has no effect on prolactin production.

At this time there are no data regarding the transfer of ondansetron to human milk; however, based on this medication's shorter half-life, larger volume of distribution and moderate oral bioavailability we predict a relatively small exposure to the infant via breast milk.

T 1/2	3-4 h	MW	365.9 Da	PB	70%-76%
Tmax	10 min, 40 min, 0.5-2 h (IV, IM, PO)	RID		Vd	2.3 L/kg
Oral	60%	M/P		pKa	

Adult Concerns: Headache, somnolence, anxiety, fever, QTc prolongation, diarrhea or constipation, changes in liver enzymes, urinary retention.

Adult Dose: 8 mg twice daily.

Pediatric Concerns: None reported via milk at this time. This medication is indicated for use in infants and children.

Infant Monitoring: Sedation, irritability, diarrhea or constipation, urinary retention.

Alternatives: Dimenhydrinate(L2)

References:
1. Pharmaceutical manufacturers prescribing information.

ORLISTAT

Trade: Alli, Xenical

Category: Antiobesity Agent

LRC: L3 - No Data-Probably Compatible

Orlistat, now available over the counter as well as prescription, is used in the management of obesity. It is a reversible inhibitor of gastric and pancreatic lipases, thus it inhibits absorption of dietary fats by 30%.[1] No studies have been performed on the transmission of orlistat to the breast milk. With high protein binding, moderately high molecular weight, and poor oral absorption, it is unlikely that orlistat would enter breast milk in clinically relevant amounts, or affect a breastfeeding infant. However, due to orlistat's effect on the absorption of fat soluble vitamins and other fats, nutritional status of a breastfeeding mother should be closely monitored.

T 1/2	1-2 h	MW	495 Da	PB	>99%
Tmax	8 h	RID		Vd	
Oral	Minimal	M/P		pKa	

Adult Concerns: Headache, oily spotting, abdominal pain, flatus with discharge, fecal urgency, fatty/oily stools, back pain.

Adult Dose: 60-120 mg three times daily.

Pediatric Concerns: Children aged 12-16 years experienced similar adverse effects as did the adult population.

Infant Monitoring: Diarrhea, fatty or oily stools, weight gain.

Alternatives:

References:
1. Pharmaceutical manufacturers prescribing information.

ORPHENADRINE CITRATE

Trade: Banflex, Disipal, Flexon, Norflex, Norgesic, Orfenace

Category: Skeletal Muscle Relaxant

LRC: L3 - No Data-Probably Compatible

Orphenadrine is an analog of diphenhydramine (Benadryl).[1] It is primarily used as a muscle relaxant although its primary effects are anticholinergic. No data are available on its secretion into breast milk. Until more is known about the transfer of this drug into human milk, use with caution in breastfeeding mothers. Observe for sedation in the breastfed infant.

T 1/2	14 h	MW	269 Da	PB	
Tmax	2-4 h	RID		Vd	
Oral	95%	M/P		pKa	

Adult Concerns: Agitation, aplastic anemia, dizziness, tremor, dry mouth, nausea, constipation.

Adult Dose: 100 mg twice daily.

Pediatric Concerns: None reported due to limited studies.

Infant Monitoring: Agitation, dizziness, tremor, dry mouth, vomiting.

Alternatives:

References:
1. Pharmaceutical manufacturers prescribing information.

OSELTAMIVIR PHOSPHATE

Trade: Tamiflu

Category: Antiviral

LRC: L2 - Limited Data-Probably Compatible

Oseltamivir is indicated for the prevention and treatment of uncomplicated acute illness due to influenza A and B infections in pediatrics and adults.[1] Oseltamivir is an oral viral neuraminidase inhibitor, which blocks or prevents viral seeding or release from infected cells and prevents viral aggregation. In a recent study of one patient who was receiving 75 mg twice daily for 5 days, the active carboxylate metabolite reached steady-state levels after 3 days and was reported to be 37-39 ng/mL.[2] Based on this data, the authors estimated the relative infant dose to be 0.5% of the maternal weight-adjusted dose. Thus, this dose is unlikely to produce clinical levels in a breastfed infant. It has recently been recommended for use in breastfeeding mothers by the CDC (Center for disease control and prevention).

In another study of oseltamivir, seven healthy patients within 48 hours of delivery were recruited. Each woman received 75 mg of oseltamivir phosphate.[3] Plasma and breast milk samples were obtained at times 0, 0.5, 1, 2, 4, 8, 12, and 24 hours after the first dose. The samples were analyzed for oseltamivir and it's active metabolite, oseltamivir carboxylate levels. Data suggested breast milk concentrations of oseltamivir phosphate peaked at 4.2 hours at an average concentration in milk of 2.8 ng/mL. Peak concentrations in milk occurred at 3.4 hours and 18.9 hours for the phosphate and carboxylate forms respectively. Levels in milk were exceedingly low.

T 1/2	6-10 h	MW	312 Da	PB	42%
Tmax		RID	0.04%-0.47%	Vd	0.37 L/kg
Oral	75%	M/P		pKa	7.75

Adult Concerns: Nausea, vomiting, abdominal pain, diarrhea.

Adult Dose: 75 mg twice daily for 5 days.

Pediatric Concerns: None reported via milk.

Infant Monitoring: Vomiting, diarrhea (unlikely due to low RID).

Alternatives:

References:
1. Center for Disease Control. Influenza Antiviral Medications: Summary for Clinicians [Online]. http://www.cdc.gov/flu/professionals/antivirals/summary-clinicians.htm
2. Wentges-van HN, van EM, van der Laan JW. Oseltamivir and breastfeeding. Int J Infect Dis. 2008;12(4):451.
3. Greer L, Leff R, Rogers V, et al. Pharmacokinetics of oseltamivir in breast milk and maternal plasma. Am J Obstet Gynecol. 2011;204:524.e521–524.

OSMOTIC LAXATIVES

Trade: Acilac, Citrate of Magnesia, Citromag, Duphalac, Milk of Magnesia, Saline laxative

Category: Laxative

LRC: L2 - No Data-Probably Compatible

Osmotic or saline laxatives comprise a large amount of magnesium and phosphate compounds, but all work similarly in that they osmotically pull and retain water in the gastrointestinal tract, thus functioning as laxatives. Because they are poorly absorbed, they largely stay in the gastrointestinal tract and are eliminated without significant systemic absorption.

Magnesium and phosphate salts absorbed systemically would be rapidly eliminated by the kidneys in normal individuals. Caution is recommended in individuals with cardiovascular or renal anomalies. Magnesium Forms (Milk of Magnesia, Citrate of Magnesia, Phillips Milk of Magnesia, etc.): magnesium citrate, magnesium hydroxide, and magnesium sulfate compose the usual forms of magnesium laxatives. Only 15%-30% of magnesium salts may be absorbed from the gastrointestinal tract, the remaining is retained in the intestinal lumen and keeps water in the intestinal lumen thus producing a laxative effect.

Phosphate Forms (Fleet, Visicol): Sodium phosphate solutions containing both dibasic sodium phosphate and monobasic sodium phosphate are used to empty the bowel prior to colonoscopy and other procedures. Approximately 1%-20% of the sodium and phosphate in such preparations is absorbed. It is very unlikely that the use of these saline laxatives would increase maternal plasma levels high enough to induce changes in electrolyte content of human milk.

While we do not have specific data on the use of higher doses of oral magnesium salts or of the phosphates, the breast cell controls the electrolyte concentrations of milk closely. Minute changes in maternal levels which could potentially occur following the use of these laxatives, would not likely alter milk content of these electrolytes.

T 1/2		MW		PB	
Tmax		RID		Vd	
Oral	Most likely poor	M/P		pKa	

Adult Concerns: Diarrhea, gut cramping, hyperphosphatemia and serious electrolyte disturbances have been reported in some patients at increased risk for electrolyte disturbances. With magnesium salts, especially in renally impaired patients, hypotension, cardiac arrhythmias or arrest, loss of deep tendon reflexes, and confusion may occur.

Adult Dose: Highly variable.

Pediatric Concerns: None reported via milk.

Infant Monitoring:

Alternatives:

References:
1. AHFS Drug Information. Bethesda, MD: American Society of Health System Pharmacists; 2003.

OXACILLIN

Trade: Bactocill, Prostaphlin

Category: Antibiotic, Penicillin

LRC: L2 - No Data-Probably Compatible

Oxacillin is a semisynthetic penicillin antibiotic indicated for the treatment of infections caused by staphylococci bacteria; oxacillin can be used in neonates, pediatrics, and adults.[1] Penicillins generally transfer into breast milk in small concentrations and are considered compatible with breastfeeding.

T 1/2	20-60 min	MW	441 Da	PB	94%
Tmax	IV: 5 min, IM: 30-60 min	RID		Vd	0.11 L/kg
Oral		M/P		pKa	

Adult Concerns: Fever, nausea, vomiting, diarrhea, changes in liver and renal function, interstitial nephritis, hematuria, leukopenia, neutropenia, thrombocytopenia.

Adult Dose: 250-1000 mg IM or IV every 4-6 hours.

Pediatric Concerns: None reported via milk at this time.

Infant Monitoring: Vomiting, diarrhea, changes in gastrointestinal flora, and rash.

Alternatives:

References:
1. Pharmaceutical manufacturers prescribing information.

OXALIPLATIN

Trade: Eloxatin, Eloxatine, O-Plat, Oxalip

Category: Antineoplastic

LRC: L5 - No Data-Hazardous

Oxaliplatin is a platinum-containing anticancer compound. Its kinetics are similar to cisplatin with a biexponential model of elimination. The decline of ultrafilterable platinum levels following oxaliplatin administration is triphasic, characterized by two relatively short distribution phases (0.43 hours and 16.8 hours) and a long-terminal elimination phase (391 hours).[1,2] Check the similar drug, cisplatin, for published milk levels. Platinum is extensively bound in peripheral tissues, which accounts for its extraordinarily long elimination half-life. While breast milk levels are unavailable, but are probably low, breastfeeding is not advisable for weeks and should probably be discontinued for this infant, unless milk platinum levels can be measured. Two options are suggested. One, breast milk should be tested for platinum levels and not used as long as they are measurable; two, without measuring platinum levels, breastfeeding should be permanently interrupted for this infant.

T 1/2	391 h	MW	397.3 Da	PB	Platinum: >90%
Tmax		RID		Vd	6.28 L/kg
Oral		M/P		pKa	1.3, 7.23

Adult Concerns: Rash, urticaria, erythema, pruritus, and, rarely, bronchospasm and hypotension.

Adult Dose:

Pediatric Concerns:

Infant Monitoring: Avoid in lactation.

Alternatives:

References:
1. Grochow LB, Ames MM. A Clinician's Guide to Chemotherapy Pharmacokinetics and Pharmacodynamics. 1st ed. Baltimore, MD: Williams & Wilkins; 1998.
2. Pharmaceutical manufacturers prescribing information.

OXAPROZIN

Trade: Daypro

Category: NSAID

LRC: L3 - No Data-Probably Compatible

Oxaprozin belongs to the NSAID family of analgesics and is reputed to have lesser gastrointestinal side effects than others.[1] Although its long half-life could prove troublesome in breastfed infants, it is probably poorly transferred to human milk. No data on transfer into human milk are available although it is known to transfer to animal milk.

T 1/2	42-50 h	MW	293 Da	PB	99%
Tmax	3-5 h	RID		Vd	
Oral	95%	M/P		pKa	4.3

Adult Concerns: Headache, dizziness, confusion, sedation, tinnitus, dyspepsia, nausea, vomiting, abdominal pain, diarrhea, constipation, gastric bleeding, anorexia, changes in liver and renal function, anemia, edema.

Adult Dose: 600-1200 mg daily.

Pediatric Concerns: None reported, but ibuprofen preferred in absence of data.

Infant Monitoring: Vomiting, diarrhea.

Alternatives: Ibuprofen (L1), naproxen (L3), ketorolac (L2).

References:
1. Pharmaceutical manufacturers prescribing information.

OXAZEPAM

Trade: Alepam, Murelax, Serax, Serepax

Category: Antianxiety

LRC: L2 - Limited Data-Probably Compatible

Oxazepam is a typical benzodiazepine and is used in anxiety disorders. Of the benzodiazepines, oxazepam is the least lipid soluble, which accounts for its low levels in milk. In one study of a patient receiving 10 mg three times daily for 3 days, the concentration of oxazepam in breast milk was relatively constant between 24 and 30 µg/L from the evening of the first day.[1] The milk/plasma ratio ranged from 0.1 to 0.33. The authors suggest that less than 1/1000th of the maternal dose was transferred to the infant. It is unlikely that significant amounts will enter the breast milk. In a study of a single mother who consumed 15-30 mg oxazepam daily, levels in breast milk were approximately 10% of maternal levels at 4 hours after the dose. In 12 milk samples collected, oxazepam levels ranged from 11 to 26 µg/L.[2]

In another study of a 22-year-old mother consuming 80 mg of diazepam and 30 mg of oxazepam, levels of diazepam and oxazepam in milk, mother's plasma and infant's plasma were reported.[3] The mean milk/plasma ratio of oxazepam was found to be 0.1, with milk concentrations ranging from 8-30 µg/L. The infant plasma concentrations on days 14 and 25 of therapy were 7.5 µg/L and 9.6 µg/L. No oxazepam was detected in milk 8 days following cessation of oxazepam. No untoward effects were noted in the infant. The authors conclude that the levels of benzodiazepines such as oxazepam in milk are minimal and are unlikely to cause untoward effects in the breastfed infant.

T 1/2	8 h	MW	287 Da	PB	97%
Tmax	3 h	RID	0.28%-1%	Vd	0.7-1.6 L/kg
Oral	97%	M/P	0.1-0.33	pKa	1.7, 11.6

Adult Concerns: Sedation, dizziness, confusion, hypotension.

Adult Dose: 10-30 mg three-four times daily.

Pediatric Concerns: None reported via milk at this time.

Infant Monitoring: Sedation, slowed breathing rate, not waking to feed/poor feeding, and weight gain.

Alternatives: Lorazepam(L3)

References:
1. Wretlind M. Excretion of oxazepam in breast milk. Eur J Clin Pharmacol. 1987;33(2):209-210.
2. Rane A, Sundwall A, Tomson G. Oxazepam withdrawal in the neonatal period. Lakartidningen. 1979;76:4416-4417.
3. Dusci LJ, Good SM, Hall RW, Ilett KF. Excretion of diazepam and its metabolites in human milk during withdrawal from combination high dose diazepam and oxazepam. Br J Clin Pharmacol. 1990;29:123-126.

OXCARBAZEPINE

Trade: Trileptal

Category: Anticonvulsant

LRC: L3 - No Data-Probably Compatible

Oxcarbazepine is a derivative of carbamazepine and is used in the treatment of partial seizures. It is rapidly metabolized to 10-monohydroxy (MHD), an active metabolite with a longer half-life (~9 hours). In a brief and somewhat incomplete study of a pregnant patient who received 300 mg three times daily while pregnant, plasma levels were studied in her infant for the first 5 days postpartum while the infant was breastfeeding.[1] While no breast milk levels were reported, plasma levels of MHD in the infant were essentially the same as the mother's immediately after delivery, suggesting complete transfer transplacentally of the drug. However, while breastfeeding for the next 5 days, plasma levels of MHD in the infant declined significantly from approximately 7 µg/mL to 0.2 µg/mL on the fifth day. The decay of MHD concentrations in neonatal plasma during the first 4 days postpartum indicated first order elimination. The plasma MHD levels on day 5 amounted to 7% of those one day postpartum (93% drop in 5 days). The authors estimated the milk/plasma ratio to be 0.5. No neonatal side effects were reported by the authors.

T 1/2	2 h ; 9 h MHD	MW	252 Da	PB	40%
Tmax	4.5 h	RID		Vd	0.7 L/kg
Oral	Complete	M/P	0.5	pKa	10.7

Adult Concerns: Headache, dizziness, drowsiness, confusion, diplopia, nystagmus, nausea, vomiting, abdominal pain, diarrhea, changes in liver function, hyponatremia, thrombocytopenia, abnormal gait, tremor, skin rashes.

Adult Dose: 300-600 mg twice daily.

Pediatric Concerns: None reported in one study.

Infant Monitoring: Sedation or irritability, not waking to feed/poor feeding, diarrhea and weight gain; if clinical symptoms arise check liver function and/or CBC.

Alternatives: Carbamazepine(L2)

References:
1. Bulau P, Paar WD, von Unruh GE. Pharmacokinetics of oxcarbazepine and 10-hydroxy-carbazepine in the newborn child of an oxcarbazepine-treated mother. Eur J Clin Pharmacol. 1988;34(3):311-313.

OXYBUTYNIN

Trade: Ditropan, Oxybutyn

Category: Renal-Urologic Agent

LRC: L3 - No Data-Probably Compatible

Oxybutynin is an anticholinergic agent used to provide antispasmodic effects for conditions characterized by involuntary bladder spasms and reduces urinary urgency and frequency. It has been used in children down to 5 years of age at doses of 15 mg daily.[1] No data on transfer of this product to human milk is available. But oxybutynin is a tertiary amine, which is poorly absorbed orally (only 6%). Further, the maximum plasma levels (Cmax) generally attained are less than 31.7 ng/mL.[2] If one were to assume a theoretical M/P ratio of 1 (which is probably unreasonably high) and a daily ingestion of 1 L of milk, then the theoretical dose to the infant would be <2 µg/day, a dose that would be clinically irrelevant to even a neonate.

T 1/2	1-2 h	MW	393 Da	PB	
Tmax	3-6 h	RID		Vd	
Oral	6%	M/P		pKa	6.96

Adult Concerns: Nausea, dry mouth, constipation, esophagitis, urinary hesitancy, flushing, and urticaria. Palpitations, somnolence, hallucinations infrequently occur.

Adult Dose: 5 mg two to four times daily.

Pediatric Concerns: Suppression of lactation has been reported by the manufacturer.

Infant Monitoring: Nausea, dry mouth, constipation, urinary hesitancy, flushing, and urticaria.

Alternatives:

References:
1. Pharmaceutical manufacturers prescribing information.
2. Douchamps J, Derenne F, Stockis A, Gangji D, Juvent M, Herchuelz A. The pharmacokinetics of oxybutynin in man. Eur J Clin Pharmacol. 1988;35(5):515-520.

OXYCODONE

Trade: Endone, Oxecta, Oxy IR, OxyContin, Oxyfast, Proladone, Supeudol

Category: Analgesic

LRC: L3 - Limited Data-Probably Compatible

Oxycodone is similar to hydrocodone and is a mild analgesic somewhat stronger than codeine. Small amounts are secreted in breast milk. Following a dose of 5-10 mg every 4-7 hours, maternal levels peaked at 1-2 hours, and analgesia persisted for up to 4 hours.[1] Reported milk levels range from <5 to 226 µg/L. Maternal plasma levels were 14-35 µg/L. The authors suggest a milk/plasma ratio of approximately 3.4. Although active metabolites were not measured, the authors suggest that an exclusively breastfed infant would receive a maximum 8% of the maternal dosage of oxycodone. No reports of untoward effects in infants were found.

In another study, 50 post-cesarean women received 30 mg oxycodone rectally, and 10 mg orally up to every 2 hours as needed. The ranges of oxycodone given in the first 0-24 hours and 24-48 hours were 30-90 mg (mode 60 mg) and 0-90 mg (mode 40 mg). The average maternal plasma levels at 0-24 hours and 24-48 hours were 18 (range

0-42) ng/mL and 12 (range 0-40) ng/mL, respectively. Average milk concentrations in samples taken during 0-24 hours and 24-48 hours were 58 (range 7-130) ng/mL and 49 (range 0-168) ng/mL, respectively. The median milk/plasma ratios were 3.2 and 3.4 at 0-24 hours and 24-28 hours. Only one infant had a detectable level of oxycodone in plasma, with a concentration of 6.6-7.4 ng/mL.[2] In addition, oxycodone was detectable in milk for up to 37 hours after the last dose in 10% of participants. These plasma and milk levels suggest that oxycodone concentrates in the milk compartment. However, the authors suggest that at doses less than 90 mg/day for up to 3 days, maternal use of oxycodone poses only a minimal threat to breastfeeding infants. This study did not measure plasma or milk concentrations at steady state or during peak plasma concentrations, therefore levels may have been higher at times.

In a recent retrospective study, the rate of CNS depression in breastfeeding infants was compared between three cohorts of breastfeeding women receiving oxycodone, codeine, and acetaminophen for alleviation of postpartum pain.[3] The mothers were receiving doses that were within the recommended adult dosages. The rates of infant CNS depression in the three groups was as follows: oxycodone group - 20.1%; codeine group - 16.7%; acetaminophen group - 0.5%. While in the oxycodone group, symptoms appeared in mothers receiving median doses of 0.4 mg/kg/day (28 mg for a 70 kg individual), symptoms in the codeine group appeared at 1.4 mg/kg/day (98 mg/day for a 70 kg individual). Although CNS depression seemed to appear over a wide range of doses, it was found that higher doses were more likely to cause symptoms in the breastfed infant. This pattern held true for both the oxycodone as well as the codeine group. Further, maternal sedation was more likely with the use of oxycodone than with the use of codeine.

There are two additional case reports regarding infant adverse effects with maternal oxycodone use in lactation.[4,5] In the first case, the mother of a full term infant reported her infant had become difficult to rouse and unable to feed on day 4 of life.[4] At the ER the infant was found to have pinpoint pupils, hypothermia, lethargy and could rouse to noxious stimuli. The mother reported taking oxycodone 10 mg the night before and 5 mg that morning for post c-section pain. After the infant was given naloxone, he woke up within 2 minutes and was able to feed. After 24 hours of observation the infant was discharged home and the mother was told to stop the oxycodone and resume breastfeeding 24 hours later.

In the second case, a 45-day-old infant was brought to the ER for slowed breathing and decreased feeds for 24 hours and an 8 day history of constipation.[5] On examination, she was reported to have pinpoint pupils, labored breathing that was shallow, slow, and irregular and sluggish movements. The mother reported taking oxycodone 5 mg every 4-6 hours for episiotomy pain. A urine drug screen on the infant revealed a hydromorphone level of > 2,000 ng/mL (cut off for positive result for opioid metabolites = 5 ng/mL). After multiple episodes of apnea and oxygen saturations at 60% she required intubation. Two days later the infant was discharged from the pediatric ICU with no long-term sequelae.

The above data suggest that oxycodone may pose a greater risk of causing infant sedation and that this risk is dose related. The use of doses greater than 40 mg/day are discouraged in opiate naive breastfeeding mothers. Higher doses maybe acceptable in breastfeeding mothers whom received opiates regularly during their pregnancy.

T 1/2	2-4 h	MW	351 Da	PB	45%
Tmax	1-2 h	RID	1.01%-4.55%	Vd	2.6 L/kg
Oral	60%-87%	M/P	3.4	pKa	8.5

Adult Concerns: Sedation, respiratory depression/apnea, nausea, vomiting, constipation, urinary retention, weakness.

Adult Dose: 5-10 mg every 6 hours as needed.

Pediatric Concerns: Multiple case reports and studies have reported sedation (20.1%), difficulty breathing, and difficulty feeding in infants exposed to oxycodone via breast milk; especially at doses higher than 30 mg/day (median = 0.4 mg/kg/day).[3-5]

Infant Monitoring: Sedation, slowed breathing rate, pallor, difficulty feeding, constipation, and appropriate weight gain.

Alternatives: Acetaminophen(L1), NSAIDs, Hydromorphone(L3)

References:

1. Marx CM, Pucin F, Carlson JD, et al. Oxycodone excretion in human milk in the puerperium. Drug Intell Clin. 1986;20:474.
2. Seaton S, Reeves M, McLean S. Oxycodone as a component of multimodal analgesia for lactating mothers after Caesarean section: relationships between maternal plasma, breast milk and neonatal plasma levels. Aust NZ J Obstet Gynaecol. 2007;47:181-185.
3. Lam J, Kelly L, Ciszkowski C, et al. Central nervous system depression of neonates breastfed by mothers receiving oxycodone for postpartum analgesia. J Pediatr. 2012 Jan;160(1):33-37.e2. Epub 2011 Aug 31.
4. Timm NL. Maternal use of oxycodone resultingin opioid intoxication in her breastfed neonate. J Pediatr. 2013;162:421-422.
5. Sulton-Villavasso C, Austin CA, Patra KP, et al. Index of suspicion. Case1. Infant who has respiratory distress. Pediatr Rev. 2012;33:279-284.

OXYMETAZOLINE

Trade: 4-Way Long Lasting, Afrin, Duramist Plus, Nasacon, Neo-Synephrine 12 Hour, Sinarest Nasal, Vicks Sinex 12 Hour, Visine L.R., Rhofade

Category: Decongestant

LRC: L3 - No Data-Probably Compatible

Oxymetazoline is a decongestant. No adequate well controlled studies exist on the use of oxymetazoline during breastfeeding; however, very little oxymetazoline is expected to reach the infant through breast milk due to its local administration and limited absorption. Oxymetazoline has been preferred over oral systemic decongestants such as pseudoephedrine during breastfeeding.[1] Oxymetazoline should only be used briefly, no more than 3 days.

Rhofade is a topical preparation of oxymetazoline used in treatment of Rosacea.

T 1/2	5-8 h	MW	260.7 Da	PB	
Tmax		RID		Vd	
Oral		M/P		pKa	7.67

Adult Concerns: Sneezing, rebound congestion, irritation, mucosa dryness, hypersensitivity.

Adult Dose: Instill 1 spray in each nostril twice daily.

Pediatric Concerns:

Infant Monitoring: Insomnia, nervousness, excitation.

Alternatives:

References:
1. Anderson PO. Decongestants and milkproduction. J Hum Lact. 2000;16:294.Letter.

OXYMORPHONE

Trade: Numorphane, Opana

Category: Analgesic

LRC: L3 - No Data-Probably Compatible

Oxymorphone is a potent opioid analgesic used to treat moderate to severe pain. On a weight basis, it is 8-10 times more potent than morphine, and it may produce more nausea and vomiting, but less constipation than morphine. It differs from morphine in its effects in that it generates less euphoria, sedation, itching, and other histamine effects and it has no antitussive properties. It is poorly absorbed orally. Milk levels are as yet unreported. However, some caution is recommended with the prolonged use of this opioid analgesic.

T 1/2	7.8 h (oral)	MW	337 Da	PB	12%
Tmax	1.9 h	RID		Vd	
Oral	10%	M/P		pKa	8.17, 9.54

Adult Concerns: Sedation, respiratory depression/apnea, nausea, vomiting, constipation, urinary retention, weakness.

Adult Dose: 10-20 every 4-6 hours.

Pediatric Concerns: None reported via milk at this time.

Infant Monitoring: Sedation, slowed breathing rate/apnea, pallor, constipation and not waking to feed/poor feeding.

Alternatives: Hydromorphone(L3), Hydrocodone(L3), Morphine(L3)

References:
1. Pharmaceutical manufacturers prescribing information.

OXYTOCIN

Trade: Pitocin, Syntocinon

Category: Pituitary Hormone

LRC: L2 - Limited Data-Probably Compatible

Oxytocin is an endogenous hormone produced by the posterior pituitary and has uterine and myoepithelial muscle cell stimulant properties, as well as vasopressive and antidiuretic effects. Prepared synthetically, it is bioavailable via IV and intranasal applications. It is destroyed orally by chymotrypsin in the stomach of adults and systemically by the liver. It is known to be secreted in small amounts into human milk.

Takeda reported that mean oxytocin concentrations in human milk at postpartum day 1 to 5 were 4.5, 4.7, 4, 3.2, and 3.3 microunits/mL respectively.[1] The oral absorption in neonates is unknown but probably minimal. Intranasal sprays (Syntocinon) contain 40 IU/mL with a recommended typical dose being one spray (3 drops) in each nostril to induce let-down. This is roughly equivalent to 2 IU per drop or a total dose of approximately 12 IU per let-down dose. Oxytocin has been used to help mother's express milk for premature infants. The efficacy was tested in a randomized trial, where 27 mothers received intranasal oxytocin and 24 received placebo. There was no difference in total milk production between the two groups, indicating that oxytocin did not improve breastmilk expression.[2] Thus this study suggests that oxytocin may not be effective in mothers "who already have oxytocin mediated let-downs." But it still may have some usefulness in mothers who apparently do not have let-downs. Although oxytocin is secreted in small amounts in breast milk, no untoward effects have been noted. However, chronic use of intranasal oxytocin may lead to dependence and should be limited to the first week postpartum.

T 1/2	3-5 min	MW	>1000 Da	PB	
Tmax		RID		Vd	
Oral	Minimal	M/P		pKa	6.56

Adult Concerns: Hypotension, hypertension, water intoxication and excessive uterine contractions, uterine hypertonicity, spasm.

Adult Dose: Varies if used for induction or postpartum hemorrhage.

Pediatric Concerns: None via breast milk.

Infant Monitoring:

Alternatives:

References:
1. Takeda S, Kuwabara Y, Mizuno M. Concentrations and origin of oxytocin in breast milk. Endocrinol Jpn. 1986;33(6):821-826.
2. Fewtrell MS, Loh KL, Blake A, Ridout DA, Hawdon J. Randomised, double blind trial of oxytocin nasal spray in mothers expressing breast milk for preterm infants. Arch Dis Child Fetal Neonatal Ed. 2006;91(3):F169-F174.

PACLITAXEL

Trade: Anzatax, Biotax, Paxene, Taxol

Category: Antineoplastic

LRC: L5 - Limited Data-Hazardous

Paclitaxel inhibits the reorganization of the microtubule network which is essential for mitotic cell functions. It is commonly used in Kaposi's sarcoma, metastatic breast cancer, and numerous other cancers. Paclitaxel is eliminated in a biphasic manner with a terminal elimination half-life of about 27 hours. It has a large molecular weight and a huge volume of distribution, which suggests extensive extravascular distribution/binding to peripheral tissues.[1]

In a study of one mother undergoing paclitaxel chemotherapy (30 mg/m² or 56.1 mg) for papillary thyroid cancer, milk levels were determined at 4, 28, 172, and 316 hours following infusion.[2] The AUC0-316h for paclitaxel was 247.9 mg.h/L. The average concentration in milk was 0.784 mg/L with a RID of 14.7%. Levels were below the limit of detection at 316 hours after final infusion. Because this dose was lower than normal, higher doses may require a longer duration of interruption.

In another study, of a mother who received injections of paclitaxel (80 mg/m²), plasma paclitaxel concentrations of 2050 ng/mL were reached 1 hour following chemotherapy, with a rapid decline in plasma concentration over the following 7.5 hours.[3] Milk samples were taken at numerous time intervals ranging from 2.75 hours to 359.75 hours. Levels in milk ranged from 111.4 ng/mL at 2.75 hours, 63.48 ng/mL at 6 hours, and undetectable (< 2.5 ng/mL) at 71.25 hours. Unfortunately, instead of calculating the RID from the AUC, the authors in this study provided an RID of 0.247% at the 27 hour sample, and 0.091% at the 72 hour sample. Levels early in the treatment cycle will be much higher.

Paclitaxel is potentially hazardous to breastfeeding infants. Mothers should withhold breastfeeding for at least 72 hours and perhaps longer depending on the dose received.

T 1/2	13-52 h	MW	853 Da	PB	89%-98%
Tmax		RID	0.79%-22.88%	Vd	5.6-17 L/kg
Oral		M/P		pKa	

Adult Concerns: Flushing, hypotension, arrhythmias, dyspnea, stomatitis, nausea, vomiting, and diarrhea, changes in liver and renal function, neutropenia, leukopenia, myalgia, arthralgia, edema.

Adult Dose: 135-175 mg/m^2 every 3 weeks.

Pediatric Concerns: None reported via milk at this time.

Infant Monitoring: Withhold breastfeeding for at least six to 10 days after treatment.

Alternatives:

References:
1. Pharmaceutical manufacturers prescribing information.
2. Griffin SJ, Milla M, Baker TE, Liu T, Wang H, Hale TW. Transfer of carboplatin and paclitaxel into breast milk. J Hum Lact. 2012 Nov;28(4):457-459. doi: 10.1177/0890334412459374. PMID: 23087196.
3. Jackson CGCA, Morris T, Hung N, Hung T. Breast milk paclitaxel excretion following intravenous chemotherapy-a case report. Br J Cancer. 2019 Aug;121(5):421-424. doi: 10.1038/s41416-019-0529-z. Epub 2019 Jul 31. PubMed 31363168.

PALIPERIDONE

Trade: Invega, Invega Sustenna

Category: Antipsychotic, Atypical

LRC: L3 - No Data-Probably Compatible

Paliperidone, 9-hydroxyrisperidone, is an atypical antipsychotic agent used in the treatment of schizophrenia, schizoaffective disorder, and as an adjunct to mood stabilizers and/or antidepressants. It is the major metabolite of risperidone.

In a study of one patient receiving 6 mg/day of risperidone at steady state, the peak plasma level of approximately 130 µg/L occurred 4 hours after an oral dose.[1] Peak milk levels of risperidone and 9-hydroxyrisperidone were approximately 12 µg/L and 40 µg/L respectively. The estimated daily dose of risperidone and metabolite (risperidone equivalents) was 4.3% of the weight-adjusted maternal dose. The milk/plasma ratios calculated from areas under the curve over 24 hours were 0.42 and 0.24, respectively for risperidone and 6-hydroxyrisperidone.

In another study, the transfer of risperidone and 9-hydroxyrisperidone to milk was studied in two breastfeeding women and one woman with risperidone-induced galactorrhea.[2] In case two (risperidone dose = 42.1 µg/kg/day), the average concentration of risperidone and 9-hydroxyrisperidone in milk (Cav) was 2.1 and 6 µg/L respectively. The relative infant dose was 2.8% of the maternal dose. In case 3 (risperidone dose = 23.1 µg/kg/day), the average concentration of risperidone and 9-hydroxyrisperidone in milk (Cav) was 0.39 and 7.06 µg/L respectively. The milk/plasma ratio determined in 2 women was <0.5 for both risperidone compounds. The relative infant doses were 2.3%, 2.8%, and 4.7% (as risperidone equivalents) of the maternal weight-adjusted doses in these three cases. Risperidone and 9-hydroxyrisperidone were not detected in the plasma of the two breastfed infants studied, and no adverse effects were noted.

Paliperidone (9-hydroxyrisperidone) is known to be secreted into human milk in low levels. Paliperidone elevates prolactin levels and therefore you must monitor patients on this drug for hyperprolactinemia.

T 1/2	Oral: 23 h, IM: 25-49 days	MW	427 Da	PB	74%
Tmax	Oral: 24 h, IM: 13 days	RID		Vd	6.95 L/kg
Oral	28%	M/P		pKa	2.6, 8.2

Adult Concerns: Somnolence, headache, tachycardia, tremor, weight gain, nausea, vomiting, injection site reactions, weakness, anxiety, hyperkinesia, orthostatic hypotension.

Adult Dose: 6 mg once daily.

Pediatric Concerns:

Infant Monitoring: Sedation or irritability, apnea, not waking to feed/poor feeding, extrapyramidal symptoms, and weight gain.

Alternatives: Quetiapine(L2)

References:
1. Hill RC, McIvor RJ, Wojnar-Horton RE, Hackett LP, Ilett KF. Risperidone distribution and excretion into human milk: case report and estimated infant exposure during breast-feeding. J Clin Psychopharmacol. 2000;20(2):285-286.
2. Ilett KF, Hackett LP, Kristensen JH, Vaddadi KS, Gardiner SJ, Begg EJ. Transfer of risperidone and 9-hydroxyrisperidone into human milk. Ann Pharmacother. 2004;38(2):273-276.

PALONOSETRON

Trade: Aloxi

Category: Antiemetic

LRC: L3 - No Data-Probably Compatible

Palonosetron hydrochloride is a selective 5HT3 receptor antagonist, blocking serotonin binding, and reducing the vomiting reflex. It is used to reduce chemotherapy induced nausea and vomiting.[1] It works similarly to ondansetron. No data are available on its transfer into human milk.

T 1/2	40 h	MW	333 Da	PB	62%
Tmax		RID		Vd	8.3 L/kg
Oral		M/P		pKa	

Adult Concerns: Headache, anxiety, dizziness, QTc prolongation, diarrhea or constipation, changes in liver enzymes, urinary retention.

Adult Dose: 0.25 mg 30 minutes before chemotherapy.

Pediatric Concerns: No data are available.

Infant Monitoring: Sedation, irritability, diarrhea or constipation, urinary retention.

Alternatives: Ondansetron(L2)

References:
1. Pharmaceutical manufacturers prescribing information.

PAMABROM

Trade: Bayer Select Maximum Strength Menstrual, Fem-1, Lurline PMS, Midol PMS, Midol Pre-Menstrual Syndrome

Category: Diuretic

LRC: L4 - No Data-Possibly Hazardous

Pamabrom is a weak diuretic used in OTC analgesics for relief of premenstrual syndrome. The active ingredient is 8-bromotheophylline. There are no adequate and well-controlled studies or case reports in breastfeeding women.[1] This a is bromide-containing product that should not be used in breastfeeding mothers.

T 1/2		MW	348 Da	PB	
Tmax		RID		Vd	
Oral		M/P		pKa	

Adult Concerns: Urine discoloration.

Adult Dose: 50 mg every 6 hours.

Pediatric Concerns:

Infant Monitoring: Observe for fluid loss, dehydration, lethargy; monitor maternal milk supply.

Alternatives:

References:
1. Pharmaceutical manufacturer drug information, 2010.

PAMIDRONATE \

Trade: Aredia

Category: Calcium Regulator

LRC: L3 - Limited Data-Probably Compatible

Pamidronate is an inhibitor of bone-resorption. Although its mechanism of action is obscure, it possibly absorbs to the calcium phosphate crystal in bone and blocks dissolution (reabsorption) of this mineral component in bone, thus reducing turnover of bone calcium.

A 39-year-old patient presented in the first month of pregnancy with reflex sympathetic dystrophy. Because she wished to continue breastfeeding, she was treated with monthly IV doses of pamidronate (30 mg) postpartum. Following the first dose, breast milk was assayed for pamidronate content. After infusion, breast milk was pumped and collected into two portions: 0-24 hours and 25-48 hours. None was detected (limit of detection, 0.4 µmol/L). The authors suggested that pamidronate could be considered safe for use in lactating women. Pamidronate is poorly absorbed (0.3% to 3% of a dose) after oral administration and thus any present in milk would not likely be absorbed by the infant.

T 1/2	21-35 h	MW	369 Da	PB	
Tmax		RID		Vd	
Oral	Very limited	M/P		pKa	

Adult Concerns: Headache, fatigue, fever, hypertension, increased parathyroid hormone, abdominal pain, nausea, dyspepsia, anorexia, hypophosphatemia, hypocalcemia, hypomagnesemia, hypokalemia, anemia, osteonecrosis, arthralgias, and myalgias.

Adult Dose: 60 to 90 mg IV monthly.

Pediatric Concerns: None reported via milk.

Infant Monitoring: Vomiting, reflux, weight gain.

Alternatives:

References:
1. Siminoski K, Fitzgerald AA, Flesch G, Gross MS. Intravenous pamidronate for treatment of reflex sympathetic dystrophy during breast feeding. J Bone Miner Res. 2000;15(10):2052-2055.

PANCRELIPASE

Trade: Cotazym, Cotazym (FM), Cotazym S Forte, Creon, Digess, Digeszyme, Enzymall, Palcaps, Pancrease (FM), Pancreaze, Pancrelipase, Pangestyme EC, Panocaps, Ultracaps, Ultrase MT20, Ultresa, Viokace, Zenpep

Category: Dietary Supplement

LRC: L3 - No Data-Probably Compatible

Pancrelipase is a pancreatic enzyme replacement product containing varying proportions of amylase, lipase, and protease, which are of porcine origin. Enzyme replacement therapy with products containing pancreatic enzymes amylase, lipase, and protease are used in conditions of exocrine pancreatic insufficiency, such as that which occurs in relation with cystic fibrosis, chronic pancreatitis or after pancreatectomy.

Amylase, lipase, and protease are pancreatic enzymes normally released from the pancreas to the upper gastrointestinal tract of humans to aid in the digestion of carbohydrates, fats, and proteins, respectively. In conditions such as cystic fibrosis or chronic pancreatitis, the pancreas lacks the ability to release these enzymes, thereby hindering the digestion and consequent absorption of carbohydrates, fats, and proteins. Malabsorption of these dietary nutrients eventually leads to malnutrition and ill-health. To avoid this, it is essential to supplement such patients with pancreatic enzyme replacement therapy.

There are no adequate or well-controlled studies on pancreatic enzyme replacement therapy in lactation.[1] But considering that the oral bioavailability of this product is negligible,[1] it can be presumed that none to minimal amounts get transferred to breast milk. Further, the high molecular weight of the individual constituents of this product also makes the possibility of transfer into human milk highly unlikely. Therefore, pancreatic enzyme replacement therapy is considered compatible with breastfeeding.

T 1/2	Amy/lipase/prot: 3 h/7-13 h/	MW	Amy/lipase/prot: 50,000/47,000/43,000 Da	PB	
Tmax	30 min	RID		Vd	
Oral	Negligible	M/P		pKa	

Adult Concerns: Headache, dizziness, fatigue, nausea, vomiting, abdominal pain, flatulence, diarrhea, rash, urticaria.

Adult Dose: 500-2500 lipase units/kg/meal. Do not exceed 6000 lipase units/kg/meal.

Pediatric Concerns:

Infant Monitoring:

Alternatives:

References:
1. Product Information. Pancreaze(TM) Delayed-Release Oral Capsules, Pancrelipase Delayed-Release Oral Capsules. Titusville, NJ: McNeil Pediatrics; 2010.

PANTOPRAZOLE

Trade: Pantoloc, Protonix

Category: Gastric Acid Secretion Inhibitor

LRC: L1 - Limited Data-Compatible

Pantoprazole is a proton-pump inhibitor similar to omeprazole. It is used primarily to suppress acid production in the stomach for treatment of gastroesophageal reflux or peptic ulcer disease. The pharmaceutical manufacturer reports 0.02% of an administered dose is excreted into milk.[1]

In a 61.6 kg patient who received a single 40 mg tablet, pantoprazole levels in milk were undetectable except at 2 hours (0.036 mg/L) and 4 hours (0.024 mg/L) after administration.[2] The pantoprazole levels in milk were estimated to be only 2.8% of the maternal plasma levels (AUC) so the M/P ratio is extraordinarily low. Using the highest concentration achieved, the relative infant dose would only be 0.95%. The daily dose would be many times lower than this as the milk levels were undetectable at 5 hours. As with all the proton-pump inhibitors, pantoprazole is completely unstable in an acid milieu and when presented in milk, it would be largely destroyed before absorption.

T 1/2	1.5 h	MW	383 Da	PB	98%
Tmax	2-4 h	RID	1%	Vd	0.32 L/kg
Oral	77% enteric-coated	M/P	0.028	pKa	3.8

Adult Concerns: Headache, dizziness, dry mouth, nausea, vomiting, diarrhea, abdominal pain, flatulence, changes in liver and renal function, rash.

Adult Dose: 40-80 mg daily.

Pediatric Concerns: None reported via milk at this time.

Infant Monitoring: Unlikely to be absorbed while dissolved in milk due to instability in acid.

Alternatives: Omeprazole(L2), Ranitidine(L2), Famotidine(L1)

References:
1. Pharmaceutical manufacturers prescribing information.
2. Plante L, Ferron GM, Unruh M, Mayer PR. Excretion of pantoprazole in human breast. J Reprod Med. 2004 Oct;49(10):825-827.

PANTOTHENIC ACID

Trade: Vitamin B5

Category: Vitamin

LRC: L1 - Limited Data-Compatible

Pantothenic acid, or vitamin B-5, is needed to form coenzyme-A, which is a carrier carbon within the cell. Pantothenic acid is often used in high doses in excess of 10 g/day for the treatment of acne.[1] The recommended daily allowance for pregnant women is 6 mg/day, while breastfeeding women need 7 mg/day. The recommended dose for infants less than 6 months of age is 1.7 mg/day, while infants over 6 months are to receive 2 mg/day. No adverse effects from oral administration of higher oral dosages of pantothenic acid were found.[3] Concentrations found in milk are between 2 and 2.5 mg/L, with a weak correlation between maternal intake and milk levels.[2] This would correspond to a daily dose of around 0.33-0.375 mg/kg/day for breastfeeding infants.

T 1/2		MW	219 Da	PB	
Tmax		RID		Vd	
Oral		M/P		pKa	4.4

Adult Concerns: Diarrhea at large doses. Skin rash.

Adult Dose:

Pediatric Concerns: Possible skin rash, or gastrointestinal symptoms including diarrhea if large doses are used by the mother.

Infant Monitoring: Diarrhea, skin rash.

Alternatives:

References:

1. Leung LH. Pantothenic acid deficiency as the pathogenesis of acne vulgaris. Med Hypotheses. 1995 Jun;44(6):490-492.
2. Picciano MF. In: Jensen RG, ed. Handbook of Milk Composition. San Diego: Academic Press; 1995.
3. Dietary Reference Intakes for Thiamin, Riboflavin, Niacin, Vitamin B6, Folate, Vitamin B12, Pantothenic Acid, Biotin, and Choline. Food and Nutrition Board. Institude of Medicine. Washington DC: National Academy Press; 1998.

PARA-AMINOSALICYLIC ACID

Trade: Nemasol, PAS, Paser, Tubasal, 4-Aminosalicylic acid

Category: Antitubercular

LRC: L3 - Limited Data-Probably Compatible

Para-aminosalicylic acid (P-ASA), also called 4-Aminosalicylic acid, inhibits folic acid synthesis and is selective for tuberculosis (TB) bacteria.[1] This medication is primarily used for multi-drug resistant TB or when typical TB therapies cannot be used.

There is one case report of a 27-year-old woman who received 4 g of P-ASA in lactation.[2] Her milk samples were collected at 0, 1, 2, 3, 4, 9, and 12 hours after her dose and showed a maximum concentration at 3 hours of 1.1 mg/L. The maximum maternal plasma concentration was 70.1 mg/L and occurred at 2 hours postdose. This medication was eventually discontinued by the woman because of gastrointestinal adverse effects. The authors note that although concentrations in milk were low, drug interactions with other medications may increase milk levels and should be considered when assessing safety of use in lactation.

T 1/2	1 h	MW	153 Da	PB	50%-60%
Tmax	6 h	RID	0.29%	Vd	
Oral	>90%	M/P	0.09-0.17	pKa	3.68

Adult Concerns: Encephalopathy, fever, vasculitis, pericarditis, hypothyroidism, nausea, vomiting, abdominal pain, diarrhea, changes in liver function, hypoglycemia, hemolytic anemia, agranulocytosis, thrombocytopenia.

Adult Dose: 8-12 g/day divided two to three times a day.

Pediatric Concerns: No known adverse events at this time.

Infant Monitoring: Changes in feeding, vomiting, diarrhea; if clinical symptoms arise check electrolytes, liver function and/or CBC.

Alternatives:

References:

1. Pharmaceutical manufacturers prescribing information.
2. Holdiness MR. Antituberculosis drugs and breast-feeding. Arch Intern Med. 1984;144(9):1888.

PARICALCITOL

Trade: Zemplar

Category: Vitamin

LRC: L3 - No Data-Probably Compatible

Paricalcitol is a vitamin D analog used in the treatment and prevention of hyperparathyroidism due to chronic kidney disease.[1] It is similar in structure to the active metabolite of vitamin D, calcitriol. There are currently no studies on the transfer of paricalcitol to human milk. The peak plasma concentrations attained after its oral administration in patients with chronic kidney disease was in the order of 0.06-0.11 ng/mL. Due to its very high protein binding and low plasma concentrations, it is unlikely that significant amounts would enter breast milk. Further, vitamin D transfers minimally to human milk. While levels of vitamin D are normally quite low in human milk (<20 IU/L), at least one study now suggests that supplementing a mother with extraordinarily high levels of vitamin D2 can elevate milk levels, and subsequently lead to hypercalcemia in a breastfed infant.[2] The same may be true with the use of paricalcitol. Therefore, while this drug is probably safe if used in clinical doses, the effects of long-term exposure to this drug are currently unknown. Use of excessive doses should be avoided.

T 1/2	14-20 h (in chronic kidney disease)	MW	416.64 Da	PB	>99.8%
Tmax	3 h	RID		Vd	0.49-0.7 L/kg
Oral	72%-86%	M/P		pKa	

Adult Concerns: Nausea, vomiting, diarrhea, edema, hypertension, hypercalcemia, hyperphosphatemia, hypercalciuria, gastrointestinal hemorrhage, hypersensitivity reaction. Its use is contra-indicated in the presence of hypercalcemia or vitamin D toxicity.

Adult Dose: 1-2 µg daily or 2-4 µg three times a week.

Pediatric Concerns: Nausea, vomiting, diarrhea, edema, hypercalcemia, hyperphosphatemia, hypercalciuria.

Infant Monitoring: Vomiting, diarrhea.

Alternatives:

References:
1. Pharmaceutical manufacturers prescribing information.
2. Greer FR, Hollis BW, Napoli JL. High concentrations of vitamin D2 in human milk associated with pharmacologic doses of vitamin D2. J Pediatr. 1984;105(1):61-64.

PAROMOMYCIN

Trade: Humatin

Category: Amebicide

LRC: L3 - No Data-Probably Compatible

Paromomycin is an aminoglycoside antibiotic used to treat acute and chronic intestinal amebiasis.[1] Paromomycin has a large molecular weight (615 Da) and is not absorbed systemically from the maternal gastrointestinal tract; therefore, paromomycin levels in breast milk are anticipated to be very low and thus this medication is thought to pose little risk to a breastfeeding infant.

T 1/2		MW	615 Da	PB	
Tmax		RID		Vd	
Oral	None	M/P		pKa	5.74, 7.55

Adult Concerns: Nausea, abdominal cramps, diarrhea.

Adult Dose: 25-35 mg/kg/day in three divided doses for 5-10 days.

Pediatric Concerns: No data available at this time; paromomycin is recommended for use in pediatrics.

Infant Monitoring:

Alternatives:

References:
1. Pharmaceutical manufacturers prescribing information.

PAROXETINE

Trade: Aropax 20, Paxil, Seroxat

Category: Antidepressant, SSRI

LRC: L2 - Limited Data-Probably Compatible

Paroxetine is a typical serotonin reuptake inhibitor. Although it undergoes hepatic metabolism, the metabolites are not active. Paroxetine is exceedingly lipophilic and distributes throughout the body with only 1% remaining in plasma. In one case report of a mother receiving 20 mg/day paroxetine at steady state[1], the breast milk level at peak (4 hours) was 7.6 µg/L. While the maternal paroxetine dose was 333 µg/kg, the maximum daily dose to the infant was estimated at 1.14 µg/kg or 0.34% of the maternal dose.

In two studies of six and four nursing mothers, respectively,[2] the mean dose of paroxetine received by the infants in the first study was 1.13% (range 0.5-1.7) of the weight adjusted maternal dose. The mean M/P (AUC) was 0.39 (range 0.32-0.51) while the predicted M/P was 0.22. In the second study, the mean dose of paroxetine received by the infants was 1.25% (range 0.38%-2.24%) of the weight adjusted maternal dose with a mean M/P of 0.96 (range

0.31-3.33). The drug was not detected in the plasma of seven of the eight infants studied and was detected (<4 mg/L) in only one infant. No adverse effects were observed in any of the infants.

In a recent study of 16 mothers by Stowe, paroxetine levels in milk were low and varied according to maternal dose.[3] Milk/plasma ratios varied from 0.056 to 1.3. Milk levels ranged from approximately 17 µg/L, 45 µg/L, 70 µg/L, 92 µg/L, and 101 µg/L in mothers receiving a dose of 10, 20, 30, 40, and 50 mg/day respectively. Levels of paroxetine were below the limit of detection (<2 ng/mL) in all 16 infants. In a study of six women receiving 20-40 mg/day, the milk/plasma ratio ranged from 0.39 to 1.11 but averaged 0.69.[4] The average estimated dose to the infants ranged from 0.7% to 2.9% of the weight-adjusted maternal dose.

In a seventh patient, and based on AUC data, the milk/plasma ratio was 0.69 at a dose of 20 mg and 0.72 at a dose of 40 mg/day.[4] The estimated dose to the infant was 1% and 2% of the weight-adjusted maternal dose at 20 and 40 mg respectively. Paroxetine levels in milk averaged 44.3 and 78.5 µg/L over 6 hours following 20 and 40 mg doses respectively. No adverse reactions or unusual behaviors were noted in any of the infants.

In another study of 24 breastfeeding mothers who received an average dose of 17.6 mg/day (range 10-40 mg/day), the average level of paroxetine in maternal serum and milk was 45.2 ng/mL and 19.2 ng/mL respectively.[5] The average milk/plasma ratio was 0.53. The authors estimated the average infant dose to be 2.88 µg/kg/day or 2.88% of the weight-adjusted maternal dose. All infant serum levels were below the limit of detection.

Yet another study of 16 mothers taking an average of 18.75 mg/day showed that paroxetine was undetectable in any of the breastfeeding infants exposed to paroxetine.[6] A pooled analysis of 68 breastfeeding mothers taking between 10-50 mg/day reported breast milk levels between 0-153 µg/mL, with an average of 28 µg/mL. No untoward effects were noted in any of these infants exposed to paroxetine through breast milk. One infant did experience lethargy and poor weight gain, but this infant had prenatal exposure.[7]

These studies generally conclude that paroxetine can be considered relatively "safe" for breastfeeding infants as the absolute dose transferred is quite low. Plasma levels in the infants were generally undetectable. Recent data suggest that a neonatal withdrawal syndrome may occur in newborns exposed in utero to paroxetine, although there is significant difficulty in differentiating between withdrawal and toxicity depending on the timing of symptom onset.[8-10] Some symptoms of SSRI withdrawal may include crying, irritability, tachypnea, poor suck or feeding difficulties, hypertonia, tremor, hypoglycemia, seizures (rare).[11] Paroxetine is a suitable SSRI for breastfeeding women simply because the clinical dose consumed by the infant via breast milk is exceedingly low. This said, due to maternal side effects and tolerability and some controversial concerns regarding heart defects in pregnancy other SSRIs are often preferred in this population (e.g., sertraline).[12]

T 1/2	21 h	MW	329 Da	PB	95%
Tmax	5-8 h	RID	1.2%-2.8%	Vd	3-28 L/kg
Oral	Complete	M/P	0.056-1.3	pKa	9.9

Adult Concerns: Sedation, insomnia, headache, dizziness, dry mouth, nausea, constipation.

Adult Dose: 20-50 mg daily.

Pediatric Concerns: None reported via milk at this time.

Infant Monitoring: Sedation or irritability, not waking to feed/poor feeding, and weight gain.

Alternatives: Sertraline(L2)

References:

1. Spigset O, Carleborg L, Norstrom A, Sandlund M. Paroxetine level in breast milk. J Clin Psychiatry. 1996;57(1):39.
2. Begg EJ, Duffull SB, Saunders DA, et al. Paroxetine in human milk. Br J Clin Pharmacol. 1999;48(2):142-147.
3. Stowe ZN, Cohen LS, Hostetter A, Ritchie JC, Owens MJ, Nemeroff CB. Paroxetine in human breast milk and nursing infants. Am J Psychiatry. 2000;157(2):185-189.
4. Ohman R, Hagg S, Carleborg L, Spigset O. Excretion of paroxetine into breast milk. J Clin Psychiatry. 1999;60(8):519-523.
5. Misri S, Kim J, Riggs KW, Kostaras X. Paroxetine levels in postpartum depressed women, breast milk, and infant serum. J Clin Psychiatry. 2000;61(11):828-832.
6. Hendrick V, Fukuchi A, Altshuler L, Widawski M, Wertheimer A, Brunhuber MV. Use of sertraline, paroxetine and fluvoxamine by nursing women. Br J Psychiatry. 2001; 179:163-166.
7. Weissman AM, Levy BT, Hartz AJ, et al. Pooled analysis of antidepressant levels in lactating mothers, breast milk, and nursing infants. Am J Psychiatry. 2004 June;161(6):1066-1078.
8. Stiskal JA, Kulin N, Koren G, Ho T, Ito S. Neonatal paroxetine withdrawal syndrome. Arch Dis Child Fetal Neonatal Ed. 2001;84(2):F134-F135.
9. Nordeng H, Lindemann R, Perminov KV, Reikvam A. Neonatal withdrawl syndrome after in utero exposure to selective serotonin reuptake inhibitors. Acta Paediatr. 2001; 90:288-291.
10. Isbister GK, Dawson A, Whyte IM, Prior FH, Clancy C, Smith AJ. Neonatal paroxetine withdrawal syndrome or actually serotonin syndrome? Arch Dis Child Fetal Neonatal Ed. 2001;85(2):F147-F148.

11. Hudak ML, Tan RC, The Committee on Drugs and The Committee on Fetus and Newborn. Neonatal drug withdrawal. Pediatics. 2012;129(2):e540-e560.
12. Diav-Citrin O, Schechetman S, Weinbaum D, et al. Paroxetine and fluoxetine in pregnancy: a multicenter, prospective, controlled observational study. Br J Clin Pharmacol. 2008;66(5):695-705.

PAZOPANIB

Trade: Votrient

Category: Antineoplastic

LRC: L5 - No Data-Hazardous

Pazopanib is a tyrosine kinase inhibitor that blocks vascular endothelial growth factor receptor mediated angiogenesis to treat multiple forms of cancer.[1] Due to its ability to profoundly block angiogenesis, it could be hazardous to a newborn infant. No data are available on its transfer to human milk, but it should be expected to enter milk in low levels. Withhold breastfeeding for 150 hours.

T 1/2	31 h	MW	473 Da	PB	>99%
Tmax	2-4 h	RID		Vd	
Oral	Good	M/P		pKa	

Adult Concerns: Headache, fatigue, insomnia, changes in hair color, alopecia, stroke, hypertension, QTc prolongation, chest pain, myocardial infarction, heart failure, dyspepsia, nausea, vomiting, abdominal pain, anorexia, changes in liver and renal function, changes in electrolytes, leukopenia, neutropenia, thrombocytopenia, hemorrhage.

Adult Dose: 800 mg once daily.

Pediatric Concerns: There are no lactation or pediatric data at this time.

Infant Monitoring: Withhold breastfeeding for 150 hours.

Alternatives:

References:
1. Product Information. Votrient Oral Tablets, Pazopanib Oral Tablets. Research Triangle Park, NC: GlaxoSmithKline; 2009.

PEGAPTANIB SODIUM

Trade: Macugen

Category: Angiogenesis Inhibitor

LRC: L3 - No Data-Probably Compatible

Pegaptanib is used in the treatment of neovascular age-related macular degeneration. Pegaptanib can bind to vascular endothelial growth factor inhibiting its binding with receptors and thus blocking neovascularization (inhibits intra-vitreal antivascular endothelial growth factor (VEGF)) and slows vision loss.[1] There have been no studies performed to measure the levels in human milk. First, the dose use for intravitreous injections is exceedingly low (0.3 mg), and levels in the plasma compartment are even lower (approximately 8 nanogram/mL). It would be exceedingly unlikely this large polymer would ever enter the milk compartment, or be orally bioavailable, or produce a clinical effect on a breastfeeding infant.

T 1/2	10 days	MW	50,000 Da	PB	
Tmax		RID		Vd	
Oral	Nil	M/P		pKa	

Adult Concerns: Adverse effects include hypertension, blurred vision, corneal edema.

Adult Dose: 0.3 mg every 6 weeks.

Pediatric Concerns: No data are available.

Infant Monitoring: Unabsorbed orally. Minimal risk.

Alternatives:

References:
1. Pharmaceutical manufacturers prescribing information.

PEGFILGRASTIM

Trade: Neulasta

Category: Hematopoietic

LRC: L3 - No Data-Probably Compatible

Pegfilgrastim, the pegylated form of filgrastim, acts on hematopoietic cells stimulating production and maturation of neutrophil precursors.[1] It is used to enhance neutrophil recovery following chemotherapy as well as to decrease infection in patients receiving myelosuppressive anticancer drugs. There are no reported levels in human milk. Due to large molecular weight of this drug, milk levels and oral bioavailability are likely to be low. Lactation studies in rodents did not show any untoward effects on growth and development of breastfed rodents.

T 1/2	15-80 h	MW	39,000 Da	PB	
Tmax		RID		Vd	
Oral	Nil	M/P		pKa	

Adult Concerns: Headache, alopecia, pyrexia, vomiting, constipation, bone pain, myalgia, weakness, peripheral edema, rarely splenic rupture.

Adult Dose: 6 mg once per chemotherapy cycle.

Pediatric Concerns: No data are available.

Infant Monitoring: If clinical symptoms arise, check CBC.

Alternatives:

References:
1. Pharmaceutical manufacturers prescribing information.

PEGINESATIDE

Trade: Omontys

Category: Hematopoietic

LRC: L3 - No Data-Probably Compatible

Peginesatide is an erythropoiesis-stimulating agent used for the treatment of anemia found in chronic kidney disease patients on dialysis. It binds to and activates the human erythropoietin receptor and stimulates production of erythrocytes (red blood cells) in human red cell precursors.[1] The transfer of Peginesatide into human milk is still not known. However, due to its large size, its transfer to human milk is unlikely.

T 1/2	17.4-32.6 h (IV), 35.3-70.7 h (SC)	MW	45,000 Da	PB	
Tmax	48 h (SC)	RID		Vd	0.021-0.048 L/kg
Oral	Minimal	M/P		pKa	

Adult Concerns: Headache, dyspnea, cough, nausea, vomiting, diarrhea, arteriovenous fistula, muscle spasms.

Adult Dose: 1-6 mg/0.5 mL once every 4 weeks.

Pediatric Concerns: The safety and efficacy in pediatric patients have not been established.

Infant Monitoring:

Alternatives:

References:
1. Pharmaceutical manufacturers prescribing information.

PENICILLAMINE

Trade: Cuprimine, D-Penamine, Depen, Distamine, Pendramine

Category: Heavy Metal Chelator

LRC: L4 - No Data-Possibly Hazardous

Penicillamine is a potent chelating agent used to chelate copper, iron, mercury, lead, and other metals.[1,2] It is also used to suppress the immune response in rheumatoid arthritis and other immunologic syndromes. Safety has not been established during lactation, but kinetics suggest it will enter milk significantly. Penicillamine is a potent drug that requires constant observation and care by attending physicians. Recommend discontinuing lactation if this drug is mandatory.

T 1/2	1.7-7 h	MW	149 Da	PB	80%
Tmax	1-3 h	RID		Vd	
Oral	40%-70%	M/P		pKa	

Adult Concerns: Anorexia, nausea, vomiting, diarrhea, alteration of taste, elevated liver enzymes, kidney damage.

Adult Dose: 250-500 mg four times daily.

Pediatric Concerns: None reported, but caution is recommended.

Infant Monitoring: Decreased feedings, vomiting, diarrhea.

Alternatives:

References:
1. Ostensen M, Husby G. Antirheumatic drug treatment during pregnancy and lactation. Scand J Rheumatol. 1985;14(1):1-7.
2. Pharmaceutical manufacturers prescribing information.

PENICILLIN G

Trade: Ayercillin, Bicillin L-A, Crystapen, Megacillin, Pfizerpen

Category: Antibiotic, Penicillin

LRC: L1 - Limited Data-Compatible

Penicillins generally penetrate into breast milk in small concentrations, largely determined by class. Following IM doses of 100,000 units, the milk/plasma ratio varied between 0.03 and 0.13.[1,2] Milk levels varied from seven units to 60 units/L. Penicillins are generally considered suitable in lactation.

T 1/2	<1.5 h	MW	372 Da	PB	60%-80%
Tmax	1-2 h	RID		Vd	
Oral	15%-30%	M/P	0.03-0.13	pKa	2.75

Adult Concerns: Nausea, vomiting, diarrhea, changes in gastrointestinal flora, changes in renal function, rash, allergic reactions.

Adult Dose: 2.5-5 million units IV every 4 hours.

Pediatric Concerns: None reported via milk.

Infant Monitoring: Vomiting, diarrhea, changes in gastrointestinal flora, and rash.

Alternatives:

References:
1. Matsuda S. Transfer of antibiotics into maternal milk. Biol Res Pregnancy Perinatol. 1984;5(2):57-60.
2. Greene H, Burkhart B, Hobby G. Excretion of penicillin human milk following partiturition. Am J Obstet Gynecol. 1946;51:732.

PENTAMIDINE ISETHIONATE

Trade: Pentam 300, Nebupent

Category: Antiprotozoal agent

LRC: L3 - No Data-Probably Compatible

It is an aromatic diamidine antiprotozoal agent that acts against Pneumocystis jiroveci (formerly known as P. carinii pneumonia or PCP). It interferes with protozoal nuclear metabolism by inhibition of DNA, RNA, phospholipid, and protein synthesis. Similarly, its excretion in human milk is not known.[1] However, it may cause serious adverse effects to infant during pregnancy or lactation so should not be given to a pregnant and lactating patient unless its potential benefits outweigh the unknown risks.

T 1/2	9-13 h	MW	592.68 Da	PB	69%
Tmax		RID		Vd	
Oral	Minimal	M/P		pKa	

Adult Concerns: Severe hypotension, hypoglycemia, acute pancreatitis, cardiac arrhythmias, nephrotoxicity, anemia, bad taste, confusion and hallucinations, hepatotoxicity, abdominal pain, diarrhea, dyspepsia.

Adult Dose: 4 mg/kg per day for 14 to 21 days.

Pediatric Concerns: Severe hypotension, hypoglycemia, acute pancreatitis, cardiac arrhythmias, nephrotoxicity, anemia, bad taste, confusion and hallucinations, hepatotoxicity, abdominal pain, diarrhea, dyspepsia.

Infant Monitoring:

Alternatives:

References:
1. Pharmaceutical manufacturers prescribing information.

PENTAZOCINE

Trade: Fortral, Talacen, Talwin

Category: Analgesic

LRC: L3 - No Data-Probably Compatible

Pentazocine is a synthetic opiate and is also an opiate antagonist. Once absorbed it undergoes extensive hepatic metabolism and only small amounts achieve plasma levels.[1] It is primarily used as a mild analgesic. No data are available on transfer to breast milk.

T 1/2	2-3 h	MW	285 Da	PB	60%
Tmax	1-3 h	RID		Vd	4.4-7.8 L/kg
Oral	18%	M/P		pKa	9

Adult Concerns: Sedation, respiratory depression, nausea, vomiting, dry mouth, taste alteration.

Adult Dose: 50-100 mg every 3-4 hours PRN.

Pediatric Concerns: None reported due to limited studies.

Infant Monitoring: Sedation, slowed breathing rate/apnea, pallor, constipation, and not waking to feed/poor feeding.

Alternatives:

References:
1. Pharmaceutical manufacturers prescribing information.

PENTOSAN POLYSULFATE

Trade: Elmiron

Category: Renal-Urologic Agent

LRC: L2 - Limited Data-Probably Compatible

Pentosan polysulfate is a negatively charged synthetic sulfated polysaccharide with heparin-like properties; however, it is used as a urinary tract analgesic for interstitial cystitis.[1] It is structurally related to dextran sulfate with a molecular weight of 4000-6000 Da. Oral bioavailability is low, only 6% is absorbed systemically. Pentosan adheres to the bladder wall mucosa and may act as a buffer to control cell permeability preventing irritating solutes in the urine from reaching the cell membrane. Although no data are available on its transfer to human milk, its large molecular weight and poor oral bioavailability would largely preclude the transfer and absorption of clinically relevant amounts in breastfed infants.

T 1/2	20-27 h	MW	4000 to 6000 Da	PB	
Tmax	3 h	RID		Vd	
Oral	6%	M/P		pKa	

Adult Concerns: Headache, dizziness, depression, insomnia, alopecia areata, dyspepsia, nausea, vomiting, diarrhea, changes in liver function, pruritus, urticaria. Weak anticoagulant and fibrinolytic effects may cause epistaxis, bleeding gums, thrombocytopenia.

Adult Dose: 100 mg three times daily.

Pediatric Concerns: None reported via milk at this time.

Infant Monitoring: Vomiting, diarrhea.

Alternatives:

References:
1. Pharmaceutical manufacturers prescribing information.

PENTOSTATIN

Trade: Nipent

Category: Antineoplastic

LRC: L5 - No Data-Hazardous

Pentostatin is indicated for the treatment of hairy cell leukemia.[1] It is poorly bound to proteins (4%) and the mean terminal half-life is reported to be 5.7 hours (increased to 18 hours with poor renal function). No data are available on the transfer of this agent to human milk. Mothers should withhold breastfeeding for a minimum of 2 days, following exposure to this agent or up to 5 days if renal function is poor.

T 1/2	3-18 h (mean 5.7 h)	MW	268.3 Da	PB	4%
Tmax		RID		Vd	0.5 L/kg
Oral		M/P		pKa	

Adult Concerns: Headache, fever, fatigue, pain, hypotension, stomatitis, nausea, vomiting, diarrhea, changes in liver function, myelosuppression, anemia, thrombocytopenia, weakness.

Adult Dose: 4 mg/m^2.

Pediatric Concerns: None reported via milk at this time.

Infant Monitoring: Withhold breastfeeding for a minimum of 2 days or up to 5 days if poor renal function.

Alternatives:

References:
1. Pharmaceutical manufacturers prescribing information.

PENTOXIFYLLINE

Trade: Trental

Category: hemorheological

LRC: L2 - Limited Data-Probably Compatible

Pentoxifylline and its metabolites improve the flow properties of blood by decreasing its viscosity. It is a methylxanthine derivative similar in structure to caffeine and is extensively metabolized although the metabolites do not have long half-lives. In a group of five breastfeeding women who received a single 400 mg dose, the mean milk/plasma ratio was 0.87 for the parent compound.[1] The milk/plasma ratios for the metabolites were lower: 0.54, 0.76, and 1.13. Average milk concentration at 2 hours following the dose was 73.9 µg/L.

T 1/2	0.4-1.6 h	MW	278 Da	PB	
Tmax	1 h	RID	0.2%	Vd	
Oral	Complete	M/P		pKa	

Adult Concerns: Dyspnea, bad taste, dyspepsia, nausea, vomiting, bloating, diarrhea, bleeding.

Adult Dose: 400 mg three times a day.

Pediatric Concerns: None reported.

Infant Monitoring:

Alternatives:

References:
1. Witter FR, Smith RV. The excretion of pentoxifylline and its metabolites into human breast milk. Am J Obstet Gynecol. 1985;151(8):1094-1097.

PERFLUTREN PROTEIN TYPE A

Trade: Definity, Optison

Category: Diagnostic Agent, Cardiac Function

LRC: L3 - No Data-Probably Compatible

Perflutren protein type A is a unique radiocontrast agent used in patients with suboptimal echocardiograms to make the left ventricular chamber opaque.[1] This product releases perflutren gas molecules that are completely eliminated in the human lung in 10 minutes. Perflutren gas is not metabolized but passes rapidly from the body. Although there are no data on levels in human milk, this product is so rapidly dissipated, that the risk to the infant would be nil. Perflutren lipid microsphere (Definity) is a new formulation of the same gas above. Again, half-life is of about 1.3 minutes. The manufacturer recommends pumping and discarding of milk once after treatment.

T 1/2	1.3 min	MW	670 Da	PB	
Tmax		RID		Vd	
Oral	Nil	M/P		pKa	

Adult Concerns: Headache, dizziness, flushing, altered taste, nausea, vomiting.

Adult Dose: 0.5 mL IV.

Pediatric Concerns: No data are available.

Infant Monitoring:

Alternatives:

References:
1. Pharmaceutical manufacturers prescribing information.

PERINDOPRIL ERBUMINE

Trade: Aceon, Coversyl

Category: ACE Inhibitor

LRC: L3 - No Data-Probably Compatible

Perindopril is an angiotensin-converting enzyme (ACE) inhibitor that is metabolized to its active metabolite perindoprilat.[1] There are no known studies on perindopril and breastfeeding. However, because of reported low levels in breast milk with similar ACE inhibitors, it is unlikely that much of this medication would be present in breast milk. Use of another ACE inhibitor that we have more information on, such as enalapril, ramipril, benazepril, or captopril, would be preferred.

Both the ACE inhibitor family and the specific angiotensin II receptor blockers are contraindicated in pregnancy and thus should be used with caution in women who are planning a subsequent pregnancy in the near future.

T 1/2	Perindoprilat 30-120 h	MW	368.47 (free acid) or 441.61 (salt form) Da	PB	Perindopril 60%/perindoprilat 10%-20%
Tmax	Perindoprilat 3-7 h	RID		Vd	Perindopril 0.22/perindoprilat 0.16 L/kg
Oral	Perindopril 75%/perindoprilat 25%	M/P		pKa	

Adult Concerns: Headache, dizziness, fatigue, hypotension, abnormal taste, cough, nausea, diarrhea, constipation, changes in renal function/urine output, hyperkalemia, rash.

Adult Dose: 2-8 mg/day.

Pediatric Concerns: None reported via milk at this time.

Infant Monitoring: Drowsiness, lethargy, pallor, poor feeding, and weight gain.

Alternatives: Enalapril(L2), Captopril(L2), Ramipril(L3), Benazepril(L2)

References:
1. Pharmaceutical manufacturers prescribing information.

PERMETHRIN

Trade: Acticin, Elimite, Nix Creme Rinse, Pronto

Category: Scabicide

LRC: L2 - Limited Data-Probably Compatible

Permethrin is a synthetic pyrethroid structure of the natural ester pyrethrum, a natural insecticide, used to treat lice, mites, and fleas. To use, it is recommended that the hair be washed with detergent and then saturated with permethrin liquid for 10 minutes before rinsing with water. One treatment is typically all that is required. At 14 days, a second treatment may be needed if viable lice are seen. Permethrin cream is generally recommended for scabies infestations and should be applied head to toe for 8-12 hours in infants, and body (not head) only in adults. Reapplication may be needed in 7 days if live mites appear.

Permethrin absorption through the skin following application of a 5% cream is reported to be less than 2%.[1] Permethrin is rapidly metabolized by serum and tissue enzymes to inactive metabolites and rapidly excreted in the urine. Overt toxicity is very low. In spite of its rapid metabolism, some residuals are sequestered in fat tissue. In a study done in South Africa, breast milk concentrations of permethrin was found to be between 1.1-1.6 µg/g milk fat. The source of exposure in this study was the use of indoor insecticide sprays containing permethrin or ingestion of food contaminated with permethrin. The authors suggest that the main route of exposure is probably from ingestion through diet, with some occurring due to skin contact. Inhalation is not recognized as a significant route of exposure to pyrethroids.[2] In another study in South Africa where 152 breast milk samples were investigated, permethrin was found in 66% (101) of the samples.[3] While most samples were exceedingly low, the highest breast milk concentration found was 14.51 µg/L. According to the authors, this suggests a daily intake of only 13.6 µg/kg, which is far lower than the set acceptable daily intake (ADI) for permethrin. The ADI for permethrin is 50 µg/kg.[3,4] Another study reported that in five infants whose mothers used permethrin during the breastfeeding period, no adverse reactions were reported.[5]

Therefore, the amounts of permethrin absorbed following topical application is far lower than the amount absorbed following oral exposure in food. Hence, the amounts ingested by the infant through milk is far lower than the acceptable daily intake for permethrin, and would therefore be unlikely to cause any significant clinical effects in the infant. The WHO considers short-term topical use of permethrin compatible with breastfeeding.[6]

T 1/2		MW	391 Da	PB	
Tmax		RID		Vd	
Oral		M/P		pKa	

Adult Concerns: Itching, rash, skin irritation. Dyspnea has been reported in one patient.

Adult Dose:

Pediatric Concerns: None via milk.

Infant Monitoring:

Alternatives:

References:
1. Pharmaceutical manufacturers prescribing information.
2. Sereda B, Bouwman H, Kylin H. Comparing water, bovine milk, and indoor residual spraying as possible sources of DDT and pyrethroid residues in breastmilk. J Toxicol Environ Health A. 2009;72(13):842-851.
3. Bouwman H, Sereda B, Meinhardt HM. Simultaneous presence of DDT and pyrethroid residues in human breast milk from a malaria endemic area in South Africa. Environ Pollut. 2006 Dec;144(3):902-917. Epub 2006 Mar 24.
4. FAO and WHO. Joint meeting of the panel of experts on pesticide residues. 2005. http://www.who.int/foodsafety/chem/jmpr/publications/en/index.html.
5. Ito S, Blajchman A, Stephenson M, et al. Prospective follow-up of adverse reactions in breast-fed infants exposed to maternal medication. Am J Obstet Gynecol. 1993;168(5):1393-1399.
6. Anon. Breastfeeding and Maternal Medication. Geneva, Switzerland: World Health Organization; 2002.

PERPHENAZINE

Trade:

Category: Antipsychotic, Typical

LRC: L3 - Limited Data-Probably Compatible

Perphenazine is a phenothiazine derivative used as an antipsychotic or sedative. In a study of one patient receiving either 16 or 24 mg/day of perphenazine divided in two doses at 12 hour intervals, milk levels were 2.1 μg/L and 3.2 μg/L, respectively.[1] The authors estimated the dose to the infant at 1.06 μg (0.3 μg/kg) or 1.59 μg (0.45 μg/kg) respective of dose. Serum perphenazine levels in the mother drawn 12 hours after doses of 16 or 24 mg/day were 2 and 4.9 ng/mL respectively. Hence milk/plasma ratios were approximately 1.1 and 0.7 respective of the dose. The authors estimate the dose to be approximately 0.1% of the weight-adjusted maternal dose. The authors report that during a 3 month period, the infant thrived and had no adverse effects from the medication.

T 1/2	8-20 h	MW	404 Da	PB	
Tmax		RID	0.1%	Vd	
Oral	40%	M/P	0.7-1.1	pKa	7.94

Adult Concerns: Amenorrhea, galactorrhea, dreams, drowsiness, headache, lethargy, bradycardia, arrhythmias, anorexia, stomach pain, nausea, hepatotoxicity, blurred vision, glycosuria, nasal congestion.

Adult Dose: 4-8 mg three times daily.

Pediatric Concerns:

Infant Monitoring: Sedation or irritability, apnea, not waking to feed/poor feeding, constipation, weight gain, and extrapyramidal symptoms.

Alternatives:

References:
1. Olesen OV, Bartels U, Poulsen JH. Perphenazine in breast milk and serum. Am J Psychiatry. 1990 Oct;147(10):1378-1379.

PERTUSSIS INFECTION

Trade: Bordetella pertussis, Whooping cough

Category: Infectious Disease

LRC: L3 - No Data-Probably Compatible

Pertussis or whooping cough is a bacterial infection caused by the bacterium *Bordetella pertussis*.[1] It is contagious and transmitted via respiratory secretions or sharing breathing space.

A recent publication reviewing pertussis in American infants less than 1 year of age found that in more than 66% of cases the source of infection has was attributable to a family member.[2] Those with pertussis can be contagious up to 2 weeks after the cough starts, thus family members or caregivers often infect infants. Symptoms typically start within 5-10 days post exposure but can occur up to 3 weeks later.

Although pertussis appears to have symptoms that resemble the common cold, pertussis can be dangerous for babies and lead to coughing fits (high pitched whoop), apneas, and fatigue.[1] Fifty percent of infants less than 1 year of age require hospitalization with this infection.

Initiating treatment as soon as possible is key to prevent worsening of symptoms and limit the spread to others. Typically treatment should start within 1-2 weeks of symptom onset.[1] The treatment of pertussis consists of supportive therapy and macrolide antibiotics (azithromycin, clarithromycin, erythromycin). Note: Antibiotics are often given to those who are a close contact of the patient.

At this time, there are no data describing the transfer of this bacterium to human milk. However, the data demonstrate that antibodies can be transmitted in breast milk.[3,4] When women were vaccinated with the Tdap (tetanus, diphtheriae, pertussis) vaccine in pregnancy, they had higher levels of select pertussis antibodies in their colostrum and milk up to 8 weeks postpartum.[5] The amount of protection the infant would receive from these antibodies in milk is controversial, further research is still required. For breastfeeding mothers diagnosed with pertussis, avoiding close contact with the infant during the first 5 days of their treatment is recommended.[1]

The best way to prevent this disease is by vaccination.[1] Speak to your physician or local public health department for timing of maternal and infant vaccination based on your local risk of infectivity.

Adult Concerns:

Adult Dose:

Pediatric Concerns:

Infant Monitoring:

Alternatives:

References:

1. Centers for Disease Control and Prevention. Pertussis (Whooping Cough) January 2016. http://www.cdc.gov/pertussis/. Online Accessed May 25, 2016.
2. Skoff TH, Kenyon C, Cocoros N, et al. Sources of infant pertussis infection in the united states. Pediatrics. 2015;136(4):635-641.
3. Pisacane A, Graziano L, Zona G, et al. Breastfeeding and acute lower respiratory tract infection. Acta Paediatr. 1994;83:714-718.
4. Maertens L, De Schutter S, Braeckman T, et al. Breastfeeding after maternal immunisation during pregnancy: providing immunological protection to the newborn: a review. Vaccine. 2014;32(16):1786-1792.
5. Abu Raya B, Srugo I, Kessel A, et al. The induction of breast milk pertussis specific antibodies following gestational tetanus-diptheria-acelluar pertussis vaccination. Vaccine. 2014;32(43):5632-5637.

PERTUSSIS VACCINE

Trade:

Category: Vaccine

LRC: L2 - Limited Data-Probably Compatible

There are two types of pertussis vaccine, whole cell and acellular.[1] Whole cell pertussis vaccine is made from inactivated B. pertussis cells. Acellular pertussis vaccines are made from inactivated components of B. pertussis cells. Acellular pertussis vaccine only comes in combination with diphtheria and tetanus vaccines.[2] Because pertussis vaccine is an inactivated bacterial product, there is no specific contraindication in breastfeeding following injection with these vaccines. It is extremely unlikely proteins of this size would be secreted in breast milk.

Adult Concerns: Local injection site reactions, irritability, fever. Rare side effects: encephalopathy, convulsions.

Adult Dose:

Pediatric Concerns:

Infant Monitoring:

Alternatives:

References:

1. Atkinson W, Wolfe S, Hamborsky J, eds. Pertussis. "Centers for Disease Control and Prevention. Epidemiology and Prevention of Vaccine-Preventable Diseases". 12th ed. Washington DC: Public Health Foundation; 2011.
2. Pharmaceutical manufacturers prescribing information.

PHENAZOPYRIDINE

Trade: Azo, Pyridium

Category: Renal-Urologic Agent

LRC: L3 - No Data-Probably Compatible

Phenazopyridine hydrochloride is an azo dye that is rapidly excreted in the urine, where it exerts a topical analgesic effect on urinary tract mucosa.[1] Pyridium is mild to moderately effective and produces a reddish-orange discoloration of the urine. It may also discolor and ruin contact lenses and clothing. It is not known if Pyridium transfers to breast milk; however, it probably does enter milk to a limited degree based on its oral bioavailability and small size. Due to this product's limited efficacy it probably should not be used in lactating women, although it is unlikely to be harmful to infants.

T 1/2		MW	250 Da	PB	
Tmax		RID		Vd	
Oral	Complete	M/P		pKa	5.1

Adult Concerns: Anemia, nausea, vomiting, diarrhea, colored urine, methemoglobinemia, hepatitis, gastrointestinal distress.

Adult Dose: 100-200 mg three times daily.

Pediatric Concerns: None reported via lactation.

Infant Monitoring: Red colored urine (normal). Vomiting, diarrhea.

Alternatives:

References:

1. Pharmaceutical manufacturers prescribing information.

PHENOBARBITAL

Trade: Barbilixir, Gardenal, Luminal, Phenobarbitone

Category: Anticonvulsant

LRC: L4 - Limited Data-Possibly Hazardous

Phenobarbital is a long half-life barbiturate frequently used as an anticonvulsant in adults and during the neonatal period. Its long half-life in infants may lead to significant accumulation and blood levels higher than mother although this is infrequent. During the first 3-4 weeks of life, phenobarbital is poorly absorbed by the neonatal gastrointestinal tract. However, protein binding by neonatal albumin is also poor, 36%-43%, as compared to the adult, 51%. Thus, the volume of distribution is higher in neonates and the tissue concentrations of phenobarbital may be significantly higher. The half-life in premature infants can be extremely long (100-500 hours).

Although varied, milk/plasma ratios vary from 0.46 to 0.6.[1-3] In one study, following a dose of 30 mg four times daily, the milk concentration of phenobarbital averaged 2.74 mg/L 16 hours after the last dose.[3] The dose an infant would receive was estimated at 2-4 mg/day.[4] Phenobarbital should be administered with caution and close observation of the infant is required, including plasma drug levels. One should generally expect the infant's plasma level to be approximately 30%-40% of the maternal level. In some reported cases, the infant plasma levels have reached twice that of the maternal plasma levels 2.5 hours after the maternal dose.[5] In general, the infant will receive one-third of mother's dose. Possibility of withdrawal symptoms such as jitteriness, irritability, crying, sweating may be expected when drug withdrawn.

T 1/2	53-140 h	MW	232 Da	PB	51%
Tmax	8-12 h	RID	24%	Vd	0.5-0.6 L/kg
Oral	80% (Adult)	M/P	0.4-0.6	pKa	7.2

Adult Concerns: Drowsiness, sedation, ataxia, respiratory depression, withdrawal symptoms.

Adult Dose: 100-200 mg daily.

Pediatric Concerns: Phenobarbital sedation has been reported, but is infrequent. Withdrawal symptoms have been reported.

Infant Monitoring: Sedation or irritability, not waking to feed/poor feeding, apneas, and weight gain. Based on clinical symptoms some infants may require monitoring of liver enzymes. Expect infant plasma levels to approximate one-third (or lower) of maternal plasma level.

Alternatives:

References:
1. Tyson RM, Shrader EA, Perlman HH. Drugs transmitted through breast milk. II Barbiturates. J Pediatr. 1938;14:86-90.
2. Kaneko S, Sato T, Suzuki K. The levels of anticonvulsants in breast milk. Br J Clin Pharmacol. 1979;7(6):624-627.
3. Nau H, Kuhnz W, Egger HJ, Rating D, Helge H. Anticonvulsants during pregnancy and lactation. Transplacental, maternal and neonatal pharmacokinetics. Clin Pharmacokinet. 1982;7(6):508-543.
4. Horning MG. Identification and quantification of drugs and drug metabolites in human milk using GC-MS-COM methods. Mod Probl Pediatr. 1975;15:73-79.
5. Pote M, Kulkarni R, Agarwal M. Phenobarbital toxic levels in a nursing neonate. Indian Pediatr. 2004;41:963-964.

PHENOL

Trade:

Category: Anesthetic, Local

LRC: L4 - No Data-Possibly Hazardous

Phenol is used in oral and topical anesthetic.[1] It is caustic at concentration of 5% or greater. There are no adequate and well-controlled studies or case reports on its use topically or in breastfeeding women. Use during lactation only if potential benefit to mother outweighs the potential risks to the infant.

T 1/2	1-4.5 h; 13.86 h with prolonged exposure	MW	94.1 Da	PB	
Tmax	19 min	RID		Vd	
Oral		M/P		pKa	9.95

Adult Concerns: Arrhythmia, epiglottitis, nausea, vomiting, urinary symptoms.

Adult Dose:

Pediatric Concerns:

Infant Monitoring:

Alternatives:

References:

1. Phenol. In: Reprotox® [Internet database]. Greenwood Village, CO: Thomson Healthcare. Updated periodically. Accessed June 8, 2011.

PHENTERMINE

Trade: Adipex-P, Duromine, Fastin, Ionamin, Zantryl

Category: Antiobesity Agent

LRC: L4 - No Data-Possibly Hazardous

Phentermine is an appetite suppressant that is similar to the amphetamine family.[1] As such, it frequently produces CNS stimulation. No data are available on its transfer to human milk. This product has a very small molecular weight (186 Da); therefore, it most likely would transfer to human milk in significant quantities. It could produce a variety of adverse effects in the infant, such as changes in sleep, irritability, hypertension, vomiting, tremor, and weight loss. The use of this product in breastfeeding mothers would be difficult to justify and is not advised.

T 1/2	20 h	MW	186 Da	PB	
Tmax	3-4.4 h	RID		Vd	
Oral	Complete	M/P		pKa	

Adult Concerns: Insomnia, headache, dizziness, paranoia/psychosis, restlessness, withdrawal syndrome, hypertension, tachycardia/palpitations, ischemic events, nausea, vomiting, diarrhea, tremors.

Adult Dose: 8 mg three times daily.

Pediatric Concerns: Growth impairment has been reported from direct use of phentermine in children aged 3-15 years.

Infant Monitoring: Not recommended in lactation

Alternatives:

References:

1. Pharmaceutical manufacturers prescribing information.

PHENYLEPHRINE

Trade: Mydfrin, Neofrin, Ocu-Phrin, Prefrin Liquifilm, Vicks Sinex

Category: Adrenergic

LRC: L3 - No Data-Probably Compatible

Phenylephrine is a sympathomimetic agent most commonly used as a nasal decongestant due to its vasoconstrictive properties, but also for treatment of ocular uveitis, inflammation, and for cardiogenic shock.[1] Phenylephrine is a potent adrenergic stimulant and systemic effects (tachycardia, hypertension, arrhythmias), although rare, have occurred following ocular administration in some sensitive individuals. Phenylephrine is most commonly added to cold mixtures and nasal sprays for use in respiratory colds, flu, and congestion.

Used ophthalmically in eye exams, the maternal dose of the medication would be very low and it is not likely to pose a problem for a breastfeeding infant. Although no data are available on its secretion into human milk, probably very small amounts will be transferred to milk.

Due to phenylephrine's poor oral bioavailability (38%), it is not likely to produce clinical effects in a breastfed infant unless the maternal doses were quite high. Because of pseudoephedrine's effect on milk production, concerns that phenylephrine may suppress milk production may arise; there is no evidence that this occurs at this time.

T 1/2	2-3 h	MW	203 Da	PB	
Tmax	10-60 min	RID		Vd	0.57 L/kg
Oral	38%	M/P		pKa	9.8, 8.8

Adult Concerns: Local ocular irritation, transient tachycardia, hypertension, and sympathetic stimulation.

Adult Dose: 10 mg orally every 4 hours as needed.

Pediatric Concerns: None reported via milk.

Infant Monitoring: Observe for excitement, poor sleep, and tremors.

Alternatives: Oxymetazoline(L3)

References:
1. Pharmaceutical manufacturers prescribing information.

PHENYLKETONURIA

Trade: PKU

Category: Metabolic Disorder

LRC: L2 - Limited Data-Probably Compatible

Phenylketonuria (PKU) is an inherited metabolic disorder characterized by a defect in the enzyme phenylalanine hydroxylase. This enzyme is necessary for the metabolism of phenylalanine to tyrosine. When phenylalanine hydroxylase activity is decreased, an abnormally high level of phenylalanine accumulates in the blood and tissues. High levels in the brain may interfere with CNS development. Therefore, those patients must be on a strict phenylalanine restricted diet.

Levels of phenylalanine in human milk were found to be lower than any formula milk.[1] Furthermore, babies with PKU who are breastfed along with formula milk containing low phenylalanine were found to have a lower phenylalanine intake and higher IQ score than infants fed only on formula containing low phenylalanine.[1]

It is advised that the mother continue breastfeeding her infant and supplement with a low phenylalanine formula.[3] The pediatrician using a special method will calculate the amount of formula the infant needs to keep the phenylalanine at appropriate levels.

In 1997, a study done on two identical twins with a phenylketonuric mother, suggested that high levels of phenylalanine in mother's serum and milk did not result in abnormal phenylalanine levels in the breastfeeding twins who did not have phenylketonuria.[1] A recent review of large numbers of mothers that breastfed an infant with PKU, suggested that a large number of women continue to breastfeed their infant successfully, and without problems in the infant.[2]

Adult Concerns:

Adult Dose:

Pediatric Concerns:

Infant Monitoring: Elevated phenylalanine levels in infant.

Alternatives:

References:
1. Riordan J, Wambach K. Breastfeeding and Human Lactation. 4th ed. Sudbury, MA: Jones and Bartlett Publishers; 2010:650-651.
2. Banta-Wright SA, Press N, Knafl KA, Steiner RD, Houck GM. Breastfeeding infants with phenylketonuria in the United States and Canada. Breastfeed Med. 2014 Apr;9(3):142-148. Epub 2013 Dec 18.
3. Kose E, Aksoy B, Kuyum P, Tuncer N, Arslan N, Ozturk Y. The effects of breastfeeding in infants with Phenylketonuria. J Pediatr Nurs. 2017 Oct;38:27-32. doi: 10.1016/j.pedn.2017.10.009. [Epub ahead of print] PubMed PMID: 29167077.

PHENYLTOLOXAMINE

Trade: Dologesic, Flextra-650, Percogesic

Category: Antihistamine

LRC: L3 - No Data-Probably Compatible

Phenyltoloxamine is an antihistamine with analgesic properties used in over-the-counter preparations. There are no reports describing the use of phenyltoloxamine during human lactation or measuring the amount, if any, of the drug excreted into milk have been located. The use of other antihistamines with more extensive data in lactation are recommended at this time.

T 1/2		MW	255 Da	PB	
Tmax	2-3 h	RID		Vd	
Oral	Well absorbed	M/P		pKa	9.1

Adult Concerns: Drowsiness, dizziness, euphoria, faintness, blurred vision, dry mouth, tachycardia, atrioventricular block with hypertension, nausea, abdominal pain.

Adult Dose:

Pediatric Concerns:

Infant Monitoring:

Alternatives: Diphenhydramine(L2), Loratadine(L1), Cetirizine(L2)

References:
1. Pharmaceutical manufacturers prescribing information.

PHENYTOIN

Trade: Dilantin, Epanutin

Category: Anticonvulsant

LRC: L2 - Limited Data-Probably Compatible

Phenytoin is an old and efficient anticonvulsant. It is secreted in small amounts into breast milk. The effect on the infant is generally considered minimal if the levels in the maternal circulation are kept in the low-normal range (10 µg/mL). Phenytoin levels peak in milk at 3.5 hours.

In one study of six women receiving 200-400 mg/day, plasma concentrations varied from 12.8 to 78.5 µmol/L, while their milk levels ranged from 1.61 to 2.95 mg/L.[1] The milk/plasma ratios were low, ranging from 0.06 to 0.18. In only two of these infants were plasma concentrations of phenytoin detectable (0.46 and 0.72 µmol/L). No untoward effects were noted in any of these infants. Others have reported milk levels of 6 µg/mL, or 0.8 µg/mL.[2,3] Although the actual concentration in milk varies significantly between studies, the milk/plasma ratio appears relatively similar at 0.13 to 0.45. Breast milk concentrations varied from 0.26 to 1.5 mg/L depending on the maternal dose. In a mother receiving 250 mg twice daily, milk levels were 0.26 and the milk/plasma ratio was 0.45.[4] The maternal plasma level of phenytoin was 0.58. In another study of two patients receiving 300-600 mg/day, the average milk level was 1.9 mg/L.[5] The maximum observed milk level was 2.6 mg/L.

In 2014 a prospective observational study looked at long-term neurodevelopment of infants exposed to antiepileptic drugs in utero and lactation.[6] This study included women taking carbamazepine, lamotrigine, phenytoin or valproate as monotherapy for epilepsy. In this study, 42.9% of the infants were breastfed for a mean of 7.2 months. The IQ of these children at 6 years of age was statistically significantly lower in children who were exposed to valproate in utero (7-13 IQ points lower). It was also noted that higher doses of medication (primarily with valproate) were associated with lower IQ scores. The children's IQ scores were found to be higher if the maternal IQ was higher, the mother took folic acid near the time of conception and if the child was breastfed (4 points higher). In addition, verbal abilities were also found to be significantly higher in children who were breastfed. Although this study has many limitations (e.g., small sample size, difficulties with patient follow-up), it does provide data up to age 6 that suggest benefits of breastfeeding are not out-weighed by risks of maternal drug therapy in milk.

The neonatal half-life of phenytoin is highly variable for the first week of life. Monitoring of the infants' plasma may be useful although it is not definitely required. All of the current studies indicate rather low levels of phenytoin in breast milk and minimal plasma levels in breastfeeding infants.

T 1/2	6-24 h	MW	252 Da	PB	89%
Tmax	4-12 h	RID	0.6%-7.7%	Vd	0.5-0.8 L/kg
Oral	70%-100%	M/P	0.18-0.45	pKa	8.3

Adult Concerns: Sedation, dizziness, confusion, nystagmus, diplopia, arrhythmias, hypotension, hypertrophied gums, changes in taste, nausea, vomiting, constipation, changes in liver function, hyperglycemia, folic acid and vitamin D deficiency, leukopenia, thrombocytopenia, ataxia, tremor, severe rash.

Adult Dose: 300 mg daily.

Pediatric Concerns: Only one case of methemoglobinemia, drowsiness, and poor sucking has been reported. Most other studies suggest no problems.

Infant Monitoring: Sedation or irritability, not waking to feed/poor feeding, and weight gain. Based on clinical symptoms some infants may require monitoring of phenytoin levels, liver function, or CBC.

Alternatives:

References:
1. Steen B, Rane A, Lonnerholm G, Falk O, Elwin CE, Sjoqvist F. Phenytoin excretion in human breast milk and plasma levels in nursed infants. Ther Drug Monit. 1982;4(4):331-334.
2. Svensmark O, Schiller PJ, Buchtahal F. 5, 5-Diphenylhydantoin (dilantin) blood levels after oral or intravenous dosage in man. Acta Pharmacol Toxicol (Copenh). 1960;16:331-346.

3. Kaneko S, Sato T, Suzuki K. The levels of anticonvulsants in breast milk. Br J Clin Pharmacol. 1979;7(6):624-627.

4. Rane A, Garle M, Borga O, Sjoqvist F. Plasma disappearance of transplacentally transferred diphenylhydantoin in the newborn studied by mass fragmentography. Clin Pharmacol Ther. 1974;15(1):39-45.

5. Mirkin BL. Diphenylhydantoin: placental transport, fetal localization, neonatal metabolism, and possible teratogenic effects. J Pediatr. 1971;78(2):329-337.

6. Meador KJ, Baker GA, Browning N, et al. Breastfeeding in children of women taking antiepileptic drugs cognitive outcomes at age 6. JAMA Pediatr. 2014;168(8):729-736.

PHOSPHATIDYLCHOLINE

Trade: Lecithin

Category: Nutritional agent

LRC: L3 - No Data-Probably Compatible

Lecithin is a generic term normally used to describe a fatty substance isolated from various oils and fats. In pure form, it consists of phosphoric acid, choline, fatty acids, glycerol. Depending on its purity, it may also contain various glycolipids, triglycerides, and other phospholipids. Found in all living tissues, this product is often used as an additive or in food preparation, it has also been suggested to help treat mastitis. The evidence for its efficacy in mastitis is lacking and is not pharmacologically realistic. Most, if not all, lecithin would be metabolized and denatured in the gastrointestinal tract long before absorption. This product is not expected to be hazardous to an infant.

T 1/2		MW		PB	
Tmax		RID		Vd	
Oral	Nil	M/P		pKa	

Adult Concerns: Possible hypersensitivity, weight gain, diarrhea.

Adult Dose: 1 to 40 grams per day.

Pediatric Concerns: None reported.

Infant Monitoring: Possible hypersensitivity, diarrhea.

Alternatives:

References:

PHYTONADIONE

Trade: AquaMEPHYTON, Konakion, Mephyton, Vitamin K1

Category: Vitamin

LRC: L1 - Limited Data-Compatible

Vitamin K1 is often used to reverse the effects of oral anticoagulants and to prevent hemorrhagic disease of the newborn.[1-3] The use of vitamin K has long been accepted primarily because it reduces the decline of the vitamin K dependent coagulation factors II, VII, IX, and X. A single IM injection of 0.5 to 1 mg during the neonatal period is recommended by the AAP. Although controversial, it is generally recognized that exclusive breastfeeding may not provide sufficient vitamin K1 to provide normal clotting factors, particularly in the premature infant or those with malabsorptive disorders. Vitamin K in breast milk is normally low (<5-20 ng/mL), and most infants are born with low coagulation factors, 30%-60% of normal. Although vitamin K is transferred to human milk, the amount may not be sufficient to prevent hemorrhagic disease of the newborn. Vitamin K requires the presence of bile and other factors for absorption, and neonatal absorption may be slow or delayed due to the lack of requisite gut factors.

Vitamin K2 (menaquinones, menatetrenone) is more orally bioavailable vitamin K. It is derived from various foods including meat, eggs, dairy, and natto. There have been some suggestions that K2 may prevent osteoporosis.

T 1/2		MW	450 Da	PB	
Tmax	12 h	RID		Vd	
Oral	Complete	M/P		pKa	

Adult Concerns: Hypotension, hemolytic anemia, thrombocytopenia, thrombosis, prothrombin abnormalities, pruritus, and cutaneous reactions. Anaphylaxis.

Adult Dose: 65 μg daily.

Pediatric Concerns: Vitamin K transfer to milk is low.

Infant Monitoring:

Alternatives:

References:
1. Olson JA. Recommended dietary intakes (RDI) of vitamin K in humans. Am J Clin Nutr. 1987;45(4):687-692.
2. Lane PA, Hathaway WE. Vitamin K in infancy. J Pediatr. 1985;106(3):351-359.
3. Vitamin and mineral supplement needs in normal children in the United States. Pediatrics. 1980;66(6):1015-1021.

PICARIDIN

Trade: Bayrepel, Cutter Advanced, OFF Clean Feel

Category: Insect Repellant

LRC: L3 - No Data-Probably Compatible

Picaridin, also known as icaridin, is a newer and potentially safer alternative to the insect repellent DEET. It works by blocking the insect's ability to locate human skin. It does not cause irritation to the skin and is odorless. Icaridin does not need to be washed off upon returning indoors. It is safe for use in children of all ages, and it will not affect plastics, synthetics, or plastic coatings. The WHO claims that icaridin is the best repellent against mosquitoes carrying malaria. The EPA suggests that icaridin has a low acute oral, inhalation, and dermal toxicity.[1] When applied to human skin, picardin was not found in plasma.[3]

One study concerning the absorption of picaridin in human skin attempted to show variations between formulations. In standard preparations, the average amount absorbed was 12.44% of the applied dose. In preparations containing sunscreens, the amount absorbed was shown to be lower, averaging 5.92%. Measures were also made to determine the total possible amount that could be absorbed, which resulted in 9.85% and 18.91% for the sunscreen and standard preparations respectively. It was noted that the amount of ethyl alcohol varied between the two formulations, with the standard having 60.6% alcohol content and the sunscreen formulation having 91.4%. In vivo studies showed significantly lower levels of absorption, with values ranging between 1.66% and 3.77%.[3]

In humans, less than 6% of the applied doses were absorbed after topical application of 14.7 or 15.0 mg of technical grade icaridin.[3] Due to its lipid solubility, it is likely it would enter milk, but plasma levels are probably low.

T 1/2		MW	229.32 Da	PB	
Tmax		RID		Vd	
Oral		M/P		pKa	

Adult Concerns: No adverse reactions noted.

Adult Dose:

Pediatric Concerns: No adverse reactions noted.

Infant Monitoring:

Alternatives:

References:
1. https://www3.epa.gov/pesticides/chem_search/reg_actions/registration/fs_PC-070705_01-May-05.pdf
2. Picaridin. In vitro dermal penetration study using human and rat skin. United States Environmental Protection Agency File R160418. https://archive.epa.gov/pesticides/chemicalsearch/chemical/foia/web/pdf/070705/070705-2008-06-26a.pdf.
3. Gervais JA, Wegner P, Luukinen B, Buhl K, Stone D. Picaridin Technical Fact Sheet. National Pesticide Information Center. Corvalis, OR: Oregon State University Extension Services; 2009.

PILOCARPINE

Trade: Akarpine, Isopto Carpine, Minims Pilocarpine Nitrate, Pilocar

Category: Antiglaucoma

LRC: L3 - No Data-Probably Compatible

Pilocarpine is a direct acting cholinergic agent used primarily in the eyes for treatment of open-angle glaucoma. The ophthalmic dose is approximately 1 mg or less per day, while the oral adult dose is approximately 15-30 mg daily.[1] It is not known if pilocarpine enters milk, but it probably does in low levels due to its minimal plasma concentration. It is not likely that an infant would receive a clinical dose via milk, but this is presently unknown.

T 1/2	0.76-1.55 h	MW	208 Da	PB	0%
Tmax	1.25 h	RID		Vd	
Oral	Good	M/P		pKa	7.15

Adult Concerns: Ophthalmic use: burning, itching, blurred vision, poor night vision, headaches. Oral use: Dizziness, flushing, hypertension, excessive salivation, nausea, diarrhea, urinary frequency, excessive sweating, weakness.

Adult Dose: 5-10 mg three times daily.

Pediatric Concerns: None reported via milk.

Infant Monitoring: Vomiting, diarrhea.

Alternatives:

References:
1. Pharmaceutical manufacturers prescribing information.

PIMECROLIMUS

Trade: Elidel

Category: Immune Modulator

LRC: L2 - No Data-Probably Compatible

Pimecrolimus is a topical agent used as a cytokine inhibitor for atopic dermatitis. While its mechanism of action is unknown, it inhibits the release of various inflammatory cytokines for T cells and many others. Systemic absorption following topical application is minimal with reported blood concentrations consistently below 0.5 ng/mL following twice-daily application of the 1% cream.[1] Oral absorption is unreported but probably low to moderate as plasma levels of 54 ng/mL have been reported following twice daily oral doses of 30 mg.[2] Pimecrolimus is cleared for use in pediatric patients 2 years and older. No data are available on its transfer to human milk, but because the maternal plasma levels are so low, it is extremely remote that this agent would penetrate milk in clinically relevant amounts. However, its use on or around the nipples should be avoided as the clinical dose absorbed orally in the infant could be significant.

T 1/2		MW	810 Da	PB	87%
Tmax		RID		Vd	
Oral	Moderate	M/P		pKa	

Adult Concerns: Headache, fever, vomiting, diarrhea, constipation, excessive skin warmth and burning, elevated risk of skin infection (varicella zoster virus, herpes simplex virus, eczema herpeticum), and skin cancer is possible. The US FDA has issued a warning concerning elevated risks of skin cancers and lymphomas in patients exposed to this product; this warning is controversial.

Adult Dose: Apply twice daily to skin.

Pediatric Concerns: None reported via milk. It is used in children 2 years of age and older. It is unlikely to penetrate milk in clinically relevant amounts. Should not be used directly on the nipple, or areola.

Infant Monitoring:

Alternatives:

References:
1. Pharmaceutical manufacturers prescribing information.
2. Harper J, Green A, Scott G, et al. First experience of topical SDZ ASM 981 in children with atopic dermatitis. Br J Dermatol. 2001;144(4):781-787.

PIMOZIDE

Trade: Orap

Category: Antipsychotic, Typical

LRC: L4 - No Data-Possibly Hazardous

Pimozide is a potent neuroleptic agent primarily used for Tourette syndrome and chronic schizophrenia, which induces a low degree of sedation.[1] No data are available on the secretion of pimozide into breast milk. This is a highly risky product and numerous other antipsychotics are available. This product is probably not worth the risk to the infant.

T 1/2	55 h	MW	462 Da	PB	
Tmax	6-8 h	RID		Vd	
Oral	>50%	M/P		pKa	7.32

Adult Concerns: Extrapyramidal symptoms, anorexia, weight loss, gastrointestinal distress, seizures.

Adult Dose: 7-16 mg daily.

Pediatric Concerns: None reported but caution is urged. No pediatric studies are found.

Infant Monitoring: Sedation or irritability, not waking to feed/poor feeding, weight gain, and extrapyramidal symptoms.

Alternatives: Risperidone(L2), Quetiapine(L2), Aripiprazole(L3)

References:
1. Pharmaceutical manufacturers prescribing information.

PINDOLOL

Trade: Visken

Category: Beta Adrenergic Blocker

LRC: L3 - Limited Data-Probably Compatible

Pindolol is a nonselective beta blocker that is used as an antihypertensives and antiarrhythmic. In one study of six hypertensive pregnant women, ages 25-35 years, with a gestational age of 37-40 weeks, patients were given 10 mg pindolol tablets every 12 hours for a minimum of 3 days during pregnancy and after delivery. A single breast milk sample was collected on the day of delivery from 11 to 14 hours postdose. Two pindolol metabolites were measured in milk, (-)-S-pindolol averaging 3.1 µg/L (range 1.5 to 3.9 µg/L) and (+)-R-pindolol averaging 1.9 µg/L (range 1.2 to 4.2 µg/L).[1] The authors estimate that a fully breastfed infant would receive an average of 0.36% of the weight-adjusted maternal dose. These data unfortunately were collected during the colostral phase and may overestimate the actual dose during regular lactation.

T 1/2	3-4 h	MW	248 Da	PB	40%
Tmax	1 h	RID	0.4%	Vd	2 L/kg
Oral	>95%	M/P		pKa	9.52

Adult Concerns: Headache, dizziness, insomnia, depression, fatigue, chest pain, bradycardia, heart block, hypotension, heart failure, wheezing, vomiting, diarrhea, changes in liver function, myalgia.

Adult Dose: 10-60 mg/day.

Pediatric Concerns: None reported at this time.

Infant Monitoring: Drowsiness, lethargy, pallor, poor feeding, and weight gain.

Alternatives:

References:
1. Goncalves PV, Cavalli RC, da Cunha SP, Lanchote VL. Determination of pindolol enantiomers in amniotic fluid and breast milk by high-performance liquid chromatography: applications to pharmacokinetics in pregnant and lactating women. J Chromatogr B Analyt Technol Biomed Life Sci. 2007 Jun;852(1-2):640-645.

PIOGLITAZONE

Trade: Actos

Category: Antidiabetic, other

LRC: L3 - No Data-Probably Compatible

Pioglitazone is a thiazolidinedione family oral antidiabetic agent similar to troglitazone and rosiglitazone. It acts primarily by increasing insulin receptor sensitivity. In essence, the insulin receptor is activated reducing insulin resistance. This family also decreases hepatic gluconeogenesis and increases insulin-dependent muscle glucose uptake.

They do not increase the release or secretion of insulin. No data are available on its entry into human milk. Due to its high plasma protein binding, transfer to milk is probably low, but there are no studies currently to confirm this. Preferably, use other antidiabetic agents on which there are more published data.

T 1/2	16-24 h	MW	392 Da	PB	>99%
Tmax	2 h	RID		Vd	0.63 L/kg
Oral		M/P		pKa	5.2, 6.8

Adult Concerns: Headache, heart failure, edema, hypoglycemia, changes in liver function, elevated CPK, anemia, weight gain or loss, myalgia.

Adult Dose: 15-30 mg once daily.

Pediatric Concerns: None reported via milk, but no data are available.

Infant Monitoring: Signs of hypoglycemia- drowsiness, lethargy, pallor, sweating, tremor.

Alternatives: Metformin(L1), Glyburide(L2), Glipizide(L2)

References:
1. Pharmaceutical manufacturers prescribing information.

PIPERACILLIN

Trade: Pipcil, Pipracil, Pipril

Category: Antibiotic, Penicillin

LRC: L2 - No Data-Probably Compatible

Piperacillin is an extended-spectrum penicillin. It is not absorbed orally and must be given IM or IV.[1] Concentrations of piperacillin secreted into milk are believed to be extremely low.[2]

T 1/2	0.6-1.3 h	MW	518 Da	PB	30%
Tmax	30-50 min	RID		Vd	
Oral	Poor	M/P		pKa	4.14

Adult Concerns: Allergic skin rash, blood dyscrasias, nausea, vomiting, diarrhea, changes in renal function.

Adult Dose: 4-5 gm 2-3 times daily.

Pediatric Concerns: None reported via milk.

Infant Monitoring: Vomiting, diarrhea, changes in gastrointestinal flora, and rash.

Alternatives:

References:
1. Pharmaceutical manufacturers prescribing information.
2. Chaplin S, Sanders GL, Smith JM. Drug excretion in human breast milk. Adv Drug React Ac Pois Rev. 1982;1:255-287.

PIPERACILLIN + TAZOBACTAM

Trade: Tazocin, Zosyn

Category: Antibiotic, Penicillin

LRC: L2 - No Data-Probably Compatible

Piperacillin and Tazobactam is a combination drug product indicated for use in pneumonia, appendicitis, pelvic inflammatory disease, peritonitis, and infections of skin and subcutaneous tissues.[1]

Piperacillin is an extended-spectrum penicillin and tazobactam is an inhibitor of different beta-lactamases. This combination is not absorbed orally and must be given IM or IV. Concentrations of piperacillin secreted into milk are believed to be extremely low and tazobactam concentrations in human milk have not been studied.[2] Studies in women suggest that this medication poses minimal risk to the infant when used during breastfeeding.

T 1/2	Pip/taz: 0.7-1.2 h	MW	Pip/taz: 539/322 Da	PB	Pip/taz: 30%/30%
Tmax		RID		Vd	Pip/taz: 0.14/0.23 L/kg
Oral	Pip/taz: Low	M/P		pKa	Pip/taz: 4.14/2.1

Adult Concerns: Headache, fever, insomnia, seizure, nausea, vomiting, diarrhea, changes in renal function, blood dyscrasias, rash, itching.

Adult Dose:

Pediatric Concerns:

Infant Monitoring: Vomiting, diarrhea, changes in gastrointestinal flora and rash.

Alternatives:

References:
1. Pharmaceutical manufacturers prescribing information.
2. Chaplin S, Sanders GL, Smith JM. Drug excretion in human breast milk. Adv Drug React Ac Pois Rev. 1982;1:255-287.

PIROXICAM

Trade: Candyl, Feldene, Mobilis, Pirox

Category: NSAID

LRC: L2 - Limited Data-Probably Compatible

Piroxicam is a typical nonsteroidal anti-inflammatory commonly used in arthritics. In one patient taking 40 mg/day, breast milk levels were 0.22 mg/L at 2.5 hours after dose.[1] In another study of long-term therapy in four lactating women receiving 20 mg/day, the mean piroxicam concentration in breast milk was 78 µg/L, which is approximately 1%-3% of the maternal plasma concentration.[2] The daily dose ingested by the infant was calculated to average 3%.4% of the weight-adjusted maternal dose of piroxicam. Even though piroxicam has a very long half-life, this report suggests its use to be safe in breastfeeding mothers.

T 1/2	30-86 h	MW	331 Da	PB	99.3%
Tmax	3-5 h	RID	3.4%-5.8%	Vd	0.31 L/kg
Oral	Complete	M/P	0.008-0.013	pKa	5.1

Adult Concerns: Headache, dizziness, tinnitus, dyspepsia, nausea, vomiting, abdominal pain, constipation, diarrhea, gastrointestinal bleed, anorexia, changes in liver and renal function, anemia, edema.

Adult Dose: 20 mg daily.

Pediatric Concerns: None reported via milk in several studies.

Infant Monitoring: Vomiting, diarrhea.

Alternatives: Ibuprofen(L1)

References:
1. Ostensen M. Piroxicam in human breast milk. Eur J Clin Pharmacol. 1983;25(6):829-830.
2. Ostensen M, Matheson I, Laufen H. Piroxicam in breast milk after long-term treatment. Eur J Clin Pharmacol. 1988;35(5):567-569.

PITOLISANT

Trade: Wakix

Category: Histamine-3 receptor agonist

LRC: L3 - No Data-Probably Compatible

Pitolisant, also known as tiprolisant, is a potent and highly selective histamine 3 (H₃) receptor antagonist/inverse agonist, representing the first commercially available medication in its class.[1] Pitolisant significantly decreased excessive daytime sleepiness versus placebo in adults with narcolepsy with or without cataplexy. Pitolisant is a small molecular weight, CNS active drug. No data are available on its entry into human milk, but low levels should be expected. Observe infant for insomnia, irritability, nausea, and abdominal pain.

T 1/2	10-12 h	MW	295.85 Da	PB	
Tmax	3 h	RID		Vd	15.7-40.3 L/kg
Oral	90%	M/P		pKa	

Adult Concerns: Headache, insomnia, irritability, nausea and abdominal pain. Pitolisant prolongs the QT interval and it should be avoided in patients with known QT prolongation or in combination with other drugs known to prolong QT interval. Do not use in patients with a history of cardiac arrhythmias, as well as other circumstances that may increase the risk of the occurrence of torsade de pointes or sudden death.

Adult Dose: 17.8 mg to 35.6 mg daily.

Pediatric Concerns:

Infant Monitoring: Observe for insomnia, irritability, nausea, and abdominal pain.

Alternatives:

References:
1. Pharmaceutical manufacturers prescribing information.

PNEUMOCOCCAL VACCINE

Trade: Pneumovax 23, Pneumovax 23 (PPSV23), Pneumo 23, Prevnar, Prevnar 13 (PCV13)

Category: Vaccine

LRC: L1 - No Data-Compatible

The pneumococcal vaccine is an inactivated product that consists of a mixture of polysaccharides from the 23 most prevalent types of *Streptococcus pneumonia*. It is non-infectious. It is available as a formulation containing seven strains (7-valent) conjugate, and a 23 strain (valent) conjugate vaccine. The 7-valent vaccine is for use in children less than 2 years. The 23-valent vaccine is for use in adults aged 50 years or older and anyone aged 2 years or older that is at risk.[1] Though no data are available regarding the safety of the polysaccharide vaccine during lactation, it is unlikely the vaccine would harm the infant, according to the CDC.

T 1/2		MW		PB	
Tmax		RID		Vd	
Oral	Nil	M/P		pKa	

Adult Concerns: Malaise, headache, nausea, vomiting, serum sickness, and fever.

Adult Dose: 0.5 mL IM.

Pediatric Concerns: Adverse reactions with the 7-valent pneumococcal conjugate vaccine include fever, irritability, drowsiness, erythema, decreased appetite, vomiting, diarrhea, and local tenderness.

Infant Monitoring:

Alternatives:

References:
1. Pharmaceutical manufacturers prescribing information.
2. www.cdc.gov/breastfeeding/recommendations/vaccinations.htm

PODOFILOX

Trade: Condylox, Podophyllotoxin

Category: Keratolytic

LRC: L3 - No Data-Probably Compatible

Podofilox (also called Podophyllotoxin) is an antimitotic agent used to treat genital warts and Condyloma acuminatum. Its transcutaneous absorption is minimal, plasma levels in 52 patients following use of 0.05 mL of 0.5% podofilox solution to external genitalia did not result in detectable serum levels. However, applications of 0.1 to 1.5 mL resulted in plasma levels of 1-17 ng/mL 1 to 2 hours post treatment. The drug does not accumulate after multiple treatments. No data are available on its transfer to human milk. It would be advisable to limit the dosage used in breastfeeding women, and to wait for a minimum of 4 hours following application before breastfeeding. The infant should be closely monitored for gastrointestinal distress. The use of this product in breastfeeding women should be avoided if possible.

T 1/2	1-4.5 h	MW	414 Da	PB	
Tmax	1-2 h	RID		Vd	
Oral		M/P		pKa	11.75

Adult Concerns: Burning, pain, inflammation, erosion and itching at site of injection. Insomnia, bleeding, tenderness, malodor, dizziness, scaring have been reported.

Adult Dose: Variable, but 0.5% solution applied topically every 12 hours is indicated for genital warts.

Pediatric Concerns: No data are available, but extreme caution is recommended if used. A brief waiting period of 4 hours or more following application is recommended.

Infant Monitoring:

Alternatives:

References:
1. Pharmaceutical manufacturers prescribing information.

POLIDOCANOL

Trade: Asclera

Category: Sclerosing agent

LRC: L3 - No Data-Probably Compatible

Polidocanol is a non-ionic detergent sclerosing agent used to treat varicose veins.[1] When injected into a vein, polidocanol locally damages the vessel endothelium. This damage is followed by platelet aggregation at the site, and subsequently by occlusion of the vessel. The varicose vein is then replaced by connective fibrous tissue. There are no adequate or well-controlled studies or case reports in breastfeeding women. The adverse effects of using polidocanol are mainly local. One-time treatment poses minimal harm to the infant, since the half-life is short and the effects are local. However, since the manufacturer has provided virtually no pharmacokinetic data, the effects are uncertain. The manufacturer recommends pumping and discarding milk for 8 hours following injections.

T 1/2	1.5 h	MW	580 Da	PB	
Tmax		RID		Vd	
Oral		M/P		pKa	6.5-8

Adult Concerns: Allergic reactions, injections site reactions, pain, thrombosis.

Adult Dose:

Pediatric Concerns: None reported.

Infant Monitoring: No known effects have been reported in breastfeeding infants. Recommend waiting period of 8 hours after injection.

Alternatives: Glycerin.

References:
1. Pharmaceutical manufacturers prescribing information.

POLIO VACCINE, INACTIVATED

Trade: Ipol

Category: Vaccine

LRC: L3 - No Data-Probably Compatible

Inactivated polio vaccine is administered for the prevention of poliomyelitis.[1] There are no adequate studies that determine the infant risk when using this medication during breastfeeding. If previously unimmunized or if traveling to an area endemic for polio, a lactating woman may receive inactivated poliovirus vaccine. Her infant should receive the inactivated polio vaccine according to the recommended childhood immunization schedule.[2]

Adult Concerns: Pain at site of injection, fever, fatigue, loss of appetite, vomiting, irritability.

Adult Dose:

Pediatric Concerns: None reported via breast milk. Adverse reactions from IPV administration: Local injection site reactions, fever, loss of appetite, vomiting, rash, irritability.

Infant Monitoring:

Alternatives:

References:
1. Pharmaceutical manufacturers prescribing information.
2. Pickering LK, Baker CJ, Long SS, McMillan JA, eds. Red Book: 2009 Report of the Committee on Infectious Diseases. 28th ed. Elk Grove Village, IL: American Academy of Pediatrics; 2009.

POLIO VACCINE, ORAL

Trade: Vaccine-Live Oral Trivalent Polio

Category: Vaccine

LRC: L3 - No Data-Probably Compatible

Oral polio vaccine is a mixture of three, live, attenuated oral polio viruses.[1] Human milk contains oral polio antibodies consistent with that of the maternal circulation.[2] Early exposure of the infant may reduce production of antibodies in the infant later on but this is not a major problem. Immunization of infant prior to 6 weeks of age is not recommended due to reduced antibody production. At this age, the effect of breast milk antibodies on the infant's development of antibodies is believed minimal. Wait until infant is 6 weeks of age before immunizing mother.

Adult Concerns: Rash, fever.

Adult Dose:

Pediatric Concerns: None reported via milk.

Infant Monitoring:

Alternatives:

References:
1. Pharmaceutical manufacturers prescribing information.
2. Adcock E, Greene H. Poliovirus antibodies in breast-fed infants. Lancet. 1971;2(7725):662-663.

POLYETHYLENE GLYCOL

Trade: Lax-A-Day, Miralax

Category: Laxative

LRC: L3 - No Data-Probably Compatible

Polyethylene glycols are derivatives of paraffins (mineral oils) and used in a large variety of applications. They are commonly used in ointments, suppositories, lubricants, plasticizers, binders, paints, polishes, paper coatings, cosmetics, hair preparations, food additives, and as a popular laxative. These agents generally exhibit little to no toxicity, and systemic absorption is unlikely when used topically or when ingested along with electrolytes for bowel cleansing purposes.

The molecular weights of these agents vary, with each preparation's molecular weight being denoted by a number after the name of the compound. For instance, polyethylene glycol 200 would consist of molecules averaging a molecular weight of 200. The weight of the chosen agent is important due to altered kinetics and incidence rates of adverse effects.[1] The popular laxative, MiraLAX, has a molecular weight of 3350. The latter, when used as a laxative is sequestered in the GI tract, and accumulates water in the GI tract, where it acts as a laxative. It would be very unlikely to enter the plasma of the mother, or milk. Although no data are available on transfer to human milk, it is highly unlikely that enough maternal absorption would occur to produce milk levels.

T 1/2		MW	Variable Da	PB	
Tmax		RID		Vd	
Oral	None	M/P		pKa	

Adult Concerns: Urticaria, nausea, bloating, cramping, diarrhea, flatulence.

Adult Dose: Variable.

Pediatric Concerns:

Infant Monitoring:

Alternatives:

References:
1. Polyethylene Glycol. TERIS. Reprotox System. Reviewed 12/06. Accessed July 21, 2011.

POLYETHYLENE GLYCOL-ELECTROLYTE SOLUTIONS

Trade: Colovage, Colyte, GoLYTELY, MoviPrep, PegLyte

Category: Laxative

LRC: L3 - No Data-Probably Compatible

Polyethylene glycol electrolyte solutions (PEG-ES) are saline laxatives.[1] It is a non-absorbable solution used as an osmotic agent to cleanse the bowel. It is completely non-absorbed from the adult gastrointestinal tract and would not likely penetrate human milk. This product is often used in children and infants prior to gastrointestinal surgery. Although no data are available on transfer to human milk, it is highly unlikely that enough maternal absorption would occur to produce milk levels.

T 1/2		MW		PB	
Tmax		RID		Vd	
Oral	None	M/P		pKa	

Adult Concerns: Diarrhea, bad taste, intestinal fullness. Do not use in gastrointestinal obstruction, gastric retention, bowel preformation, toxic colitis, megacolon, or ileus.

Adult Dose: 240 mL every 10 minutes up to 4 L.

Pediatric Concerns: None reported via milk.

Infant Monitoring:

Alternatives:

References:
1. Pharmaceutical manufacturers prescribing information.

POLYMYXIN B SULFATE

Trade:

Category: Antibiotic, Other

LRC: L2 - No Data-Probably Compatible

Polymyxin B is a commonly used topical, ophthalmic, and rarely injectable antibiotic. Most commonly used with other antibiotics, including neomycin and corticosteroids (hydrocortisone), it is commonly used to treat conjunctivitis, blepharitis, keratitis, and other topical infections.[1] It primarily covers most gram-negative bacteria and some gram-positive. It has been used in infants via injection (40,000 units/kg/day) but this is extremely rare. When applied ophthalmically, it is almost completely unabsorbed in surrounding tissues. No data are available on its transfer to human milk. However, when used topically it is very unlikely enough would be absorbed transcutaneously to produce plasma or milk levels. Orally, it would be largely destroyed by the gastric acid in the infant as it is very unstable in acidic milieu. When applied topically to nipples in small amounts, it is unlikely to produce problems in a breastfed infant.

T 1/2	6 h	MW	Large Da	PB	Low
Tmax	2 h	RID		Vd	
Oral		M/P		pKa	

Adult Concerns: Plasma concentrations exceeding 5 µg/mL in adults may produce paresthesia, dizziness, weakness, drowsiness, ataxia, etc. But these are only seen following IM, IV, or intrathecal injections, not via topical application.

Adult Dose: Topical: 10,000-25,000 units/mL.

Pediatric Concerns:

Infant Monitoring:

Alternatives:

References:
1. Pharmaceutical manufacturers prescribing information.

POSACONAZOLE

Trade: Noxafil

Category: Antifungal

LRC: L3 - No Data-Probably Compatible

Posaconazole is an antifungal medication used in the treatment of oropharyngeal candidiasis. The drug is also used in the treatment of chromoblastomycosis, invasive aspergillosis, mycetoma infections, fusariosis, and coccidioidomycosis. There is no increase in plasma concentration with daily doses above 800 mg. Steady-state is reached in 7 to 10 days. The pharmacokinetics are linear with a high fat meal. The drug is absorbed slowly from the gastrointestinal tract. The drug also has a large volume of distribution. Elimination is 77% via feces and 14% via urine. Sixty-six percent is excreted unchanged in the feces. Posaconazole has been found to be excreted in rat milk, but no human studies have been conducted on excretion into breast milk.[1-2] This drug's kinetic parameters suggest that significant transfer to breast milk is unlikely, however, caution is still advised due to its relatively long half-life.

T 1/2	35 h	MW	700.8 Da	PB	98%
Tmax	5 h	RID		Vd	Large L/kg
Oral		M/P		pKa	3.6, 4.6

Adult Concerns: Headache, fever, hypertension, QTc prolongation, nausea, vomiting, abdominal pain, diarrhea, changes in liver and renal function, hypokalemia, anemia, thrombocytopenia.

Adult Dose:

Pediatric Concerns:

Infant Monitoring: Vomiting, diarrhea.

Alternatives:

References:
1. Moton A, Krishna G, Ma L, et al. Pharmacokinetics of a single dose of the antifungal posaconazole as oral suspension in subjects with hepatic impairment. Curr Med Res Opin. 2010 Jan;26(1):1-7.
2. Courtney R, Pai S, Laughlin M, Lim J, Batra V. Pharmacokinetics, safety, and tolerability of oral posaconazole administered in single and multiple doses in healthy adults. Antimicrob Agents Chemother. 2003 Sep;47(9):2788-2795.

POTASSIUM IODIDE

Trade: SSKI, Iodide-potassium

Category: Antithyroid Agent

LRC: L4 - Limited Data-Possibly Hazardous

Potassium iodide is frequently used to suppress thyroxine secretion in hyperthyroid patients (thyroid storm). About 30% of the oral dose administered is taken up by the thyroid gland, 20% goes to fecal excretion, the rest is cleared renally. Thus the biological half-lives are: blood, 6 hours; thyroid gland, 80 days; rest of the body, 12 days.[1] Most of a dose administered is rapidly cleared from the body via feces and urine. Part (30%) is sequestered for long periods in the thyroid gland. Because plasma iodine is the only source of iodine uptake in breast milk, and it is cleared rapidly with a 6 hour half-life, mothers could theoretically return to breastfeeding after exposure to potassium iodide within approximately 24-48 hours. Iodide salts are known to be secreted into milk in high concentrations.[2,3] Milk/plasma ratios as high at 15-23 have been reported. Iodides are sequestered in the thyroid gland at high levels and can potentially cause severe thyroid depression in a breastfed infant.[1] Use with extreme caution if at all in breastfeeding mothers. Combined with the fact that it is a poor expectorant and that it is concentrated in breast milk, it is not recommended in breastfeeding mothers. However, following treatment of thyroid storm, mothers should pump and discard milk for at least 24-48 hours.

T 1/2	6 h (blood)	MW	166 Da	PB	
Tmax		RID		Vd	
Oral	Complete	M/P	23	pKa	

Adult Concerns: Thyroid depression, goiter, gastrointestinal distress, rash, gastrointestinal bleeding, fever, weakness.

Adult Dose: Varies by indication, RDA= 150 µg (iodine).

Pediatric Concerns: Thyroid suppression may occur. Do not use doses higher than RDA.

Infant Monitoring: Not recommended in lactation.

Alternatives:

References:

1. Kramer GH, Hauck BM, Chamberlain MJ. Biological half-life of iodine in adults with intact thyroid function and in athyreotic persons. Radiat Prot Dosimetry. 2002;102(2):129-135.
2. Delange F, Chanoine JP, Abrassart C, Bourdoux P. Topical iodine, breastfeeding, and neonatal hypothyroidism. Arch Dis Child. 1988;63(1):106-107.
3. Postellon DC, Aronow R. Iodine in mother's milk. JAMA. 1982;247(4):463.

POVIDONE IODIDE

Trade:

Category: Antiseptic

LRC: L4 - Limited Data-Possibly Hazardous

Povidone iodide is a chelated form of iodine. It is primarily used as an antiseptic and antimicrobial. When placed on the adult skin, very little is absorbed. When used intravaginally, significant and increased plasma levels of iodine have been documented. In a study of 62 pregnant women who used povidone-iodine douches, significant increases in plasma iodine were noted, and a seven-fold increase in fetal thyroid iodine content was reported.[1] Topical application to infants has resulted in significant absorption through the skin. Once plasma levels are attained in the mother, iodide rapidly sequesters in human milk at high milk/plasma ratios.[2,3] High oral iodine intake in mothers is documented to produce thyroid suppression in breastfed infants.[2] Use with extreme caution or not at all. Repeated use of povidone iodide is not recommended in nursing mothers or their infants.

T 1/2		MW		PB	
Tmax		RID		Vd	
Oral	Complete	M/P	>23	pKa	

Adult Concerns: Iodine toxicity, hypothyroidism, goiter, neutropenia.

Adult Dose:

Pediatric Concerns: Transfer of absorbed iodine could occur leading to neonatal thyroid suppression.

Infant Monitoring: Avoid if possible.

Alternatives:

References:

1. Mahillon I, Peers W, Bourdoux P, Ermans AM, Delange F. Effect of vaginal douching with povidone-iodine during early pregnancy on the iodine supply to mother and fetus. Biol Neonate. 1989;56(4):210-217.
2. Delange F, Chanoine JP, Abrassart C, Bourdoux P. Topical iodine, breastfeeding, and neonatal hypothyroidism. Arch Dis Child. 1988;63(1):106-107.
3. Postellon DC, Aronow R. Iodine in mother's milk. JAMA. 1982;247(4):463.

PRAMLINTIDE ACETATE

Trade: Symlin

Category: Antidiabetic, other

LRC: L3 - No Data-Probably Compatible

Pramlintide acetate is an antihyperglycemic agent used in diabetics.[1] Pramlintide is a synthetic analog of human amylin, a naturally occurring peptide created by the pancreatic beta cells that contributes to glucose control during the postprandial period. Amylin is co-located in beta cells and is co-secreted with insulin in response to food intake. Amylin has a number of biologic functions including; slowing gastric emptying and suppressing glucagon secretion, which reduces glucose output by the liver. It also reduces appetite by action in the CNS. In diabetics both insulin and amylin secretion are reduced in response to food. Pramlintide is a small peptide with a molecular weight of 3949 Da and is administered subcutaneously. Although we do not have data on its transfer to milk, this product is probably far too large to enter milk in clinically relevant amounts after the first 3-7 days postpartum. Being a small peptide, it is also unlikely to be absorbed orally in infants. Even when injected subcutaneously it is only 30%-40% bioavailable. It would probably not be contraindicated in breastfeeding mothers, but we have no data yet and some caution is certainly recommended.

T 1/2	48 min		MW	3949 Da		PB	
Tmax	20 min		RID			Vd	
Oral	40%		M/P			pKa	

Adult Concerns: Pramlintide in combination with insulin may lead to hypoglycemia. Nausea, headache, anorexia, vomiting, dizziness have been reported.

Adult Dose: Highly variable, consult prescribing information.

Pediatric Concerns: None reported via milk.

Infant Monitoring: Vomiting, weight gain and signs of hypoglycemia- drowsiness, lethargy, pallor, sweating, tremor.

Alternatives:

References:
1. Pharmaceutical manufacturers prescribing information.

PRAMOXINE

Trade: Curasore, PramoxGel, Prax, Proctofoam, Proctofoam-NS, Sarna Sensitive, Tronolane

Category: Anesthetic, Local

LRC: L3 - No Data-Probably Compatible

Pramoxine is a topical anesthetic used for the treatment of pruritus, and inflammation secondary to hemorrhoids, proctitis, cryptitis, and fissures.[1] Because this agent is used topically, it is not likely to be absorbed systemically. Do not use directly on the nipple. There are no adequate and well-controlled studies or case reports in breastfeeding women.

T 1/2			MW	293 Da		PB	
Tmax	3-5 min		RID			Vd	
Oral			M/P			pKa	7.1

Adult Concerns: Contact dermatitis, stinging, eczema, angioedema.

Adult Dose:

Pediatric Concerns:

Infant Monitoring:

Alternatives:

References:
1. Pharmaceutical manufacturers prescribing information.

PRASUGREL

Trade: Effient

Category: Platelet Aggregation Inhibitor

LRC: L4 - Limited Data-Possibly Hazardous

Prasugrel hydrochloride binds irreversibly to platelet receptors preventing platelet aggregation. Prasugrel reduces ischemic events seen (such as stent thrombosis) in acute coronary syndrome in patients who are undergoing percutaneous coronary intervention.[1] Prasugrel is a prodrug that is metabolized to both active and inactive chemicals. Approximately 68% of the drug is excreted in urine and 27% in feces. Most patients have a 50% decrease in platelet aggregation within 1 hour of dosing. Steady state was reached following 3 to 5 days of a 10 mg daily dose after loading with 60 mg. Platelet aggregation was inhibited 70%. Bleeding time was prolonged when administered with warfarin.

No studies on the transfer of prasugrel into breast milk are available. Because prasugrel produces an irreversible inhibition of platelet aggregation, any present in milk could inhibit an infant's platelet function for a prolonged period. Because aspirin affects platelet aggregation similarly, and its milk levels are quite low, it would appear to be an ideal alternative (see acetylsalicylic acid monograph for details). Prasugrel and aspirin are often given together to prevent thrombotic complications after placement of coronary stents. Caution is urged while using this drug in lactating women.

T 1/2	7 h (range 2-15 h)	MW	409.9 Da	PB	98%
Tmax	30 min	RID		Vd	0.62-0.97 L/kg
Oral	>79 %	M/P		pKa	5.1

Adult Concerns: Headache, dizziness, fatigue, hyper or hypotension, arrhythmias, nausea, diarrhea, leukopenia, anemia, bruising, bleeding, peripheral edema.

Adult Dose: 10 mg daily.

Pediatric Concerns: None reported.

Infant Monitoring: Rare-bruising on the skin, blood in urine, vomit, or stool.

Alternatives: Aspirin (low dose).

References:
1. Pharmaceutical manufacturers prescribing information.
2. Armani AM. Prasugrel: an efficacy and safety review of a new antiplatelet therapy option. Crit Pathw Cardiol. 2010 Dec;9(4):199-202.

PRAVASTATIN

Trade: Lipostat, Pravachol

Category: Antihyperlipidemic

LRC: L3 - No Data-Probably Compatible

Pravastatin belongs to the HMG-CoA reductase family of cholesterol lowering drugs.[1] Small amounts are believed to be secreted into human milk, but the levels are unreported. The effect on the infant is unknown and statins could reduce cholesterol synthesis. Cholesterol and other products of cholesterol biosynthesis are essential components for neonatal development; therefore, it is not clear if it would be safe for use in a breastfed infant who needs high levels of cholesterol. Caution is recommended until more data are available.

T 1/2	77 h	MW	446 Da	PB	50%
Tmax	1-1.5 h	RID		Vd	
Oral	17%	M/P		pKa	4.7

Adult Concerns: Headache, fatigue, dizziness, chest pain, dyspepsia, nausea, vomiting, changes in liver function, hemolytic anemia, myalgia.

Adult Dose: 10-20 mg daily.

Pediatric Concerns: None reported via milk but studies are limited.

Infant Monitoring: Weight gain, growth.

Alternatives:

References:
1. Pharmaceutical manufacturers prescribing information.

PRAZIQUANTEL

Trade: Biltricide

Category: Anthelmintic

LRC: L2 - Limited Data-Probably Compatible

Praziquantel is a trematodicide used for treatment of schistosome infections and infestations of liver flukes. In a study of 10 women who received 1) a single dose of 50 mg/kg; or 2) 20 mg/kg three times daily, milk and plasma levels were determined at multiple time intervals over the next 32 hours.[1] In group 1, the average milk concentration was 0.19 mg/L. In group 2, the average milk concentration was 0.198 mg/L. Throughout the duration of this study, the infants in group 1 ingested 27.4 µg and those in group 2 ingested 25.6 µg of praziquantel. On average, the maternal plasma concentrations were four times higher than milk concentrations. Using this data, the relative infant dose would be approximately 0.05% of the maternal dose in both groups. These values are probably too low to harm an infant.

T 1/2	0.8-1.5 h, metabolite 4.5 h	MW	312 Da	PB	80%
Tmax	1-3 h	RID	0.05%-0.06%	Vd	
Oral	80%	M/P	0.25%	pKa	

Adult Concerns: Fever, dizziness, headache, abdominal pain, drowsiness, and malaise.

Adult Dose: 10-25 mg/kg BID-TID X 1 day.

Pediatric Concerns: None reported via milk.

Infant Monitoring:

Alternatives:

References:
1. Leopold G, Ungethum W, Groll E, Diekmann HW, Nowak H, Wegner DH. Clinical pharmacology in normal volunteers of praziquantel, a new drug against schistosomes and cestodes. An example of a complex study covering both tolerance and pharmacokinetics. Eur J Clin Pharmacol. 1978;14(4):281-291.

PRAZOSIN

Trade: Hypovasl, Minipress, Pressin

Category: Alpha-Adrenergic Blocker

LRC: L3 - No Data-Probably Compatible

Prazosin is a selective alpha-1-adrenergic antagonist used to control hypertension. It is structurally similar to doxazosin and terazosin.[1] While we have no data on prazosin levels in milk, doxazosin is shown to have minimal milk levels.

T 1/2	2-3 h	MW	383 Da	PB	92%-97%
Tmax	2-3 h	RID		Vd	0.5 L/kg
Oral	43%-82%	M/P		pKa	6.5

Adult Concerns: Headache, dizziness, drowsiness, hypotension, palpitations, dry mouth, constipation, urinary frequency, weakness, edema.

Adult Dose: 3-7.5 mg twice daily.

Pediatric Concerns: None reported via milk at this time.

Infant Monitoring: Drowsiness, low blood pressure, lethargy, pallor, poor feeding, and weight gain.

Alternatives: Doxazosin(L3), Labetalol(L2)

References:
1. Pharmaceutical manufacturers prescribing information.

PREDNICARBATE

Trade: Dermatop, Rayos

Category: Corticosteroid

LRC: L3 - No Data-Probably Compatible

Prednicarbate is a high potency steroid ointment.[1] Its absorption via skin surfaces is exceedingly low, even in infants. Its oral absorption is not reported but would probably be equivalent to prednisolone, or higher. If recommended for topical application on the nipple, other less potent steroids should be suggested, including hydrocortisone or triamcinolone. If applied to the nipple, only extremely small amounts should be applied.

T 1/2		MW	488 Da	PB	
Tmax		RID		Vd	
Oral		M/P		pKa	

Adult Concerns: Symptoms of adrenal steroid suppression, fluid retention, gastric ulcers.

Adult Dose:

Pediatric Concerns: None reported via milk.

Infant Monitoring: Feeding, growth, and weight gain.

Alternatives:

References:
1. Pharmaceutical manufacturers prescribing information.

PREDNISONE-PREDNISOLONE

Trade: Prednisolone, Prednisone

Category: Corticosteroid

LRC: L2 - Limited Data-Probably Compatible

Small amounts of most corticosteroids are secreted into breast milk. Following a 10 mg oral dose of prednisone, peak milk levels of prednisolone and prednisone were 1.6 µg/L and 2.67 µg/L, respectively.[1] In a group of 10 women who received 10-80 mg/day prednisolone, the milk levels were only 5%-25% of the maternal serum levels.[2]

In one patient who received 80 mg/day prednisolone, the peak plasma concentration at 1 hour was 317 µg/L. The AUC average milk concentration in this mother was 156 µg/L over 6 hours.[2] This is significantly less than 2% of the weight-normalized maternal dose. Because this last estimate was only determined over 6 hours and this dose was administered once each 24 hours, the total daily estimate would be much less than the 2% estimate.

In another study of a single patient who received 120 mg prednisone/day, the total combined steroid levels (predni-sone + prednisolone) peaked at 2 hours.[3] The peak level of combined steroid was 627 µg/L, we used this peak value to calculate an RID of 5.3%, this is most likely an overestimate. Assuming the infant received 120 mL of milk every 4 hours, the total possible ingestion would only be 47 µg/day.

In a group of seven women who received radioactive labeled prednisolone 5 mg, the total recovery per liter of milk during the 48 hours after the dose was 0.14%.[4]

In small doses, most steroids are certainly not contraindicated in nursing mothers. Whenever possible use low-dose alternatives such as aerosols or inhalers. With high doses (>40 mg/day), particularly for long periods, steroids could potentially produce problems in infant growth and development, although we have absolutely no data in this area, or which doses would pose problems. Brief applications of high dose steroids are not contraindicated as the overall exposure is low. With prolonged high dose therapy, the infant should be closely monitored. Following extremely high dose administration for prolonged periods, the mother could wait at least 4 hours prior to feeding her infant to reduce exposure.

T 1/2	2-3 h	MW	358 Da	PB	>90%
Tmax	1-2 h (maternal plasma) 1 h (milk)	RID	1.8%-5.3%	Vd	
Oral	Complete	M/P	0.25	pKa	12.58

Adult Concerns: Headache, changes in mood, insomnia, nervousness, hypertension, heart failure, edema, vomiting, peptic ulcers, weight gain, changes in liver function, hyperglycemia, changes in electrolytes, leukocytosis, muscle weakness, osteoporosis.

Adult Dose: 5-120 mg/day.

Pediatric Concerns: None reported via milk.

Infant Monitoring: Feeding, growth, and weight gain; could consider a CBC with prolonged exposure. Try to limit degree and duration of exposure if possible. Short-term use is suitable.

Alternatives:

References:
1. Katz FH, Duncan BR. Letter: Entry of prednisone into human milk. N Engl J Med. 1975;293(22):1154.
2. Ost L, Wettrell G, Bjorkhem I, Rane A. Prednisolone excretion in human milk. J Pediatr. 1985;106(6):1008-1011.
3. Berlin CM, Kaiser DG, Demmers L. Excretion of prednisone and prednisolone in human milk. Pharmacologist. 1979;21:264.
4. McKenzie SA, Selley JA, Agnew JE. Secretion of prednisolone into breast milk. Arch Dis Child. 1975;50(11):894-896.

PREGABALIN

Trade: Lyrica

Category: Anticonvulsant

LRC: L3 - Limited Data-Probably Compatible

Pregabalin is an anticonvulsant with multiple clinical indications, including partial seizures, fibromyalgia and neuropathic pain.[1] In a study of 10 healthy women (median 35 weeks postpartum) given pregabalin 150 mg twice daily for four doses, milk levels peaked at 4.63 hours.[2] The average C_{max} was 2.47 µg/mL, the C_{avg} was 2.05 µg/mL and the mean milk/plasma ratio was 0.53. The RID and absolute infant dose were 7.18% and 0.31 mg/kg/day, respectively. It should be noted that the infants in this study were not breastfed.

T 1/2	6 h	MW	159 Da	PB	Unbound
Tmax	1.5 h	RID	7.18%	Vd	0.5 L/kg
Oral	90%	M/P	0.34-0.76	pKa	4.8

Adult Concerns: Dizziness, somnolence, confusion, insomnia, blurred vision, dry mouth, constipation, edema, weakness, tremor.

Adult Dose: 150-600 mg/day in divided doses.

Pediatric Concerns: No data available in infants at this time.

Infant Monitoring: Sedation, slowed breathing rate/apnea, constipation, and not waking to feed/poor feeding.

Alternatives:

References:
1. Pharmaceutical manufacturers prescribing information.
2. Lockwood PA, Pauer L, Scavone JM, et al. The pharmacokinetics of pregabalin in breast milk, plasma, and urine of healthy postpartum women. J Hum Lact. 2016;32(3):NP1-NP8.

PRIMAQUINE PHOSPHATE

Trade: Primaquine

Category: Antimalarial

LRC: L2 - Limited Data-Probably Compatible

Primaquine is a typical antimalarial medication that is primarily used as chemoprophylaxis after the patient has returned from the region of exposure with the intention of preventing relapses of *plasmodium vivax* and/or *ovale*. It is used in pediatric patients at a dose of 0.3 mg/kg/day for 14 days.[1-3]

In a recent study, 21 breastfeeding mothers received a dose of 0.5 mg/kg daily for up to 14 days.[4] Maternal plasma T_{max} occurred at 2 hours and 2.99 hours at day zero and day 13 respectively. T_{max} levels in milk occurred at 3.42 and 3.87 hours on day zero and day 13, respectively. C_{max} levels of primaquine in milk were 44.0 ng/mL and 43.9 ng/mL at day zero and day 13, respectively. Capillary blood samples were taken from infants on day 0, 3, 7, and 13 of therapy. Primaquine concentration exceeded the lower limit of detection in only one infant plasma sample, and this level was low at 2.59 ng/mL. The authors reported cumulative infant exposure to primaquine in breast milk of 0.042 mg/kg over 14 days, or 2.98 µg/kg/day. They estimated the RID at 0.618% on day 0 and 0.517% on day 13.

The authors reported concentrations of primaquine in breast milk were very low and therefore very unlikely to cause adverse effects in the breastfeeding infant. Primaquine should not be withheld from mothers breastfeeding infants or young children.

T 1/2	4-7 h	MW	259 Da	PB	
Tmax	2 h	RID	0.517%-0.618%	Vd	3.84 L/kg
Oral	96%	M/P		pKa	

Adult Concerns: Headache, changes in vision, arrhythmias, vomiting, diarrhea, agranulocytosis, anemia, leukopenia, leukocytosis, methemoglobinemia, pruritus.

Adult Dose: 15 mg daily.

Pediatric Concerns: None reported from milk at this time.

Infant Monitoring: A recent study suggests concentrations of primaquine in breast milk are very low and therefore very unlikely to cause adverse effects in the breastfeeding infant. No infants in a study of 23 mothers displayed side effects. Primaquine should not be withheld from mothers breastfeeding infants or young children.

Alternatives:

References:
1. Mihaly GW, Ward SA, Edwards G, Orme ML, Breckenridge AM. Pharmacokinetics of primaquine in man: identification of the carboxylic acid derivative as a major plasma metabolite. Br J Clin Pharmacol. 1984;17(4):441-446.

2. Mihaly GW, Ward SA, Edwards G, Nicholl DD, Orme ML, Breckenridge AM. Pharmacokinetics of primaquine in man. I. Studies of the absolute bioavailability and effects of dose size. Br J Clin Pharmacol. 1985;19(6):745-750.

3. Bhatia SC, Saraph YS, Revankar SN, et al. Pharmacokinetics of primaquine in patients with P. vivax malaria. Eur J Clin Pharmacol. 1986;31(2):205-210.

4. Gilder ME, Hanpithakphong W, Hoglund RM, et al. Primaquine pharmacokinetics in lactating women and breastfed infant exposures. Clin Infect Dis. 2018 Sep;67(7):1000-1007. doi: 10.1093/cid/ciy235. PMID: 29590311; PubMed Central PMCID: PMC6137118.

PRIMIDONE

Trade: Misolyne, Mysoline, Sertan

Category: Anticonvulsant

LRC: L4 - Limited Data-Possibly Hazardous

Primidone is a barbiturate and an anticonvulsant with sedative/hypnotic properties. It is metabolized in adults to several derivatives including phenobarbital. After chronic therapy, levels of phenobarbital rise to a therapeutic range. Hence, problems for the infant would not only include primidone but, subsequently, phenobarbital. In one study of two women receiving primidone, the steady-state concentrations of primidone in neonatal serum via ingestion of breast milk were 0.7 and 2.5 µg/mL.[1] The steady-state phenobarbital levels in neonatal serum were between 2 to 13 µg/mL. The calculated dose of phenobarbital per day received by each infant ranged from 1.8 to 8.9 mg/day. Some sedation has been reported, particularly during the neonatal period. In another group of 4 women receiving 7.3 mg/kg/day primidone, levels in milk averaged 4.2 mg/L.[2] In another patient receiving 750 mg/day primidone and valproic acid 2.4 grams/day, breast milk levels of primidone averaged 6 mg/L.[3]

Please also review phenobarbital monograph.

T 1/2	5-18 h (primidone), 75-120 h metabolite	MW	218 Da	PB	25%
Tmax	1-2 h	RID	8.4%-8.6%	Vd	0.5-1 L/kg
Oral	90%	M/P	0.72	pKa	

Adult Concerns: Sedation, ataxia, drowsiness, vertigo, nystagmus, diplopia, anorexia, nausea, vomiting, hematologic changes.

Adult Dose: 250 mg three times daily.

Pediatric Concerns: Some sedation, during neonatal period.

Infant Monitoring: Sedation or irritability, not waking to feed/poor feeding, and weight gain. Based on clinical symptoms some infants may require monitoring of liver enzymes or CBC. Infant phenobarbital plasma levels approximate one-third (or lower) of maternal plasma levels.

Alternatives:

References:

1. Kuhnz W, Koch S, Helge H, Nau H. Primidone and phenobarbital during lactation period in epileptic women: total and free drug serum levels in the nursed infants and their effects on neonatal behavior. Dev Pharmacol Ther. 1988;11(3):147-154.

2. Nau H, Rating D, Hauser I, et al. Placental transfer and pharmacokinetics of primidone and its metabolites phenobarbital, PEMA, and hydroxyphenobarbital in neonates and infants of epileptic mothers. Eur J Clin Pharmacol. 1980;18:31-42.

3. Espir MLE, Benton P, Will E, et al. Sodium valproate - some clinical and pharmacological aspects. In: Legg NJ, ed. Clinical and Pharmacological Aspects of Sodium Valproate in the Treatment of Epilepsy: Proceedings of a Symposium; 1976;145-151.

PROBENECID

Trade: Apurina, Benecid, Benemid, Probanalan, Proben, Uricosid

Category: Other

LRC: L2 - Limited Data-Probably Compatible

Probenecid is a uricosuric agent which accelerates the urinary excretion of uric acid by inhibiting the reabsorption of uric acid in the proximal convoluted tubule in the kidney. Hence it dramatically reduces plasma uric acid. It is also used to prevent the elimination of various penicillins and cephalosporins and is used to prolong their elimination half-lives.

In a case report of a mother taking cephalexin 500 mg 4x/day along with probenecid 500 mg 4x/day (to prolong half-life of cephalexin), the baby had gastrointestinal adverse effects.[1] It was noted that while the mother was receiving IV cephalothin, her infant had a green liquid stool with severe diarrhea, discomfort, and crying. These symptoms continued when the mother was switched to oral cephalexin + probenecid. The infant did not have signs of dehydration; however, on day 13, the infant began supplementation with 15% of its daily intake as goat's milk formula. By day 20, the symptoms had resolved. The average milk concentration of probenecid 964 μg/L, this corresponds to a relative infant dose of 0.7%.

T 1/2	6-12 h	MW	285 Da	PB	75%-95%
Tmax	2-4 h	RID	0.7%	Vd	
Oral	Complete	M/P	0.03	pKa	

Adult Concerns: Headache, dizziness, hepatic necrosis, vomiting, nausea, anorexia and sore gums. Nephrotic syndrome may occur with presence of uric acid stones, renal colic, and urinary frequency. Anaphylaxis, fever, urticaria, pruritus, aplastic anemia, leukopenia, neutropenia, and thrombocytopenia have been reported.

Adult Dose: 500 mg four times daily or less.

Pediatric Concerns: Although milk levels are quite low, the renal excretion of many drugs is significantly impeded by probenecid. Thus when used in combination with other medications, the infant may have complications from altered half-lives of other medications.

Infant Monitoring: Vomiting, diarrhea, changes in feeding.

Alternatives:

References:
1. Ilett KF, Hackett LP, Ingle B, Bretz PJ. Transfer of probenecid and cephalexin into breast milk. Ann Pharmacother. 2006 May;40(5):986-989.

PROBIOTICS

Trade:

Category: Gastrointestinal Agent

LRC: L3 - Limited Data-Probably Compatible

Probiotics are micro-organisms that are identical or similar to natural microflora that are found in the gut. They are defined as living organisms that may elicit a beneficial health effect when ingested or applied to the body. The evidence for use of these products is controversial and potential benefits are often minimal when compared to cost.[1,2] While most of these products are used orally, there have been some instances of vaginal administration. Common organisms found in these products are Lactobacillus, Bifidobacterium, and Saccharomyces species.[1]

When ingested or used vaginally, these products are typically well tolerated; however, there has been ongoing concerns that, due to the activity of these preparations, the organisms could penetrate the blood stream and cause a systemic infection in the individual taking the product.[1] While there are few reports of such problems occurring, it should be noted that such infections have occurred; the estimated incidences are very low, less than 1 per 1 million for Lactobacillus, and 1 per 5.6 million for Saccharomyces.[3-5] No reports of Bifidobacterium infection have been reported from probiotic use.[6] Potential risk factors that could increase the chance of systemic infection include immunosuppression, severe illness, central catheters, and injury to the gut.[4]

There are limited data regarding the transfer of probiotics to breast milk. In one study, 232 women were randomized to L reuteri or placebo supplementation for the last 4 weeks of pregnancy, the authors found that the colostrum of women taking the supplement isolated the bacteria more frequently than the placebo group (12% vs. 2% of samples).[7] There are currently no published data with adequate sample sizes that specifically address adverse effects in breastfed infants whose mothers were actively taking probiotics.[1]

With new research being published daily regarding the effects of the microbiome on the developing infants' immune system and risk for disease later in life, it is difficult to determine the benefits and risks of introducing a new bacterial strain into this complicated system.[8]

We recommend caution with use in women with a premature infant whom would be at greatest risk of infection and necrotizing enterocolitis.

Adult Concerns: Endocarditis, burping, vomiting, gas, bloating, constipation, septicemia, fungemia, rash.

Adult Dose: Dosing varies, most often taken 1-4 times daily.

Pediatric Concerns:

Infant Monitoring:

Alternatives:

References:

1. Bozzo P, Einarson A, Elias J. Are probiotics safe for use during pregnancy and lactation? Can Fam Physician. 2011 Mar;57:299–301.
2. Therapeutic Research Center. Comparison of common probiotic products. Pharmacists Lett. 2012 July;19(7):280707.
3. Snydman DR. The safety of probiotics. Clin Infect Dis. 2008;46(Suppl 2):S104-S111.
4. Borriello SP, Hammes WP, Holzapfel W, et al. Safety of probiotics that contain lactobacilli or bifidobacteria. Clin Infect Dis. 2003;36(6):775-780. Epub 2003 Mar 5.
5. Karpa KD. Probiotics for clostridium difficile diarrhea: putting it into perspective. Ann Pharmacother. 2007;41(7):1284-1287. Epub 2007 Jun 26.
6. Boyle RJ, Robins-Browne RM, Tang ML. Probiotic use in clinical practice: what are the risks? Am J Clin Nutr. 2006;83(6):1256-1264.
7. Abrahamsson TR, Sinkiewicz G, Jakobsson T, Fredrikson M, Björkstén B. Probiotic lactobacilli in breast milk and infant stool in relation to oral intake during the first year of life. J Pediatr Gastroenterol Nutr. 2009;49(3):349-354.
8. Backhed F, Roswall J, Peng Y, et al. Dynamics and stabilization of the human gut microbiome during the first year of life. Cell Host Microbe. 2015;17(5):690-703.

PROCAINAMIDE

Trade: Procan, Procan SR, Pronestyl

Category: Antiarrhythmic

LRC: L3 - Limited Data-Probably Compatible

Procainamide is an anti-arrhythmic agent. Procainamide and its active metabolite are secreted into breast milk in moderate concentrations. In one patient receiving 500 mg four times daily, the breast milk levels of procainamide at 0, 3, 6, 9, and 12 hours were 5.3, 3.9, 10.2, 4.8, and 2.6 mg/L respectively.[1] The milk/serum ratio varied from 1 at 12 hours to 7.3 at 6 hours postdose (mean 4.3). The milk levels averaged 5.4 mg/L for parent drug and 3.5 mg/L for metabolite. Although levels in milk are still too small to provide significant blood levels in an infant, use with caution.

T 1/2	3 h	MW	235 Da	PB	15%-20%
Tmax	0.75-2.5 h	RID	5.4%	Vd	2 L/kg
Oral	75%-90%	M/P	1-7.3	pKa	9.2

Adult Concerns: Dizziness, changes in mood, hypotension, arrhythmias, changes in taste, nausea, vomiting, anorexia, changes in liver function, agranulocytosis, myalgia, rash.

Adult Dose: 500-1000 mg every 6 hours.

Pediatric Concerns: None reported via milk.

Infant Monitoring: Drowsiness, lethargy, arrhythmias, poor feeding, vomiting, diarrhea, weight gain; if clinical symptoms arise check liver function.

Alternatives:

References:

1. Pittard WB III, Glazier H. Procainamide excretion in human milk. J Pediatr. 1983;102(4):631-633.

PROCAINE HCL

Trade: Novocain

Category: Anesthetic, Local

LRC: L3 - No Data-Probably Compatible

Procaine is an ester-type local anesthetic with low potential for systemic toxicity and short duration of action.[1] Procaine is generally used for infiltration or local anesthesia, peripheral nerve block, or rarely, spinal anesthesia. Procaine is rapidly metabolized by plasma pseudocholinesterase to p-aminobenzoic acid. No data are available on its transfer to human milk, but it is unlikely. Most other local anesthetics (see bupivacaine, lidocaine) penetrate milk only poorly and it is likely that procaine, due to its brief plasma half-life, would produce even lower milk levels. Due to its ester bond, it would be poorly bioavailable.

T 1/2	7.7 min	MW	236 Da	PB	5.8%
Tmax		RID		Vd	
Oral	Poor	M/P		pKa	9.1

Adult Concerns: High plasma concentrations of procaine due to excessive dosage, or inadvertent intravascular injection may result in systemic adverse effects involving the cardiovascular and central nervous systems including nervousness, drowsiness, or blurred vision.

Adult Dose: 350-600 mg X 1.

Pediatric Concerns: None reported via milk.

Infant Monitoring:

Alternatives:

References:
1. Pharmaceutical manufacturers prescribing information.

PROCHLORPERAZINE

Trade: Buccastem, Compazine, Nu-Prochlor, Prorazin, Stemetil

Category: Antiemetic

LRC: L3 - No Data-Probably Compatible

Prochlorperazine is a phenothiazine primarily used as an antiemetic in adults and pediatric patients.[1] There are no data yet concerning breast milk levels but other phenothiazine derivatives enter milk in small amounts. Because infants are extremely hypersensitive to these compounds, we suggest caution in mothers with younger infants. This product may also increase prolactin levels.[2] We recommend the use of other alternatives with more data in lactation when suitable for the maternal condition (e.g., ondansetron, dimenhydrinate, metoclopramide).

T 1/2	6-10 h (single dose), 14-22 h (repeated dose)	MW	374 Da	PB	90%
Tmax	4-8 h	RID		Vd	20-22.1 L/kg
Oral	12.5% oral	M/P		pKa	

Adult Concerns: Sedation, dizziness, agitation, seizure, hypotension, arrhythmias, dry mouth, vomiting, constipation, increased appetite, changes in liver function, leukopenia, thrombocytopenia, extrapyramidal effects, weight gain.

Adult Dose: 5-10 mg three to four times daily.

Pediatric Concerns: None reported via milk, but caution is recommended.

Infant Monitoring: Sedation or irritability, apneas, not waking to feed/poor feeding, dry mouth, weight gain, and extrapyramidal symptoms.

Alternatives: Dimenhydrinate(L2), Metoclopramide(L2), Ondansetron(L2)

References:
1. Pharmaceutical manufacturers prescribing information.

PROGUANIL + ATOVAQUONE

Trade: Malarone

Category: Antimalarial

LRC: L3 - No Data-Probably Compatible

Proguanil is used in combination with atovaquone to treat and prevent malaria.[1,2] Due to increasing resistance, atovaquone and proguanil are always given together to treat malaria (combination tablet available commercially).[1] According to the manufacturer only trace quantities of proguanil have been found in human milk (details not specified). At this time, this medication combination is not recommended by the WHO for malaria in lactation.[3] Please see atovaquone monograph for further details.

Please note that regardless of maternal malaria therapy, concentrations achieved in human milk are too low to be therapeutic in the infant.[3] Therefore, a nursing infant should be assessed and given appropriate prophylaxis or treatment for malaria based on their individual needs.

T 1/2	12-21 h	MW	254 Da	PB	75%
Tmax	2-4 h	RID		Vd	27-42 L/kg
Oral	60%	M/P		pKa	

Adult Concerns: When given in combination with atovaquone: Headache, dizziness, anorexia, nausea, vomiting, abdominal pain, diarrhea, changes in liver enzymes, weakness, anemia, pancytopenia, pruritus, rash.

Adult Dose: 100-400 mg/day (varies by indication).

Pediatric Concerns: No data in lactation. Proguanil is recommended for prevention of malaria in children > 11 kg and has limited data for treatment of malaria in infants greater than 5 kg.[3]

Infant Monitoring: Weakness, vomiting, diarrhea, decreased feeding/poor weight gain. If clinical signs of jaundice check liver enzymes or if ongoing infection check CBC.

Alternatives:

References:

1. Pharmaceutical manufacturers prescribing information.
2. Product Information. Paludrine (R), Proguanil. Plankstadt: Zeneca GmbH; 1995.
3. World Health Organization (WHO). Chapter 7 Malaria. International Travel and Health 2010. http://www.who.int/ith/ITH_chapter_7.pdf

PROMETHAZINE

Trade: Avomine, Histanil, Phenergan, Promethegan

Category: Antiemetic

LRC: L3 - No Data-Probably Compatible

Promethazine is a phenothiazine that is primarily used for nausea, vomiting, and motion sickness.[1] It has been used for many years in adult and pediatric patients for vomiting, particularly associated with pregnancy.[2] No data are available on the transfer of promethazine to milk, but small amounts probably do transfer. We recommend the use of other alternatives with more data in lactation when suitable for the maternal condition (e.g., ondansetron, dimenhydrinate, metoclopramide).

T 1/2	9-16 h	MW	321 Da	PB	76%-93%
Tmax	2-3 h	RID		Vd	13.9 L/kg
Oral	25%	M/P		pKa	9.1

Adult Concerns: Sedation, dizziness, agitation, confusion, seizure, blurred vision, hypotension, arrhythmias, QTc prolongation, dry mouth, vomiting, constipation, changes in liver function, leukopenia, thrombocytopenia, extrapyramidal symptoms, weight gain.

Adult Dose: 12.5-25 mg every 4-6 hours as needed.

Pediatric Concerns: None reported via breast milk; some caution is recommended as this medication has been associated with CNS depression and apneas in children less than 1 year of age.[3]

Infant Monitoring: Sedation or irritability, apneas, not waking to feed/poor feeding, dry mouth, weight gain, extrapyramidal symptoms.

Alternatives: Ondansetron(L2), Dimenhydrinate(L2), Metoclopramide(L2)

References:

1. Pharmaceutical manufacturers prescribing information.
2. Kris EB. Children born to mothers maintained on pharmacotherapy during pregnancy and postpartum. Recent Adv Biol Psychiatry. 1961;4:180-187.
3. Pollard AJ, Rylance G. Inappropriate prescribing of promethazine in infants. Arch Dis Child. 1994;70(4):357.

PROPAFENONE

Trade: Arythmol, Rythmol

Category: Antiarrhythmic

LRC: L2 - Limited Data-Probably Compatible

Propafenone is a class 1C antiarrhythmic agent with structural similarities to propranolol.[1] In a mother receiving 300 mg three times daily and at 3 days postpartum, maternal serum levels of propafenone and 5-OH-propafenone (active metabolite) were 219 µg/L and 86 µg/L respectively. The breast milk level of propafenone and 5-OH-propafenone was 32 µg/L and 47 µg/L respectively.[2] The milk/plasma ratios for drug and metabolite were 0.15 and 0.54 respectively. The authors estimate that the daily intake of drug and active metabolite in the infant (3.3 kg) would have been 16 µg and 24 µg per day respectively.

T 1/2	2-10 h, 10-32 h (poor metabolizer)	MW	341 Da	PB	85%-97%
Tmax	2-3 h	RID	0.09%	Vd	3.6 L/kg
Oral	5%-50%	M/P	0.15	pKa	14.09

Adult Concerns: Dizziness, headache, insomnia, anxiety, unusual taste, dry mouth, hypotension, arrhythmias, heart failure, chest pain, dyspnea, nausea, vomiting, constipation, changes in liver function, agranulocytosis, leukopenia, tremor.

Adult Dose: 150-225 mg three times daily.

Pediatric Concerns: None reported via milk at this time.

Infant Monitoring: Drowsiness, lethargy, insomnia, pallor, arrhythmias, dry mouth, poor feeding, vomiting, weight gain, tremor.

Alternatives:

References:
1. Pharmaceutical manufacturers prescribing information.
2. Libardoni M, Piovan D, Busato E, Padrini R. Transfer of propafenone and 5-OH-propafenone to foetal plasma and maternal milk. Br J Clin Pharmacol. 1991;32(4):527-528.

PROPOFOL

Trade: Diprivan

Category: Sedative-Hypnotic

LRC: L2 - Limited Data-Probably Compatible

Propofol is an IV sedative hypnotic agent for induction and maintenance of anesthesia. It is particularly popular in various pediatric procedures. Although the terminal half-life is long, it is rapidly distributed out of the plasma compartment to other peripheral compartments (adipose) so that anesthesia is short (3-10 minutes). Propofol is incredibly lipid soluble. However, only very low concentrations of propofol have been found in breast milk.

In one study of four women who received propofol 2.5 mg/kg IV followed by a continuous infusion, the breast milk levels at 4 hours ranged from 0.04 to 0.24 mg/L during the induction phase only.[1] Following continued infusion of propofol in some patients at 5 mg/kg/h, milk samples at 4 hours ranged from 0.04 to 0.74 mg/L. The second breast milk level, obtained 24 hours after delivery, contained only 6% of the 4-hour sample. Similar levels (0.12-0.97 mg/L) were noted by Schmitt in colostrum samples obtained 4-8 hours after induction with propofol.[2]

In another study of five women undergoing surgery with midazolam premedication and induction with propofol and fentanyl, milk samples were obtained at 5, 7, 9, 11, and 24 hours post propofol administration.[3] These women were on average 11 weeks postpartum and produced about 325 mL/day of milk. The median amount of propofol recovered in milk within 24 hours postdose was 26 μg or 0.015% of the median maternal dose (180 mg). The weight-normalized infant dose was 5.2 μg/kg (1.5-29.6 μg/kg). None of the infants were given their mothers milk during this study.

In a publication with four women undergoing surgery with propofol and remifentanil induction and remifentanil and xenon maintenance, milk samples were taken from two women at 90 and 300 minutes postdose.[4] The women in this study were breastfeeding newborns to babies 5 months of age and resumed feeding their infants 90 minutes to 5 hours post-procedure (once alert, eating, and discharged from recovery). All infants were watched during their first feed and no signs of drowsiness were reported. In case 3, the mother was given 350 mg of IV propofol and her milk contained 19.5 μg/150 mL of milk at 300 minutes. In case 4, the women was given 443 mg of IV propofol and her milk contained 417 μg/150 mL of milk at 90 minutes and 126 μg/150 mL of milk at 300 min

There is one case report of a woman with green breast milk after an infusion of 474 mg of propofol.[5] The patient collected milk for the first time 8 hours post-op and the milk was bluish/green; the milk then remained green throughout the day and normalized over 48 hours. The authors of this case report were unable to determine the reason/mechanism for this change in milk color but speculated propofol may have been the cause. Additional perioperative medications included: fentanyl, remifentanil, mivacurium, metamizole, dimenhydrinate, piritramide, butylscopolamine, and metoclopramide.

From these data, it is apparent that only minimal amounts of propofol are transferred to human milk.[1-4] No data are available on the oral absorption of propofol. Propofol is rapidly cleared from the neonatal circulation.[1]

T 1/2	1-3 days	MW	178 Da	PB	99%
Tmax	Instant (IV)	RID	4.44%	Vd	60 L/kg
Oral		M/P		pKa	11

Adult Concerns: Sedation, agitation, delirium, hyper or hypotension, arrhythmias, apnea, hypertriglyceridemia, changes in electrolytes, propofol-related infusion syndrome.

Adult Dose: 3-6 mg/kg/hour maintenance anesthesia.

Pediatric Concerns: None have been reported via milk at this time.

Infant Monitoring: Sedation, slowed breathing rate, not waking to feed/poor feeding.

Alternatives: Midazolam(L2)

References:

1. Dailland P, Cockshott ID, Lirzin JD, et al. Intravenous propofol during cesarean section: placental transfer, concentrations in breast milk, and neonatal effects. A preliminary study. Anesthesiology. 1989;71(6):827-834.
2. Schmitt JP, Schwoerer D, Diemunsch P, Gauthier-Lafaye J. Passage of propofol in the colostrum. Preliminary data. Ann Fr Anesth Reanim. 1987;6(4):267-268.
3. Nitsun M, Szokol JW, Saleh HJ, et al. Pharmacokinetics of midazolam, propofol, and fentanyl transfer to human breast milk. Clin Pharmacol Ther. 2006;79(6):549-557.
4. Stuttmann R, Schafer C, Hilbert P, et al. The breast feeding mother and xenon anaesthesia: four case reports. Breast feeding and xenon anaesthesia. BMC Anesthesiol. 2010;10:1-5.
5. Torsten B, Eckardt G, Renner S, et al. Green breast milk after propofol administration. Anesthesiology. 2009;111(5):1168-1169.

PROPRANOLOL

Trade: Cardinol, Deralin, Inderal

Category: Beta Adrenergic Blocker

LRC: L2 - Limited Data-Probably Compatible

Propranolol is a popular beta-blocker used in treating hypertension, cardiac arrhythmias, migraine headache, and numerous other syndromes. In general, the maternal plasma levels are exceedingly low, hence the milk levels are low as well. Milk/plasma ratios are generally less than 1. In one study of three patients, the average milk concentration was only 35.4 µg/L after multiple dosing intervals. The milk/plasma ratio varied from 0.33 to 1.65.[1] Using this data, the authors suggest that an infant would receive only 70 µg/L of milk per day, which is <0.1% of the maternal dose.

In another patient who was receiving 20 mg orally every 8 hours, levels of propranolol ranged from 0 to 5 µg/L.[2] In another study of a patient receiving 20 mg twice daily, milk levels varied from 4 to 20 µg/L with an estimated average dose to infant of 3 µg/day.[3] In another patient receiving 40 mg four times daily, the peak concentration occurred at 3 hours after dosing.[4] Milk levels varied from 0 to 9 µg/L. After a 30 day regimen of 240 mg/day propranolol, the predose and postdose concentrations in breast milk was 26 and 64 µg/L respectively.[4] No symptoms or signs of beta-blockade were noted in this infant. The above amounts in milk would likely be clinically insignificant. Long-term exposure has not been studied, and caution is urged. Of the beta blocker family, propranolol is probably preferred in lactating women. Use with great caution, if at all, in mothers or infants with asthma.

T 1/2	3-5 h	MW	259 Da	PB	90%
Tmax	60-90 min	RID	0.3%-0.5%	Vd	3-5 L/kg
Oral	30%	M/P	0.5	pKa	9.5

Adult Concerns: Headache, dizziness, insomnia, depression, fatigue, chest pain, bradycardia, arrhythmias, hypotension, heart failure, wheezing, vomiting, diarrhea, constipation, anorexia, changes in liver and renal function, thrombocytopenia, myalgia.

Adult Dose: 160-240 mg daily.

Pediatric Concerns: None reported via breast milk in numerous studies.

Infant Monitoring: Drowsiness, lethargy, pallor, poor feeding, and weight gain.

Alternatives: Metoprolol(L2)

References:

1. Smith MT, Livingstone I, Hooper WD, Eadie MJ, Triggs EJ. Propranolol, propranolol glucuronide, and naphthoxylactic acid in breast milk and plasma. Ther Drug Monit. 1983; 5(1):87-93.
2. Lewis AM, Patel L, Johnston A, Turner P. Mexiletine in human blood and breast milk. Postgrad Med J. 1981 Sep;57(671):546-547.
3. Taylor EA, Turner P. Anti-hypertensive therapy with propranolol during pregnancy and lactation. Postgrad Med J. 1981;57(669):427-430.
4. Bauer JH, Pape B, Zajicek J, Groshong T. Propranolol in human plasma and breast milk. Am J Cardiol. 1979; 43(4):860-862.

PROPYLHEXEDRINE

Trade: Benzedrex

Category: Decongestant

LRC: L5 - No Data-Hazardous

Propylhexedrine is a stimulant with similar structure to methamphetamine, which is commonly used as a nasal decongestant but can also be used as a drug of abuse when taken orally or IV. There are no adequate and well-controlled studies or case reports in breastfeeding women. Systemic effects include headache, hypertension, nervousness, and tachycardia. There have been fatalities due to myocardial infarction, pulmonary hypertension, and psychosis.

T 1/2		MW	155.3 Da	PB	
Tmax		RID		Vd	
Oral		M/P		pKa	

Adult Concerns: Sneezing, stinging, burning, rebound congestion. Systemic side-effects are hypertension, headache, tachycardia, nervousness.

Adult Dose: Two inhalations per nostril every 2 hours.

Pediatric Concerns:

Infant Monitoring:

Alternatives: Oxymetazoline(L3)

References:

PROPYLTHIOURACIL

Trade: PTU, Propyl-Thyracil

Category: Antithyroid Agent

LRC: L2 - Limited Data-Probably Compatible

Propylthiouracil (PTU) reduces the production and secretion of thyroxine by the thyroid gland. Only small amounts are secreted into breast milk. Reports thus far suggest that levels absorbed by infant are too low to produce side effects.[1] In one study of nine patients given 400 mg doses, mean serum and milk levels were 7.7 mg/L and 0.7 mg/L, respectively.[2] No changes in infant thyroid have been reported. PTU is the best of antithyroid medications for use in lactating mothers. Monitor infant thyroid function (T4, TSH) carefully during therapy.

T 1/2	1.5-5 h	MW	170 Da	PB	80%-95%
Tmax	1 h	RID	1.8%	Vd	0.87 L/kg
Oral	50%-95%	M/P	0.1	pKa	8.09

Adult Concerns: Hypothyroidism, liver toxicity, aplastic anemia, anemia.

Adult Dose: 100 mg three times daily.

Pediatric Concerns: None reported.

Infant Monitoring: Signs of hypothyroidism. Monitor thyroid function if clinical symptoms present.

Alternatives:

References:
1. Cooper DS. Antithyroid drugs: to breast-feed or not to breast-feed. Am J Obstet Gynecol. 1987;157(2):234-235.
2. Kampmann JP, Johansen K, Hansen JM, Helweg J. Propylthiouracil in human milk. Revision of a dogma. Lancet. 1980;1(8171):736-737.

PRUCALOPRIDE

Trade: Resotran

Category: Laxative

LRC: L3 - No Data-Probably Compatible

Prucalopride is approved in the European Union and Canada for the symptomatic relief of chronic constipation in females whom laxatives fail to provide relief. It is a selective 5-HT4 receptor agonist that has enterokinetic properties that target impaired gastrointestinal motility.[1] No data are available on the transfer of prucalopride to human milk.

T 1/2	24-30 h	MW	367.9 Da	PB	28-33%
Tmax	2-3 h	RID		Vd	8.1 L/kg
Oral	90%	M/P		pKa	

Adult Concerns: Headache, nausea, diarrhea, abdominal pain, vomiting, flatulence, and dizziness.

Adult Dose: 2 mg daily.

Pediatric Concerns: None reported via milk, but caution recommended.

Infant Monitoring: Diarrhea.

Alternatives:

References:

1. Frampton, J. Prucalopride. vol 69. Aukland, New Zealand: Adis International International limited; 2009.

PSEUDOEPHEDRINE

Trade: 12 Hour Cold Maximum Strength, Biofed, Cenafed, Dimetapp Decongestant, Simply Stuffy, Sudafed

Category: Decongestant

LRC: L3 - Limited Data-Probably Compatible

Pseudoephedrine is an adrenergic compound primarily used as a nasal decongestant. It is secreted into breast milk but in low levels. In a study of three lactating mothers who received 60 mg of pseudoephedrine, the milk/plasma ratio was as high as 2.6-3.9.[1] The average pseudoephedrine milk level over 24 hours was 264 µg/L. The calculated dose that would be absorbed by the infant was still very low (0.4% to 0.6% of the maternal dose).

In a study of eight lactating women who received a single 60 mg dose of pseudoephedrine, the 24 hour milk production was reduced by 24% from 784 mL/day in the placebo period to 623 mL/day in the pseudoephedrine period.[2] The authors speculate that this may have been due to a 13.5% reduction in prolactin (greater in those in late stage lactation, beyond 60 weeks); however, this change was not statistically significant compared to placebo. While this study was done with a single 60 mg dose, if the typical dosing regimen of 60 mg four times a day was used, the authors' estimated that the infant dose of pseudoephedrine would have been 4.3% of the weight-adjusted maternal dose.

While these results are preliminary, it is apparent that mothers in late-stage lactation may be more sensitive to pseudoephedrine and have greater loss in milk production. Therefore, breastfeeding mothers with poor or marginal milk production should be cautious in using pseudoephedrine. While there are anecdotal reports of its use in mothers with engorgement, we do not know if it is effective, or recommend its use for this purpose at this time.

T 1/2	9-16 h	MW	165 Da	PB	
Tmax	1-3 h	RID	4.7%	Vd	
Oral	90%	M/P	2.6-3.3	pKa	9.7

Adult Concerns: Irritability, agitation, anorexia, stimulation, insomnia, hypertension, tachycardia.

Adult Dose: 60 mg every 4-6 hours.

Pediatric Concerns: One case of irritability via milk.

Infant Monitoring: Irritability, poor sleep, poor feeding, tremor, weight loss. Potentially, reduced breast milk production.

Alternatives: Oxymetazoline(L3)

References:

1. Findlay JW, Butz RF, Sailstad JM, Warren JT, Welch RM. Pseudoephedrine and triprolidine in plasma and breast milk of nursing mothers. Br J Clin Pharmacol. 1984;18(6):901-906.

2. Aljazaf K, Hale TW, Ilett KF, et al. Pseudoephedrine: effects on milk production in women and estimation of infant exposure via breastmilk. Br J Clin Pharmacol. 2003;56(1):18-24.

PSYLLIUM

Trade: Cilium, Konsyl, Metamucil, Reguloid

Category: Laxative

LRC: L2 - Limited Data-Probably Compatible

Psyllium is a bulk-forming fiber. It is not absorbed systemically. In one report, 20 postpartum mothers were given a laxative containing psyllium daily on days 2 to 4 postpartum. Of the 11 breastfed infants, none had loose stools.[1]

T 1/2		MW		PB	
Tmax		RID		Vd	
Oral	Not absorbed	M/P		pKa	

Adult Concerns: Abdominal distension, obstruction of bowel or esophagus, hypersensitivity.

Adult Dose: 5-10 g one to three times a day.

Pediatric Concerns:

Infant Monitoring:

Alternatives:

References:
1. Faber P, Strenge-Hesse A. Relevanceof rhein excretion into breast milk. Pharmacology. 1988;36 (Suppl 1):212-20.

PYRANTEL

Trade: Ascarel, Early Bird, Pamix, Pin-X, Pinworm

Category: Anthelmintic

LRC: L3 - No Data-Probably Compatible

Pyrantel is an anthelmintic used to treat pinworm, hookworm, and round worm infestations.[1] It is only minimally absorbed orally, with the majority being eliminated in feces. Peak plasma levels are generally less than 0.05 to 0.13 µg/mL and occur prior to 3 hours. Reported side effects are few and minimal. No data are available on transfer of pyrantel to human milk, but due to minimal oral absorption, and low plasma levels, it is unlikely that breast milk levels would be clinically relevant. Generally, it is administered as a single dose.

T 1/2		MW	206 Da	PB	
Tmax	<3 h	RID		Vd	
Oral	<50%	M/P		pKa	

Adult Concerns: Side effects are generally minimal and include headache, dizziness, somnolence, insomnia, nausea, vomiting, abdominal cramps, diarrhea, and pain. Only moderate changes in liver enzymes have been noted, without serious hepatotoxicity.

Adult Dose: 11 mg/kg X 2 over two weeks.

Pediatric Concerns: None reported via milk.

Infant Monitoring:

Alternatives:

References:
1. Pharmaceutical manufacturers prescribing information.

PYRAZINAMIDE

Trade: Pyrazinamide, Tebrazid, Zinamide

Category: Antitubercular

LRC: L3 - Limited Data-Probably Compatible

Pyrazinamide is an antitubercular antibiotic used in the treatment of tuberculosis infections. There is one case report of a 29-year-old woman who received 1 g of pyrazinamide in lactation.[1] Her milk samples were collected at 0, 1, 2, 3, 4, 9, and 12 hours after her dose and showed a maximum concentration at 3 hours of 1.5 mg/L. The maximum maternal plasma concentration was 42 mg/L and occurred at 2 hours post-dose. Using this peak milk concentration, the relative infant dose was estimated to be 1.5%.

T 1/2	9-10 h	MW	123 Da	PB	5%-10%
Tmax	2 h	RID	1.5%	Vd	0.75-1.65 L/kg
Oral	Complete	M/P		pKa	

Adult Concerns: Malaise, vomiting, anorexia, changes in liver function, hyperuricemia including gout, changes in coagulation, thrombocytopenia, anemia, arthralgias, angioedema, and rash.

Adult Dose: 15-30 mg/kg daily.

Pediatric Concerns: None reported via milk.

Infant Monitoring: Drowsiness, lethargy, vomiting, and weight gain. If clinical symptoms arise (e.g., yellowing of the skin or eyes) check liver function tests.

Alternatives:

References:
1. Holdiness MR. Antituberculosis drugs and breast-feeding. Arch Intern Med. 1984;144(9):1888.

PYRETHRUM EXTRACT + PIPERONYL BUTOXIDE

Trade: A200 Maximum Strength, A200 Time-Tested Formula, Lice-X, Licide, Medi-Lice Maximum Strength, Pronto Maximum Strength, Pronto Plus, Rid, Tisit

Category: Pediculicide

LRC: L3 - No Data-Probably Compatible

This is a shampoo that contains pyrethrum extract (equivalent to 0.33% pyrethrins) and piperonyl butoxide (4%) used for the treatment of head and body lice.[1] Pyrethrins are natural insecticides derived from chrysanthemum plants. They have minimal systemic toxicity. Topical absorption through the skin is negligible, so levels in milk are likely nil. However, there are no adequate and well-controlled studies or case reports in breastfeeding women.

T 1/2		MW	316 Da	PB	
Tmax		RID		Vd	
Oral	Poor topically	M/P		pKa	

Adult Concerns: Dermatitis.

Adult Dose:

Pediatric Concerns:

Infant Monitoring:

Alternatives:

References:
1. Pharmaceutical manufacturers prescribing information.

PYRIDOSTIGMINE

Trade: Mestinon, Regonol

Category: Cholinergic

LRC: L2 - Limited Data-Probably Compatible

Pyridostigmine is a potent cholinesterase inhibitor used in myasthenia gravis to stimulate muscle strength. In a group of two mothers receiving from 120-300 mg/day, breast milk concentrations varied from 5 to 25 µg/L.[1] The calculated milk/plasma ratios varied from 0.36 to 1.13. No cholinergic side effects were noted in the infants and no pyridostigmine was found in the infants' plasma. Because the oral bioavailability is so poor (10%-20%), the actual dose received by the breastfed infant would be significantly less than the above concentrations. Please note the dosage is highly variable and may be as high as 600 mg/day in divided doses. The authors estimated total daily intake at 0.1% or less of the maternal dose.

T 1/2	3.3 h	MW	261 Da	PB	None
Tmax	1-2 h	RID	0.09%	Vd	0.53-1.76 L/kg
Oral	10%-20%	M/P	0.36-1.13	pKa	

Adult Concerns: Headache, dizziness, drowsiness, loss of consciousness, seizure, arrhythmias, bronchospasm, abdominal cramps, vomiting, diarrhea, urinary urgency, weakness.

Adult Dose: 60-180 mg 2-4 times daily.

Pediatric Concerns: None reported in one study of two infants.

Infant Monitoring: Poor sleep, irritability, excessive salivation, vomiting, diarrhea, poor weight gain, weakness.

Alternatives:

References:

1. Hardell LI, Lindstrom B, Lonnerholm G, Osterman PO. Pyridostigmine in human breast milk. Br J Clin Pharmacol. 1982;14(4):565-567.

PYRIDOXINE

Trade: Vitamin B6, Hexa-Betalin, Pyroxin

Category: Vitamin

LRC: L2 - Limited Data-Probably Compatible

The recommended daily allowance of pyridoxine (vitamin B6) for non-pregnant women is 1.3 mg/day.[1] Pyridoxine is required in slight excess during pregnancy (1.9 mg/day) and lactation (2 mg/day) and most prenatal vitamin supplements contain 10 mg/day.[2]

Pyridoxine is secreted in milk in direct proportion to maternal intake.[3] In a study of 20 women breastfeeding term infants, 14 women were supplemented with a prenatal vitamin (2 mg/day pyridoxine) and six were supplemented with 27 mg/day of pyridoxine. Maternal blood and milk were collected on day 0, 7, 14, and 28 days after birth. In this study, total vitamin B6 concentrations in milk ranged from 75-120 ng/mL (450-700 nmol/L) in the 2 mg/day group and from 390-525 ng/mL (2300-3100 nmol/L) in the 27 mg/day group. It should be noted that vitamin B6 levels in the infants were 10 ng/mL in the maternal prenatal vitamin group and 49 ng/mL in the maternal 27 mg/day group on day 28. It was also reported that in this study milk volumes were higher on day 28 in the 2 mg/day maternal supplement group.

In one study, which compared pyridoxine (600 mg/day x 6 days) to stilboestrol and placebo for cessation of lactation in women 2-3 days postpartum, pyridoxine was found to be superior.[4] More women were symptom free within 10-12 hours of starting therapy and 93% of women ceased producing milk within one week of starting therapy. A second study that administered a combination tablet of Vitamin B1, B6, and B12 to postpartum women starting on the day of delivery reported that pyridoxine (300 mg/day x 7 days) inhibited lactation in 96% of patients given the vitamin compared to 76.5% of those given placebo when started before lactation was established.[5]

However, this data has been refuted in two studies where high doses of pyridoxine failed to suppress prolactin levels and lactation.[6,7] In the first study, pyridoxine (600 mg/day x 7 days) was given to nine women starting immediately postpartum. The prolactin levels of these women were compared to nine women who were breastfeeding their infants.[6] There were no differences in the serum prolactin levels at baseline and on day 5 when the treatment group had prolactin levels that were 53% of their baseline level and the control group had prolactin levels that were 68% of their baseline level. In addition, lactation was not suppressed in the treatment group. In the second study, 14 women given pyridoxine (450 mg/day x 7 days) starting on the day of delivery were compared to 20 women given bromocriptine (7.5 mg/day x 7 days).[7] In this study, pyridoxine had no effect on prolactin levels or engorgement when compared to bromocriptine.

In summary, one study clearly indicates that pyridoxine readily transfers into breast milk and that levels in milk correlate closely with maternal intake, thus excessive maternal doses of pyridoxine in lactation are not recommended.[3] At this time, the use of pyridoxine supplementation at doses similar to those found in prenatal vitamins would seem reasonable in lactation.

T 1/2	0.5 h (active metabolite days)	MW	169 Da	PB	
Tmax	1-2 h	RID		Vd	
Oral	Well absorbed	M/P		pKa	

Adult Concerns: Sedation, sensory neuropathy, ataxia, nausea, changes in liver enzymes. Seizures at high IV doses.

Adult Dose: Supplement 1-10 mg/day; 40 mg/day or less for NVP.

Pediatric Concerns: Excessive oral doses have been reported to produce sedation, hypotonia, and respiratory distress in infants, although none have been reported via breast milk.

Infant Monitoring: Sedation, seizures, vomiting.

Alternatives:

References:

1. 2015 Dietary Guidelines Advisory Committee. Appendix 7: Nutritional goals for age-sex groups based on dietary reference intakes and dietary guidelines recommendations. Dietary Guidelines for Americans 2015-2020. 8th ed. Washington, DC: Department of Health and Human Services; 2015. https://health.gov/dietaryguidelines/2015/guidelines/appendix-7/.
2. National Institutes of Health (NIH) Office of Dietary Supplements. Vitamin B6 dietary supplement fact sheet. Last Updated February 2016. https://ods.od.nih.gov/factsheets/VitaminB6-HealthProfessional/#disc
3. Kang-Yoon SA, Kirksey A, Giacoia G, West K. Vitamin B-6 status of breast-fed neonates: influence of pyridoxine supplementation on mothers and neonates. Am J Clin Nutr. 1992;56(3):548-558.
4. Foukas MD. An antilactogenic effect of pyridoxine. J Obstet Gynaecol Br Commonw. 1973;80(8):718-720.
5. Marcus RG. Suppression of lactation with high doses of pyridoxine. S Afr Med J. 1975;49(52):2155-2156.
6. de Waal JM, Steyn AF, Harms JHK, Slabber CF, Pannall PR. Failure of pyridoxine to suppress raised serum prolactin levels. S Afr Med J. 1978;53(8):293-294.
7. Canales ES, Soria J, Zarate A, Mason M, Molina M. The influence of pyridoxine on prolactin secretion and milk production in women. Br J Obstet Gynaecol. 1976;83(5):387-388.

PYRILAMINE

Trade: Corzall, Dextrophenylpril, Polyhist

Category: Antihistamine

LRC: L3 - No Data-Probably Compatible

Pyrilamine is an antihistamine that blocks the H1 receptor.[1] It is used in many over-the-counter products. Antihistamines in this class may cause excitement or sleeplessness in children. Pyrilamine also has anticholinergic (drying) effects as well. Use of these older antihistamines in pregnant and breastfeeding mothers should be avoided. Use the newer non-sedating antihistamines, such as loratadine or cetirizine.

T 1/2		MW	401 Da	PB	
Tmax		RID		Vd	
Oral	Complete	M/P		pKa	

Adult Concerns: Sedation, incoordination, anticholinergic effects, excitement in children, CNS depression.

Adult Dose: 75-200 mg per day in four divided doses.

Pediatric Concerns:

Infant Monitoring: Sedation, dry mouth.

Alternatives: Cetirizine(L2), Loratadine(L1)

References:

1. Pharmaceutical manufacturers prescribing information.

PYRIMETHAMINE

Trade: Daraprim, Fansidar, Maloprim

Category: Antimalarial

LRC: L4 - Limited Data-Possibly Hazardous

Pyrimethamine is a folic acid antagonist that has been used for prophylaxis of malaria.[1] Pyrimethamine is secreted into human milk and maternal peak plasma levels occur around 2-6 hours postdose.[1,2] In a group of mothers given 25, 50, or 75 mg single doses of pyrimethamine, milk levels ranged from 2650 to 3325 µg/L 6 hours following the dose and 660 to 1000 µg/L forty eight hours following the dose. The peak concentration was 3325 µg/L.[2] An infant would receive an estimated dose of 3-4 mg in a 24-hour period on the day of drug administration (following 75 mg maternal dose).

In another study, three women were given a single oral dose of 12.5 mg pyrimethamine + 100 mg dapsone + 300 mg chloroquine within 2-5 days of delivery.[3] Blood and milk samples were then collected over the next 9 days; the three infants were reported to receive about 140, 210, and 340 µg pyrimethamine over the study period of about 9 days if they each consumed about 1 L of milk a day. The authors estimate the relative infant dose to be 46% of the maternal dose or 0.09 mg/kg over 9 days. No adverse effects were reported in any of the infants.

T 1/2	96 h	MW	249 Da	PB	87%
Tmax	2-6 h	RID	13.86%-111.31%	Vd	
Oral	Complete	M/P	0.2-0.43	pKa	7.2

Adult Concerns: Arrhythmias, atrophic glossitis, vomiting, anorexia, hematuria, leukopenia, eosinophilia, thrombocytopenia, anemia, severe rash.

Adult Dose: 25 mg every week.

Pediatric Concerns: None reported via milk at this time but limited data available.

Infant Monitoring: Vomiting, poor feeding, weight gain, if clinical symptoms arise, check CBC.

Alternatives:

References:
1. Pharmaceutical manufacturers prescribing information.
2. Clyde DF, Press J, Shute GT. Transfer of pyrimethamine in human milk. J Trop Med Hyg. 1956;59(12):277-284.
3. Edstein MD, Veenendaal JR, Newman K, et al. Excretion of chloroquine, dapsone and pyrimethamine in human milk. Br J Clin Pharmacol. 1986;22:733-735.

PYRITHIONE ZINC

Trade:

Category: Dermatologic Agents

LRC: L3 - No Data-Probably Compatible

Pyrithione zinc is an antibacterial and antifungal agent used in dandruff treatment. Animal studies suggested that systemic absorption from topical administration of pyrithione zinc is low, in the order of 1%-2%.[1] Because of minimal systemic absorption from topical administration, pyrithione zinc is unlikely to be present in milk. There are no adequate and well-controlled studies or case reports in breastfeeding women.

T 1/2		MW	318 Da	PB	
Tmax		RID		Vd	
Oral		M/P		pKa	

Adult Concerns: Peripheral neuritis, irritation to mucous membranes. If accidentally ingested, hypernatremia, tachycardia, hypotension, nausea, vomiting, diarrhea.

Adult Dose:

Pediatric Concerns:

Infant Monitoring:

Alternatives:

References:
1. Zinc pyrithione. In: REPROTOX® Database [Internet database]. Greenwood Village, CO: Thomson Reuters (Healthcare) Inc. Updated periodically. Accessed July 1, 2011.

QUAZEPAM

Trade: Doral, Dormalin

Category: Sedative-Hypnotic

LRC: L2 - Limited Data-Probably Compatible

Quazepam is a long half-life benzodiazepine medication used as a sedative and hypnotic. It is selectively metabolized to several metabolites that have even longer half-lives. In a study of four breastfeeding mothers who received a single 15 mg dose of quazepam, the average milk/plasma ratio (AUC) was 4.18.[1] The Cmax of quazepam in milk occurred at 3 hours and was 95.8 µg/L and over the 48 hours, only 11.59 µg quazepam was recovered. The average concentration (AUC) of quazepam equivalents over 48 hours was 19.6 µg/L. However, including metabolites, the authors suggest that 17.1 µg of quazepam equivalents or 0.11% of the administered dose was recovered in milk. The authors estimated that 28.7 µg quazepam equivalents, or 0.19% of the quazepam dose would be excreted in breast milk every 24 hours. These estimates were not weight-adjusted. Observe for sedation in the breastfed infant.

T 1/2	39 h	MW	387 Da	PB	>95%
Tmax	2 h	RID	1.4%	Vd	5-8.6 L/kg
Oral	Complete	M/P	4.18	pKa	

Adult Concerns: Drowsiness, sedation.

Adult Dose: 15 mg daily.

Pediatric Concerns: None reported via milk at this time.

Infant Monitoring: Sedation, slowed breathing rate, not waking to feed/poor feeding, and weight gain.

Alternatives: Lorazepam(L3), Alprazolam(L3)

References:

1. Hilbert JM, Gural RP, Symchowicz S, Zampaglione N. Excretion of quazepam into human breast milk. J Clin Pharmacol. 1984;24(10):457-462.

QUETIAPINE

Trade: Seroquel, Seroquel XR

Category: Antipsychotic, Atypical

LRC: L2 - Limited Data-Probably Compatible

Quetiapine is indicated for the treatment of many psychiatric disorders including depression, mania, and schizophrenia.[1] It has some affinity for histamine receptors, which may account for its sedative properties. It has been shown to increase the incidence of seizures, increase prolactin levels, and lower thyroid levels in adults.

In a patient (92 kg) receiving 200 mg/day of quetiapine throughout pregnancy and postpartum, milk samples were expressed just before dosing, and at 1, 2, 4, and 6 hours postdose.[2] The average milk concentration of quetiapine over the 6 hours was 13 µg/L, with a maximum concentration of 62 µg/L at 1 hour. Levels of quetiapine rapidly fell to almost pre-dose levels by 2 hours. The authors report that an exclusively breastfed infant would ingest only 0.09% of the weight-adjusted maternal dose. At maximum, the infant would ingest 0.43% of the weight-adjusted maternal dose. Although only one patient was studied, the data suggests levels in milk are minimal at this maternal dose.

One study of six mothers taking a combination of quetiapine +/- paroxetine, clonazepam, trazodone, or venlafaxine to help augment their antidepressant therapy to treat obsessive compulsive disorder or panic disorder showed that no medication was detectable in three of the mothers' milk.[3] In two of the other mothers, quetiapine levels were low and the infant doses were estimated to be 0.01 mg/kg/day, while the final mother had an infant dose of less than 0.1 mg/kg/day. The mothers' doses of quetiapine ranged from 25-400 mg. The infants' motor, mental, and behavioral development was assessed in this study using the Bayley Scales of Infant Development (BSID-II). This scale assesses cognitive, language, personal-social, fine, and gross motor development. In four cases the babies showed normal development; however, two of the infants with undetectable quetiapine breast milk samples showed some signs of developmental delay. In the first case, the scores were in the "slightly delayed" range on the mental and motor scales, but were within normal limits on the behavioral scale. In the second case, the scores were within 1 point of normal on the mental development and all other scales were within normal limits. The authors concluded that there was no correlation between quetiapine exposure and developmental outcomes in this study.

In another study of one mother receiving 400 mg quetiapine per day 3 months postpartum, expressed milk contained an average drug concentration of 41 µg/L, and a milk/plasma ratio of 0.29.[4] The relative infant dose reported was 0.09% of the mother's dose. The infant's plasma concentration was 1.4 µg/L, or 6% of the mother's plasma concentration. No adverse effects were reported in the infant.

A publication in 2015, described the case of a 33-year-old women who 2 days after delivering her twins was initiated on sodium valproate for bipolar maintenance therapy.[5] On days 18 to 20 postpartum, she developed both psychotic and manic symptoms, thus olanzapine 15 mg and quetiapine 200 mg were added daily at 11 pm. The patient was advised to start breastfeeding 8 hours after her bedtime doses, and to pump and discard her milk accumulated overnight around 7 am each day. Three breast milk samples were collected and saved by the patient at 4 a.m., 8 a.m., and 11 p.m. (before taking her medications) for 27 days within a 48-day period. The median daily concentration of quetiapine was 3.7 ng/mL. The absolute infant dose for quetiapine was 0.38 µg/kg, this corresponded to a relative infant dose of 0.02%. The infants were breastfed using this routine for 15 months, no adverse effects or concerns with development were reported by the pediatrician.

T 1/2	6 h	MW	883 Da	PB	83%
Tmax	1.5 h	RID	0.02%-0.1%	Vd	10 L/kg
Oral	100%	M/P	0.29	pKa	

Adult Concerns: Sedation, dizziness, agitation, dry mouth, orthostatic hypotension, QTc prolongation, increased appetite, constipation, changes in liver function, hypertriglyceridemia, hypercholesterolemia, hyperglycemia, hyper-prolactinemia, extrapyramidal symptoms, weight gain.

Adult Dose: 300-800 mg a day.

Pediatric Concerns: None reported via milk at this time.

Infant Monitoring: Sedation or irritability, apnea, not waking to feed/poor feeding, extrapyramidal symptoms, and weight gain.

Alternatives: Risperidone(L2), Olanzapine(L2)

References:
1. Pharmaceutical manufacturers prescribing information.
2. Lee A, Giesbrecht B, Dunn E, Ito S. Excretion of quetiapine in breast milk. Am J Psychiatry. 2004;161(9):1715-1716.
3. Misri S, Corral M, Wardrop AA, Kendrick K. Quetiapine Augmentation in lactation: a series of case reports. J Clin Psychopharmacol. 2006;26(5):508-511.
4. Rampono J, Kristensen JH, Ilett KF, Hackett P, Kohan R. Quetiapine and breast feeding. Ann Pharmacother. 2007;41:711-714.
5. Aydin B, Nayir T, Sahin S, Yildiz A. Olanzapine and quetiapine use during breastfeeding excretion into breast milk and safe breast-feeding strategy. J Clin Psychopharmacol. 2015;35(2):206-208.

QUINAPRIL

Trade: Accupril, Accupro, Accuretic, Asig

Category: ACE Inhibitor

LRC: L2 - Limited Data-Probably Compatible

Quinapril is an angiotensin converting enzyme inhibitor (ACE) used as an antihypertensive. Once in the plasma, quinapril is rapidly converted to its active metabolite quinaprilat. In a study of six women who received 20 mg a day, the milk/plasma ratio for quinapril was 0.12.[1] Quinapril was not detected in milk after 4 hours. No quinaprilat (metabolite) was detected in any of the milk samples. The estimated "dose" of quinapril that would be received by an infant was 1.6% of the maternal dose. The authors suggest that quinapril appears to be "safe" during breastfeeding although, as always, the risk-benefit ratio should be considered when it is given to a nursing mother. The drug is not recommended early postpartum in preterm infants.

Both the ACE inhibitor family and the specific Angiotensin II receptor blockers are contraindicated in pregnancy and thus should be used with caution in women who are planning a subsequent pregnancy in the near future.

T 1/2	2 h	MW	474 Da	PB	97%
Tmax	2 h	RID	1.6%	Vd	
Oral	Complete	M/P	0.12	pKa	

Adult Concerns: Headache, dizziness, fatigue, hypotension, abnormal taste, cough, nausea, diarrhea, constipation, changes in renal function/urine output, hyperkalemia, rash.

Adult Dose: 20-80 mg daily.

Pediatric Concerns: None reported via milk at this time.

Infant Monitoring: Drowsiness, lethargy, pallor, poor feeding, and weight gain.

Alternatives: Captopril(L2), Enalapril(L2), Ramipril(L3)

References:
1. Begg EJ, Robson RA, Gardiner SJ, et al. Quinapril and its metabolite quinaprilat in human milk. Br J Clin Pharmacol. 2001;51(5):478-481.

QUINIDINE

Trade: Cardioquin, Kiditard, Kinidin Durules, Quinaglute, Quinidex

Category: Antiarrhythmic

LRC: L3 - Limited Data-Probably Compatible

Quinidine is used to treat cardiac arrhythmias. Three hours following a dose of 600 mg, the level of quinidine in the maternal serum was 9 mg/L and the concentration in her breast milk was 6.4 mg/L.[1] Subsequently, a level of 8.2 mg/L was noted in breast milk. Quinidine is selectively stored in the liver.

T 1/2	6-8 h	MW	324 Da	PB	87%
Tmax	1-2 h	RID	14.4%	Vd	1.8-3 L/kg
Oral	80%	M/P	0.71	pKa	13.89

Adult Concerns: Dizziness, headache, changes in sleep, arrhythmias, nausea, vomiting, diarrhea, changes in liver function, hemolysis (in patients with G6PD deficiency), weakness, tremor, skin rash.

Adult Dose: 200-400 mg three to four times daily.

Pediatric Concerns: None reported.

Infant Monitoring: Drowsiness, lethargy, pallor, poor feeding, diarrhea, weight gain, tremor; if symptoms arise check liver function and/or CBC.

Alternatives:

References:
1. Hill LM, Malkasian GD Jr. The use of quinidine sulfate throughout pregnancy. Obstet Gynecol. 1979;54(3):366-368.

QUININE

Trade: Biquinate, Myoquin, Quinamm, Quinate, Quinbisul

Category: Antimalarial

LRC: L2 - Limited Data-Probably Compatible

Quinine is a cinchona alkaloid primarily used in malaria prophylaxis and treatment. Small to trace amounts are secreted into milk. No harmful effects have been reported in breastfed infants; however, extreme caution should be taken in infants with G6PD deficiencies.

In a study of six women receiving 600-1300 mg/day, the concentration of quinine in breast milk ranged from 0.4 to 1.6 mg/L at 1.5 to 6 hours postdose.[1] The authors suggest these levels are clinically insignificant.

Another study investigated the suitability of quinine for falciparum malaria in pregnancy and lactation.[2] Severely ill women were given a quinine loading dose of 10-20 mg/kg IV followed by 10 mg IV every 8 hours (mean weight 54.8 kg). Those with uncomplicated malaria were given 10 mg/kg orally every 8 hours for up to 10 days. Thirty women provided breast milk samples, five of whom were given IV therapy. The breast milk concentrations for IV quinine ranged from 0.5-3.6 mg/L (mean 2.6 mg/L), most women had received between two to seven does of the IV medication prior to sample collection. The breast milk samples of women who had taken the oral dosage form were 0.5-8 mg/L (mean 3.4 mg/L). The milk/plasma ratios taken throughout lactation ranged between 0.11 to 0.53 (mean 0.31). In addition, three patients had samples taken while producing colostrum, their levels were 0.4, 0.9 and 1.9 mg/L. The milk/plasma ratios with colostrum were 0.11, 0.26 and 0.25. The study estimated that infants would receive less than 2-3 mg/day of quinine in breast milk. Although no adverse events were reported in the breastfed infants, the authors do suggest that adverse events such as thrombocytopenia could occur at these doses.

T 1/2	11 h	MW	324 Da	PB	93%
Tmax	1-3 h	RID	0.26% - 5.11%	Vd	1.8-3 L/kg
Oral	76%	M/P	0.11-0.53	pKa	4.3, 8.4

Adult Concerns: Headache, dizziness, confusion, restlessness, seizure, changes in vision and hearing, flushing, hypotension, arrhythmias, dyspnea, vomiting, diarrhea, anorexia, hypoglycemia, changes in liver and renal failure, aplastic anemia, leukopenia, neutropenia, thrombocytopenia.

Adult Dose: 650 mg every 8 hours.

Pediatric Concerns: None reported via breast milk in several studies.

Infant Monitoring: Vomiting, diarrhea, weight gain. With prolonged exposure monitor vision.

Alternatives:

References:
1. Terwillinger WG, Hatcher RA. The elimination of morphine and quinine in human milk. Surg Gynecol Obstet. 1934;58:823.
2. Phillips RE, Looareesuwan S, White NJ, Silamut K, Kietinun S, Warrell DA. Quinine pharmacokinetics and toxicity in pregnant and lactating women with falciparum malaria. Br J Clin Pharmacol. 1986;21(6):677-683.

RABEPRAZOLE

Trade: Aciphex, Pariet

Category: Gastric Acid Secretion Inhibitor

LRC: L3 - No Data-Probably Compatible

Rabeprazole is an antisecretory proton pump inhibitor similar to omeprazole. Rodent studies suggest a high milk/plasma ratio, but as we know, these do not correlate well with humans. No data are available in humans. Further, rabeprazole is only 52% bioavailable in adults even when enteric coated due to its instability in gastric acids.[1] When presented in milk, it would be virtually destroyed in the infant's stomach prior to absorption.

T 1/2	1-2 h	MW	381 Da	PB	96.3
Tmax	2-5 h	RID		Vd	
Oral	52% (enteric)	M/P		pKa	

Adult Concerns: Headache, dizziness, dry mouth, nausea, vomiting, diarrhea, constipation, abdominal pain, flatulence, changes in liver and renal function, anemia.

Adult Dose: 20 mg daily.

Pediatric Concerns: None reported via milk.

Infant Monitoring: Unlikely to be absorbed while dissolved in milk due to instability in acid.

Alternatives: Omeprazole(L2), Ranitidine(L2), Famotidine(L1)

References:
1. Pharmaceutical manufacturers prescribing information.

RABIES INFECTION

Trade:

Category: Infectious Disease

LRC: L3 - No Data-Probably Compatible

Rabies is an acute rapidly progressing illness caused by an RNA-containing virus that is usually fatal. Infection occurs via exposure to infected saliva, usually following animal bites. Incubation is prolonged and can be up to 4-6 weeks.[1] The virus multiplies locally, passes into local neurons and progressively ascends to the central nervous system. The virus is seldom found in the plasma compartment. The issue of breastfeeding following exposure to an animal bite is contentious and somewhat obscure. Person to person transmission has not been documented, nor has there been documentation of transmission of the rabies virus into human milk.[2,3] If a breastfeeding woman is exposed to the rabies virus, she should receive the human rabies immune globulin and begin the vaccination series.[4] Most sources agree that once immunization has begun, the mother can continue breastfeeding. For a thorough review, see reference 4.

Adult Concerns:

Adult Dose:

Pediatric Concerns:

Infant Monitoring: Seizures.

Alternatives:

References:
1. American Academy of Pediatrics. In: Pickering LK, ed. Red Book: Report of the Committee on Infectious Diseases. 25th ed. Elk Grove Village, IL: American Academy of Pediatrics; 2000.
2. Lawrence RA. Breastfeeding: A Guide for the Medical Profession. St. Louis: Mosby Publishers; 1994.
3. Hall TG. Diseases Transmitted from Animal to Man. Springfield, IL: Thomas; 1963.
4. Merewood A, Philipp B. Breastfeeding: Conditions and Diseases. 1st ed. Amarillo, TX: Pharmasoft Publishing L.P.; 2001.

RABIES VACCINE

Trade: Imovax Rabies Vaccine, RabAvert

Category: Vaccine

LRC: L3 - No Data-Probably Compatible

Rabies vaccine is prepared from inactivated rabies virus. No data are available on transmission to breast milk. Even if transferred to breast milk, it is unlikely to produce untoward effects.[1] The CDC does not have data regarding the inactivated virus during lactation however this vaccine is commonly given to nursing women without harm to the infant.

T 1/2		MW		PB	
Tmax	30-60 days	RID		Vd	
Oral		M/P		pKa	

Adult Concerns: Rash, anaphylactoid reactions, nausea, vomiting, diarrhea, etc.

Adult Dose: 1 mL X 3 over 21-28 days.

Pediatric Concerns: No untoward effect reported.

Infant Monitoring:

Alternatives:

References:
1. Pharmaceutical manufacturers prescribing information. www.cdc.gov/breastfeeding/recommendations/vaccinations.htm

RALOXIFENE

Trade: Evista

Category: Antiestrogen

LRC: L4 - No Data-Possibly Hazardous

Raloxifene hydrochloride is a selective estrogen receptor modulator (SERM) that has estrogenic actions on bone and anti-estrogenic actions on the uterus and breast. It blocks such estrogen effects as those that lead to breast cancer and uterine cancer. In addition, it also prevents bone loss and improved lipid profiles. It is used to prevent osteoporosis in postmenopausal women.[1] It is poorly absorbed orally (2%). While we do not have data on its transfer into human milk, levels are probably quite low. That present in milk would not be orally absorbed to any degree in infants. While the manufacturer suggests it is contraindicated in breastfeeding women, short-term exposure may not be overtly hazardous. Small levels of estrogen are required for milk production, hence exposure to raloxifene will potentially suppress milk production. Long-term exposure should be avoided, short-term exposure is probably of minimal risk.

T 1/2	27-32 h	MW	510 Da	PB	>95%
Tmax		RID		Vd	2348 L/kg
Oral	2%	M/P		pKa	

Adult Concerns: Headache, hot flashes, arthralgia, leg cramps, thrombosis (DVT, PE, retinal vein thrombosis), flu-like syndrome, infection.

Adult Dose: 60 mg/day.

Pediatric Concerns: No data are available.

Infant Monitoring: Not recommended in lactation long-term.

Alternatives:

References:
1. Pharmaceutical manufacturers prescribing information.

RALTEGRAVIR

Trade: Isentress

Category: Antiviral

LRC: L5 - No Data-Hazardous if Maternal HIV Infection

Raltegravir is an antiretroviral drug used to treat HIV infection.[1] This medication exerts its effect by inhibiting the enzyme integrase, which is responsible for integrating the viral genetic material into human DNA. It is not known if raltegravir transfers to human milk; however, raltegravir transfers avidly to milk of lactating rats. Mean drug concentrations in rodent milk were approximately three times greater than those in maternal plasma. No effects in rat offspring were attributable to exposure via milk.

Note: This medication is an L5 to highlight the contraindication of breastfeeding when the mother is known to be infected with HIV; this medication is not an L5 based on its risk to the infant in breast milk (no data available at this time). The Centers for Disease Control and Prevention recommend that HIV-1 infected mothers do not breastfeed their infants to avoid postnatal transmission of HIV-1.

T 1/2	9-12 h	MW	482.5 Da	PB	83%
Tmax	3 h	RID		Vd	
Oral	32%	M/P		pKa	

Adult Concerns: Headache, insomnia, dizziness, fatigue, nausea, vomiting, abdominal pain, gastritis, dyspepsia, changes in liver and renal function, nephrolithiasis, myopathy, rhabdomyolysis.

Adult Dose: 400 mg orally twice a day.

Pediatric Concerns: Safety and effectiveness in children under 2 years of age have not been established.

Infant Monitoring: Breastfeeding is not recommended in mothers who have HIV.

Alternatives:

References:
1. Pharmaceutical manufacturers prescribing information.

RAMELTEON

Trade: Rozerem

Category: Sedative-Hypnotic

LRC: L3 - No Data-Probably Compatible

Ramelteon is a melatonin receptor agonist and is used for insomnia. It assists in the synchronization of the circadian rhythm and induces sleep.[1] Unlike the benzodiazepines, ramelteon does not bind to the GABA receptors. There have been no studies of levels of ramelteon in human milk. However, small amounts would be present in milk, and would only be 1.8% bioavailable. It is unlikely to sedate an infant.

T 1/2	1-2.6 h	MW	259 Da	PB	82%
Tmax	0.5-1.5 h	RID		Vd	1.06 L/kg
Oral	1.8%	M/P		pKa	

Adult Concerns: Headache, fatigue, somnolence, dizziness, nausea.

Adult Dose: 8 mg nightly.

Pediatric Concerns: No data are available.

Infant Monitoring: Sedation, slowed breathing rate, not waking to feed/poor feeding, and weight gain.

Alternatives:

References:
1. Pharmaceutical manufacturers prescribing information.

RAMIPRIL

Trade: Altace, Tritace

Category: ACE Inhibitor

LRC: L3 - Limited Data-Probably Compatible

Ramipril is rapidly metabolized to ramiprilat, which is a potent ACE inhibitor with a long half-life.[1] It is used to control hypertension. According to the manufacturer, after ingestion of a single 10 mg oral dose levels in breast milk were undetectable.[1] However, animal studies have indicated that ramiprilat is transferred to milk in concentrations about one-third of those found in serum; animal lactation studies typically have higher concentrations of drug in milk and do not correlate well with human data. In this case only 0.25% of the total dose was estimated to penetrate into rat milk.[2]

Both the ACE inhibitor family and the specific angiotensin II receptor blockers are contraindicated in pregnancy and thus should be used with caution in women who are planning a subsequent pregnancy in the near future.

T 1/2	13-17 h	MW	417 Da	PB	56%
Tmax	2-4 h	RID		Vd	
Oral	60%	M/P		pKa	

Adult Concerns: Headache, dizziness, fatigue, hypotension, abnormal taste, cough, nausea, diarrhea, constipation, changes in renal function/urine output, hyperkalemia, rash.

Adult Dose: 2.5-20 mg daily.

Pediatric Concerns: None reported via milk at this time.

Infant Monitoring: Drowsiness, lethargy, pallor, poor feeding, and weight gain.

Alternatives: Captopril(L2), Enalapril(L2), Benazepril(L2)

References:
1. Pharmaceutical manufacturers prescribing information.
2. Ball SG, Robertson JI. Clinical pharmacology of ramipril. Am J Cardiol. 1987;59(10):23D-27D.

RANIBIZUMAB

Trade: Lucentis

Category: Angiogenesis Inhibitor

LRC: L3 - No Data-Probably Compatible

Ranibizumab binds to and inhibits human vascular endothelial growth factor A, inhibiting it from binding to its receptor and suppressing neovascularization and slowing vision loss.[1] It is used in the treatment of macular degeneration. No data are available on the transfer of ranibizumab to the milk compartment, however, due to the large molecular weight, it is unlikely that this drug would pose a threat to a breastfeeding infant after the first week postpartum.

T 1/2	9 days	MW	48,000 Da	PB	
Tmax		RID		Vd	
Oral	Nil	M/P		pKa	

Adult Concerns: Headache, arthralgia, conjunctival hemorrhage, eye pain, increased intraocular pressure, nasopharyngitis, and upper respiratory tract infection.

Adult Dose: 0.5 mg every month intravitreally.

Pediatric Concerns: No data are available.

Infant Monitoring:

Alternatives: Pegaptanib.

References:
1. Pharmaceutical manufacturers prescribing information.

RANITIDINE

Trade: Deprizine, Taladine, Zantac

Category: Gastric Acid Secretion Inhibitor

LRC: L2 - Limited Data-Probably Compatible

Ranitidine is a prototypic histamine-2 blocker used to reduce acid secretion in the stomach. It has been widely used in pediatrics without significant side effects primarily for gastroesophageal reflux (GER). Following four 150 mg doses given every 12 hours, concentrations in breast milk were 0.72, 2.6, and 1.5 mg/L at 1.5, 5.5, and 12 hours, respectively.[1] The milk/serum ratios varied from 6.81, 8.44 to 23.77 at 1.5, 5.5, and 12 hours, respectively. Although the milk/plasma ratios are quite high, using this data, an infant would ingest about 0.4 mg/kg/day. This amount is quite small considering the pediatric dose currently recommended is 2-10 mg/kg/24 hours.

T 1/2	2-3 h	MW	314 Da	PB	15%
Tmax	2-3 h	RID	2.53%-9.14%	Vd	1.4 L/kg
Oral	50%	M/P	1.9-6.7	pKa	2.3, 8.2

Adult Concerns: Headache, dizziness, insomnia, nausea, vomiting, diarrhea, constipation, changes in liver and renal function, hemolytic anemia.

Adult Dose: 150 mg twice daily.

Pediatric Concerns: None reported via milk.

Infant Monitoring:

Alternatives: Famotidine(L1)

References:
1. Kearns GL, McConnell RF Jr, Trang JM, Kluza RB. Appearance of ranitidine in breast milk following multiple dosing. Clin Pharm. 1985;4(3):322-324.

REGADENOSON

Trade: Lexiscan

Category: Diagnostic Agent, Cardiac Function

LRC: L4 - No Data-Possibly Hazardous

Regadenoson is a pharmacologic stress agent (adenosine receptor agonist) that is used for myocardial perfusion imaging in patients unable to undergo stress from exercise. It is most often administered in a dose of 5 mL by rapid intravenous injection. This dose is quickly followed by a saline flush and radiopharmaceutical agent.[1] It is currently unknown if regadenoson is excreted into human milk. Due to the potential for serious adverse effects in infants, the necessity of the drug to the mother must be evaluated to determine if the interruption of nursing or the cessation of regadenoson is the appropriate choice. Based on the pharmacokinetics of regadenoson, it should be cleared after 10 hours. It is recommended that nursing women wait 10 hours before resuming breastfeeding.[1]

T 1/2	Initial phase: 2-4 min, Intermediate phase: 30 min, Terminal phase: 2 h	MW	408.37 Da	PB	27%-33%
Tmax	1-4 min	RID		Vd	1.04 L/kg
Oral		M/P		pKa	

Adult Concerns: Dyspnea, headache, flushing, chest discomfort, angina pectoris, ST segment depression, dizziness, chest pain, nausea, abdominal discomfort, dysgeusia, feeling hot, heart block, asystole, marked hypertension, symptomatic hypertension, seizure, syncope, arrhythmias.

Adult Dose: 5 mL by rapid IV injection.

Pediatric Concerns:

Infant Monitoring:

Alternatives:

References:
1. Pharmaceutical manufacturers prescribing information

REMDESIVIR

Trade:

Category: Antiviral

LRC: L3 - No Data-Probably Compatible

Remdesivir is a prodrug that is metabolized to an active form. It is an adenosine triphosphate analog recently of interest as a potential treatment for Ebola and Covid-1 virus. In 2017, its activity against the coronavirus family of viruses was also demonstrated.[1] Recently, there has been interest in its potential, but undocumented activity against COVID-19. Remdesivir was originally investigated for activity against Ebola virus, but was poorly active. It is a nucleoside analog that is theorized to inhibit the action of RNA polymerase. It is rather large in molecular weight (602.585 Da). Structurally it is unlikely to be absorbed orally, which is why it is administered intravenously. Its transfer into milk is unlikely, and it is unlikely to be orally absorbed by the infant.

T 1/2	20 h (triphosphate metabolite)	MW	602.585 Da	PB	
Tmax		RID		Vd	
Oral	Nil	M/P		pKa	10.2

Adult Concerns: None reported as of yet.

Adult Dose: 200 mg STAT, followed by 100 mg daily.

Pediatric Concerns:

Infant Monitoring:

Alternatives:

References:
1. Sheahan TP, Sims AC, Graham RL, et al. Broad-spectrum antiviral GS-5734 inhibits both epidemic and zoonotic coronaviruses. Sci Transl Med. 2017 Jun;9(396). pii: 9/396/eaal3653. doi: 10.1126/scitranslmed.aal3653. PubMed:28659436.

REMIFENTANIL

Trade: Ultiva

Category: Analgesic

LRC: L3 - No Data-Probably Compatible

Remifentanil is a new opioid analgesic similar in potency and use as fentanyl. It is primarily metabolized by plasma and tissue esterases (in adults and neonates) and has an incredibly short elimination half-life of only 10-20 minutes, with an effective biological half-life of only 3 to 10 minutes.[1] Unlike other fentanyl analogs, the half-life of remifentanil does not increase with prolonged administration. Although remifentanil has been found in rodent milk, no data are available on its transfer into human milk. It is cleared for use in children >2 years of age. As an analog of fentanyl, breast milk levels should be similar and probably exceedingly low. In addition, remifentanil metabolism is not dependent on liver function and should be exceedingly short even in neonates. Due to its kinetics and brief half-life and its poor oral bioavailability, it is unlikely this product will produce clinically relevant levels in human breast milk.

T 1/2	3-6 min	MW	412 Da	PB	70%
Tmax		RID		Vd	0.1 L/kg
Oral	Poor	M/P		pKa	7.07

Adult Concerns: Nausea, hypotension, sedation, vomiting, bradycardia.

Adult Dose: 0.25-0.4 µg/kg/minute.

Pediatric Concerns: None reported via milk. Not orally bioavailable.

Infant Monitoring: Sedation, slowed breathing rate/apnea, pallor, constipation, and not waking to feed/poor feeding.

Alternatives:

References:
1. Pharmaceutical manufacturers prescribing information.

REPAGLINIDE

Trade: Gluconorm, Novonorm, Prandin

Category: Antidiabetic, other

LRC: L3 - No Data-Probably Compatible

Repaglinide is a non-sulfonylurea hypoglycemic agent that lowers blood glucose levels in type 2 non-insulin dependent diabetics by stimulating the release of insulin from functional beta cells.[1] No data are available on its transfer to human milk, but rodent studies suggest that it may transfer to milk and induce hypoglycemic and skeletal changes in young animals via milk. Unfortunately, no dosing regimens were mentioned in these studies, so it is not known if normal therapeutic doses would produce such changes in humans. Dosing of repaglinide is rather unique, with doses taken prior to each meal due to its short half-life and according to the need of each patient. At this point, we do not know if it is safe for use in breastfeeding patients. But if it is used, the infant should be closely monitored for hypoglycemia and should not be breastfed until at least several hours after the dose to reduce exposure.

T 1/2	1 h	MW		PB	98%
Tmax	1 h	RID		Vd	0.44 L/kg
Oral	56%	M/P		pKa	

Adult Concerns: Headache, chest pain, ischemia, diarrhea or constipation, hypoglycemia, arthralgia.

Adult Dose: 0.5 mg to 4 mg before meals, with a maximum daily dose of 16 mg

Pediatric Concerns: Hypoglycemia in animal studies via milk, but doses were not mentioned.

Infant Monitoring: Signs of hypoglycemia - drowsiness, lethargy, pallor, sweating, tremor.

Alternatives:

References:
1. Pharmaceutical manufacturers prescribing information.

RESORCINOL

Trade: R A Acne, Resinol

Category: Antiacne

LRC: L3 - No Data-Probably Compatible

Resorcinol is a topical agent used to treat a wide variety of dermatologic disorders, including acne, seborrheic dermatitis, eczema, and psoriasis. It is a benzene alcohol that is fully absorbed by the oral route, but has only limited bioavailability when absorbed through intact skin. Approximately 1.64% of a topical dose reaches the systemic circulation.[1] Information regarding excretion into breast milk is limited, though studies in rats have shown no untoward effects in either the lactating mother or the offspring. Decreases in weight were noted at a dose of 3000 mg/L of drinking water, but lower doses did not carry the same effect.[2] Exposure is likely minimal due to low topical absorption.

T 1/2	8-10 h	MW	110.1 Da	PB	
Tmax	15 min	RID		Vd	
Oral	100%	M/P		pKa	

Adult Concerns: Headache, dizziness, drowsiness, nervousness, abdominal pain, vomiting, diarrhea, skin irritation, weakness. All adverse effects other than skin irritation are associated with resorcinol poisoning, which is unlikely unless dosed with extremely high amounts.

Adult Dose: Apply to affected area no more than three to four times daily.

Pediatric Concerns:

Infant Monitoring:

Alternatives:

References:
1. Yeung D, Kantor S, Nacht S, Gans EH. Percutaneous absorption, blood levels, and urinary excretion of resorcinol applied topically in humans. Int J Dermatol. 1983;22:321-324.
2. Welsch F, Nemec MD, Lawrence WB. Two-generation reproductive toxicity study of resorcinol administered via drinking water to Crl:CD(SD) rats. Int J Toxicol. 2008 Jan;27(1):43-57.

RESPIRATORY SYNCYTIAL VIRUS

Trade: RSV

Category: Infectious Disease

LRC: L3 - No Data-Probably Compatible

Respiratory Syncytial Virus (RSV) is a member of the genus Pneumovirus in the family Paramyxoviridae that usually infects human epithelial cells in the nasopharynx.[1] It is a thermolabile virus and only survives on the skin, tissues, and hands for a short amount of time. It survives longer on hard, nonporous surfaces such as tables, crib rails, and toys for much longer (up to 30 hours at room temperature).[1-3]

RSV appears to cause infection via the eyes and nose but not so much through the mouth.[3-4] It is mainly transmitted through close contact with direct inoculation of large droplets or by indirect contact with infectious secretions by touching contaminated surfaces and then rubbing the nose or eyes.[1-4] RSV has an incubation period of 2 to 8 days.[1] However, some infants and immunocompromised individuals can be contagious for as long as 4 weeks.[2] Symptoms of RSV infection usually start 4 to 6 days after exposure with a runny nose and decrease in appetite. Coughing, sneezing, and fever typically develop 1 to 3 days later. Wheezing may also occur. Very young infants may only present with non-specific symptoms like irritability, decreased activity, and breathing difficulties.[2]

No studies describing the transfer of RSV to the breast milk or RSV transmission from mother to child via breast milk were located. If a nursing mother is infected with RSV, isolation from the child till she is no longer contagious may be considered to prevent transmission of RSV infection through close contact although it is not clear this is beneficial. However, it is likely that the infant would be exposed to the virus long before the mother knows she is infected with RSV, thus separation of mother and child seems illogical. It is clear that breastfeeding is highly beneficial to an infant infected with RSV. Thus the infant should probably remain with the mother, or if advised by healthcare officials, the child could be fed from expressed breast milk.

Adult Concerns: Respiratory congestion, fever, headache, cough, rhinorrhea.

Adult Dose:

Pediatric Concerns: Respiratory congestion, fever, headache, cough, rhinorrhea.

Infant Monitoring:

Alternatives:

References:

1. Respiratory Syncytial Virus. Public Health Agency of Canada Website. November, 2010. http://www.phac-aspc.gc.ca/lab-bio/res/psds-ftss/pneumovirus-eng.php#endnote1. Accessed February 1, 2017
2. Respiratory Syncytial Virus Infection (RSV). Centers for Disease Control and Prevention Website. December 4, 2014. https://www.cdc.gov/rsv/about/index.html. Accessed February 1, 2017
3. Hall CB, Douglas RG Jr. Modes of transmission of respiratory syncytial virus. J Pediatr. 1981 Jul;99(1):100-103.
4. Hall CB, Douglas RG Jr, Schnabel KC, Geiman JM. Infectivity of respiratory syncytial virus by various routes of inoculation. Infect Immun. 1981 Sep;33(3):779-783.

RETAPAMULIN

Trade: Altabax

Category: Antibiotic, Other

LRC: L3 - No Data-Probably Compatible

Retapamulin is a topical antibacterial used to treat impetigo caused by S. aureus (not MRSA) in both children and adults. It is only minimally absorbed systemically when applied topically.[1] No data are available on the transfer of retapamulin to human milk; however, since systemic absorption is quite low, and this medication is used in children, retapamulin would probably be safe for use in breastfeeding mothers.

T 1/2		MW	517.8 Da	PB	94%
Tmax		RID		Vd	
Oral		M/P		pKa	

Adult Concerns: Headache, pruritus, application site irritation.

Adult Dose: Apply to affected area twice daily.

Pediatric Concerns: Adverse effects seen in pediatric patients over 9 months of age include itching, eczema, and diarrhea. No data on transfer into milk.

Infant Monitoring:

Alternatives: Mupirocin.

References:

1. Pharmaceutical manufacturers prescribing information.

rhBMP-2

Trade: INFUSE bone graft

Category: Other

LRC: L3 - Limited Data-Probably Compatible

Recombinant human bone morphogenetic protein-2 (rhBMP-2) is a growth factor used to stimulate bone and cartilage growth. Implantable bone graft kits may contain rhBMP-2 soaked collagen sponge that is designed to disappear after a certain amount of time. RhBMP-2 is a very large molecule (26,000 Da) and unlikely to be absorbed and secreted in breast milk. In one case study, rhBMP-2 was not detected in breast milk (minimum detection level of 62.5 pg/mL) after implantation of the Infuse bone graft kit which contains rhBMP-2.[1]

T 1/2		MW	26,000 Da	PB	
Tmax		RID		Vd	
Oral		M/P		pKa	

Adult Concerns: Ectopic bone formation, hematoma, swelling, dysphagia.

Adult Dose:

Pediatric Concerns:

Infant Monitoring:

Alternatives:

References:

1. Tzeng ST, Liao JC, Murray SS, Brochmann EJ, Carlson GD, Wang JC. Absence of bone morphogenetic protein-2 in human breast milk after spinal surgery. Spine J. 2010 Jun;10(6):e17-e20.

RHO (D) IMMUNE GLOBULIN

Trade: Gamulin RH, Hyprho-D, Mini-Gamulin RH, Rhogam

Category: Immune Serum

LRC: L2 - Limited Data-Probably Compatible

Rho(D) immune globulin is an immune globulin prepared from human plasma containing high concentrations of Rh antibodies. Only trace amounts of anti-Rh are present in colostrum and none in mature milk in women receiving large doses of Rh immune globulin. No untoward effects have been reported. Most immunoglobulins are destroyed in the gastric acidity of the newborn infant. Rh immune globulins are not contraindicated in breastfeeding mothers.[1]

T 1/2	24 days	MW		PB	
Tmax		RID		Vd	
Oral	None	M/P		pKa	

Adult Concerns: Infrequent allergies, discomfort at injection site.

Adult Dose: 300 μg X 1-2.

Pediatric Concerns: None reported via milk.

Infant Monitoring:

Alternatives:

References:

1. Lawrence RA. Breastfeeding: A Guide for the Medical Profession. St. Louis: Mosby Publishers; 1994.

RIBAVIRIN

Trade: Copegus, Rebetol, Virazide, Virazole

Category: Antiviral

LRC: L4 - No Data-Possibly Hazardous

Ribavirin is a synthetic nucleoside used as an antiviral agent and is effective in a wide variety of viral infections.[1] It has been used acutely in respiratory syncytial virus (RSV) infections in infants without major complications. However, its current use in breastfeeding patients for treatment of hepatitis C infections when combined with interferon-alfa (Rebetron) for periods up to 1 year may be more problematic as high concentrations of ribavirin could accumulate in the breastfed infant.

No data are available on its transfer to human milk, but it is probably low and its oral bioavailability is low as well. However, ribavirin concentrates in peripheral tissues and in the red blood cells in high concentrations over time

(Vd= 40 L/kg).[2] Its elimination half-life at steady state averages 298 hours, which reflects slow elimination from non-plasma compartments. Red cell concentrations on average are 60 fold higher than plasma levels and may account for the occasional hemolytic anemia. It is likely the acute exposure of a breastfed infant would produce minimal side effects. However, chronic exposure over 6-12 months may be more risky, so caution is recommended.

T 1/2	298 h at steady state	MW	244 Da	PB	None
Tmax	1.5 h	RID		Vd	40 L/kg
Oral	64%	M/P		pKa	

Adult Concerns: Seizures, conjunctivitis, bronchospasm, pulmonary edema, congestive heart failure, hypotension, bradycardia, nausea, vomiting, anorexia, increases in bilirubin, hemolytic anemia, weakness, rash.

Adult Dose: 800-1200 mg daily.

Pediatric Concerns: None yet reported via breast milk.

Infant Monitoring: Not recommended for chronic exposure via breast milk.

Alternatives:

References:
1. Pharmaceutical manufacturers prescribing information.
2. Lertora JJ, Rege AB, Lacour JT, et al. Pharmacokinetics and long-term tolerance to ribavirin in asymptomatic patients infected with human immunodeficiency virus. Clin Pharmacol Ther. 1991;50(4):442-449.

RIBOFLAVIN

Trade: Vitamin B-2

Category: Vitamin

LRC: L1 - Limited Data-Compatible

Riboflavin is a B complex vitamin, also called vitamin B2. Riboflavin is absorbed by the small intestine by a well-established transport mechanism. It is easily saturable, so excessive levels are not usually absorbed. Riboflavin is transported to human milk in concentrations proportional to dietary intake, generally averaging 32-848 µg/L.[1] These data were derived without an estimated assessment of daily intake.

High-dose riboflavin (400 mg per day) has been proposed for migraine prophylaxis, although the evidence regarding efficacy is controversial.[2-4] No studies have been published examining this dosage in breastfeeding women. However, no toxic dose of this vitamin has been established in humans.[5] Adult, adolescent, and pediatric participants in efficacy trials for migraine using similar doses reported no side effects.[2-4]

One breastfeeding mother who communicated with InfantRisk stated that her baby had no apparent symptoms after she began taking 400 mg per day, and that the baby's urine never turned the characteristic bright yellow color associated with riboflavin. No untoward effects have been reported via milk at this time.

The US RDA for all ages is 0.6 mg/1000 kcal, with an additional 0.5 mg per day in lactating women.[5]

T 1/2	14 h	MW	376 Da	PB	
Tmax	Rapid	RID		Vd	
Oral	Complete	M/P		pKa	

Adult Concerns: Yellow colored urine.

Adult Dose: 1-4 mg daily.

Pediatric Concerns: None reported via milk.

Infant Monitoring: Yellow colored urine.

Alternatives:

References:
1. Deodhar AD, Hajalakshmi R, Ramakrishnan CV. Studies on human lactation. III. Effect of dietary vitamin supplementation on vitamin contents of breastfmilk. Acta Paediatr. 1964;53:42-48.
2. Condo M, Posar A, Arbizzani A, Parmeggiani A. Riboflavin prophylaxis in pediatric and adolescent migraine. J Headache Pain. 2009 Oct;10(5):361-365.
3. MacLennan SC, Wade FM, Forrest KM, Ratanayake PD, Fagan E, Antony J. High-dose riboflavin for migraine prophylaxis in children: a double-blind, randomized, placebo-controlled trial. J Child Neurol. 2008 Nov;23(11):1300-1304.

4. Maizels M, Blumenfeld A, Burchette R. A combination of riboflavin, magnesium, and feverfew for migraine prophylaxis: a randomized trial. Headache. 2004 Oct;44(9):885-890.
5. Select Committee on GRAS Substances (SCOGS) Opinion: Riboflavin. U.S. Food and Drug Administration. http://www.fda.gov/food/ingredientspackaginglabeling/gras/scogs/ucm261091.htm

RIFAMPIN

Trade: Rifadin, Rifampicin, Rimactane, Rimycin, Rofact

Category: Antitubercular

LRC: L2 - Limited Data-Probably Compatible

Rifampin is a broad-spectrum antibiotic with particular activity against tuberculosis. It is secreted into breast milk in very small levels. One report indicates that following a single 450 mg oral dose, maternal plasma levels averaged 21.3 mg/L and milk levels averaged 3.4-4.9 mg/L.[1] Vorherr reported that after a 600 mg dose of rifampin, peak plasma levels were 50 mg/L while milk levels were 10-30 mg/L.[2] These studies suggest a milk dose 0.45-0.75 mg/kg/day, far lower than the generally recommended clinical doses (10-20 mg/kg/day). Therefore, the amounts of rifampin ingested through breast milk are most likely not clinically relevant.

T 1/2	3.5 h	MW	823 Da	PB	80%
Tmax	2-4 h	RID	5.3%-11.5%	Vd	
Oral	90%-95%	M/P	0.16-0.23	pKa	

Adult Concerns: Headache, dizziness, drowsiness, behavioral changes, vomiting diarrhea, anorexia, changes in liver function, changes in renal function, hemolytic anemia, agranulocytosis.

Adult Dose: 600 mg daily.

Pediatric Concerns: No adverse effects in breastfed infants have been reported.

Infant Monitoring: Drowsiness, lethargy, vomiting, diarrhea, and weight gain. If clinical symptoms arise (e.g., yellowing of the skin or eyes) check liver function tests.

Alternatives:

References:
1. Lenzi E, Santuari S. Preliminary observations on the use of a new semi-synthetic rifamycin derivative in gynecology and obstetrics. Atti Accad Lancisiana Roma. 1969;13(suppl 1):87-94.
2. Vorherr H. Drug excretion in breast milk. Postgrad Med. 1974;56(4):97-104.

RIFAXIMIN

Trade: Xifaxan

Category: Antibiotic, Other

LRC: L3 - No Data-Probably Compatible

Rifaximin is a new antibiotic used for the treatment of traveler's diarrhea. It is poorly absorbed orally and plasma levels are extremely low.[1] While we do not have data in breastfeeding mothers, it is unlikely enough would enter the maternal plasma compartment to produce clinically relevant levels in milk, or that any in milk would be orally absorbed by the infant.

T 1/2	2-5 h	MW	785.9 Da	PB	68%
Tmax	1.25 h	RID		Vd	
Oral	Low	M/P		pKa	

Adult Concerns: Flatulence, headache, nausea, increased sweating, abdominal pain have been reported in adults.

Adult Dose: 200 mg three times daily for 3 days.

Pediatric Concerns: Maternal plasma levels are extremely low. It is unlikely enough would enter the plasma compartment to produce clinically relevant levels in milk.

Infant Monitoring: Vomiting, diarrhea, changes in gastrointestinal flora, and rash.

Alternatives:

References:
1. Pharmaceutical manufacturers prescribing information.

RILUZOLE

Trade: Riluzole

Category: Glutamate antagonist

LRC: L2 - Limited Data-Probably Compatible

Riluzole is the disease-modifying therapy presently approved by the US Food and Drug Administration for use in ALS patients. Theories behind the pathogenesis of ALS primarily include glutamate-induced neurotoxicity. Excessive levels of glutamate apparently predispose patients to prolonged depolarization, ultimately causing calcium-mediated cell lysis.[1] The glutamate antagonist, riluzole, is the only neuroprotective drug found to be effective for the treatment of patients suffering from ALS.[2,3]

In a study of a healthy 34-year-old mother with ALS taking 50 mg orally twice daily, milk samples were collected at 0, 1, 2, 4, 8, and 12 hours on the third day of her treatment.[4] The 12-hour collection period was based on the dose interval before taking the second dose. During this study period, she received no medications other than riluzole. Elevated levels observed at 0 hr (33.8 ng/ml) suggested steady state levels. The relative infant dose was calculated to be 1.6% based on average infant milk intake of 150 ml/kg/day, the reported maternal weight of 59 kg, and the dose administered of 50 mg. The peak concentration(Tmax) of riluzole occurred at 2 hours post-ingestion, and maximum concentration (Cmax) observed was 229.5 ng/ml. Levels of riluzole in milk were found to be exceedingly low, as the average concentration Cavg was only 94.4 ng/ml (0.094 µg/ml).[4] The calculated infant dose was 14.1 µg/kg/day, and relative infant dose was 1.6%, which is far below the 10% theoretical level of concern for medications in human milk.

T 1/2	12 h	MW	234.19 Da	PB	97%
Tmax		RID	1.68%	Vd	
Oral	60%	M/P		pKa	

Adult Concerns: Asthenia, nausea, deceased lung function, abdominal pain, vomiting, arthralgia, insomnia.

Adult Dose: 50 mg BID

Pediatric Concerns:

Infant Monitoring: Nausea, vomiting, breathing difficulties.

Alternatives:

References:

1. Bensimon G, Lacomblez L, Meininger V. A controlled trial of riluzole in amyotrophic lateral sclerosis. ALS/Riluzole Study Group. N Engl J Med. 1994; 330(9):585-591. doi:10.1056/NEJM199403033300901
2. Doble A. The pharmacology and mechanism of action of riluzole. Neurology. 1996;47(6, Suppl. 4):S233-S241.
3. Dyer AM, Smith A. Riluzole 5 mg/mL oral suspension: for optimized drug delivery in amyotrophic lateral sclerosis. Drug Des Dev Ther. 2017;11:59-64. doi:10.2147/DDDT.S123776
4. Datta P, Rewers-Felkins K, Aurora N, Baker T, Hale TW. Estimation of riluzole levels in human milk and infant exposure during its use in a patient with ALS. J Hum Lact. 2017 Nov:890334417737042. doi: 10.1177/0890334417737042. PMID: 29100479.

RIMANTADINE

Trade: Flumadine

Category: Antiviral

LRC: L3 - No Data-Probably Compatible

Rimantadine hydrochloride is an antiviral agent primarily used for prevention and treatment of influenza A infections.[1,2] Rimantadine has been indicated for prophylaxis of influenza A in pediatric patients >1 year of age; however, due to the increasing resistance of the influenza A virus to this medication its use is declining. This medication is known to be concentrated in rodent milk.[1] Levels in animal milk 2-3 hours after administration were approximately twice those of the maternal serum, suggesting a milk/plasma ratio of about 2. No side effects have been reported in breastfeeding infants at this time.

T 1/2	25.4 h	MW	179 Da	PB	40%
Tmax	6 h	RID		Vd	
Oral	92%	M/P	2	pKa	

Adult Concerns: Headache, fatigue, seizure, insomnia, nervousness, dry mouth, heart failure, arrhythmias, vomiting, anorexia, weakness.

Adult Dose: 100 mg twice daily.

Pediatric Concerns: None reported via milk.

Infant Monitoring: Dry mouth, vomiting, diarrhea, weight gain.

Alternatives:

References:
1. Pharmaceutical manufacturers prescribing information.
2. Center for Disease Control. Antiviral Dosage Guidance on the Use of Influenza Antiviral Agents [Online]. http://www.cdc.gov/flu/professionals/antivirals/antiviral-dosage.htm

RISANKIZUMAB-RZAA

Trade: Skyrizi

Category: Monoclonal Antibody

LRC:

Risankizumab-rzaa, is a humanized immunoglobulin G1 (IgG1) monoclonal antibody. It is an interleukin-23 antagonist indicated for the treatment of moderate-to-severe plaque psoriasis in adults who are candidates for systemic therapy or phototherapy. As a large molecular weight immunoglobulin, it is unlikely to enter milk. In the GI tract, it would be rapidly metabolized by proteases in the infant's stomach and intestines.

T 1/2	28 days	MW		PB	
Tmax		RID		Vd	0.16 L/kg
Oral		M/P		pKa	

Adult Concerns: Upper respiratory infections, headache, fatigue, injections site reactions, tinea (fungal) infections.

Adult Dose: 150 mg SC Week 0, 4, and every 12 weeks thereafter.

Pediatric Concerns:

Infant Monitoring: Upper respiratory infections, fatigue, fungal infections.

Alternatives:

References:

RISEDRONATE

Trade: Actonel

Category: Calcium Regulator

LRC: L3 - No Data-Probably Compatible

Risedronate is a bisphosphonate that slows the dissolution of hydroxyapatite crystals in the bone, thus reducing bone calcium loss in certain syndromes such as Paget's syndrome.[1] Its penetration into milk is possible due to its small molecular weight, but it has not yet been reported except in rats. However, due to the presence of fat and calcium in milk, its oral bioavailability in infants would be exceedingly low. However, the presence of this product in an infant's growing bones is concerning, and due caution is recommended.

T 1/2	480 h	MW	305 Da	PB	24%
Tmax	1 h	RID		Vd	6.3 L/kg
Oral	0.63%	M/P		pKa	

Adult Concerns: Headache, hypertension, increased parathyroid hormone, abdominal pain, nausea, diarrhea or constipation, hypophosphatemia, hypocalcemia, arthralgias, and back pain. There are reports of osteonecrosis of the jaw, esophagitis, and esophageal ulceration.

Adult Dose: 30 mg/day for 2 months.

Pediatric Concerns: None via milk.

Infant Monitoring: Vomiting, reflux, constipation.

Alternatives:

References:

1. Pharmaceutical manufacturers prescribing information.

RISPERIDONE

Trade: Risperdal

Category: Antipsychotic, Atypical

LRC: L2 - Limited Data-Probably Compatible

Risperidone is a potent antipsychotic agent belonging to a new chemical class and is a dopamine and serotonin antagonist. Risperidone is metabolized to an active metabolite, 9-hydroxyrisperidone. In a study of one patient receiving 6 mg/day of risperidone at steady state, the peak plasma level of approximately 130 µg/L occurred 4 hours after an oral dose.[1] Peak milk levels of risperidone and 9-hydroxyrisperidone were approximately 12 µg/L and 40 µg/L respectively. The estimated daily dose of risperidone and metabolite (risperidone equivalents) was 4.3% of the weight-adjusted maternal dose. The milk/plasma ratios calculated from areas under the curve over 24 hours were 0.42 and 0.24 respectively for risperidone and 6-hydroxyrisperidone.

In another study, the transfer of risperidone and 9-hydroxyrisperidone to milk was measured in two breastfeeding women and one woman with risperidone-induced galactorrhea.[2] In case two (risperidone dose = 42.1 µg/kg/day), the average concentration of risperidone and 9-hydroxyrisperidone in milk was 2.1 and 6 µg/L, respectively. The relative infant dose was 2.8% of the maternal dose. In case three (risperidone dose = 23.1 µg/kg/day), the average concentration of risperidone and 9-hydroxyrisperidone in milk was 0.39 and 7.06 µg/L, respectively. The milk/plasma ratio determined in two women was <0.5 for both risperidone compounds. The relative infant doses were 2.3%, 2.8%, and 4.7% (as risperidone equivalents) of the maternal weight-adjusted doses in these three cases. Risperidone and 9-hydroxyrisperidone were not detected in the plasma of the two breastfed infants studied, and no adverse effects were noted.

A recent case reports hypersomnia, poor feeding, and slowing in motor movements in an infant whose mother was consuming risperidone and haloperidol. These symptoms arose following addition of haloperidol.[3]

T 1/2	20 h	MW	410 Da	PB	90%
Tmax	3-17 h	RID	2.8%-9.1%	Vd	1-2 L/kg
Oral	70%-94%	M/P	0.42	pKa	

Adult Concerns: Sedation, insomnia, anxiety, dizziness, blurred vision, dry mouth, arrhythmias, QTc prolongation, hypotension, increased appetite, nausea, vomiting, constipation, changes in liver function, hyperglycemia, anemia, neutropenia, extrapyramidal symptoms.

Adult Dose: 3 mg twice daily.

Pediatric Concerns: None reported via milk at this time.

Infant Monitoring: Sedation or irritability, apnea, not waking to feed/poor feeding, extrapyramidal symptoms, and weight gain.

Alternatives: Quetiapine(L2)

References:

1. Hill RC, McIvor RJ, Wojnar-Horton RE, Hackett LP, Ilett KF. Risperidone distribution and excretion into human milk: case report and estimated infant exposure during breast-feeding. J Clin Psychopharmacol. 2000;20(2):285-286.
2. Ilett KF, Hackett LP, Kristensen JH, Vaddadi KS, Gardiner SJ, Begg EJ. Transfer of risperidone and 9-hydroxyrisperidone into human milk. Ann Pharmacother. 2004;38(2):273-276.
3. Uguz F. Adverse events in a breastfed infant exposed to risperidone and haloperidol. Breastfeed Med. 2019 Nov;14(9):683-684. PubMed: 31135176.

RITODRINE

Trade: Pre-Par, Yutopar

Category: Adrenergic

LRC: L3 - No Data-Probably Compatible

Ritodrine is primarily used to reduce uterine contractions in premature labor due to its beta-2 adrenergic effect on uterine receptors.[1] No data are available on its transfer to human milk. Its pharmacokinetic parameters suggest that transfer to milk is likely, but low oral bioavailability suggests that little would be absorbed in the infant's gut. Nevertheless, caution is advised with its use. Use only if potential benefit to mother outweighs potential risk to breastfed infant.

T 1/2	15 h	MW	287 Da	PB	32%
Tmax	40-60 min	RID		Vd	0.7 L/kg
Oral	30%	M/P		pKa	9

Adult Concerns: Fetal and maternal tachycardia, hypertension, lethargy, sleepiness, ketoacidosis, pulmonary edema.

Adult Dose: 10-20 mg every 4-6 hours.

Pediatric Concerns: None reported via milk.

Infant Monitoring: Observe for excitement, poor sleep, and tremors.

Alternatives:

References:

1.   Gandar R, de Zoeten LW, van der Schoot JB. Serum level of ritodrine in man. Eur J Clin Pharmacol. 1980;17(2):117-122.

RITONAVIR

Trade: Norvir

Category: Antiviral

LRC: L5 - Limited Data-Hazardous if Maternal HIV Infection

Ritonavir is an antiretroviral agent used in the treatment of HIV infection.[1] A study that evaluated the safety of maternal antiretrovirals for prophylaxis against HIV transmission to the infant during lactation also reported the milk levels of ritonavir (n = 23 samples).[2] This study tested maternal serum and breast milk on the day of delivery and at months 1, 3, and 6 postpartum. Infant levels were also taken at months 1, 3, and 6 of age. The median drug concentrations of ritonavir in maternal serum, breast milk and the infant were 422 ng/mL (160-982 ng/mL), 79 ng/mL (31-193 ng/mL), and 7 ng/mL (0-138 ng/mL), respectively. The milk to plasma ratio was 0.2. The relative infant dose that we calculated using the maternal dose of 100 mg twice a day and median milk level was 0.42%. This study also reported other infant adverse events (e.g., pneumonia, diarrhea, changes in liver function, neutropenia, thrombocytopenia), but was unable to determine which medication caused the effects based on drug levels, please see study for adverse event details.

In 2014, a study was published that looked at HIV RNA in milk and the pharmacokinetics of maternal medications in milk to prevent transmission of HIV to the infant during lactation.[3] In this study, 30 women were given 1 Combivir tablet twice a day (zidovudine 300 mg + lamivudine 150 mg/tab) with two tablets of Aluvia twice a day (lopinavir 200 mg + ritonavir 50 mg) starting post delivery until breastfeeding was stopped or 28 weeks. Samples were taken pre-dose (time 0) and then at 2, 4 and 6 hours post-dose when the women were enrolled at either 6, 12, or 24 weeks postpartum. The median drug concentrations of ritonavir in maternal serum, breast milk, and the infant were 364 ng/mL (280-489 ng/mL), 79 ng/mL (47-112 ng/mL), and undetectable, respectively. The milk to plasma ratio was 0.195. The RID that we calculated using the maternal dose of 100 mg twice a day and median milk level was 0.42%.

Note: This medication is an L5 to highlight the contraindication of breastfeeding when the mother is known to be infected with HIV; this medication is not an L5 based on its risk to the infant in breast milk. The Centers for Disease Control and Prevention recommend that HIV infected mothers do not breastfeed their infants to avoid postnatal transmission of HIV.[4]

T 1/2	3-5 h	MW	720.95 Da	PB	98%-99%
Tmax	2-4 h	RID	0.42%	Vd	0.16-0.56 L/kg
Oral	80%	M/P		pKa	13.68

Adult Concerns: Headache, dyspepsia, diarrhea, nausea, vomiting, abdominal pain, asthenia.

Adult Dose: 600 mg twice a day.

Pediatric Concerns:

Infant Monitoring: Breastfeeding is not recommended in mothers who have HIV.

Alternatives:

References:
1. Pharmaceutical manufacturers prescribing information.
2. Palombi L, Pirillo MF, Andreotti M, et al. Antiretroviral prophylaxis for breastfeeding transmission in Malawi: drug concentrations, virological efficacy and safety. Antivir Ther. 2012;17:1511-1519.
3. Corbett AH, Kayira D, White NR,et al. Antiretroviral pharmacokinetics in mothers and breastfeeding infants from 6 to 24 weeks postpartum: results of the BAN study. Antivir Ther. 2014;19(6):587-595.
4. World Health Organization. Global Programme on AIDS. Consensus Statement from the WHO/UNICEF Consultation on HIV Transmission and Breast-Feeding. Geneva: WHO; 1992.

RITUXIMAB

Trade: Rituxan

Category: Monoclonal Antibody

LRC: L3 - Limited Data-Probably Compatible

Rituximab, an IgG1 antibody, binds to the CD20 antigen found on the surface of B lymphocytes.[1] It is used in the treatment of non-Hodgkin's lymphoma, rheumatoid arthritis, and lymphoid leukemia. Due to its large molecular weight, it is unlikely this drug will enter milk in clinically relevant concentrations. In addition, the low oral bioavailability of this protein suggests little absorption in the infant's gut.

In a recent case report of a 34-year-old mother who received 1000 mg IV rituximab, milk samples were collected 7 days after the initial infusion.[2] Samples were collected daily for 4 consecutive days. Rituximab levels in milk ranged from 0.4 to 0.6 µg/mL with an average of 0.5 µg/mL. In this study, maternal plasma levels were 240 times higher than milk levels. From this report, levels appear too low to produce clinical effects in breastfed infants.

T 1/2	9-49 days	MW	145,000 Da	PB	
Tmax		RID	0.53%	Vd	0.06 L/kg
Oral	Nil	M/P		pKa	

Adult Concerns: Headache, insomnia, fatigue, fever, chills, hypo or hypertension, edema, nausea, abdominal pain, diarrhea, changes in liver function, hyperglycemia, weight gain, leukopenia, neutropenia, thrombocytopenia, myalgia.

Adult Dose: 375 mg/m^2 IV.

Pediatric Concerns: None reported via milk at this time.

Infant Monitoring: Fever, frequent infections, poor feeding/poor weight gain.

Alternatives:

References:
1. Pharmaceutical manufacturers prescribing information.
2. Bragnes Y, Boshuizen R, de Vries A, Lexberg Å, Østensen M. Low level of Rituximab in human breast milk in a patient treated during lactation. Rheumatology (Oxford). 2017 Jun;56(6):1047-1048. doi: 10.1093/rheumatology/kex039. PubMed PMID: 28339781.

RIVAROXABAN

Trade: Xarelto

Category: Anticoagulant

LRC: L3 - Limited Data-Probably Compatible

Rivaroxaban is a Factor Xa inhibitor with a crucial role in the coagulation cascade.[1] Rivaroxaban has multiple indications including the prevention of postoperative deep vein thrombosis (DVT), prevention of strokes in nonvalvular atrial fibrillation and the treatment of DVT and pulmonary embolism (PE). In a single case report of a postpartum woman with a PE given rivaroxaban 15 mg twice daily, milk samples were taken on day 3 at 3, 6, and 10 hours after the morning dose.[2] The peak milk concentration was 86.4 µg/L at 3 hours postdose, the average milk concentration was 38.4 µg/L and the milk/plasma ratio was 0.4. The relative infant dose was 1.3% using the Cavg from the 10 hour collection period. It should be noted that this infant was not breastfed, thus safety data in lactation are still unavailable.

In a recent study, milk samples were collected from two lactating mothers consuming 15 mg twice daily.[3] After 21 days, each mother transitioned to 20 mg once daily. The maximum concentration of rivaroxaban observed for the 15 mg dose was 0.3 ± 0.02 µg/mL and that for the 20 mg dose was 0.26 ± 0.01 µg/mL. The relative infant dose (RID) was calculated to be 5% and 4%, respectively. This relatively low infant dose is probably explained by the high plasma protein binding of rivaroxaban and its subsequent poor penetration into human milk. The results indicate that rivaroxaban decreased to a minimum concentration over a period of 12 hours. In these two cases, levels of rivaroxaban in milk were quite low, with a RID of 4% of the maternal dose. Although the levels detected were low, rivaroxaban does transfer to breast milk. Caution should be exercised until further studies are conducted and report the safety profile of rivaroxaban in breastfeeding infants.

A 38-year-old female diagnosed with the antiphospholipid syndrome had received rivaroxaban (15 mg/day) after delivery.[4] The infant was partially breastfed until the age of 18 months. The mean minimum and maximum rivaroxaban concentrations in breast milk were 9.73 ng/mL before each dose and 53.9 ng/mL at 6 hours after each dose, respectively. In this study with a 15 mg dose at 18 months postpartum, the mean daily infant dose was 0.0034 mg/kg and the mean relative infant dose (RID) via breast milk was 1.79%.

T 1/2	5-9 h	MW	435 Da	PB	92%-95%
Tmax	2-4 h	RID	0.68%-3.78%	Vd	0.7 L/kg
Oral	66%-100%	M/P	0.4	pKa	

Adult Concerns: Headache, dizziness, syncope, fatigue, nausea, vomiting, diarrhea, constipation, changes in liver and renal function, bruising, hemorrhage (blood in vomit, stool, urine), anemia.

Adult Dose: 10-20 mg once daily (varies by indication).

Pediatric Concerns:

Infant Monitoring: Rare - bruising on the skin, blood in urine, vomit, or stool.

Alternatives: Warfarin(L2), LMWH, Heparin(L2)

References:

1. Pharmaceutical manufacturers prescribing information.
2. Wiesen MHJ, Blaich C, Muller C, et al. The direct factor Xa inhibitor rivaroxaban passes into human breast milk. Chest. 2016;150(1):e1-e4.
3. Muysson M, Marshall K, Datta P, Rewers-Felkins K, Baker T, Hale TW. Rivaroxaban treatment in two breastfeeding mothers: a case series. Breastfeed Med. 2019 Sep;15(1):41-43. doi: 10.1089/bfm.2019.0124. PMID: 31532233.
4. Saito J, Kaneko K, Yakuwa N, Kawasaki H, Yamatani A, Murashima A. Rivaroxaban Concentration in Breast Milk During Breastfeeding: A Case Study. Breastfeed Med. 2019;14(10):748-751. doi:10.1089/bfm.2019.0230

RIZATRIPTAN

Trade: Maxalt, Rizalt, Rizamelt

Category: Antimigraine

LRC: L3 - No Data-Probably Compatible

Rizatriptan is a 5-HT1B/1D (serotonin) receptor agonist used to treat migraine headaches.[1] Activating these receptors is believed to constrict cranial blood vessels and block the release of pro-inflammatory neuropeptides from the trigeminal nerve. The oral bioavailability of rizatriptan (45%) has not been found to be affected by the presence of a migraine and is greater than sumatriptan (14%).

No studies examining rizatriptan secretion into human breast milk or adverse effects in infants have been published. Some transfer is likely based on this medications small size and low protein binding; however, the clinical significance of this is unknown. Consider sumatriptan as the preferred alternative.

T 1/2	2-3 h	MW	269 Da	PB	14%
Tmax	1-1.5 h	RID		Vd	1.6-2 L/kg
Oral	45%	M/P		pKa	

Adult Concerns: Dizziness, fatigue, flushing, hot tingling sensations, dry mouth, jaw pain, chest pain, feeling of heaviness, arrhythmias, nausea, vomiting, abdominal pain, weakness, paresthesia.

Adult Dose: 5-10 mg orally, may repeat in 2 hours if needed.

Pediatric Concerns: None reported via milk at this time.

Infant Monitoring: Drowsiness, vomiting, poor feeding.

Alternatives: Sumatriptan(L3), NSAIDs, Acetaminophen(L1)

References:

1. Pharmaceutical manufacturers prescribing information.

ROCKY MOUNTAIN SPOTTED FEVER

Trade: Rocky Mountain Spotted Fever, Rickettsia Rickettsia

Category: Infectious Disease

LRC: L4 - No Data-Possibly Hazardous

Rocky mountain spotted fever is a severe tick-borne fever following infection with *Rickettsia rickettsia* a member of the spotted fever group of rickettsiae. It is a coccobacillary, obligate, intracellular organism. The rickettsia is generally transferred to the host only after attachment for 6-10 hours. Following a tick bite, myalgia severe headache, nausea/vomiting and a rash that begins with 6 days following exposure. Patients typically present with symptoms four to ten days after exposure to the Rickettsia via tick bite. The rash (80% of patients only) initially appears on wrists and ankles, subsequently spreading to trunk. As this syndrome has a high degree of mortality, immediate treatment is mandatory. Doxycycline is considered the drug of choice for the treatment of Rocky mountain spotted fever in adults and children of all ages.[1,2] This would include children. Treatment should extend for 7-10 days. The risk of dental staining following 10 days of therapy is nil. The dose for children under 45 kg (100 lbs) is 2.2 mg/kg body weight given twice a day orally or IV.[1]

There are no data on the transfer of RMSP to human milk. In general, according the CDC, it is not spread from person to person. However, there are no data at all on its transmission via human milk. Some should be expected and infection via milk may be possible. Breastfeeding should be withheld upon diagnosis or at least until after initiation of doxycycline therapy in the mother.

Adult Concerns: Fever, headache, and muscle aches, rash with blackened or crusted skin at the site of a tick bite.

Adult Dose:

Pediatric Concerns:

Infant Monitoring: Nausea, vomiting, loss of appetite, and rash.

Alternatives:

References:
1. www.cdc.gov/rmsf/
2. American Academy of Pediatrics. Committee on Infectious diseases, 2016

ROMIPLOSTIM

Trade: Nplate

Category: Platelet Stimulator

LRC: L3 - No Data-Probably Compatible

Romiplostim is a fusion protein analog of thrombopoietin that increases platelet production when it binds to the thrombopoietin receptor.[1] It is indicated for the treatment of chronic idiopathic (immune) thrombocytopenic purpura (ITP). It is administered subcutaneously at weekly intervals to maintain the platelet count at an adequate level. Currently, there are no data available reporting the transfer of romiplostim to human milk. However, its transfer to human milk is probably limited as this medication has a very high molecular weight (59,000 Da) and must be administered subcutaneously due to its poor oral absorption.

T 1/2	1 to 34 days	MW	59,000 Da	PB	
Tmax	7 to 50 h	RID		Vd	
Oral	Nil	M/P		pKa	

Adult Concerns: Dizziness, insomnia, dyspepsia, abdominal pain, myalgia, arthralgia, pain in the extremities, bone marrow reticulin deposition, worsening thrombocytopenia on discontinuation and antibody formation. If the dose is not adjusted or overdose occurs, there could be an increased risk of thromboembolism if the platelet count rises above normal.

Adult Dose: Initial dose: 1 µg/kg sc weekly then adjust dose by 1 µg/kg/week until target platelet count achieved.

Pediatric Concerns: Currently no data are available in the pediatric population.

Infant Monitoring:

Alternatives:

References:
1. Pharmaceutical manufacturers prescribing information.

ROMOSOZUMAB

Trade: Evenity

Category: Monoclonal Antibody

LRC: L3 - No Data-Probably Compatible

Romosozumab is a monoclonal antibody that binds with and inhibits sclerostin, a growth factor in bone metabolism. Romosozumab decreases bone resorption, and thus increases bone mineralization. Indicated for osteoporosis patients at high risk for fracture. It is primarily indicted for elderly women but could be used in younger individuals off protocol. Romosozumab is a large IgG2 molecule of 149,000 Da, which is probably metabolized in the stomach and small intestine long before any is absorbed. No levels in human milk have yet been reported.

T 1/2	12.8 days	MW	149,000 Da	PB	
Tmax		RID		Vd	0.056 L/kg
Oral	Nil	M/P		pKa	

Adult Concerns: Upper respiratory infections, headaches, injection site reactions, arthralgia, diarrhea, gastroenteritis, tinea infection, herpes simplex infections.

Adult Dose: 210 mg every 4 weeks

Pediatric Concerns:

Infant Monitoring: Increased risk of upper respiratory infections, headaches, injection site reactions, arthralgia, diarrhea, gastroenteritis, tinea infection, herpes simplex infections.

Alternatives:

References:
1. Pharmaceutical manufacturers prescribing information.

ROPINIROLE

Trade: Requip

Category: Antiparkinsonian

LRC: L4 - No Data-Possibly Hazardous

Ropinirole is a non-ergoline dopamine agonist. It is used to treat Parkinson's and restless leg syndromes.[1] While it has not been studied in breastfeeding mothers, it should not be used. Ropinirole is known to reduce prolactin levels, even in men, and would likely reduce milk production in breastfeeding mothers.

T 1/2	6 h	MW	297 Da	PB	40%
Tmax	1-2 h	RID		Vd	7.5 L/kg
Oral	55%	M/P		pKa	

Adult Concerns: Dizziness, daytime sleepiness, syncope, orthostatic hypotension, dry mouth, nausea, vomiting, constipation, anorexia, changes in liver function, sweating.

Adult Dose: 0.25-1 mg three times daily.

Pediatric Concerns: None reported.

Infant Monitoring: Can reduce breast milk production - not recommended in lactation.

Alternatives:

References:
1. Pharmaceutical manufacturers prescribing information.

ROPIVACAINE

Trade: Naropin

Category: Anesthetic, Local

LRC: L2 - Limited Data-Probably Compatible

Ropivacaine is a newer local anesthetic commonly used as a regional anesthetic and for epidural infusions. It is believed to produce less hypotension when compared to bupivacaine.

In a recent study that included 25 women with cesarean deliveries who were given a spinal epidural with 7.5-10 mg of 0.5% ropivacaine + 20 μg fentanyl, patient controlled epidural anesthesia (PCEA) was used postoperatively for 24 hours: ropivacaine 0.15% + fentanyl 2 μg/mL at a basal rate of 6 mL/hour, plus 4 mL doses as requested (max every 20 minutes).[1] All women chose to breastfeed during this study. The mean initial dose of ropivacaine given via the epidural was 8.6 mg. The mean accumulated doses of ropivacaine at 18 and 24 hours were 187.7 mg (range, 69-295.5 mg) and 248.3 mg (range, 131.3-378 mg), respectively. The mean concentrations in maternal plasma were 979 ng/mL at 18h and 1282 ng/mL at 24h.

The breast milk concentrations were 246 ng/mL at 18 hours and 301 ng/mL at 24 hours. The milk/plasma ratios were similar at 0.25 and 0.23 at 18 and 24 hours. Using these cumulative doses and breast milk concentrations the relative infant doses at 18 hours and 24 hours were estimated to be 1.4% and 1.3%, respectively.

The median APGAR scores at 1 and 5 minutes were both 10 (range 8-10) and the median NACS at 24 hours was 39 (range 38-40). However, one newborn developed respiratory distress 2 hours after birth and was transferred to another hospital, the cause of this was not reported but the authors did comment that no adverse effects were attributed to the medications in mothers or neonates.

T 1/2	4.2 h (epidural)	MW	328 Da	PB	94%
Tmax	43 min (epidural)	RID		Vd	0.58 L/kg
Oral		M/P		pKa	8.07

Adult Concerns: Following epidural administration- headache, hypotension, bradycardia or tachycardia, shivering, nausea, vomiting, urinary retention, back pain.

Adult Dose: Varies by indication.

Pediatric Concerns: None reported in breast milk.

Infant Monitoring: This agent is commonly used in obstetrics and is unlikely to affect the infant via milk.

Alternatives: Bupivacaine(L2)

References:
1. Matsota PK, Markantonis SL, Fousteri MZF, et al. Excretion of ropivacaine in breast milk during patient controlled epidural analgesia after caesarean delivery. Reg Anesth Pain Med. 2009;34:126-129.

ROSIGLITAZONE

Trade: Avandia

Category: Antidiabetic, other

LRC: L3 - No Data-Probably Compatible

Rosiglitazone is an oral antidiabetic agent which acts primarily by increasing insulin sensitivity. In essence, the insulin receptor is activated reducing insulin resistance. It also decreases hepatic gluconeogenesis and increases insulin-dependent muscle glucose uptake. It does not increase the release of or secretion of insulin. No data are available on its entry into human milk. The maximum plasma concentration following a 2 mg dose is only 156 ng/mL.[1]

T 1/2	3-4 h	MW	357 Da	PB	99.8%
Tmax	1 h	RID		Vd	0.25 L/kg
Oral	99%	M/P		pKa	6.8

Adult Concerns: Headache, hypertension, heart failure, edema, myocardial infarction, increased cholesterol, diarrhea, changes in liver function, hypoglycemia, anemia, weight gain.

Adult Dose: 2-8 mg daily.

Pediatric Concerns: None via milk, but it has not been studied.

Infant Monitoring: Signs of hypoglycemia - drowsiness, lethargy, pallor, sweating, tremor.

Alternatives:

References:
1. Pharmaceutical manufacturers prescribing information.

ROSUVASTATIN CALCIUM

Trade: Crestor

Category: Antihyperlipidemic

LRC: L3 - Limited Data-Probably Compatible

Rosuvastatin, like other statins, is used to reduce cholesterol synthesis in patients with hypercholesterolemia. It works by blocking HMG-CoA reductase, the rate limiting enzyme in cholesterol synthesis.[1] At this time only one case report exists regarding the transfer of statins to human milk.[2] A young woman taking rosuvastatin 40 mg/day (starting 33 days postpartum) for familial hypercholesterolemia had milk samples drawn on day 4, 24, and 80 of treatment. The rosuvastatin milk concentration rose from 15.2-29.4 µg/L 1-7 hours postdose and peaked at about 10 hours. The rosuvastatin concentrations in milk drawn 3-21 hours post dose ranged from 21.9 to 22.8 µg/L, using this data the RID is < 1%. In this study it appears that the infant was not given the maternal milk and the authors comment that the safety of statins in breast milk is still unknown.

In a more recent study of a single 38-year-old breastfeeding mother who was consuming 20 mg/day rosuvastatin, milk samples were collected over a 24 hour period.[3] The average concentration of rosuvastatin in breast milk was 30.84 ng/mL with a peak concentration at 17 hours of 58.59 ng/mL. The relative infant dose was estimated to be 1.5%.

While atherosclerosis is a chronic process, the discontinuation of lipid-lowering medications while breastfeeding should have little effect on the overall treatment of hypercholesterolemia for most women. However, two studies now suggest that the relative infant dose is minimal, and it is unlikely that this dose would compromise development in the infant.

T 1/2	19 h	MW	1001 Da	PB	88%
Tmax	3-5 h	RID	0.6%-1.5%	Vd	1.9 L/kg
Oral	20%	M/P		pKa	

Adult Concerns: Headache, dizziness, nausea, abdominal pain, constipation, changes in liver function, weakness, myalgia.

Adult Dose: 5-40 mg/day.

Pediatric Concerns: No data are available.

Infant Monitoring: Weight gain, growth.

Alternatives:

References:

1. Pharmaceutical manufacturers prescribing information.
2. Schutte AE, Symington EA, du Preez JL. Rosuvastatin is transferred into human breast milk: a case report. Am J Med. 2013:126(9):e7-e8.
3. Lwin EMP, Leggett C, Ritchie U, et al. Transfer of rosuvastatin into breast milk: liquid chromatography-mass spectrometry methodology and clinical recommendations. Drug Des Devel Ther. 2018 Oct;12:3645-3651. doi: 10.2147/DDDT.S184053. eCollection 2018. PubMed PMID: 30464396.

ROTAVIRUS VACCINE

Trade: Rotarix, RotaTeq

Category: Vaccine

LRC: L3 - No Data-Probably Compatible

Rotavirus vaccine for oral administration, is a live, attenuated rotavirus vaccine derived from the human 89-12 strain that belongs to G1P[8] type. The rotavirus strain is propagated on Vero cells. While the use of rotavirus vaccines in infants is generally recommended in certain areas of the world, the impact of breastfeeding in the seroconversion in the infants is argued.

Rotavirus infections are a prominent cause of viral gastroenteritis in infants and young children. Numerous studies have suggested that breastfeeding protects infants from contracting rotavirus infections; however, many other studies suggest breastfeeding provides no protective effect from rotavirus infections. There is a huge literature arguing one way or the other as to the benefit of breastfeeding in the severity of this disease in breastfed infants. A new meta analysis of 17 such studies with 10,841 participants suggests that breastfeeding does not actually reduce the risk of seroconversion in immunized breastfed infants.[1] As to the use of rotavirus vaccines in breastfeeding infants, the preponderance of evidence clearly suggests that there is no change in the rate of seroconversion in breastfed infants.[2,3,4]

In mothers who have received various monoclonal antibodies during pregnancy (Infliximab, etanercept, and others) that suppress the immune response, the infants born of these mothers should probably NOT receive rotavirus or BCG for at least 6 months after birth.[5] The exception to this rule is certolizumab, which does not transfer to the fetus during gestation. Milk levels of certolizumab are minimal as well.

In breastfeeding mothers who have received the above monoclonal antibodies, it is probably advisable that their infants NOT receive oral Rotavirus vaccines or BCG as well. Some monoclonal IgG has been documented to be transferred to human milk. It is not advisable that breastfed infants receive oral live vaccines.

Adult Concerns: Fussiness, irritability, cough, runny nose, fever, loss of appetite, vomiting, diarrhea.

Adult Dose:

Pediatric Concerns: Fussiness, irritability, cough, runny nose, fever, loss of appetite, vomiting, diarrhea.

Infant Monitoring: Fussiness, irritability, cough, runny nose, fever, loss of appetite, vomiting, diarrhea.

Alternatives:

References:

1. Shen J, Zhang BM, Zhu SG, Chen JJ. No direct correlation between rotavirus diarrhea and breast feeding: a meta-analysis. Pediatr Neonatol. 2017 Aug;59(2):129-135. pii:S1875-9572(17)30522-3. doi: 10.1016/j.pedneo.2017.06.002. PMID: 28958831.
2. Vesikari T, Prymula R, Schuster V, et al. Efficacy and immunogenicity of live-attenuated human rotavirus vaccine in breast-fed and formula-fed European infants. Pediatr Infect Dis J. 2012;31:509-513. PMID: 22228235
3. Groome MJ, Moon SS, Velasquez D, et al. Effect of breastfeeding on immunogenicity of oral live-attenuated human rotavirus vaccine: a randomized trial in HIV-uninfected infants in Soweto, South Africa. Bull World Health Organ. 2014;92:238-245. PMID: 24700991
4. Rongsen-Chandola T, Strand TA, Goyal N, et al. Effect of withholding breastfeeding on the immune response to a live oral rotavirus vaccine in North Indian infants. Vaccine. 2014;32 (Suppl 1):A134-A139. PMID: 25091668
5. Pharmaceutical manufacturers prescribing information, Remicade, 2018.

ROTIGOTINE

Trade: Neupro

Category: Antiparkinsonian

LRC: L4 - No Data-Possibly Hazardous

Rotigotine is a dopamine agonist used to treat the signs and symptoms of Parkinson's disease. It is thought to stimulate postsynaptic dopamine D2-type auto receptors in the brain, leading to improved dopaminergic transmission in the motor areas of the basal ganglia.[1] No data are available on the transfer of rotigotine to human milk. According to the manufacturer, rotigotine stimulates dopamine and thus reduces prolactin secretion from the pituitary. It is possible that this medication could significantly decrease prolactin release and in turn, decrease milk production. Therefore, milk production should be monitored carefully if this medication is used in a lactating mother.

T 1/2	5-7 h	MW	315.48 Da	PB	90%
Tmax	15-18 h	RID		Vd	84 L/kg
Oral		M/P		pKa	

Adult Concerns: Somnolence, dizziness, headache, nausea, vomiting, and application site reactions.

Adult Dose: 1-2 mg/24-hour patch daily.

Pediatric Concerns: No data are available.

Infant Monitoring: Can reduce breastmilk production - not recommended in lactation.

Alternatives:

References:

1. Pharmaceutical manufacturers prescribing information.

RUBELLA VIRUS VACCINE, LIVE

Trade: Meruvax, Rubella Vaccine

Category: Vaccine

LRC: L2 - Limited Data-Probably Compatible

Rubella virus vaccine contains a live attenuated virus. The American College of Obstetricians and Gynecologists (ACOG) and the CDC currently recommends the early postpartum immunization of women who show no or low antibody titers to rubella. At least four studies have found rubella virus to be transferred via milk although presence of clinical symptoms was not evident.[1-3] Rubella virus has been cultured from the throat of one infant while another infant was clinically ill with minor symptoms and serologic evidence of rubella infection after maternal vaccination.[4] In general, the use of rubella virus vaccine in breastfeeding mothers of full-term, normal infants has not been associated with untoward effects and is generally recommended.[5]

Adult Concerns: Burning, stinging, lymphadenopathy, rash, malaise, sore throat, etc.

Adult Dose: 0.5 mL X 1.

Pediatric Concerns: One case report of rash, vomiting, and mild rubella infection.

Infant Monitoring:

Alternatives:

References:
1. Buimovici-Klein E, Hite RL, Byrne T, Cooper LZ. Isolation of rubella virus in milk after postpartum immunization. J Pediatr. 1977;91(6):939-941.
2. Losonsky GA, Fishaut JM, Strussenberg J, Ogra PL. Effect of immunization against rubella on lactation products. I. Development and characterization of specific immunologic reactivity in breast milk. J Infect Dis. 1982;145(5):654-660.
3. Losonsky GA, Fishaut JM, Strussenberg J, Ogra PL. Effect of immunization against rubella on lactation products. II. Maternal-neonatal interactions. J Infect Dis. 1982;145(5):661-666.
4. Landes RD, Bass JW, Millunchick EW, Oetgen WJ. Neonatal rubella following postpartum maternal immunization. J Pediatr. 1980;97(3):465-467.
5. Lawrence RA. Breastfeeding: A Guide for the Medical Profession. St. Louis: Mosby Publishers; 1994.

SAGE

Trade:

Category: Herb

LRC: L4 - No Data-Possibly Hazardous

Salvia officinalis L. (Dalmatian sage) and Salvia lavandulaefolia Vahl (Spanish sage) are most common of the species. Extracts and teas have been used to treat digestive disorders (antispasmodic), as an antiseptic and astringent, for treating diarrhea, gastritis, sore throat, and other maladies.[1] The dried and smoked leaves have been used for treating asthma symptoms. These uses are largely unsubstantiated in the literature. Sage extracts have been found to be strong antioxidants and with some antimicrobial properties (*Staphylococcus aureus*) due to the phenolic acid salvin content. Sage oil has antispasmodic effects in animals, and this may account for its moderating effects on the gastrointestinal tract. For the most part, sage is relatively nontoxic and nonirritating. Ingestion of significant quantities may lead to cheilitis, stomatitis, dry mouth, or local irritation.[2] Due to drying properties and pediatric hypersensitivity to anti-cholinergics, sage should be used with some caution in breastfeeding mothers.

Adult Concerns: Typical anticholinergic effects such as cheilitis, stomatitis, dry mouth or local irritation.

Adult Dose:

Pediatric Concerns: None reported.

Infant Monitoring: Drying mouth, stomatitis, cheilitis.

Alternatives:

References:
1. Leung AY. Encyclopedia of Common Natural Ingredients used in Food, Drugs and Cosmetics. New York, NY: John Wiley & Sons; 1980.
2. Bissett NG. Herbal Drugs and Phytopharmaceuticals. Boca Raton: Medpharm Scientific Publishers, CRC Press; 1994.

SALICYLAMIDE

Trade:

Category: NSAID

LRC: L3 - No Data-Probably Compatible

Salicylamide is not hydrolyzed to salicylate. It is well absorbed; however, its bioavailability is very low due to first pass metabolism. Only 1 µg/mL is in the plasma after ingesting a 650 mg dose.[1] Its purported use is as an analgesic and antipyretic. There are no data on transfer of salicylamide to breast milk. Since salicylamide is similar to aspirin, it may have similar issues as aspirin. Avoid the use of salicylamide if the infant has a viral syndrome.

T 1/2		MW	137 Da	PB	40%-55%
Tmax	1.5-2 h	RID		Vd	
Oral	Good	M/P		pKa	8.21

Adult Concerns: Dizziness, dry mouth, heartburn, nausea, vomiting, diarrhea, rash.

Adult Dose: 325-650 mg 3-4 times daily.

Pediatric Concerns:

Infant Monitoring: Vomiting, diarrhea.

Alternatives:

References:

1. Salicylamide. Available in: Lexi-Comp OnlineTM ,AHFS-DI , Hudson, Ohio: Lexi-Comp, Inc.; 2011; Updated May 26, 2011.

SALICYLIC ACID, TOPICAL

Trade: Avosil, Compound W, Duofilm, Mediplast, Occlusal-HP, Sal-Plant Gel, Stri-Dex, Trans-Ver-Sal

Category: Keratolytic

LRC: L3 - No Data-Probably Compatible

Salicylic acid,[1] is often used in anti-acne preparations, as well as in many wart and corn removal products. It produces desquamation of hyperkeratotic epithelium by dissolving the intercellular cement, thus leading to softening, maceration of the tissue, and ultimately desquamation. Concentrations vary, ranging from 0.5% to 60%, in gels, shampoos, ointments and creams. Salicylic acid acts as a keratolytic at concentrations of 3%-6%, and above 6% becomes destructive. Systemic absorption depends on the concentration of the product used, the amount applied, the surface area treated, and duration of use. Absorption increases with the duration of use. The systemic absorption following topical administration has been found to range from 9.3% to 25.1%. Due to significant systemic absorption, prolonged use of topical salicylic acid should be used with some caution. Salicylic acid is not known to be associated with Reye syndrome in infants and children.

T 1/2	2-3 h	MW	138.12 Da	PB	50%-80%
Tmax		RID		Vd	0.17 L/kg
Oral	Complete	M/P		pKa	

Adult Concerns: Burning and stinging, as well as redness around the application area.

Adult Dose: Topical.

Pediatric Concerns: No data are available in breastfeeding women.

Infant Monitoring:

Alternatives: Azelaic acid(L3)

References:

1. Pharmaceutical manufacturers prescribing information.

SALMETEROL XINAFOATE

Trade: Serevent

Category: Antiasthma

LRC: L2 - No Data-Probably Compatible

Salmeterol is a long acting beta-2 adrenergic stimulant used as a bronchodilator in asthmatics. Maternal plasma levels of salmeterol after inhaled administration are very low (85-200 pg/mL), or undetectable.[1] Studies in animals have shown that plasma and breast milk levels are very similar. Oral absorption of both salmeterol and the xinafoate moiety are good. The terminal half-life of salmeterol is 5.5 hours, xinafoate is 11 days. No reports of use in lactating women are available.

T 1/2	5.5 h	MW		PB	98%
Tmax	10-45 min	RID		Vd	
Oral	Complete	M/P	1	pKa	10.12

Adult Concerns: Headache, dizziness, anxiety, insomnia, dry mouth, throat irritation, hypertension, tremor.

Adult Dose: 50 µg twice daily.

Pediatric Concerns: None reported via milk.

Infant Monitoring: Irritability, insomnia, arrhythmias, weight loss, tremor.

Alternatives:

References:
1. Pharmaceutical manufacturers prescribing information.

SALSALATE

Trade: Amigesic, Disalcid, Salflex

Category: NSAID

LRC: L4 - Limited Data-Possibly Hazardous

Salsalate is a nonsteroidal anti-inflammatory drug used to treat minor pain or fever and arthritis. Salsalate is a dimer of salicylic acid, that when ingested releases pure salicylic acid.[1] Absorption of salicylic acid (SA) is complete. SA inhibits prostaglandin synthesis and acts on the hypothalamus heat-regulating center to reduce fever. Salicylic acid is excreted in breast milk (see aspirin) and chronic use of salicylates should be avoided. Therefore, salsalate should not be used while breastfeeding. Avoid its use in a lactating mother if the infant has a viral illness.

T 1/2	7-8 h	MW	258 Da	PB	80%-90%
Tmax		RID		Vd	
Oral	Complete	M/P		pKa	

Adult Concerns: Vertigo, tinnitus, hypotension, dyspnea, dyspepsia, nausea, abdominal pain, diarrhea, gastrointestinal bleed, changes in liver and renal function, edema, serious rash.

Adult Dose: 3000 mg/day in 2-3 divided doses.

Pediatric Concerns: Avoid use in breastfeeding mothers due to the risk of Reye syndrome in infants. One case of neonatal metabolic acidosis has been reported in a mother consuming aspirin.[2]

Infant Monitoring: Vomiting, diarrhea.

Alternatives: Acetaminophen(L1), Ibuprofen(L1)

References:
1. Pharmaceutical manufacturers prescribing information.
2. Clark JH, Wilson WG. A 16-day-old breast-fed infant with metabolic acidosis caused by salicylate. Clin Pediatr. 1981;20:53-54.

SAQUINAVIR

Trade: Fortovase, Invirase

Category: Antiviral

LRC: L5 - No Data-Hazardous if Maternal HIV infection

Saquinavir is an antiretroviral agent used for HIV infections.[1] There are no data regarding the amount of drug transfer in human milk at this time; however, due to this medications large size (767 Da) and high protein binding (97%), milk levels will probably be low. In addition, oral bioavailability is poor at about 4%.

Note: This medication is an L5 to highlight the contraindication of breastfeeding when the mother is known to be infected with HIV; this medication is not an L5 based on its risk to the infant in breast milk (no data are available at this time). The Centers for Disease Control and Prevention recommend that HIV-1 infected mothers do not breastfeed their infants to avoid postnatal transmission of HIV-1.[2,3]

T 1/2	9-15 h	MW	767 Da	PB	97%
Tmax	3 h	RID		Vd	10 L/kg
Oral	4%	M/P		pKa	

Adult Concerns: Headache, fatigue, insomnia, anxiety, chest pain, abnormal heart rhythms (QTc prolongation), nausea, vomiting, abdominal pain, diarrhea, changes in liver and renal function, elevated blood glucose, neutropenia, thrombocytopenia, anemia, skin rash.

Adult Dose: 1000 mg twice daily but is highly variable.

Pediatric Concerns: None reported via milk at this time.

Infant Monitoring: Breastfeeding is not recommended in mothers who have HIV.

Alternatives:

References:
1. Pharmaceutical manufacturers prescribing information.
2. World Health Organization. Global Programme on AIDS. Consensus Statement from the WHO/UNICEF Consultation on HIV Transmission and Breast-Feeding. Geneva: WHO; 1992.
3. Latham MC, Greiner T. Breastfeeding versus formula feeding in HIV infection. Lancet. 1998;352:737.

SARECYCLINE

Trade: Seysara

Category: Antibiotic, Tetracycline

LRC: L4 - No Data-Possibly Hazardous

Sarecycline is a new formulated tetracycline primarily indicated for the treatment of inflammatory lesions of non-nodular moderate-to-severe acne vulgaris in patients 9 years of age and older.[1] No data are available on the transmission to human milk, but other tetracyclines are known to transfer minimally. Dental abnormalities and staining are well-known complications of tetracyclines and this product should not be used in breastfeeding mothers.

T 1/2	21-22 h	MW	523.96 Da	PB	62.5%-74.7%
Tmax	1.5-2 h	RID		Vd	1.38 L/kg
Oral	Significant	M/P		pKa	

Adult Concerns: Central nervous system side effects, including light-headedness, dizziness or vertigo, intracranial hypertension.

Adult Dose: 100 mg for patients who weigh 55-84 kg.

Pediatric Concerns:

Infant Monitoring: Diarrhea, GI distress.

Alternatives:

References:
1. Pharmaceutical manufacturers prescribing information.

SCOPOLAMINE

Trade: Benacine, Buscopan, Scopoderm TTS, Transderm Scop, Transderm-V

Category: Cholinergic Antagonist

LRC: L3 - No Data-Probably Compatible

Scopolamine (also called hyoscine) is a muscarinic antagonist structurally similar to the acetylcholine and blocks the muscarinic acetylcholine receptors.

It is a typical anticholinergic used primarily for motion sickness and preoperatively to produce amnesia and decrease salivation.[1] Scopolamine is structurally similar to atropine but is known for its prominent CNS effects, including reducing motion sickness. There are no reports on its transfer to human milk, but due to its poor oral bioavailability it is generally believed to have minimal absorption in the infant. However, following prolonged exposure in a newborn, some anticholinergic symptoms could appear, and include constipation and urinary retention.

T 1/2	2.9 h	MW	303 Da	PB	
Tmax	1 h	RID		Vd	1.4 L/kg
Oral	8%	M/P		pKa	7.55

Adult Concerns: Drowsiness, confusion, blurred vision, dry mouth, hypotension, bradycardia, constipation, urinary retention, dermatitis.

Adult Dose: 0.3-0.6 mg IV or IM once; apply one patch transdermally every 3 days as needed.

Pediatric Concerns: None via milk.

Infant Monitoring: Sedation or irritability, drying of oral and ophthalmic secretions, urinary retention, constipation.

Alternatives:

References:
1. Pharmaceutical manufacturers prescribing information.

SECNIDAZOLE

Trade: Solosec

Category: Antibiotic, Other

LRC: L4 - No Data-Possibly Hazardous

Secnidazole is a 5-nitroimidazole antimicrobial similar to metronidazole and tinidazole and was recently released for a single dose treatment of bacterial vaginosis, anaerobic microorganisms, including amoebiasis, giardiasis, and trichomoniasis. [1] At present no data are available on transfer to human milk. Should be similar to metronidazole. Manufacturer recommends delay of 96 hours for breastfeeding. Because its structure is virtually identical to metronidazole, this new drug's transfer to breast milk should be somewhat equivalent to metronidazole.

T 1/2	17-30 h	MW	185.18 Da	PB	15%
Tmax	1-3 h	RID		Vd	0.70 L/kg
Oral	Complete	M/P		pKa	2.62

Adult Concerns: Gastric upset, headache, nausea, itching, vomiting, dizziness, and bloody vomiting.

Adult Dose: 2 gm oral granules single dose.

Pediatric Concerns: None.

Infant Monitoring:

Alternatives:

References:
1. Gillis JC, Wiseman LR. Secnidazole. A review of its antimicrobial activity, pharmacokinetic properties and therapeutic use in the management of protozoal infections and bacterial vaginosis. Drugs. 1996 Apr;51(4):621-638. Review. PMID: 8706597.

SELEGILINE

Trade: Eldepryl, Emsam, Zelapar

Category: Antiparkinsonian

LRC: L4 - No Data-Possibly Hazardous

Selegiline is a selective irreversible inhibitor of monoamine oxidase, which in turn increases dopaminergic activity.[1] It is used to treat parkinsonian patients, major depressive disorder, and ADHD. It is available in a capsule form, an orally disintegrating tablet, as well as a transdermal system. The transdermal application has a half-life of 18-25 hours, and an absorption of 25%-30% over 24 hours. The orally disintegrating tablet concentration peaks at 10-15 minutes, and has a half-life of 10 hours. No data are available on the transfer of selegiline to human milk. However, monoamine oxidase inhibitors require extraordinarily careful use and have many food-drug and drug-drug interactions that could be dangerous. These products should not be used in breastfeeding mothers.

T 1/2	10 h	MW	187 Da	PB	99.5%
Tmax		RID		Vd	
Oral	5.5%	M/P		pKa	

Adult Concerns: Headache, insomnia, dizziness, confusion, hypotension, dry mouth, nausea, diarrhea, constipation, urinary retention, bruising, rash.

Adult Dose: 10 mg daily (capsule).

Pediatric Concerns: Do not use in breasfeeding mothers.

Infant Monitoring: Not recommended in lactation.

Alternatives:

References:
1. Pharmaceutical manufacturers prescribing information.

SELENIUM

Trade: SE-Aspartate, Se-100, Selenicaps, Selenimin

Category: Dietary Supplement

LRC: L3 - No Data-Probably Compatible

Selenium is an essential trace element which is needed for antioxidant enzymes. Selenium is often found in the form of various selenoproteins and is involved in various biochemical and physiological including the enhancement of immunity and oxidation resistance. Blood Selenium concentrations generally increase from birth until the age of 6 months in breastfed infants and then remain stable in the long-term.[1] Recommended dietary allowance of selenium for breastfeeding women is 70 µg/day.[2] Foods that are rich is selenium includes tuna, brazil nuts, beef, cod, chicken, turkey, egg, cheese, rice, oatmeal, bread, and walnut. Interestingly, formula levels are often deficient in this important trace element.

T 1/2		MW	79 Da	PB	
Tmax		RID		Vd	
Oral		M/P		pKa	

Adult Concerns: Abdominal pain, fatigue, tremor, excessive sweating.

Adult Dose: 20-40 µg/day.

Pediatric Concerns:

Infant Monitoring:

Alternatives:

References:
1. Victora CG, Bahl R, Barros AJ, et al. Breastfeeding in the 21st century: epidemiology, mechanisms, and lifelong effect. Lancet. 2016;387:475-490. doi: 10.1016/s0140-6736(15)01024-7.
2. Selenium. Dietary Supplement Fact Sheet. Washington, DC: Office of Dietary Supplements. National Institute of Health, November 12, 2009

SELENIUM SULFIDE

Trade: Dandrex, Selenos, Selseb, Selsun Blue Medicated Treatment, Tersi Foam

Category: Antiseborrheic

LRC: L3 - No Data-Probably Compatible

Selenium sulfide is an anti-infective compound with mild antibacterial and antifungal activity. Selenium sulfide appears to have a cytostatic effect on cells of the epidermis and follicular epithelium, reducing corneocyte production. It is commonly used for tinea versicolor and seborrheic dermatitis such as dandruff. Selenium is not apparently absorbed significantly through intact skin but is absorbed by damaged skin or open lesions.[1] There are no data on its transfer to human milk. If used properly on undamaged skin, it is very unlikely that enough would be absorbed systemically to produce untoward effects in a breastfed infant. Do not apply directly to nipple as enhanced absorption by the infant could occur.

Adult Concerns: Changes in hair color and loss of hair have been reported. Extensive washing of hair reduces the incidence of these problems. Extensive systemic absorption can occur with application to broken skin. Nausea, vomiting, diarrhea.

Adult Dose: Apply topically twice weekly.

Pediatric Concerns: None reported via milk. Do not apply directly to nipple.

Infant Monitoring:

Alternatives: Topical Clotrimazole(L2), Itraconazole(L3)

References:
1. Pharmaceutical manufacturers prescribing information.

SENNA LAXATIVES

Trade: Senokot

Category: Laxative

LRC: L3 - Limited Data-Probably Compatible

Senna is a potent, proven laxative. Anthraquinones, its key ingredient, are believed to increase bowel activity due to secretion of anthraquinones into the colon. Side effects such as abdominal cramping and colic are unpredictable with homemade varieties of this plant. Most sources recommend taking a standardized formulation commonly available. This product is only recommended for short use, such as 10 days. Do not use for intestinal obstruction, or appendicitis, or abdominal pain of unknown origin. Senna laxatives are occasionally used in postpartum women to alleviate constipation. In one study of 23 women who received Senokot (100 mg containing 8.602 mg of sennosides A and B), no sennoside A or B was detectable in their milk.[1] Of 15 mothers reporting loose stools, two infants had loose stools.

Adult Concerns: Diarrhea, abdominal cramps, dark colored urine, chronic diarrhea, fluid loss.

Adult Dose: 15 mg once daily.

Pediatric Concerns: Several infants had loose stools, although no drug was detected in milk.

Infant Monitoring: Diarrhea.

Alternatives:

References:
1. Werthmann MW Jr, Krees SV. Quantitative excretion of Senokot in human breast milk. Med Ann Dist Columbia. 1973;42(1):4-5.

SERRATIA MARCESCENS

Trade: Red diaper syndrome, Pink milk Syndrome, Pink breast milk, Chromobacteria violaceum

Category: Infectious Disease

LRC: L2 - Limited Data-Probably Compatible

"Pink milk syndrome", or breastmilk that exhibits a yellow to bright pink pigmentation upon exposure to oxygen, is the result of colonization with the gram-negative bacterium *Serratia marcescens*, a member of the Enterobacteriaceae family.[1] The reddish pigment, prodigiosin, is produced by some strains of *S. marcescens* after incubation at room temperature and may be present without any overt signs of infection.[2,3] It is unlikely that the pigment itself poses a danger to the infant.[4] S. marcescens is commonly found in the environment and can act as an opportunistic pathogen. While outbreaks are rare, they are most likely to occur in neonates or young infants.[5] The organism persists in moist environments and can be spread via hand-to-hand transmission or via contaminated medical equipment.[3,6-8] There have been several reports of hospital outbreaks and serious, nosocomial infections among critically ill neonates,[6,7] but the majority of infections (65%) caused by S. marcescens are community-based.[5] Such infections may be preceded by the appearance of pink milk.

Colonization or infection of the newborn with *S. marcescens* is likely to occur after delivery, as there appears to be no reports of in-utero transmission. At delivery, the infant's GI tract is sterile until exposure to fecal flora in the birth canal.[6] Typically, newborns delivered vaginally do not acquire S. marcescens as part of their normal gut flora. In contrast, those infants delivered via cesarean section or those receiving immediate critical care after birth, are more likely to be colonized by bacteria present in the hospital environment, including S. marcescens.[6] Infants without significant risk factors for nosocomial infection (e.g. low birth weight, prematurity, etc) may become asymptomatic carriers.[7] This bacterial reservoir may allow the organism to be transmitted repeatedly to the breast tissue or feeding bottle where it can contaminate breast pumps and stored milk supplies. Breast pumps have been implicated in numerous infections with S. marcescens. Contaminated milk is marked by a conspicuous pink residue that is often alarming to mothers.[9-10] Expressed breast milk is an excellent culture medium for S. marcescens and the bacteria will continue to multiply in storage.[9]

Pink milk may be present in the absence of illness. Commonly, both mother and infant lack signs of infection or fever. Because the organism has a propensity for moist environments and an ability to survive decontamination efforts with many soaps, disinfectants, or cleansers, the organism may flourish in the patient's breast pump and its parts.[7] Discoloration may occur between washing sessions, after pumping, or even appear on cloths or breast pads used while nursing.[1,2] The discoloration may not appear until sometime after feeding or pumping because the pigment requires time to react with oxygen.[1] The infant's diapers may have pink stains as well (referred to as "red diaper syndrome"), indicating a colonization of the gastrointestinal tract.[1] After the discovery of pink stains, both mother and infant should be evaluated for the presence of any infection. If cultures are positive for S. marcescens in the absence of overt infection, there are no clear guidelines on the use of antibiotics. Conservative management, without antibiotics, is possible with proper patient training and education on sterilization techniques to be performed at home on breast pump equipment.[1] Those parts that cannot be sterilized should be replaced. A decrease of the findings of pink stains should be expected with proper infection control measures. Consider using a countertop steam sterilizer on breast pump equipment.[1]

There is a lack of expert consensus regarding breastfeeding during maternal colonization with *S. marcescens*. Some physicians recommend empiric antibiotic therapy while withholding breast milk until the organism is cleared[2] while others encourage mothers to continue breastfeeding while on antibiotic therapy.[1] Other researchers suggest that the presence of organisms excreted into the milk may lead to feeding intolerance or even illness,[5] however, there appears to be a lack of evidence for this risk among healthy infants. In the presence of overt infection in the mother (mastitis) or infant (bacteremia), antibiotic therapy should be prescribed and both should be followed until the infection has resolved and repeat cultures are clear.[2,5] Asymptomatic colonization of the infant's gut tract may persist after resolution of infection or contamination of breast pump equipment. This should not be cause for alarm in a normal, thriving infant and breastfeeding should be continued.[9]

Adult Concerns: Mastitis: pink milk, localized erythema, warmth, pain, fever, cracked or chapped nipples, breast engorgement, or difficulty breastfeeding.

Adult Dose:

Pediatric Concerns: Bacteremia: fever, chills, rigor, malaise, irritability, mild respiratory distress, or feeding intolerance.

Infant Monitoring: Fever, feeding intolerance, irritability.

Alternatives:

References:

1. Jones J, Crete J, Neumeier R. A case report of pink breast milk. J Obstet Gynecol Neonatal Nurs: JOGNN/NAACOG. 2014 Sep-Oct;43(5):625-630.
2. Faro J, Katz A, Berens P, Ross PJ. Premature termination of nursing secondary to Serratia marcescens breast pump contamination. Obstet Gynecol. 2011 Feb;117(2 Pt 2):485-486.
3. Yu VL. Serratia marcescens: historical perspective and clinical review. N Engl J Med. 1979 Apr;300(16):887-893.
4. Frolov VM, Rychnev VE. Use of prodigiozan in the combined therapy of infectious diseases (a review of the literature). Vrachebnoe delo. 1986 Feb;2:111-114
5. Valle CA, Salinas ET. Pink breast milk: serratia marcescens colonization. AJP Rep. 2014 Nov;4(2):e101-e104.
6. Berthelot P, Grattard F, Amerger C, et al. Investigation of a nosocomial outbreak due to Serratia marcescens in a maternity hospital. Infect Control Hosp Epidemiol. 1999 Apr;20(4):233-236.
7. Jones BL, Gorman LJ, Simpson J, et al. An outbreak of Serratia marcescens in two neonatal intensive care units. J Hosp Infect. 2000 Dec;46(4):314-319.
8. Cullen MM, Trail A, Robinson M, Keaney M, Chadwick PR. Serratia marcescens outbreak in a neonatal intensive care unit prompting review of decontamination of laryngoscopes. J Hosp Infect. 2005 Jan;59(1):68-70.
9. Clifford V, Dyson K, Jarvis M, Erac O, Jacobs SE, Daley AJ. My expressed breast milk turned pink! J Paediatr Child Health. 2014 Jan;50(1):81-82.
10. Moloney AC, Quoraishi AH, Parry P, Hall V. A bacteriological examination of breast pumps. J Hosp Infect. 1987 Mar;9(2):169-174.

SERTRALINE

Trade: Lustral, Zoloft

Category: Antidepressant, SSRI

LRC: L2 - Limited Data-Probably Compatible

Sertraline is a typical serotonin reuptake inhibitor similar to fluoxetine; however, the longer half-life metabolite of sertraline, desmethylsertraline, is only marginally active. In one study of a single patient taking 100 mg of sertraline daily for 3 weeks postpartum, the concentration of sertraline in milk was 24, 43, 40, and 19 µg/L of milk at 1, 5, 9, and 23 hours, respectively following the dose.[1] The maternal plasma levels of sertraline after 12 hours was 48 ng/mL. Sertraline plasma levels in the infant at 3 weeks were below the limit of detection (<0.5 ng/mL) at 12 hours postdose. Routine pediatric evaluation after 3 months revealed a neonate of normal weight who had achieved the appropriate developmental milestones.

In another study of three breastfeeding patients who received 50-100 mg sertraline daily, the maternal plasma levels ranged from 18.4 to 95.8 ng/mL, whereas the plasma levels of sertraline and its metabolite, desmethylsertraline, in the three breastfed infants were below the limit of detection (<2 ng/mL).[2] Milk levels were not measured. One of the three infants was reported to have developed benign neonatal sleep myoclonus at 4 months of age, which resolved by 6 months of age; the authors reported the cause if this condition was unknown.

Another recent publication reviewed the changes in platelet serotonin levels in breastfeeding mothers and their infants who received up to 100 mg of sertraline daily.[3] Mothers treated with sertraline had significant decreases in their platelet serotonin levels, which is expected. However, there was no change in platelet serotonin levels in breastfed infants of mothers consuming sertraline, suggesting that only minimal amounts of sertraline are actually transferred to the infant. This confirms other studies. Studies by Stowe of 11 mother/infant pairs (maternal dose = 25-150 mg/day) further suggest minimal transfer of sertraline to human milk.[4] From this good study, the concentration of sertraline peaked in the milk at 7-8 hours and the metabolite (desmethylsertraline) at 5-11 hours. The reported concentrations of sertraline and desmethylsertraline in breastmilk were 17-173 µg/L and 22-294 µg/L respectively. The reported dose of sertraline to the infant via milk varied from undetectable (5 of 11) to 0.124 mg/day in one infant. The infant's serum concentration of sertraline varied from undetectable to 3 ng/mL but was undetectable in 7 of 11 patients. No developmental abnormalities were noted in any of the infants studied.

In a study of eight women taking sertraline (1.05 mg/kg/day) the mean milk/plasma ratio was 1.93 and 1.64 for sertraline and N-desmethylsertraline.[5] Infant exposure estimated from actual milk produced was 0.2% and 0.3% of the weight-adjusted maternal dose for sertraline and N-desmethylsertraline (sertraline equivalents) respectively. Assuming a 150 mL/kg/day intake, infant exposure was significantly greater at 0.9% and 1.32% for sertraline and N-desmethylsertraline respectively. Neither sertraline nor its N-desmethyl metabolite could be detected in plasma samples from the four infants tested. No adverse effects were observed in any of the eight infants and all had achieved normal developmental milestones.

Sertraline is a potent inhibitor of 5-HT transporter function both in the CNS and platelets. One recent study assessed the effect of sertraline on platelet 5-HT transporter function in 14 breastfeeding mothers (25-200 mg/day) and their infants to determine if even low levels of sertraline exposure could perhaps lead to changes in the infant's blood platelet 5-HT levels and, therefore, CNS serotonin levels.[6] While a significant reduction in platelet levels of 5-HT were noted in the mothers, no changes in 5-HT levels were noted in the 14 infants. Thus, it appears that at typical clinical doses, maternal sertraline has a minimal effect on platelet 5-HT transport in breastfeeding infants.

These studies generally confirm that the transfer of sertraline and its metabolite to the infant is minimal, and that attaining clinically relevant plasma levels in infants is remote at maternal doses less than 150 mg/day. Thorough reviews of antidepressant use in breastfeeding mothers are available.[7-9]

A 2015 review of sertraline levels in breastfed infants confirmed that drug levels in breast milk are low.[10] This review reported that of 167 infant sertraline levels, 146 (87%) were undetectable and of 150 desmethylsertraline levels, 105 (70%) were undetectable. The authors of this analysis reported that no adverse events occurred in the 167 infants included in the drug level analysis, even in those with detectable levels (median 5 ng/mL for both sertraline and its metabolite). The authors of this review do comment on two case reports of neonatal adverse events that could be associated with sertraline exposure in milk. The Australian Adverse Drug Reactions Advisory Committee reported these two cases in a brief letter in 1997.[11] The first case was of a 5-month-old who initially became agitated for a few days while her mother was on sertraline, this resolved spontaneously. The second case was of a woman who started sertraline 10 days postpartum and continued therapy for about 3 months. During this time, the baby was reported to be "somnolent, with low muscle tone, hearing problems, and suspected development difficulties." It was reported that all concerns resolved when the mother stopped this medication. Based on the brief report, it is difficult to determine how likely sertraline contributed to these concerns.

T 1/2	26 h	MW	306 Da	PB	98%
Tmax	7-8 h	RID	0.4%-2.2%	Vd	20 L/kg
Oral	Complete	M/P	0.89	pKa	

Adult Concerns: Headache, dizziness, insomnia, nervousness, dry mouth, dyspepsia, nausea, diarrhea, anorexia, tremor, increased sweating, galactorrhea in non-pregnant and non-nursing adults.

Adult Dose: 50-200 mg daily.

Pediatric Concerns: Three side effects related to sertraline have been reported. Benign neonatal sleep myoclonus at 4 months which spontaneously resolved at 6 months; its relationship to sertraline is unknown.[2] A 5-month-old who initially became agitated for a few days while her mother was on sertraline, this resolved spontaneously.[11] Baby was reported to be "somnolent, with low muscle tone, hearing problems, and suspected development difficulties." It was reported that all concerns resolved when the mother stopped this medication.[11]

Infant Monitoring: Sedation or irritability, not waking to feed/poor feeding, and weight gain.

Alternatives: Escitalopram(L2), Citalopram(L2), Fluoxetine(L2)

References:

1. Altshuler LL, Burt VK, McMullen M, Hendrick V. Breastfeeding and sertraline: a 24-hour analysis. J Clin Psychiatry. 1995;56(6):243-245.
2. Mammen OK, Perel JM, Rudolph G, Foglia JP, Wheeler SB. Sertraline and norsertraline levels in three breastfed infants. J Clin Psychiatry. 1997;58(3):100-103.
3. Epperson CN, Anderson GM, McDougle CJ. Sertraine and breastfeeding. NEJM. 1997;336(16):1189-1190.
4. Stowe ZN, Owens MJ, Landry JC, et al. Sertraline and desmethylsertraline in human breast milk and nursing infants. Am J Psychiatry. 1997;154(9):1255-1260.
5. Kristensen JH, Ilett KF, Dusci LJ, et al. Distribution and excretion of sertraline and N-desmethylsertraline in human milk. Br J Clin Pharmacol. 1998;45(5):453-457.
6. Epperson N, Czarkowski KA, Ward-O'Brien D, et al. Maternal sertraline treatment and serotonin transport in breast-feeding mother-infant pairs. Am J Psychiatry. 2001;158(10):1631-1637.

7. Wisner KL, Perel JM, Findling RL. Antidepressant treatment during breast-feeding. Am J Psychiatry. 1996; 153(9):1132-1137.

8. Stowe ZN, Hostetter AL, Owens MJ, et al. The pharmacokinetics of sertraline excretion into human brest milk: determinants of infant serum concentrations. J Clin Psychiatry. 2003;64(1):73-80.

9. Weissman AM, Levy BT, Hartz AJ, et al. Pooled analysis of antidepressant levels in lactating mothers, breast milk, and nursing infants. Am J Psychiatry. 2004 June;161(6):1066-1078.

10. Pinheiro W, Bogen DL, Hoxha D, et al. Sertraline and breastfeeding: review and meta-analysis. Arch Womens Ment Health. 2015;18:139-146.

11. Rohan A. Drug distribution in human milk. Aust Prescriber. 1997;20:84.

SEVELAMER HYDROCHLORIDE

Trade: Renagel, Renvela

Category: Other

LRC: L3 - No Data-Probably Compatible

Sevelamer is a chelating resin that is used to treat elevated plasma phosphate levels in patients with chronic kidney disease who are on dialysis. Sevelamer hydrochloride is not systemically absorbed and is retained in the gastrointestinal tract.[1] Hence, it would not readily enter milk at all.

T 1/2		MW	High Da	PB	
Tmax		RID		Vd	
Oral	Nil	M/P		pKa	

Adult Concerns: Dyspepsia, peritonitis, diarrhea, nausea, constipation, pruritus.

Adult Dose: 800-1600 mg three times a day with meals.

Pediatric Concerns: This product unabsorbed from the gastrointestinal tract and would not pose a hazard to a breastfeeding infant.

Infant Monitoring:

Alternatives:

References:
1. Pharmaceutical manufacturers prescribing information.

SEVOFLURANE

Trade: Ultane

Category: Anesthetic

LRC: L3 - No Data-Probably Compatible

Sevoflurane is a gaseous halogenated general anesthetic drug that is particularly popular because of its rapid wash-out.[1] Average patient time to emergence is approximately 8.2 minutes. It is commonly used in adult and pediatric patients, and is used in cesarean sections. The manufacturer states that while the concentration of sevoflurane has not been measured in breast milk, it is probably of no clinical importance 24 hours after anesthesia. Because of its rapid wash-out, sevoflurane concentrations in milk are predicted to be below those found with many other volatile anesthetics. Sevoflurane follows a three term exponential decay with half-lives of 11 minutes (18% of the dose in plasma compartment), 1.8 hours (15% from muscle compartment), and 20 hours (6% from fat compartment).[2] Small (3%) amounts of sevoflurane are metabolized and result in plasma levels that average 36 µmol/L. Levels reported are temporary and completely dissipate by 6 days. The fluoride ion released is not high enough to be a contraindication to breastfeeding. Further, the oral absorption of fluoride in infants is believed poor as it is chelated with calcium ions orally in milk.

While no data on levels of sevoflurane in breast milk are available, this product, due to its rapid clearance from the body (100-fold drop in 120 minutes), should not pose a problem for continued breastfeeding soon after exposure. The mother should resume breastfeeding after the procedure once she is alert, orientated and able to feed her infant or pump on her own.

T 1/2	1.8-3.8 h	MW	200 Da	PB	None
Tmax		RID		Vd	0.5 L/kg
Oral		M/P		pKa	

Adult Concerns: Malignant hyperthermia, bradycardia, agitation, laryngospasm, shivering, hypotension.

Adult Dose: Variable.

Pediatric Concerns: None reported via milk. Milk levels are likely insignificant, and oral bioavailability is unlikely.

Infant Monitoring: Observe for sedation, irritability, poor feeding.

Alternatives:

References:
1. Pharmaceutical manufacturers prescribing information.
2. Holaday DA, Smith FR. Clinical characteristics and biotransformation of sevoflurane in healthy volunteers. Anesthesiology. 1981;54:100-106.

SILDENAFIL

Trade: Revatio, Viagra

Category: Vasodilator

LRC: L3 - No Data-Probably Compatible

Sildenafil is a phosphodiesterase type 5 (PDE-5) inhibitor. It has vasodilating and smooth muscle relaxing properties. It is used in the treatment of pulmonary hypertension and in erectile dysfunction in men.[1] No data are available on the transfer of sildenafil into human milk, but due to its pharmacokinetic parameters, it is unlikely that significant transfer will occur. However, caution is recommended in breastfeeding mothers. Oral sildenafil has been used successfully in infants for the management of pulmonary hypertension.[2,3] No untoward effects were reported in these infants.

T 1/2	4 h	MW	666 Da	PB	96%
Tmax	1 h	RID		Vd	1.5 L/kg
Oral	40%	M/P		pKa	

Adult Concerns: Headache, insomnia, dizziness, blurred vision, changes in color vision, flushing, hypotension, dyspepsia, diarrhea, changes in liver function.

Adult Dose: Pulmonary hypertension: 20 mg three times daily; 10 mg IV three times daily.

Pediatric Concerns: None reported via milk.

Infant Monitoring: Drowsiness, lethargy, pallor or flushing, poor feeding, and weight gain.

Alternatives:

References:
1. Pharmaceutical manufacturers prescribing information.
2. Palma G, Giordano R, Russolillo V, et al. Sildenafil therapy for pulmonary hypertension before and after pediatric congenital heart surgery. Tex Heart Inst J. 2011;38(3):238-242.
3. Humpl T, Reyes JT, Erickson S, Armano R, Holtby H, Adatia I. Sildenafil therapy for neonatal and childhood pulmonary hypertensive vascular disease. Cardiol Young. 2011 Apr;21(2):187-193.

SILICONE BREAST IMPLANTS

Trade:

Category: Other

LRC: L3 - No Data-Probably Compatible

Augmentation mammoplasty with silicone implants has only recently been available in the United States. Millions of women have silicone implants for various esthetic reasons. In general, placement of the implant behind the breast seldom produces interruption of vital ducts, nerve supply, or blood supply. Periareolar incisions should be avoided, as they might interrupt nerves vital to prolactin production. Most women have been able to breastfeed. Breast reduction surgery, on the other hand, has been found to produce significant interruption of the nervous supply (particularly the ductile tissue), leading to a reduced ability to lactate. Other reports suggesting autoimmune diseases such as scleroderma with esophageal dysfunction in breastfed infants[1,2] have failed to be confirmed.

Silicone transfer to breast milk has been studied in one group of 15 lactating mothers with bilateral silicone breast implants.[3] Silicon levels were measured in breast milk, whole blood, cow's milk, and 26 brands of infant formula. Comparing implanted women to controls, mean silicon levels were not significantly different in breast milk (55.45 +/- 35 and 51.05 +/- 31 ng/mL respectively) or in blood (79.29 +/- 87 and 103.76 +/- 112 ng/mL respectively).

Mean silicon level measured in store-bought cow's milk was 708.94 ng/mL and that for 26 brands of commercially available infant formula was 4402.5 ng/mL (ng/mL = parts per billion). The authors concluded that lactating women with silicone implants are similar to control women with respect to levels of silicon in their breast milk and blood. From these studies, silicon levels are 10 times higher in cow's milk and even higher in infant formulas. It is not known for certain if ingestion of leaking silicone by a nursing infant is dangerous. Although one article has been published showing esophageal strictures, it has subsequently been recalled by the author. Silicone by nature is extremely inert and is unlikely to be absorbed in the gastrointestinal tract by a nursing infant although good studies are lacking. Silicone is a ubiquitous substance, found in all foods, liquids, etc.

Adult Concerns:

Adult Dose:

Pediatric Concerns: None reported via milk.

Infant Monitoring:

Alternatives:

References:

1. Spiera RF, Gibofsky A, Spiera H. Scleroderma in women with silicone breast implants: comment on the article by Sanchez-Guerrero et al. Arthritis Rheum. 1995 May;38(5):719-721.
2. Spiera H, Kerr LD. Scleroderma following silicone implantation: a cumulative experience of 11 cases. J Rheumatol. 1993 Jun;20(6):958-961.
3. Semple JL, Lugowski SJ, Baines CJ, Smith DC, McHugh A. Breast milk contamination and silicone implants: preliminary results using silicon as a proxy measurement for silicone. Plast Reconstr Surg. 1998;102(2):528-533.

SILODOSIN

Trade: Rapaflo

Category: Alpha-Adrenergic Blocker

LRC: L3 - No Data-Probably Compatible

Silodosin is an alpha-1 adrenergic receptor antagonist used for the treatment of benign prostatic hyperplasia. Silodosin relaxes the smooth muscles of the bladder neck and prostate. The drug is not indicated for the treatment of hypertension. Side effects include postural hypotension, dizziness, diarrhea, headache, nasopharyngitis, and nasal congestion. In one animal study, administration of silodosin 300 mg/kg/day did not suggest physical and development abnormalities in offspring of rats.[1] There are no studies on the transfer of silodosin to human milk. Due to the pharmacokinetic properties, little of the drug is expected to transfer to milk. Observe baby for nasal congestion and hypotension.

T 1/2	13 h	MW	495.5 Da	PB	97%
Tmax	2.6 h	RID		Vd	0.71 L/kg
Oral	32%	M/P		pKa	

Adult Concerns: Dizziness, diarrhea, orthostatic hypotension, headache, nasopharyngitis, and nasal congestion.

Adult Dose: 8 mg once daily.

Pediatric Concerns: Observe baby for nasal congestion and hypotension.

Infant Monitoring: Drowsiness, low blood pressure, lethargy, pallor, poor feeding, and weight gain.

Alternatives:

References:

1. Physicians Total Care, Inc. manufacturer product information, 11/2009

SILVER SULFADIAZINE

Trade: Dermazin, Flamazine, SSD Cream, Silvadene, Thermazene

Category: Antibiotic, Other

LRC: L3 - No Data-Probably Compatible

Silver sulfadiazine is a topical antimicrobial cream primarily used for reducing sepsis in burn patients. The silver component is not absorbed from the skin.[1] Sulfadiazine is partially absorbed. After prolonged therapy of large areas, sulfadiazine levels in plasma may approach therapeutic levels. Although sulfonamides such as sulfadiazine, are known to be secreted into human milk, they are not particularly problematic except in the newborn period when they may produce kernicterus. The WHO considers silver sulfadiazine as compatible with breastfeeding.[2]

T 1/2	10 h (sulfa)	MW		PB	
Tmax		RID		Vd	
Oral	Complete	M/P		pKa	

Adult Concerns: Allergic rash, renal failure, crystalluria.

Adult Dose:

Pediatric Concerns: None reported, but studies are limited. Observe caution during the neonatal period.

Infant Monitoring:

Alternatives:

References:
1. Pharmaceutical manufacturers prescribing information.
2. Anon. Breastfeeding and Maternal Medication. Geneva, Switzerland: World Health Organization; 2002.

SILVER, COLLOIDAL, NITRATE, OTHER

Trade: Silver nitrate liquid, Silver pellet

Category: Antiseptic

LRC: L4 - No Data-Possibly Hazardous

There are many different forms of silver such as colloidal silver, silver nitrate, and silver sulfadiazine. Colloidal silver solution is normally labeled by silver content in parts per million. Silver ions are present in humans at low concentrations (2.3 µg/L) from environmental exposure (inhaled, food and drinking water contamination, etc).[1] One study suggests that less than 4% of topical silver nitrate administration is absorbed transcutaneously.[1] Another in vitro study suggests that nanoparticulate silver absorption is very low, in the order of 0.46 ng/cm² for intact skin and 2.32 ng/cm² for damaged skin. The oral bioavailability of silver is estimated to be less than 10%.

Silver toxicity occurs when excessive exposure over a long period of time exceeds the capacity of liver or kidney excretion. The NOAEL (Human No Observable Adverse Effect Level) for silver is 10 grams of lifetime intake. Silver is not acutely toxic; however, accumulation of silver can cause adverse effects such as argyria, argyrosis, leukopenia, and anemia. In one case, ingestion of 30 mg/day of silver nitrate for an extended period with total intake of 6.4 grams caused generalized argyria. Argyria is a blue/greenish discoloration of the skin that is irreversible. There have been reported cases of argyria with total silver exposure of 3.8-6 grams. Another study of 30 healthy volunteers did not suggest significant adverse effects after ingesting 50 mg/day of silver leaf for 20 days (total dose of 1 gram).[2] There is one case of argyria (limited to finger nails) after ingesting 550 mg of silver colloidal over two years.[3]

There are no studies regarding silver transfer to breast milk, however the long-term use of this drug should be avoided in all humans, particularly breastfeeding mothers.

T 1/2	52 days	MW	108 Da	PB	
Tmax		RID		Vd	
Oral	Poor	M/P		pKa	

Adult Concerns: Silver toxicity: Argyria, argyrosis, leukopenia, and anemia.

Adult Dose:

Pediatric Concerns:

Infant Monitoring:

Alternatives:

References:
1. Lansdown AB. A pharmacological and toxicological profile of silver as an antimicrobial agent in medical devices. Adv Pharmacol Sci. 2010;2010:910686. Epub 2010 Aug 24.
2. Sharma DC, Sharma P, Sharma S. Effect of silver leaf on circulating lipids and cardiac and hepatic enzymes. Indian J Physiol Pharmacol. 1997 Jul;41(3):285-288. Abstract.
3. McKenna JK, Hull CM, Zone JJ. Argyria associated with colloidal silver supplementation. Int J Dermatol. 2003 Jul;42(7):549.

SIMEPREVIR

Trade: Galexos, Olysio

Category: Antiviral

LRC: L3 - No Data-Probably Compatible

Simeprevir is an inhibitor of hepatitis C virus (HCV) protease indicated for the treatment of chronic hepatitis C infection; this medication can be used in combination with peginterferon alfa and ribavirin or sofosbuvir alone.[1,2] At this time there are no data regarding the transfer of simeprevir to human milk. Based on this medication's large molecular weight and high protein binding, it is unlikely to enter milk readily; however, it does have a long half-life in patients with hepatitis C.

Simeprevir in combination with ribavirin is not recommended for use in breastfeeding patients at this time. While Ribavirin lacks lactation data, it has the potential to accumulate in breast milk because of its long half-life (298 hours at steady-state). See ribavirin monograph for more details.

T 1/2	10-13 h healthy patients; 41 h HCV infected patients	MW	749.94 Da	PB	99%
Tmax	4-6 h	RID		Vd	
Oral		M/P		pKa	

Adult Concerns: Headache, dizziness, insomnia, dyspnea, nausea, diarrhea, changes in liver function and increased bilirubin, myalgia, numerous skin reactions including photosensitivity.

Adult Dose: 150 mg once daily when part of combination therapy.

Pediatric Concerns: None reported via milk at this time, pediatric data are also limited.

Infant Monitoring: Changes in sleep or feeding, diarrhea, weight gain; if clinical symptoms arise, consider checking liver function and bilirubin.

Alternatives:

References:
1. Pharmaceutical manufacturers prescribing information.
2. Spera AM, Eldin TK, Tosone G, et al. Antiviral therapy for hepatitis C: has anything changed for pregnant/lactation women? World J Hepatol. 2016;8(12):557-565.

SIMETHICONE

Trade: Alka-Seltzer Anti-Gas, Gas-X, Genasyme, Maalox Anti-Gas, Mylanta Gas, Mylicon, Mytab Gas, Phazyme

Category: Antiflatulant

LRC: L3 - No Data-Probably Compatible

Simethicone is an antiflatulent, used to relieve upper gastrointestinal gas and also used as an adjunct in ultrasonography. Because the drug is not absorbed, the risk to a nursing infant from maternal use of simethicone is thought to be negligible.[1] There was no evidence of medication-related adverse effects in the neonate with simethicone exposure.[2] Simethicone is not systemically absorbed, so none would enter milk.

T 1/2		MW		PB	
Tmax		RID		Vd	
Oral	Unabsorbed orally	M/P		pKa	

Adult Concerns: Rash, diarrhea, nausea, vomiting, pharyngitis.

Adult Dose: 40-360 mg daily.

Pediatric Concerns: None reported. Commonly used in pediatric patients.

Infant Monitoring:

Alternatives:

References:
1. Briggs GG, Freeman RK, Yaffe SJ. Drugs in Pregnancy and Lactation: A Reference Guide to Fetal and Neonatal Risk. Philadelphia: Lippincott Williams & Wilkins; 2008.
2. Hodgkinson R, Glassenberg R, Joyce TH 3rd, Coombs DW, Ostheimer GW, Gibbs CP. Comparison of cimetidine (Tagamet) with antacid for safety and effectiveness in reducing gastric acidity before elective cesarean section. Anesthesiology. 1983;59:86-90.

SIMVASTATIN

Trade: Lipex, Zocor

Category: Antihyperlipidemic

LRC: L3 - No Data-Probably Compatible

Simvastatin is an HMG-CoA reductase inhibitor that reduces the production of cholesterol in the liver. Other medications in the statin family are known to be secreted into human and rodent milk, but no data are available on simvastatin.[1] It is likely that milk levels will be low and oral bioavailability is poor; however, the effect on the infant is unknown and statins could reduce cholesterol synthesis. Cholesterol and other products of cholesterol biosynthesis are essential components for neonatal development; therefore, it is not clear if it would be safe for use in a breastfed infant who needs high levels of cholesterol. Caution is recommended until more data are available.

T 1/2	4.85 h	MW	419 Da	PB	95%
Tmax	1.3-2.4 h	RID		Vd	
Oral	<5%	M/P		pKa	

Adult Concerns: Headache, dizziness, nausea, abdominal pain, constipation, changes in liver function, weakness, myalgia.

Adult Dose: 20-40 mg daily.

Pediatric Concerns: None reported.

Infant Monitoring: Weight gain, growth.

Alternatives:

References:
1. Pharmaceutical manufacturers prescribing information.

SINCALIDE

Trade: Kinevac

Category: Gastrointestinal Agent

LRC: L3 - No Data-Probably Compatible

Sincalide is a synthetically prepared, C-terminal octapeptide fragment of cholecystokinin (CCK).[1] When injected intravenously, it produces a substantial contracture of the gall bladder. Sincalide is therefore used for diagnostic purposes to assess biliary and gall bladder function. A reduction in radiographic gall bladder size of up to 40% is considered satisfactory contraction.[2,3] The half-life of sincalide was found to be approximately 1.3 minutes, with a high molecular weight of 1143 Da. Data from a study conducted in rats reveal that sincalide has a large volume of distribution and tends to concentrate in the liver, pancreas, upper digestive tract and in the thyroid. It does not penetrate the blood-brain barrier.

No data are available on the transfer of this peptide to human milk, but due to its high molecular weight, brief plasma half-life and extensive volume of distribution, it is extremely unlikely significant quantities would reach the milk compartment. Therefore, sincalide may be considered compatible with breastfeeding. A brief interruption of breastfeeding (1-2 hours) would preclude any possible side effects.

T 1/2	1.3 min	MW	1143 Da	PB	
Tmax	5-15 min	RID		Vd	
Oral	Nil	M/P		pKa	

Adult Concerns: Flushing, dizziness, nausea, gastrointestinal and abdominal pain, cramping, the urge to defecate.

Adult Dose: 0.02 µg/kg over 30 seconds.

Pediatric Concerns: None reported via milk.

Infant Monitoring: While it is unlikely to enter milk, a brief interruption of breastfeeding (1-2 hours) would preclude any possible side effects.

Alternatives:

References:

1. Pharmaceutical manufacturers prescribing information.
2. Sturdevant RAL, Stern DH, Resin H, et al. Effect of graded doses of octapeptide of cholecystokinin on gallbladder size in man. Gastroenterology. 1973;64(3):452-456
3. Sargent EN, Meyers HI, Hubsher J. Cholecystokinetic cholecystography: efficacy and tolerance study of sincalide. Am J Roentgenol. 1976;127:267-271.

SINECATECHINS

Trade: Veregen

Category: Neutraceutical

LRC: L3 - No Data-Probably Compatible

Sinecatechins is a topical ointment used to treat external genital and perianal warts in adults.[1] Sinecatechins has an unknown mechanism of action; however, it is thought that the drug has anti-oxidative activity as the four main catechins in the medication are derived from green tea leaves. In addition to the catechins, this product also contains gallic acid, caffeine, theobromine and other components of green tea leaves. It is not known whether topically applied sinecatechins are excreted in breast milk.

In one study, systemic exposure of the four main catechins (Epigallocatechin gallate [EGCg], Epicatechin [EC], Epigallocatechin [EGC], Epicatechin gallate [ECg]), were undetectable on day 1 of topical use.[1] However, one catechin (EGCg) was measurable in the plasma after 7 days of topical use in two of the 20 patients. The C_{max} was 10.1 ng/mL and the AUC was 52.2 ng*h/mL. In comparison, these values were substantially lower than the control group of adults who drank green tea (500 mL three times a day for 7 days). The green tea group had measurable concentrations of EGCg in all subjects on both days 1 and 7, with a mean C_{max} of 23 ng/mL and an AUC of 104.6 ng*h/mL on day 7.

Adult Concerns: Mainly local skin and application site reactions- redness, swelling, burning, itching, pain, sores or blisters and infections. Other regional reactions included enlargement of the lymph nodes, pelvic pain, and cervical dysplasia.

Adult Dose: Apply topically three times a day.

Pediatric Concerns: Safety and effectiveness in pediatric patients have not been established.

Infant Monitoring: Oral and GI irritation.

Alternatives:

References:

1. Pharmaceutical manufacturers prescribing information.

SIROLIMUS

Trade: Rapamune, Rapamycin

Category: Immune Suppressant

LRC: L4 - No Data-Possibly Hazardous

Sirolimus is an immunosuppressant sometimes used in combination with cyclosporine in renal transplants. No data are available on its transfer to human milk. Average plasma levels are quite low (264 ng x hr/mL) and the drug is strongly attached to cellular components and plasma levels are low. It is not likely it will penetrate milk in levels that are significant. However, it is a potent inhibitor of the enzyme 70 K S6 kinase, which is stimulated in breast tissue by prolactin. This agent, in rodent mammary tissue, strongly inhibits milk component production.[1] It could potentially suppress milk production in lactating mothers and caution is recommended.

T 1/2	57-63 h	MW	914 Da	PB	
Tmax	1-3 h	RID		Vd	12 L/kg
Oral	15%	M/P		pKa	

Adult Concerns: Headache, insomnia, hypertension, edema, hyperglycemia, hyperlipidemia, diarrhea or constipation, changes in liver and renal function, leukopenia, thrombocytopenia, anemia, arthralgia.

Adult Dose: 2 mg/day.

Pediatric Concerns: None via milk.

Infant Monitoring: Changes in sleep, vomiting, diarrhea, weight gain; reduced maternal milk production.

Alternatives:

References:
1. Hang J, Rillema JA. Effect of rapamycin on prolactin-stimulated S6 kinase activity and milk product formation in mouse mammary explants. Biochim Biophys Acta. 1997;1358(2):209-214.

SITAGLIPTIN PHOSPHATE

Trade: Januvia

Category: Antidiabetic, other

LRC: L3 - No Data-Probably Compatible

Sitagliptin phosphate is a dipeptidyl peptidase IV inhibitor resulting in prolonged active incretin levels, thus increasing insulin release from pancreatic beta cells in type II diabetics and decreasing glucagon secretion from pancreatic alpha cells, and ultimately decreasing blood glucose levels.[1] It does not lower blood glucose or cause hypoglycemia in healthy subjects. There are no data available on the transfer of sitagliptin to human milk. Levels will probably be quite low due to its size and kinetics. Some caution is recommended until we have data.

T 1/2	12 h	MW	523 Da	PB	38%
Tmax	1-4 h	RID		Vd	2.8 L/kg
Oral	87%	M/P		pKa	

Adult Concerns: Headache, diarrhea, upper respiratory tract infection, and nasopharyngitis.

Adult Dose: 100 mg once daily.

Pediatric Concerns: No data are available.

Infant Monitoring: Signs of hypoglycemia - drowsiness, lethargy, pallor, sweating, tremor.

Alternatives: Metformin(L1), Insulin(L2)

References:
1. Pharmaceutical manufacturers prescribing information.

SMALLPOX VACCINE

Trade: Dryvax, Smallpox Vaccine

Category: Vaccine

LRC: L4 - No Data-Possibly Hazardous

Smallpox is a viral syndrome caused by infection with the vaccinia virus. The smallpox vaccine contains a live but attenuated (weakened) preparation of vaccinia virus. The reconstituted vaccine contains approximately 100 million infectious vaccinia viruses per mL. Introduction of potent smallpox vaccine into the superficial layers of the skin results in viral multiplication, immunity, and cellular hypersensitivity. With the primary vaccination, a papule appears at the site of vaccination on the second to fifth day. It then becomes a pustule surrounded by erythema and induration. The erythema and swelling then subside after about 10 days and the crust forms. Secretions from the lesions are capable of inoculating other individuals and care should be exercised around pregnant women, infants, and particularly premature infants.

No data are available suggesting the degree of transmission to human milk, but it is likely to enter milk to some degree. Infants are at increased risk from vaccinia infections and the use of smallpox vaccine in infants is contraindicated unless it is an emergency situation. Although the use of the smallpox vaccine in children is not recommended in non-emergent situations, it was safely used in the past. The product information suggests that pregnant and breastfeeding mothers should not receive the vaccination under non-emergent conditions. However, there are no absolute contraindications regarding vaccination of a person with a high-risk exposure to smallpox. In breastfeeding mothers who are not at high risk, the use of smallpox live attenuated vaccinations is not justified (Centers for Disease Control).

Adult Concerns: Fever, lymphedema, urticaria, secondary pyogenic infections, vesicular rash.

Adult Dose:

Pediatric Concerns: No data are available on its use in breastfeeding mothers or its transfer to human milk. However, vaccinia virus is likely transmitted via milk and is probably minimally infectious. Its use in breastfeeding mothers is generally not recommended in non-emergent situations.

Infant Monitoring:

Alternatives:

References:
1. Pharmaceutical manufacturers prescribing information.
2. www.cdc.gov/breastfeeding/recommendatins/vaccinations.htm

SODIUM OXYBATE

Trade: Xyrem

Category: Sedative-Hypnotic

LRC: L4 - No Data-Possibly Hazardous

Sodium oxybate is a salt of gamma hydroxybutyrate. It is a rapidly acting central nervous system depressant used in patients with narcolepsy to treat excessive daytime sleepiness and cataplexy. Its mechanism of action is unknown, but theorized to involve interactions with GABA-B receptors in the brain.[1] No data are available on the transfer of oxybate to breast milk, but due to the low molecular weight and low protein binding, it is likely this medication will be secreted into milk and passed to a breastfeeding infant. Due to the sedative properties of this drug, this product should be used very cautiously in breastfeeding mothers, if at all.

T 1/2	0.5-1 h	MW	126.09 Da	PB	<1%
Tmax	0.5-1.25 h	RID		Vd	0.19-0.384 L/kg
Oral	25%	M/P		pKa	

Adult Concerns: Dizziness, headache, confusion, hallucinations, psychosis, vertigo, and nightmares, pain, nausea, vomiting, confusion, hyperglycemia, hypernatremia, peripheral edema.

Adult Dose: 4.5-9 g/day.

Pediatric Concerns: No data are available but caution recommended.

Infant Monitoring: Sedation, slowed breathing rate, not waking to feed/poor feeding, and weight gain.

Alternatives:

References:
1. Pharmaceutical manufacturers prescribing information.

SODIUM TETRADECYL SULFATE

Trade: Sotradecol

Category: Sclerosing agent

LRC: L3 - No Data-Probably Compatible

Varicose veins can be ablated by injecting an irritant into the vein, which then scars down and closes. Sodium tetradecyl sulfate is a modified version of sodium lauryl sulfate, a common ingredient in toothpaste, shampoo, and dish soap.[1] With smaller veins, many physicians rarely need to compress the vessel to keep the STS in place, instead relying on it being caustic in high concentrations at the needle point and harmless once diluted further down in the bloodstream. No data on STS excretion into breast milk are available, but toxicity is expected to be low. Breastfeeding can be resumed a few hours after the procedure.

T 1/2		MW	316 Da	PB	
Tmax		RID		Vd	
Oral		M/P		pKa	

Adult Concerns: Local injection site reactions, pain, urticaria, ulceration, permanent discoloration, necrosis, allergic reactions.

Adult Dose: 0.5-1 mL IV.

Pediatric Concerns: None reported

Infant Monitoring:

Alternatives: Glycerin, Polidocanol(L3)

References:
1. Pharmaceutical manufacturers prescribing information.

SOFOSBUVIR

Trade: Sovaldi, Harvoni (with ledipasvir)

Category: Antiviral

LRC: L3 - No Data-Probably Compatible

Sofosbuvir is a hepatitis C virus (HCV) nucleotide analog NS5B polymerase inhibitor indicated for the treatment of chronic hepatitis C infection. Previously, this medication was always used in combination with peginterferon alfa and ribavirin. Due to the ribavirin content it was rated hazardous for lactation.[1] However, recently sofosbuvir has been introduced in another combination and is rated here independently. There are no studies regarding the transfer of sofosbuvir to human milk. However, the manufacturer found that in rodent studies the predominant component recovered in rodent milk was the main inactive metabolite of sofosbuvir (GS-331007; half-life 27 hours). This inactive metabolite was not found to have any effect on the nursing pups.

In addition, this medication may in some instances be used in combination with ribavirin, which also lacks lactation data and has the potential to accumulate in breast milk because of its long half-life (298 hours at steady state). In combination with ribavirin, it should not be used in breastfeeding mothers. However, when used independently from ribavirin, it is apparently far less hazardous.

T 1/2	0.4 h, 27 h (primary inactive metabolite)	MW	529.45 Da	PB	61%-65%
Tmax	0.5-2 h, 2-4 h (primary inactive metabolite)	RID		Vd	
Oral		M/P		pKa	

Adult Concerns: Fatigue, headache, insomnia, irritability, nausea, decreased appetite, diarrhea, change in liver and renal function, anemia, neutropenia, myalgia, rash, pruritus.

Adult Dose: 400 mg once daily when part of triple therapy.

Pediatric Concerns: None reported via milk at this time, pediatric data are also limited.

Infant Monitoring: Changes in sleep or feeding, diarrhea, weight gain; if clinical symptoms arise consider checking liver function.

Alternatives: None.

References:
1. Pharmaceutical manufacturer prescribing information.

SOLIFENACIN SUCCINATE

Trade: VESIcare

Category: Renal-Urologic Agent

LRC: L4 - No Data-Possibly Hazardous

Solifenacin is a muscarinic agonist drug that reduces the symptoms of overactive bladder disorder (OAB) and has a high affinity for the M3 muscarinic receptor.[1] OAB is a medical condition that causes the bladder muscle (known as the detrusor muscle) to contract while the bladder is filling with urine, rather than when the bladder is full. Patients with OAB feel the urge to urinate more often (urgency), without advance warning, and when the bladder isn't completely full.

Solifenacin is an unusual anticholinergic, structurally different but similar in effect to atropine. We do not have data on its use in breastfeeding mothers. However, the potency of this product, its effect on numerous important organs, the sensitivity of infants to anticholinergic agents, and its long half-life make this product problematic for breastfeeding infants. It is likely that milk levels will ultimately be low (due to its structure), no data are available at present, and caution is recommended. This product should be used with significant caution in breastfeeding mothers, if at all.

T 1/2	45-68 h	MW	480 Da	PB	98%
Tmax	3-8 h	RID		Vd	8.57 L/kg
Oral	90%	M/P		pKa	

Adult Concerns: Dry mouth, constipation, nausea, dyspepsia, blurred vision, tachycardia, and drowsiness.

Adult Dose: 5-10 mg daily.

Pediatric Concerns: None reported but caution is recommended due to the anticholinergic effects and long half-life of this product.

Infant Monitoring: Dry mouth, urinary retention, constipation.

Alternatives: Tolterodine(L3)

References:
1. Pharmaceutical manufacturers prescribing information.

SOMATREM, SOMATROPIN

Trade: Genotropin, Growth Hormone, Human Growth Hormone, Humatrope, Norditropin, Nutropin, Omnitrope, Protropin, Saizen, Serostim, Zorbtive

Category: Pituitary Hormone

LRC: L3 - No Data-Probably Compatible

Somatrem and somatropin are purified anterior pituitary hormones of recombinant DNA origin. It is a large protein. They are structurally similar or identical to the human growth hormone (hGH). One study in 16 women indicates that hGH treatment for 7 days stimulated breastmilk production by 18.5% (verses 11.6% in controls) in a group of normal lactating women.[1] No adverse effects were noted. Leukemia has occurred in a small number of children receiving hGH, but the relationship is uncertain. Because it is a peptide of 191 amino acids and its molecular weight is so large, its transfer to milk is very unlikely. Further, its oral absorption would be minimal to nil.

T 1/2		MW	22,124 Da	PB	
Tmax	7.5 h	RID		Vd	
Oral	Poor	M/P		pKa	

Adult Concerns: Dizziness, fatigue, flu-like symptoms, hypertension, hyper and hypoglycemia, changes in thyroid and liver function, acne, myalgia, edema.

Adult Dose: 0.1-0.3 mg/kg every week.

Pediatric Concerns: None reported via milk. Some fatalities have been reported in pediatric patients with Prader-Willi syndrome.

Infant Monitoring: Changes in feeding, growth; if clinical symptoms arise, check thyroid function.

Alternatives:

References:
1. Milsom SR, Breier BH, Gallaher BW, Cox VA, Gunn AJ, Gluckman PD. Growth hormone stimulates galactopoiesis in healthy lactating women. Acta Endocrinol (Copenh). 1992;127(4):337-343.

SORAFENIB

Trade: Nexavar

Category: Antineoplastic

LRC: L4 - No Data-Possibly Hazardous

Sorafenib is a multikinase inhibitor that reduces tumor cell proliferation; this medication is used to treat unresectable hepatocellular carcinoma and advanced renal cell carcinoma.[1] There are no human data regarding the transfer of this medication to milk; however, the pharmaceutical company reported that about 27% of a radio-labeled dose entered rat milk. In addition, the milk/plasma ratio was determined in rat milk to be 5:1. Based on this medications larger size (637 Da) and high protein binding (99.5%), very little of this medication is anticipated to enter human milk. Caution is still recommended at this time due to the lack of human milk data. Adverse effects have been seen in animal studies with medication exposures in young/growing dogs.

T 1/2	25 to 48 h	MW	637 Da	PB	99.5%
Tmax	3 h	RID		Vd	
Oral	38-49%	M/P		pKa	

Adult Concerns: Headache, fatigue, fever, hypertension, myocardial infarction, changes in thyroid function (increased TSH), anorexia, nausea, vomiting, diarrhea or constipation, abdominal pain, weight loss, changes in liver and renal function, lymphocytopenia, thrombocytopenia, neutropenia, hemorrhage, peripheral sensory neuropathy, painless swelling, and serious skin reactions of the hand and foot - with blistering, ulceration and moist desquamation that can impair activities of daily living.

Adult Dose: 400 mg twice daily.

Pediatric Concerns: No adverse events reported via milk at this time. The safety and efficacy of this medication has not been studied in pediatrics.[1] Animal data using young/growing dogs found concerns with irregular thickening of the femoral growth plate and changes in the composition of dentin at an AUC of 0.3 times that of what would be expected at the recommended human dose. In addition, they found hypocellularity of the bone marrow adjoining the growth plate at an AUC of 0.1 times that of what would be expected at the recommended human dose.

Infant Monitoring: AVOID use in lactation.

Alternatives:

References:
1. Pharmaceutical manufacturer prescribing information.

SOTALOL

Trade: Betapace, Cardol, Rylosol, Sotacor

Category: Beta Adrenergic Blocker

LRC: L4 - Limited Data-Possibly Hazardous

Sotalol is a typical beta blocker antihypertensive with low lipid solubility. It is secreted into milk in high levels. Sotalol concentrations in milk ranged from 4.8 to 20.2 mg/L (mean = 10.5 mg/L) in five mothers.[1] The mean maternal dose was 433 mg/day. Although these milk levels appear high, no evidence of toxicity was noted in 12 infants. Another study of a 22-year-old mother taking 120 to 240 mg daily reported an infant dose of 20%-23% of the weight adjusted maternal dose in milk. This would relate to an infant dose of 0.41 to 0.58 mg/kg. However, there were no untoward effects noted in the infant.[2] It is suggested that if a mother decides to breastfeed while taking sotalol, the baby should receive close monitoring for side effects.

T 1/2	12 h	MW	272 Da	PB	0%
Tmax	2.5-4 h	RID	25.5%	Vd	1.6-2.4 L/kg
Oral	90%-100%	M/P	5.4	pKa	8.3, 9.8

Adult Concerns: Headache, dizziness, insomnia, depression, fatigue, chest pain, palpitations, arrhythmias (bradycardia, prolonged QTc, torsade's de pointes), hypotension, heart failure, wheezing, vomiting, diarrhea, myalgia, weakness.

Adult Dose: 80-160 mg twice daily.

Pediatric Concerns: None reported via milk at this time.

Infant Monitoring: Drowsiness, lethargy, pallor, poor feeding, and weight gain.

Alternatives: Propranolol(L2), Metoprolol(L2)

References:
1. O'Hare MF, Murnaghan GA, Russell CJ, Leahey WJ, Varma MP, McDevitt DG. Sotalol as a hypotensive agent in pregnancy. Br J Obstet Gynaecol. 1980;87(9):814-820.
2. Hackett LP, Wojnar-Horton RE, Dusci LJ, Ilett KF, Roberts MJ. Excretion of sotalol in breast milk. Br J Clin Pharmacol. 1990;29:277-279.

SPICE

Trade: Legal highs, Legal weed, Spice gold

Category: Drugs of Abuse

LRC: L4 - No Data-Possibly Hazardous

Spice is a new class of designer drug and is an alternative to marijuana, characterized as "legal highs." The psychoactive effects are mainly due to delta-9-tetrahydrocannabinol, which acts with high affinity as a full agonist at CB1 receptor in CNS and CB2 receptors in the periphery. However, marijuana is only a partial agonist at CB1 and CB2 receptors. All of synthetic cannabinoids are lipid-soluble, non-polar, highly volatilized compounds and because they are a full agonist and with high affinity for CB1 receptors in the brain, they are stronger than marijuana. However some synthetic cannabinoids also show high affinity for CB2 receptors present in the spleen, tonsils, and immune system so they can affect the immune system.

Tetrahydrocannabinol can accumulate in human breast milk to high concentrations and infants exposed to this milk will excrete THC in their urine.[1-11] There is increasing concern about the use of marijuana or other cannabis products, in breastfeeding mothers. Both human and animal studies suggest that early exposure to cannabis may not be benign, and that cannabis exposure in the perinatal period may produce long-term changes in mental and motor development. While this data poses numerous limitations, and does not directly examine the benefits of breast milk versus risks of exposure to marijuana in milk, cannabis and similar products should be strongly discouraged in breastfeeding mothers at this time. Healthcare professionals should encourage alternative treatment options for maternal health conditions requiring the use of this product. See Cannabis monograph for details.

Adult Concerns: Psychosis, seizures, anxiety, agitation, irritability, memory changes, sedation, confusion, tachycardia, cardiotoxicity, chest pain, nausea, vomiting, appetite changes, dilated pupils, brisk reflexes.

Adult Dose:

Pediatric Concerns: Limited information in lactation and pediatrics at this time. Infants may eliminate drug in urine for weeks after exposure.[10]

Infant Monitoring: Sedation, not waking to feed/poor feeding, weight gain, potential neurobehavioral or psychomotor delays.

Alternatives:

References:

1. Grotenhermen F. Pharmacokinetics and pharmacodynamics of cannabinoids. Clin Pharmacokinet. 2003;42(4):327-360.
2. Ranganathan M, Braley G, Pittman B, et al. The effects of cannabinoids on serum cortisol and prolactin in humans. Pyschopharmacology (Berl.). 2009;203(4):737-744.
3. Mendelson JH, Mello NK, Ellingboe J. Acute effects of marihuana smoking on prolactin levels in human females. J Pharmacol Exp Ther. 1985;232(1):220-222.
4. Perez-Reyes M, Wall ME. Presence of delta9-tetrahydrocannabinol in human milk. N Engl J Med. 1982;307(13):819-820.
5. Marchei E, Escuder D, Pallas CR, et al. Simultaneous analysis of frequently used licit and illicit psychoactive drugs in breast milk by liquid chromatography tandem mass spectrometry. J Pharm Biomed Anal. 2011;55:309–316.
6. Ahmad GR, Ahmad N. Passive consumption of marijuana through milk: a low level chronic exposure to delta-9-tetrahydrocannabinol (THC). J Toxicol Clin Toxicol. 1990;28(2):255-260.
7. Chao FC, Green DE, Forrest IS, Kaplan JN, Winship-Ball A, Braude M. The passage of 14C-delta-9-tetrahydrocannabinol into the milk of lactating squirrel monkeys. Res Commun Chem Pathol Pharmacol. 1976;15(2):303-317.
8. Tennes K, Avitable N, Blackard C, et al. Marijuana: prenatal and postnatal exposure in the human. NIDA Res Monogr. 1985;59:48-60.
9. Astley SJ, Little RE. Maternal marijuana use during lactation and infant development at one year. Neurotoxicol Teratol. 1990;12:161-168.
10. Jutras-Aswad D, DiNieri JA, Harkany T, Hurd YL. Neurobiological consequences of maternal cannabis on human fetal development and its neuropsychiatric outcome. Eur Arch Psychiatry Clin Neurosci. 2009 Oct;259(7):395-341.
11. Liston J. Breastfeeding and the use of recreational drugs-alcohol, caffeine, nicotine and marijuana. Breastfeed Rev. 1998;6(2):27-30.

SPINOSAD

Trade: Natroba, ParaPro Natroba Topical Suspension

Category: Pediculicide

LRC: L3 - No Data-Probably Compatible

Spinosad is an insecticide used in the treatment of pediculosis capitis (head lice). Spinosad causes neuronal excitation in lice followed by paralysis and death. Spinosad topical suspension is a mixture of spinosyn A and spinosyn D in a 5:1 ratio. Spinosad is approved for children older than 4 years. The drug should not be used in infants, especially preterm infants as it contains benzoyl alcohol. One study of 14 pediatric patients using one application to the scalp of 1.8% topical suspension of spinosad for 10 minutes revealed no drug detected in the plasma of the patients. No studies have been located on the use of spinosad during lactation.[1] Spinosad is not absorbed systemically when used in topical preparations. The benzyl alcohol in spinosad formulations may be absorbed and mothers may wish to pump and discard for 8 hours to avoid any benzyl alcohol exposure to the child.[1]

Adult Concerns: Skin erythema, skin irritation, ocular erythema, ocular irritation, ocular hyperemia.

Adult Dose: Apply on scalp and hair, leave on for 10 minutes.

Pediatric Concerns:

Infant Monitoring:

Alternatives:

References:

1. Pharmaceutical manufacturers prescribing information.

SPIRONOLACTONE

Trade: Aldactone, Spiractin

Category: Diuretic

LRC: L2 - Limited Data-Probably Compatible

Spironolactone is an aldosterone receptor antagonist used as a diuretic in various edematous conditions, as well as in the treatment of hypertension, hypokalemia, and primary aldosteronism. Spironolactone is metabolized to canrenone, which is known to be secreted into breast milk. In one mother receiving 25 mg of spironolactone, at 2 hours postdose the maternal serum and milk concentrations of canrenone were 144 and 104 µg/L respectively.[1] At 14.5 hours, the corresponding values for serum and milk were 92 and 47 µg/L respectively. Milk/plasma ratios varied from 0.51 at 14.5 hours, to 0.72 at 2 hours. Based on these values, the calculated relative infant dose is 2%-4%. The amounts ingested by the infant through breast milk are probably too low to be clinically significant.

T 1/2	10-35 h	MW	417 Da	PB	>90%
Tmax	3-4 h	RID	2%-4.3%	Vd	
Oral	70%	M/P	0.51-0.72	pKa	

Adult Concerns: Headache, dizziness, nausea, vomiting, diarrhea, changes in liver function, changes in renal function, hyperkalemia, irregular menses, gynecomastia, and rash.

Adult Dose: 50-100 mg daily.

Pediatric Concerns: None reported via milk at this time.

Infant Monitoring: Signs of dehydration, lethargy; monitor maternal milk supply.

Alternatives:

References:

1. Phelps DL, Karim Z. Spironolactone: relationship between concentrations of dethioacetylated metabolite in human serum and milk. J Pharm Sci. 1977;66(8):1203.

ST. JOHN'S WORT

Trade: SJW, Hypericum perforatum, Klamath weed, Remotiv, Tipton's weed

Category: Herb

LRC: L3 - Limited Data-Probably Compatible

St. John's Wort (hypericum perforatum) consists of the whole fresh or dried plant or its components containing not less than 0.04% naphthodianthrones of the hypericin group. Hypericum contains many biologically active compounds and most researchers consider its effect due to a combination of constituents rather than any single component.[1] St. John's wort is primarily used for the treatment of mild to moderate depression as it has shown to have benefit when compared to placebo and other antidepressant therapies.[2] In a recent systematic review that evaluated the efficacy of St. John's wort, the most commonly used hypericum extract contained 0.3% hypericin and 1%-4% hyperforin.

In one case report, a breastfeeding woman who had taken St. John's wort in pregnancy (900 mg/day - stopped 1 day prior to delivery) restarted her therapy 20 days postpartum (300 mg/day).[3] This woman continued to breastfeed her infant with no concerns; the behavioral assessments at 4 and 33 days of life were normal.

In another study of a single patient receiving St. John's wort starting 5 months postpartum, hypericin levels in milk were undetectable (<0.2 ng/mL).[4] Hyperforin levels in milk ranged from 0.58 to 18.2 ng/mL. Maternal plasma levels of hypericin and hyperforin were 10.71 and 151 ng/mL, respectively. Both components were undetectable in the plasma of the infant. No side effects of any kind were noted in the infant and the Denver Developmental Screen was normal.

A prospective, observational, cohort study of the safety of St. John's wort in lactation compared 33 breastfeeding mothers (group 1), to 101 condition-matched (group 2) and 33 age and parity-matched women (group 3).[5] No significant differences were found in maternal adverse effects or changes in milk production following treatment with

St. John's wort. The mean dose of St. John's wort taken in group 1 was 705 mg/day, the mean timing of initiation of therapy was 4.5 months postpartum and the mean duration of therapy was 1.5 months. Although, one infant in group 2 and one infant in group 3 were reported to be colicky, there were two cases of colic, two cases of drowsiness and one case of lethargy reported in group 1.

Please be aware that many products may be of poor quality and contain little or no St. John's wort; users should only purchase standardized or assayed products from reputable sources. In addition, St. John's wort is a strong inducer of liver enzymes, and may increase or decrease therapeutic levels of numerous drugs. Patients are advised to consult their pharmacist or physician for information prior to initiating therapy.

T 1/2	26.5 h	MW	504 Da	PB	
Tmax	5.9 h	RID		Vd	
Oral		M/P		pKa	

Adult Concerns: Dizziness, confusion, fatigue, vivid dreams, anxiety, irritability, dry mouth, nausea, vomiting, diarrhea, constipation, skin rash.

Adult Dose: Varies by formulation.

Pediatric Concerns: Two cases of colic, two cases of drowsiness and one case of lethargy reported in one lactation study.[5]

Infant Monitoring: Drowsiness or insomnia, irritability, dry mouth, vomiting, diarrhea, or constipation.

Alternatives: Sertraline(L2), Citalopram(L2)

References:
1. Upton R. St. John's Wort. American Herbal Pharmacopoeia and Therapeutic Compendium. Rocklin, CA: Prima Publishing; 1997.
2. Apaydin EA, Maher AR, Shanman R, et al. A systematic review of St. John's wort for major depressive disorder. Syst Rev. 2016;5(1):148. doi: 10.1186/s13643-016-0325-2
3. Grush LR, Nierenberg A, Keefe B, et al. St John's wort during pregnancy [letter]. JAMA. 1998;280(18):1566.
4. Klier CM, Schafer MR, Schmid-Siegel B, et al. St. John's wort (Hypericum perforatum) - is it safe during breastfeeding? Pharmacopsychiatry. 2002;35:29-30.
5. Lee A, Minhas R, Matsuda N, et al. The safety of St. John's wort (Hypericum perforatum) during breastfeeding. J Clin Psychiatry. 2003;64:966-968.

STAVUDINE

Trade: Zerit

Category: Antiviral

LRC: L5 - Limited Data-Hazardous if Maternal HIV Infection

Stavudine is an antiretroviral agent used in HIV infection.[1] A study that evaluated the safety of maternal antiretrovirals for prophylaxis against transmission to the infant during lactation also reported the milk levels of stavudine (n = 93 samples).[2] This study tested maternal serum and breast milk on the day of delivery and at months 1, 3, and 6 postpartum. Infant levels were also taken at months 1, 3, and 6 of age. The median drug concentrations of stavudine in maternal serum, breast milk, and the infant were 109 ng/mL (37-225 ng/mL), 105 ng/mL (34-117 ng/mL) and 0 ng/mL (0-2.5 ng/mL), respectively. The milk to plasma ratio was 1.14. The relative infant dose that we calculated using the maternal dose of 30 mg twice a day and median milk level was 1.8%. In this study seven of 28 stavudine exposed infants had severe anemia and one infant had a severe skin rash. This study also reported other infant adverse events (e.g., pneumonia, diarrhea, changes in liver function, neutropenia, thrombocytopenia), but was unable to determine which medication caused the effects based on drug levels, please see study for adverse event details.

Fatal lactic acidosis has occurred in patients treated with stavudine in combination with other antiretroviral agents.[1] Caution is recommended.

Note: This medication is an L5 to highlight the contraindication of breastfeeding when the mother is known to be infected with HIV; this medication is not an L5 based on its risk to the infant in breast milk. The Centers for Disease Control and Prevention recommend that HIV infected mothers do not breastfeed their infants to avoid postnatal transmission of HIV.[3,4]

T 1/2	2.3 h	MW	224 Da	PB	Low
Tmax		RID	1.84%	Vd	0.73 L/kg
Oral	86%	M/P		pKa	

Adult Concerns: Headache, nausea, vomiting, diarrhea, changes in liver function, jaundice, increase in amylase and lipase, peripheral neurologic symptoms/neuropathy, rash.

Adult Dose: 40 mg twice daily.

Pediatric Concerns: In one study, seven of 28 stavudine breast milk exposed infants had severe anemia and one infant had a severe skin rash.[2] Please see study for further adverse event details.

Infant Monitoring: Breastfeeding is not recommended in mothers who have HIV.

Alternatives:

References:
1. Pharmaceutical manufacturers prescribing information.
2. Palombi L, Pirillo MF, Andreotti M, et al. Antiretroviral prophylaxis for breastfeeding transmission in Malawi: drug concentrations, virological efficacy and safety. Antivir Ther. 2012;17:1511-1519.
3. World Health Organization. Global Programme on AIDS. Consensus Statement from the WHO/UNICEF Consultation on HIV Transmission and Breast-Feeding. Geneva: WHO; 1992.
4. Latham MC, Greiner T. Breastfeeding versus formula feeding in HIV infection. Lancet. 1998;352:737.

STREPTOMYCIN

Trade: Streptobretin, Streptotriad

Category: Antibiotic, Aminoglycoside

LRC: L3 - Limited Data-Probably Compatible

Streptomycin is an aminoglycoside antibiotic from the same family as gentamicin. It is primarily administered IM or IV, although it is seldom used today with exception of the treatment of tuberculosis. One report suggests that following a 1 g dose (IM), levels in breast milk were 0.3 to 0.6 mg/L (2%-3% of plasma level).[1] Another report suggests that only 0.5% of a 1 g IM dose is excreted in breast milk within 24 hours.[2] Because the oral absorption of streptomycin is very poor, absorption by infant is probably minimal (unless premature or early neonate).

T 1/2	2.6 h	MW	582 Da	PB	34%
Tmax	1-2 h (IM)	RID	0.3%-0.6%	Vd	
Oral	Poor	M/P	0.12-1	pKa	

Adult Concerns: Headache, ototoxicity, paresthesia of the face, nausea, vomiting, diarrhea, changes in renal function, hematologic changes.

Adult Dose: 1-2 g daily.

Pediatric Concerns: None reported via milk.

Infant Monitoring: Vomiting, diarrhea, changes in gastrointestinal flora, and rash.

Alternatives:

References:
1. Wilson J. Drugs in Breast Milk. New York: ADIS Press; 1981.
2. Snider DE Jr, Powell KE. Should women taking antituberculosis drugs breast-feed? Arch Intern Med. 1984;144(3):589-590.

SUCCIMER, DIMERCAPTOSUCCINIC ACID

Trade: Chemet, DMSA

Category: Heavy Metal Chelator

LRC: L3 - No Data-Probably Compatible

Succimer is a chelating agent containing dimercaptosuccinic acid. It is commonly used to chelate and increase the urinary excretion of lead.[1] While removing lead is important, some chelators (EDTA) are noted for increasing the plasma levels of lead and promoting its migration to neural and other tissues. In the instance of a breastfeeding woman, this could theoretically increase milk lead levels. However, succimer as studied in rodents has been found to increase the urinary elimination of lead without redistribution of lead to other compartments (this would theoretically include milk).[2] While we do not have studies of succimer transfer to human milk, due to its low pKa of succimer, it is unlikely that lead, chelated to succimer, would transfer to human milk. But this is not known for sure. Clinical studies in succimer-treated patients indicate that lead levels reach their lowest point after 4-5 days of therapy with succimer.[3] If breastfeeding patients were to pump and discard milk for 5 days while under therapy with succimer, it would significantly remove the risk of lead transfer to milk (if this occurs). However, more data are required before breastfeeding can be recommended following the use of succimer.

T 1/2	2-48 h	MW	182 Da	PB	
Tmax	1-2 h	RID		Vd	
Oral	Complete	M/P		pKa	3

Adult Concerns: Nausea, vomiting, diarrhea, appetite loss, thrombocytosis, intermittent eosinophilia, arrhythmias, neutropenia, drowsiness, dizziness, neuropathies, headache, rash, and paresthesias.

Adult Dose: 30 mg/kg/day for 5 days.

Pediatric Concerns: None reported.

Infant Monitoring: Nausea, vomiting, diarrhea.

Alternatives:

References:
1. Pharmaceutical manufacturers prescribing information.
2. Graziano JH, Lolacono NJ, Moulton T, Mitchell ME, Slavkovich V, Zarate C. Controlled study of meso-2,3-dimercaptosuccinic acid for the management of childhood lead intoxication. J Pediatr. 1992;120(1):133-139.
3. Graziano JH, Lolacono NJ, Meyer P. Dose-response study of oral 2,3-dimercaptosuccinic acid in children with elevated blood lead concentrations. J Pediatr. 1988;113(4):751-757.

SUCRALFATE

Trade: Antepsin, Carafate, Sulcrate, Ulcyte

Category: Antiulcer

LRC: L1 - No Data-Compatible

Sucralfate is a sucrose aluminum complex used for stomach ulcers. When administered orally, sucralfate forms a complex that physically covers stomach ulcers.[1] Less than 5% is absorbed orally. At these plasma levels it is very unlikely to penetrate into breast milk.

T 1/2		MW	2087 Da	PB	
Tmax		RID		Vd	
Oral	<5%	M/P		pKa	

Adult Concerns: Constipation.

Adult Dose: 1 gram four times a day.

Pediatric Concerns: None reported via milk. Absorption is very unlikely.

Infant Monitoring:

Alternatives:

References:
1. Pharmaceutical manufacturers prescribing information.

SULCONAZOLE NITRATE

Trade: Exelderm

Category: Antifungal

LRC: L3 - No Data-Probably Compatible

Sulconazole nitrate is a broad-spectrum antifungal topical cream.[1] Although no data exist on transfer to human milk, it is unlikely that the degree of transdermal absorption would be high enough to produce significant milk levels. Only 8.7% of the topically administered dose is transcutaneously absorbed.

Adult Concerns: Rash, skin irritation, burning, stinging.

Adult Dose: Applied topically twice daily.

Pediatric Concerns: None reported via milk.

Infant Monitoring:

Alternatives:

References:
1. Pharmaceutical manufacturers prescribing information.

SULFACETAMIDE SODIUM OPHTHALMIC DROPS

Trade: Bleph-10, Isopto Cetamide, Sulf-10

Category: Antibiotic, sulfonamide

LRC: L2 - Limited Data-Probably Compatible

Sulfacetamide is one of the N-acetyl derivatives of sulfanilamide.[1] Sodium sulfacetamide is a bacteriostatic medication that inhibits the bacterial enzyme system. It provides coverage for many gram-positive organisms but does not provide coverage for Neisseria species, *Serratia marcescens* or *Pseudomonas aeruginosa*. Sulfanilamide, when given orally, has been found to be excreted into breast milk in large quantities but because sodium sulfacetamide is instilled topically, the amount of the drug excreted in milk would be expected to be minimal. Because sulfonamides, as a drug class, may increase the risk of kernicterus in the first few weeks of life, sodium sulfacetamide should not be used during the neonatal period. Avoid in premature infants and in neonates.

T 1/2	7-13 h	MW	214.2 Da	PB	
Tmax		RID		Vd	
Oral		M/P		pKa	

Adult Concerns: May cause burning and stinging.

Adult Dose: One to two drops every 3 hours for 7 to 10 days.

Pediatric Concerns:

Infant Monitoring:

Alternatives:

References:
1. Pharmaceutical manufacturers prescribing information.

SULFAMETHOXAZOLE

Trade:

Category: Antibiotic, sulfonamide

LRC: L3 – Limited Data-Probably Compatible

Sulfamethoxazole is a common and popular sulfonamide antimicrobial. It is secreted in breast milk in small amounts.

In a study of 40 women less than 6 days postpartum who received doses of 800 mg twice daily, and in an additional 10 women who received 800 mg three times daily, milk levels were measured at random times during the day.[1] The average levels of sulfamethoxazole were 4.71 mg/L (n = 718). These milk levels would produce relative infant doses of sulfamethoxazole of 2% to 3.09% of the maternal dose, respectively, far too low to produce clinical effects in an infant. However, use with caution in premature infants, neonates with hyperbilirubinemia, infants with G6PD deficiency, or those in the first month of life (especially first 22 days). Sulfonamides displace bilirubin off its albumin binding site and could leave to higher free plasma bilirubin in infants early postpartum. Ito reports poor feeding in some infants following exposure to sulfamethoxazole.[2] However, use with caution in premature infants and neonates with hyperbilirubinemia, and avoid in infants with G6PD deficiency or those in the first month of life (especially first 22 days).

T 1/2	10.1 h	MW	253 Da	PB	62%
Tmax	1-4 h	RID	2.06%-3.09%	Vd	
Oral	Complete	M/P	0.06	pKa	

Adult Concerns: Headache, vertigo, fever, nausea, vomiting, abdominal pain, diarrhea, changes in liver and renal function, hyperkalemia, hyponatremia, hemolytic anemia, blood dyscrasias, allergic reaction, severe rash.

Adult Dose: 400 to 800 mg 1-2 times daily.

Pediatric Concerns: Poor feeding by infants in two cases.[2]

Infant Monitoring: Yellowing of the skin and eyes, check bilirubin; CBC if risk of hemolytic anemia.

Alternatives:

References:

1. Miller RD, Salter AJ. The passage of trimethoprim/sulfamethoxazole into breast milk and its significance. In: Daikos GK, ed. Progress in Chemotherapy, Proceedings of the Eight International Congress of Chemotherapy, Athens, 1973. Athens: Hellenic Society for Chemotherapy; 1974.
2. Ito S, Blajchman A, Stephenson M, Eliopoulos C, Koren G. Prospective follow-up of adverse reactions in breast-fed infants exposed to maternal medication. Am J Obstet Gynecol. 1993 May;168(5):1393-1399.

SULFAMETHOXAZOLE + TRIMETHOPRIM

Trade: Bactrim, Cotrim, Cotrimox, Resprim-Forte, Septra, Sulfatrim, Cotrimoxazole

Category: Antibiotic, sulfonamide

LRC: L3 - Limited Data-Probably Compatible

Sulfamethoxazole and Trimethoprim is a combined drug product. It is used as an antibiotic in conditions such as acute otitis media, pneumocystis pneumonia, traveler's diarrhea, shigellosis, and urinary tract infections.

Sulfamethoxazole is secreted in breast milk in small amounts.[1] It has a longer half-life than other sulfonamides. Use with caution in premature infants, neonates with hyperbilirubinemia, G6PD deficiency or those in the first month of life (but especially first 22 days). Pediatric half-life = 14.7-36.5 hours (neonate), 8-9 hours (older infants).

In one study of 50 patients, average milk levels of trimethoprim were 2 mg/L.[2] Milk/plasma ratio was 1.25. In another group of mothers receiving 160 mg two to four times daily, concentrations of 1.2 to 5.5 mg/L were reported in milk. Because it may interfere with folate metabolism, its long-term use should be avoided in breastfeeding mothers, or the infant should be supplemented with folic acid. However, trimethoprim apparently poses few problems in full term or older infants where it is commonly used clinically.[3] The relative infant dose is 4%-9%.

T 1/2	Sulfa/trim: 10.1 h/8-10 h	MW	Sulfa/trim: 253/290 Da	PB	SSulfa/trim: 62%/44%
Tmax	Sulfa/trim: 1-4 h/1-4 h	RID		Vd	
Oral	Sulfa/trim: complete/complete	M/P	Sulfa/trim: 0.06/1.25	pKa	Sulfa/trim: /6.6

Adult Concerns: Headache, vertigo, fever, nausea, vomiting, abdominal pain, diarrhea, changes in liver and renal function, hyperkalemia, hyponatremia, hemolytic anemia, blood dyscrasias, allergic reaction, severe rash.

Adult Dose: Sulfa/trim: 400-800 mg/80-160 mg one to two times daily.

Pediatric Concerns: None reported via milk at this time.

Infant Monitoring: Yellowing of the skin and eyes, check bilirubin; CBC if risk of hemolytic anemia.

Alternatives:

References:

1. Rasmussen F. Mammary excretion of sulphonamides. Acta Pharmacol Toxicol. 1958;15:138-148.
2. Miller RD, Salter AJ. The passage of trimethoprim/sulphamethoxazole into breast milk and its significance. In: Daikos GK, ed. Progress in Chemotherapy, Proceedings of the Eight International Congress of Chemotherapy, Athens, 1973. Athens: Hellenic Society for Chemotherapy; 1974.
3. Pagliaro L. Problems in Pediatric Drug Therapy. Hamilton, IL: Drug Intelligence Publications; 1979.

SULFASALAZINE

Trade: Azulfidine, SAS-500, Salazopyrin

Category: Anti-Inflammatory

LRC: L3 - Limited Data-Probably Compatible

Sulfasalazine is a conjugate of sulfapyridine and 5-aminosalicylic acid (5-ASA) and is used as an anti-inflammatory, immunosuppressant and bacteriostatic agent for treatment of ulcerative colitis.[1] Only 20% of the sulfasalazine dose is orally absorbed in the mother's small intestine. Some of the absorbed drug and the drug which stays in the gastrointestinal tract is cleaved by bacteria into two metabolites: sulfapyridine and 5-ASA.[1] Secretion of sulfapyridine into milk is estimated to be about 30-60% of maternal serum levels; secretion of 5-ASA (active compound) and its inactive metabolite (acetyl -5-ASA) in milk are very low.

In one study of 12 women receiving 1 to 3 g/day of sulfasalazine, the amount of sulfasalazine in milk was below the limit of detection (1 mg/L) for 26 samples; in the remaining 5 samples it was approximately 2 mg/L.[2] The concentrations of sulfapyridine in milk were about 40% of maternal levels and ranged from 1-32 mg/L. It was estimated by the authors that breastfed infants would receive approximately 3-4 mg/kg/day of sulfapyridine (if maternal dose 2 g/day). The authors comment that this very small amount may be regarded as negligible when considering risk of kernicterus because sulfapyridine and sulfadiazine are known to have a poor bilirubin-displacing capacity.

Esbjorner et al followed women taking sulfasalazine in pregnancy and lactation and measured both the breast-milk and infant serum concentrations of sulfasalazine and sulfapyridine.[3] This study obtained samples from 8 of 9 mother-infant pairs. The women took an average of 2.6 grams of sulfasalazine/day. The maternal milk levels for sulfasalazine and sulfapyridine ranged from < 0.52 mg/L to 4.1 mg/L and undetectable to 30 mg/L, respectively. The infant serum samples of sulfasalazine and sulfapyridine ranged from <0.52 mg/L to 1.72 mg/L and 1 mg/L to 5 mg/L. The authors of this study feel that these levels of medication in milk do not pose a risk for displacing neonatal bilirubin in otherwise healthy infants.

Berlin reported a case of a women treated with salicylazosulfapyridine (Azulfidine) 500 mg four times a day for ulcerative colitis.[4] No 5-ASA was found in milk; however, the sulfapyridine levels were approximately 3 to 6 mg/L. The authors estimated that an infant would ingest about 4 mg or 0.3% of the maternal dose of sulfapyridine via breastmilk. The infant in this case was exclusively breastfed, the mother started this medication when the infant was 4.5 months of age and the infant was reported to have no adverse effects from the medication in milk.

In a study of a patient receiving 1 g of 5-ASA three times daily, the milk levels for 5-ASA and acetyl-5-ASA were 0.1 µg/mL and 12.3 µg/mL respectively at 11 days postpartum.[5] The authors estimated the infant would receive about 0.015 mg/kg/day of 5-ASA and 2-3 mg/kg/day of acetyl-5-ASA. These results suggest that even with high doses (3 g/day) the amount of 5-ASA transferred is minimal.

In another study of 3 mothers receiving 0.5 g of sulfasalazine four times per day, the average maternal serum concentration of sulfasalazine and sulfapyridine were 8.8 and 19 mg/L, respectively.[6] The milk concentrations were 2.7 and 10 mg/L, respectively. The authors reported sulfasalazine and sulfapyridine levels in breastmilk are approximately 30% and 50% of maternal serum levels, respectively. No adverse reactions were noted in the infants.

In one patient receiving 500 mg mesalamine orally three times daily, the concentration of 5-ASA in breastmilk was 0.11 mg/L, and the acetyl-5-ASA metabolite was 12.4 mg/L of milk.[7] Using these numbers, the weight-adjusted RID was about 8.8%.

Few adverse effects have been observed in most nursing infants; however, a 3 month old infant exposed to sulfasalazine in breastmilk experienced bloody diarrhea.[8] The mother was taking 3 g/day of sulfasalazine and the infant was exclusively breastfed. At 2 months of age the infant had its first episode of bloody diarrhea, this recurred 2 weeks later and then persisted until 3 months of age. The diarrhea occurred up to 6 times per a day; all investigations were considered normal, except sulfapyridine was measurable in the infants blood (5.3 mg/L). When the mother's therapy was stopped, the infant's symptoms resolved 48-72 hours later.

There is an additional case report, where a woman was taking 5-ASA 500 mg rectally twice daily and her infant had multiple episodes of diarrhea.[9] This woman stopped and started her medication multiple times due to her infants diarrhea and each time the diarrhea started 8-12 hours after she took the medication and resolved 8-12 hours she stopped. No further episodes occurred after breastfeeding ceased.

T 1/2	8 h	MW	398 Da	PB	99% sulfasalazine; 70% sulfapyridine
Tmax	3-5 h; 3-12 h delayed release	RID	0.26%-2.73%	Vd	0.11 L/kg
Oral	20%	M/P	0.09-0.17 (5-ASA)	pKa	

Adult Concerns: Headache, dizziness, fever, nausea, vomiting, anorexia, abdominal pain, watery diarrhea, bloody diarrhea, leukopenia, thrombocytopenia, hemolytic anemia, skin rash, pruritus.

Adult Dose: 1 g two to three times daily.

Pediatric Concerns: One reported case of hypersensitivity. Multiple case reports of infants with bloody stools and diarrhea; additional case reports of pediatric patients taking the medication have also found bloody diarrhea.[10] Most studies showed minimal effects via milk. Caution in infants with G6PD deficiency.[3]

Infant Monitoring: Vomiting, diarrhea, bloody diarrhea.

Alternatives:

References:
1. Pharmaceutical manufacturers prescribing information
2. Jarnerot G, Into-Malmberg MB. Sulphasalazine treatment during breast feeding. Scand J Gastroenterol. 1979; 14(7):869-871.
3. Esbjorner E, Jarnerot G, Wranne L. Sulphasalazine and sulphapyridine serum levels in children to mothers treated with sulphasalazine during pregnancy and lactation. Acta Paediatr Scand. 1987;76(1):137-142.
4. Berlin CM Jr, Yaffe SJ. Disposition of salicylazosulfapyridine (Azulfidine) and metabolites in human breast milk. Dev Pharmacol Ther. 1980;1(1):31-39.
5. Klotz U, Harings-Kaim A. Negligible excretion of 5-aminosalicylic acid in breast milk. Lancet. 1993; 342(8871):618-619.
6. Khan AK, Truelove SC. Placental and mammary transfer of sulphasalazine. Br Med J. 1979;2(6204):1553.

7. Jenss H, Weber P, Hartmann F. 5-Aminosalicylic acid and its metabolite in breast milk during lactation. Am J Gastroenterol. 1990 Mar;85(3):331.
8. Branski D, Kerem E, Gross-Kieselstein E, Hurvitz H, Litt R, Abrahamov A. Bloody diarrhea--a possible complication of sulfasalazine transferred through human breast milk. J Pediatr Gastroenterol Nutr. 1986;5(2):316-317.
9. Nelis GF. Diarrhoea due to 5-aminosalicylic acid in breast milk. Lancet. 1989;1(8634):383.
10. Werlin SL, Grand RJ. Bloody diarrhea-a new complication of sulfasalazine. J Pediatri. 1978 Mar;92:450.

SULFISOXAZOLE

Trade: Gantrisin, Sulfizole

Category: Antibiotic, sulfonamide

LRC: L2 - Limited Data-Probably Compatible

Sulfisoxazole is a popular sulfonamide antimicrobial. It is secreted in breast milk in small amounts although the actual levels are somewhat controversial.[1] Kauffman (1980) reports the total amount of sulfisoxazole recovered over 48 hours following a dose of 1 gm every 6 hours (total = 4gm) was 0.45% of the total dose.[2] The milk/plasma ratio was quite low for sulfisoxazole, only 0.06, and for n-acetyl sulfisoxazole, 0.22. The infant secreted 1104 µg total sulfisoxazole in his urine over 24 hours, compared to the 1142 µg secreted in milk. Less than 1% of the maternal dose is secreted into human milk. This is probably insufficient to produce problems in a normal newborn. Sulfisoxazole appears to be best choice with lowest milk/plasma ratio. Use with caution in weakened infants or those with hyperbilirubinemia.

T 1/2	4.6-7.8 h	MW	267 Da	PB	91%
Tmax	2-4 h	RID	0.3%	Vd	
Oral	100%	M/P	0.06	pKa	

Adult Concerns: Elevated bilirubin, rash.

Adult Dose: 1-4 g every 4-6 hours.

Pediatric Concerns: None reported via milk. Use with caution in hyperbilirubinemia neonates and in infants with G6PD.

Infant Monitoring:

Alternatives:

References:

1. Rasmussen F. Mammary excretion of sulphonamides. Acta Pharmacol Toxicol. 1958;15:138-148.
2. Kauffman RE, O'Brien C, Gilford P. Sulfisoxazole secretion into human milk. J Pediatr. 1980;97(5):839-841.

SULPIRIDE

Trade: Dolmatil, Sulparex, Sulpitil

Category: Antidepressant, other

LRC: L3 - Limited Data-Probably Compatible

Sulpiride is a selective dopamine antagonist used as an antidepressant and antipsychotic. Sulpiride is a strong neuroleptic antipsychotic drug; however, several studies using smaller doses have found it to significantly increase prolactin levels and breast milk production in smaller doses that do not produce overt neuroleptic effects on the mother.[1] In a study with 14 women who received sulpiride (50 mg three times daily), and in a subsequent study with 36 breastfeeding women, Ylikorkala found major increases in prolactin levels and significant but only moderate increases in breast milk production.[2,3] In a group of 20 women who received 50 mg twice daily, breast milk samples were drawn 2 hours after the dose.[4] The concentration of sulpiride in breast milk ranged from 0.26 to 1.97 mg/L. No effects on breastfed infants were noted. The authors concluded that sulpiride, when administered early in the postpartum period, is useful in promoting initiation of lactation. In a study by McMurdo, sulpiride was found to be a potent stimulant of maternal plasma prolactin levels.[5] Interestingly, it appears that the prolactin response to sulpiride is not dose-related and reached a maximum at 3-10 mg and thereafter, further increased doses did not further increase prolactin levels. Sulpiride is not available in the United States.

T 1/2	6-8 h	MW	341 Da	PB	
Tmax	2-6 h	RID	2.7%-20.7%	Vd	2.7 L/kg
Oral	27%-34%	M/P		pKa	

Adult Concerns: Tardive dyskinesia, extrapyramidal symptoms, sedation, neuroleptic malignant syndrome, cholestatic jaundice.

Adult Dose: 50 mg twice daily.

Pediatric Concerns: None reported via milk.

Infant Monitoring:

Alternatives: Metoclopramide(L2), Domperidone(L3)

References:

1. Wiesel FA, Alfredsson G, Ehrnebo M, Sedvall G. The pharmacokinetics of intravenous and oral sulpiride in healthy human subjects. Eur J Clin Pharmacol. 1980;17(5):385-391.
2. Ylikorkala O, Kauppila A, Kivinen S, Viinikka L. Sulpiride improves inadequate lactation. Br Med J (Clin Res Ed). 1982;285(6337):249-251.
3. Ylikorkala O, Kauppila A, Kivinen S, Viinikka L. Treatment of inadequate lactation with oral sulpiride and buccal oxytocin. Obstet Gynecol. 1984;63(1):57-60.
4. Aono T, Shioji T, Aki T, Hirota K, Nomura A, Kurachi K. Augmentation of puerperal lactation by oral administration of sulpiride. J Clin Endocrinol Metab. 1979;48(3):478-482.
5. McMurdo ME, Howie PW, Lewis M, Marnie M, McEwen J, McNeilly AS. Prolactin response to low dose sulpiride. Br J Clin Pharmacol. 1987;24(2):133-137.

SUMATRIPTAN

Trade: Alsuma, Imigran, Imitrex, Sumavel DosePro, Onzetra Xsail

Category: Antimigraine

LRC: L3 - Limited Data-Probably Compatible

Sumatriptan is a 5-HT1B/1D (serotonin) receptor agonist used to treat migraine and cluster headaches. Activating these receptors is believed to constrict cranial blood vessels and block the release of proinflammatory neuropeptides from the trigeminal nerve.[1]

Sumatriptan is the best-studied drug in its class and is suitable for use in breastfeeding women. One trial measured drug levels in the plasma and milk of five women given a 6 mg subcutaneous injection.[2] Milk levels were 4.9 times higher than plasma levels and peaked at 87.2 µg/L at 2.6 hours postdose.[2] The mean half-life of elimination from the milk was 2.2 hours. Total recovery of the drug via milk was calculated to be about 14.4 µg, or 0.24% of the 6 mg dose. This equates to a relative infant dose of 3.5%. Given that triptans are not given continuously and that the drug has such poor oral bioavailability (14%), the amount of sumatriptan that reaches the infant's circulation is expected to be exceedingly low (less than 1%).

At this time, sumatriptan is the preferred triptan for use in lactation.

T 1/2	2-3 h	MW	413 Da	PB	14%-21%
Tmax	12 min (SC), 2-2.5 h (oral)	RID	3.5% (single dose)	Vd	2.4 L/kg
Oral	14%	M/P	4.9	pKa	9.63

Adult Concerns: Dizziness, flushing, hot or cold sensation, diaphoresis, chest pain, feeling of heaviness, nausea, vomiting, weakness, paresthesia.

Adult Dose: 25-100 mg orally, may repeat in 2 hours if needed.

Pediatric Concerns: None reported via milk at this time.

Infant Monitoring: Drowsiness, vomiting, poor feeding.

Alternatives: NSAIDs, Acetaminophen(L1)

References:

1. Pharmaceutical manufacturers prescribing information.
2. Wojnar-Horton RE, Hackett LP, Yapp P, Dusci LJ, Paech M, Ilett KF. Distribution and excretion of sumatriptan in human milk. Br J Clin Pharmacol. 1996;41(3):217-221.

SUNITINIB

Trade: Sutent

Category: Anticancer

LRC: L4 - No Data-Possibly Hazardous

It is a tyrosine kinase inhibitor used in gastrointestinal stromal tumor (GIST), renal cell carcinoma (RCC), well-differentiated pancreatic neuroendocrine tumors (pNET). It is not known whether this drug or its primary active metabolite are excreted in human milk. In lactating female rats sunitinib and its metabolites were extensively excreted in milk at concentrations up to 12 times higher than plasma.[1] Because of the potential for serious adverse reactions in nursing infants, a decision should be made whether to discontinue nursing or to discontinue the drug taking into account the importance of the drug to the mother.

T 1/2	40-60 h, active metabolites 80-110 h	MW	398 Da	PB	95%
Tmax	6-12 h	RID		Vd	
Oral		M/P		pKa	

Adult Concerns: Fatigue, hypertension, QT prolongation, hypothyroidism, altered taste, stomatitis, nausea, diarrhea, constipation, anorexia, changes in blood sugar, changes in liver and renal function, changes in electrolytes, leukopenia, neutropenia, anemia, severe skin reactions.

Adult Dose: GIST and RCC: 50 mg orally once daily ; pNET: 37.5 mg orally once daily.

Pediatric Concerns: The safety and efficacy of SUTENT in pediatric patients have not been established.

Infant Monitoring: AVOID in lactation.

Alternatives:

References:
1. Pharmaceutical manufacturers prescribing information.

SUVOREXANT

Trade: Belsomra

Category: Sedative-Hypnotic

LRC: L3 - No Data-Probably Compatible

Suvorexant is a new medication used for insomnia.[1] This medication is part of a new class of medications that are orexin receptor antagonists. The orexin neuropeptide signaling system promotes wakefulness, thus this medication blocks the orexin receptor from wake-promoting peptides. At this time, it is unknown if suvorexant will enter human milk, the manufacturer reports it enters rodent milk at levels about 9 times greater than maternal plasma. Until human data is available, we recommend the use of other sleep agents with more safety data in lactation such as lorazepam, oxazepam or zopiclone.

T 1/2	12 h	MW	450.9 Da	PB	99%
Tmax	2 h	RID		Vd	0.7 L/kg
Oral	82%	M/P		pKa	

Adult Concerns: Headache, drowsiness, dizziness, abnormal dreams, amnesia, anxiety, exacerbation of depression, dry mouth, diarrhea, increases in cholesterol, weakness.

Adult Dose: 10 mg orally at bedtime.

Pediatric Concerns:

Infant Monitoring: Sedation, irritability, dry mouth, diarrhea.

Alternatives: Oxazepam(L2), Lorazepam(L3), Zopiclone(L2)

References:
1. Pharmaceutical manufacturers prescribing information.

SYNEPHRINE

Trade: Advantra, Bitter Orange, Oxedrine

Category: Anti-obesity Agent

LRC: L4 - No Data-Possibly Hazardous

Synephrine (or oxedrine) is commonly used as an ephedrine-free weight loss agent. There are little to no data on its use during lactation. Its effectiveness as a weight-loss agent is highly speculative and debated. It is likely transferred to breast milk due to its small molecular weight and chemical structure. This product should be used with caution as little is known about its pharmacology.

T 1/2	2-3 h	MW	167 Da	PB	
Tmax	90 min	RID		Vd	376 L/kg
Oral	22%	M/P		pKa	9.3

Adult Concerns: Cardiovascular toxicity, myocardial infarction, arrhythmia, excitement.

Adult Dose:

Pediatric Concerns:

Infant Monitoring: Not recommended in lactation.

Alternatives:

References:

SYPHILIS

Trade:

Category: Infectious Disease

LRC: L4 - No Data-Possibly Hazardous

Syphilis is a sexually transmitted disease that is caused by a bacterium called *Treponema pallidum*, which belongs to the family of spirochetes.[1] Syphilis is caused due to sexual contact with infected lesions. Primary syphilis is characterized by the appearance of painless skin ulcers or chancres in the genital area. These chancres are infectious and disappear spontaneously without treatment within a few weeks. This is followed by secondary syphilis characterized by the appearance of a generalized rash that involves the palms and soles, and also the appearance of warts in the genital area called condyloma lata. This stage also resolves spontaneously to cause latent syphilis years later, characterized by neurological and cardiac manifestations.

The treatment of syphilis is with parenteral penicillin G or azithromycin. Doxycycline is an alternative choice. When a lactating mother has been diagnosed with syphilis, treatment should be instituted immediately. The infant should be immediately tested for syphilis as well and treatment instituted if positive for the disease. Any wet sores on the body may be infectious and should be adequately covered during breastfeeding to avoid contact with the infant. If there are wet sores on one breast, breastfeeding should be avoided from that breast and the infant may breastfeed from the opposite breast. Breastfeeding should be avoided from the affected breast until the skin sores completely heal.

Adult Concerns: Primary syphilis is characterized by the appearance of painless skin ulcers or chancres in the genital area. These chancres are infectious and disappear spontaneously without treatment within a few weeks. This is followed by secondary syphilis characterized by the appearance of a generalized rash that involves the palms and soles, and also the appearance of warts in the genital area called condyloma lata. This stage also resolves spontaneously to cause latent syphilis years later, characterized by neurological and cardiac manifestations.

Adult Dose:

Pediatric Concerns:

Infant Monitoring: Rash.

Alternatives:

References:
1. American Academy of Pediatrics. Pediatric Infectious Disease Red Book, 2015. Elk Grove Village, IL: American Academy of Pediatrics.

TACROLIMUS

Trade: Prograf, Protopic

Category: Immune Suppressant

LRC: L3 - Limited Data-Probably Compatible

Tacrolimus is an immunosuppressant used to reduce rejection of transplanted organs including the liver and kidney.[1] In one report of 21 mothers who received tacrolimus while pregnant, milk concentrations in colostrum averaged 0.79 ng/mL and varied from 0.3 to 1.9 ng/mL.[2] Maternal oral doses ranged from 9.8 to 10.3 mg/day. Milk/blood ratio averaged 0.54. Using this data and an average daily milk intake of 150 mL/kg, the average dose to the infant per day via milk would be <0.1 µg/kg/day. Because the oral bioavailability is poor (<32%), an infant would likely ingest less than 100 ng/kg/day. The usual pediatric oral dose for preventing rejection varies from 0.15 to 0.2 mg/kg/day (equivalent to 150,000-200,000 ng/kg/day).

In a 32-year-old woman who took tacrolimus 0.1 mg/kg/day throughout pregnancy, samples were manually expressed postpartum at 0 (trough), 1, 6, 9, 11, and 12 hours after the morning dose.[3] The C_{max} occurred at 1 hour and was 0.57 µg/L. Using AUC data, the mean milk concentration was calculated to be 0.429 ng/mL. From these measurements, the exclusively breastfed infant would ingest, on average, 0.06 µg/kg/day, which corresponds to 0.06% of the mother's weight-normalized dose. Given the low oral bioavailability of tacrolimus, the maximum amount the baby would receive is 0.02% of the mother's weight-adjusted dose. The milk/blood ratios of tacrolimus at pre-dosing and 1 hour post-dosing concentrations were calculated to be 0.08 and 0.09, respectively. At 2.5 months of age, the infant was developing well both physically and neurologically. The authors suggest that maternal therapy with tacrolimus for liver transplant may be compatible with breastfeeding.

In a more recent study, a 29-year-old woman with a 3-month-old breastfed infant, was receiving 2 mg tacrolimus twice daily, azathioprine 100 mg, prednisone 5 mg, diltiazem 180 mg, atenolol 100 mg, and furosemide 20 mg daily.[4] The milk-to-blood ratio was 0.23, and the average tacrolimus concentration in milk was 1.8 µg/L. The authors estimated the daily intake in the infant to be 0.5% of the maternal weight-adjusted dose (RID) or 0.27 µg/kg/day. This is less than 0.2% of the recommended pediatric dose for renal or liver transplant. The concentration-time profile of tacrolimus in milk was essentially flat. The highest concentration of tacrolimus in milk was at 4 and 8.5 hours post-dose.

In a cohort of 14 women who used tacrolimus in pregnancy, nine attempted to breastfeed; however, three had to discontinue within 2 weeks due to breastfeeding difficulties or the addition of other medications.[5] Of the remaining six mothers who took tacrolimus to prevent solid organ transplant rejection, their average daily dose was 9.6 mg (4.5-15 mg). The infants (born at 34- 41 weeks) were breastfed for a median of 3 months (1.5- 6), and four were exclusively breastfed. Four of the infants had tacrolimus levels drawn between days 15 and 27 of life; all of the levels were below the limit of detection (<19 µg/L). The infants were followed between 2 to 30 months of age with no adverse effects found to be due to the medication. One infant did have thrombocytopenia at 20 days of life; however, this resolved without cessation of breastfeeding and was not attributed to the medication.

In another cohort study of 15 women who took tacrolimus during pregnancy and lactation, a total of 14 women and 15 infants were observed in the lactation phase (11 exclusively breastfed; one female delivered two infants during study period; one female excluded- no breastmilk samples).[6] The infants' tacrolimus blood levels decreased by about 15% per day after birth; there was no difference in this decline if the infant was breastfed or given formula. Three women provided four peak (4 h post dose) and trough breast milk samples that demonstrated no significant changes in the tacrolimus milk levels. Using the highest breast milk concentration (1.56 µg/L) and a maternal dose of 6 mg/day, the authors estimated the relative infant dose to be 0.23%.

One additional case report was published in 2013, in this case breast milk samples were drawn from a woman who was 45 weeks and 1 day postpartum who was taking tacrolimus 1.5 mg orally every 12 hours.[7] The milk samples were collected over one full dosing interval (0-12 hours); the peak breast milk concentration occurred around 6 hours after the dose and was 1.11 ng/mL. The average concentration in breast milk was 0.93 ng/mL. The authors calculated that the average 3-month-old would ingest about 0.14 µg/kg/day of tacrolimus via breast milk or about 0.3% of the maternal dose.

In addition, there is a topical form of tacrolimus (Protopic) for use in moderate to severe eczema, in those for whom standard eczema therapies are deemed inadvisable because of potential risks, or who are not adequately treated by, or who are intolerant to standard eczema therapies. Absorption via skin is minimal. In a study of 46 adult patients after multiple doses, plasma levels ranged from undetectable to 20 ng/mL, with 45 of the patients having peak blood concentrations less than 5 ng/mL.[1] In another study, the peak blood levels averaged 1.6 ng/mL, which is significantly less than the therapeutic range in kidney transplantation (7-20 ng/mL). While the absolute transcutaneous bioavailability is unknown, it is apparently very low. Combined with the poor oral bioavailability of this product, it is not likely a breastfed infant will receive enough following topical use (maternal) to produce adverse effects.

T 1/2	34.2 h	MW	822 Da	PB	99%
Tmax	1.6 h	RID	0.1% - 0.53%	Vd	2.6 L/kg
Oral	14-32%	M/P	0.54	pKa	

Adult Concerns: Headache, insomnia, hypertension, edema, nausea, diarrhea, abdominal pain, changes in kidney and liver function, leukopenia (increase in risk of infection), thrombocytopenia.

The US FDA has issued a warning concerning elevated risks of skin cancers and lymphomas in patients exposed to this product. This warning is highly controversial and is not supported by many dermatologic organizations.

Adult Dose: 0.15-0.3 mg/kg daily.

Pediatric Concerns: None reported.

Infant Monitoring: Changes in sleep, vomiting, diarrhea, weight gain; if clinical symptoms arise, consider checking CBC.

Alternatives:

References:

1. Pharmaceutical manufacturers prescribing information.
2. Jain A, Venkataramanan R, Fung JJ, et al. Pregnancy after liver transplantation under tacrolimus. Transplantation. 1997;64(4):559-565.
3. French AE, Soldin SJ, Soldin OP, Koren G. Milk transfer and neonatal safety of tacrolimus. Ann Pharmacother. 2003;37(6):815-818.
4. Gardiner SJ, Begg EJ. Breastfeeding during tacrolimus therapy. Obstet Gynecol. 2006;107:453-455.
5. Gouraud A, Bernard N, Millaret M, Paret N, Descotes J, Vial T. Follow-up of tacrolimus breastfed babies. Transplantation. 2012;94(6):e38-e40.
6. Bramham K, Chusney G, Lee J, Lightstone L, Nelson-Piercy C. Breastfeeding and tacrolimus: serial monitoring in breast-fed and bottle-fed infants. Clin J Am Soc Nephrol. 2013;8:563-567.
7. Zheng A, Easterling TR, Hays K, et al. Tacrolimus placental transfer at delivery and neonatal exposure through breast milk. Br J Clin Pharmacol. 2013;76(6):988-996.

TADALAFIL

Trade: Adcirca, Cialis

Category: Phosphodiesterase Type 5 Inhibitors

LRC: L3 - No Data-Probably Compatible

Tadalafil is a phosphodiesterase-5 inhibitor primarily used for erectile dysfunction, benign prostatic hyperplasia, and pulmonary hypertension.[1] The transfer of tadalafil to human milk is still not known. Although tadalafil was found in rodent milk, these levels do not normally predict levels in human milk. This product is not overtly hazardous and minimal levels in milk would probably be tolerated by an infant.

T 1/2	17.5 h	MW	389.4 Da	PB	94%
Tmax	30 min - 6 h	RID		Vd	0.9 L/kg
Oral	Unknown	M/P		pKa	

Adult Concerns: Headache, dyspepsia, back pain, myalgia, nasal congestion, flushing.

Adult Dose: 2.5 - 20 mg/ day.

Pediatric Concerns: None have been published.

Infant Monitoring: Drowsiness, lethargy, pallor or flushing, poor feeding, and weight gain.

Alternatives: Sildenafil(L3)

References:

1. Pharmaceutical manufacturers prescribing information.

TAMOXIFEN

Trade: Eblon, Genox, Noltam, Nolvadex, Tamofen, Tamone, Tamoxen

Category: Antiestrogen

LRC: L5 - Significant Data-Hazardous

Tamoxifen is a nonsteroidal anti-estrogen. It attaches to the estrogen receptor and produces only minimal stimulation, thus preventing estrogen from stimulating the receptor. Aside from this, it also produces a number of other effects within the cytoplasm of the cell and some of its anticancer effects may be mediated by its effects at sites other than the estrogen receptor. Tamoxifen is metabolized by the liver and has an elimination half-life of greater than 7 days (range 3-21 days).[1] It is well absorbed orally, and the highest tissue concentrations are in the liver (60-fold). It is 99% protein-bound and normally reduces plasma prolactin levels significantly (66% after 3 months).

At present, there are no data on its transfer into breast milk; however, it has been shown to inhibit lactation early postpartum in several studies. In one study, doses of 10-30 mg twice daily early postpartum, completely inhibited postpartum engorgement and lactation.[2] In a second study, tamoxifen doses of 10 mg four times daily significantly reduced serum prolactin and inhibited milk production as well.[3] We do not know the effect of tamoxifen on established milk production. It has a pKa of 8.85 which may suggest some trapping in milk compared to the maternal plasma levels. This product has a very long half-life, and the active metabolite is concentrated in the plasma (2-fold). This drug has all the characteristics that would suggest a concentrating mechanism in breastfed infants over time. Its prominent effect on reducing prolactin levels will inhibit early lactation and may ultimately inhibit established lactation. In this instance, the significant risks to the infant from exposure to tamoxifen probably outweigh the benefits of breastfeeding. Mothers receiving tamoxifen should not breastfeed until we know more about the levels transferred into milk and the plasma/tissue levels found in breastfed infants.

T 1/2	3-21 days	MW	371 Da	PB	99%
Tmax	2-3 h	RID		Vd	
Oral	Complete	M/P		pKa	8.85

Adult Concerns: Hot flashes, nausea, vomiting, vaginal bleeding/discharge, menstrual irregularities, amenorrhea.

Adult Dose: 10-20 mg twice daily.

Pediatric Concerns: None reported but caution is urged.

Infant Monitoring: Not recommended in lactation

Alternatives:

References:
1. Pharmaceutical manufacturers prescribing information.
2. Shaaban MM. Suppression of lactation by an antiestrogen, tamoxifen. Eur J Obstet Gynecol Reprod Biol. 1975; 4(5):167-169.
3. Masala A, Delitala G, Lo DG, Stoppelli I, Alagna S, Devilla L. Inhibition of lactation and inhibition of prolactin release after mechanical breast stimulation in puerperal women given tamoxifen or placebo. Br J Obstet Gynaecol. 1978; 85(2):134-137.

TAMSULOSIN HYDROCHLORIDE

Trade: Flomax, Flomax CR

Category: Alpha-Adrenergic Blocker

LRC: L3 - No Data-Probably Compatible

Tamsulosin is indicated for treatment of benign prostatic hyperplasia,[1] but it is also used in women who have difficulty voiding and in patients to facilitate kidney stone passage.[2,3] This drug selectively blocks alpha-1A adrenergic receptors in the ureter and bladder neck, thus reducing smooth muscle tone in those regions. No breastfeeding data are presently available but, due to its high protein binding and larger molecular weight, it is unlikely that tamsulosin would be present in the milk in clinically relevant amounts.

T 1/2	13 h	MW	445 Da	PB	94-99%
Tmax	4-7 h	RID		Vd	0.23 L/kg
Oral	90%	M/P		pKa	

Adult Concerns: Headache, dizziness, insomnia, orthostatic hypotension, nausea, diarrhea, weakness.

Adult Dose: 0.4 mg once daily.

Pediatric Concerns: No data are available.

Infant Monitoring: Drowsiness, lethargy, poor feeding, and weight gain.

Alternatives:

References:
1. Pharmaceutical manufacturers prescribing information
2. Singh SK, Pawar DS, Griwan MS, Indora JM, Sharma S. Role of tamsulosin in clearance of upper ureteral calculi after extracorporeal shock wave lithotripsy: a randomized controlled trial. Urol J. 2011 Winter;8(1):14-20.
3. Vincendeau S, Bellissant E, Houlgatte A, et al. Tamsulosin hydrochloride vs placebo for management of distal ureteral stones: a multicentric, randomized, double-blind trial. Arch Intern Med. 2010 Dec;170(22):2021-2027.

TAPENTADOL

Trade: Nucynta

Category: Analgesic

LRC: L3 - No Data-Probably Compatible

Tapentadol is an opiate analgesic and norepinephrine reuptake inhibitor.[1] There have been no studies done on the effects of tapentadol in breastfeeding mothers. However, from a pharmacokinetic standpoint, we believe it is likely that tapentadol is secreted in breast milk. Tapentadol has a relatively small molecular weight of 258 Da and it is only 20% protein-bound; these factors facilitate transfer of drug to breast milk. Since the pKa of the drug is quite basic, ion trapping may occur which leads to concentration of the drug within the milk. Also, the oil:water partition coefficient log P value is 2.87, which is very lipophilic; this means tapentadol may cross easily into milk. However, tapentadol undergoes extensive first-pass metabolism and has a short half-life. Thus, this may limit the effects of tapentadol on mother's milk. Nonetheless, caution is advised.

T 1/2	6 h	MW	257.8 Da	PB	20%
Tmax	1.25 h	RID		Vd	6.3-9.1 L/kg
Oral	32%	M/P		pKa	9.34 and 10.45

Adult Concerns: Dizziness, somnolence, abnormal dreams, insomnia, anxiety, hypotension, dry mouth, dyspepsia, nausea, vomiting, constipation.

Adult Dose: 50-100 mg every 4-6 hours PRN.

Pediatric Concerns: None reported via milk at this time.

Infant Monitoring: Sedation, slowed breathing rate/apnea, pallor, dry mouth, constipation and not waking to feed/poor feeding, vomiting.

Alternatives: Hydrocodone(L3), Hydromorphone(L3), Morphine(L3)

References:
1. Pharmaceutical manufacturers prescribing information.

TAVABOROLE

Trade: Kerydin

Category: Antifungal

LRC: L3 - No Data-Probably Compatible

Tavaborole is a boron-containing antifungal used in the treatment of onychomycosis. Used topically on the nail for many months, levels in plasma are barely detectable and hence dose transfer to milk is likely exceedingly low. Boron is a naturally occurring ion and present in many foods and even water systems with a suggested upper limit of 20 mg/day. [1] Adverse effect for humans, including anorexia, digestive disruption, and dermatitis with a long-term intake of 5.0 mg B/kg/day. This far exceeds the amount present in tavaborole.[2] Following a 2-week daily topical application of 5% tavaborole to all 10 toenails, steady state occurred after 14 days. After a single dose, the mean plasma peak concentration (C_{max}) of tavaborole was 3.54 ± 2.26 ng/mL. After 2 weeks of daily dosing, the mean plasma C_{max} was 5.17 ± 3.47 ng/mL. These plasma levels are quite low and would not likely produce significant milk levels.

T 1/2	28.5 h (boron only)	MW	151.9 Da	PB	
Tmax		RID		Vd	
Oral		M/P		pKa	

Adult Concerns: Persistent local irritation, erythema, exfoliation, or dermatitis may develop.

Adult Dose: Apply to nails daily.

Pediatric Concerns:

Infant Monitoring: Observe for vomiting, diarrhea.

Alternatives:

References:
1. Farfán-García ED, Castillo-Mendieta NT, Ciprés-Flores FJ, Padilla-Martínez II, Trujillo-Ferrara JG, Soriano-Ursúa MA. Current data regarding the structure-toxicity relationship of boron-containing compounds. Toxicol Lett. 2016 Sep;258:115-125. doi: 10.1016/j.toxlet.2016.06.018. Epub 2016 Jun 18. Review. PubMed PMID: 27329537.
2. Pharmaceutical manufacturers prescribing information.

TAZAROTENE

Trade: Tazorac, Zorac

Category: Antipsoriatic

LRC: L3 - No Data-Probably Compatible

Tazarotene is a specialized retinoid for topical use and is used for the topical treatment of stable plaque psoriasis and acne.[1] Applied daily, it is indicated for treatment of stable plaque psoriasis of up to 20% of the body surface area. Only 2-3% of the topically applied drug is absorbed transcutaneously. Tazarotene is metabolized to the active ingredient, tazarotenic acid. At steady state, plasma levels were only 0.09 ng/mL although this value is largely a function of surface area treated. When applied to large surface areas, systemic absorption is increased. Data on transmission to breast milk are not available. The manufacturer reports some is transferred to rodent milk, but it has not been tested in humans.

T 1/2	18 h (metabolite)	MW	351 Da	PB	99%
Tmax	8 h	RID		Vd	
Oral	Complete	M/P		pKa	1.5

Adult Concerns: Hypertriglyceridemia, peripheral edema, pruritus, erythema, burning, contact dermatitis have been reported.

Adult Dose: Apply daily.

Pediatric Concerns: None via milk. Some caution is recommended if used over large surface areas (20-30%).

Infant Monitoring:

Alternatives:

References:
1. Pharmaceutical manufacturers prescribing information.

TECHNETIUM-99m

Trade: Technetium-99m, Sestamibi

Category: Diagnostic Agent, Radiopharmaceutical Imaging

LRC: L3 - Limited Data-Probably Compatible

Metastable technetium-99 (Tc-99m) is a man-made radioisotope used as a tracer in a wide variety of diagnostic medical procedures.[1] Tc-99m decays to Tc-99 via gamma emission of photons that have a wavelength similar to conventional X-rays.[1] The many different diagnostic medical formulations that contain Tc-99m use conjugate molecules to control the spread of radioactivity and to target the organ system of interest.[1] These synthetic conjugates also affect the biological half-life of the tracer product. Regardless of the formulation, the radioactive half-life of Tc-99m is fixed at 6 hours.[1] The average American adult is exposed to 3.1 mSv per year from natural sources and an additional 3.1 mSv from man-made sources (primarily routine medical procedures).[2]

The American Academy of Pediatrics (AAP) and the International Commission on Radiological Protection recommend different periods of breastfeeding cessation depending on which formulation of Tc-99m is used (see list below).[3-5] These recommendations still permit a minimal amount of radiation transfer to the infant (<1 mSv or 100 mrem).[3]

For the following salts do not breastfeed for 4 hours: DMSA, DTPA, DISDA, ECD, gluconate, glucoheptonate, HM-PAO, sulfur colloids, MAG3, MIBI, PYP, phosphonates (MDP), Technegas, tetrofosmin

For the following salts do not breastfeed for 12-24 hours: Pertechnetate, MAA, microspheres (HAM), radiolabeled RBCs, radiolabeled WBCs

Note: For a more conservative approach, breast milk pumped between 0 and 5 half-lives (30 hours) after the procedure may be stored until radio decay is effectively complete at 30 hours post-procedure. The stored milk should be safe to use after this period. All forms of Tc-99m not specifically mentioned above should be handled in this way.

As with radioactive iodine (I-131, I-125), the Academy of Pediatrics and the US Nuclear Regulatory Commission do not recommend any form of close contact (<10 cm) isolation following technetium use; however, the close-contact recommendations are based on a mathematical model that assumes women hold their babies for about 35 minutes out of every hour while practicing a typical pattern of breastfeeding.[2-8] We advise avoiding extended close contact, such as co-sleeping or carrying the baby in a sling, for the first 24 hours after the procedure. Limiting close contact to 20 minutes every 4 hours for the first 24 hours after the procedure further reduces infant radiation exposure by 67%.[7,8]

In a case report published in 2004, a breastfeeding woman had been given a typical dose of Tc-99 sestamibi (33.8 mCi); the woman was advised not to breastfed for 24 hours.[9] The estimated amount of the maternal dose excreted in breast milk was about 0.03% (0.01 mCi) and the anticipated infant dose of radiation based on this dose in breast milk was 0.0052 rem (effective dose in infants is anticipated to be 0.52 rem/mCi) Based on the information described in this report, we believe it would be reasonable to resume breastfeeding 6 hours after Tc-99 sestamibi administration to the mother.

In an older case report from 1978, a mother received 15 mCi of Tc-99m pertechnetate for a brain scan and expressed breast milk containing 0.1, 0.02, and 0.006 μCi/mL, at 8.5, 20, and 60 hours respectively.[10] The breast milk at 4 hours, which she gave to her infant, would have contained 0.5 μCi/mL. Assuming that this 10-week-old infant consumed 180 mL per feeding and accounting for the pharmacokinetics of Tc-99m in infants, the authors estimated that a one-time feeding at 4 hours post-injection resulted in radiation doses of 300, 100, and 68 mRad to the infant thyroid, stomach, and large intestine respectively. It was also estimated that if the infant had been breastfed within 30 minutes of the test, the infant would have received 10 times the dose (728 μCi).

In another study, following a dose of 10 mCi of Tc-99m pertechnetate in a breastfeeding mother, breast milk levels were 5.7, 1.5, 0.015 μCi/mL at 3.25, 7.5, and 24 hours respectively. The estimated dose to infant was 1,036, 284, and 2.7 μCi/180 mL milk.[11]

In another study using Tc-99 MAG3 in two mothers receiving 150 MBq (4 mCi) of radioactivity, the total percent of ingested radioactivity ranged from 0.7 to 1.6% of the total.[12]

Of the radioisotopes, Tc-99 is perhaps one of the safest to use in breastfeeding mothers, primarily because 1) it is a weak emitter, and 2) it has a brief 6-hour half-life. Some authorities suggest a brief 3-6 hour interruption, followed by pumping and discarding once. After 24 hours, almost all the radiation has decayed away.

T 1/2	<6 h	MW		PB	
Tmax		RID		Vd	
Oral	Complete	M/P		pKa	

Adult Concerns: Headache, malaise, hypersensitivity reactions, hypotension, edema, nausea, vomiting, arthralgia, rash.

Adult Dose: 4-20 mCi X 1.

Pediatric Concerns: None reported via milk at this time.

Infant Monitoring:

Alternatives:

References:

1. Technetium-99m (99mTc) Fact Sheet 320-083. Division of Environmental Health Office of Radiation Protection Washington State Department of Health. July 2002. http://www.doh.wa.gov/Portals/1/Documents/Pubs/320-083_tc99_fs.pdf
2. Fact Sheet on Biological Effects of Radiation. United States Nuclear Regulatory Comission; October 2011. http://www.nrc.gov/reading-rm/doc-collections/fact-sheets/bio-effects-radiation.html, 2014.
3. Sachs HC, Committee On Drugs. The transfer of drugs and therapeutics into human breast milk: an update on selected topics. Pediatrics. 2013;132(3):e796-e809.
4. International Commission on Radiological Protection. Annex D. Recommendations on breast-feeding interruptions. Ann ICRP. 2008;38(1-2):163-184.
5. Stabin MG. Radiating dose concerns for the pregnant or lactating patient. Semin Nucl Med. 2014;44:479-488.
6. Regulatory Guide 8.39. Release of patients administered radioactive materials. U.S. Nuclear Regulatory Commission; 1997.
7. Mountford PJ. Estimation of close contact doses to young infants from surface dose rates on radioactive adults. Nucl Med Commun. 1987 Nov;8(11):857-863.
8. Mountford PJ, O'Doherty MJ, Forge NI, Jeffries A, Coakley AJ. Radiation dose rates from adult patients undergoing nuclear medicine investigations. Nucl Med Commun. 1991 Sep;12(9):767-777.
9. Ramakrishna G, Miller TD. Significant breast uptake of Tc-99m sestamibi in an actively lactating woman during SPECT myocardial perfusion imaging. J Nucl Cardiol. 2004 Mar-Apr;11(2):222-223.
10. Rumble WF, Aamodt RL, Jones AE, Henkin RI, Johnston GS. Accidental ingestion of Tc-99m in breast milk by a 10-week-old child. J Nucl Med. 1978;19(8):913-915.
11. Maisels MJ, Gilcher RO. Excretion of technetium in human milk. Pediatrics. 1983;71(5):841-842.
12. Evans JL, Mountford AN, Herring AN, Richardson MA. Secretion of radioactivity in breast milk following administration of 99Tcm-MAG3. Nucl Med Comm. 1993;14:108-111.

TEDIZOLID

Trade: Sivextro

Category: Antibiotic, Other

LRC: L3 - No Data-Probably Compatible

Tedizolid is a new oxazolidinone antibiotic (similar to linezolid) primarily used for the treatment of bacterial skin infections.[1] It is active against many strains, including resistant *Staphylococcus aureus* (MRSA) and *Enterococcus faecium*. At this time there are no data regarding the transfer of tedizolid to human milk. Based on this medication's small volume of distribution and longer half-life, some medication is expected to enter human milk.

T 1/2	12 h	MW	450 Da	PB	70-90%
Tmax	3 h (oral); 1-1.5 h (IV)	RID		Vd	0.95-1.14 L/kg
Oral	91%	M/P		pKa	

Adult Concerns: Headache, insomnia, dizziness, palpitations, nausea, vomiting, diarrhea, changes in liver function, anemia, thrombocytopenia, leukopenia, neutropenia. Serotonin syndrome when used with other pro-serotonergic medications (e.g. SSRIs, SNRIs).

Adult Dose: 200 mg once daily given oral or IV.

Pediatric Concerns: No safety data in breastfed infants or pediatrics is available at this time.[1]

Infant Monitoring: Vomiting, diarrhea, changes in gastrointestinal flora and rash; if clinical symptoms arise a CBC or liver function tests may be warranted.

Alternatives: Vancomycin(L1), Clindamycin(L2), Linezolid(L3)

References:
1. Pharmaceutical manufacturers prescribing information.

TELAVANCIN

Trade: Vibativ

Category: Antibiotic, Other

LRC: L3 - No Data-Probably Compatible

Telavancin is a semi-synthetic derivative of vancomycin. It is a bactericidal lipoglycopeptide.[1] This antibiotic can be used to treat severe skin infections and hospital- or ventilator-associated pneumonia caused by Gram-positive bacteria. Based on this medication's large size (1755 Da) and high protein binding, clinically significant levels are not anticipated in human milk. At this time, the use of alternative antibiotics with more data in lactation would be recommended when possible (e.g. vancomycin).

T 1/2	6.6-9.6 h	MW	1755.6 Da	PB	90%
Tmax		RID		Vd	0.13 L/kg
Oral		M/P		pKa	

Adult Concerns: Headache, dizziness, insomnia, shortness of breath, metallic taste, nausea, vomiting, diarrhea, changes in renal function, proteinuria, hypokalemia, thrombocytopenia, skin rashes, paresthesia.

Adult Dose: 10 mg/kg IV every 24 hours.

Pediatric Concerns: None reported via milk at this time. Pediatric data is unavailable at this time.

Infant Monitoring: Vomiting, diarrhea.

Alternatives: Vancomycin(L1)

References:
1. Pharmaceutical manufacturers prescribing information.

TELBIVUDINE

Trade: Tyzeka

Category: Antiviral

LRC: L3 - Limited Data-Probably Compatible

Telbivudine is a thymidine nucleoside analog that inhibits reverse transcriptase and DNA polymerase in hepatitis B virus infections. It was recently removed from the US market. It does not inhibit human cellular polymerase. Telbivudine is used to treat hepatitis B virus in pregnant women that are at high risk of transmitting the virus to their fetus (e.g. Hepatitis B e (HbeAg) antigen positive, high viral load).[1,2] This medication has a small molecular weight and low protein binding; therefore, its transfer into milk is likely, but probably not clinically relevant. At this time there are no data confirming the amount of drug that transfers into human milk. A recent study published in 2015, which evaluated the use of telbivudine for preventing vertical transmission of hepatitis B in pregnancy reported that 83 women in the telbivudine group breastfed their infants.[2] In this study women were able to stop therapy at delivery or continue for up to 4 weeks postpartum, and details regarding the number of women which breastfeed while taking the medication postpartum were not reported; however, the authors suggested that breastfeeding while taking telbivudine could be an option for women requiring this medication. Maternal benefits of therapy and risk to infant need to be determined prior to use in lactation as safety data is limited.

T 1/2	40-49 h	MW	242 Da	PB	3%
Tmax	1-4 h	RID		Vd	
Oral		M/P		pKa	9.61

Adult Concerns: Headache, fatigue, fever, dyspepsia, nausea, abdominal pain, diarrhea, changes in liver function, neutropenia, muscle pain, increased creatine phosphokinase.

Adult Dose: 600 mg daily.

Pediatric Concerns: No data are available.

Infant Monitoring: Not recommended for long-term use in lactation.

Alternatives:

References:
1. Pharmaceutical manufacturers prescribing information.
2. Wu Q, Huang H, Sun X, et al. Telbivudine prevents vertical transmission of hepatitis B virus from women with high viral loads: a prospective long-term study. Clin Gastroenterol Hepatol. 2015;13(6):1170-1176.

TELMISARTAN

Trade: Micardis, Micardis HCT

Category: Angiotensin II Receptor Antagonist

LRC: L4 - No Data-Possibly Hazardous

Telmisartan is a potent antihypertensive that blocks the angiotensin II receptor site.[1] No data are available on its use in lactating mothers, thus other medications should be used if suitable for the maternal medical condition (e.g. ramipril, labetalol, nifedipine). In addition, its use early postpartum in lactating mothers should be approached with caution, particularly in mothers with premature infants.

Both the ACE inhibitor family and the specific angiotensin II receptor blockers are contraindicated in pregnancy and thus should be used with caution in women who are planning a subsequent pregnancy in the near future.

T 1/2	24 h	MW	514 Da	PB	99.5%
Tmax	1 h	RID		Vd	7.14 L/kg
Oral	42-58%	M/P		pKa	3.83

Adult Concerns: Headache, dizziness, fatigue, hypotension, nausea, diarrhea, constipation, changes in renal function/urine output, hyperkalemia.

Adult Dose: 40 mg daily.

Pediatric Concerns: None reported via milk at this time.

Infant Monitoring: Drowsiness, lethargy, pallor, poor feeding, and weight gain.

Alternatives: Ramipril(L3), Enalapril(L2), Captopril(L2)

References:
1. Pharmaceutical manufacturers prescribing information.

TEMAZEPAM

Trade: Euhypnos, Nocturne, Normison, Restoril, Temtabs

Category: Sedative-Hypnotic

LRC: L3 - Limited Data-Probably Compatible

Temazepam is a short-acting benzodiazepine primarily used as a nighttime sedative. In a study of 10 breastfeeding mothers (<15 days postpartum) who received doses of 10-20 mg at bedtime for 2 days prior to the study, the milk/plasma ratio varied from <0.09 to <0.63 (mean 0.18).[1] Levels of temazepam were undetectable (<5 µg/L) in nine out of 10 subjects. The tenth mother had plasma levels of temazepam of 234 µg/L and milk levels that ranged from 26-28 µg/L. Temazepam is relatively water-soluble and therefore partitions poorly into breast milk. Levels of temazepam were undetectable in the infants studied although these studies were carried out 15 hours postdose. Although the study shows low neonatal exposure to temazepam via breast milk, the infant should be monitored carefully.

T 1/2	9.5-12.4 h	MW	301 Da	PB	96%
Tmax	2-4 h	RID		Vd	0.8-1 L/kg
Oral	90%	M/P	0.18	pKa	1.6

Adult Concerns: Sedation, confusion, vertigo, blurred vision, vomiting, diarrhea.

Adult Dose: 7.5-30 mg daily.

Pediatric Concerns: None reported via milk at this time.

Infant Monitoring: Sedation, slowed breathing rate, not waking to feed/poor feeding, and weight gain.

Alternatives: Lorazepam(L3), Alprazolam(L3)

References:
1. Lebedevs TH, Wojnar-Horton RE, Yapp P, et al. Excretion of temazepam in breast milk. Br J Clin Pharmacol. 1992;33(2):204-206.

TEMOZOLOMIDE

Trade: Temodal, Temodar

Category: Antineoplastic

LRC: L5 - No Data-Hazardous

Temozolomide is an alkylating agent used to treat refractory anaplastic astrocytoma and glioblastoma multiforme.[1] No studies have been performed regarding the transmission of this drug to milk; however, it is highly likely that temozolomide would transfer to the milk compartment, due to the low volume of distribution, low protein binding, and low molecular weight. Temozolomide would be orally bioavailable to an infant and thus should not be used in a nursing mother. Temozolomide is an extremely toxic agent, and infants should be withdrawn from the breast for a prolonged period of at least 7 days after a dose.

T 1/2	1.8 h	MW	194 Da	PB	15%
Tmax	1-2.25 h	RID		Vd	0.4 L/kg
Oral	100%	M/P		pKa	10.5

Adult Concerns: Alopecia, headache, fatigue, seizures, insomnia, dizziness, nausea, vomiting, diarrhea or constipation, anorexia, hemiparesis, changes in coordination, viral infection, weakness.

Adult Dose: Highly variable.

Pediatric Concerns: No data in breastfed infants at this time.

Infant Monitoring: Withhold breastfeeding for at least 7 days.

Alternatives:

References:
1. Pharmaceutical manufacturers prescribing information.

TENIPOSIDE

Trade: Vehem, Vumon

Category: Antineoplastic

LRC: L4 - No Data-Possibly Hazardous

Teniposide is a semi-synthetic derivative of podophyllotoxin. It is similar to etoposide chemically. Teniposide has a broad spectrum of in vivo antitumor activity against murine tumors, including hematologic malignancies and various solid tumors. Plasma drug levels declined biexponentially following intravenous infusion (155 mg/m^2 over 1 to 2.5 hours) of teniposide given to eight children (4-11 years old) with newly diagnosed acute lymphoblastic leukemia (ALL). The terminal elimination half-life was 5.4 hours. The average volumes of distribution at steady state were low and ranged from 0.2-1.09 L/kg. Teniposide is highly protein-bound (99%), has a large molecular weight, and does not readily enter the CNS. Most of these kinetics suggest milk levels are probably exceedingly low. However, no data are yet available on the transfer of this product to human milk. Withhold breastfeeding for a minimum of 36-48 hours.

T 1/2	5-21 h	MW	656.7 Da	PB	>99%
Tmax		RID		Vd	0.2-1.09 L/kg
Oral		M/P		pKa	

Adult Concerns: Alopecia, headache, confusion, fever, hypotension, mucositis, vomiting, diarrhea, neutropenia, leukopenia, anemia, thrombocytopenia, bleeding, infection, skin rash.

Adult Dose: Varies according to cancer type/treatment.

Pediatric Concerns: No data in lactation at this time.

Infant Monitoring: Withhold breastfeeding for a minimum of 48 hours.

Alternatives:

References:
1. Pharmaceutical manufacturers prescribing information.

TENOFOVIR DISOPROXIL FUMARATE

Trade: Viread

Category: Antiviral

LRC: L5 - Limited Data-Hazardous if Maternal HIV Infection

Tenofovir is used in the management of HIV and hepatitis B infections. It interferes with the viral RNA-dependent DNA polymerase, inhibiting viral replication.[1] In a recent study in two Rhesus macaques given a subcutaneous dose of 30 mg/kg tenofovir, peak plasma levels were reported to be 18.3 and 30.3 µg/mL.[2] Peak levels in milk were reported to be 0.808 and 0.610 µg/mL. The AUC levels were 68.9 and 12.8 µg.h/mL for plasma and milk in one animal and 56.2 and 12.1 µg.h/mL for plasma and milk in the second animal. Using this peak data, the relative infant dose in monkeys would only be 0.4% of the maternal dose. In addition, the oral bioavailability of tenofovir (non-salt form) is negligible (5%). Thus, the overall risk to a breastfeeding infant would probably be low.

In 2011, a study was published that determined the concentrations of tenofovir and emtricitabine in breast milk when given in labor and postpartum to prevent resistance after nevirapine is given in labor for prevention of mother-to-child transmission of HIV.[3] These women were treated with tenofovir 600 mg/emtricitabine 400 mg at the time of delivery, followed by tenofovir 300 mg/emtricitabine 200 mg daily for 7 days postpartum. In this study, milk samples were collected on days 1, 2, 3, and 7 postpartum (10 min to 21 hours postdose). The maximum milk concentrations occurred 4-5 hours postdose and the lowest concentration was about 19 hours postdose. The median maximum and minimum tenofovir concentrations in milk were 14.1 ng/mL (11.6-16.25 ng/mL) and 6.8 ng/mL (5.83-8.75 ng/mL). The authors of this study estimated the infant dose to be 4.2 µg/day (0.03% of an infant dose) based on the median of the maximum and minimum levels and a daily infant intake of 500 mL. The infant intake of tenofovir in milk correlated to levels well below the lowest IC50 for this medication. Due to unknown details of exact sampling times and corresponding concentrations in milk the relative infant dose could not be calculated.

In 2014, a pharmacokinetic study was published determining the appropriate dose of tenofovir that should be given to women during labor and the infant during the first week of life when studying the efficacy of tenofovir to prevent mother-to-child transmission of HIV during delivery.[4] During this study there were four cohorts with different maternal and infant dose regimens. Twenty-five milk samples were taken from cohort 1 (maternal doses of 600 mg during labor) and cohort 2 (no maternal doses given in labor). Three of the four milk samples taken within 2 days of delivery had detectable levels of tenofovir, and the concentrations reported were 6.3-17.8 ng/mL. Only one of 21 samples collected 4-6 days postpartum still had a detectable level at 15.7 ng/mL. Due to unknown details of exact sampling times and corresponding concentrations in milk, the relative infant dose could not be calculated.

In 2014, a study that evaluated tenofovir use in pregnancy to prevent vertical transmission of Hepatitis B reported that 36 infants were breastfed in this study while their mothers took this medication for 12 weeks postpartum; no adverse events were reported.[5]

Note: This medication is an L5 to highlight the contraindication of breastfeeding when the mother is known to be infected with HIV, this medication is not an L5 based on its risk to the infant in breast milk. The Centers for Disease Control and Prevention recommend that HIV-1 infected mothers do not breastfeed their infants to avoid postnatal transmission of HIV-1.

T 1/2	17 h	MW	636 Da	PB	7%
Tmax	36-144 min	RID	0.02% - 0.03%	Vd	1.2-1.3 L/kg
Oral	25-40%	M/P		pKa	3.75

Adult Concerns: Headache, fatigue, fever, dizziness, insomnia, pain, abdominal pain, vomiting, anorexia, hematuria, increase in triglycerides and creatine kinase, neutropenia, weakness, rash.

Adult Dose: 300 mg daily.

Pediatric Concerns: None reported via breastmilk at this time.

Infant Monitoring: Insomnia, vomiting, poor weight gain. With some exceptions, breastfeeding is not recommended in mothers who have HIV.

Alternatives:

References:
1. Pharmaceutical manufacturers prescribing information.
2. Van Rompay K, Hamilton M, Kearney B, Bischofberger N. Pharmacokinetics of tenofovir in breast milk of lactating rhesus macaques. Antimicrob Agents Chemother. 2005;49: 2093-2094.
3. Benaboud S, Pruvost A, Coffie PA, et al. Concentrations of tenofovir and emtricitabine in breast milk of HIV-1-infected women in abidjan, Cote d'Ivoire, in the ANRS 12109 TEmAA study, step 2. Antimicrob Agents Chemother. 2011;55(3):1315-1317.
4. Mirochnick M, Taha T, Kreitchmann R, et al. Pharmacokinetics and safety of tenofovir in HIV-infected women during labor and their infants during the first week of life. J Acquir Immune Defic Syndr. 2014;65:33-41.
5. Greenup AJ, Tan PK, Nguyen V, et al. Efficacy and safety of tenofovir disoproxil fumarate in pregnancy to prevent perinatal transmission of hepatitis B virus. J Hepatol. 2014;61:501-507.

TERAZOSIN HCL

Trade: Hytrin

Category: Alpha-Adrenergic Blocker

LRC: L4 - No Data-Possibly Hazardous

Terazosin is an antihypertensive that belongs to the alpha-1 blocking family. This family is generally very powerful, producing significant orthostatic hypotension and other side effects.[1] Terazosin has rather powerful effects on the prostate and testes producing testicular atrophy in some animal studies (particularly newborn) and is therefore not preferred in pregnant or in lactating women. No data are available on transfer to human milk.

T 1/2	9-12 h	MW	423 Da	PB	94%
Tmax	1-2 h	RID		Vd	
Oral	90%	M/P		pKa	7.1

Adult Concerns: Hypotension, bradycardia, sedation.

Adult Dose: 1-10 mg daily.

Pediatric Concerns: None reported, but extreme caution is recommended.

Infant Monitoring: Drowsiness, lethargy, pallor, poor feeding, and weight gain.

Alternatives:

References:
1. Pharmaceutical manufacturers prescribing information.

TERBINAFINE

Trade: Lamisil, Terbinex

Category: Antifungal

LRC: L3 - Limited Data-Probably Compatible

Terbinafine is an antifungal agent primarily used for tinea species such as athlete's foot and ringworm. Systemic absorption following topical therapy is minimal.[1] Following an oral dose of 500 mg in two volunteers, the total dose of terbinafine secreted in breast milk during the 72-hour postdosing period was 0.65 mg in one mother and 0.15 mg in another.[2] The total excretion of terbinafine in breast milk ranged from 0.13% to 0.03% of the total maternal dose respectively. In a study of two mothers with limited milk production, they were administered 500 mg terbinafine orally. The highest reported concentrations occurred at 6 hours and were 7.3 and 7.9 mg/L. After 18 hours, terbinafine was undetectable in milk. Using these peak concentrations, the RID was 15.35% to 16.61%. Due to the poor milk production in these mothers, this data may not clearly indicate the transfer of this drug in normal fully breastfeeding mothers. Some caution is recommended due to the high RID following oral administration.

T 1/2	26 h	MW	291 Da	PB	99%
Tmax	1-2 h	RID	15.35% - 16.61%	Vd	>28 L/kg
Oral	70% absorbed 40% bio-available after first pass	M/P		pKa	7.1

Adult Concerns: Topical: burning, pruritus. Oral: fatigue, headache, gastrointestinal distress, elevated liver enzymes, alopecia.

Adult Dose: 250 mg daily.

Pediatric Concerns: None reported via milk.

Infant Monitoring: Caution, levels in infants could be significant.

Alternatives: Fluconazole(L2)

References:
1. Pharmaceutical manufacturers prescribing information.
2. Schatz F, Haberl H. Analytical methods for the determination of terbinafine and its metabolites in human plasma, milk and urine. Arzneimittelforschung. 1989;39:527-532.

TERBUTALINE

Trade: Brethine, Bricanyl

Category: Antiasthma

LRC: L2 - Limited Data-Probably Compatible

Terbutaline is a beta-2 adrenergic receptor agonist used for bronchodilation in asthmatics. It is secreted in breast milk but in low quantities. Following doses of 7.5 to 15 mg/day of terbutaline, milk levels averaged 3.37 µg/L.[1] Assuming a daily milk intake of 165 mL/kg, these levels would suggest a daily intake of less than 0.5 µg/kg/day, which corresponds to 0.2 to 0.7% of maternal dose. In another study of a patient receiving 5 mg three times daily, the mean milk concentrations ranged from 3.2 to 3.7 µg/L.[2] The author calculated the daily infant dose to be 0.4-0.5 µg/kg. Terbutaline was not detectable in the infant's serum. No untoward effects have been reported in breastfeeding infants.

T 1/2	14 h	MW	225 Da	PB	20%
Tmax	5-30 min	RID	0.2% - 0.3%	Vd	1-2 L/kg
Oral	33-50%	M/P	<2.9	pKa	10.1

Adult Concerns: Tremors, nervousness, tachycardia.

Adult Dose: 5 mg three times daily.

Pediatric Concerns: None reported via milk.

Infant Monitoring: Irritability, insomnia, arrhythmias, weight loss, tremor.

Alternatives:

References:
1. Lindberg C, Boreus LO, De Chateau P, Lindstrom B, Lonnerholm G, Nyberg L. Transfer of terbutaline into breast milk. Eur J Respir Dis Suppl. 1984;134:87-91.
2. Lonnerholm G, Lindstrom B. Terbutaline excretion into breast milk. Br J Clin Pharmacol. 1982;13(5):729-730.

TERCONAZOLE

Trade: Terazol, Terazol 3, Terazol 7

Category: Antifungal

LRC: L3 - No Data-Probably Compatible

Terconazole is an antifungal primarily used for vaginal candidiasis. It is similar to fluconazole and itraconazole. When administered intravaginally, only a limited amount (5-16%) is absorbed systemically (mean peak plasma level= 6 ng/mL).1,2 It is well absorbed orally. At high doses, terconazole is known to enter rodent milk, although no data are available in human milk. The milk levels are probably too small to be clinically relevant.

T 1/2	4-11.3 h	MW	532 Da	PB	
Tmax		RID		Vd	
Oral	Complete	M/P		pKa	7.23

Adult Concerns: Vaginal burning, itching, flu-like symptoms.

Adult Dose: 5 gm daily.

Pediatric Concerns: None reported due to minimal studies.

Infant Monitoring:

Alternatives: Fluconazole(L2)

References:
1. Pharmaceutical manufacturers prescribing information.
2. McEvoy GE, ed. AHFS Drug Information. Bethesda, MD: American Society of Health-System Pharmacists; 2003.

TERIFLUNOMIDE

Trade: Aubagio

Category: Immune Modulator

LRC: L5 - No Data-Hazardous

Teriflunomide (Aubagio) is a pyrimidine synthesis inhibitor indicated for the treatment of patients with relapsing forms of multiple sclerosis. It is the active metabolite of leflunomide. No direct human studies have been conducted regarding this drug's ability to pass into human milk. Animal studies have identified teriflunomide in rat milk after a single dose. In humans, teriflunomide has an extensive half-life due to gastrointestinal reabsorption.[1] Given this drug's toxicity in adults, its likely presence in milk, and its long half-life, teriflunomide should be used with great caution in breastfeeding mothers.

T 1/2	19 days	MW	270 Da	PB	99%
Tmax	1-4 h	RID		Vd	0.157 L/kg
Oral		M/P		pKa	

Adult Concerns: Decreased WBC count, infections, peripheral neuropathy, renal failure, hyperkalemia, skin reactions, hyper-/hypotension.

Adult Dose: 7 mg or 14 mg orally once daily.

Pediatric Concerns: None reported.

Infant Monitoring: Diarrhea, nausea, liver toxicity.

Alternatives:

References:
1. Pharmaceutical manufacturer Prescribing Information. Genzyme Corp, 2012.

TERIPARATIDE

Trade: Forteo

Category: Calcium Regulator

LRC: L3 - No Data-Probably Compatible

Teriparatide is the identical peptide hormone secreted by the parathyroid gland in humans. This leads to an increase in skeletal mass, markers of bone formation and resorption, and bone strength. Teriparatide is used to treat osteoporosis.[1] No studies are available on the levels in breast milk; however, due to the high molecular weight and poor oral bioavailability, it is unlikely that teriparatide will cross into the milk or be absorbed by an infant.

T 1/2	1 h	MW	4118 Da	PB	
Tmax		RID		Vd	0.12 L/kg
Oral	Nil	M/P		pKa	

Adult Concerns: Dizziness, insomnia, hypotension, syncope, hyperuricemia, hypercalcemia, nausea, gastritis, dyspepsia, arthralgias, weakness.

Adult Dose: 20 µg subcutaneous daily.

Pediatric Concerns: No data are available, but this is the normal human parathyroid hormone.

Infant Monitoring: Changes in sleep, hypotension, vomiting, reflux, weakness.

Alternatives:

References:
1. Pharmaceutical manufacturers prescribing information.

TESTOSTERONE

Trade: Androderm, Androgel, Axiron, Delatestryl, Depo-testosterone, Fortesta

Category: Androgen

LRC: L4 - Limited Data-Possibly Hazardous

Testosterone is a male sex hormone used to treat testosterone deficiency in males, reverse delayed puberty in males, improve libido, and as part of female-to-male gender reassignment. It is available in oral, injectable, and topical forms, all of which are dosed with the intent to reach a specific blood level of testosterone.

Testosterone is contraindicated in breastfeeding women. It is not known how much testosterone transfers to human milk; however even small amounts may affect nursing infants. Testosterone can be absorbed through the skin and infants exposed indirectly to residues of testosterone gel or patches, such as via unwashed clothing, can receive a significant dose. Infants exposed to external androgens may experience accelerated bone maturation without a proportional gain in linear growth, thereby compromising their adult stature. Androgens like testosterone may adversely affect milk supply.[1]

Testosterone and other androgens can appear in homeopathic products not regulated by the FDA. Caution should be advised when using these products.

T 1/2	10-100 min	MW	288 Da	PB	98%
Tmax	24 h (IM)	RID		Vd	75-122 L/kg
Oral	Poor	M/P		pKa	

Adult Concerns: Gynecomastia, polycythemia, worsening of benign prostatic hyperplasia, hepatitis, hirsuitism.

Adult Dose: 50-400 mg IM.

Pediatric Concerns: Aggressive behavior, virilization of genitalia, advanced bone age, hirsuitism.

Infant Monitoring: Virilization of genitalia, advanced bone age, hirsuitism.

Alternatives:

References:
1. Pharmaceutical manufacturers prescribing Information. Watson Pharma, 2012.

TETANUS TOXOID VACCINE

Trade: TE Anatoxal Berna

Category: Vaccine

LRC: L1 - No Data-Compatible

Tetanus toxoid contains a large molecular weight protein. Tetanus vaccine is made from inactivated tetanus toxoid by formaldehyde.[1] Tetanus vaccine is part of Tdap, DT, Td, DTaP, Pediarix, Pentacel, and DTP vaccines. Because tetanus vaccine is an inactivated bacterial product, there is no specific contraindication in breastfeeding following injection with this vaccine. It is extremely unlikely proteins of this size would be secreted in breast milk.

Adult Concerns: Local injection site reactions, fever, pain, hypotension. Rare cases: Peripheral neuropathy, Guillain-Barre syndrome.

Adult Dose:

Pediatric Concerns:

Infant Monitoring:

Alternatives:

References:

1. Atkinson W, Wolfe S, Hamborsky J, eds. Tetanus. In: Centers for Disease Control and Prevention. Epidemiology and Prevention of Vaccine-Preventable Diseases- The Pink Book. 12th ed. Washington DC: Public Health Foundation; 2011:341-352.

THALLIUM-201

Trade: Thallium-201, Thallous chloride Tl 201

Category: Diagnostic Agent, Radiopharmaceutical Imaging

LRC: L4 - Limited Data-Possibly Hazardous

Thallium-201 in the form of thallous chloride is used extensively for myocardial perfusion imaging to delineate ischemic myocardium. Following infusion, almost 85% of the administered dose is extracted into the heart on the first pass. Less than 5% of the dose remains free in the plasma in as little as 5 minutes after administration. Whereas thallium-201 has a radioactive half-life of only 73 hours, the terminal elimination half-life of the thallium ion from the body is about 10 days. Almost all radiation will be decayed in 5-6 half-lives (15 days). In a study of one breastfeeding patient who received 111MBq (3 mCi) for a brain scan, the amount of thallium-201 in breast milk at 4 hours was 326 Bq/mL and subsequently dropped to 87 Bq/mL after 72 hours.[1] Even without interrupting breastfeeding, the infant would have received less than the NCRP radiation safety guideline dose for infrequent exposure for a 1-year-old infant. However, a brief interruption of breastfeeding was nevertheless recommended. The length of interrupted breastfeeding is dependent on age of infant and dose of thallium. With an interruption time varying from 2, 24, 48, to 96 hours, the respective thallium dose to the infant would be 0.442, 0.283, 0.197, and 0.101 MBq compared to the maternal dose of 111 MBq. In another study of a breastfeeding mother who received 111 MBq (3 mCi), the calculated dose an infant would receive (without any interruption of breastfeeding and assuming the consumption of 1000 mL of milk daily) is approximately 0.81 MBq, which is presently less than the maximal allowed radiation dose (NCRP) for an infant.[2] The authors therefore recommend that breastfeeding be discontinued for at least 24-48 hours following the administration of 111 MBq of thallium-201. The amount of infant exposure from close contact with the mother was also measured and found to be very small in comparison to the orally ingested dose via milk.

Thus the interruption of breastfeeding largely depends on the dose and the volume of milk consumed by the infant. Most authors recommend interruption for 24 up to 96 hours[1,2,3], although the Nuclear Regulatory commission (NRC) recommends interruption for 2 weeks.[4] International Commission of Radiological Protection (ICRP) recommends interruptions of breastfeeding for 48 hours.[5] Estimated radiation exposure from breast milk is 0.63 mSv after administration of 3 mCi with 48 hours interruption.[1]

Breastfeeding restrictions:

201-Tl-chloride (Brain scan): 3 mCi dose: 48 hours interruption.[1,5]

201-Tl-chloride (Cardiac perfusion and stress test): 2.5-3.5 mCi: 2 weeks interruption.[4]

Close-contact restrictions (6 feet separation from infant) for 201-Tl-chloride at a dose of 3 mCi or less: Avoid close contact for the first 4 hours. Limit close contact to 35 min every 2-3 hours.[1]

Note: These recommendations still permit a minimal amount of <1mSv of radiation transfer to the infant. Exposure of 1 mSv has a cancer incidence risk of 1 in 10,000 people. This amount of exposure is less than the amount an average American is exposed to from the natural environment (6.2 mSv/year). The only way to avoid all radiation exposure is to wait for 5-10 half-lives, until all of the radioisotope decays (15-30 days).

T 1/2	73 h	MW		PB	
Tmax	<60 min	RID		Vd	
Oral		M/P		pKa	

Adult Concerns: Anaphylaxis, flushing, hypotension, rash, nausea, vomiting, fever, chills, blurred vision, shortness of breath.

Adult Dose:

Pediatric Concerns: None reported in one case, but a brief interruption for 24-48 hours (depending on dose) is advised.

Infant Monitoring:

Alternatives:

References:

1. Johnston RE, Mukherji SK, Perry RJ, Stabin MG. Radiation dose from breastfeeding following administration of thallium-201. J Nucl Med. 1996;37(12):2079-2082.
2. Murphy PH, Beasley CW, Moore WH, Stabin MG. Thallium-201 in human milk: observations and radiological consequences. Health Phys. 1989;56(4):539-541.

3. Stabin MG, Breitz HB. Breast milk excretion of radiopharmaceuticals: mechanisms, findings, and radiation dosimetry. J Nucl Med. 2000 May;41(5):863-873.
4. U.S. Nuclear Regulatory Commission. Regulatory Guide 8.39. Release of Patients administered radioactive materials, April 1997. http://www.orau.org/ptp/PTP%20Library/library/NRC/Reguide/08-039.pdf
5. ICRP. Radiation dose to patients from radiopharmaceuticals - addendum 3 to ICRP publication 53. ICRP publication 106. Ann ICRP. 2008;38 (1-2).

THEOPHYLLINE

Trade: Aminophylline, Austyn, Nuelin, Pulmophylline, Quibron, Quibron-T/SR, Theo-Dur

Category: Antiasthma

LRC: L3 - Limited Data-Probably Compatible

Theophylline is a methylxanthine bronchodilator. It has a prolonged half-life in neonates, which may cause retention. Milk concentrations are approximately equal to the maternal plasma levels. If a mother is maintained at 10-20 µg/mL, the milk concentrations are closely equivalent. Estimates generally indicate that less than 1% of the dose is absorbed by infant. Assuming maternal plasma levels of 10-20 µg/mL, the theophylline levels in a neonate would range from 0.9 to 3.6 µg/mL.[1] In another study of 12 patients receiving 300 mg theophylline, followed 5 hours later by 200 mg, the reported milk concentration was 2.8 mg/L and the milk/plasma ratio ranged from 0.6 to 0.89.[2] The reported maximum concentration was 6 mg/L. The relative infant dose would be approximately 5.8% of the weight-normalized maternal dose. One reported case of irritability and fretful sleeping was reported in an infant exposed to breast milk only on days when the mother reported taking theophylline. The average milk concentration of theophylline in this case was 0.7 mg/L.[3]

T 1/2	3-12.8 h	MW	180 Da	PB	56%
Tmax	1-2 h (oral)	RID	5.9%	Vd	0.3-0.7 L/kg
Oral	76%	M/P	0.67	pKa	8.6

Adult Concerns: Headache, insomnia, irritability, seizures, tachycardia, nausea, vomiting, tremor.

Adult Dose: 3 mg/kg every 8 hours.

Pediatric Concerns: One case of irritability and fretful sleeping on days when the mother took this medication.

Infant Monitoring: Irritability, insomnia, arrhythmias, vomiting, weight loss, tremor.

Alternatives:

References:
1. Stec GP, Greenberger P, Ruo TI, et al. Kinetics of theophylline transfer to breast milk. Clin Pharmacol Ther. 1980; 28(3):404-408.
2. Reinhardt D, Richter O, Brandenburg G. Pharmacokinetics of drugs from the breast-feeding mother passing into the body of the infant, using theophylline as an example. Monatsschr Kinderheilkd. 1983;131(2):66-70.
3. Yurchak AM, Jusko WJ. Theophylline secretion into breast milk. Pediatrics. 1976;57(4):518-520.

THIABENDAZOLE

Trade: Mintezol

Category: Anthelmintic

LRC: L3 - No Data-Probably Compatible

Thiabendazole is an antiparasitic agent for the treatment of roundworm, pinworm, hookworm, whipworm, and other parasitic infections.[1] After absorption, it is completely eliminated from the plasma by 48 hours although most is excreted by 24 hours. Although it is effective in pinworms, other agents with fewer side effects are preferred. No reports on its transfer to breast milk have been found.

T 1/2		MW	201 Da	PB	
Tmax	1-2 h	RID		Vd	
Oral	Complete	M/P		pKa	4.7

Adult Concerns: Headache, dizziness, seizures, psychiatric reactions (hallucinations, delirium), nausea, vomiting, rash, pruritus, intrahepatic cholestasis, liver toxicity.

Adult Dose: 1.5 g twice daily.

Pediatric Concerns: None reported. Can be used in pediatrics.

Infant Monitoring:

Alternatives: Pyrantel(L3)

References:
1. Pharmaceutical manufacturers prescribing information.

THIAMINE

Trade: Betaxin, Vitamin B1

Category: Vitamin

LRC: L1 - Limited Data-Compatible

Thiamine, also known as Vitamin B1, is used to treat thiamine deficiency. It is an essential coenzyme in carbohydrate metabolism, combining with adenosine triphosphate to form thiamine pyrophosphate. Thiamine has been shown to cross into human milk, with average concentrations in milk of 5 - 66 µg/L under normal circumstances.[1] Thiamine deficiency causes beriberi, which presents with weight loss, mental changes, muscle weakness, or cardiovascular effects. The recommended daily allowance for infants 0 to 12 months is 0.03 mg/kg/day. The recommended daily intake for pregnant and lactating females is 1.2 mg/day. The concentration of thiamine in human milk increases with the progression of lactation, with an average milk level of 200 µg/L.[2] We do not know what milk levels would be following the use of extraordinarily large oral doses, although it appears that it would be a linear increase in milk levels. Supratherapeutic doses should be avoided in breastfeeding mothers. Long-term high doses (3 g/day) have been associated with adult toxicity.

T 1/2		MW	265 Da	PB	
Tmax		RID		Vd	
Oral	Adequate	M/P		pKa	

Adult Concerns: Cyanosis, restlessness, nausea, edema, pruritus, weakness.

Adult Dose: 1.4 mg daily.

Pediatric Concerns: No data are available.

Infant Monitoring:

Alternatives:

References:
1. Deodhar AD, Hajalakshmi R, Ramakrishnan CV. Studies on human lactation. III. Effect of dietary vitamin supplementation on vitamin contents of breastfmilk. Acta Paediatr. 1964;53:42-48.
2. Picciano MF. In: Jensen RG, ed. Handbook of milk composition. San Diego: Academic Press; 1995.

THIOPENTAL SODIUM

Trade: Pentothal

Category: Anesthetic

LRC: L3 - Limited Data-Probably Compatible

Thiopental is an ultra-short-acting, barbiturate sedative. Used in the induction phase of anesthesia, it rapidly redistributes from the brain to adipose and muscle tissue; hence, the plasma levels are small, and the sedative effects are virtually gone in 20 minutes. Thiopental sodium is secreted into milk in low levels.

In a study of two groups of eight women who received from 5 to 5.4 mg/kg thiopental sodium, the maximum concentration in breast milk was 0.9 mg/L in mature milk and in colostrum was 0.34 mg/L.[1] The milk/plasma ratio was 0.3 for colostrum and 0.4 for mature milk. The maximum daily dose to the infant would be 0.135 mg/kg or approximately 2.5% of the adult dose.

In a second study, 40 women were given either a single IV dose of etomidate (0.3 mg/kg) or thiopentone (5 mg/kg) for induction of anesthesia prior to cesarean section. The mean maternal plasma concentrations of thiopentone at 2, 4, 9, and 12 hours after the dose were 2640 µg/L, 1350 µg/L, 860 µg/L, and 590 µg/L. The concentrations in colostrum at 30 min, 4 hours, and 9 hours postdose were 1980 µg/L, 910 µg/L, and 590 µg/L. We estimated the relative infant dose to be 1.8-6%. We used the 30-min, 4-hour, and 9-hour concentrations and a maternal dose of 350 mg (5 mg/kg x 70 kg female); thus this RID calculation over estimates the amount of drug that would enter milk in a 24-hour period after a single dose.

This medication appears to be suitable for use in lactation. The mother should resume breastfeeding after her procedure only once she is alert, orientated, and able to feed her infant or pump on her own.

T 1/2	3-8 h	MW	264 Da	PB	60-96%
Tmax	1-2 min	RID	1.77% - 5.94%	Vd	1.4 L/kg
Oral	Variable	M/P	0.3-0.4	pKa	7.6

Adult Concerns: Hemolytic anemia has been reported. Respiratory depression, renal failure, delirium, nausea, vomiting, pruritus.

Adult Dose: 50-100 mg X 2.

Pediatric Concerns: None reported in a study of 16 women receiving induction doses.

Infant Monitoring: Observe for sedation, irritability, lethargy, poor feeding, weight loss.

Alternatives:

References:
1. Andersen LW, Qvist T, Hertz J, Mogensen F. Concentrations of thiopentone in mature breast milk and colostrum following an induction dose. Acta Anaesthesiol Scand. 1987;31(1):30-32.
2. Esener Z, Sarihasan B, Guven H, Ustun E. Thiopentone and etomidate concentrations in maternal and umbilical plasma, and in colostrum. Br J Anaesth. 1992;69:586-588.

THIORIDAZINE

Trade: Aldazine, Mellaril

Category: Antipsychotic, Typical

LRC: L4 - No Data-Possibly Hazardous

Thioridazine is a potent phenothiazine tranquilizer. It has a high volume of distribution and long half-life. No data are available on its secretion in human milk, but it should be expected.[1] Pediatric indications (2-12 years of age) are available although neonatal apnea is associated with this family of drugs.

T 1/2	21-24 h	MW	371 Da	PB	95%
Tmax	2-4 h	RID		Vd	1.8-6.7 L/kg
Oral	60%	M/P		pKa	9.5

Adult Concerns: Blood dyscrasias, arrhythmias, sedation, gynecomastia, nausea, vomiting, constipation, dry mouth, retinopathy.

Adult Dose: 100-400 mg daily.

Pediatric Concerns: None reported due to limited studies. Neonatal apnea is common in this family of drugs.

Infant Monitoring: Sedation or irritability, apnea, not waking to feed/poor feeding, constipation, weight gain, and extrapyramidal symptoms.

Alternatives:

References:
1. O'Brien TE. Excretion of drugs in human milk. Am J Hosp Pharm. 1974;31(9):844-854.

THYROID SCAN

Trade: Thyroid Scan

Category: Diagnostic Agent, Thyroid Function

LRC: L5 - Significant Data-Hazardous

Thyroid scanning with radioiodine (I-131) or technetium-99m is useful in delineating structural abnormalities of the thyroid, e.g., to distinguish Graves' disease from multinodular goiter and a single toxic adenoma or to determine the functional state of a single nodule ("hot" vs. "cold"). In one procedure, the radiologist uses radioactive technetium-99m pertechnetate, which has a short half-life of 6.02 hours. At least 97% of the radioactivity would be decayed in 5 half-lives (30.1 hours), after which it would be presumably safe to breastfeed. In the second procedure (an uptake scan) radioactive iodine-131 is used. The radioactive half-life of I-131 is 8.1 days. Five half-lives in this situation is 40.5 days. Although the biologic half-life of iodine would be less than the 40.5 days, it is not known with certainty how long is required before breast milk samples are at background levels. For safety in this case, breast milk samples should be counted by a gamma counter prior to restarting breastfeeding. I-131 is sequestered in high concentrations in breast milk, and breast milk levels could be exceedingly high. Excessive exposure of the infant's thyroid to I-131 is exceedingly dangerous.[1-6]

Following exposure to I-131, prolonged interruption of breastfeeding is recommended and is a function of dose. Following exposure to technetium-99m, only 24 hours of interruption is required.

T 1/2	8 days (radioactive)	MW	131 Da	PB	
Tmax		RID		Vd	
Oral	Complete	M/P		pKa	

Adult Concerns: High radioactive exposure to the patient's thyroid gland. High radioactive exposure to the breasts of breastfeeding mothers if iodine-131 is used.

Adult Dose:

Pediatric Concerns: Possible thyroid suppression is possible if high levels of I-131 are used. Count breast milk samples to determine radiation levels.

Infant Monitoring:

Alternatives:

References:
1. American Academy of Pediatrics, Committee on Drugs. Transfer of drugs and other chemicals into human milk. Pediatrics. 2001;108(3):776-789.
2. Palmer KE. Excretion of 125I in breast milk following administration of labelled fibrinogen. Br J Radiol. 1979;52(620):672-673.
3. Karjalainen P, Penttila IM, Pystynen P. The amount and form of radioactivity in human milk after lung scanning, renography and placental localization by 131 I labelled tracers. Acta Obstet Gynecol Scand. 1971;50(4):357-361.
4. Hedrick WR, Di Simone RN, Keen RL. Radiation dosimetry from breast milk excretion of radioiodine and pertechnetate. J Nucl Med. 1986;27(10):1569-1571.
5. Romney B, Nickoloff EL, Esser PD. Excretion of radioiodine in breast milk. J Nucl Med. 1989;30(1):124-126.
6. Robinson PS, Barker P, Campbell A, Henson P, Surveyor I, Young PR. Iodine-131 in breast milk following therapy for thyroid carcinoma. J Nucl Med. 1994;35(11):1797-1801.

THYROTROPIN

Trade: TSH, Thyrogen, Thyrotropin, Thytropar

Category: Pituitary Hormone

LRC: L1 - Limited Data-Compatible

Thyrotropin (TSH) is known to be secreted in breast milk, but in low levels. Virtually none of it would be orally bioavailable or transferred to human milk. Because TSH is significantly elevated in hypothyroid mothers, if present in milk at high levels, it could theoretically cause a hyperthyroid condition in the breastfeeding infant. In a 34-year-old breastfeeding mother with severe hypothyroidism, maternal plasma levels of TSH were measured at 110 mU/L. Milk levels of TSH were 1.4 mU/L.[1] The author suggests that breast milk TSH was too low to affect thyroid function in a breastfeeding infant, even with milk from a mother with extremely elevated TSH.

Thyrotropin is most often used to detect malignant thyroid nodules. In this situation, it is often used with radioactive iodine-131. Radioactive iodine is absolutely contraindicated in breastfeeding women. Be sure that radioactive iodine-131 is NOT being concomitantly used with this therapy, and if it is, stop breastfeeding completely.

T 1/2		MW	359 Da	PB	
Tmax		RID		Vd	
Oral	Poor	M/P		pKa	

Adult Concerns: Headache, dizziness, insomnia, paresthesia, vomiting, diarrhea, changes in cholesterol, weakness.

Adult Dose: 10 units daily.

Pediatric Concerns: None reported via milk. Breastfeeding by hypothyroid mother is permissible.

Infant Monitoring: If clinical symptoms arise check for elevated levels of thyroxine.

Alternatives:

References:
1.   Robinson P, Hoad K. Thyrotropin in human breast milk. Aust N Z J Med. 1994;24(1):68.

TICAGRELOR

Trade: Brilinta

Category: Anticoagulant

LRC: L4 - No Data-Possibly Hazardous

Ticagrelor is an anticoagulant similar to clopidogrel and prasugrel. Unlike these other agents, ticagrelor exerts a reversible effect and is not a direct ADP antagonist, but rather prevents ADP from binding to the platelet through allosteric action. There are currently no studies of this drug in breastfeeding women, though it is known to be excreted in the milk of lactating rats. In animal studies, ticagrelor was found to be in greater concentrations in milk than in the maternal plasma. The majority of the radiation was from unchanged drug, while small amounts were from several different metabolites, of which one, AR-C124910XX, is pharmacologically active. Ticagrelor and its active metabolites are highly protein-bound and do not exhibit extensive oral bioavailability.[1,2]

T 1/2	6.2-6.9 h	MW	522.27 Da	PB	99.7%
Tmax	1.5-3 h	RID		Vd	1.26 L/kg
Oral	30-42%	M/P		pKa	4.12

Adult Concerns: Bleeding, atrial fibrillation, arrhythmia, chest pain, hyper/hypotension, syncope, diarrhea, nausea, vomiting, backache, dizziness, headache, cough.

Adult Dose: 180 mg loading dose, followed by 90 mg twice daily.

Pediatric Concerns:

Infant Monitoring: Rare- bruising on the skin, blood in urine, vomit, or stool.

Alternatives:

References:
1.   Li Y, Landqvist C, Scott GW. Disposition and metabolism of ticagrelor, a novel P2Y12 receptor antagonist, in mice, rats, and marmosets. Drug Metab Dispos. 2011 Jun;39(9):1555-1567.
2.   Product Information. BRILINTA(TM) Oral Tablets, Ticagrelor Oral Tablets. Wilmington, DE: AstraZeneca LP (per manufacturer); 2011.

TICLOPIDINE

Trade: Ticlid, Tilodene

Category: Platelet Aggregation Inhibitor

LRC: L4 - No Data-Possibly Hazardous

Ticlopidine is useful in preventing thromboembolic disorders, increased cardiovascular mortality, stroke, infarcts, and other clotting disorders. Ticlopidine is reported to be excreted in rodent milk.[1] No data are available on penetration into human breast milk. However it is highly protein-bound, and the levels of ticlopidine in plasma are quite low.

T 1/2	12.6 h	MW	264 Da	PB	98%
Tmax	2 h	RID		Vd	
Oral	80%	M/P		pKa	

Adult Concerns: Bleeding, neutropenia, maculopapular rash.

Adult Dose: 250 mg twice daily.

Pediatric Concerns: None reported via milk, but caution is recommended.

Infant Monitoring: Rare-bruising on the skin, blood in urine, vomit, or stool.

Alternatives:

References:
1.   Pharmaceutical manufacturers prescribing information.

TIGECYCLINE

Trade: Tygacil

Category: Antibiotic, Other

LRC: L4 - No Data-Possibly Hazardous

Tigecycline is a glycylcycline antibiotic similar to tetracyclines.[1] Tigecycline is not affected by the major mechanisms of resistance, and thus is effective against a broad spectrum of bacterial pathogens. Tigecycline may cause fetal harm when administered to a pregnant woman, as well as discoloration of the bone and teeth (yellow gray-brown) when used during tooth development in pediatric patients. Tigecycline is known to enter rat milk but was not found systemically in rat pups; this was attributed to the low oral bioavailability of the medication. There have been no studies performed on the transmission of tigecycline to human breast milk; however, it would be unlikely that the infant would absorb clinically relevant levels over a brief exposure. Prolonged exposure (>3 weeks) is not recommended.

T 1/2	27-42 h	MW	586 Da	PB	71-89%
Tmax		RID		Vd	7-9 L/kg
Oral	Nil	M/P		pKa	4.37

Adult Concerns: Headache, dizziness, dyspepsia, vomiting, diarrhea, hypoproteinemia, changes in liver and renal function, anemia, weakness.

Adult Dose: Initial 100 mg IV, then 50 mg IV every 12 hours.

Pediatric Concerns: Use during tooth development (fetus-age 8) has resulted in tooth discoloration and safety data has not been established in the pediatric population.

Infant Monitoring: Vomiting, diarrhea, changes in gastrointestinal flora and rash.

Alternatives:

References:
1. Pharmaceutical manufacturers prescribing information.

TIMOLOL

Trade: Betim, Betimolol, Blocadren, Tenopt, Timoptic, Timoptol, Timpilo

Category: Antiglaucoma

LRC: L2 - Limited Data-Probably Compatible

Timolol is a beta-blocker used for treating hypertension and glaucoma. It is secreted in milk. Following a dose of 5 mg three times daily, milk levels averaged 15.9 µg/L.[1] Both oral and ophthalmic drops produce modest levels in milk. Breast milk levels following ophthalmic use of 0.5% timolol drops was 5.6 µg/L at 1.5 hours after the dose.[2] Untoward effects on the infant have not been reported. These levels are probably too small to be clinically relevant.

T 1/2	4 h	MW	316 Da	PB	10%
Tmax	1-2 h	RID	1.1%	Vd	1-3 L/kg
Oral	50%	M/P	0.8	pKa	9.21

Adult Concerns: Hypotension, bradycardia, depression, sedation.

Adult Dose: 10-20 mg twice daily.

Pediatric Concerns: None reported via milk at this time.

Infant Monitoring: Drowsiness, lethargy, pallor, poor feeding, and weight gain.

Alternatives: Propranolol(L2), Metoprolol(L2)

References:
1. Fidler J, Smith V, De Swiet M. Excretion of oxprenolol and timolol in breast milk. Br J Obstet Gynaecol. 1983;90(10):961-965.
2. Lustgarten JS, Podos SM. Topical timolol and the nursing mother. Arch Ophthalmol. 1983;101(9):1381-1382.

TINIDAZOLE

Trade: Fasigyn, Tindamax

Category: Antibiotic, Other

LRC: L3 - Limited Data-Probably Compatible

Tinidazole is an antimicrobial agent that is sometimes used for the treatment of anaerobic infections and protozoal infections such as intestinal amebiasis, giardiasis, and trichomoniasis. It is similar to metronidazole. Tinidazole is highly lipophilic and passes membranes easily attaining high concentrations in virtually all body tissues. Concentrations in saliva and bile are equivalent to that of the plasma compartment.

In a study of 24 women, who received a single IV infusion immediately postpartum of 500 mg, aliquots of milk and serum were collected at 12, 24, 48, 72, and 96 hours after the injection.[1] At 48 and 72 hours, foremilk and hindmilk samples were also taken, whereas at 12 and 24 hours only mixed-milk samples were collected. Milk levels at 12 and 24 hours were 5.8 and 3.5 mg/L respectively. Serum levels at 12 and 24 hours averaged 6.1 and 3.7 mg/L respectively. The milk/serum ratios at 12 and 24 hours were 0.94 and 0.95 respectively, further suggesting the high lipid solubility of this product. At 48 and 72 hours, the foremilk levels were 1.28 and 0.32 mg/L respectively. Hindmilk levels at these same times were 1.2 and 0.3 respectively. At 96 hours only trace amounts were present in milk and none in serum. As this study was done early postpartum when milk lipid content is low, it should be presumed that milk levels in mature, more lipid-rich milk might actually be higher than reported in this study. The maximum relative infant dose (12 hours) would be 12.1%, but this is assuming milk intake of 150 mL/kg/day. One other study of five women taking a dose of 1600 mg IV reported milk-to-plasma ratios of between 0.62 and 1.39. After 72 hours, the majority of the milk samples were below 0.5 µg/mL. The authors therefore concluded that breastfeeding should be withheld for 72 hours after a 1600-mg IV dose of tinidazole.[2]

Following the oral use of a 2-g dose, maternal levels at 30 hours are exceedingly low. With this dosage regimen, recommend withholding breastfeeding for 30 hours.

T 1/2	11-14.7 h	MW		PB	12%
Tmax	2 h	RID	12.2%	Vd	0.8 L/kg
Oral	100%	M/P	1.28	pKa	4.7

Adult Concerns: Headaches, confusion, dizziness, drowsiness, insomnia, seizure, confusion, flushing, palpitations, metallic taste, tongue discoloration, vomiting, constipation, changes in liver function, darkened urine, anorexia, weakness.

Adult Dose: 2 grams daily for 1 to 3 days.

Pediatric Concerns: No untoward effects were reported in breastfed infants at this time.

Infant Monitoring: Drowsiness, insomnia, vomiting, constipation, changes in feeding, darkened urine, weight gain.

Alternatives: Metronidazole(L2)

References:

1. Mannisto PT, Karhunen M, Koskela O, et al. Concentrations of tinidazole in breast milk. Acta Pharmacol Toxicol (Copenh). 1983;53:254-256.
2. Evaldson GR, Lindgren S, Nord CE, Rane AT. Tinidazole milk excretion and pharmacokinetics in lactating women. Br J Clin Pharmacol. 1985;19:503-507.

TINZAPARIN SODIUM

Trade: Innohep, Logiparin

Category: Anticoagulant

LRC: L3 - No Data-Probably Compatible

Tinzaparin is a depolymerized heparin (low molecular weight heparin)[1] similar to several others such as dalteparin, enoxaparin, or nadroparin. The average molecular weight range of tinzaparin is approximately one-half that of regular (unfractionated) heparin (5500-7500 vs 12,000 Da). No data are available on the transfer of this anticoagulant to human milk but it is likely low. In studies with dalteparin none was found in milk in one study, and only small amounts in another (see dalteparin). In studies with enoxaparin, no changes in anti-Xa activity were noted in breastfed infants. It is very unlikely any would be orally bioavailable.

T 1/2	3-4 h	MW	<7500 Da	PB	None
Tmax	4-5 h (SC)	RID		Vd	3.1-5 L/kg
Oral	Nil	M/P		pKa	

Adult Concerns: Bruising on the skin, hemorrhage, blood in urine or stool, thrombocytopenia, and pain/bruising at injection site.

Adult Dose: 175 IU/kg/day (highly variable).

Pediatric Concerns: None reported via milk at this time.

Infant Monitoring: Rare bruising on the skin, blood in urine, vomit, or stool.

Alternatives: Dalteparin(L2), Enoxaparin(L2)

References:
1. Pharmaceutical manufacturers prescribing information.

TIOCONAZOLE

Trade: Monistat 1, Tioconazole 1, Vagistat-1

Category: Antifungal

LRC: L3 - No Data-Probably Compatible

Tioconazole is an anti-fungal agent used in the treatment of candida vulvovaginitis.[1] There are no adequate and well-controlled studies or case reports in breastfeeding women. Oral bioavailability following topical or vaginal application is minimal to nil. Therefore, it is unlikely that any exposure through breast milk would be clinically significant in the infant.

T 1/2		MW	387.7 Da	PB	
Tmax		RID		Vd	
Oral	2.9% (topical), negligible (vaginal)	M/P		pKa	6.42

Adult Concerns: Burning, itching, rash, erythema.

Adult Dose:

Pediatric Concerns:

Infant Monitoring:

Alternatives:

References:
1. Pharmaceutical manufacturers prescribing information.

TIOPRONIN

Trade: Thiola

Category: Heavy Metal Chelator

LRC: L4 - No Data-Possibly Hazardous

Tiopronin is a reducing agent used in the treatment of cystinuria. It has similar structure with penicillamine such that it may have similar adverse reactions.[1] Tiopronin has been approved for children aged 9 years or older. Tiopronin is excreted in urine, up to 48% after 4 hours and 78% after 72 hours. There are no data on its transfer to breast milk. Recommend discontinuing lactation if this drug is mandatory.

T 1/2	53 h	MW	163 Da	PB	
Tmax	3-6 h	RID		Vd	6.5 L/kg
Oral	63%	M/P		pKa	

Adult Concerns: Fatigue, fever, rash, pruritus, anemia, leukopenia, jaundice, Goodsposture's syndrome, hematuria, loss of smell, bronchiolitis, dyspnea.

Adult Dose: 1000 mg/day in 3 divided dose.

Pediatric Concerns:

Infant Monitoring: Drowsiness, fever, blood in urine, rash.

Alternatives:

References:
1. Thiola. Full Prescribing Information. San Antonio, TX: Mission Pharmacal Company.

TIOTROPIUM BROMIDE MONOHYDRATE

Trade: Spiriva

Category: Anticholinergic

LRC: L3 - No Data-Probably Compatible

Tiotropium is a muscarinic anticholinergic used via inhaled powder.[1] It is indicated for the long-term maintenance of bronchospasm associated with chronic obstructive pulmonary disease (COPD), and for reducing COPD exacerbations. Following dry powder inhalation by young healthy volunteers, the absolute bioavailability of 19.5% suggests that the fraction reaching the lung is highly bioavailable. Due to its quaternary ammonium compound structure, tiotropium is poorly absorbed from the gastrointestinal tract. Oral solutions of tiotropium have a bioavailability of only 2% to 3%. This product has an enormous volume of distribution (32 L/kg) indicating that the drug binds extensively to peripheral tissues, thus plasma levels are exceedingly low (3-4 pg/mL). While the terminal half-life is long (5-6 days), the plasma levels, and probably the levels in milk, are exceedingly low.

T 1/2	5-6 days	MW	490.4 Da	PB	72%
Tmax	1 h	RID		Vd	32 L/kg
Oral	2-3%: Inhaled 19.5%	M/P		pKa	

Adult Concerns: Worsening of narrow angle glaucoma and urinary retention. Observe for paradoxical bronchospasm.

Adult Dose: 18 µg dry powder inhaled daily.

Pediatric Concerns: None reported via milk at this time.

Infant Monitoring: Irritability, insomnia, arrhythmias, dry mouth, constipation, urinary retention, weight loss, tremor.

Alternatives:

References:
1. Pharmaceutical manufacturers prescribing information.

TIZANIDINE

Trade: Zanaflex

Category: Skeletal Muscle Relaxant

LRC: L4 - No Data-Possibly Hazardous

Tizanidine is a centrally acting muscle relaxant. It has demonstrated efficacy in the treatment of tension headache and spasticity associated with multiple sclerosis. It is not known if it is transferred into human milk although the manufacturer states that due to its lipid solubility, it likely penetrates milk.[1] This product has a long half-life, high lipid solubility, and significant CNS penetration, all factors that would increase milk penetration. While the half-life of the conventional formulation is only 4-8 hours, the half-life of the sustained release formulation is 13-22 hours.[2] Further, 48% of patients complain of sedation. Use caution if used in a breastfeeding mother.

T 1/2	13-22 h	MW		PB	30%
Tmax	1.5 h	RID		Vd	2.4 L/kg
Oral	40%	M/P		pKa	7.47

Adult Concerns: Hypotension (49%), sedation (48%), dry mouth, asthenia, dizziness, and other symptoms have been reported. Nausea and vomiting have been reported. A high risk of elevated liver enzymes (5%).

Adult Dose: 8 mg every 6 hours PRN.

Pediatric Concerns: None reported via milk, but caution is recommended.

Infant Monitoring: Sedation, weakness, dry mouth, vomiting.

Alternatives:

References:
1. Pharmaceutical manufacturers prescribing information.
2. Wagstaff AJ, Bryson HM. Tizanidine. A review of its pharmacology, clinical efficacy and tolerability in the management of spasticity associated with cerebral and spinal disorders. Drugs. 1997;53(3):435-452.

TOBRAMYCIN

Trade: Nebcin, Tobi, Tobralex, Tobrex

Category: Antibiotic, Aminoglycoside

LRC: L2 - Limited Data-Probably Compatible

Tobramycin is an aminoglycoside antibiotic similar to gentamicin.[1] Although small levels of tobramycin are known to transfer to milk, they probably pose few problems. In one study of five patients, following an 80-mg IM dose, tobramycin levels in milk ranged from undetectable to 0.5 mg/L in only one patient.[2] In a case report of a mother receiving 150 mg three times daily for 14 days (IV), milk concentrations were determined on day 4, before administration, and 60, 120, 180, 240, and 300 minutes after dosing. Tobramycin was undetectable in all samples. The limit of detection was >0.18 mg/L. No untoward effects were noted in the infant.[3] In another study of one mother who received 80 mg every 8 hours (IM), milk levels ranged from 0.6 mg/L at 1 hour to 0.58 mg/L at 8 hours postdose.[4] Levels in milk are generally low, but could produce minor changes in gut flora. As oral tobramycin is not absorbed orally, systemic levels in an infant would be unexpected.

T 1/2	2-3 h	MW	468 Da	PB	<5%
Tmax	30-90 min (IM)	RID	2.63% - 6.57%	Vd	0.22-0.31 L/kg
Oral	Nil	M/P		pKa	12.54

Adult Concerns: Headache, ototoxicity, nausea, vomiting, diarrhea, changes in liver and renal function, hematologic changes.

Adult Dose: 1 mg/kg every 8 hours.

Pediatric Concerns: None reported via milk.

Infant Monitoring: Vomiting, diarrhea, changes in gastrointestinal flora, and rash.

Alternatives:

References:
1. Pharmaceutical manufacturers prescribing information.
2. Takase Z. Laboratory and clinical studies on tobramycin in the field of obstetrics and gynecology. Chemotherapy (Tokyo). 1975;23:1402.
3. Festini F, Ciuti R, Taccetti G, Repetto T, Campana S, Martino M. Breast feeding in a woman with cystic fibrosis undergoing antibiotic intravenous treatment. J Matern Fetal Neonatal Med. 2006;19(6):375-376.
4. Uwaydah M, Bibi S, Salman S. Therapeutic efficacy of tobramycin--a clinical and laboratory evaluation. J Antimicrob Chemother. 1975;1:429-437.

TOCILIZUMAB

Trade: Actemra

Category: Immune Modulator

LRC: L3 - No Data-Probably Compatible

Tocilizumab is an interleukin 6 (IL-6) receptor inhibitor used in the treatment of rheumatoid arthritis (RA). Tocilizumab is used in severe cases of RA or in cases where the RA had a subclinical response to TNF antagonists.[1] The dose starts at 4 mg/kg and is increased to 8 mg/kg depending on clinical response. There are no studies on the passage of tocilizumab into human milk. Tocilizumab has a large molecular weight of 148,000 Da and is unlikely to pass into breast milk.

Although the molecular weight of this medication is very large and the amount in breast milk is expected to be exceptionally low, there are no long-term data concerning the safety of using immune-modulating medications in breastfeeding mothers. Further there are current data that suggest that some IgG drugs do transfer to milk, and perhaps the breastfed infant. Therefore, some caution is recommended, and each woman should understand the benefits and risk of using this type of medication in lactation.

T 1/2	6.3 days (single dose); 13 days (steady state)	MW	148,000 Da	PB	
Tmax		RID		Vd	0.09 L/kg
Oral		M/P		pKa	

Adult Concerns: Headache, dizziness, hypertension, edema, diarrhea, stomatitis, changes in liver enzymes, increases in cholesterol, leukopenia, neutropenia, thrombocytopenia, increased frequency of infection, and infusion reactions.

Adult Dose: 4-8 mg/kg IV every 4 weeks.

Pediatric Concerns: None reported via milk at this time.

Infant Monitoring: Fever, diarrhea, weight gain, frequent infections.

Alternatives: Infliximab(L3)

References:
1. Pharmaceutical manufacturers prescribing information.

TOFACITINIB CITRATE

Trade: Xeljanz

Category: Antirheumatic

LRC: L4 - No Data-Possibly Hazardous

Tofacitinib is a Janus kinase inhibitor that is used to treat patients with moderate to severe rheumatoid arthritis.[1] It is usually used in patients who have shown inadequate response or were unable to tolerate methotrexate. Tofacitinib may be used in combination with methotrexate or a non-biologic disease modifying antirheumatic drug.

The transfer of Tofacitinib to human milk is still unknown. However, because of serious side effects that may occur in nursing infants it is advised to not use during breastfeeding.

T 1/2	3 h	MW	312.3 Da	PB	40%
Tmax	0.5 - 1 h	RID		Vd	1.24 L/kg
Oral	74%	M/P		pKa	

Adult Concerns: Headache, hypertension, diarrhea, changes in renal and liver function, increased risk of infection.

Adult Dose: 5 mg twice daily.

Pediatric Concerns: None reported.

Infant Monitoring: Fever, diarrhea, weight gain, frequent infections.

Alternatives: Infliximab(L3), certolizumab.

References:
1. Pharmaceutical manufacturers prescribing information.

TOLBUTAMIDE

Trade: Glyconon, Mobenol, Oramide, Orinase, Rastinon

Category: Antidiabetic, Sulfonylurea

LRC: L3 - Limited Data-Probably Compatible

Tolbutamide is a short-acting sulfonylurea used to stimulate insulin secretion in type II diabetics. Only low levels are secreted in breast milk. Following a dose of 500 mg twice daily, milk levels in two patients were 3 and 18 μg/L respectively.[1] Maternal serum levels averaged 35 and 45 μg/L.

T 1/2	4.5-6.5 h	MW	270 Da	PB	93%
Tmax	3.5 h	RID	0.004% - 0.02%	Vd	0.1-0.15 L/kg
Oral	Complete	M/P	0.09-0.4	pKa	5.3

Adult Concerns: Headache, nausea, taste alteration, changes in liver function and hypoglycemia.

Adult Dose: 250-2000 mg daily.

Pediatric Concerns: None reported via milk at this time.

Infant Monitoring: Signs of hypoglycemia- drowsiness, lethargy, pallor, sweating, tremor.

Alternatives:

References:
1. Moiel RH, Ryan JR. Tolbutamide orinase in human breast milk. Clin Pediatr (Phila). 1967;6(8):480.

TOLNAFTATE

Trade: Absorbine Jr. Antifungal, Aftate, Blis-To-Sol, Dermasept Antifungal, Fungi-Guard, Podactin, Q-Naftate, Tinactin

Category: Antifungal

LRC: L3 - No Data-Probably Compatible

Tolnaftate is a topical antifungal agent that is used in over-the-counter products. There are no adequate and well-controlled studies of tolnaftate use in breastfeeding women. In an in vitro study, dermal absorption of 1% tolnaftate from topical application is 0.92 $\mu g/cm^2$.[1] It is not recommended for use on the nipple or areas that may be in direct contact with the infant. Water-based creams, liquid, and gels are preferred compared to ointment bases because of possible infant ingestion of mineral paraffins.[2]

T 1/2		MW	307 Da	PB	
Tmax		RID		Vd	
Oral		M/P		pKa	

Adult Concerns: Local irritation, contact dermatitis, pruritus.

Adult Dose: 1-3 drops or small amount of cream twice a day.

Pediatric Concerns:

Infant Monitoring:

Alternatives:

References:
1. Kezutyte T, Kornysova O, Maruska A, Briedis V. Assay of tolnaftate in human skin samples after in vitro penetration studies using high performance liquid chromatography. Acta Pol Pharm. 2010 Jul-Aug;67(4):327-334.
2. Noti A, Grob K, Biedermann M, et al. Exposure of babies to C(15)-C(45) mineral paraffins from human milk and breast salves. Regul Toxicol Pharmacol. 2003;38:317-325.

TOLTERODINE

Trade: Detrol, Detrusitol

Category: Renal-Urologic Agent

LRC: L3 - No Data-Probably Compatible

Tolterodine is a muscarinic anticholinergic agent similar in effect to atropine but is more selective for the urinary bladder.[1] Tolterodine levels in milk have been reported in mice, where offspring exposed to extremely high levels had slightly reduced body weight gain, but no other untoward effects. While it is more selective for the urinary bladder, preclinical trials still showed adverse effects including blurred vision, constipation, and dry mouth in adults. While we have no data on human milk, it is unlikely concentrations will be high enough to produce untoward effects in infants.

T 1/2	1.9-3.7 h	MW		PB	96%
Tmax	1-2 h	RID		Vd	1.6 L/kg
Oral	77%	M/P		pKa	9.87

Adult Concerns: Blurred vision, dry mouth, urinary retention, constipation.

Adult Dose: 2 mg twice daily.

Pediatric Concerns: None reported via milk.

Infant Monitoring: Dry mouth, decreased urinary output, constipation.

Alternatives:

References:
1. Pharmaceutical manufacturers prescribing information.

TOPIRAMATE

Trade: Topamax, Trokendi XR

Category: Anticonvulsant

LRC: L3 - Limited Data-Probably Compatible

Topiramate is an anticonvulsant used in the long-term management of seizure disorders and migraines.[1] Its exact mechanism of action remains poorly described.

Only a handful of case reports have been published, but they consistently indicate that exposure to topiramate via breast milk produces subtherapeutic plasma levels in infants. There are no published studies examining the long-term neurodevelopmental outcomes of infants exposed to topiramate in lactation. In a small report of nine preschool-aged children with in utero exposure to topiramate, an association with significant alterations in motor and cognitive function were found when these children were compared to a control group.[2]

A group of three women receiving topiramate 150-200 mg/day were followed from 14-97 days postpartum.[3] The milk concentrations ranged from 0.5-4.7 μg/mL (1.6-13.7 μmol). The mean milk/plasma ratio at day 21 was 0.86 (range=0.67-1.1). The absolute infant dose and RID ranged from 0.1-0.7 mg/kg/day and 3-23%, respectively. Plasma concentrations in the infants were 10-20% of the maternal plasma level and ranged from undetectable to 2.1 μmol up to 3 months after delivery. It should be noted that milk and plasma concentrations were taken prior to the morning maternal dose (10-15 h post last dose) and thus may underestimate the amount transferred in milk. No adverse effects were reported in the three breastfed infants.

In contrast, a 2014 case report described a 2-month-old infant who developed persistent, watery diarrhea (8-10 stools/day) at 40 days of life.[4] The mother was taking 100 mg/day of topiramate and had replaced two feeds per day with formula to reduce medication exposure. After 18 days of diarrhea and weight loss, topiramate was blamed for the symptom (testing was negative for infectious causes). The diarrhea resolved over 2 days once breastfeeding was ceased. A sample of the mother's milk yielded a topiramate concentration of 5.3 μg/mL (15.7 μmol). No details were provided regarding the timing of this sample; however, we used this concentration to calculate the RID (55.6%) and absolute infant dose (0.8 mg/kg/day) and found that although the RID was high, the absolute infant dose was similar to previous reports.

Another case report describes a healthy male infant exposed in utero and via exclusive breastfeeding to a maternal dose of 300 mg/day.[5] The infant appeared to have normal neurodevelopment and no reported side effects as of 8 months postpartum.

T 1/2	21 h	MW	339.4 Da	PB	15-41%
Tmax	1.5-4 h	RID	24.68% - 55.65%	Vd	0.7 L/kg
Oral	80%	M/P	0.86	pKa	8.7

Adult Concerns: Sedation, cognitive dysfunction especially in older patients (memory, speech, behavior), paresthesia, diarrhea, weight loss (7%).

Adult Dose: 200 mg twice daily.

Pediatric Concerns: One case report of persistent watery diarrhea in a breastfed infant.[4]

Infant Monitoring: Sedation or irritability, not waking to feed/poor feeding, diarrhea, weight loss.

Alternatives:

References:
1. Pharmaceutical manufacturers prescribing information.
2. Rihtman T, Parush S, Ornoy A. Preliminary findings of the developmental effects of in utero exposure to topiramate. Reprod Toxicol. 2012;34(3):308-311.
3. Ohman I, Vitols S, Luef G, et al. Topiramate kinetics during delivery, lactation, and in the neonate: preliminary observations. Epilepsia. 2002;43(10):1157-1160.
4. Westergren T, Hjelmeland K, Kristoffersen B, et al. Probable topiramate-induced diarrhea in a 2-month-old breast-fed child - a case report. Epilepsy Behav Case Rep. 2014;2:22-23.
5. Gentile S. Topiramate in pregnancy and breastfeeding. Clin Drug Investig. 2009;29(2):139-141.

TOREMIFENE

Trade: Fareston

Category: Antineoplastic

LRC: L4 - No Data-Possibly Hazardous

Toremifene is a nonsteroidal agent that binds to estrogen receptors without producing an estrogenic response, hence blocking estrogenic activity. It is well absorbed orally (100%).[1] The plasma concentration time profile of toremifene declines biexponentially after absorption, with a mean distribution half-life of about 4 hours and an elimination half-life of about 5 days. Toremifene has an apparent volume of distribution of 8.3 L/kg and binds extensively (>99.5%) to serum proteins, mainly to albumin No data are available on its transfer to milk, but its molecular weight of 580 and high protein binding will probably reduce its entry into milk. However, the potential for severe interruption of estrogen levels in breastfed infants would largely suggest this agent should not be used in breastfeeding mothers. Breastfeeding mothers should withhold breastfeeding for a minimum of 25-30 days.

T 1/2	5 days	MW	598.1 Da	PB	99.5%
Tmax	3-6 h	RID		Vd	8.3 L/kg
Oral	Complete	M/P		pKa	8

Adult Concerns: Nausea, sudden sweating and feeling of warmth, blurred vision, change in vaginal discharge, changes in vision, confusion, increased urination, loss of appetite, pain or feeling of pressure in pelvis, tiredness, vaginal bleeding.

Adult Dose: 60 mg once daily.

Pediatric Concerns:

Infant Monitoring: Withhold breastfeeding for a minimum of 25-30 days.

Alternatives:

References:
1. Pharmaceutical manufacturers prescribing information.

TORSEMIDE

Trade: Demadex

Category: Diuretic

LRC: L3 - No Data-Probably Compatible

Torsemide is a potent loop diuretic generally used in congestive heart failure and other conditions that require a strong diuretic.[1] There are no reports of its transfer to human milk. Its extraordinarily high protein binding would likely limit its transfer to human milk. As with many diuretics, reduction of plasma volume and hypotension may adversely reduce milk production although this is rare.

T 1/2	3.5 h	MW	348 Da	PB	>99%
Tmax	1 h	RID		Vd	0.21 L/kg
Oral	80%	M/P		pKa	5.92

Adult Concerns: Headache, dizziness, hypotension, hypokalemia, volume depletion/excessive urination, muscle weakness.

Adult Dose: 5-10 mg daily.

Pediatric Concerns: None reported via milk at this time.

Infant Monitoring: Observe for fluid loss, dehydration, lethargy.

Alternatives: Furosemide(L3)

References:
1. Pharmaceutical manufacturers prescribing information.

TOXOPLASMA GONDII

Trade: Toxoplasmosis

Category: Infectious Disease

LRC: L4 - No Data-Possibly Hazardous

Toxoplasmosis is an infection caused by the parasite Toxoplasma gondii commonly spread by eating undercooked meat of infected animals, by contact with the feces of infected cats, or through contact with infected soil or insects in the soil. The infection can get into the blood causing a parasitemia that can get into the placenta and cause fetal infection. Although the disease seems to be self-limited in healthy adults, it can affect the infants of affected mothers. Some of the clinical signs of infection in infants include hearing loss, developmental delay, rash, and seizures. According to the CDC, there are no studies documenting breast milk transmission of Toxoplasma gondii in humans. Even though the breastfeeding infant was probably exposed to this parasite long before the diagnosis was made, it still may be advisable to withhold breastfeeding until treatment has been initiated.

Adult Concerns: Symptoms in adults include cervical lymphadenopathy, fever, night sweats, myalgias, and hepatosplenomegaly.

Adult Dose:

Pediatric Concerns:

Infant Monitoring: Fever, myalgia.

Alternatives:

References:

TRAMADOL

Trade: ConZip, Dromadol, Nycodol, Rybix ODT, Ryzolt, Tramake, Tramal, Ultram, Ultram ER, Zamadol, Zydol

Category: Analgesic

LRC: L3 - Limited Data-Probably Compatible

Tramadol is an analgesic from a new class that most closely resembles the opiates, although it is not a controlled substance. It appears to be slightly more potent than codeine. After oral use, its onset of analgesia is within 1 hour and reaches a peak in 2-3 hours. Following a single IV 100 mg dose of tramadol, the cumulative excretion in breast milk within 16 hours was 100 µg of tramadol (0.1% of the maternal dose) and 27 µg of the M1 metabolite.[1]

In a study of 75 mothers who received 100 mg of tramadol every 6 hours for cesarean section pain; milk samples were taken on days 2-4 postpartum.[2] At steady state, the milk/plasma ratio averaged 2.4 for rac-tramadol and 2.8 for rac-O-desmethyltramadol. The estimated absolute infant doses were 112 µg/kg/day and 30 µg/kg/day for rac-tramadol and its desmethyl metabolite. The authors estimated the relative infant doses were 2.24% and 0.64% for rac-tramadol and its desmethyl metabolite, respectively. No significant neurobehavioral adverse effects were noted between controls and exposed infants.

Caution is recommended as this medication also has an active metabolite via CYP 2D6 metabolism (like codeine) and experience with this medication in pediatric patients has not yet demonstrated adverse effects.[5]

T 1/2	7 h	MW	263 Da	PB	20%
Tmax	2 h	RID	2.86%	Vd	2.9 L/kg
Oral	60%	M/P	2.4	pKa	9.4

Adult Concerns: Seizure, sedation, respiratory depression, nausea, vomiting, constipation, hypoglycemia, hyponatremia.[3,4]

Adult Dose: 50-100 mg every 4-6 hours as needed.

Pediatric Concerns: None reported via milk at this time. This product is not recommended for use in those under 18 years of age.[5] There have been nine cases of breathing problems with three reports of death that were associated with the use of this medication in the pediatric population.

Infant Monitoring: Sedation, slowed breathing rate/apnea, pallor, constipation, not waking to feed/poor feeding.

Alternatives: Acetaminophen(L1), NSAIDs, Hydromorphone(L3)

References:
1. Pharmaceutical manufacturers prescribing information.
2. Ilett KF, Paech MJ, Page-Sharp M, et al. Use of a sparse sampling study design to assess transfer of tramadol and its O-desmethyl metabolite into transitional breast milk. Br J Clin Pharmacol. 2008;65(5):661-666.
3. Fournier JP, Azoulay L, Yin H, et al. Tramadol use and the risk of hospitalization for hypoglycemia in patients with noncancer pain. JAMA Intern Med. 2015;175(2):186-193.
4. Fournier JP, Yin H, Nessim SJ, et al. Tramadol for noncancer pain and the risk of hyponatremia. Am J Med. 2015;128(4):418-425.
5. U.S. Food & Drug Administration. FDA drug safety communication: FDA restricts use of prescription codeine pain and cough medicines and tramadol pain medicines in children; recommends against the use in breastfeeding women. https://www.fda.gov/Drugs/DrugSafety/ucm549679.htm

TRANDOLAPRIL

Trade: Mavik, Tarka

Category: ACE Inhibitor

LRC: L3 - No Data-Probably Compatible

Trandolapril is an ACE inhibitor used to control blood pressure and improve heart function.[1] According to the manufacturer this medication has been found in rodent milk (amount not quantified); however, no human milk data are available at this time. Based on this medication's size, small volume of distribution (0.26 L/kg), and moderately high protein binding it should be expected that some of this medication will enter breast milk. In addition, trandolapril has an active metabolite, trandolaprilat, with a long half-life of 22.5 hours.

At this time it would be preferred to use ACEI with human data available such as captopril, ramipril, and enalapril.

Please note: Both the ACE inhibitor family and the specific Angiotensin II receptor blockers are contraindicated in pregnancy and thus should be used with caution in women who are planning a subsequent pregnancy in the near future.

T 1/2	6 h as trandolapril; 22.5 h as trandolaprilat	MW	430.54 Da	PB	80%
Tmax	6 h	RID		Vd	0.26 L/kg
Oral	10% as trandolapril; 70% as trandolaprilat	M/P		pKa	

Adult Concerns: Headache, dizziness, fatigue, hypotension, bradycardia, abnormal taste, cough, nausea, diarrhea, constipation, changes in renal function/urine output, hyperkalemia, rash.

Adult Dose: 2 to 8 mg once daily.

Pediatric Concerns: None reported via milk at this time.

Infant Monitoring: Drowsiness, lethargy, pallor, poor feeding, and weight gain.

Alternatives: Ramipril(L3), Captopril(L2), Enalapril(L2), Benazepril(L2)

References:
1. Pharmaceutical manufacturers prescribing information.

TRANEXAMIC ACID

Trade: Cyklokapron, Lysteda

Category: Hemostatic

LRC: L3 - Limited Data-Probably Compatible

Tranexamic acid is used to reduce the risks of hemorrhage in patients with bleeding disorders. In the United States, this drug is only approved for short-term applications such as tooth extraction or menorrhagia. Tranexamic acid binds to multiple sites within the plasminogen/plasmin molecule and reduces its ability to destabilize a fibrin clot.[1] Unpublished data from the manufacturer reports that tranexamic acid is excreted in human milk minimally, and is present in the mother's milk at a concentration of about one-hundredth of the corresponding maternal serum concentration.

A prospective, observational study of 21 mother-infant pairs was published in 2014, which assessed the suitability of tranexamic acid in lactation.[2] In this study, women were contacted 1-3 years after they phoned an information line to ask if they could breastfeed while taking tranexamic acid and were asked questions regarding possible infant adverse effects from using this medication in lactation. The women were taking between 1500 mg and 4000 mg per day.

The authors reported one of 21 infants in the tranexamic acid group had restlessness. When compared to a non-exposed mother-infant pair cohort, more women reported lactation issues during or just after drug use (9.5% vs 4.7%) and there were no significant differences in infant growth or development at follow-up.

T 1/2	11 h	MW	157.2 Da	PB	3%
Tmax	3 h	RID		Vd	0.39 L/kg
Oral	45%	M/P		pKa	4.77

Adult Concerns: Headache, fatigue, visual changes, nausea, vomiting, abdominal pain, diarrhea, changes in renal function, thrombosis (DVT, PE), pain in muscles and joints.

Adult Dose: 1300 mg orally three times a day for up to 5 days during menstruation.

Pediatric Concerns: One infant reported to have restlessness.

Infant Monitoring: Restlessness, vomiting, diarrhea.

Alternatives:

References:
1. Pharmaceutical manufacturer prescribing information.
2. Gilad O, Merlob P, Stahl B, Klinger G. Outcome following tranexamic acid exposure during breastfeeding. Breastfeed Med. 2014;9(8):407-410.

TRASTUZUMAB

Trade: Herceptin

Category: Monoclonal Antibody

LRC: L4 - No Data-Possibly Hazardous

Trastuzumab is a therapy for women with metastatic breast cancer, whose tumors have too much HER2 protein.[1] For patients with this disease, herceptin is approved for first-line use in combination with paclitaxel. Trastuzumab is a recombinant DNA-derived monoclonal antibody that selectively binds to the extracellular receptor domain of the human epidermal growth factor protein (HER2). The antibody is an IgG1 kappa antibody that binds to HER2 receptors. The manufacturer reports conducting a study in lactating cynomolgus monkeys at doses 25 times the weekly human maintenance dose of 2 mg/kg, which demonstrated that trastuzumab is secreted in milk (no levels reported). The presence of trastuzumab in the serum of infant monkeys was not associated with any adverse effects on their growth or development from birth to 3 months of age.

It is not known whether trastuzumab is secreted in human milk. IgG levels in colostrum are much higher, but IgG is normally present in mature human milk only at low levels, only 4 mg/dL. After a dose of 2 mg/kg trastuzumab, only one in approximately every 432 molecules of IgG would be this drug, thus the daily dose to infant would be infinitesimally small. It is unlikely that levels in mature human milk will be high enough to produce untoward symptoms in human infants, but this has not yet been demonstrated.

Although the molecular weight of this medication is very large and the amount in breast milk is expected to be exceptionally low, there are no long-term data concerning the safety of using immune-modulating medications in breastfeeding mothers. Further there are current data that suggest that some IgG drugs do transfer to milk, and perhaps the breastfed infant. Therefore, some caution is recommended, and each woman should understand the benefits and risk of using this type of medication in lactation.

T 1/2	5.8 days	MW	185,000 Da	PB	
Tmax		RID		Vd	0.044 L/kg
Oral	Nil	M/P		pKa	

Adult Concerns: Pain, insomnia, headache, asthenia, fever, chills, cough, dyspnea, rhinitis, abdominal pain, nausea, vomiting, diarrhea, rash.

Adult Dose: 2 mg/kg/week.

Pediatric Concerns: No adverse events have been reported at this time.

Infant Monitoring: Fever, frequent infections, poor feeding/poor weight gain.

Alternatives:

References:
1. Pharmaceutical manufacturers prescribing information.

TRAVOPROST

Trade: Travatan, Travatan Z

Category: Prostaglandin

LRC: L3 - No Data-Probably Compatible

Travoprost is a prostaglandin analog that is used to treat intraoccular hypertension and open-angle glaucoma. Travoprost is undetectable in plasma 1 hour after eye drops are instilled. The drug appears in rat milk after oral administration but there were no studies located on the use of travoprost and human lactation.[1] Due to its use as an ophthalmic agent, it is unlikely to be absorbed systemically and thus unlikely to enter milk.

T 1/2	45 min	MW	500.5 Da	PB	
Tmax	0.5 h	RID		Vd	
Oral		M/P		pKa	13.95

Adult Concerns: May cause increased pigmentation of iris & eyelid along with increased growth & pigmentation of eyelashes. Has caused macular edema. Plasma levels undetectable within 1 hour of application to the eye.

Adult Dose: One drop in affected eye once daily.

Pediatric Concerns:

Infant Monitoring: Vomiting, diarrhea, flushing.

Alternatives:

References:
1. Pharmaceutical manufacturers prescribing information.

TRAZODONE

Trade: Molipaxin, Desyrel, Oleptro, Trazorel

Category: Antidepressant, other

LRC: L2 - Limited Data-Probably Compatible

Trazodone is an antidepressant whose structure is dissimilar to the tricyclics and to the other antidepressants. In six mothers who received a single 50-mg dose, the milk/plasma ratio averaged 0.14.[1] Peak milk concentrations occurred at 2 hours and were approximately 110 µg/L (taken from graph) and declined rapidly thereafter. On a weight basis, an adult would receive 0.77 mg/kg whereas a breastfeeding infant, using this data, would consume 0.005 mg/kg. The authors estimate that about 0.6% of the maternal dose was ingested by the infant over 24 hours. Milk levels are probably too low to be clinically relevant in the breastfed infant.

T 1/2	4-9 h	MW	372 Da	PB	85-95%
Tmax	1-2 h	RID	2.8%	Vd	0.9-1.5 L/kg
Oral	65%	M/P	0.142	pKa	6.74

Adult Concerns: Dry mouth, sedation, hypotension, blurred vision.

Adult Dose: 150-400 mg daily.

Pediatric Concerns: None reported via milk at this time.

Infant Monitoring: Sedation or irritability, not waking to feed/poor feeding, and weight gain.

Alternatives:

References:
1. Verbeeck RK, Ross SG, McKenna EA. Excretion of trazodone in breast milk. Br J Clin Pharmacol. 1986;22(3):367-370.

TREPROSTINIL

Trade: Remodulin

Category: Vasodilator

LRC: L3 - No Data-Probably Compatible

Treprostinil causes direct vasodilation of pulmonary and systemic arterial vasculature and inhibits platelet aggregation.[1] It is used to treat symptoms related to exercise in patients with concomitant pulmonary arterial hypertension and heart failure. Although there are no data at this time about the transfer of treprostinil to human milk, the oral bioavailability of this product is low (18%); therefore, systemic concentrations in breastfed infants would most likely be low.[2]

T 1/2	4 h	MW	390 Da	PB	91%
Tmax		RID		Vd	0.2 L/kg
Oral	18%	M/P		pKa	

Adult Concerns: Headache, dizziness, anxiety, jaw pain, vasodilation, nausea, vomiting, abdominal pain, diarrhea, edema, injection site pain and reactions.

Adult Dose: Subcutaneous or IV infusion starts at 1.25 ng/kg/min, then increased by 1.25 ng/kg/min/week for first four weeks then 2.5 ng/kg/min/week (little experience with doses greater than 40 ng/kg/min).

Pediatric Concerns: No pediatric efficacy or safety data available at this time.

Infant Monitoring: Drowsiness, lethargy, pallor, poor feeding, and weight gain.

Alternatives:

References:
1. Pharmaceutical manufacturers prescribing information.
2. de Jesus Perez VA. Understanding the pharmacokinetics of oral treprostinil in patients with pulmonary arterial hypertension. J Cardiovasc Pharmacol. 2013;61(6):471-473.

TRETINOIN

Trade: Renova, Retin-A, Stieva-A, Vesanoid, Vitamin A Acid

Category: Antiacne

LRC: L3 - No Data-Probably Compatible

Tretinoin is a retinoid derivative similar to Vitamin A. It is primarily used topically for acne and wrinkling and sometimes administered orally for leukemias and psoriasis. Used topically, tretinoin stimulates epithelial turnover and reduces cell cohesiveness.[1] Blood concentrations measured 2-48 hours following application are essentially zero. Absorption of Retin-A via topical sources is reported to be minimal, and breast milk would likely be minimal to none.[2]

However, if it is used orally, transfer to milk is likely and use in lactation is cautioned. If taken orally the lactation risk would significantly increase (L4- No data- possibly hazardous).

T 1/2	2 h	MW	300 Da	PB	
Tmax		RID		Vd	0.44 L/kg
Oral	70%	M/P		pKa	4.79

Adult Concerns: Headache, fatigue, fever, changes in blood pressure, chest pain, peripheral edema, increased serum cholesterol and triglycerides, abdominal pain, mucositis, diarrhea, weight loss, changes in liver function, hemorrhage, leukocytosis, weakness, dry skin, pruritus, rash.

Adult Dose: Variable.

Pediatric Concerns: None reported via milk. Do not breastfeed if used orally.

Infant Monitoring: Caution if used orally- diarrhea, weight loss.

Alternatives:

References:
1. Zbinden G. Investigation on the toxicity of tretinoin administered systemically to animals. Acta Derm Verereol Suppl(Stockh). 1975;74:36-40.
2. Lucek RW, Colburn WA. Clinical pharmacokinetics of the retinoids. Clin Pharmacokinet. 1985;10(1):38-62.

TRIAMCINOLONE ACETONIDE

Trade: Adcortyl, Aristocort, Azmacort, Cinolar, Kenalog, Kenalone, Nasacort, Oralone, Tri-Nasal, Triaderm, Triamcot, Trianex, Triesence

Category: Corticosteroid

LRC: L3 - No Data-Probably Compatible

Triamcinolone is a typical corticosteroid that is available for topical, intranasal, injection, inhalation, and oral use. When administered intranasally to the nose or by inhalation to the lungs, only minimal doses are used and plasma levels are exceedingly low to undetectable.[1] When applied topically, absorption varies between 1-36% depending on amount used and surface area covered on application.[2] Absorption after topical application is promoted with use of higher doses, increased dosing frequency, and use of occlusive dressings.[3,4] Derendorf[5] found that absorption was complete within 2-3 weeks after intra-articular injection and low systemic levels of corticosteroid were attained. Although no data are available on triamcinolone secretion in human milk, it is likely that the milk levels would be exceedingly low and not clinically relevant when administered via inhalation or intranasally. There is virtually no risk to the infant following use of the intranasal or aerosol products in breastfeeding mothers. With topical application such as to the nipple, use with caution, and limit the dose and frequency of use.

T 1/2	Intranasal/inhalation/oral: 88 min; IM/joint: 18-36 h	MW	434 Da	PB	IM: 68%
Tmax	IM: 8-10 h	RID		Vd	1.42 L/kg
Oral	Complete	M/P		pKa	13.4

Adult Concerns: Intranasal and inhaled: nasal irritation, dry mucous membranes, sneezing, throat irritation, hoarseness, candida overgrowth.

Adult Dose: 220 μg/day (intranasal), 200 μg 3-4 times daily (inhaled), 4-48 mg/day(oral), 2.5-15 mg (intra-articular), 40-80 mg (IM).

Pediatric Concerns: None reported via milk.

Infant Monitoring: Feeding, growth, and weight gain.

Alternatives:

References:
1. Pharmaceutical manufacturers prescribing information.
2. Kelly R, Keipert JA. Selecting a topical corticosteroid. Curr Ther. 1979;20:89,90,93-95.
3. Pellanda C, Strub C, Figueiredo V, Rufli T, Imanidis G, Surber C. Topicalbioavailability of triamcinolone acetonide: effect of occlusion. Skin Pharmacol Physiol. 2007;20(1):50-56.
4. Pellanda C, Ottiker E, Strub C, et al. Topical bioavailability of triamcinolone acetonide: effect of dose andapplication frequency. Arch Dermatol Res. 2006 Oct;298(5):221-230.
5. Derendorf H, Möllmann H, Grüner A, Haack D, Gyselby G. Pharmacokinetics and pharmacodynamics of glucocorticoid suspensions after intra-articular administration. Clin Pharmacol Ther. 1986 Mar;39(3):313-317.

TRIAMTERENE

Trade: Dyrenium, Hydrene

Category: Diuretic

LRC: L3 - No Data-Probably Compatible

Triamterene is a potassium-sparing diuretic, commonly used in combination with thiazide diuretics such as hydrochlorothiazide. Plasma levels average 26-30 ng/mL.[1] No data are available on the transfer of triamterene into human milk, but it is known to transfer to animal milk. Because of the availability of other less dangerous diuretics, triamterene should be used as a last resort in breastfeeding mothers.

T 1/2	1.5-2.5 h	MW	253 Da	PB	55%
Tmax	1.5-3 h	RID		Vd	
Oral	30-70%	M/P		pKa	6.2

Adult Concerns: Headache, dizziness, hypotension, bradycardia, nausea, constipation, edema, rash.

Adult Dose: 25-100 mg daily.

Pediatric Concerns: None reported via milk at this time.

Infant Monitoring: Observe for fluid loss, dehydration, lethargy.

Alternatives: Hydrochlorothiazide(L2)

References:
1. Mutschler E, Gilfrich HJ, Knauf H, Mohrke W, Volger KD. Pharmacokinetics of triamterene. Clin Exp Hypertens A. 1983;5(2):249-269.

TRIAZOLAM

Trade: Halcion

Category: Sedative-Hypnotic

LRC: L3 - No Data-Probably Compatible

Triazolam is a typical benzodiazepine used as a nighttime sedative. Animal studies indicate that triazolam is secreted in milk although levels in human milk have not been reported.[1] As with all the benzodiazepines, some penetration into breast milk is likely.

T 1/2	1.5-5.5 h	MW	343 Da	PB	89%
Tmax	0.5-2 h	RID		Vd	1.1-2.7 L/kg
Oral	85%	M/P		pKa	1.5

Adult Concerns: Sedation, confusion, dizziness, incoordination, worsening depression, nervousness, nausea, vomiting, changes in liver function.

Adult Dose: 0.125-0.25 mg daily.

Pediatric Concerns: None reported via milk at this time.

Infant Monitoring: Sedation, slowed breathing rate, not waking to feed/poor feeding, and weight gain.

Alternatives: Lorazepam(L3), Midazolam(L2)

References:
1. Pharmaceutical manufacturers prescribing information.

TRIFLURIDINE OPHTHALMIC DROPS

Trade: Viroptic

Category: Other

LRC: L3 - No Data-Probably Compatible

Trifluridine, also known as trifluorothymidine, is a fluorinated pyrimidine nucleoside used in the treatment of both epithelial keratitis and keratoconjunctivitis of the eye which is caused by herpes simplex viruses 1 and 2. The drug interferes with DNA synthesis in cultured mammalian cells, but the actual mechanism of action is unknown. The major metabolite is 5-carboxy-2'-deoxyuridine. If the corneal epithelium is not intact, there is a twofold increase in penetration of the drug into the eye. Trifluridine is not effective against infections of the cornea by chlamydia, bacteria, or fungi. Trifluridine should not be used longer than 21 days. Systemic absorption of trifluridine ophthalmic preparation following therapeutic dosing appears to be negligible. No detectable concentrations of trifluridine or 5-carboxy-2'-deoxyuridine were found in the sera of adult healthy normal subjects who had trifluridine instilled into their eyes seven times daily for 14 consecutive days. Trifluridine ophthalmic drops are unlikely to be excreted in human milk after ophthalmic instillation because of the relatively small dosage (<5 mg/day), its dilution in body fluids, and its extremely short half-life (approx. 12 minutes).

T 1/2	12 min	MW	296.2 Da	PB	
Tmax		RID		Vd	
Oral		M/P		pKa	7.6

Adult Concerns: Transient burning or stinging, eyelid edema, contact dermatitis, impaired stomal wound healing, and increased ocular pressure.

Adult Dose: 1 drop every 2 hours, total 9 drops/day until corneal ulcer is healed; followed by 1 drop every 4 hours, total 5 drops/day for 7 days. Treatment should not exceed 21 days.

Pediatric Concerns:

Infant Monitoring:

Alternatives:

References:
1. NLM. Daily Med. US Dept of Health and Human Services; June 1, 2010. daily.nlm.nih.gov/dailymed/about.cfm. Accessed March 30, 2011.
2. Carmine AA, Brogden RN, Heel RC, Speight TM, Avery GS. Trifluridine: a review of its antiviral activity and therapeutic use in the topical treatment of viral eye infections. Drugs. 1982 May;23(5):329-353.

TRIHEXYPHENIDYL

Trade: Artane

Category: Anticholinergic

LRC: L3 - No Data-Probably Compatible

It is an antiparkinsonian agent of the antimuscarinic class, which binds to the M1 muscarinic receptor.[1] It is used to treat both Parkinson's disease and extrapyramidal symptoms (EPS) caused by some medications (e.g. phenothiazines, thioxanthenes). It is not known whether it is excreted in human milk. Therefore, trihexyphenidyl should only be used if the expected benefit to the mother outweighs the potential risk to the infant.

T 1/2	3.3-4 h	MW	337.9 Da	PB	
Tmax	2-3 h	RID		Vd	
Oral		M/P		pKa	

Adult Concerns: Drowsiness, vertigo, headache, agitation, anxiety, delirium, confusion, blurred vision, tachycardia, hypotension, dry mouth, abdominal discomfort, constipation, impaired sweating.

Adult Dose: 5-15 mg/day in 3-4 divided doses.

Pediatric Concerns:

Infant Monitoring: Agitation, drowsiness, dry mouth, constipation, urinary retention, weakness, weight gain.

Alternatives:

References:
1. Pharmaceutical manufacturers prescribing information.

TRIMEBUTINE MALEATE

Trade: Debridat, Modulon, Polybutin, Recutin, Timotor

Category: Opioid agonist

LRC: L3 - No Data-Probably Compatible

Trimebutine is a spasmolytic agent with some opioid agonistic action and some antiserotonergic activity; it is used to treat irritable bowel syndrome and to normalize intestinal transit time following abdominal surgery.[1] No data are available on the use of this product in breastfeeding mothers. However, a review of its pharmacokinetic properties suggests that transfer to breast milk is likely. Therefore, use of this drug during lactation is best avoided and should be used only if the potential benefits to the mother outweigh the potential risks to the infant.

T 1/2	10-12 h	MW	387 Da	PB	<5%
Tmax	1 h	RID		Vd	
Oral		M/P		pKa	

Adult Concerns: Headache, anxiety, dizziness, drowsiness, changes in hearing, dry mouth, dyspepsia, constipation, diarrhea, urinary retention, gynecomastia, hot or cold sensations.

Adult Dose: 200 mg three times daily.

Pediatric Concerns: None reported via milk; not recommended for use in pediatrics.

Infant Monitoring: Drowsiness, dry mouth, constipation or diarrhea, urinary retention.

Alternatives:

References:
1. Pharmaceutical manufacturers prescribing information.

TRIMETHADIONE

Trade: Tridione

Category: Anticonvulsant

LRC: L4 - No Data-Possibly Hazardous

Trimethadione is an oxazolidinedione compound used as an anticonvulsant.[1] There are no adequate and well-controlled studies or case reports in breastfeeding women. Due to its numerous side effects and toxicities, including significant risks of blood dyscrasias, this is not a preferred anticonvulsant for breastfeeding mothers.

T 1/2		MW	143 Da	PB	90%
Tmax	0.5 to 2 h	RID		Vd	
Oral	Complete	M/P		pKa	

Adult Concerns: Nausea, vomiting, abdominal pain, anorexia, weight loss, gastric distress. Observe for blood dyscrasias including aplastic anemia, neutropenia, agranulocytosis, and bleeding disorders. Hepatitis and jaundice have been reported.

Adult Dose: 900 mg/day in 3-4 divided doses.

Pediatric Concerns:

Infant Monitoring: Sedation or irritability, not waking to feed/poor feeding, vomiting, diarrhea, weight loss, jaundice.

Alternatives:

References:
1. Pharmaceutical manufacturers prescribing information.

TRIMETHOPRIM

Trade: Alprim, Monotrim, Primsol, Triprim

Category: Antibiotic, sulfonamide

LRC: L2 - Limited Data-Probably Compatible

Trimethoprim is an inhibitor of folic acid production in bacteria. In one study of 50 patients, average levels of trimethoprim in milk were 1.97 mg/L.[1] The milk/plasma ratio was 1.25. In another group of mothers receiving 160 mg two to four times daily, concentrations of 1.2 to 5.5 mg/L were reported in milk.

In a group of 40 women who received cotrimoxazole (320 mg daily), average milk levels ranged from 2-3 mg/L after 5 days.[2] In a separate group of 10 women, who received 480 mg/day, milk levels were approximately 2-3 mg/L as well.

Because trimethoprim may interfere with folate metabolism, its long-term use in young infants should be avoided in breastfeeding mothers, or the infant should be supplemented with folic acid. However, trimethoprim apparently poses few problems in full-term or older infants where it is commonly used clinically.

T 1/2	8-10 h	MW	290 Da	PB	44%
Tmax	1-4 h	RID	3.94% - 9.86%	Vd	
Oral	Complete	M/P	1.25	pKa	6.6

Adult Concerns: Rash, pruritus nausea, vomiting, anorexia, altered taste sensation.

Adult Dose: 100 mg twice daily.

Pediatric Concerns: None reported via milk.

Infant Monitoring:

Alternatives:

References:
1. Miller RD, Salter AJ. The passage of trimethoprim/sulphamethoxazole into breast milk and its significance. In: Daikos GK, ed. Progress in Chemotherapy, Proceedings of the Eight International Congress of Chemotherapy, Athens, 1973. Athens: Hellenic Society for Chemotherapy; 1974.
2. Miller RD, Salter AJ. The passage of trimethoprim/sulfamethoxazole into breast milk and its significance. In: Daikos CK, ed. Progress in chemotherapy. Antibacterial Chemother. 1974;1:687-691.

TRIPROLIDINE

Trade: Tripohist, Zymine

Category: Antihistamine

LRC: L1 - Limited Data-Compatible

Triprolidine is an antihistamine. It is secreted in milk but in very small levels and is marketed with pseudoephedrine as Actifed. In a study of three patients who received 2.5 mg triprolidine, the average concentration in milk ranged from 1.2 to 4.4 µg/L over 24 hours.[1] The relative infant dose is less than 1.8% of the weight-normalized maternal dose. This dose is far too low to be clinically relevant.

T 1/2	5 h	MW	278 Da	PB	
Tmax	2 h	RID	1.8%	Vd	
Oral	Complete	M/P	0.5-1.2	pKa	6.5

Adult Concerns: Sedation, dry mouth, anticholinergic side effects.

Adult Dose: 2.5 mg every 4-6 hours.

Pediatric Concerns: None reported.

Infant Monitoring: Sedation, dry mouth, constipation.

Alternatives:

References:
1. Findlay JW, Butz RF, Sailstad JM, Warren JT, Welch RM. Pseudoephedrine and triprolidine in plasma and breast milk of nursing mothers. Br J Clin Pharmacol. 1984;18(6):901-906.

TROLAMINE

Trade: Arthricream, Asper-Flex, FlexPower, Joint-Ritis, Mobisyl, Myoflex

Category: Analgesic

LRC: L3 - No Data-Probably Compatible

Trolamine is the salt formed by combining salicylic acid and triethanolamine.[1] It is used in sunscreens, analgesic topical balms, and cosmetics. Because trolamine is used topically for a local effect, it is unlikely to be absorbed systemically or produce problems for a breastfeeding mother or her infant. Topical absorption is estimated to be <10%. There are no adequate and well-controlled studies or case reports in breastfeeding women.

T 1/2	1-2 h	MW	287 Da	PB	50% to 90%
Tmax		RID		Vd	
Oral	Significant	M/P		pKa	7.8

Adult Concerns: Allergic reaction, rash, hives, nausea, vomiting.

Adult Dose: Apply topically three to four times a day.

Pediatric Concerns:

Infant Monitoring:

Alternatives: Ibuprofen(L1), Acetaminophen(L1)

References:
1. Pharmaceutical manufacturers prescribing information.

TROPICAMIDE

Trade: Diotrope, Mydral, Mydriacyl, Tropicacyl

Category: Mydriatic-Cycloplegic

LRC: L3 - No Data-Probably Compatible

Tropicamide is used as a short-acting pupil dilator used in diagnostic procedures. It is an antimuscarinic agent that produces competitive antagonism of the actions of acetylcholine, thus preventing the sphincter muscle of the iris and the muscle of the ciliary body from responding to cholinergic stimulation.[1] It is unlikely that systemic levels in adults will be sufficient to produce clinically relevant levels in milk. A brief waiting period of 3-4 hours would eliminate most risks.

T 1/2		MW	284 Da	PB	45%
Tmax		RID		Vd	
Oral		M/P		pKa	5.2

Adult Concerns: Sedation, dry mouth, blurred vision, corneal irritation, increased intraocular pressure, cardiorespiratory collapse, tachycardia.

Adult Dose: 1-2 drops 15-20 minutes before exam.

Pediatric Concerns: Pediatric patients may require smaller doses to avoid systemic effects. Levels in milk are probably too low to affect an infant.

Infant Monitoring: Sedation, mydriasis, dry mouth, vomiting.

Alternatives:

References:
1. Pharmaceutical manufacturers prescribing information.

TROSPIUM CHLORIDE

Trade: Sanctura XR

Category: Anticholinergic

LRC: L3 - No Data-Probably Compatible

Trospium chloride is a muscarinic antagonist used for the treatment of overactive bladder (OAB).[1,2] Although there are no human data regarding the excretion of this medication in breast milk, there are data from rodent studies; less than 1% of trospium chloride was excreted in the milk of lactating rats when given at doses of 2 mg/kg orally and 50 μg/kg intravenously.[2] This medication is less than 10% orally absorbed and when given with a high-fat meal the oral absorption is further reduced; therefore, a very limited systemic concentration would be expected in a breastfed infant.[2]

T 1/2	35 h	MW	428 Da	PB	50 to 85%
Tmax	5 h	RID		Vd	5.6 to 8.6 L/kg
Oral	< 10 %	M/P		pKa	

Adult Concerns: Dizziness, confusion, dry eyes, dry nose, dry mouth, tachycardia, dyspepsia, nausea, abdominal pain, constipation, urinary tract infections.

Adult Dose: 60 mg extended release once daily in the morning.

Pediatric Concerns: No data available in the pediatric population at this time.

Infant Monitoring: Drowsiness, dry mouth, constipation, urinary retention, weight loss, tremor.

Alternatives:

References:
1. Guay DR. Trospium chloride: an update on a quaternary anticholinergic for treatment of urge urinary incontinence. Ther Clin Risk Manag. 2005 Jun;1(2):157–167.
2. Pharmaceutical manufacturers prescribing information.

TROVAFLOXACIN MESYLATE

Trade: Alatrofloxacin, Trovan

Category: Antibiotic, Quinolone

LRC: L4 - Limited Data-Possibly Hazardous

Trovafloxacin mesylate is a synthetic broad-spectrum fluoroquinolone antibiotic for oral use. Its IV form is called alatrofloxacin mesylate, which is metabolized to trovafloxacin in vivo. Trovafloxacin was found in measurable but low concentrations in breast milk of three breastfeeding mothers.[1] Following an IV dose of 300 mg trovafloxacin equivalent and repeated oral 200 mg doses of trovafloxacin, breast milk levels averaged 0.8 mg/L and ranged from 0.3 to 2.1 mg/L. This would average less than 4% of the weight-normalized maternal dose. New data on this antibiotic, documents a higher risk of hepatotoxicity and its use is restricted. This agent has been withdrawn from the US market due to risk of acute liver failure.

Because fluoroquinolones have limited safety data in pediatric and breastfeeding patients, use in lactation is not recommended if alternative therapies exist.[1]

T 1/2	12.2 h	MW	512 Da	PB	76%
Tmax	1.2 h	RID	4.2%	Vd	1.3 L/kg
Oral	88%	M/P		pKa	8.09

Adult Concerns: Dizziness, nausea, headache, vomiting, diarrhea have been reported.

Adult Dose: 200-300 mg daily.

Pediatric Concerns: None reported via milk.

Infant Monitoring: Vomiting, diarrhea, changes in gastrointestinal flora, and rash.

Alternatives: Norfloxacin, Ofloxacin(L2), Ciprofloxacin(L3)

References:
1. Pharmaceutical manufacturers prescribing information.

TUBERCULIN PURIFIED PROTEIN DERIVATIVE

Trade: Aplisol, Mantoux, PPD, Sclavo, Tubersol

Category: Diagnostic Agent, Other

LRC: L1 - No Data-Compatible

Tuberculin (also called Mantoux, PPD, Tine test) is a skin test using antigen derived from the concentrated, sterile, soluble products of growth of *mycobacterium tuberculosis* or *mycobacterium bovis*. Small amounts of this purified product, when placed intradermally, produce a hypersensitivity reaction at the site of injection in those individuals with antibodies to *mycobacterium tuberculosis*.[1,2] Preliminary studies also indicate that breastfed infants may passively acquire sensitivity to mycobacterial antigens from mothers who are sensitized. There are no contraindications to using PPD tests in breastfeeding mothers as the proteins are sterilized and unlikely to penetrate milk.

Adult Concerns: Local vesiculation, irritation, bruising, and rarely hypersensitivity.

Adult Dose: 5 units X 1.

Pediatric Concerns: None via milk.

Infant Monitoring:

Alternatives:

References:
1. Pharmaceutical manufacturers prescribing information.
2. www.cdc.gov/breastfeeding/recommendations/vaccinations.htm

TUBERCULOSIS

Trade: Tuberculosis, Mycobacterium tuberculosis

Category: Infectious Disease

LRC: L3 - Limited Data-Probably Compatible

Mycobacterium tuberculosis is a bacterial species in the Mycobacteriaceae family and is the causative agent in pulmonary tuberculosis. Tuberculosis cannot be spread by personal contact such as shaking hands, toilet seats, sharing toothbrushes, or kissing. It can only be spread via air droplets from a person (not an infant) who has the disease and via coughing, sneezing, singing, or speaking. One of the highest potentials for spreading the disease to an infant is during the early stages of the disease in the mother in close respiratory contact with the infant. Breast milk does not contain *mycobacterium tuberculosis*. Mothers with an active tuberculin skin test, without evidence of disease, can continue to breastfeed. Mothers with newly active and untreated tuberculosis should be isolated from the infant. Once treatment has been instituted, and sputum samples are negative, the mothers can resume close contact and breastfeeding of the infant. Breastfeeding in women undergoing treatment with anti-tubercular drugs should not be discouraged for women. The concentrations of these drugs in breast milk are too small to produce toxicity in the nursing newborn. For the same reason, drugs in breast milk are not an effective treatment for TB disease or LTBI in a nursing infant. Breastfeeding women taking INH should also take pyridoxine (vitamin B6) supplementation.[1]

Adult Concerns: Bloody cough.

Adult Dose:

Pediatric Concerns:

Infant Monitoring: Remove infant from mother or other infected individuals, until oral antitubercular therapy has been instituted.

Alternatives: Isoniazid(L3), Rifampin(L2), Ethambutol(L3), Pyrazinamide(L3)

References:
1. https://www.cdc.gov/tb/topic/populations/pregnancy/

TYPHOID FEVER

Trade: Salmonella enterica serotype typhi

Category: Infectious Disease

LRC: L3 - No Data-Probably Compatible

Typhoid fever is caused by *Salmonella enterica serotype typhi*, a Gram-negative bacterium. Typhoid fever occurs primarily through the ingestion of contaminated food. The organisms invade through intestinal mucosa, multiply, and subsequently transfer to the blood. The incubation period is 7-14 days. The clinical presentation varies from mild illness with low-grade fever, malaise, and slight, dry cough to a severe clinical picture with high (typically over 103 degrees Fahrenheit) fever and severe diarrhea.

Some people may develop rash on the abdomen and chest called "rose spots." Complications include intestinal hemorrhage, intestinal perforation, kidney failure, and peritonitis. Some individuals rarely may become an asymptomatic carrier of typhoid fever, suffering no symptoms, but capable of infecting others.[1] The diagnosis of typhoid fever is made by culture of the causative microorganism in the setting of a compatible clinical illness. Blood cultures are positive in 40-80% of patients. Bone marrow culture is the most sensitive routinely available diagnostic tool.[2]

The treatment of typhoid fever with antibiotics include the use of ceftriaxone as main drug of choice, and fluoroquinolones like ciprofloxacin as an alternative.[1]

There are no data on the transfer of this infectious agent to human milk, but thus far there is no reported transmission of this agent via milk itself. Mothers should be advised to continue breastfeeding, but using frequent hand washing, and other hygienic control measures to reduce transmission from other foods, or objects (pacifier). It usually takes 7-10 days to make a diagnosis of typhoid fever during which the infant has already been breastfeeding. This is the time period when the typhoid organisms found most abundantly in the blood. Breast milk has many antibodies that probably protect the infant from infections such as this.

Adult Concerns: The clinical presentation varies from mild illness with low-grade fever, malaise, and slight, dry cough to a severe clinical picture with high (typically over 103 degrees Fahrenheit) fever and severe diarrhea.

Adult Dose:

Pediatric Concerns: No complications from breastfeeding with this syndrome have been found.

Infant Monitoring: Fever, malaise, dry cough, diarrhea.

Alternatives:

References:

1. Parry CM, Hien TT, Dougan G, White NJ, Farrar JJ. Typhoid fever. N Engl J Med. 2002 Nov;347(22):1770-1782.
2. Gasem MH, Dolmans WM, Isbandrio BB, Wahyono H, Keuter M, Djokomoeljanto R. Culture of Salmonella typhi and Salmonella paratyphi from blood and bone marrow in suspected typhoid fever. Trop Geogr Med. 1995;47(4):164-167.
3. Lanata CF, Levine MM, Ristori C, et al. Vi serology in detection of chronic Salmonella typhi carriers in an endemic area. Lancet. 1983 Aug 20;2(8347):441-443.

TYPHOID VACCINE

Trade: Typhim Vi, Vivotif Berna

Category: Vaccine

LRC: L3 - No Data-Probably Compatible

Typhoid vaccine promotes active immunity against typhoid fever. It is available in an oral form, Ty21a, which is a live attenuated vaccine for oral administration.[1] The parenteral (injectable) form is derived from acetone-treated killed and dried bacteria, phenol-inactive bacteria, or a special capsular polysaccharide vaccine extracted from killed *Salmonella typhi* Ty21a strains. Due to a limited lipopolysaccharide coating, the Ty21a strains are limited in their ability to produce infection. No data are available on its transfer to human milk. If immunization is required, the injectable form would be preferred, as infection of the neonate would be unlikely. According to the CDC, the polysaccharide (ViCPS) and live bacterial Ty21a should only be used when risk of exposure is high as there is no safety data available during lactation.

Adult Concerns: Following oral administration, nausea, abdominal cramps, vomiting, urticaria. IM preparations may produce soreness at injection site, tenderness, malaise, headache, myalgia, fever.

Adult Dose: 0.5 mL X 2 over 4 weeks.

Pediatric Concerns: None reported, but injectable killed vaccine suggested.

Infant Monitoring:

Alternatives:

References:
1. Pharmaceutical manufacturers prescribing information.
2. www.cdc.gov/breastfeeding/recommendations/vaccinations.htm

TYROPANOATE

Trade: Bilopaque

Category: Diagnostic Agent, Radiological Contrast Media

LRC: L3 - No Data-Probably Compatible

Tyropanoate is an oral contrast agent used for examining the gallbladder, when gallstones are suspected. It contains 57.4% bound iodine and is only used in adults.[1] Safety in pediatrics has not been established. There have been no studies done on the transfer of tyropanoate to human milk. It is possible that minimal drug would transfer to the milk compartment; however, levels are unknown.

T 1/2	45% gone in 24 h	MW	641 Da	PB	Moderate
Tmax		RID		Vd	
Oral	Well absorbed	M/P		pKa	

Adult Concerns: Hypotension, tachycardia, fever, chills, perspiration, nausea, vomiting, diarrhea, pain, and cramping of extremities. Rarely allergic reactions occur including rash, urticaria, pruritus, dysphagia, syncope, shock and chest pain, conjunctivitis.

Adult Dose:

Pediatric Concerns:

Infant Monitoring:

Alternatives:

References:
1. Pharmaceutical manufacturers prescribing information.

ULIPRISTAL ACETATE

Trade: Ella, Fibristal

Category: Contraceptive

LRC: L3 - Limited Data-Probably Compatible

Ulipristal acetate is a selective progesterone receptor modulator with two indications. In certain countries, such as the United States, a single dose can be used for emergency contraception within 120 hours of unprotected intercourse.[1] In others countries, such as Canada, it can be used for the treatment of uterine fibroids. The manufacturer reports that after this medication was given to 12 breastfeeding women for emergency contraception the mean concentration of ulipristal and its metabolite monodemethyl-ulipristal acetate in milk were 22.7 ng/mL and 4.49 ng/mL in the first 24 hours.[1] Using this mean ulipristil concentration in the first 24 hours of therapy, the relative infant dose was 0.8%. The mean concentration of drug then declined at 24-48 hours, 48-72 hours, 72-96 hours and 96-120 hours to 2.96 ng/mL, 1.56 ng/mL, 1.04 ng/mL and 0.69 ng/mL, respectively. The manufacturer did not report any neonatal outcomes as the infants in this report were not breastfed.

T 1/2	32-38 h	MW	475.6 Da	PB	>98%
Tmax	1 h	RID	0.79%	Vd	
Oral	100%	M/P		pKa	

Adult Concerns: Headache, fatigue, dizziness, acne, nausea, abdominal pain, dysmenorrhea.

Adult Dose: 30 mg within 120 hours of intercourse; 5 mg daily for 3 months for fibroids.

Pediatric Concerns:

Infant Monitoring:

Alternatives: Levonorgestrel (L3)

References:
1. Pharmaceutical manufacturer prescribing information.

UNDECYLENIC ACID

Trade: Cruex, Desenex, Trifungol

Category: Antifungal

LRC: L3 - No Data-Probably Compatible

Undecylenic acid and its derivatives are fatty acids that are used topically in the treatment of fungal infections, most often in tinea pedis, tinea cruris, and ringworm. This medication exerts a fungistatic action, though fungicidal properties have been observed at extremely high doses. Undecylenic acid is found naturally in human sweat, and is absorbed orally.[1] Presently, there are no data regarding the use of undecylenic acid or its derivatives in breastfeeding women. As a topical agent it is unlikely that undecylenic acid will be absorbed systemically in a high enough concentration to have an adverse effect on breastfeeding infants.

T 1/2		MW	184.27 Da	PB	
Tmax		RID		Vd	
Oral		M/P		pKa	

Adult Concerns: Rash, skin irritation, stinging, sensitization.

Adult Dose: Apply as needed twice daily for 2-4 weeks.

Pediatric Concerns:

Infant Monitoring:

Alternatives:

References:
1. Gomez I. The teratogenic effect of unsaturated short-chain fatty acids in Rhodnium prolixus. Mem Inst Oswaldo Cruz. 1985;80:375-385.

UREA

Trade:

Category: Other

LRC: L3 - No Data-Probably Compatible

Urea is a chemical that is formed from protein breakdown. It is a large source of nitrogen in urine. It acts as a humectant in creams to improve hydration of the skin. Urea is naturally found in human milk[1]. Urea comprises approximately 15% of milk nitrogen, and some of this urea may be used by gut bacteria as a source of nitrogen.[1,2]

T 1/2		MW	60 Da	PB	
Tmax		RID		Vd	
Oral	Rapid	M/P		pKa	

Adult Concerns: Local irritation, stinging.

Adult Dose: Apply one to three times/day (topical).

Pediatric Concerns:

Infant Monitoring:

Alternatives:

References:
1. Harzer G, Franzke V, Bindels JG. Human milk nonprotein nitrogen components:changing patterns of free amino acids and urea in the course of early lactation. Am J Clin Nutr. 1984 Aug;40(2):303-309.
2. Jackson AA. Urea as a nutrient: bioavailability and role in nitrogen economy. Arch Dis Child. 1994 Jan;70(1):3-4.

URSODIOL

Trade: Actigall, Combidol, Destolit, Lithofalk, Urdox, Urso, Ursodeoxycholic acid, Ursogal

Category: Gastrointestinal agent

LRC: L3 - No Data-Probably Compatible

Ursodiol (ursodeoxycholic acid) is a bile salt found in small amounts in humans that is used to dissolve cholesterol gallstones. It is almost completely absorbed orally via the portal circulation and is extracted almost completely by the liver. Ursodiol suppresses hepatic synthesis and excretion of cholesterol. Following extraction by the liver, it is conjugated with glycine or taurine and is resecreted into the hepatic bile duct. Only trace amounts are found in the plasma and it is not likely significant amounts would be present in milk.[1] While no breastfeeding data are available, only small amounts of bile salts are known to be present in milk.[2] It is not likely with the low levels of ursodiol in the maternal plasma, that clinically relevant amounts would enter milk.

T 1/2		MW	392 Da	PB	
Tmax		RID		Vd	
Oral	90%	M/P		pKa	4.76

Adult Concerns: Insomnia, headache, dizziness, nausea, vomiting, abdominal pain, flatulence, constipation, diarrhea, rash.

Adult Dose: 8-10 mg/kg/day in 3 divided doses.

Pediatric Concerns: None via breast milk.

Infant Monitoring: Vomiting, diarrhea, constipation.

Alternatives:

References:
1. Bachrach WH, Hofmann AF. Ursodeoxycholic acid in the treatment of cholesterol cholelithiasis. part I. Dig Dis Sci. 1982;27(8):737-761.
2. Forsyth JS, Ross PE, Bouchier IA. Bile salts in breast milk. Eur J Pediatr. 1983;140(2):126-127.

USTEKINUMAB

Trade: Stelara

Category: Monoclonal Antibody

LRC: L3 - No Data-Probably Compatible

Ustekinumab is a human IgG1 monoclonal antibody against the p40 subunit of the IL-12 and IL-23 cytokines. It is comprised of 1326 amino acids and has an estimated molecular weight of 149,000 Da.[1] It is used in the treatment of severe plaque psoriasis patients who are candidates for phototherapy or systemic therapy. The drug has also been used in treating rheumatoid arthritis. Ustekinumab is excreted in the milk of lactating monkeys.[2] While some IgG is excreted into human milk, levels of ustekinumab are probably exceedingly low. It is not known if ustekinumab is absorbed systemically after ingestion.

Although the molecular weight of this medication is very large and the amount in breast milk is very low, there are no long-term data concerning the safety of using immune modulating medications in breastfeeding mothers. Further there are current data that suggest that some IgG drugs do transfer to milk, and perhaps the breastfed infant. Therefore, some caution is recommended, and each woman should understand the benefits and risk of using this type of medication in lactation.

T 1/2	14.9-45.6 days	MW	148,079 Da	PB	
Tmax	13.5 days	RID		Vd	0.161 L/kg
Oral	Nil	M/P		pKa	

Adult Concerns: Headache, fatigue, dizziness, infection, antibody development, injection site reaction, pruritus.

Adult Dose: 45-90 mg every 12 weeks.

Pediatric Concerns: No studies available.

Infant Monitoring: Fever, frequent infections, poor feeding/poor weight gain.

Alternatives: Etanercept(L2), Infliximab(L3)

References:
1. Pharmaceutical manufacturers prescribing information.
2. Martin PL, Sachs C, Imai N, et al. Development in the cynomolgus macaque following administration of ustekinumab, a human anti-IL-12/23p40 monoclonal antibody, during pregnancy and lactation. Birth Defects Res B Dev Reprod Toxicol. 2010 Oct;89(5):351-363.

VALACYCLOVIR

Trade: Valaciclovir, Valtrex

Category: Antiviral

LRC: L2 - Limited Data-Probably Compatible

Valacyclovir is a prodrug that is rapidly metabolized in the plasma to acyclovir. In a study of five women who received 500 mg twice daily for 7 days after delivery, the median peak acyclovir concentration in breast milk was 4.2 mg/L at 4 hours while the average concentration (AUC) was 2.24 mg/L if 12 hour dosing intervals were used.[1] Thus the relative infant dose would be 4.7% of the weight-normalized maternal dose. The milk/serum ratio was highest 4 hours after the initial dose at 3.4 and then reached a steady state ratio at 1.85. Valacyclovir is rapidly converted to acyclovir, which transfers into breast milk. However, the amount of acyclovir in breast milk after valacyclovir administration is considerably less than that used in therapeutic dosing of neonates.

T 1/2	2.5-3 h	MW	324.3 Da	PB	9%-33%
Tmax	1.5 h	RID	4.7%	Vd	
Oral	54%	M/P	0.6-4.1	pKa	

Adult Concerns: Nausea, vomiting, diarrhea, sore throat, edema, and skin rashes.

Adult Dose: 500-1000 mg two to three times daily.

Pediatric Concerns: None reported via milk.

Infant Monitoring: Vomiting, diarrhea.

Alternatives: Acyclovir(L2)

References:
1. Sheffield JS, Fish DN, Hollier LM, Cadematori S, Nobles BJ, Wendel GD, Jr. Acyclovir concentrations in human breast milk after valaciclovir administration. Am J Obstet Gynecol. 2002;186(1):100-102.

VALERIAN OFFICINALIS

Trade: All-heal, Garden heliotrope, Garden valerian

Category: Herb

LRC: L4 - No Data-Possibly Hazardous

Valerian root is most commonly used as a sedative/hypnotic. Of the numerous chemicals present in the root, the most important chemical group appears to be the valepotriates. This family consists of at least a dozen or more related compounds and is believed responsible for the sedative potential of this plant although it is controversial. The combination of numerous components may inevitability account for the sedative response. Controlled studies in man have indicated a sedative/hypnotic effect with fewer night awakenings and significant somnolence.[1-3] The toxicity of valerian root appears to be low, with only minor side effects reported. However, the valepotriates have been found to be cytotoxic, with alkylating activity similar to other nitrogen mustard-like anticancer agents. Should this prove to be so in vivo, it may preclude the use of this product in humans. No data are available on the transfer of valerian root compounds to human milk. However, the use of sedatives in breastfeeding mothers is generally discouraged; if required, medications with lactation data are preferred.

Adult Concerns: Ataxia, hypothermia, muscle relaxation. Headaches, excitability, cardiac disturbances.

Adult Dose:

Pediatric Concerns: None reported via human milk.

Infant Monitoring: Sedation.

Alternatives: Oxazepam(L2), Lorazepam(L3), Zopiclone(L2)

References:
1. Leathwood PD, Chauffard F, Heck E, Munoz-Box R. Aqueous extract of valerian root (Valeriana officinalis L.) improves sleep quality in man. Pharmacol Biochem Behav. 1982;17(1):65-71.

2. von Eickstedt KW, Rahman S. Psychopharmacologic effect of valepotriates. Arzneimittelforschung. 1969;19(3):316-319.
3. Leathwood PD, Chauffard F. Aqueous extract of valerian reduces latency to fall asleep in man. Planta Med. 1985;51(2):144-148.

VALGANCICLOVIR

Trade: Valcyte

Category: Antiviral

LRC: L3 - No Data-Probably Compatible

Valganciclovir is a prodrug that is rapidly metabolized to the active antiviral drug ganciclovir.[1] It is used for cytomegalovirus infections particularly in HIV infected patients. The oral bioavailability of valganciclovir is 60% while only 6% with its active metabolite ganciclovir. Further, it is very water soluble and lipophobic, which would suggest milk levels will be low. No data are available on its use in breastfeeding mothers but its oral absorption in the infant is likely low.

Please note: The Centers for Disease Control and Prevention recommend that HIV-1 infected mothers do not breastfeed their infants to avoid postnatal transmission of HIV-1.

T 1/2	4 h	MW	390 Da	PB	1%-2%
Tmax	1-3 h	RID		Vd	0.7 L/kg
Oral	60%	M/P		pKa	7.6

Adult Concerns: Headache, insomnia, nausea, abdominal pain, diarrhea, neutropenia, anemia, catheter-related infections.

Adult Dose: 450-900 mg daily.

Pediatric Concerns: None data in breastfeeding at this time.

Infant Monitoring: Insomnia, diarrhea, neutropenia.

Alternatives:

References:
1. Pharmaceutical manufacturers prescribing information.

VALPROIC ACID

Trade: Convulex, Depacon, Depakene, Depakote, Deproic, Epilim, Stavzor, Valpro, Divalproex

Category: Anticonvulsant

LRC: L4 - Limited Data-Possibly Hazardous

Valproic acid is a popular anticonvulsant used in grand mal, petit mal, myoclonic, temporal lobe seizures, and for treatment of manic disorders. In a study of 16 patients receiving 300-2400 mg/day, valproic acid concentrations ranged from 0.4 to 3.9 mg/L (mean 1.9 mg/L).[1] The milk/plasma ratio averaged 0.05. In a study of one patient receiving 250 mg twice daily, milk levels ranged from 0.18 to 0.47 mg/L. The milk/plasma ratio ranged from 0.01 to 0.02.[2]

There are also two case reports of mothers who took valproate during lactation.[3] The first mother took 750 mg once daily and her infant had serum levels of 4 µg/mL and the second mother took 250 mg twice daily and her infant had serum levels of 1 µg/mL. Both infants had normal complete blood counts and liver function tests. Development was reported to be normal at 18 months of age for the first infant and at 12 months of age for the second infant.

Four mothers who took 1200-1500 mg a day of sodium valproate for seizure control were followed during pregnancy and the postpartum period.[4] The concentration of valproate in milk was 5%-10% of the maternal dose (estimated to be about 6 mg/L breast milk). There were no reports of infant side effects from breastfeeding.

There are two additional cases where mothers were given sodium valproate for seizure control. In the first case the mother took 1000 mg a day, milk samples were drawn on day 6, 7, and 17 after delivery and the milk levels were 3, 2.3, and 1.4 µg/mL, respectively.[5] The maternal concentration was 104 µg/mL on day 118 after delivery. In the second case, the mother took 1400 mg a day, breast milk samples were drawn on day 1, 3, 15, 29, and 43, the milk levels were 2, 1.4, 3.5, 2.3, and 2.8 µg/mL respectively. The maternal level in case 2 was 108 µg/mL on day 43 postpartum.

Alexander reports milk levels of 5.1 mg/L following a larger dose of up to 1600 mg/day.[6] In a study of six women receiving 9.5 to 31 mg/kg/day valproic acid, milk levels averaged 1.4 mg/L while serum levels averaged 45.1 mg/L.[7] The average milk/serum ratio was 0.027.

There is also a report of six mother-infant pairs that were exposed to divalproex sodium (valproate) in breast milk.[8] Five of the mothers began therapy within 24 hours of delivery and doses were titrated to achieve a therapeutic level between 50-100 μg/mL (doses ranged from 750-1000 mg/day). Four weeks after initiation of therapy (infants 4-19 weeks old) maternal and infant serum levels were drawn and the maternal levels ranged from 56.2-79 μg/mL (one patient sub-therapeutic 39.4 μg/mL) and infant serum levels ranged from 0.7-1.5 μg/mL. These data also demonstrated that breast milk drug exposure is low as infants achieved 0.9%-2.3% of maternal drug levels.

Although most authors agree that the amount of valproic acid transferring to the infant via milk is low and breast-feeding would appear safe, there has been one report of an infant having had thrombocytopenic purpura. Valproic acid may have been the cause; however, viral illness was not able to be ruled out.[9] Therefore, if clinically indicated the infant may need monitoring of liver and platelet changes.

A Norwegian study published in 2013 assessed the adverse effects of antiepileptic medications via breast milk in infants who were also exposed in utero.[10] The study evaluated maternal reports of their child's behavior, motor, social and language skills at 6, 18, and 36 months using validated screening tools. At age 6 months, infants of mothers using antiepileptic drugs in utero had a significantly higher risk of impaired fine motor skills when compared to control group infants. In addition, infants exposed to multiple antiepileptics also had a greater risk of fine motor and social impairment when compared to control group infants. However, it was noted that continuous breastfeeding in the first 6 months did demonstrate a trend toward improvement in all of the developmental domains.

In addition, the study demonstrated that continuous breastfeeding (daily for more than 6 months) in children of women using antiepileptic drugs in utero reduced the impairment in development at 6 and 18 months when compared with those who did not breastfeed or breastfed for less than 6 months. At 18 months, children in the drug-exposed group had an increased risk of impaired development compared with the reference group; the risks were highest in children who stopped breastfeeding early. Within the drug-exposed group, this impairment was statistically significant for autistic traits, 22.4% with discontinued breastfeeding were affected compared with 8.7% with prolonged breastfeeding. By 36 months, prenatal antiepileptic drug exposure was associated with impaired development such as autistic traits, reduced sentence completeness and aggressive symptoms, regardless of breastfeeding during the first year of life. The authors concluded that women with epilepsy should be encouraged to breastfeed regardless of their antiepileptic medication. However, the use of valproic acid should be discouraged, as there are other anticonvulsants without these neurobehavioral complications.

In 2014, a prospective observational study looked at long-term neurodevelopment of infants exposed to antiepileptic drugs in utero and lactation.[11] This study included women taking carbamazepine, lamotrigine, phenytoin or valproate as monotherapy for epilepsy. In this study 42.9% of the infants were breastfed for a mean of 7.2 months. The IQ of these children at 6 years of age was statistically significantly lower in children who were exposed to valproate in utero (7-13 IQ points lower). It was also noted that higher doses of medication (primarily with valproate) were associated with lower IQ scores. The children's IQ scores were found to be higher if the maternal IQ was higher, the mother took folic acid near the time of conception and if the child was breastfed (4 points higher). In addition, verbal abilities were also found to be significantly higher in children that were breastfed. Although this study has many limitations (e.g., small sample size, difficulties with patient follow-up) it does provide data up to age 6 that suggest benefits of breastfeeding are not out-weighed by risks of maternal drug therapy in milk.

T 1/2	14 h	MW	144 Da	PB	94%
Tmax	1-4 h	RID	0.99%-5.6%	Vd	0.1-0.4 L/kg
Oral	Complete	M/P	0.42	pKa	4.8

Adult Concerns: Sedation, thrombocytopenia, tremor, nausea, diarrhea, liver toxicity.

Adult Dose: 10-30 mg/kg daily.

Pediatric Concerns: One report of an infant having had thrombocytopenic purpura; however, viral illness was not ruled out in this case.[9]

Infant Monitoring: Sedation or irritability, not waking to feed/poor feeding and weight gain. Based on clinical symptoms some infants may require monitoring of liver enzymes or platelets.

Alternatives:

References:

1. von Unruh GE, Froescher W, Hoffmann F, Niesen M. Valproic acid in breast milk: how much is really there? Ther Drug Monit. 1984;6(3):272-276.
2. Dickinson RG, Harland RC, Lynn RK, Smith WB, Gerber N. Transmission of valproic acid (Depakene) across the placenta: half-life of the drug in mother and baby. J Pediatr. 1979;94(5):832-835.
3. Wisner K, Perel J. Serum levels of valproate and carbamazepine in breastfeeding mother-infant pairs. J Clin Psychopharmacol. 1998;18:167-169.
4. Philbert A, Pedersen B, Dam M. Concentration of valproate during pregnancy, in the newborn and in breast milk. Acta Neurol Scand. 1985;72:460-463.
5. Tsuru N, Maeda T, Tsuruoka M. Three cases of delivery under sodium valproate- placental transfer, milk transfer and probable teratogenicity of sodium valproate. Jpn J Psychiatr Neurol. 1988;42:89-96.

6. Alexander FW. Sodium valproate and pregnancy. Arch Dis Child. 1979;54(3):240.
7. Nau H, Rating D, Koch S, Hauser I, Helge H. Valproic acid and its metabolites: placental transfer, neonatal pharmacokinetics, transfer via mother's milk and clinical status in neonates of epileptic mothers. J Pharmacol Exp Ther. 1981;219(3):768-777.
8. Piontek CM, Baab S, Peindl KS, Wisner KL. Serum valproate levels in 6 breastfeeding mother-infant pairs. J Clin Psychiatry. 2000;61(3):170-172.
9. Stahl MM, Neiderud J, Vinge E. Thrombocytopenic purpura in a breast-fed infant whose mother was treated with valproic acid. J Pediatr. 1997;130(6):1001-1003.
10. Veiby G, Engelsen BA, Gilhus NE. Early child development and exposure to antiepileptic drugs prenatally and through breastfeeding A prospective cohort study on children of women with epilepsy. JAMA Neurol. 2013;70(11):1367-1374.
11. Meador KJ, Baker GA, Browning N, et al. Breastfeeding in children of women taking antiepileptic drugs cognitive outcomes at age 6. JAMA Pediatr. 2014;168(8):729-736.

VALSARTAN

Trade: Diovan

Category: Angiotensin II Receptor Antagonist

LRC: L3 - No Data-Probably Compatible

Valsartan is an angiotensin-II receptor antagonist used to treat hypertension.[1] Other medications should be used if suitable for the maternal medical condition (e.g., ramipril, labetalol, nifedipine). In addition, its use early postpartum in lactating mothers should be approached with caution, particularly in mothers with premature infants.

Both the ACE inhibitor family and the specific angiotensin II receptor blockers are contraindicated in pregnancy and thus should be used with caution in women who are planning a subsequent pregnancy in the near future.

T 1/2	6 h	MW	435.5 Da	PB	95%
Tmax	2-4 h	RID		Vd	0.24 L/kg
Oral	23%	M/P		pKa	8.15

Adult Concerns: Headache, dizziness, fatigue, hypotension, nausea, diarrhea, constipation, changes in renal function/urine output, hyperkalemia.

Adult Dose: 80-320 mg daily.

Pediatric Concerns: None reported via milk at this time.

Infant Monitoring: Drowsiness, lethargy, pallor, poor feeding, and weight gain.

Alternatives: Ramipril(L3), Enalapril(L2), Captopril(L2)

References:
1. Pharmaceutical manufacturers prescribing information.

VANCOMYCIN

Trade: Vancocin, Vancoled

Category: Antibiotic, Other

LRC: L1 - Limited Data-Compatible

Vancomycin is an antimicrobial agent used intravenously to treat staphylococcal and streptococcal infections, and orally to treat clostridium difficile infections (not absorbed orally, only treats organisms in gut).[1] Due to this medication's large molecular weight (1449 Da), very little drug is anticipated enter milk. This medication also has very low oral bioavailability; therefore, any medication that enters breast milk would have difficulty being absorbed by the infant's gut.

In an older study, which followed pregnant women given vancomycin, a single postpartum milk sample was obtained.[2] This woman received vancomycin 1 gram IV every 12 hours from 35-38 weeks gestation. The woman's vancomycin peak level was reported to be 36.1 mg/L (30 min after end of infusion) and her trough was 12.5 mg/L. At the time of birth, a cord blood sample was taken from the neonate, this level was 2.5 hours after the end of infusion of the last maternal dose of vancomycin and was 13.2 mg/L. The breast milk sample was taken about 4 hours after the end of the infusion of the last maternal dose before delivery and was 12.7 mg/L. Using this level, the relative infant dose was 6.7% and the infant dose was 1.9 mg/kg/day. This level was drawn during the colostrol phase (within hours after delivery) so levels in mature milk are expected to be even lower. In addition, its poor absorption from the infant's gastrointestinal tract limit its ability to have systemic adverse effects in the breastfed infant.

T 1/2	5-11 h	MW	1,449 Da	PB	20%-50%
Tmax		RID	6.57%-6.67%	Vd	0.3-0.7 L/kg
Oral	Negligible	M/P		pKa	8.78

Adult Concerns: Headache, drug fever, ototoxicity, hypotension and flushing during infusion, nausea, vomiting, diarrhea, changes in kidney function, neutropenia, thrombocytopenia.

Adult Dose: 1000 mg IV every 8-12 hours.

Pediatric Concerns: None reported via milk.

Infant Monitoring: Vomiting, diarrhea, changes in gastrointestinal flora.

Alternatives:

References:
1. Pharmaceutical manufacturers prescribing information.
2. Reyes MP, Ostrea EM Jr, Cabinian AE, Schmitt C, Rintelmann W. Vancomycin during pregnancy: does it cause hearing loss or nephrotoxicity in the infant? Am J Obstet Gynecol. 1989;161(4):977-981.

VARENICLINE

Trade: Champix, Chantix

Category: Smoking Cessation Agent

LRC: L4 - No Data-Possibly Hazardous

Varenicline is used to assist smoking cessation. It is a partial alpha-4-beta-2-nicotinic receptor agonist that binds to nicotine receptors in the brain, thus preventing nicotine stimulation. It stimulates dopamine activity, but to a lesser extent than nicotine, thus reducing craving and withdrawal symptoms.[1] There have been no studies performed on the transfer of varenicline to human milk; however, based on this medications long half-life, poor protein binding and small molecular weight it is anticipated to transfer to human milk. Caution should be used in breastfeeding mothers until more data are available.

T 1/2	24 h	MW	361 Da	PB	Less than 20%
Tmax	3-4 h	RID		Vd	
Oral	90%	M/P		pKa	9.73

Adult Concerns: Headache, insomnia, abnormal dreams, agitation, changes in mood, chest pain, dry mouth, decreased appetite, nausea, vomiting, constipation, flatulence.

Adult Dose: 1 mg twice daily.

Pediatric Concerns: No data are available at this time.

Infant Monitoring: Changes in sleep, changes in feeding, vomiting, constipation.

Alternatives:

References:
1. Pharmaceutical manufacturers prescribing information.

VARICELLA VACCINE

Trade: Varivax

Category: Vaccine

LRC: L2 - No Data-Probably Compatible

A live attenuated varicella vaccine was recently approved for marketing by the US Food and Drug Administration. Although effective, it does not apparently provide the immunity attained from infection with the parent virus and may not provide life-long immunity. The Oka/Merck strain used in the vaccine is attenuated by passage in human and embryonic guinea pig cell cultures. It is not known if the vaccine-acquired VZV is secreted in human milk, nor its infectiousness to infants. Interestingly, in two women with varicella-zoster infections, the virus was not culturable from milk. The antibody from the varicella zoster vaccine has been isolated in breast milk along with the DNA.[2] Both the AAP and the Centers for Disease Control approve the use of varicella-zoster vaccines in breastfeeding mothers, if the risk of infection is high.[3] Consult pediatrician prior to maternal vaccination for risks/benefits discussion if infant is known to be immunocompromised; caution is recommended.

Adult Concerns: Tenderness and erythema at the injection site in about 25% of patients and a sparse generalized maculopapular rash occurring within one month after immunization in about 5%. Spread of the vaccine virus to others has been reported. Susceptible, immunodeficient individuals should be protected from exposure.

Adult Dose: 0.5 mL X 2 over 4-8 weeks.

Pediatric Concerns: None reported via milk, but no studies are available.

Infant Monitoring:

Alternatives:

References:

1. Frederick IB, White RJ, Braddock SW. Excretion of varicella-herpes zoster virus in breast milk. Am J Obstet Gynecol. 1986;154(5):1116-1117.
2. Yoshida M, Yamagami N, Tezuka T, Hondo R. Case report: detection of varicella-zoster virus DNA in maternal breast milk. J Med Virol. 1992;38(2):108-110.
3. American Academy of Pediatrics. Committee on Infectious Diseases. Elk Grove Village, IL: Red Book; 1997.

VARICELLA-ZOSTER INFECTION

Trade: Chickenpox, Shingles

Category: Infectious Disease

LRC: L4 - Limited Data-Possibly Hazardous

The varicella-zoster virus (VZV) belongs to the family of herpes viruses. Mode of transmission includes aerosol droplet transmission, contact with the infected vesicular rash, and transplacental passage.[1] The incubation period is generally 14-16 days after exposure. In the unimmunized or in those exposed for the first time, VZV establishes a primary infection, otherwise known as chickenpox. It is characterized by a generalized rash and mild flu-like symptoms. Following the primary infection, VZV tends to remain latent in the dorsal root ganglia and may become re-activated later in life causing herpes zoster infection, popularly known as shingles.

Chickenpox virus has been reported to be transferred via breast milk in one 27-year-old mother who developed chickenpox postpartum.[2] Her 2-month old son also developed the disease 16 days after the mother. Chickenpox virus was detected in the mother's milk and may suggest that transmission can occur via breast milk. However, in a study of two breastfeeding patients who developed varicella-herpes zoster infections, in neither case was the virus isolated and cultured from their milk.[3]

An additional paper from Turkey described the case of a 27-year-old woman who breastfed her 4-month-old baby during a primary VZV infection. Varicella IgM was found in her blood and VZV DNA in her milk. The baby was exclusively breastfed for 3 weeks despite open sores on the mother's areola. The infant developed an apparent VZV-related pneumonia. There being no commercial Varicella-Zoster Immune Globulin available. The baby showed no signs of disease after the 3-week follow-up period.[4]

According to the American Academy of Pediatrics, airborne and contact precautions are recommended for neonates born to mothers with varicella and, if still hospitalized, should be continued until 21 or 28 days of age if they received Varicella-Zoster Immune Globulin or IGIV. Infants with varicella embryopathy do not require isolation if they do not have active lesions.[5] More recently, many infectious disease physicians now (2020) recommend treatment of the infant with an antiviral and continued breastfeeding.

Candidates for VZIG include; immunocompromised children, pregnant women, and a newborn infant whose mother has onset of VZV within 5 days before or 48 hours after delivery. For an excellent review of VZV and breastfeeding see Merewood and Philipp.[6]

Adult Concerns:

Adult Dose:

Pediatric Concerns: Varicella-zoster virus transfers into human milk. Infants should not breastfeed unless protected with VZIG.

Infant Monitoring: High fever, rash.

Alternatives:

References:

1. AAP CoID. Varicella-Zoster Infections. In: Red Book: 2009 Report of the Committe on Infectious Diseases. Edited by Pickering LK BC, Kimberlin DW, Long SS, 28 ed. Elk Grove Village, IL: American Academy of Pediatrics; 2009:714-727.
2. Yoshida M, Yamagami N, Tezuka T, Hondo R. Case report: detection of varicella-zoster virus DNA in maternal breast milk. J Med Virol. 1992;38(2):108-110.
3. Frederick IB, White RJ, Braddock SW. Excretion of varicella-herpes zoster virus in breast milk. Am J Obstet Gynecol. 1986;154(5):1116-1117.
4. Karabayir N, Yasa B, Gokcay G. Chickenpox infection during lactation. Breastfeed Med. 2015;10(1):71-72.

5. Committee on Infectious Diseases, American Academy of Pediatrics. In: Larry K. Pickering, MD, ed. FAAP Red Book 29th ed. Elk Grove Village, IL: American Academy of Pediatrics; 2012.

6. Merewood A, Philipp B. Breastfeeding: Conditions and Diseases. 1st ed. Amarillo, TX: Pharmasoft Publishing L.P.; 2001.

VASOPRESSIN

Trade: Pitresin, Pitressin, Pressyn

Category: Vasopressor

LRC: L3 - No Data-Probably Compatible

Vasopressin, also known as the antidiuretic hormone, is a small peptide (8 amino acids) that is normally secreted by the posterior pituitary.[1] It reduces urine production by the kidney. Although it probably passes to some degree to human milk, it is rapidly destroyed in the gastrointestinal tract by trypsin and must be administered by injection or intranasally. Hence, oral absorption by a nursing infant is very unlikely. Desmopressin is virtually identical and milk levels have been reported to be very low.

T 1/2	10-20 min	MW		PB	
Tmax	1 h	RID		Vd	
Oral	None	M/P		pKa	8

Adult Concerns: Increased blood pressure, water retention and edema, sweating, tremor, and bradycardia.

Adult Dose: 5-10 units daily.

Pediatric Concerns: None reported via milk.

Infant Monitoring:

Alternatives:

References:

1. Cobaugh, ed. AFHS Drug Information. New York, NY: McGraw-Hill;2018.

VEDOLIZUMAB

Trade: Entyvio

Category: Monoclonal Antibody

LRC: L3 - Limited Data-Probably Compatible

Vedolizumab is a humanized immunoglobulin G1 monoclonal antibody directed against the human lymphocyte integrin $\alpha 4\beta 7$.[1] It is indicated for the treatment of ulcerative colitis and Crohn's disease. It blocks the migration of T-lymphocytes into swollen gastrointestinal tissues. As an IgG molecule, it is large in molecular weight (147,000 Da) with a serum half-life of 25 days. In a study of five women receiving vedolizumab 300 mg IV on maintenance therapy every 8 weeks.[2] Others received loading doses at 0, 2, and 6 weeks. Five mothers were studied at trough levels prior to infusion. Milk levels of vedolizumab appear to peak at 3-4 days post infusion with a range of 108 to 478 ng/mL. In one patient who was studied over 15 days, C_{max} levels were 405 ng/mL at 3 days and 101 ng/mL at 15 days. The authors suggest that levels in milk are minuscule and probably unabsorbed orally by the infant.

In another group of five women who received repeated 300 mg IV infusions, vedolizumab levels in milk ranged from 0.124-0.228 µg/mL immediately before each subsequent infusions. Following new infusions, vedolizumab levels peaked at 0.196-0.318 µg/mL on days 3 through 7. The highest level reported was 0.318 µg/mL. All infants reportedly followed normal immunization protocols without problems.[3]

Although the molecular weight of this medication is very large and the amount in breast milk is expected to be exceptionally low, there are no long-term data concerning the safety of using immune modulating medications in breastfeeding mothers. Some caution is recommended, and each woman should understand the benefits and risk of using this type of medication in lactation.

T 1/2	25 days	MW	147,000 Da	PB	
Tmax	72 h	RID	0.38%-1.68%	Vd	0.07 L/kg
Oral	Nil	M/P		pKa	

Adult Concerns: Headache, fever, fatigue, nasopharyngitis, cough, nausea, changes in liver enzymes, arthralgia, skin rashes, infection, and infusion-related reactions.

Adult Dose: 300 mg IV at 0, 2, and 6 weeks, then every 8 weeks.

Pediatric Concerns: Levels in milk exceedingly low. No complications in one study.

Infant Monitoring: Fever, frequent infections, poor feeding/poor weight gain.

Alternatives: Certolizumab

References:

1. Pharmaceutical manufacturer's prescribing information, 2014.
2. Lahat A, Shitrit AB, Naftali T, et al. Vedolizumab levels in breast milk of nursing mothers with inflammatory bowel disease. J Crohns Colitis. 2017 Aug;12:120–123.
3. Julsgaard M, Kjeldsen J, Bibby BM, Brock B, Baumgart DC. Vedolizumab concentrations in the breast milk of nursing mothers with inflammatory bowel disease. Gastroenterology. 2018;154(3):752–754.e1. doi:10.1053/j.gastro.2017.08.067

VENLAFAXINE

Trade: Effexor

Category: Antidepressant, other

LRC: L2 - Limited Data-Probably Compatible

Venlafaxine is a newer antidepressant that is both a serotonin and norepinephrine reuptake inhibitor. It is somewhat similar in mechanism to other antidepressants such as fluoxetine, but has fewer anticholinergic side effects. In an excellent study of three mothers (mean age 34.5 years, 84.5 kg) receiving venlafaxine (225-300 mg/day), the mean milk/plasma ratios for venlafaxine (V) and its active metabolite O-desmethylvenlafaxine (ODV) were 2.5 and 2.7, respectively.[1] The mean maximum concentrations of V and ODV in milk were 1.16 mg/L and 0.796 mg/L. The peak concentrations in milk occurred at 2.25 hours. The mean infant exposure was 3.2% for V and 3.2% for ODV of the weight-adjusted maternal dose. Venlafaxine was detected in the plasma of one of the seven infants while ODV was detected in four of the seven infants. The infants were healthy and showed no acute adverse effects.

In a study of 11 women consuming an average of 194.3 mg/day of venlafaxine, the theoretical infant dose of venlafaxine and desvenlafaxine was 0.208 mg/kg/day, or a relative infant dose of 8.1% of the maternal dose. The maximum level in milk occurred at 8 hours after maternal ingestion. Infant plasma levels for V + ODV were 37.1% of maternal levels. No adverse effects were noted in any of the infants.[2]

One woman receiving high dose venlafaxine (300 mg daily) in pregnancy (reduced to mono-therapy at 20 weeks) and lactation had an infant with signs of poor neonatal adaptation, poor feeding and failure to thrive at 1 month of age.[3] On day 3 of life the infant was thought to have seizure activity, uncoordinated suck and was easily fatigued. The infant had ongoing concerns with poor feeding (interruptions due to fatigue and distress) and poor weight gain. It should be noted that this infant was initially breastfed with additional formula given via a nasogastric tube. Once breast milk was stopped, the infant was noted to be more alert and demonstrated weight gain within 7 days. Thus the authors of this case report question if the ongoing breast milk exposure contributed to the poor weight gain and failure to thrive by 1 month of age or if these concerns should only be attributed to the poor neonatal adaptation from in-utero exposure.

However, recent data (MedWatch, FDA) have suggested that infants exposed in utero to various serotonin reuptake inhibitors such as venlafaxine, may have adverse effects immediately upon delivery. These include; respiratory distress, cyanosis, apnea, seizures, temperature instability, etc. It is not known if these adverse events are due to a direct toxic effect of venlafaxine on the fetus, or due to a discontinuation (withdrawal) syndrome. Studies have shown that these adverse effects may be partially relieved with venlafaxine received through breast milk.[4]

T 1/2	5 h	MW	313 Da	PB	27%
Tmax	2.25 h	RID	6.8%-8.1%	Vd	4-12 L/kg
Oral	45%	M/P	2.75	pKa	9.4

Adult Concerns: Headache, somnolence, dizziness, insomnia, dry mouth, hypertension (at higher doses), nausea/vomiting, weakness.

Adult Dose: 75-225 mg/day Extended Release.

Pediatric Concerns: One case report of an infant with ongoing sedation, poor feeding, and inadequate weight gain at 1 month of life; this infant was exposed to venlafaxine in utero and in lactation.[3]

Infant Monitoring: Sedation or irritability, not waking to feed/poor feeding, and weight gain.

Alternatives: Sertraline(L2), Fluoxetine(L2)

References:

1. Ilett KF, Kristensen JH, Hackett LP, Paech M, Kohan R, Rampono J. Distribution of venlafaxine and its O-desmethyl metabolite in human milk and their effects in breastfed infants. Br J Clin Pharmacol. 2002;53(1):17-22.
2. Newport DJ, Ritchie JC, Knight BT, Glover BA, Zach EB, Stowe ZN. Venlafaxine in human breast milk and nursing infant plasma: determination of exposure. J Clin Psychiatry. 2009 Sep;70(9):1304-1310.
3. Tran MM, Fancourt N, Ging JM, et al. Failure to thrive potentially secondary to maternal venlafaxine use. Australas Psychiatry. 2016;24(1):98-99.
4. Koren G, Moretti, Kapur B. Can venlafaxine in breast milk attenuate the norepinephrine and serotonin reuptake neonatal withdrawal syndrome? JOGC. 2006 Apr;28(4):299-302.

VERAPAMIL

Trade: Berkatens, Calan, Covera-HS, Isoptin, Veracaps SR

Category: Calcium Channel Blocker

LRC: L2 - Limited Data-Probably Compatible

Verapamil is a typical calcium channel blocker used as an antihypertensive. It is secreted into milk but in very low levels, which are highly controversial. Anderson reports that in one patient receiving 80 mg three times daily, the average steady-state concentrations of verapamil and norverapamil in milk were 25.8 and 8.8 µg/L respectively.[1] The respective maternal plasma level was 42.9 µg/L. The milk/plasma ratio for verapamil was 0.60. No verapamil was detected in the infant's plasma. Inoue reports that in one patient receiving 80 mg four times daily, the milk level peaked at 300 µg/L at approximately 14 hours.[2] These levels are considerably higher than the aforementioned. In another study of a mother receiving 240 mg daily, the concentrations in milk were never higher than 40 µg/L.[3]

From these three studies, the relative infant doses were 0.15%, 0.98%, and 0.18% respectively. Regardless of the variability, the relative amount transferred to the infant is still quite small.

T 1/2	3-7 h	MW	455 Da	PB	90%
Tmax	1-2 h	RID	0.2%	Vd	3.89 L/kg
Oral	20%-35%	M/P	0.94	pKa	8.8

Adult Concerns: Headache, dizziness, fatigue, hypotension, dyspepsia, constipation, peripheral edema.

Adult Dose: 80-100 mg three times daily.

Pediatric Concerns: None reported via milk at this time.

Infant Monitoring: Drowsiness, lethargy, pallor, poor feeding, and weight gain.

Alternatives: Nifedipine(L2), Nimodipine(L2)

References:

1. Anderson P, Bondesson U, Mattiasson I, Johansson BW. Verapamil and norverapamil in plasma and breast milk during breast feeding. Eur J Clin Pharmacol. 1987;31(5):625-627.
2. Inoue H, Unno N, Ou MC, Iwama Y, Sugimoto T. Level of verapamil in human milk. Eur J Clin Pharmacol. 1984;26(5):657-658.
3. Andersen HJ. Excretion of verapamil in human milk. Eur J Clin Pharmacol. 1983;25(2):279-280.

VERTEPORFIN

Trade: Visudyne

Category: Photosensitizing Agent

LRC: L4 - Limited Data-Possibly Hazardous

Verteporfin is a photosensitizing agent used in the treatment of neovascularization associated with macular degeneration. When administered, verteporfin is transported to the neovascular endothelium, where it needs to be activated by nonthermal red light, resulting in local damage to the endothelium. This leads to temporary choroidal vessel occlusion.[1] The manufacturer reports verteporfin and its metabolites have been found in the breast milk of one woman after a 6 mg/m² infusion.[1] Milk levels were up to 66% of the corresponding plasma levels. Verteporfin was undetectable after 12 hours but its metabolites were present for up to 48 hours. A waiting period of 24 hours is recommended.

T 1/2	5-6 h	MW	718 Da	PB	
Tmax		RID		Vd	
Oral	Nil	M/P		pKa	

Adult Concerns: Headache, vertigo, changes in hearing, blurred vision, decreased visual acuity, visual disturbances, hypertension, arrhythmias, change in liver function, hematologic changes.

Adult Dose: 6 mg/m² IV.

Pediatric Concerns: Milk levels are significant but brief.

Infant Monitoring: Breastfeeding should be interrupted for 24 hours.

Alternatives:

References:
1. Pharmaceutical manufacturers prescribing information.

VIGABATRIN

Trade: Sabril

Category: Anticonvulsant

LRC: L3 - Limited Data-Probably Compatible

Vigabatrin is an anticonvulsant. It is a mixture consisting of 50% active S-enantiomer and 50% inactive R-enantiomer. This drug acts by inhibiting the metabolism of the inhibitory neurotransmitter GABA, thereby raising its levels in the human brain.[1] It is an effective adjunctive anticonvulsant for the treatment of multi-drug resistant complex partial seizures. It has also shown efficacy in controlling seizures and spasms in infants 3 months and older.

Milk levels of vigabatrin were estimated in two mothers who had been on 2000 mg/day vigabatrin therapy during pregnancy.[2] Case 1 had been on therapy since third trimester and case 2 had taken vigabatrin throughout her pregnancy. The milk levels of both enantiomers were assessed in this study. Milk samples were collected from case 1 and case 2 on the seventh and eighth day postpartum, respectively, at pre-dose and then at 3 and 6 hours postdose. Assuming that the infants consumed 0.15 L/kg/day of breast milk, it was found that the doses received by the infants through milk of the active S-enantiomer were 108 µg/kg/day and 160 µg/kg/day, respectively for case 1 and 2. Likewise, the absolute infant doses for the inactive R-enantiomer for case 1 and 2 were 333 µg/kg/day and 601 µg/kg/day respectively. The relative infant doses for the active S-enantiomer were <0.06% and 0.96% for case 1 and 2, respectively. The relative infant doses for the inactive R-enantiomer for case 1 and 2 were <2% and 3.6% respectively. The milk/plasma ratio at all times throughout the study were always <1. The authors suggest that the maximum relative infant dose for vigabatrin (R- + S-enantiomer) will barely exceed 4%. The total relative infant dose of the active S-enantiomer in this study barely exceeded 1%.

Vigabatrin enters milk in small amounts and is not likely to be clinically relevant in the breastfed infant. However, since this drug acts by raising the levels of inhibitory GABA in the brain, the effect of this property on neonatal development is unknown.[1] As with all CNS depressants, the risk of apnea also exists, especially in the premature and newborn infants. Some caution is recommended.

T 1/2	10.5 h	MW	129 Da	PB	None
Tmax	0.5-2 h	RID	1.5%-2.7%	Vd	1.1 L/kg
Oral	50%	M/P	<1	pKa	

Adult Concerns: Headache, sedation, dizziness, confusion, irritability, nystagmus, blurry vision, potential vision loss, tinnitus, decreased appetite, nausea, vomiting, diarrhea, constipation, anemia, tremor, weakness.

Adult Dose: 1-4 g daily.

Pediatric Concerns: None reported via milk.

Infant Monitoring: Sedation or irritability, not waking to feed/poor feeding, and weight gain.

Alternatives:

References:
1. Dichter MA, Brodie MJ. New antiepileptic drugs. N Engl J Med. 1996;334(24):1583-1590.
2. Tran A, O'Mahoney T, Rey E, Mai J, Mumford JP, Olive G. Vigabatrin: placental transfer in vivo and excretion into breast milk of the enantiomers. Br J Clin Pharmacol. 1998 Apr;45(4):409-411.

VILAZODONE

Trade: Viibryd

Category: Antidepressant, SSRI

LRC: L3 - No Data-Probably Compatible

Vilazodone is a selective serotonin reuptake inhibitor that has high affinity for 5-HT1 alpha receptors and is a 5-HT1 alpha partial agonist.[1] It is indicated for the treatment of depression. At present there are no data on its transfer to human milk; however, this medication has high protein binding (96%-99%) and a relatively larger molecular weight (477 Da), which may limit the amount that enters human milk. The manufacturer reports this medication is known to be excreted into rodent milk.

T 1/2	25 h	MW	477.99 Da	PB	96%-99%
Tmax	4-5 h	RID		Vd	
Oral	72%	M/P		pKa	

Adult Concerns: Dizziness, insomnia, abnormal dreams, drowsiness, sweating, palpitations, dry mouth, nausea, vomiting, diarrhea, tremor.

Adult Dose: 40 mg once daily.

Pediatric Concerns: None reported via milk at this time.

Infant Monitoring: Sedation or irritability, not waking to feed/poor feeding, diarrhea, and weight gain.

Alternatives: SSRIs, SNRIs.

References:
1. Pharmaceutical manufacturers prescribing information.

VILDAGLIPTIN

Trade: Galvus

Category: Antidiabetic, other

LRC: L3 - No Data-Probably Compatible

Vildagliptin is a dipeptidyl peptidase IV inhibitor resulting in prolonged active incretin levels, thus increasing insulin release from pancreatic beta cells in type II diabetics, decreasing glucagon secretion from pancreatic alpha cells, and ultimately decreasing blood glucose levels.[1] It does not lower blood glucose or cause hypoglycemia in healthy subjects. There are no data available on the transfer of vildagliptin to human milk; however, the manufacturer reports that this medication is known to enter rodent milk. Based on this medication's smaller size (303.4 Da), minimal protein binding (9.3%) and small volume of distribution (1.01 L/kg) it is expected that this medication will enter human milk. Some caution is recommended until we have human milk data.

T 1/2	3 h	MW	303.4 Da	PB	9.3%
Tmax	1.75 h fasting; 2.5 h with food	RID		Vd	1.01 L/kg
Oral	85%	M/P		pKa	

Adult Concerns: Headache, dizziness, constipation, changes in liver function, hypoglycemia (uncommon), peripheral edema.

Adult Dose: 50 mg once to twice daily.

Pediatric Concerns: None reported via milk at this time. Safety has not been established in pediatric patients.

Infant Monitoring: Signs of hypoglycemia - drowsiness, lethargy, pallor, sweating, tremor.

Alternatives: Metformin(L1), Glyburide(L2), Insulin(L2).

References:
1. Pharmaceutical manufacturer prescribing information.

VINBLASTINE

Trade: Lemblastine, Velban, Velbe, Velsar

Category: Antineoplastic

LRC: L5 - No Data-Hazardous

Vinblastine is an antineoplastic agent derived from the Catharanthus alkaloids family. It is commonly used in numerous cancers including breast cancer, Kaposi's sarcoma, Hodgkin's, choriocarcinoma, and many others. Vinblastine has a triphasic elimination with half-lives of 3.7 minutes, 1.6 hours, and 24.8 hours respectively.[1] No data are available on its transfer to human milk, but its levels are probably low due to a relatively higher molecular weight of 909 Da. However, mothers should be advised to withhold breastfeeding for a minimum of 10 days following treatment.

T 1/2	24.8 h (range 3-29 h)	MW	909 Da	PB	99%
Tmax		RID		Vd	18.9-27.3 L/kg
Oral		M/P		pKa	10.87

Adult Concerns: Headache, depression, vertigo, seizure, alopecia, fever, malaise, deafness, hypertension, constipation, anorexia, urinary retention, leukopenia, bone pain.

Adult Dose: Given once weekly for duration of treatment; dosage amounts vary according to body surface area and duration of treatment.

Pediatric Concerns:

Infant Monitoring: Withhold breastfeeding for a minimum of 10 days after treatment.

Alternatives:

References:
1. Grochow LB, Ames MM. A Clinician's Guide to Chemotherapy Pharmacokinetics and Pharmacodynamics. 1st ed. Baltimore, MD: Williams & Wilkins; 1998.

VINCRISTINE

Trade: Citomid, Farmistin, Ifavin, Marqibo, Norcristine, Oncovin, Vincasar PFS, Vincizina

Category: Antineoplastic

LRC: L5 - No Data-Hazardous

Vincristine is an antineoplastic agent derived from the Catharanthus alkaloids familly. It is commonly used in numerous cancers including breast cancer, Kaposi's sarcoma, non-Hodgkin's, lymphoma, and many others. Vincristine has a molecular weight of 923 Da. The kinetic studies thus far are highly variable and exact data are lacking. Vincristine exhibits a large and variable volume of distribution and ranges from 8.4 to 10.8 L/kg.[1] Studies in patients suggest it has a triphasic elimination pattern with initial, middle, and terminal half-lives of five minutes, 2.3 hours, and 85 hours respectively. However, the terminal elimination half-live sometimes ranges from 19-155 hours depending on the individual patient. No data are available on its transfer into human milk, but its levels are probably low due to the relatively higher molecular weight. However, mothers should be advised to withhold breastfeeding for a minimum of 35 days following treatment, as this product is slowly eliminated from the body.[2]

T 1/2	19-55 h	MW	923 Da	PB	
Tmax		RID		Vd	8.4-10.8 L/kg
Oral		M/P		pKa	10.85

Adult Concerns: Seizures, vertigo, alopecia, changes in vision and hearing, hypertension, edema, abdominal pain, constipation, anorexia, urinary retention, changes in liver function, bone pain, myalgia, motor difficulties.

Adult Dose: A maximum of 2 mg/dose; amount of medication varies according to treatment plan.

Pediatric Concerns:

Infant Monitoring: Withhold breastfeeding for a minimum of 35 days after treatment.

Alternatives:

References:
1. Grochow LB, Ames MM. A Clinician's Guide to Chemotherapy Pharmacokinetics and Pharmacodynamics. 1st ed. Baltimore, MD: Williams & Wilkins; 1998.
2. Pharmaceutical manufacturers prescribing information.

VINORELBINE

Trade: Biovelbin, Navelbine

Category: Antineoplastic

LRC: L5 - No Data-Hazardous

Vinorelbine is a close congener of vincristine. It is used for the treatment of advanced breast cancer, non-small cell lung cancer, non-Hodgkin's lymphoma, Hodgkin's disease, and ovarian carcinoma.[1] In a number of studies, the terminal elimination half-life ranged from 31.2 to 80 hours. The volume of distribution in these studies ranged from 25 to 40 L/kg.[2] No data are available on the transfer of this agent to human milk. Mothers should abstain from breastfeeding for a minimum of 30 days.

T 1/2	31.2-80 h	MW	1079.1 Da	PB	80%-91%
Tmax		RID		Vd	25-40 L/kg
Oral		M/P		pKa	10.87

Adult Concerns: Alopecia, fatigue, nausea, vomiting, diarrhea, constipation, changes in liver or renal function, hematologic changes, peripheral neuropathy, weakness, increased risk of infection.

Adult Dose: 30 mg/m²/weekly.

Pediatric Concerns:

Infant Monitoring: Withhold breastfeeding for a minimum of 30 days after treatment.

Alternatives:

References:
1. Grochow LB, Ames MM. A Clinician's Guide to Chemotherapy Pharmacokinetics and Pharmacodynamics. 1st ed. Baltimore, MD: Williams & Wilkins; 1998.
2. Pharmaceutical manufacturers prescribing information.

VITAMIN A

Trade: A-25, A-Natural, A-Natural-25, Aquasol A

Category: Vitamin

LRC: L3 - No Data-Probably Compatible

Vitamin A (retinol) is a typical retinoid. It is a fat-soluble vitamin that is secreted into human milk and primarily sequestered in high concentrations in the liver (90%).[1] Retinol is absorbed in the small intestine by a selective carrier-mediated uptake process. Levels in infants are generally unknown. The overdose of Vitamin A is extremely dangerous and is characterized by nausea, vomiting, headache, vertigo, and muscular incoordination. Acute toxicity generally occurs at doses of 25,000 IU/kg. Chronic exposure to levels of 4,000 IU/kg daily for 6 or more months is hazardous.

Liver damage can occur at doses as low as 15,000 IU per day. In infants, a bulging fontanel is also indicative of vitamin A toxicity. The suggested adult female dose is listed at 700 μg or 2300 IU. Upper limit is normally 3000 μg or 10,000 IU. Adults should never exceed 5000 units/day unless under the direct supervision of a physician and for specific diseases. Use normal doses in breastfeeding mothers if at all possible. Mature human milk is rich in retinol and contains 750 μg/L (2800 units). At this point we do not know if vitamin A levels in milk correlate with maternal plasma levels, but they probably do. Caution is recommended in supratherapeutic dosing in breastfeeding mothers.

T 1/2		MW	286 Da	PB	
Tmax		RID		Vd	
Oral	Complete	M/P		pKa	

Adult Concerns: Liver toxicity in overdose. Numerous other symptoms are possible including drying of mucous membranes, alopecia, fever, fatigue, weight loss, etc.

Adult Dose: <5000 IU daily.

Pediatric Concerns: None reported via milk.

Infant Monitoring:

Alternatives:

References:
1. McEvoy GE, ed. AFHS Drug Information. New York, NY: McGraw-Hill; 2005.

VITAMIN B12

Trade: Anacobin, B12, Cyanocobalamin, Cytacon, Rubramin

Category: Vitamin

LRC: L1 - Limited Data-Compatible

Vitamin B-12 is also called cyanocobalamin and is used for the treatment of pernicious anemia. It is an essential vitamin that is secreted in human milk at concentrations of 0.1 µg/100 mL. B-12 deficiency is very dangerous (severe brain damage) to an infant. Vegan mothers and certain other vegetarians should be supplemented during pregnancy. Milk levels vary in proportion to maternal serum levels.[1] Vegetarian mothers may have low levels unless supplemented. Supplementation of nursing mothers is generally recommended.

Following the maternal administration of radiolabeled cyanocobalamin during a Schilling test, peak concentrations occur at 24 hours postdose. However, the amount absorbed by an infant is less than the current regulatory limit at any time. Therefore, discarding the first feed at 4 hours after administration (as advised by the Administration of Radioactive Substances Advisory Committee) is not warranted.[2] B-12 is now available in many forms, including injections, oral tablets, and intranasal gels, all of which are safe in breastfeeding mothers and infants.

T 1/2		MW	1355 Da	PB	
Tmax	2 h	RID		Vd	
Oral	Variable	M/P		pKa	

Adult Concerns: Itching, skin rash, mild diarrhea, megaloblastic anemia in vegetarian mothers.

Adult Dose: 25 µg daily.

Pediatric Concerns: None reported with exception of B-12 deficiency states.

Infant Monitoring:

Alternatives:

References:

1. Lawrence RA. Breastfeeding: A Guide for the Medical Profession. St. Louis: Mosby Publishers; 1994.
2. Pomeroy KM, Sawyer LJ, Evans MJ. Estimated radiation dose to breast feeding infant following maternal administration of 57Co labelled to vitamin B12. Nucl Med Commun. 2005 Sep;26(9):839-841.

VITAMIN D

Trade: Bio-D-Mulsion, Ergocalciferol, Cholecalciferol, Calciferol, D3-50

Category: Vitamin

LRC: L1 - Limited Data-Compatible

Vitamin D is secreted into human milk and is somewhat proportional to maternal serum levels. A 1982 study done in South African winter included women given placebo, vitamin D 500 units, 1000 units or nothing (control) during lactation for 6 weeks.[1] The control group infants were given vitamin D 400 units daily. The authors noted that in this area the commercial milk supply was not fortified with vitamin D. The maternal 25-OHD blood levels at 6 weeks were 10, 13.8, 14.7, and 11 ng/mL in the placebo, 500 units, 1000 units, and a control group, respectively. The corresponding infant 25-OHD blood levels at 6 weeks were 1.1, 10.2, 9.4, and 15.2 ng/mL in the placebo, 500 units, 1000 units and control group, respectively. The control infants had significantly higher levels of vitamin D, thus the authors recommend that direct infant supplementation with vitamin D is superior to maternal supplementation in lactation.

In one case report of a mother taking vitamin D 50,000 units daily for hypoparathyroidism, the author reported that breast milk analysis showed a high content of 25-OHD in milk.[2] No details regarding the exact amount of vitamin D in milk were provided.

In a second case report of a woman with hypoparathyroidism taking high dose vitamin D2 100,000 units/day, milk levels were quantified.[3] In this case the mother's milk was sampled 2 weeks postpartum and contained 126-155 ng/mL of Vitamin D2, < 1 ng/mL of Vitamin D3, 7.3-8.3 ng/mL of 25-OHD2, < 0.01 ng/mL of 25-OHD3. The authors estimated this was equivalent to 7000 units of vitamin D per liter of milk (normal ~20-40 units/L).[3,4] The infant was exclusively breastfed for 25 days (weaned by 2 months of age) with no signs or symptoms of hypercalcemia or vitamin D toxicity. The authors of this report recommend avoiding high doses of vitamin D in lactation.

In addition, there are two publications by Hollis et al. that have reviewed high dose maternal supplementation with vitamin D in lactation.[4] In the first study published in 2004, breastfeeding women (n = 18) were randomized

1 month after birth to receive 1600 units vitamin D2 + 400 units vitamin D3 (prenatal) or 3600 units vitamin D2 + 400 units vitamin D3 (prenatal) for 3 months. Supplementation at these higher levels increased circulating 25-hydroxyvitamin D [25(OH)D] concentrations for both groups. The vitamin D activity of milk from mothers receiving 2000 units/day vitamin D increased by 34.2 units/L, on average, whereas the activity in the 4000 units/day group increased by 94.2 units/L. Infants of mothers receiving 2000 units/day exhibited increases in circulating 25(OH)D3 and 25(OH)D2 concentrations from 7.9 to 21.9 ng/mL and from <0.5 to 6 ng/mL, respectively. Total circulating 25(OH)D concentrations increased from 7.9 to 27.8 ng/mL. Infants of mothers receiving 4000 units/day exhibited increases in circulating 25(OH)D3 and 25(OH)D2 concentrations from 12.7 to 18.8 ng/mL and from 0.8 to 12 ng/mL, respectively. Total circulating 25(OH)D concentrations increased from 13.4 to 30.8 ng/mL. This latter study clearly shows that increasing the maternal intake of vitamin D significantly increases both the maternal milk and infant vitamin D levels.

In the second study by Hollis et al. published in 2015, breastfeeding women were randomized 4-6 weeks postpartum to either 400, 2400, or 6400 units of vitamin D3/day for 6 months.[5] The infants in the 400 units maternal dose group received an additional 400 units orally, while all other infants were not supplemented. The 2400 units/day group stopped the study early as more infants had vitamin D deficiency. When infant vitamin D levels were compared, no differences were found between the maternal 400 units/day group and the 6400 units/day group. Although this study has interesting results, numerous limitations (sample size, lack of maternal and neonatal safety data, etc.) and concern with maternal compliance mean that direct infant supplementation is still preferred.[6]

In 2016, another study (n = 107) was published which looked at foremilk and hindmilk concentrations of vitamin D2 and D3 at 2 weeks, 4 months and 9 months postpartum.[7] In this study vitamin D levels were undetectable in 46% of foremilk and 27% of hindmilk samples. In addition, the milk levels were dependent on maternal plasma concentrations and were higher in women who took vitamin D supplements (average maternal dose 400 units/day). Breastfed infants in this study received about 77 units/day, less than 20% of the recommended daily dose for infants less than 1 year of age from milk. Most infants in this study were given 400 units/day as per the national health guidelines where this study took place.

In 2003, the American Academy of Pediatrics, responding to increased reports of rickets in breastfeeding infants, published a recommendation that all US infants should consume 200 IU of vitamin D per day by supplementation if needed.[8] In 2008, the American Academy of Pediatrics changed this recommendation to 400 IU of vitamin D per day, based on evidence that vitamin D deficiency can occur early in life, vitamin D levels in infants are lower if breastfed and that this increase in supplementation increased these serum levels. Based on the evidence to date, direct infant supplementation is recommended over maternal supplementation in lactation.[4-8] See the American Academy of Pediatrics guideline for the most up to date vitamin D dose recommendation for breastfed infants.

Maternal use of vitamin D supplementation is not contraindicated in lactation as long as doses are not supra-therapeutic, less than 5000-6000 units/day.[4,5]

T 1/2		MW	396 Da	PB	
Tmax		RID		Vd	
Oral	Variable	M/P		pKa	

Adult Concerns: Elevated calcium levels in the plasma following chronic high doses (>10,000 IU/day).

Adult Dose: RDA = 400 units/day.

Pediatric Concerns: None reported via milk. The AAP recommends an infant dose of 400 IU/day.

Infant Monitoring:

Alternatives:

References:
1. Rothberg AD, Pettifor JM, Cohen DF, Sonnendecker EW, Ross FP. Maternal-infant vitamin D relationships during breast-feeding. J Pediatr. 1982;101(4):500-503.
2. Goldberg LD. Transmission of a vitamin-D metabolite in breast milk. Lancet. 1972;2(7789):1258-1259.
3. Greer FR, Searcy JE, Levin RS, Steichen JJ, Asch PS, Tsang RC. Bone mineral content and serum 25-hydroxyvitamin D concentration in breast-fed infants with and without supplemental vitamin D. J Pediatr. 1981;98(5):696-701.
4. Hollis BW, Wagner CL. Vitamin D requirements during lactation: high-dose maternal supplementation as therapy to prevent hypovitaminosis D for both the mother and the nursing infant. Am J Clin Nutr. 2004 Dec;80(6 Suppl):1752S-1758S.
5. Hollis BW, Wagner CL, Howard CR, et al. Maternal versus infant vitamin D supplementation during lactation: a randomized controlled trial. Pediatrics. 2015;136(4):625-634.
6. Furman L. Maternal vitamin D supplementation for breastfeeding infants: will it work? Pediatrics. 2015;136(4):763-764.
7. vio Streym S, Hojskov CS, Moller UK, et al. Vitamin D content in human breast milk: a 9-mo follow-up study. Am J Clin Nutr. 2016;103:107-114.
8. Wagner CL, Greer FR. Prevention of rickets and vitamin D deficiency in infants, children, and adolescents. Pediatrics. 2008;122(5):1142-1152.

VITAMIN E

Trade: Alpha-Tocopherol, Bio E

Category: Vitamin

LRC: L2 - Limited Data-Probably Compatible

Vitamin E is a collective name for a group of eight naturally occurring compounds: alpha-, beta-, gamma-, delta-tocopherol, and alpha-, beta-, gamma-, delta-tocotrienol.[1] While the gut absorbs all of these forms, only alpha-tocopherol appears to be biologically useful and is selectively maintained by the liver. The remaining compounds are rapidly metabolized and excreted. The presence of these other forms results in a substantial difference in activity between natural and synthetic formulations of vitamin E.

Vitamin E secretion into breast milk appears to be regulated. Alpha-tocopherol levels in milk vary with the stage of lactation and between individuals.[2] Concentrations are highest during the first 2 weeks postpartum but, overall, can vary between 0.1 to 0.9 mg/dL.[2,3]

The effect of maternal supplementation with vitamin E is not well characterized. In one study, supplementing with as little as 50 mg/day did not increase vitamin E content in human milk.[4] Another study randomized breastfeeding women to no treatment, 400 units of natural vitamin E, and 400 units of synthetic vitamin E.[5] Maternal blood and milk samples were drawn 12 hours postpartum, supplements were given and then samples were repeated again 24 hours later. The milk concentrations of vitamin E in the natural and synthetic groups increased by 57.6% and 39%, respectively. No change was noted in the control group and no correlation was found between maternal concentrations in blood and milk. In a case report of a woman who supplemented with Vitamin E at 245% the RDA, the vitamin E milk level at 38 days postpartum was 1.1 mg/dL.[6]

In a study which applied vitamin E capsules to the nipples (400 IU/feeding) after each infant feed, Vitamin E plasma levels in these breastfed infants were about 40% higher than controls in only 6 days.[7]

Supplementation beyond the recommended dietary intake and direct application of vitamin E to the nipple is not recommended.

T 1/2		MW	431 Da	PB	
Tmax		RID		Vd	
Oral	Variable	M/P		pKa	10.8

Adult Concerns: Fatigue, headache, nausea, cramping, diarrhea, changes in renal function, muscle weakness, contact dermatitis (topical).

Adult Dose: 22.4 IU daily.

Pediatric Concerns: None reported via milk, but caution is recommended. Do not use highly concentrated vitamin E oils directly on nipple. Necrotizing enterocolitis has been associated with high oral doses given to low birth weight infants.

Infant Monitoring:

Alternatives:

References:

1. National Institutes of Health Office of Dietary Supplements. Vitamin E fact sheet for health professionals, 2013. http://ods.od.nih.gov/about/error.aspx-500?aspxerrorpath=/factsheets/VitaminE-HealthProfessional/
2. Lammi-Keefe CJ. Vitamins D and E in Human Milk. In: Jensen R, ed. Handbook of Milk Composition. New York: Academic Press; 1995:710-717.
3. Kobayashi H, Kanno C, Yamauchi K, Tsugo T. Identification of alpha-, beta-, gamma-, and delta-tocopherols and their contents in human milk. Biochim Biophys Acta. 1975 Feb;380(2):282-290.
4. Lammi-Keefe CJ. Tocopherols in human milk: analytical method using high-performance liquid chromatography. J Pediatr Gastroenterol Nutr. 1986 Nov;5(6):934-937.
5. Clemente HA, Ramalho HMM, Lima MSR, et al. Maternal supplementation with natural or synthetic vitamin E and its levels in human colostrum. JPGN. 2015;60(4):533-537.
6. Anderson DM, Pittard WB III. Vitamin E and C concentrations in human milk with maternal megadosing: a case report. J Am Diet Assoc. 1985 Jun;85(6):715-717.
7. Marx CM, Izquierdo A, Driscoll JW, Murray MA, Epstein MF. Vitamin E concentrations in serum of newborn infants after topical use of vitamin E by nursing mothers. Am J Obstet Gynecol. 1985 Jul;152(6 Pt 1):668-670.

VORICONAZOLE

Trade: VFEND

Category: Antifungal

LRC: L3 - No Data-Probably Compatible

It is a triazole antifungal drug indicated for use in the treatment of: 1) Invasive aspergillosis, 2) Candidemia and disseminated candidiasis, 3) Serious infections caused by *Scedosporium apiospermum* and *Fusiarium*.[1] It is not known if voriconazole is excreted in human milk, but levels are probably low. Voriconazole has proved very effective for candidemia, and may be a replacement for amphotericin B with far fewer side effects, particularly less renal toxicity. While the half-life is dose-dependent, it is totally eliminated via hepatic metabolism, and subsequently renally excreted. The majority (94%) is excreted within 94 hours after oral and IV dosing. Pediatric dosing regimens are available which suggests this product is probably safe to use in a breastfeeding mother. Suggest a 4 hour wait before feeding following high dose IV regimens to reduce infant exposure.

T 1/2	Dose dependent	MW	349 Da	PB	58%
Tmax	1-2 h	RID		Vd	4.6 L/kg
Oral	96%	M/P		pKa	

Adult Concerns: Headache, hallucinations, visual disturbances, tachycardia, prolongation of QTc interval, nausea, vomiting, changes in liver and renal function, changes in electrolytes.

Adult Dose: Loading dose: 6 mg/kg IV q 12 hours for first 24 hours. Maintenance dose: 4 mg/kg IV q 12 hours or 200 mg orally q 12 hours.

Pediatric Concerns: Safety and effectiveness below 12 years has not yet been established, although there have been reports of pancreatitis in pediatric patients.

Infant Monitoring: Vomiting, diarrhea.

Alternatives: Fluconazole(L2), Itraconazole(L3), Miconazole(L2)

References:
1. Pharmaceutical manufacturers prescribing information.

VORTIOXETINE

Trade: Trintellix

Category: Antidepressant, other

LRC: L3 - No Data-Probably Compatible

Vortioxetine is a serotonin modulator and stimulator (SMS) that enhances serotonergic activity in the brain.[1] This medication has similar effects as other well-known antidepressant classes (e.g., SSRIs, SNRIs) but works differently at the receptor level. The manufacturer reports that vortioxetine is present in rodent milk (did not report quantity present) and that it is unknown if this drug would appear in human milk.

This medication has a small molecular weight and long half-life; however, its large volume of distribution (37 L/kg) and high protein binding (98%) suggest it will most likely enter milk at levels similar to other antidepressants. Tentative unpublished data from our laboratories suggest a RID ranging from 1.24% to 3.29%, which would make it one of the lowest transferred of the antidepressants.[2]

T 1/2	66 h	MW	379.36 Da	PB	98%
Tmax	7-11 h	RID	1.24 - 3.29%	Vd	37.14 L/kg
Oral	75%	M/P		pKa	

Adult Concerns: Dizziness, abnormal dreams, dry mouth, dyspepsia, nausea, vomiting, diarrhea or constipation, sexual dysfunction, serotonin syndrome, hyponatremia, pruritus.

Adult Dose: 20 mg per day.

Pediatric Concerns: None reported via milk at this time.

Infant Monitoring: Sedation or irritability, not waking to feed/poor feeding, and weight gain.

Alternatives: Sertraline(L2), Escitalopram(L2)

References:
1. Pharmaceutical manufacturers prescribing information.
2. Marshall K, Datta P, Rewers-Felkins L, Baker T, Hale T. Serotonin modulator vortioxetine transfer into human milk. 2020, Unpublished data.

WARFARIN

Trade: Coumadin, Marevan, Warfilone

Category: Anticoagulant

LRC: L2 - Limited Data-Probably Compatible

Warfarin is a potent anticoagulant. Warfarin is highly protein bound (99%) in the maternal circulation and therefore very little is secreted into human milk. Although very small and insignificant amounts are secreted into milk, it depends to some degree on the dose administered. In one study of two patients who were anticoagulated with warfarin, no warfarin was detected in maternal milk (case 1), and no changes in coagulation were detectable in either infant.[1] The infant in case one was followed for 56 days and the infant in case two was followed for 131 days after birth with no reported adverse effects.

In another study of 13 mothers receiving 2-12 mg of warfarin a day, the breast milk samples were also undetectable (less than 0.08 µmol/L or 25 ng/mL).[2] Warfarin was undetectable in the plasma of the seven infants that were breastfed. The anticoagulant effect was measured in four of the breastfed infants using the British Corrected Ratio (BCR) and were all within normal range. No adverse events such as bleeding occurred in the breastfed infants in this study. According to the authors, maternal warfarin use is suitable in lactation.

T 1/2	1-2.5 days	MW	308 Da	PB	99%
Tmax	5-7 days for full therapeutic effect	RID		Vd	0.14 L/kg
Oral	Complete	M/P		pKa	4.5

Adult Concerns: Abdominal pain, diarrhea, changes in liver function, anemia, bruising on the skin, hemorrhage (blood in vomit, stool, urine, etc.).

Adult Dose: 2-10 mg daily.

Pediatric Concerns: None reported via milk at this time.

Infant Monitoring: Rare bruising on the skin, blood in vomit, stool, or urine.

Alternatives:

References:
1. McKenna R, Cole ER, Vasan U. Is warfarin sodium contraindicated in the lactating mother? J Pediatr. 1983;103(2):325-327.
2. Orme ML, Lewis PJ, De Swiet M, et al. May mothers given warfarin breast-feed their infants? Br Med J. 1977;1(6076):1564-1565.

WEST NILE FEVER

Trade:

Category: Infectious Disease

LRC: L4 - Limited Data-Possibly Hazardous

West Nile Virus (WNV), which belongs to the flaviviridae family, is transmitted to humans from infected birds via the bite of culex mosquito. Although prevalent in many parts of the world, there have been increasing reports of WNV infection in the United States since 1999. Several modes of transmission have been reported which includes air-borne, blood-borne, trans-placental, organ transplantation and also possible transmission through breast milk. Mosquitoes, largely bird-feeding species, are the principal vectors of West Nile Virus. The virus has been isolated from 43 mosquito species, predominantly of the genus Culex.[1-3] West Nile fever in humans usually is a febrile, influenza-like illness characterized by an abrupt onset (incubation period is 3 to 6 days) of moderate to high fever (3 to 5 days, infrequently biphasic, sometimes with chills), headache (often frontal), sore throat, backache, myalgia, arthralgia, fatigue, conjunctivitis, retrobulbar pain, maculopapular or roseolar rash, lymphadenopathy, anorexia, nausea, abdominal pain, diarrhea, and respiratory symptoms.

Only one established case of transmission of WNV in breast milk occurred in Michigan in 2002 when a mother was transfused with WNV-contaminated blood one day after delivering a healthy infant. The mother started breastfeeding her baby on the day of delivery. Twelve days after delivery, the mother developed WNV illness and her serum tested positive for WNV-specific IgM antibody. Sixteen days after delivery her breast milk sample tested positive for WNV-RNA as well as for WNV specific IgM antibodies. Although the infant's serum also tested positive for IgM antibodies, the infant did not develop WNV illness and remained healthy.[4] In 2003, six infants known to have breastfed from WNV infected mothers were studied.[5] Of the six, five remained healthy without any serological evidence of WNV infection. One infant did develop a rash, but breast milk transmission could not be established since neither infant serum nor breast milk samples were collected. Therefore, although WNV transmission by breast milk could be a possibility, it is rare.[5] The American Academy of Pediatrics states, "Because the benefits of breastfeeding seem to outweigh the risk of any WNV illness in breastfeeding infants, mothers should be encouraged to breastfeed even in areas of ongoing WNV transmission."[6]

For answers to questions about West Nile Virus, please see the CDC web site http://www.cdc.gov/ncidod/dvbid/westnile/q&a.htm.

Adult Concerns: Febrile influenza-like illness, characterized by an abrupt onset of moderate to high fever, headache (often frontal), sore throat, backache, myalgia, arthralgia, fatigue, conjunctivitis, retrobulbar pain, maculopapular or roseolar rash, lymphadenopathy, anorexia, nausea, abdominal pain, diarrhea, and respiratory symptoms.

Adult Dose:

Pediatric Concerns: No transmission reported via milk but it has not been studied.

Infant Monitoring: Fever, sore throat, myalgia, fatigue.

Alternatives:

References:
1. Hayes C. West Nile fever. In: Monath TP, ed. The Arboviruses: Epidemiology and Ecology. vol 5. Boca Raton, FL: CRC Press; 1989.
2. Shope RE. Other flavivirus infections. In: Guerrant RL, Walker DH, Weller PF, eds. Tropical Infectious Diseases: Principals, Pathogens, and Practice. Philadelphia, PA: Churchill Livingstone; 2004.
3. Hubalek Z, Halouzka J. West Nile fever--a reemerging mosquito-borne viral disease in Europe. Emerg Infect Dis. 1999;5(5):643-650.
4. Centers for Disease Control and Prevention (CDC). Possible West Nile virustransmission to an infant through breast-feeding--Michigan, 2002. MMWR MorbMortal Wkly Rep. 2002 Oct;51(39):877-878.
5. Hinckley AF, O'Leary DR, Hayes EB. Transmission of West Nile virus throughhuman breast milk seems to be rare. Pediatrics. 2007 Mar;119(3):e666-e671.
6. AAP CoID. West Nile virus. In: Pickering LK BC, Kimberlin DW, Long SS, eds. Red Book: 2009 Report of the Committe on Infectious Diseases. 28th ed. Elk. Grove Village, IL: American Academy of Pediatrics; 2009:730-732.

XYLOMETAZOLINE

Trade: Aqua Maris, Sinosil

Category: Decongestant

LRC: L3 - No Data-Probably Compatible

Xylometazoline is a vasoconstrictive agent used both nasally and ophthalmically. No reports are available regarding the use of xylometazoline during lactation and effects on the infant with exposure of the drug in human milk are unknown. Xylometazoline is a direct acting sympathomimetic adrenergic alpha-agonist used to induce systemic vasoconstriction, thereby decreasing nasal congestion for a prolonged period of 8-12 hours. Generally, use of topical agents possess less risk than systemically absorbed agents. However, xylometazoline may be absorbed systemically when used nasally. Caution is warranted when contemplating use of xylometazoline while breastfeeding.

T 1/2		MW	244.37 Da	PB	
Tmax		RID		Vd	
Oral	Good (nasal)	M/P		pKa	

Adult Concerns: With excessive use or dose, hypertension and arrhythmias are possible. Headache, insomnia, and dizziness have been reported.

Adult Dose: Two to three drops of a 0.1% solution every 12 hours.

Pediatric Concerns:

Infant Monitoring: Agitation, excitement, tremors.

Alternatives: Oxymetazoline(L3), Pseudoephedrine(L3)

References:

YELLOW FEVER VACCINE

Trade: Arilvax, Stamaril, YF-Vax

Category: Vaccine

LRC: L4 - Limited Data-Possibly Hazardous

Yellow fever is an acute viral illness caused by a mosquito-borne flavivirus. The clinical spectrum of yellow fever is highly variable, from subclinical infection to overwhelming pansystemic disease. Yellow fever has an abrupt onset after an incubation period of 3 to 6 days, and usually includes fever, prostration, headache, photophobia, lumbosacral pain, extremity pain, epigastric pain, vomiting, and anorexia. The illness may progress to liver and renal failure, and hemorrhagic symptoms caused by thrombocytopenia and abnormal clotting. The case-fatality rate of yellow fever varies widely in different studies and may be different for Africa compared to South America, but is typically 20% or higher. Jaundice or other signs of severe liver disease is associated with higher mortality rates.[1] Yellow fever occurs only in Africa, Central, and South America. Those reported in the United States are usually imported cases.[2] Based on 2013 data, the World Health Organization (WHO) estimated about 170,000 severe cases of yellow fever occurred and 29,000-60,000 deaths could be attributed to this disease.[3]

Yellow fever vaccine is a live, attenuated virus preparation made from the 17D yellow fever virus strain.[1] Historically, the 17D vaccine has been considered to be one of the safest and most effective live virus vaccines ever developed. Being a live attenuated vaccine, there is significant risk to the infant following breast milk exposure to this vaccine. A report of possible yellow fever virus transmission in breast milk occurred in Brazil 2009 when a 23-day-old breastfed infant developed fever and seizures 8 days after the mother received the yellow fever vaccine. The infant's CSF tested positive for yellow fever vaccine virus (17D). A case of yellow fever viral meningoencephalitis was established.[4,5] The Canadian Medical Association Journal recently published a report of a 5-week-old breastfed infant who developed yellow fever encephalitis 30 days after his mother received the yellow fever vaccine. The infant presented with fever, focal seizures, irritability, and vomiting. The infant's serum tested positive for yellow fever-specific IgM antibody, and more importantly the cerebrospinal fluid (CSF) of the infant demonstrated the presence of yellow fever antigen.[6] Although in both cases breast milk samples were not tested, breast milk was the most likely route of transmission. In both cases, the infants recovered fully with no neurological sequelae at their 5- and 6-month follow-ups, respectively.[4-6]

According to CDC recommendations, all persons aged >9 months, traveling to, or living in areas of high yellow fever transmission should be vaccinated. According to CDC, immunization of lactating mothers with infants <9 months of age, should preferably be avoided. However, if travel of a lactating mother to an endemic area cannot be avoided or postponed, or in situations where exposure to the yellow fever virus is high, then the potential benefits of the vaccine outweigh the potential risks, and immunization should be considered.[7]

Studies have found that in up to 80%-100% of cases, the 17D vaccine virus is no longer present in serum 10-13 days following vaccination.[7,8] This would suggest that breastfeeding poses minimal risk to an infant 2 weeks after immunization.

Adult Concerns: Headaches, myalgia, low-grade fever. Local reactions include edema, hypersensitivity, and pain at the injection site.

Adult Dose:

Pediatric Concerns: One reported case of severe seizures and vaccine encephalitis in an infant whose mother received yellow fever vaccination 8 days prior. While not adequately documented that the infection was via milk, the CDC strongly suggests that this infant probably received the virus via its mother's breast milk. Risks in infants and children can be severe and include vaccine-induced encephalitis, most of which have occurred in infants <4 months of age (n = 14), and in children >3 years (n = 7).

Infant Monitoring:

Alternatives:

References:

1. Pharmaceutical manufacturers prescribing information.
2. AAP CoID. In: Pickering LK BC, Kimberlin DW, Long SS, eds. Red Book: 2009 Report of the Committee on Infectious Diseases. 29th ed. Elk Grove Village: American Academy of Pediatrics; 2009.
3. World Health Organization (WHO). Yellow fever fact sheet, May 2016 [Online]. http://www.who.int/mediacentre/factsheets/fs100/en/.
4. Chen LH, Zeind C, Mackell S, LaPointe T, Mutsch M, Wilson ME. Yellow fever virus transmission via breastfeeding: follow-up to the paper on breastfeeding travelers. J Travel Med. 2010,17(4):286-287.
5. Couto AMSM. Transmission of Yellow fever vaccine virus through breast-feeding - Brazil, 2009. MMWR Morbidity and Mortality Weekly Report. 2010;59(5):130-132.
6. Kuhn S, Twele-Montecinos L, MacDonald J, Webster P, Law B. Case report: probable transmission of vaccine strain of yellow fever virus to an infant via breast milk. CMAJ. 2011;183(4):E243-E245.

7. Staples JE, Gershman M, Fischer M. Yellow fever vaccine: recommendations of the Advisory Committee on Immunization Practices (ACIP). MMWR Recomm Rep. 2010;59(RR-7):1-27.
8. Reinhardt B, Jaspert R, Niedrig M, Kostner C, L'Age-Stehr J. Development of viremia and humoral and cellular parameters of immune activation after vaccination with yellow fever virus strain 17D: a model of human flavivirus infection. J Med Virol. 1998 Oct;56(2):159-167.
9. Shealy, KR. International Travel with Infants & Children: Travel and Breastfeeding. Centers for Disease Control and Prevention July 2015 [Online]. http://wwwnc.cdc.gov/travel/yellowbook/2016/international-travel-with-infants-children/travel-breastfeeding

ZAFIRLUKAST

Trade: Accolate

Category: Antiasthma

LRC: L3 - No Data-Probably Compatible

Zafirlukast is a new competitive receptor antagonist of leukotriene D4, which is a mediator of bronchoconstriction in asthmatic patients. Zafirlukast is not a bronchodilator and should not be used for acute asthma attacks. Zafirlukast is excreted into milk in low concentrations. Following repeated 40 mg doses twice daily (please note: average adult dose is 20 mg twice daily), the average steady-state concentration in breast milk was 50 µg/L compared to 255 ng/mL in maternal plasma.[1] Zafirlukast is poorly absorbed when administered with food. It is likely the oral absorption via ingestion of breast milk would be low.

T 1/2	10-13 h	MW	575 Da	PB	>99%
Tmax	3 h	RID	0.7%	Vd	
Oral	Poor	M/P	0.15	pKa	4.01

Adult Concerns: Headache, dizziness, fever, dyspepsia, nausea, vomiting, diarrhea, abdominal pain, changes in liver enzymes, myalgia.

Adult Dose: 20 mg twice daily.

Pediatric Concerns: None reported.

Infant Monitoring: Irritability, diarrhea.

Alternatives:

References:
1. Pharmaceutical manufacturers prescribing information.

ZALEPLON

Trade: Sonata, Zaplon

Category: Sedative-Hypnotic

LRC: L2 - Limited Data-Probably Compatible

Zaleplon is a sleep medication that interacts at the GABA receptor; however, it is not a benzodiazepine. In a study of five lactating mothers given one 10 mg dose of zaleplon milk was sampled until 8 hours after the dose. The peak milk level occurred at 1.2 hours postdose and averaged 14 µg/L.[1] Milk levels decreased rapidly and were less than 5 µg/L 4 hours postdose. The infants in this study were not breastfed during this study. While the authors estimated infant dose at 0.0128% to 0.0166%, we calculate the Relative Infant Dose at 0.4%.

T 1/2	1 h	MW	305 Da	PB	45%-75%
Tmax	1 h	RID	0.4%	Vd	1.4 L/kg
Oral	30%	M/P	0.5	pKa	

Adult Concerns: Headache, drowsiness, peripheral edema, dizziness have been reported.

Adult Dose: 10 mg nightly.

Pediatric Concerns: None reported via milk.

Infant Monitoring: Sedation, not waking to feed.

Alternatives: Zopiclone(L2), Lorazepam(L3), Oxazepam(L2)

References:
1.   Darwish M, Martin PT, Cevallos WH, Tse S, Wheeler S, Troy SM. Rapid disappearance of zaleplon from breast milk after oral administration to lactating women. J Clin Pharmacol. 1999;39(7):670-674.

ZANAMIVIR

Trade: Relenza

Category: Antiviral

LRC: L2 - No Data-Probably Compatible

Zanamivir is a viral neuraminidase inhibitor that blocks or prevents viral seeding or release from infected cells and prevents viral aggregation.[1] Zanamivir is indicated for the prevention and treatment of illness due to influenza A and B infections in pediatrics and adults.[1,2] It is administered via inhalation using a diskhaler device. Only 4%-17% of the inhaled drug is systemically absorbed. Peak plasma concentrations are only 17-142 ng/mL within 2 hours of administration and then rapidly decline. The manufacturer reports that it is present in the milk of rodents although no human data are available. Due to the poor oral or inhaled absorption and the incredibly low plasma levels, it is unlikely to produce untoward effects in breastfed infants.

T 1/2	2.5-5.1 h	MW	332.3 Da	PB	<10%
Tmax	1-2 h	RID		Vd	
Oral	4%-17%	M/P		pKa	3.25

Adult Concerns: Headache, fatigue, throat discomfort, bronchospasm, cough, urticaria.

Adult Dose: 10 mg twice daily for 5 days.

Pediatric Concerns: None reported via milk.

Infant Monitoring: Vomiting, diarrhea (unlikely due to low bioavailability).

Alternatives:

References:
1.   Pharmaceutical manufacturers prescribing information.
2.   Center for Disease Control. Influenza Antiviral Medications: Summary for Clinicians [Online]. http://www.cdc.gov/flu/professionals/antivirals/summary-clinicians.htm

ZIDOVUDINE

Trade: Combivir, Retrovir

Category: Antiviral

LRC: L5 - Limited Data-Hazardous if Maternal HIV Infection

Zidovudine in an antiretroviral agent used in the treatment of HIV. In a study of 18 women receiving 300 mg twice daily at steady state, median zidovudine levels at 5.4 hours postdose in maternal serum, breast milk, and infant serum were 58 ng/mL, 207 ng/mL and 123 ng/mL, respectively.[1] The milk/serum ratio was 3.21. The median infant serum concentration of zidovudine (123 ng/mL) was at least 25 times the 50% inhibitory concentration for HIV. Infant serum concentrations of zidovudine were a median of 2.5 times higher than the respective maternal concentration of zidovudine. The elevated infant serum levels are somewhat inexplicable. In adults, and apparently infants, zidovudine has a delayed terminal phase half-life (4.8 hours) longer than its initial half-life (<3 hours). The rather high serum levels in infants is worrisome and some caution is recommended although no untoward effects were reported in this study of 18 patients.

In 2007, 40 women were given zidovudine, lamivudine, and nevirapine from 28 weeks gestational age to 1 month postpartum to evaluate the potential efficacy of using these medications to prevent the transmission of perinatal HIV.[2] All women in this study were instructed not to breastfeed their infants. Milk samples were collected five times a day from delivery to day 7 postpartum, blood samples were collected on day 3 (time 0) and day 7 (time 7); the samples were used to quantify the amount of HIV RNA and DNA in milk and the concentrations of each medication in maternal plasma and milk. The mean concentrations of zidovudine at time 0 and 7 in maternal plasma were 130 μg/L and 220 μg/L. The mean concentrations of zidovudine at time 0 and 7 in milk were 130 μg/L and 150 μg/L. The milk plasma ratios were 1 at time 0 and 7. We used the milk levels from time 0 and 7 to estimate the relative infant dose for zidovudine to range from 0.23% to 0.26%. Although the RID is still remarkably low, the concentrations of zidovudine in milk were much higher in this study when compared to the 2009 and 2013 publications, we believe this could be related to the fact that these levels were drawn during the colostral phase.

In 2009, a study was published that assessed 67 women taking combination antiretroviral therapy from 34 to 36 weeks through 6 months postpartum.[3] These women took one Combivir tablet twice daily (lamivudine 150 mg + zidovudine 300 mg/tab) with nevirapine 200 mg x 14 days then 200 mg twice a day. Zidovudine milk samples were taken within 24 hours of delivery, then at weeks 2, 6, 14, and 24 postpartum. The median values for each parameter were estimated across all study visits, the maternal concentration was 23 ng/mL (12-59 ng/mL), the milk concentration was 9 ng/mL (below detection to 26 ng/mL) and the milk/plasma ratio was 0.44. The authors of this study estimated that an infant would receive about 1.35 µg/kg/day of zidovudine if they consumed about 150 mL/kg/day of breast milk. We calculated the relative infant dose to be 0.015% which is equivalent to the infant dose estimated by the authors of this study. The authors also noted that zidovudine was not detectable in any of the infant plasma samples beyond the day of delivery.

Another study that evaluated the safety of maternal antiretrovirals for prophylaxis against transmission to the infant during lactation reported milk levels of zidovudine (n = 114 samples).[4] This study tested maternal serum and breast milk on the day of delivery and at months 1, 3, and 6 postpartum. Infant levels were also taken at months 1, 3, and 6 of age. The median drug concentrations of zidovudine in maternal serum, breast milk and the infant were 43 ng/mL (15-167 ng/mL), 33 ng/mL (5-117 ng/mL), and 0 ng/mL (0-2.5 ng/mL), respectively. The milk to plasma ratio was 0.64. The RID that we calculated using the maternal dose of 300 mg twice a day and median milk level was 0.06%. In this study 11 of 38 zidovudine exposed infants had severe anemia and one infant had a severe skin rash. This study also reported other infant adverse events (e.g., pneumonia, diarrhea, changes in liver function, neutropenia, thrombocytopenia), but was unable to determine which medication caused the effects based on drug levels, please see study[4] for adverse event details.

A publication in 2013, followed women taking antivirals in pregnancy and breastfeeding and studied maternal milk samples 30 days postpartum.[5] Twelve breast milk samples were available, the median milk concentration was 0.007 µg/mL. No milk to plasma ratio was reported. The relative infant dose calculated using this median milk sample and a maternal dose of zidovudine 300 mg twice a day was 0.012%.

In 2014, a study was published that looked at HIV RNA in milk and the pharmacokinetics of maternal medications in milk to prevent transmission of HIV to the infant during lactation.[6] In this study 30 women were given one Combivir tablet twice a day (zidovudine 300 mg + lamivudine 150 mg/tab) with two tablets of Aluvia twice a day (lopinavir 200 mg + ritonavir 50 mg) starting postpartum until breastfeeding was stopped or 28 weeks. Samples were taken pre-dose (time 0) and then at 2, 4, and 6 hours postdose when the women were enrolled at either 6, 12, or 24 weeks postpartum. The median drug concentrations of zidovudine in maternal serum, breast milk, and the infant were 143 ng/mL (107-192 ng/mL), 200 ng/mL (119-263 ng/mL), and undetectable, respectively. The milk to plasma ratio was 1.35. The RID that we calculated using the maternal dose of 300 mg twice a day and median milk level was 0.35%.

Note: This medication is an L5 to highlight the contraindication of breastfeeding when the mother is known to be infected with HIV, this medication is not an L5 based on its risk to the infant in breast milk. The Centers for Disease Control and Prevention recommend that HIV infected mothers do not breastfeed their infants to avoid postnatal transmission of HIV.

T 1/2	<3 h	MW	267 Da	PB	<38%
Tmax	1.5 h	RID	0.01%-0.36%	Vd	1.6 L/kg
Oral	61%	M/P	3.21	pKa	9.96

Adult Concerns: Headache, fever, heart failure, dyspnea, cough, esophageal ulcer, nausea, vomiting, anorexia, changes in liver function, gynecomastia, lactic acidosis, anemia, neutropenia, thrombocytopenia.

Adult Dose: 300 mg twice daily.

Pediatric Concerns: In one study, 11 of 38 zidovudine breast milk exposed infants had severe anemia and one infant had a severe skin rash.[4] Please see study for further adverse event details.

Infant Monitoring: Breastfeeding is not recommended in mothers who have HIV.

Alternatives: Nevirapine(L5), Lamivudine(L5)

References:

1. Shapiro RL, Holland DT, Capparelli E, et al. Antiretroviral concentrations in breast-feeding infants of women in Botswana receiving antiretroviral treatment. J Infect Dis. 2005 Sep;192(5):720-727.
2. Giuliano M, Guidotti G, Andreotti M, et al. Triple antiviral prophylaxis administered during pregnancy and after delivery significantly reduces breast milk viral load. J Acquir Immune Defic Syndr. 2007;44:286-291.
3. Mirochnick M, Thomas T, Capparelli E, et al. Antiretroviral concentrations in breast-feeding infants of mothers receiving highly active antiretroviral therapy. Antimicrob Agents Chemother. 2009;53(3);1170-1176.
4. Palombi L, Pirillo MF, Andreotti M, et al. Antiretroviral prophylaxis for breastfeeding transmission in Malawi: drug concentrations, virological efficacy and safety. Antivir Ther. 2012;17:1511-1519.
5. Shapiro RL, Rossi S, Ogwu A, et al. Therapeutic levels of lopinavir in late pregnancy and abacavir passage into breast milk in the Mma Bana Study, Botswana. Antivir Ther. 2013;18(4):585-590.
6. Corbett AH, Kayira D, White NR, et al. Antiretroviral pharmacokinetics in mothers and breastfeeding infants from 6 to 24 weeks postpartum: results of the BAN study. Antivir Ther. 2014;19(6):587-595.

ZIKA VIRUS

Trade: Zika Virus

Category: Infectious Disease

LRC: L3 - Limited Data-Probably Compatible

Zika virus is a member of the Flaviviridae virus family and is transmitted to humans via a bite from the Aedes mosquito. Person-to-person transmission has been documented by sexual contact, blood transfusions, and perinatally. The Zika virus has been identified in breast milk, but active Zika virus transmission via human milk has not yet been definitively associated with breastfeeding.[1]

In a review of two Zika-infected mothers, Zika virus RNA was present in breast milk although it was was not replicative.[2] In addition, both mothers and their infants had positive PCR results from at least one serum sample, which confirmed Zika infection. In the first case, the mother had an itchy rash (with no fever) that started 2 days before delivery and continued for 2 days postpartum; her infant was breastfed and no concerns were reported up to 5 days of life. In the second case, the woman had a fever, itchy rash, and myalgia starting 3 days after delivery. This mother breastfed her infant starting 3 days postpartum and the infant was reported to have a rash on day 4 of life along with thrombocytopenia from day 3 to 7. The authors do report the rash was discovered after a session of phototherapy for neonatal jaundice. Although transmission in these cases were suspected to be transplacental or at the time of delivery, the authors conclude that due to the high Zika RNA load detected in breast milk that Zika virus transmission via breastfeeding should be considered.

In another series of 4 breastfeeding mothers who were rt-RT-PCR positive for Zika virus, none of their breastfed infants tested positive for Zika virus.[3] At this time it is clear that Zika virus readily transfers transplacentally, but not clear it transfers via milk.

In a very recent study, researchers described the presence of Zika virus in a Venezuela mother, her breast milk, and her infected infant.[5] As above, the virus has been found in breast milk before, but the infants were apparently not infected. While the source of the child's infection in this recent study was not determinable, the authors strongly suggest the occurrence of postnatal transmission of Zika virus from mother to child via breast milk.

At present, the CDC and the World Health Organization still recommend that the benefits of breastfeeding outweigh the theoretical risks of Zika virus infection from breast milk.[1,4] As the data regarding Zika virus infection in children, pregnant women and adults is rapidly changing and case reports to date are limited, consult the CDC and WHO websites for the most up to date recommendations regarding breastfeeding and the risks of Zika transmission.

Adult Concerns: Many people have no symptoms. Other symptoms associated with Zika infection include; fever, rash, joint pain, conjunctivitis (red eyes), muscle pain, headache.

Adult Dose:

Pediatric Concerns:

Infant Monitoring: Zika virus RNA is present in human milk, although it is not know if it is infectious. The CDC and the WHO recommend continued breastfeeding with maternal infection with Zika virus.

Alternatives:

References:

1. Centers for Disease Control and Prevention. Zika virus transmission & risks. http://www.cdc.gov/zika/transmission/index.html.
2. Besnard M, Lastere S, Teissier A, Cao-Lormeau V, Musso D. Evidence of perinatal transmission of Zika virus, French Polynesia, December 2013 and February 2014. Euro Surveill. 2014 Apr;19(13). pii: 20751.
3. Cavalcanti MG, Cabral-Castro MJ, Gonçalves JL, Santana LS, Pimenta ES, Peralta JM. Zika virus shedding in human milk during lactation: an unlikely source of infection? Int J Infect Dis. 2017 Apr;57:70-72.
4. World Health Organization. Infant feeding in areas of Zika virus transmission. Summary or rapid advice guideline; June 29, 2016. http://reliefweb.int/sites/reliefweb.int/files/resources/WHO_ZIKV_MOC_16%205_eng.pdf
5. Blohm GM, Lednicky JA, Márquez M, et al. Evidence for mother-to-child transmission of Zika virus through breast milk. Clin Infect Dis. 2017 Dec;66(7):1120-1121. doi: 10.1093/cid/cix968. PMID: 29300859.

ZILEUTON

Trade: Zyflo

Category: Antiasthma

LRC: L3 - No Data-Probably Compatible

Zileuton is used for chronic treatment of asthma. It inhibits leukotriene formation, which in turn inhibits neutrophil and eosinophil migration, neutrophil and monocyte aggregation, and leukocyte adhesion, minimizing inflammation and bronchoconstriction in the airways.[1] No data are available on its transfer to human milk at this time.

T 1/2	3 h	MW	236 Da	PB	93%
Tmax	1.7 h	RID		Vd	1.2 L/kg
Oral		M/P		pKa	9.96

Adult Concerns: Headache, dizziness, insomnia, pain, dyspepsia, nausea, abdominal pain, diarrhea, changes in liver function, leukopenia, weakness.

Adult Dose: 600 mg four times daily.

Pediatric Concerns: No data are available.

Infant Monitoring: Irritability, insomnia, diarrhea.

Alternatives:

References:
1. Pharmaceutical manufacturers prescribing information.

ZINC OXIDE

Trade:

Category: Metals

LRC: L2 - Limited Data-Probably Compatible

Zinc oxide is a metal compound found in a number of topical preparations and dietary supplements. Studies in rats show that the administration of dietary zinc oxide or other organic zinc salts at levels not exceeding 38 mg per day had no effect on breastfeeding pups.[1] A sign of zinc toxicity, metal fume fever, which can be identified by fever, chills, myalgias, vomiting, and malaise, may decrease milk production.[2] Dermal absorption of zinc oxide is minimal.[3] No statistically significant increases in zinc levels occurred in the serum following administration of 40% zinc oxide ointment.[4]

T 1/2		MW		PB	
Tmax		RID		Vd	
Oral	41%	M/P		pKa	

Adult Concerns: Dermal preparations of zinc may result in irritation and skin sensitivity. Gastrointestinal upset (nausea, vomiting, diarrhea) may result from oral intake.

Adult Dose: Dermal: Apply to affected area several times each day; Oral: 25-50 mg/day.

Pediatric Concerns:

Infant Monitoring: Gastritis.

Alternatives:

References:
1. Thompson PK, Marsh M, Drinker KR. The effect of zinc administration upon reproduction and growth in the albino rat, together with a demonstration of the constant concentration of zinc in a given species, regardless of age. Am J Physiol. 1927;80:65-74.
2. HSDB. Hazardous Substances Data Bank. Bethesda, MD: National Library of Medicine. (Internet Version). Edition expires 2001; provided by Greenwood Village, CO: Thomson Healthcare Inc.
3. TERIS. Teratogen Information System database. CD-ROM Version. 28. Seattle, WA: University of Washington.(Internet Version). Edition expires 4/30/1996; provided by Greenwood Village, CO: Thomson Healthcare Inc.
4. Derry JE, McLean WM, Freeman JB. A study of percutaneous absorption from topically applied zinc oxide ointment. J Parent Enteral Nutr. 1983;7:131-135.

ZINC SALTS

Trade:

Category: Metals

LRC: L2 - Limited Data-Probably Compatible

Zinc is an essential element that is required for enzymatic function within the cell. Zinc deficiencies have been documented in newborns and premature infants with symptoms such as anorexia nervosa, arthritis, diarrhea, eczema, recurrent infections, and recalcitrant skin problems. The Recommended Daily Allowance (RDA) for adults is 12-15 mg/day. The average oral dose of supplements is 25-50 mg/day; higher doses may lead to gastritis. Doses used for treatment of cold symptoms averaged 13.3 mg (lozenges) every 2 hours while awake for the duration of cold symptoms. The acetate or gluconate salts are preferred due to reduced gastric irritation and higher absorption. Zinc sulfate should not be used.

Excessive intake is detrimental. Eleven healthy males who ingested 150 mg twice daily for 6 weeks showed significant impairment of lymphocyte and polymorphonuclear leukocyte function and a significant reduction of HDL cholesterol. Intranasal zinc salts should not be used as their use was recently implicated in damage to the olfactory cells, leading the complete loss of smell.

Interestingly, absorption of dietary zinc is nearly twice as high during lactation as before conception. In 13 women studied, zinc absorption at preconception averaged 14% and during lactation, 25%.[1] There was no difference in serum zinc values between women who took iron supplements and those who did not although iron supplementation may reduce oral zinc absorption. Zinc absorption by the infant from human milk is high, averaging 41%, which is significantly higher than from soy or cow formulas (14% and 31%, respectively). Minimum daily requirements of zinc in full term infants vary from 0.3 to 0.5 mg/kg/day. Daily ingestion of zinc from breast milk has been estimated to be 0.35 mg/kg/day and declines over the first 17 weeks of life as older neonates require less zinc due to slower growth rate.

Supplementation with 25-50 mg/day is probably safe, but excessive doses are discouraged. Another author has shown that zinc levels in breast milk are independent of maternal plasma zinc concentrations or dietary zinc intake.[2] Other body pools of zinc (i.e., liver and bone) are perhaps the source of zinc in breast milk. Therefore, higher levels of oral zinc intake probably have minimal effect on zinc concentrations in milk but excessive doses above the Recommended Daily Allowance (RDA) are not recommended.

T 1/2		MW		PB	
Tmax		RID		Vd	
Oral	41%	M/P		pKa	

Adult Concerns: Nausea, vomiting, diarrhea.

Adult Dose: 15 mg daily. Gluconate salts, and lower doses are preferred.

Pediatric Concerns: None reported via milk.

Infant Monitoring: Gastritis.

Alternatives:

References:

1. Fung EB, Ritchie LD, Woodhouse LR, Roehl R, King JC. Zinc absorption in women during pregnancy and lactation: a longitudinal study. Am J Clin Nutr. 1997;66(1):80-88.
2. Krebs NF, Reidinger CJ, Hartley S, Robertson AD, Hambidge KM. Zinc supplementation during lactation: effects on maternal status and milk zinc concentrations. Am J Clin Nutr. 1995;61(5):1030-1036.

ZIPRASIDONE

Trade: Geodon

Category: Antipsychotic, Atypical

LRC: L2 - Limited Data-Probably Compatible

Ziprasidone is an atypical antipsychotic agent chemically unrelated to phenothiazines or butyrophenones.[1] In a brief case report of one patient receiving a dose of 160 mg/day with a plasma level of 177 ng/mL, milk levels were undetectable until day 10 of therapy which was 11 ng/mL and 170 ng in maternal plasma.[2] Milk/plasma ratio was 0.06. The authors estimated the relative infant dose to be 1.2% of the weight-normalized maternal dose. No untoward effects were noted in the infant.

In another case report of an infant exposed throughout pregnancy and subsequently breastfed for 6 months, the infant (2.64 kg) was delivered at 39-weeks, and did not exhibit withdrawal symptoms or any other drug-related symptoms.[3] While milk levels were not determined, no adverse effects of ziprasidone were noted. The infant developed normally over the following 6 months.

T 1/2	7 h	MW	419 Da	PB	99%
Tmax	4-5 h	RID	0.07%-1.2%	Vd	1.5 L/kg
Oral	60%	M/P	0.06	pKa	13.18

Adult Concerns: Somnolence, headache, dizziness, prolonged QTc, hypotension, dyspepsia, nausea, constipation, changes in liver function, hyperglycemia, increased serum prolactin, weight gain, extrapyramidal symptoms (low risk).

Adult Dose: 20-80 mg twice daily.

Pediatric Concerns: None reported via milk at this time.

Infant Monitoring: Sedation or irritability, apnea, not waking to feed/poor feeding, extrapyramidal symptoms, and weight gain.

Alternatives: Risperidone(L2), Olanzapine(L2)

References:

1. Pharmaceutical manufacturers prescribing information.
2. Schlotterbeck P, Saur R, Hiemke C, et al. Low concentration of ziprasidone in human milk: a case report. Int J Neuropsychopharmacol. 2009 Apr;12(3):437-438.
3. Werremeyer A. Ziprasidone and citalopram use in pregnancy and lactation in a woman with psychotic depression. Am J Psychiatry. 2009 Nov;166(11):1298.

ZOLMITRIPTAN

Trade: Zomig, Zomigon, Zomigoro

Category: Antimigraine

LRC: L3 - No Data-Probably Compatible

Zolmitriptan is a 5-HT1B/1D (serotonin) receptor agonist used to treat migraine headaches.[1] Activating these receptors is believed to constrict cranial blood vessels and block the release of proinflammatory neuropeptides from the trigeminal nerve. Although the oral bioavailability of zolmitriptan (40%) is greater than sumatriptan (14%), it has been found that a moderate to severe migraine attack can reduce absorption by up to 40%.

No studies examining zolmitriptan secretion into human breast milk or adverse effects in infants have been published. Some transfer is likely based on this medication's small size and low protein binding; however, the clinical significance of this is unknown. Zolmitriptan has an active metabolite with 2-6 times the potency for 5-HT receptors. Consider sumatriptan as the preferred alternative.

T 1/2	3 h	MW	287 Da	PB	25%
Tmax	1.5-3 h	RID		Vd	7 L/kg
Oral	40%	M/P		pKa	9.64

Adult Concerns: Dizziness, drowsiness, flushing, hot tingling sensations, facial edema, jaw pain, unpleasant taste, dry mouth, chest pain, arrhythmias, hypertension, nausea, vomiting, abdominal pain, weakness, paresthesia.

Adult Dose: 2.5 mg orally, may repeat in 2 hours if needed.

Pediatric Concerns: None reported via milk at this time.

Infant Monitoring: Drowsiness, vomiting, poor feeding.

Alternatives: Sumatriptan(L3), NSAIDs, Acetaminophen(L1)

References:

1. Pharmaceutical manufacturers prescribing information.

ZOLPIDEM TARTRATE

Trade: Ambien, Ambien CR, Edluar, Intermezzo

Category: Sedative-Hypnotic

LRC: L3 - Limited Data-Probably Compatible

Zolpidem, although not a benzodiazepine, interacts with the same GABA-BZ receptor site and shares some of the same pharmacologic effects of the benzodiazepine family.[1] It is used for the treatment of insomnia and difficulty falling asleep after middle of the night awakening.

In a study of five lactating mothers receiving 20 mg daily, the maximum plasma concentration occurred between 1.75 and 3.75 hours and ranged from 90 to 364 µg/L.[2] The authors suggest that the amount of zolpidem recovered in breast milk 3 hours after administration ranged between 0.76 and 3.88 µg or 0.004% to 0.019% of the total dose administered. Breast milk clearance of zolpidem is very rapid, and none was detectable (below 0.5 ng/mL) by 4-5 hours postdose.

One case of infant sedation and poor appetite related to zolpidem use has been reported following the nightly use of sertraline (100 mg) and 10 mg zolpidem.[3] Upon discontinuation of zolpidem, the infant regained appetite and became more alert.

T 1/2	2.5-5 h	MW	307 Da	PB	93%
Tmax	1.6 h	RID	0.02%-0.18%	Vd	0.54 L/kg
Oral	70%	M/P	0.13-0.18	pKa	

Adult Concerns: Sedation, dizziness, headache, anxiety, hypertension, dry mouth, changes in appetite, dyspepsia, vomiting, constipation.

Adult Dose: 5-10 mg daily.

Pediatric Concerns: One case of infant drowsiness and poor feeding.

Infant Monitoring: Sedation, slowed breathing rate, dry mouth, not waking to feed/poor feeding, and weight gain.

Alternatives: Zopiclone(L2), Eszopiclone(L3), Lorazepam(L3), Oxazepam(L2)

References:
1. Pharmaceutical manufacturers prescribing information.
2. Pons G, Francoual C, Guillet P, et al. Zolpidem excretion in breast milk. Eur J Clin Pharmacol. 1989;37(3):245-248.
3. A.K. Personnal communication, 1999.

ZONISAMIDE

Trade: Zonegran

Category: Anticonvulsant

LRC: L4 - Limited Data-Possibly Hazardous

Zonisamide is a broad-spectrum anticonvulsant medication chemically classified as a sulfonamide.[1] It is especially effective in partial seizures and in patients whose seizures are drug resistant. It has a long half-life and high pKa, which from the data below leads to high maternal milk and plasma concentrations.

In a study of one patient receiving 100 mg three times daily of zonisamide on postpartum days 0, 3, 6, 14, and 30, the reported milk levels were drawn at 1.5 to 2.5 hours following administration of the medication.[2] The reported milk levels ranged from 8.25 to 10.5 mg/L (mean 9.5 mg/L), while the maternal plasma levels ranged from 9.52 to 10.6 mg/L (mean 10.13 mg/L). The milk/plasma ratio averaged 0.93. Using the highest reported milk level, the average relative infant dose would be about 33% of the maternal dose.

In another study in a patient receiving 400 mg zonisamide during and after pregnancy, the plasma levels of zonisamide at delivery were 15.7 µg/mL in the mother and 14.4 µg/mL in the infant at birth.[3] Thus the placental transfer was 92%. Levels in maternal plasma and maternal milk were similar, 10.7-13.3 µg/mL. The authors suggested the rate of breast milk transfer was 41%-57%. The breastfed infant plasma level of zonisamide at day 24 was 3.9 µg/mL. While significantly less than the cord blood level of 14.4 µg/mL at birth, these levels are still quite high and are equal to that of an adult receiving 300 mg/day (C_{max} 3.479 µg/mL).[4]

In 2014, two case reports were published in Japan regarding zonisamide use in lactation.[5] In the first case report, a 35-year-old female taking 100 mg in the morning and 200 mg at night (300 mg/day) breastfed her full-term baby boy. Breast milk samples were taken on days 4 and 5 postpartum and the concentrations of zonisamide were found to be 16.2 and 18 µg/mL, respectively. These levels produced an estimated infant dose of 2.7 mg/kg/day (typical infant starting dose 1-2 mg/kg/day, usual dose 5-8 mg/kg/day) and an RID of 44%. Based on these levels, the mother was instructed to partially breastfeed twice a day (starting on day 9 postpartum). The infant's serum was tested on day 34 and found to be undetectable; the RID at the time of this infant's level was estimated to be about 8% (based on two feeds a day). This infant was also reported to be healthy with no adverse effects from the medication in breast milk. This study was done during the colostral period and levels may be excessively high during this transitional period.

The second case report, in the 2014 publication, was a 32-year-old female taking 100 mg/day of zonisamide while breastfeeding her healthy term baby girl.[5] Milk samples were taken immediately before dosing (trough) and at the peak maternal plasma concentration and were found to be 3.4 µg/mL on day 3 postpartum and 5.1 µg/mL on day 5 postpartum. These levels produced an infant dose of 0.77 mg/kg/day and a relative infant dose of 36%. Again, the woman was advised to partially breastfeed her infant; however, due to low milk supply lactation ceased at 2 weeks postpartum. In this case the infant was also noted to have no adverse effects while exposed to the medication in breast milk.

Significant caution is recommended with this medication as a number of pediatric adverse effects have been noted in older children such as somnolence, anorexia, and severe skin rashes.[5] In addition, a few cases of heat stroke have resulted from zonisamide-induced dysfunction of the sweat glands.[1]

T 1/2	63 h	MW	212 Da	PB	40%
Tmax	2-6 h	RID	28.88%-44.1%	Vd	1.45 L/kg
Oral		M/P	0.93	pKa	10.2

Adult Concerns: Somnolence, dizziness, headache, agitation, confusion, speech abnormalities, diplopia, kidney stones, nausea, anorexia, abnormal gait, paresthesias, leukopenia, Steven-Johnson syndrome; abrupt withdrawal can lead to seizures in epilepsy patients (wean slowly).

Adult Dose: 100-200 mg/day.

Pediatric Concerns: None via breastmilk, but levels are extremely high. Oligohidrosis and hyperthermia has been reported in pediatric patients given the medication.[6]

Infant Monitoring: Sedation or irritability, agitation, nausea, poor appetite, elevated temperature. Hazardous.

Alternatives:

References:
1. Pharmaceutical manufacturer prescribing information.
2. Shimoyama R, Ohkubo T, Sugawara K. Monitoring of zonisamide in human breast milk and maternal plasma by solid-phase extraction HPLC method. Biomed Chromatogr. 1999;13(5):370-372.
3. Kawada K, Itoh S, Kusaka T, Isobe K, Ishii M. Pharmacokinetics of zonisamide in perinatal period. Brain Dev. 2002 Mar;24(2):95-97.
4. Maanen R, Bentley D. Bioequivalence of zonisamide orally dispersible tablet and immediate-release capsule formulations: results from two open-label, randomized-sequence, single-dose, two-period, two-treatment crossover studies in healthy male volunteers. Clin Ther. 2009 Jun;31(6):1244-1255.
5. Ando H, Matsubara S, Oi A, et al. Two nursing mothers treated with zonisamide: should breastfeeding be avoided? J Obstet Gynaecol Res. 2014;40(1):275-278.
6. Low PA, James S, Peschel T, et al. Zonisamide and associated oligohidrosis and hyperthermia. Epilepsy Res. 2004;62(1):27-34.

ZOPICLONE

Trade: Imovane, Rhovan, Zileze, Zimovane

Category: Sedative-Hypnotic

LRC: L2 - Limited Data-Probably Compatible

Zopiclone is a sedative/hypnotic that, although structurally dissimilar to the benzodiazepines, shares their pharmacologic profile.[1] In a group of 12 women who received 7.5 mg of zopiclone, the average peak milk concentration at 2.4 hours was 34 µg/L[2], but the average milk concentration was 10.92 µg/L. The milk half-life was 5.3 hours compared to the maternal plasma half-life of 4.9 hours. The milk/plasma AUC ratio was 0.51 and ranged from 0.4 to 0.7. The authors report that the average infant dose of zopiclone via milk would be 1.4% of the weight adjusted dose ingested by the mother.

T 1/2	4-5 h	MW	388 Da	PB	45%
Tmax	1.6 h	RID	1.5%	Vd	1.51 L/kg
Oral	75%	M/P	0.51	pKa	6.7

Adult Concerns: Sedation, confusion, agitation, dry mouth, bitter taste, anorexia, vomiting, constipation, changes in liver function.

Adult Dose: 7.5 mg orally.

Pediatric Concerns: None reported via milk at this time.

Infant Monitoring: Sedation, slowed breathing rate, not waking to feed/poor feeding and weight gain.

Alternatives: Lorazepam(L3), Oxazepam(L2)

References:
1. Gaillot J, Heusse D, Hougton GW, Marc AJ, Dreyfus JF. Pharmacokinetics and metabolism of zopiclone. Pharmacology. 1983;27 Suppl 2:76-91.
2. Matheson I, Sande HA, Gaillot J. The excretion of zopiclone into breast milk. Br J Clin Pharmacol. 1990;30(2):267-271.

ZOSTER VACCINE RECOMBINANT ADJUVANTED

Trade: Shingrix

Category: Vaccine

LRC: L3 - No Data-Probably Compatible

Zoster vaccine recombinant adjuvanted is a vaccine indicated for prevention of herpes zoster (shingles) in adults aged 50 years and older. However, it has been used in younger individuals. This vaccine is not live, nor can it induce herpes zoster infections. Shingrix vaccine contains a vial of lyophilized recombinant varicella zoster virus surface glycoprotein E (gE) antigen component. It does not contain live or attenuated live virus, hence there should be no risk if it is used in breastfeeding or even for that matter if used in an immunocompromised patient. It requires two injections at 2-4 months apart.

Adult Concerns: Local adverse reactions, pain, redness, swelling, myalgia, fatigue, headache, shivering, GI disturbances.

Adult Dose: Administer two doses (0.5 mL each) at 0 and 2 to 6 months.

Pediatric Concerns:

Infant Monitoring: Gi distress, but unlikely.

Alternatives:

References:
1. Pharmaceutical manufacturers prescribing information.

ZOSTER VACCINE, LIVE

Trade: Zostavax

Category: Vaccine

LRC: L3 - No Data-Probably Compatible

The varicella zoster virus (VZV) belongs to the family of herpes viruses. Primary VZV infection is commonly called chickenpox and occurs usually in childhood. After the primary illness subsides, this virus remains latent in the ganglia and may get reactivated decades later to cause herpes zoster, or shingles. The infectivity of shingles to other susceptible individuals is 15%. Transmission can be reduced by covering the lesions of shingles, until they dry up and form crusts.

The zoster vaccine is prepared from a live, attenuated VZV strain. This vaccine is routinely recommended for all those older than 60 years of age. There is currently no established evidence of transmission of the zoster virus vaccine in breast milk. This vaccine is not contraindicated in breastfeeding.[1,2]

Adult Concerns: Redness, pain, tenderness, swelling at the site of injection, varicella-like rash, hypersensitivity reactions. Avoid in those with an ongoing viral illness, and those with immunodeficiency disorders.

Adult Dose: 0.65 mL, subcutaneous, in the deltoid.

Pediatric Concerns: None reported via milk, but no studies are available. Consult pediatrician prior to maternal vaccination for risks/benefits discussion if infant is known to be immunocompromised; caution is recommended.

Infant Monitoring:

Alternatives:

References:
1. National Center for Immunization and Respiratory Diseases. General recommendations on immunization - recommendations of the Advisory Committee on Immunization Practices (ACIP). MMWR Recomm Rep. 2011 Jan;60(2):1-64.
2. Schaefer C. Drugs During Pregnancy and Lactation. Amsterdam, The Netherlands: Elsevier Science B.V.; 2001.

ZUCLOPENTHIXOL

Trade: Clopixol, Clopixol Depot, Clopixol-Acuphase

Category: Antipsychotic, Typical

LRC: L3 - Limited Data-Probably Compatible

Zuclopenthixol is a typical antipsychotic agent used in the management of schizophrenia. It is not available in the United States. It works by blocking the postsynaptic dopaminergic receptors.[1] In a study of a single patient who initially received 24 mg zuclopenthixol for 4 days and then 14 mg/day thereafter, levels in milk averaged 20 µg/L following the 24 mg dose, and 5 µg/L at the 14 mg dose.[2] Based on these concentrations, the authors estimated the absolute infant doses to be 0.8 to 3 µg/kg/day and the relative infant doses to be 0.3% to 0.8% of the maternal dose (used maternal weight of 60 kg). We found very similar results with a relative infant dose of 0.4%-0.87% (standard maternal weight 70 kg and mean concentration (20 and 5 µg/L). In addition, we also calculated the relative infant dose using the peak zuclopenthixol concentration of 35 µg/L and still only found a RID of 1.5%. This infant was partially breastfed until the mother's condition improved and she was able to fully breastfeed. At this time the medication was gradually tapered off. No adverse effects were reported in the infant.

In a group of six patients ranging from 3 days to 10 months postpartum, the dose ranged from 4 mg/day to 72 mg/2 weeks (IM).[3] In all instances, milk levels were much lower than plasma. Zuclopenthixol levels in milk averaged 29% of the maternal plasma levels. The daily dose to an infant was estimated to be 0.5-5 µg/day which roughly corresponds to a relative infant dose of 0.03%-0.38% of the weight-adjusted maternal dose.

The plasma levels of zuclopenthixol in infants were low in both studies. No untoward effects were noted in the infants although some caution is recommended with prolonged exposure to this medication.

T 1/2	20 h	MW	443-555 Da	PB	98%
Tmax	4 h	RID	0.4%-1.55%	Vd	15-20 L/kg
Oral	49%	M/P	0.29	pKa	

Adult Concerns: Drowsiness, anxiety, insomnia, tachycardia, hypotension, dry mouth, constipation, anorexia, extrapyramidal symptoms, weakness.

Adult Dose: 10-100 mg/day (oral): 50-150 mg every 48-72 h (IM).

Pediatric Concerns: No untoward effects were noted in seven infants studied thus far.

Infant Monitoring: Sedation or irritability, apnea, dry mouth, not waking to feed/poor feeding, weight gain, extrapyramidal symptoms.

Alternatives: Risperidone(L2), Olanzapine(L2)

References:
1. Pharmaceutical manufacturers prescribing information.
2. Matheson I, Skjaeraasen J. Milk concentrations of flupenthixol, nortriptyline and zuclopenthixol and between-breast differences in two patients. Eur J Clin Pharmacol. 1988;35(2):217-220.
3. Aaes-Jorgensen T, Bjorndal F, Bartels U. Zuclopenthixol levels in serum and breast milk. Psychopharmacology (Berl). 1986;90(3):417-418.

APPENDIX

Using Radiopharmaceutical Products in Breastfeeding Mothers

The use of radioactive products in breastfeeding mothers must be approached with great care. Invariably, the administration of a radiopharmaceutical to a lactating mother will result in some transfer of radioactivity into her milk. The relative dose received by the infant is dependent on a number of factors, but most importantly by the radioactive dose administered, the absorption and distribution of the radioisotope, the biological and radioactive half-life of the product, and the amount that enters milk. The following table presents data from some of the best sources in the world and provides their recommendations on interrupting breastfeeding to allow for the decay and/or clearance of the radiopharmaceutical. Most of their decisions were based on the probable radioactive "dose" transferred to the infant, and whether or not it was considered hazardous. Please note that some of their recommendations conflict. Ultimately the mother and her radiologist will have to assess the relevance of these data in their specific situation.

When evaluating radiopharmaceuticals, it is important to understand that all of these products have "two" half-lives. One is the radioactive half-life of the isotope. This half-life is set and invariable. While we prefer shorter half-life products like ^{99m}Technetium (6.02 h), many other isotopes have important uses in medicine. The second half-life is the "biological" or "effective" half-life of the specific product. Many of these products are rapidly eliminated from the body via the kidney, some within minutes to hours. Thus, the "biological" or "effective" half-life is critical and sometimes is so fast that the radiopharmaceutical is gone from the body long before its isotope is decayed (see ^{111}In-Octreotide). However, some isotopes, such as the radioactive iodides (^{131}I, ^{125}I), may be retained in the body for long periods and present extraordinary hazards to the breastfeeding infant.

Lastly, two units of radioactivity are commonly used by differing sources. Just remember that 1 mCi (millicurie) is equal to 37 MBq (megabecquerel). Regardless of the unit you are given, you can now convert them easily.

Some Important Points to Remember About Evaluating These Products in Breastfeeding Mothers:

- Use the shortest half-life product permitted such as ^{99m}Technetium. Its half-life is so short, and its radioactive emissions are so weak, that it poses little risk (but this depends on dose). While the table that follows often does not even require interrupting breastfeeding, we still suggest that waiting even 12-24 hours before breastfeeding would virtually eliminate all possible risks associated with this isotope.

- Regardless of the isotope used, if the dose is extremely high, then withholding breastfeeding for a minimum of 5 to as many as 10 radioactive half-lives is probably advisable.

- Measuring the radioactivity present in milk is the most accurate way to determine risk. This often requires sophisticated equipment not available in most hospitals, but it is the "final" determinant of risk to the infant. If the isotope present in milk approaches "background" levels, there is no risk to the infant.

- Use great caution before returning to breastfeeding if the radioactive iodides are used. Iodine is selectively concentrated in the thyroid gland, the lactating breast (27% of dose), and breast milk, and high doses could potentially lead to thyroid cancer in the infant. ^{131}I and ^{125}I are potentially high risk due to their long radioactive half-lives and their affinity for thyroid tissues. ^{123}I has a much shorter half-life, and brief interruptions may eliminate most risks. In mothers who have had their thyroid removed, the return to breastfeeding will be much quicker. Further, even close contact can produce high radiation exposure to an individual in close contact with the individual. Thus, we have added comments regarding close contact restrictions under the breastfeeding interruption section in the Radioisotope table.

- Because radioactivity decays at a set rate, milk can be stored in the freezer for at least 8 to 10 half-lives and then fed to the infant without problem. All of the radioactivity will be gone.

Typical Radioactive Half-Lives

Radioactive Element	Radioactive Half-Life
^{99}Mo	2.75 Days
^{201}TI	3.05 Days
^{201}TI	73.1 Hours
^{67}Ga	3.26 Days
^{67}Ga	78.3 Hours
^{131}I	8.02 Days
^{133}Xe	5.24 Days
^{111}In	2.80 Days
^{51}Cr	27.7 Days
^{125}I	60.1 Days
^{89}Sr	50.5 Days
^{99}mTc	6.02 Hours
^{123}I	13.2 Hours
^{153}Sm	47.0 Hours

Radioisotopes in Lactation

When assessing the use of a radioisotope in lactation it is important to know that the International Commission on Radiological Protection (ICRP) recommends to limit the infants exposure to less than 1 millisievert (mSv) of radiation. To put this exposure in context, the average American adult is exposed to 6.2 mSv of radiation per year from their environment. Please be advised that these recommendations still permit a minimal amount of radiation transfer to the infant; to avoid any radiation to the infant it is best to wait for all of the radiopharmaceutical to decay (5–10 radioactive half-lives). The physician may use discretion in their recommendation based on maternal and infant health and increase the duration of interruption. In addition, please follow any further instructions regarding limitations of close contact (proximity to the infant) and duration of contact as per your healthcare provider (procedure/radioisotope dependent). For more individual information, call the InfantRisk Center.

Radiopharmaceutical	Activity administered to women in lactation studies (MBq)	Effective half-time (h)	Total fraction excreted in milk: % injected activity	Infant dose in milk ($mSv_{infant}/MBq_{mother}$)	Mean infant dose via milk and/or contact	Breastfeeding interruption
^{11}C-Way 100635	526	0.3			2.7 μSv milk	No
^{11}C-Raclopride	384	0.3			0.6 μSv milk	No[¶]
^{111}In-Octreotide						No
^{111}In-WBC						No[§]
^{133}Xe Gas						No
^{11}C-labeled						No
^{11}N-labeled						No
^{11}O-labeled						No
^{13}N-labeled						No

(continued)

Radioisotopes in Lactation (continued)

Radiopharmaceutical	Activity administered to women in lactation studies (MBq)	Effective half-time (h)	Total fraction excreted in milk: % injected activity	Infant dose in milk ($mSv_{infant}/MBq_{mother}$)	Mean infant dose via milk and/or contact	Breastfeeding interruption
^{15}O-labeled						No
^{22}Na						> 3 weeks
^{75}Se-labeled						> 3 weeks
^{18}F-FDG	277, 422	1.8 (1.7–1.8)	0.07 (0.068–0.071)	6.7×10^{-4}		No
^{201}Tl-chloride						48 h
^{51}Cr-EDTA	3.7	6.1 (4.9–7.2)	0.065 (0.018–0.11)	2.1×10^{-4}		No
^{123}I-BMIPP						> 3 weeks
^{123}I-HSA						> 3 weeks
^{123}I-Iodohippurate						12 h
^{123}I-IPPA						> 3 weeks
^{123}I MIBG						> 3 weeks
^{123}I-NaI						> 3 weeks
^{125}I-HSA						> 3 weeks
^{123}I-Iodohippurate	0.4	5	2	1		12 h; pump and discard milk at least 3 times during this period.
^{131}I-Iodohippurate	0.28–0.66	6.3 (4.5–7.6)	2.4 (1.1–4.3)	5.3		12 h; pump and discard milk at least 3 times during this period.

(continued)

Radioisotopes in Lactation (continued)

Radiopharmaceutical	Activity administered to women in lactation studies (MBq)	Effective half-time (h)	Total fraction excreted in milk: % injected activity	Infant dose in milk ($mSv_{infant}/MBq_{mother}$)	Mean infant dose via milk and/or contact	Breastfeeding interruption
^{131}I MIBG						> 3 weeks
^{131}I-NaI	1-1.85	14 (10-17)	31 (13-48)	68		**Cessation:** see I^{131} close contact restrictions table; Consider cessation of breastfeeding at least 6 weeks – 3 weeks prior as lactating breast will concentrate iodide.
^{131}I-NaI	40				3930.4 mSv milk / 0.68 mSv contact	
^{131}I-NaI	5200	11.02	23.12		510952 mSv milk / 88.18 mSv contact	
^{67}Ga Citrate	185	51.12 (15.92-64.78)	7.23 (3.16-9.89)	77.75 mSv milk / 0.97 mSv contact		> 3-4 weeks; When possible, consider monitoring milk activity before re-starting
^{14}C-Glycocholic acid (GCA)	0.2	143	9.2	6.9×10^{-1}		No
^{14}C-Triolein	0.065	15	14	4.1		No
^{14}C-Urea						No
^{99m}Tc Diisopropyl imino-diacetic acid (DISDA)	150	5.51(3.76-9.14)	0.16 (0.1-0.28)		0.14 mSv milk / 0.11 mSv contact	No^ ; consider discarding 1st feeds

(continued)

Radioisotopes in Lactation (continued)

Radiopharmaceutical	Activity administered to women in lactation studies (MBq)	Effective half-time (h)	Total fraction excreted in milk: % injected activity	Infant dose in milk ($mSv_{infant}/MBq_{mother}$)	Mean infant dose via milk and/or contact	Breastfeeding interruption
99mTc Dimercaptosuccinic acid (DMSA)						No[*][^]
99mTc Diethylenetriamine-pentaacetic acid (DTPA)	151, 190, 600	4.53 (3.13-5)	0.12 (0.01-0.24)	2.2×10^{-5}	0.48 mSv milk 0.7 mSv contact One outlying case: 16.12 mSv milk 0.7 mSv contact	Yes (0-6 h)[*][^]; due to one outlying case with an exceptionally high effective dose (16.12 mSv) consider monitoring milk activity before re-starting
99mTc Ethylenedicysteine diester (ECD)						No[^]; consider discarding first feed
99mTc Phosphonates (MDP)						No[*][^]
99mTc Gluconate	600	3.63	0.14		0.28 mSv milk 0.7 mSv contact	No[^]; consider discarding first feed
99mTc Glucoheptonate						No[^]
99mTc Sulphur colloids	100	6.23 (5.12-8.3)	0.67 (0.16-1.48)		0.5 mSv milk 0.12 mSv contact	Yes (0-6 h)[†][^]
99mTc RBC (in vivo)	545, 602 when pre-treated	6.7	0.0057	6.7×10^{-6}		Yes (12 h)[†]; Limit close contact to 5 h in 24 h
99mTc RBC (in vitro)	800	8.37 (7.76-8.99)	0.02 (0.02-0.03)		0.08 mSv milk 1.25 mSv contact	No[^]; consider discarding 1st feed
99mTc WBC						12 h[‡]

(continued)

Radioisotopes in Lactation (continued)

Radiopharmaceutical	Activity administered to women in lactation studies (MBq)	Effective half-time (h)	Total fraction excreted in milk: % injected activity	Infant dose in milk ($mSv_{infant}/MBq_{mother}$)	Mean infant dose via milk and/or contact	Breastfeeding interruption
^{99m}Tc HMPAO-leucocytes	228	7.5	0.11	2×10^{-4}		No^; consider discarding 1st feed
^{99m}Tc Microspheres (HAMs)	100	5.31 (3.02-7.01)	4.33 (0.88-11.34)		3.87 mSv milk 0.08 mSv contact	Yes (12-24 h)‡
^{99m}Tc-Macroaggregated albumin (MAA)	60-104	4 (3.5-4.7)	3.7 (0.51-8.5)	7×10^{-3}		Yes (12 h); pump and discard milk at least 3 times during this period.
^{99m}Tc MAG3	52-68	4.2 (3.6-4.9)	0.073 (0.02-0.1)	1.4×10^{-4}		No^; consider discarding 1st feed
^{99m}Tc MDP (not blocked)	600	3.6	0.027	5.2×10^{-5}		No^; consider discarding 1st feed
^{99m}Tc MDP (blocked)	360-379	4.9 (4.6-5.2)	0.01 (0.0084-0.011)	1.2×10^{-5}		No^; consider discarding 1st feed
^{99m}Tc MIBI	480, 586, 900	5.5 (4.49-6.73)	0.048 (0.01-0.056)	9×10^{-5}	0.08 mSv milk 1.4 mSv contact	No^; limit close contact to 5 h in 24 h
^{99m}Tc Perchnetate (not blocked)	102-207	4.15 (2.23-8.26)	12.18 (0.56-24.36)	1.9×10^{-2}	8.28 mSv milk 0.012 mSv contact	Yes (12-30 h)‡; pump and discard milk at least 3 times during this period.
^{99m}Tc Perchnetate (blocked)	360, 500	5.2 (4.5-5.9)	0.82 (0.68-0.95)	9.6×10^{-4}		Yes (12 h)‡; pump and discard milk at least 3 times during this period.

(continued)

Radioisotopes in Lactation (continued)

Radiopharmaceutical	Activity administered to women in lactation studies (MBq)	Effective half-time (h)	Total fraction excreted in milk: % injected activity	Infant dose in milk ($mSv_{infant}/MBq_{mother}$)	Mean infant dose via milk and/or contact	Breastfeeding interruption
^{99m}Tc Pyrophosphate (PYP)	600	4.86 (3.54-6.83)	0.28 (0.15-0.44)		0.91 mSv milk 0.47 mSv contact	Yes (0-8 h)[*^] ; suggest feed interruption to reduce exposure without limiting contact
^{99m}Tc Tetrofosmin	556	4.8	0.082	1.5×10^{-4}		No[*^]
^{99m}Tc Technegas						No[^] ; consider discarding first feed

[*]AAP recommends 0-4 hours as long as no free pertechnetate; could discard first feed after procedure
[†]AAP recommends 6 hours
[‡]AAP recommends 12-24 hours
[§]AAP recommends 1 week
[¶]AAP recommends expressing first feed to avoid direct contact
[]Interruption for 2 h would eliminate almost all risk
[^]An interruption of 4 hours (one feed) may not be necessary for all 99mTc products (as long as there is no free pertechnetate) but could be advised

Selected Sources on Radioisotopes in Breastfeeding Mothers:

1. Mattsson S, Johansson L, Svegborn S et al. Radiation dose to patients from radiopharmaceuticals: a compendium of current information related to frequently used substances. Annex D. Recommendations on breast-feeding interruptions. Ann ICRP 2015;44(2Suppl):319-21.
2. Rubow S, Klopper J, Wasserman H et al. The excretion of radiopharmaceuticals in human breast milk: additional data and dosimetry. European Journal of Nuclear Medicine 1994;21:144-53.
3. Moses-Kolko EL, Meltzer CC, Helsel JC et al. No interruption of lactation in needed after (11)C-WAY 100635 or (11)C-raclopride PET. J Nucl Med 2003 Oct;46(10):1765.
4. Pullar M, Hartkamp A. Excretion of radioactivity in breastmilk following administration of an 113-Indium labeled chelate complex. Br J Radial 1977; 50:846.
5. Leide-Svegborn S, Ahlgren L, Johansson L et al. Excretion of radiopharmaceuticals in human breast milk after nuclear medicine examinations. Biokinetic and dosimetric data and recommendations on breastfeeding interruption. Eur J Nucl Med Mol Imaging 2015: DOI 10.1007/s00259-016-3326-4.
6. Mountford PJ, O'Doherty MJ, Forge NI, Jeffries A, Coakley AJ. Radiation dose rates from adult patients undergoing nuclear medicine investigations. Nucl Med Commun. 1991 Sep;12(9):767-77.
7. U.S. Nuclear Regulatory Commission. Regulatory Guide 8.39. Release of Patients administered radioactive materials. April 1997.
8. American Academy of Pediatrics, Committee on Drugs. Transfer of drugs and other chemicals into human milk. Pediatrics 2001; 108(3):776-89.
9. American Academy of Pediatrics Committee on Drugs. The transfer of drugs and therapeutics into human breast milk: an update on selected topics. Pediatrics 2013;132(3):796-809.
10. International Commission on Radiological Protection, Radiation Dose to Patients from Radiopharmaceuticals. Annex D. Recommendations on breastfeeding interruptions. ICRP Publication 106, Annals of the ICRP 38(1-2):163-165, 2008.
11. Sisson JC, Freitas J, McDougall IR et al. Radiation safety in the treatment of patients with thyroid diseases by radioiodine 1311: Practice recommendations of the American thyroid association. Thyroid 2011;21(4):335-46.

Radioactive ^{131}Iodine Close Contact Restrictions

Treatment of Hyperthyroidism (Assuming 50% Uptake)*, **				
Radiation dose	370 MBq (10 mCi)	555 MBq (15 mCi)	740 MBq (20 mCi)	1110 MBq (30 mCi)
Sleeping restriction (6 feet separation sleeping arrangement) for adult.	3 nights	6 nights	8 nights	11 nights
Sleeping restriction (6 feet separation of sleeping arrangement) for infant, children, and pregnant women.	15 nights	18 nights	20 nights	23 nights
Close contact restriction (6 feet separation) from children and pregnant women.	1 day	1 day	2 days	5 days

Treatment of Thyroid Cancer Remnant Ablation (Assuming 2% Uptake) (No Thyroid)*, **				
Radiation dose	1850 MBq (50 mCi)	3700 MBq (100 mCi)	5550 MBq (150 mCi)	7400 MBq (200 mCi)
Sleeping restriction (6 feet separation sleeping arrangement) for adult.	1 night	1 night	2 nights	4 nights
Sleeping restriction (6 feet separation of sleeping arrangement) for infant, children, and pregnant women.	6 nights	13 nights	18 nights	21 nights
Close contact restriction (6 feet separation) from children and pregnant women.	1 day	1 day	1 day	1 day

Adapted from American Thyroid Association Taskforce on Radioiodine Safety, Sisson JC, Freitas J, McDougall IR, Dauer LT, Hurley JR, Brierley JD, Edinboro CH, Rosenthal D, Thomas MJ, Wexler JA, Asamoah E, Avram AM, Milas M, Greenlee C. Radiation safety in the treatment of patients with thyroid diseases by radioiodine ^{131}I: practice recommendations of the American Thyroid Association. Thyroid. 2011 Apr;21(4): 335-346.

* IMPORTANT: The recommendations in the previous table were derived by calculating the dose and time required to limit the effective dose to the infant below 1 mSv. Please be advised, these recommendations still permit a minimal amount of radiation transfer to the infant that is considered safe by the authorities. An average adult American is exposed to 6.2 mSv/year according to the Nuclear Regulatory Commission. The only way to totally avoid any radiation is to wait for all of it to decay (5-10 half-lives). Exposure of 1 mSv slightly increases the incidence of cancer to 1 in 10,000 people.

** The half-life of ^{131}I is around 8 days. To avoid all radiation exposure to the breastfed infant, close contact must be avoided for at least 5 half-lives (i.e., 40 days).

Commonly Used Antidepressants—Suitability in Lactation

Drug Name	Half-Life	Adult Dose	RID	Lactation Risk Category
AMITRIPTYLINE	31-46 h	10-300 mg daily (varies by indication)	1.9-2.8%	L2 - Limited Data-Probably Compatible
BUPROPION	8-24 h	150 mg twice a day sustained release	0.1-2%	L3 - Limited Data-Probably Compatible
CITALOPRAM	36 h	20-40 mg a day	3.6-5.4%	L2 - Limited Data-Probably Compatible
DESVENLAFAXINE	11 h	50 mg a day	5.9-9.3%	L3 - Limited Data-Probably Compatible
DULOXETINE	12 h	40-60 mg a day	0.1-1.1%	L3 - Limited Data-Probably Compatible
ESCITALOPRAM	27-32 h	10-20 mg a day	5.2-7.9%	L2 - Limited Data-Probably Compatible
FLUOXETINE	2-3 days	20-60 mg a day	1.6-14.6%	L2 - Limited Data-Probably Compatible
FLUVOXAMINE	15.6 h	50-300 mg a day	0.3-1.4%	L2 - Limited Data-Probably Compatible
PAROXETINE	21 h	20-50 mg a day	1.2-2.8%	L2 - Limited Data-Probably Compatible
SERTRALINE	26 h	50-200 mg a day	0.4-2.2%	L2 - Limited Data-Probably Compatible
VENLAFAXINE	5 h	75-225 mg a day extended release	6.8-8.1%	L2 - Limited Data-Probably Compatible

Commonly Used Atypical Antipsychotics—Suitability in Lactation

Drug Name	Half-Life	Adult Dose	RID	Lactation Risk Category
ARIPIPRAZOLE	75 h	10-15 mg a day	0.7-6.4%	L3 - Limited Data-Probably Compatible *Caution: May suppress prolactin levels*
OLANZAPINE	21-54 h	5-10 mg a day	0.3-2.2%	L2 - Limited Data-Probably Compatible
PALIPERIDONE	Oral 23 h; IM 25-49 days	6 mg a day	Unknown	L3 - No Data-Probably Compatible
QUETIAPINE	6 h	300-800 mg a day	0.02-1%	L2 - Limited Data-Probably Compatible
RISPERIDONE	20 h	3 mg twice a day	2.8-9.1%	L2 - Limited Data-Probably Compatible
ZIPRASIDONE	7 h	20-80 mg twice a day	0.07-1.2%	L2 - Limited Data-Probably Compatible

Commonly Used Benzodiazepines—Suitability in Lactation

Drug Name	Half-Life	Adult Dose	RID	Lactation Risk Category
ALPRAZOLAM	12-15 h	0.5-1 mg three times a day	8.5%	L3 - Limited Data-Probably Compatible
CLOBAZAM	17-31 h	20-30 mg a day	Unknown	L3 - No Data-Probably Compatible
CLONAZEPAM	18-50 h	0.5-1 mg three times a day	2.8%	L3 - Limited Data-Probably Compatible
DIAZEPAM	43 h	2-10 mg two-four times a day	0.88-7.14%	L3 - Limited Data-Probably Compatible
LORAZEPAM	12 h	1 mg two-three times a day	2.6-2.9%	L3 - Limited Data-Probably Compatible
MIDAZOLAM	3 h	1-2.5 mg IV (varies by indication and route of administration)	0.63%	L2 - Limited Data-Probably Compatible
NITRAZEPAM	30 h	5-10 mg a day	2.9%	L2 - Limited Data-Probably Compatible
OXAZEPAM	8 h	10-30 mg three-four times a day	0.28-1%	L2 - Limited Data-Probably Compatible

Commonly Used Opioid Analgesic Medications—Suitability in Lactation

Drug Name	Half-Life	Adult Dose	RID	Lactation Risk Category
CODEINE	2.9 h	15-60 mg orally every 4-6 h as needed	0.6-8.1%	L3 - Limited Data-Probably Compatible
HYDROCODONE	3.8 h	5-10 mg orally every 6 h as needed	2.2-3.7%	L3 - Limited Data-Probably Compatible
HYDROMORPHONE	2-3 h IV & oral immediate release	2-4 mg orally every 4-6 h as needed or 0.2-1 mg IV every 2-3 hours as needed	0.67%	L3 - Limited Data-Probably Compatible
MORPHINE	1.5-2 h	10-30 mg orally or 5-15 mg IM or 2.5-5 mg IV every 4 h as needed	9-35%	L3 - Limited Data-Probably Compatible
OXYCODONE	2-4 h	5-10 mg orally every 6 h as needed	1-8%	L3 - Limited Data-Probably Compatible
FENTANYL	2-4 h	25-35 µg IV every 30-60 min as needed	2.9-5%	L2 - Limited Data-Probably Compatible
TRAMADOL	7 h	50-100 mg orally every 4-6 h as needed	2.86%	L3 - Limited Data-Probably Compatible

*When possible, acetaminophen and nonsteroidal anti-inflammatories (NSAIDs) should be given regularly for pain control and narcotics taken just as needed.

Iodine Content From Various Natural Sources

Iodine Sources	Descriptions	Quantity	Dose Form	Iodine Contents (Mcg)	Percent of Daily Recommended Value
Bread[2]	White enriched	2 slices		45	30%
Cheese[2]	Cheddar	1 oz		12	8%
Cod[2]		3 oz		99	66%
Corn[2]	Creamy (canned)	1/2 cup		14	9%
Egg[2]		1 large		24	16%
Fish sticks[2]		3 oz		54	36%
Fruit cocktail[2]	Heavy syrup	1/2 cup		42	28%
Ice cream[2]	Chocolate	1/2 cup		30	20%
Macaroni[2]	Enriched	1 cup		27	18%
Milk[2]		1 cup		56	37%
Prunes[2]	Dried	5		13	9%
Iodized salt[2]		3 g		142	94%
Sea weed[1]		1 g		16-8165	11-540%
Sea weed[1]	Arame	1 g		586 ± 56	391%
Sea weed[1]	Bladderwrack	1 g		276 ± 82	184%
Sea weed[1]	Dulse	1 g		72 ± 23	48%
Sea weed[1]	Fingered tangle	1 g		1997 ± 563	[133]1%
Sea weed[1]	Fingered tangle	1 g	Granules	8165 ± 373	5443%
Sea weed[1]	Hijiki	1 g		629 ± 153	419%
Sea weed[1]	Horsetail tangle	1 g		30 ± 1	20%
Sea weed[1]	Kelp	1 g	Capsule	1259 ± 200	839%
Sea weed[1]	Kelp	1 g		1513 ± 117	1009%
Sea weed[1]	Kelp (wild)	1 g	Capsule	1356 ± 665	904%
Sea weed[1]	Kelp Oarweed	1 g		746 ± 26	497%
Sea weed[1]	Knotted wrack	1 g		646 ± 153	431%
Sea weed[1]	Kombu	1 g		1350 ± 362	900%
Sea weed[1]	Mekabu	1 g	Tablet	22 ± 1	15%
Sea weed[1]	Mekabu	1 g	Powder	53 ± 3	35%
Sea weed[1]	Mitthsuishi-kombu	1 g	Powder	2353 ± 65	1569%
Sea weed[1]	Nori	1 g	Sheet	16 ± 2	11%
Sea weed[1]	Oarweed	1 g		1862 ± 520	1241%
Sea weed[1]	Paddle weed	1 g		2123 ± 352	1415%
Sea weed[1]	Sea palm	1 g		871 ± 231	581%
Sea weed[1]	Wakame	1 g		32-431	21-287%
Selenum[3]		1 tablet	Tablet	215	143%
Shrimp[2]		3 oz		35	23%
Tuna[2]	Canned in oil	3 oz		17	11%
Yogurt[2]		1 cup		75	50%

References:

1. Teas J, Pino S, Critchley A, Braverman LE. Variability of iodine content in common commercially available edible seaweeds. Thyroid. 2004 Oct; 14(10): 836-841.

2. Iodine: Dietary Supplement Fact Sheet. National Institutes of Health, Office of Dietary Supplements. Updated 4/18/2011. Accessed 5/27/2011.

3. Arum SM, He X, Braverman LE. Excess iodine from an unexpected source. N Engl J Med. 2009 Jan 22; 360(4): 424-426.

Hormonal Contraception
See Contraception Hormonal Monograph for Details

Trade Name	Type	Estrogen	Progestin	Formulation	Comment
Alesse, Aviane, Lessina, Levlite, Lutera, Sronyx	Monophasic	Ethinyl estradiol 20 mcg	Levonorgestrel 0.1 mg	Oral	Avoid
Angeliq	Monophasic	Estradiol 1 mg	Drospirenone 0.5 mg	Oral	Avoid
Annovera	Combination	Estradiol	Segesterone acetate	Vaginal Ring	Avoid
Apri, Desogen, Emoquette, Ortho-Cept, Reclipsen, Solia	Monophasic	Ethinyl estradiol 30 mcg	Desogestrel 0.15 mg	Oral	Avoid
Aranelle, Leena, Tri-Norinyl	Triphasic	Ethinyl estradiol 35 mcg	Norethindrone 0.5 mg (days 1-7), 1 mg (days 8-16), 0.5 mg (days 17-21)	Oral	Avoid
Azurette, Kariva, Mircette	Biphasic	Ethinyl estradiol 20 mcg (days 1-21), 10 mcg (days 24-28)	Desogestrel 0.15 mg	Oral	Avoid
Balziva-28, Briellyn 28, Ovcon-35, Zenchent, Zeosa	Monophasic	Ethinyl estradiol 35 mcg	Norethindrone 0.4 mg	Oral	Avoid
Beyaz, Gianvi, Loryna, Yaz	Monophasic + levomefolate calcium 0.451 mg	Ethinyl estradiol 20 mcg (days 1-24)	Drospirenone 3 mg (days 1-24)	Oral	Avoid
Brevicon, Modicon, Necon 0.5/35, Nortrel 0.5/35	Monophasic	Ethinyl estradiol 35 mcg	Norethindrone 0.5 mg	Oral	Avoid
Camila, Errin, Jolivette, Micronor, Nora-BE, Norethindrone, Nor-QD, Ortho-Micronor	Progestin only		Norethindrone 0.35 mg	Oral	Acceptable
Caziant, Cesia, Cyclessa, Velivet	Triphasic	Ethinyl estradiol 25 mcg	Desogestrel 0.1 mg (days 1-7), 0.125 (days 8-14), 0.15 mg (days 15-21)	Oral	Avoid
Cryselle, Lo/Ovral, Low-Ogestrel	Monophasic	Ethinyl estradiol 30 mcg	Norgestrel 0.3 mg	Oral	Avoid
Demulen 1/35, Kelnor, Zovia 1/35	Monophasic	Ethinyl estradiol 35 mcg	Ethynodiol diacetate 1 mg	Oral	Avoid
Depo-Provera	Progestin only		Medroxyprogesterone 150 mg every 3 months	IM injection	Acceptable

(continued)

Hormonal Contraception (*continued*)
See Contraception Hormonal Monograph for Details

Trade Name	Type	Estrogen	Progestin	Formulation	Comment
Depo-SubQ Provera	Progestin only		Medroxyprogesterone 104 mg every 3 months	SQ injection	Acceptable
Enpresse, Levonest, Trivora	Triphasic	Ethinyl estradiol 30 mcg (days 1-6), 40 mcg (days 7-11), 30 mcg (days 12– 21)	Levonorgestrel 0.05 mg (days 1-6), 0.075 mg (days 8-14), 0.15 mg (days 15-21)	Oral	Avoid
Triphasil	Triphasic	Ethinyl estradiol 30 mcg (days 1-6), 40 mcg (days 7-11), 30 mcg (days12– 21)	Levonorgestrel 0.05 mg (days 1-6), 0.075 mg (days 8-14), 0.125 mg (days 15-21)	Oral	Avoid
Estrostep 21, Tilia	Triphasic	Ethinyl estradiol 20 mcg (days 1-5), 30 mcg (days 6-12), 35 mcg (days 13-21)	Norethindrone 1 mg	Oral	Avoid
Estrostep Fe, Tilia Fe, Tri-Legest Fe	Triphasic/ iron days 22-28	Ethinyl estradiol 20 mcg (days 1-5), 30 mcg (days 6-12), 35 mcg (days 13-21)	Norethindrone 1mg	Oral	Avoid
Femcon Fe, Zeosa Fe	Monophasic/ iron days 22-28	Ethinyl estradiol 35 mcg	Norethindrone 0.4 mg	Oral	Avoid
Gildess Fe, Junel FE 1/20, Loestrin 24 FE 1/20, Microgestin Fe 1/20	Monophasic/ iron days 25-28	Ethinyl estradiol 20 mcg (days 1-24)	Norethindrone acetate 1 mg (days 1-24)	Oral	Avoid
Gildess Fe 1.5/30, Junel Fe 1.5/30, Loestrin Fe 1.5/30, Microgestin Fe 1.5/30	Monophasic/ iron days 22-28	Ethinyl estradiol 30 mcg	Norethindrone acetate 1.5 mg	Oral	Avoid
Implanon	Progestin only		Etonogestrel 60-70 mcg/day(year 1), 35-45 mcg/day (year 2), 30-40 mcg/day (year 3)	Subdermal implant	Acceptable
Camrese Lo	Continuous cycle regimen	Ethinyl estradiol 20 mcg (days 1-84), 10 mcg (days 85-91)	Levonorgestrel 0.10 mg (days 1-84)	Oral	Avoid
Introvale, Jolessa, Quasense, Seasonale	Continuous cycle regimen	Ethinyl estradiol 30 mcg (days 1-84)	Levonorgestrel 0.15 mg (days 1-84)	Oral	Avoid
Camrese	Continuous cycle regimen	Ethinyl estradiol 30 mcg (days 1-84), 10 mcg (days 85-91)	Levonorgestrel 0.15 mg (days 1-84)	Oral	Avoid

(*continued*)

Hormonal Contraception (continued)
See Contraception Hormonal for Details

Trade Name	Type	Estrogen	Progestin	Formulation	Comment
Junel-21 1/20, Loestrin 21 1/20, Microgestin 1/20	Monophasic	Ethinyl estradiol 20 mcg	Norethindrone acetate 1 mg	Oral	Avoid
Junel-21 1.5/30, Loestrin-21 1.5/30, Microgestin 1.5/30	Monophasic	Ethinyl estradiol 30 mcg	Norethindrone acetate 1.5 mg	Oral	Avoid
Levlen, Levora, Nordette, Portia	Monophasic	Ethinyl estradiol 30 mcg	Levonorgestrel 0.15 mg	Oral	Avoid
Lo Loestrin Fe	Monophasic/iron days 26-28	Ethinyl estradiol 10 mcg (days 1-26)	Norethindrone acetate 1 mg (days 1-24)	Oral	Avoid
LoSeasonique	Continuous cycle regimen	Ethinyl estradiol 20 mcg (days 1-84), 10 mcg (days 85-91)	Levonorgestrel 0.1 mg (days 1-84)	Oral	Avoid
Lybrel	Continuous	Ethinyl estradiol 20 mcg	Levonorgestrel 90 mcg	Oral	Avoid
Mirena	Progestin only		Levonorgestrel 20 mcg/day for 5 years	Intrauterine device (IUD)	Acceptable
MonoNessa, Ortho-Cyclen, Previfem, Sprintec	Monophasic	Ethinyl estradiol 35 mcg	Norgestimate 0.25 mg	Oral	Avoid
Natazia	Quadrephasic	Estradiol valerate 3 mg (days 1-2), 2 mg (days 3-24), 1 mg (days 25-26)	Dienogest none (days 1-2), 2 mg (days 3-7), 3 mg (days 8-24), none (days 25-28)	Oral	Avoid
Necon 1/35, Norinyl 1+35, Nortrel 1/35, Ortho-Novum 1/35	Monophasic	Ethinyl estradiol 35 mcg	Norethindrone 1 mg	Oral	Avoid
Necon 1/50, Norinyl 1+50, Ortho-Novum 1/50	Monophasic	Mestranol 50 mcg	Norethindrone 1 mg	Oral	Avoid
Necon 7/7/7, Nortrel 7/7/7, Ortho-Novum 7/7/7	Triphasic	Ethinyl estradiol 35 mcg	Norethindrone 0.5 mg (days 1-7), 0.75 mg (days 8-14), 1 mg (days 15-21)	Oral	Avoid
Necon 10/11, Ortho-Novum 10/11	Biphasic	Ethinyl estradiol 35 mcg	Norethindrone 0.5 mg (days 1-10), 1 mg (days 11-21)	Oral	Avoid
Next Choice, Next Step, Plan B	Emergency contraception		Levonorgestrel 0.75 mg	Oral	Acceptable
NuvaRing	Combination	Ethinyl estradiol 0.015 mg/day	Etonogestrel 0.12 mg/day	Vaginal ring	Avoid

(continued)

Hormonal Contraception (continued)
See Contraception Hormonal Monograph for Details

Trade Name	Type	Estrogen	Progestin	Formulation	Comment
Ocella, Syeda, Yasmin	Monophasic	Ethinyl estradiol 30 mcg	Drospirenone 3 mg	Oral	Avoid
Ogestrel	Monophasic	Ethinyl estradiol 50 mcg	Norgestrel 0.5 mg	Oral	Avoid
Low-Ogestrel	Monophasic	Ethinyl estradiol 30 mcg	Norgestrel 0.3 mg	Oral	Avoid
Ortho Evra	Combination	Ethinyl estradiol 20 mcg/day	Norelgestromin 150 mcg/day	Transdermal patch	Avoid
Ortho-Tri-Cyclen, TriNessa, Tri-Previfem, Tri-Sprintec	Triphasic	Ethinyl estradiol 35 mcg	Norgestimate 0.18 mg (days 1-7), 0.215 mg (days 8-14), 0.25 mg (days 15-21)	Oral	Avoid
Ortho-Tri-Cyclen Lo, Tri-Lo-Sprintec	Triphasic	Ethinyl estradiol 25 mcg	Norgestimate 0.18 mg (days 1-7), 0.215 mg (days 8-14), 0.25 mg (days 15-21)	Oral	Avoid
Ovcon-50	Monophasic	Ethinyl estradiol 50 mcg	Norethindrone 1 mg	Oral	Avoid
Ovrette	Progestin only		Norgestrel 0.075 mg	Oral	Acceptable
ParaGard	Non-hormonal (copper)			Intrauterine device (IUD)	Acceptable
Plan B One Step	Emergency contraception		Levonorgestrel 1.5 mg	Oral	Acceptable
Prefest	Multiphasic	Ethinyl estradiol 1 mg (days 1-6)	Norgestimate 0.09 mg (days 4-6)	Oral	Avoid
Preven	Emergency contraception	Ethinyl estradiol 50 mcg	Levonorgestrel 0.25 mg	Oral	Avoid
Safyral	Monophasic + levomefolate calcium 0.451 mg days 22-28	Ethinyl estradiol 30 mcg	Drospirenone 3 mg	Oral	Avoid
Seasonique	Continuous cycle regimen	Ethinyl estradiol 30 mcg (days 1-84), 10 mcg (days 85-91)	Levonorgestrel 0.15 mg (days 1-84)	Oral	Avoid
Tri-Norinyl	Triphasic	Ethinyl estradiol 35 mcg	Norethindrone 0.5 mg (days 1-7), 1 mg (days 8-16), 0.5 mg (days 17-21)	Oral	Avoid
Zarah	Monophasic	Ethinyl estradiol 30 mcg	Drospirenone 3 mg	Oral	Avoid
Zovia 1/50	Monophasic	Ethinyl estradiol 50 mcg	Ethynodiol diacetate 1 mg	Oral	Avoid

Foul Tasting Drugs That Might Alter the Taste of Milk	
Common Foul Tasting Drugs	**Trade Names**
Acyclovir	Aciclover, Acyclo-V, Aviraz, Lipsovir, Zovirax, Zyclir
Amlodipine	Istin, Norvasc
Azelastine	Astelin, Astepro, Azep, Optilast, Optivar, Rhinolast
Azithromycin	Zithromax
Captopril	Acepril, Capoten
Cetirizine	Zyrtec
Cholecalciferol	
Ciprofloxacin	Ciloxan, Cipro, Ciproxin
Clarithromycin	Biaxin, Klacid, Klaricid
Clindamycin	Cleocin, Clindacin
Clomipramine	Anafranil, Placil
Cod liver oil	
Desipramine	Norpramin, Pertofran
Dextromethorphan	Babee Cof Syrup, Creomulsion, Dexalone, Hold DM, Robitussin, Vicks 44 Cough Relief
Didanosine	Videx
Diethylpropion	Dospan, Tenuate, Tepanil
Diltiazem	Adizem, Britiazim, Cardcal, Cardizem, Cartia XT, Coras, Dilacor-XR
Disulfiram	Antabuse
Donepezil	Aricept
Doxepin	Adapin, Deptran, Silenor, Sinequan
Doxycycline	Doryx, Doxychel, Doxycin, Doxylar, Doxylin, Periostat, Vibra-Tabs, Vibramycin
Efavirenz	Atripla, Sustiva
Emedastine	
Enalapril	Amprace, Innovace, Renitec, Vasotec
Enoxacin	Comprecin, Enoxin, Penetrex
Erythromycin	Ceplac, E-Mycin, EES, Emu-V E, Ery-Tab, Eryc, Erycen, Erythrocin, Erythromide, Ilosone
Famotidine	Pepcid, Pepcid AC
Flecainide	Tambocor
Hydrochlorothiazide	Direma, Diuchlor H, Esidrex, Esidrix, Hydrodiuril, Modizide, Oretic, Tekturna HCT
Imipramine	Impril, Melipramine, Tofranil
Indinavir	Crixivan
Labetalol	Labrocol, Normodyne, Presolol, Trandate
Lamivudine	3TC, Epivir-HBV, Heptovir
Metronidazole	Flagyl, Metrocream, Metrolotion, Metrozine, Neo-Metric
Mexiletine	Mexitil
Nedocromil	Tilade
Oxypentifylline	

(*continued*)

Foul Tasting Drugs That Might Alter The Taste Of Milk (*continued*)	
Common Foul Tasting Drugs	**Trade Names**
Penicillins	
Phentermine	Adipex-P, Duromine, Fastin, Ionamin, Zantryl
Potassium chloride	Micro-K, K-Dur, Slow-K
Potassium iodide	SSKI
Prednisolone powder	Prednisolone, Prednisone
Procainamide	Procan, Procan SR, Pronestyl
Propafenone	Arythmol, Rythmol
Propranolol	Cardinol, Deralin, Inderal
Ritonavir	Norvir
Saquinanir	Fortovase
Stavudine	Zerit
Sulfamethoxazole + Trimethoprim	Bactrim, Cotrim, Resprim-Forte, Septra, Sulfatrim
Tinidazole	Fasigyne, Tindamax
Valacyclovir	Valtrex
Zidovudine	Combivir, Retrovir

Foul smelling/tasting drugs when introduced to an infant in breastmilk may cause alteration in the taste of breastmilk and could possibly cause a "breastfeeding strike" in an infant.

Combination Drugs	
Trade Name	**Drugs**
Acanya	Benzoyl Peroxide, Clindamycin
Accuretic	Hydrochlorothiazide, Quinapril
Advair	Fluticasone, Salmeterol Xinafoate
Advair Diskus	Fluticasone, Salmeterol Xinafoate
Advair Diskus 100/50	Fluticasone, Salmeterol Xinafoate
Advair Diskus 250/50	Fluticasone, Salmeterol Xinafoate
Advair Diskus 500/50	Fluticasone, Salmeterol Xinafoate
Advair HFA	Fluticasone, Salmeterol Xinafoate
Advair Inhalation Aerosol	Fluticasone, Salmeterol Xinafoate
Altafluor	Benoxinate, Fluorescein
Anexsia	Hydrocodone, Acetaminophen
Articadent Dental with Ephinephrine	Articaine, Epinephrine
Astracaine	Articaine, Epinephrine
Astracaine Dental with Epinephrine	Articaine, Epinephrine
Atripla	Emtricitabine, Tenofovir Disoproxil Fumarate
Azor	Amlodipine Besylate, Olmesartan Medoxomil
Bancap	Acetaminophen, Butalbital, Caffeine
Benicar HCT	Hydrochlorothiazide, Olmesartan Medoxomil
Benzaclin	Benzoyl Peroxide, Clindamycin
Ceta Plus	Acetaminophen, Hydrocodone
Chlorax	Chlordiazepoxide, Clidinium Bromide
Clinoxide	Chlordiazepoxide, Clidinium Bromide
Combivent	Albuterol, Ipratropium Bromide
Duac	Benzoyl Peroxide, Clindamycin
Duac CS	Benzoyl Peroxide, Clindamycin
Dulera	Formoterol, Mometasone
DuoNeb	Albuterol, Ipratropium Bromide
Dyazide	Hydrochlorothiazide, Triamterene
Elavil Plus	Amitriptyline, Perphenazine
Endocet	Acetaminophen, Oxycodone
Endodan	Acetylsalicylic Acid, Oxycodone
Entrafon	Amitriptyline, Perphenazine
Etrafon	Amitriptyline, Perphenazine
Etrafon 2-10	Amitriptyline, Perphenazine
Etrafon A	Amitriptyline, Perphenazine
Fioricet	Acetaminophen, Butalbital, Caffeine
Fiorinal	Acetylsalicylic Acid, Butalbital, Caffeine
Fiorinal Codeine	Butalbital, Caffeine, Codeine
Flurate	Benoxinate, Fluorescein
Fluress	Benoxinate, Fluorescein

(continued)

Combination Drugs (*continued*)	
Trade Name	**Drugs**
Flurox	Benoxinate, Fluorescein
Glucovance	Glyburide, Metformin
Harvoni	Ledipasvir + Sofosbuvir
Hycodan	Homatropine, Hydrocodone
Hydrene	Hydrochlorothiazide, Triamterene
Hyzaar	Hydrochlorothiazide, Losartan
Janumet	Metformin, Sitagliptin Phosphate
Jentadueto	Linagliptin, Metformin
Librax	Chlordiazepoxide, Clidinium Bromide
Lorcet	Acetaminophen, Hydrocodone
Lortab	Acetaminophen, Hydrocodone
Lotrel	Amlodipine Besylate, Benazepril
Magnacet	Acetaminophen, Oxycodone
Malarone	Atovaquone, Proguanil
Maxidone	Acetaminophen, Hydrocodone
Maxzide	Hydrochlorothiazide, Triamterene
Metaglip	Glipizide, Metformin
Mutabon D	Amitriptyline, Perphenazine
Narvox	Acetaminophen, Oxycodone
Norco	Acetaminophen, Hydrocodone
Oxycocet	Acetaminophen, Oxycodone
Percocet	Acetaminophen, Oxycodone
Percodan	Acetylsalicylic Acid, Oxycodone
Perloxx	Acetaminophen, Oxycodone
Prevpac	Amoxicillin, Clarithromycin, Lansoprazole
Primalev	Acetaminophen, Oxycodone
Qsymia	Phentermine, Topiramate
Rebetron	Interferon Alfa-2B, Ribavirin
Roxicet	Acetaminophen, Oxycodone
Roxilox	Acetaminophen, Oxycodone
Septanest	Articaine, Epinephrine
Septocaine	Articaine, Epinephrine
Seretide	Fluticasone, Salmeterol Xinafoate
Symbicort	Budesonide, Formoterol
Tramacet	Acetaminophen, Tramadol
Treximet	Naproxen, Sumatriptan
Triamco	Hydrochlorothiazide, Triamterene
Triamzide	Hydrochlorothiazide, Triamterene
Triavil	Amitriptyline, Perphenazine
Triazide	Hydrochlorothiazide, Triamterene

(*continued*)

Trade Name	Drugs
Tribenzor	Amlodipine Besylate, Hydrochlorothiazide, Olmesartan Medoxomil
Tri-Luma	Fluocinolone, Hydroquinone, Tretinoin
Truvada	Emtricitabine, Tenofovir Disoproxil Fumarate
Two-Dyne	Acetaminophen, Butalbital, Caffeine
Tylox	Acetaminophen, Oxycodone
Ultracaine Ds	Articaine, Epinephrine
Ultracaine Ds Forte	Articaine, Epinephrine
Ultracet	Acetaminophen, Tramadol
Veltin	Clindamycin, Tretinoin
Vicodin	Acetaminophen, Hydrocodone
Vimovo	Esomeprazole, Naproxen
Ziac	Bisoprolol, Hydrochlorothiazide
Ziana	Clindamycin, Tretinoin
Zydone	Acetaminophen, Hydrocodone
Zylet	Loteprednol, Tobramycin

Combination Drugs (continued)

INDEX